Tennis Medicine

"In my career, I have witnessed firsthand the key role that sports medicine has had in both treating the injuries that I have had and preventing further injuries from occurring. I am very happy that a book edited by Dr. Di Giacomo, Todd S. Ellenbecker from ATP, and Dr. Kibler has been developed to further the methods and education for sports medicine professionals who work with tennis players to enhance their performance and prevent injuries. The ability to have a long and extended career is very important to all players and the advances in sports medicine are allowing this to happen for many players throughout the sport of tennis. I have always worked closely with my entire team including my doctors and physios who have assisted me in my career and for whom I am very thankful for their great work."

—Rafael NADAL

Giovanni Di Giacomo
Todd S. Ellenbecker · W. Ben Kibler
Editors

Tennis Medicine

A Complete Guide to Evaluation, Treatment, and Rehabilitation

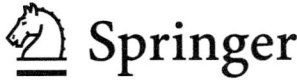

Editors
Giovanni Di Giacomo
Dept of Orthopaedics and Trauma
Concordia Hospital
Rome
Italy

Todd S. Ellenbecker
ATP World Tour
Rehab Plus Sports Therapy Scottsdale
Scottsdale, Arizona
USA

W. Ben Kibler
Lexington Clinic Orthopedics
Lexington, Kentucky
USA

ISBN 978-3-319-71497-4   ISBN 978-3-319-71498-1 (eBook)
https://doi.org/10.1007/978-3-319-71498-1

Library of Congress Control Number: 2018950140

© Springer International Publishing AG, part of Springer Nature 2018
This work is subject to copyright. All rights are reserved by the Publisher, whether the whole or part of the material is concerned, specifically the rights of translation, reprinting, reuse of illustrations, recitation, broadcasting, reproduction on microfilms or in any other physical way, and transmission or information storage and retrieval, electronic adaptation, computer software, or by similar or dissimilar methodology now known or hereafter developed.
The use of general descriptive names, registered names, trademarks, service marks, etc. in this publication does not imply, even in the absence of a specific statement, that such names are exempt from the relevant protective laws and regulations and therefore free for general use.
The publisher, the authors and the editors are safe to assume that the advice and information in this book are believed to be true and accurate at the date of publication. Neither the publisher nor the authors or the editors give a warranty, express or implied, with respect to the material contained herein or for any errors or omissions that may have been made. The publisher remains neutral with regard to jurisdictional claims in published maps and institutional affiliations.

This Springer imprint is published by the registered company Springer Nature Switzerland AG
The registered company address is: Gewerbestrasse 11, 6330 Cham, Switzerland

To our wives (Gail and Betty) (daughter Jacqueline) and families for their love and tremendous unwavering support, as well as our mentors who trained us and helped us develop.

We are thankful to all the authors who gave their time and expertise to this book and for the countless players whom we have treated and examined that have led us to this project to enhance Tennis Medicine by all who practice it.

Special mention to Sonia Errera for her conscientious effort in coordinating the project.

We also dedicate this book to an unbelievable friend and truly respected colleague in Tennis Medicine—Dr. Javier Maquirrian, who died earlier this year.

We would also like to acknowledge the commitment and insight of Elisa Geranio who assisted in the initial development of the book and also died earlier this year.

Foreword

This book highlights the key role sports medicine and sport science play in the sport of tennis. As a former player, tournament director, and now an Executive Chairman & President of the ATP, I have witnessed first-hand the important role Medical Services plays in elite-level tennis. I have benefited from the treatments and evaluations provided to me while playing that both prevented further injury and allowed me to return to play. I have also worked with tournament physicians, physios, and massage therapists while serving as the Tournament Director for the ATP tournament at the Queen's Club in London, as well as the ATP Finals at the O2, for many years. The role they play in facilitating player health and recovery, as well as injury and illness management, is critical to the success of any tournament. Lastly, in my role with the ATP, we have developed an extensive Medical Services department providing critically important sports medicine and recovery care to our players on both the ATP World Tour and ATP Challenger Tour. It is hoped that the information provided in this book by Di Giacomo, Ellenbecker, and Kibler will advance the clinical knowledge of clinicians who work with tennis players and lead to continued improvements in player care.

Chris Kermode
Monte Carlo, Monaco

Contents

Part I Biomechanics and Pathophysiology

1 **Biomechanics of the Tennis Serve** 3
   Caroline Martin

2 **Biomechanics of Groundstrokes and Volleys** 17
   Bruce Elliott, Machar Reid, and David Whiteside

3 **Epidemiology of Tennis Injuries** 43
   Babette M. Pluim and Gary Windler

4 **Pathophysiology of Tennis Injuries: The Kinetic Chain** 53
   Natalie L. Myers and W. Ben Kibler

5 **Tennis Equipment and Technique Interactions
   on Risk of Overuse Injuries** 61
   Tom Allen, Sharon Dixon, Marcus Dunn, and Duane Knudson

Part II Player Evaluation

6 **Evaluation of the Shoulder and Elbow
   in the Elite Tennis Player** 83
   David Dines, Todd S. Ellenbecker, and Jonathan Berkowitz

7 **Physical Evaluation of the Hip** 101
   Paul K. Herickhoff and Marc R. Safran

8 **Spine Injuries in Tennis** 111
   Stephan N. Salzmann, Javier Maquirriain, Jennifer Shue,
   and Federico P. Girardi

9 **Imaging of the Shoulder, Hip and Pelvis** 119
   Giuseppe Monetti, Gianluca Rampino, Giuseppe Rusignuolo,
   and Serena Tripoli

10 **Musculoskeletal Screening for the Elite
   and Developing Tennis Player** 131
   Todd S. Ellenbecker

11 **The Preparticipation Physical: The WTA Experience and Findings** 147
Walter C. Taylor, Brian Adams, Kathy Martin,
Susie Parker-Simmons, Marc Safron, Belinda Herde,
and Kathleen Stroia

12 **Assessment of Physical Performance for Individualized Training Prescription in Tennis**.............................. 167
Alexander Ferrauti, Alexander Ulbricht,
and Jaime Fernandez-Fernandez

Part III Shoulder Injuries

13 **Diagnosis and Management of Partial- and Full-Thickness Rotator Cuff Tears in Tennis Players** 191
Christopher L. Camp, David M. Dare, and David W. Altchek

14 **Labral Injury and Posterior Impingement in Elite Tennis Players**................................ 203
Giovanni Di Giacomo and Nicola de Gasperis

15 **Scapulothoracic Evaluation and Treatment in Tennis Players** 215
Natalie L. Myers and W. Ben Kibler

16 **Rehabilitation of the Shoulder in Tennis Players**............ 231
Todd S. Ellenbecker and Ann Cools

17 **Osteoarthritis and the Senior Tennis Player**................ 249
Keith T. Corpus, Evan W. James, Javier Maquirriain,
and David M. Dines

Part IV Elbow Wrist and Hand Injuries

18 **Pathophysiology of Tendinopathy: Implications for Tennis Elbow** 263
Per Renstrom and Paul W. Ackermann

19 **Humeral Epicondylitis in Elite Tennis Players and Indications for Elbow Arthroscopy** 277
David M. Dare, Christopher L. Camp, Ioonna Felix,
and Joshua S. Dines

20 **Minimally Invasive Treatment of Wrist and Hand Lesions in Tennis Players** 293
Alejandro Badia

21 **Pathophysiology of Wrist and Hand Injuries in Tennis Players: Tendons, Ligaments and TFCC Lesions** ... 313
Andrea De Vita, R. A. Purnachandra Tejaswi,
and Paolo Scarso

22	**Wrist and Hand Rehabilitation** 327
	Belinda Herde and Kathleen A. Stroia

Part V   Lower Extremity Injuries

23	**Principles of Hip Arthroscopy in Elite Tennis Players** 361
	J. W. Thomas Byrd
24	**Treatment of Femoroacetabular Impingement and Labral Injuries in Tennis Players** 369
	Marc R. Safran and Alberto Costantini
25	**Tennis Injuries of the Hip and Thigh** 381
	Ioonna Félix, Pete Draovitch, Todd S. Ellenbecker, and Joshua Dines
26	**Physiotherapy Management of Patellar Tendinopathy in Tennis Players** 401
	Hio Teng Leong, Jill Cook, Sean Docking, and Ebonie Rio
27	**Rehabilitation of Knee Injuries** 415
	Robert C. Manske and Mark V. Paterno
28	**The Foot and Ankle at Risk of Injury in Tennis Players** 439
	Luca Avagnina
29	**Acute Management of Common Foot and Ankle Injuries** 449
	Clay Sniteman and Shuhei Suzuki

Part VI   Spinal Injury

30	**Spondylolysis** 473
	Carles Pedret, Ramon Balius, and Angel Ruiz-Cotorro
31	**Spinal Rehabilitation Strategies for the Elite Tennis Player** . . . 487
	Hugo Gravil and Luke Fuller
32	**Core Stability in Tennis Players** 531
	Natalie L. Myers and W. Ben Kibler

Part VII   Medical Issues

33	**Key Medical Issues for Tennis Players** 549
	Bradley G. Changstrom, Babette M. Pluim, and Neeru Jayanthi
34	**Sports Nutrition for Tennis Players** 563
	Susie Parker-Simmons and Page Love
35	**Heat Stress, Hydration, and Heat Illness in Elite Tennis Players** 573
	Julien D. Périard and Olivier Girard

36	**On-Site Management and Coverage for Tournament Physicians in Professional Tennis** .... Mark E. Batt, Philip A. Bell, and Ian M. McCurdie	589
37	**Dermatologic Conditions in Elite Tennis Players**............ Walter C. Taylor and Brian Adams	599

Part VIII Special Topics

38	**Strength and Conditioning in Developmental Tennis Players** .... Jaime Fernandez-Fernandez and Mark Kovacs	611
39	**Strength and Conditioning of the Hips and Core (Practical Applications)** .... Carl Petersen and Nina Nittinger	627
40	**The Role of Scheduling and Periodization in Competitive Tennis Players** .... Mark Kovacs	679

Part I
Biomechanics and Pathophysiology

Biomechanics of the Tennis Serve

Caroline Martin

1.1 Introduction

In the professional male game, the serve has been reported to be the most important stroke [1]. From a strategy and tactics perspective, the main keys to a successful serve are velocity, spin, and placement. Statistics from the 2009 US Open show that for the men's draw, five of the top ten ranked players also had the highest serve speed [2]. Indeed, the ability for tennis players to produce highball velocity during the serve is a crucial element of a successful play because it puts the opponent under stress and may hinder its return. Consequently, if you ask tennis coaches what are their main priorities when teaching tennis serve, their responses could be "improving performance, especially ball velocity" but also "preventing injury." Indeed, previous studies have associated the serve with overuse injuries in the upper limb and back joints [3–5], which are a common medical problem in all competitive levels in tennis [6, 7]. The purpose of this review is to assimilate all the available scientific research on tennis serve biomechanics related to performance and upper limb joint injuries.

C. Martin
M2S Laboratory "Movement, Sport, Health",
University of Rennes 2, Bruz Cedex, France
e-mail: caromartin@numericable.fr

1.2 Ball Velocity and Tennis Serve Kinematics

In tennis, the serve is a sequence of motions referred to as a "kinetic chain" that begins with the lower limb action and is followed by the trunk and the upper limb. Fleisig et al. [8] have shown that tennis players produce a rapid sequence of segment rotations (Table 1.1). The order of maximal angular velocities is trunk tilt (280°/s), upper torso longitudinal rotation (870°/s), pelvis rotation (440°/s), elbow extension (1510°/s), wrist flexion (1950°/s), and shoulder internal rotation (2420°/s) [8]. These joint and segmental rotation contributions to racket velocity in the serve are of great interest in the literature [9–12]. The major contributors to the mean linear velocity of the racket at impact are internal rotation of the shoulder, flexion of the hand, horizontal flexion and abduction of the shoulder, and trunk flexion (Table 1.2).

The proficiency of these rotations through the kinetic chain involves a transfer of linear and angular momentum from the legs to the trunk and then to the arm and the racket [14]. Although the concept of angular momentum transfer is frequently reported to be critical in producing explosive serves, few studies have studied angular momentum during the tennis serve [14, 15]. Only Bahamonde [14] has described, quantified, and explained the evolution of angular momentum during the tennis serve about the three orthogonal axes (transverse or "cartwheel,"

Table 1.1 Peak values of joint rotations during the tennis serve

References	Knee extension (°/s)	Pelvis rotation (°/s)	Shoulder rotation (°/s)	Shoulder internal rotation (°/s)	Elbow extension (°/s)	Wrist flexion (°/s)
[9]	–	–	–	2090 ± 330	1230 ± 180	1720 ± 580
[8]	800 ± 400	440 ± 90	870 ± 120	2420 ± 590	1510 ± 310	1950 ± 510
[13]	–	510 ± 110	–	5580 ± 2350	1670 ± 380	–

Table 1.2 Segment contributions to linear racket velocity in the tennis serve

References	10	12	13
Number of players	11	1	66
Trunk flexion	9.7 ± 1.8	7.4	–
Shoulder internal rotation	54.2 ± 4.1	30	41.1 ± 14.7
Shoulder horizontal flexion and abduction	12.9 ± 5.9	24	6.4 ± 11.7
Elbow extension	−14.2 ± 6.4	–	3.2 ± 6.0
Elbow pronation	5.2 ± 4.1	15	3.6 ± 5.0
Wrist flexion	30.6 ± 9.1	26	31.7 ± 7.5
Wrist ulnar deviation	0.6 ± 1.2	–	0.8 ± 5.9

anteroposterior or "shoulder-over-shoulder," longitudinal or "twist") in five collegiate tennis players. It has been reported that most of the clockwise angular momentum about the transverse axis is concentrated in the trunk and the racket arm. The angular momentum about the longitudinal axis of rotation is small and lacked a consistent pattern. Moreover, Bahamonde [14] has noticed that the difference between the players with the highest ball speeds (51.0, 46.3, and 50.4 m/s) and the players with the lowest ball speeds (39.8 and 43.9 m/s) is the contribution of the trunk to the total anteroposterior axis angular momentum. A recent study has identified the relationships between segmental angular momentum and ball velocity in professional players [15]. The results of this study indicate that from maximal elbow flexion to ball impact, the players with the highest values of trunk and racket-arm angular momentums about the transverse axis are those with the highest ball velocity. As a consequence, it seems that the ability of a player to produce high upper body segmental angular momentum values about the transverse axis during the serve increases ball velocity. For the cocking, and acceleration phases of the serve, there were significant correlations between the trunk angular momentum values about the anteroposterior axis and ball velocity. In other words, the more the players produce trunk angular momentum about the anteroposterior axis between maximal elbow flexion and ball impact, the higher the ball velocity will be. These strong relationships confirm the results of Bahamonde [14] suggesting that the rotation of the trunk about the anteroposterior axis (also called "shoulder-over-shoulder" rotation) differentiates players with the highest ball speeds from players with the lowest ball speeds.

1.3 Ball Velocity and Tennis Serve Kinetics

Elliott et al. [16] demonstrated that male professional players commonly recorded higher torques and forces at the shoulder and elbow joints than their female counterparts. According to them, these higher kinetic measures are an important factor in producing the significantly higher serve velocity for this group of players [16]. Davis et al. [17] proposed efficiency measurements for the baseball pitch about the relationship between ball velocity and kinetics. They divided joint loadings by ball velocity in order to better understand the pitcher's efficiency [17]. Indeed, a highly efficient pitcher or server is one who can maximize output (ball velocity) with the least joint load [18]. Martin et al. [19] showed that advanced tennis players are less "efficient" than professional ones since they increase both their shoulder and elbow kinetics compared to professional players without reaching higher ball velocity. It is assumed that the low efficiency measured in advanced players could be related to improper mechanics of the kinetic chain. It has been indicated that any disruption to the kinetic chain caused by improper mechanics could result in increased loading of upper limb joints in the sequence of movements [20]. As a consequence, it can be supposed that advanced players tried to compensate for the kinetic chain disruption caused by improper serve mechanics by increasing segment activation and loading [21].

1.4 Upper Limb Joint Injuries, Tennis Serve Biomechanics, and Energy Flow

Overuse injuries in sport can result from a complex interaction between various risk factors such as age, gender, muscle weakness and imbalance, poor equipment, number of repetitions during trainings and competitions, and excessive joint loadings [22]. Among all the risk factors in overhand throwing and striking activities, excessive joint loadings (forces and torques) are known to be a crucial risk factor causing repetitive microtrauma that is responsible for overuse upper limb joint injuries [20–22]. Indeed, it appears logical that players subjected to higher loadings might be more likely to sustain joint overuse injury. Concerning tennis, the serve has been reported to be a traumatic skill, as it causes high loads on the upper limb joints in professional and advanced tennis players [16, 19, 23] (Table 1.3).

The traumatic effect of the tennis activity is also linked to the repetitive nature of the serve movement throughout the player's competitive career. Interestingly, tennis players hit between 50 and 150 serves during a match. This result is increased by the number of single matches played by the players during a competitive season (around 60 matches), without considering double matches and training sessions [25]. This repetition of serves inflicted on the upper limb joints in competitive tennis players may explain why overuse injuries of the upper limb joints are a common medical problem in all competitive levels in tennis [26]. Indeed, these overuse injuries concern not only professional tennis players but also recreational and advanced competitive players [6]. Tennis is a world-class competitive sport attracting tens of millions of players all around the world, and the majority of them is presumed to be recreational or advanced rather than elite. Consequently, Martin et al. [19] have compared the joint kinetics and stroke production efficiency for the shoulder, elbow, and wrist during the serve between professionals and advanced tennis players. Peaks of shoulder inferior force, shoulder anterior force, shoulder horizontal abduction torque, and elbow medial force are significantly higher in advanced players. Ball velocity is significantly faster for the professional players (177.8 ± 17.3 km/h) compared to the advanced players (143.3 ± 14.4 km/h). Consequently, professional players are more efficient than advanced players, as they maximize ball velocity with lower or similar joint kinetics. Since advanced players are subjected to higher joint kinetics, the results suggest that they appear more susceptible to high risk of shoulder and elbow injuries than professionals, especially during the cocking and deceleration phases of the serve.

According to Fortenbaugh [27], changes in kinematics can increase or decrease velocity or not affect it at all. Clearly, any kinematic pattern that significantly increases kinetics values without increasing velocity is pathomechanical. Indeed, even minor technical and temporal errors, which are continually repeated throughout a match, a competitive season, or a career, may affect the performance, increase joint kinetics, and consequently cause tendon overuse microinstability problems [22, 28].

Table 1.3 Peak values of joint kinetics measured for the tennis serve

References	Population	Shoulder internal rotation torque (N/m)	Shoulder horizontal adduction torque (N/m)	Elbow varus torque (N/m)	Elbow flexion torque (N/m)	Shoulder anterior force (N)	Shoulder proximal force (N)
[16]	8 professional tennis players	71 ± 15	108 ± 25	78 ± 12	37 ± 23	292 ± 120	608 ± 110
[24]	12 elite tennis players	23 ± 8	/	/	/	167 ± 47	229 ± 52

Conversely, it has been suggested that proper temporal mechanics may enable athletes to achieve maximum performance with minimum chances of injury. Concerning the tennis serve, it has been reported that a poor leg drive decreases ball velocity [29] and increases shoulder and elbow kinetics during the tennis serve (+15% for the peak of shoulder internal rotation torque and +18% for the peak of elbow varus moment) [16]. Moreover, it has been shown that the type of backswing influences shoulder anterior force [16]. Indeed, higher normalized anterior force at the shoulder joint was noticed for those players with an abbreviated swing compared with those players who used a full backswing (+34%) [16]. In baseball, it is believed that the safest and most efficient pitching depends on the correct timing and sequence of motions as much as the quality of the motions themselves [17]. In such a sequence of motions, the timing of trunk and shoulder rotations seems to be crucial because the trunk and the shoulder are links that considerably contribute to the body angular momentum and can affect tennis performance [15]. Consequently, research has focused on the effects of trunk rotation timing on upper limb joint kinetics during the tennis serve [30]. The purposes of this study were to measure the effects of temporal parameters on both ball velocity and upper limb joint kinetics to identify pathomechanical factors during the tennis serve and to validate these pathomechanical factors by comparing upper limb joint injured and non-injured players. The later timing of peak trunk angular velocities and the improper timing between the shoulder horizontal adduction and the external rotation are indeed associated to higher upper limb joint kinetics and lower ball velocity [30]. Non-injured players are able to maximize ball velocity and reduce upper limb joint kinetics by rotating their trunk at maximal velocities earlier than injured players, allowing the energy to pass from the trunk to the shoulder at precisely the right timing within the correct sequence of movements. Moreover, during the cocking and acceleration phases of the tennis serve, the arm moves from horizontal abduction to adduction and to extreme angles of external rotation. The correlation analyses show that the more the instant of shoulder external rotation precedes the instant of shoulder horizontal adduction, the more the shoulder anterior force ($r = 0.40$, $p < 0.001$) and horizontal abduction torque increase ($r = 0.40$, $p < 0.001$) and the more the ball velocity decreases ($r = -0.26$, $p < 0.05$). According to the results, non-injured players are more effective because they achieve shoulder horizontal adduction just before extreme positions of external rotation. As a consequence, they are able to maximize ball velocity and limit upper limb joint loadings by using proper temporal parameters during the serve. Conversely, injured players "leave" their arm in horizontal abduction for too long during the shoulder external rotation phase. Consequently, injured players reach significantly lower ball velocities and demonstrated higher joint kinetics. Excessive shoulder horizontal abduction that occurs during the late cocking phase of the throwing motion has been reported to be critical for internal impingement [31] caused by a translation of the humeral head relative to the glenoid [32], which may lead to rotator cuff tears, shoulder tendinopathies, and labral lesions.

Energy flow has been hypothesized to be one of the most critical biomechanical concepts related to tennis serve performance and overuse injuries. Martin et al. [19] investigated the relationships among the quality and magnitude of energy flow, the ball velocity, and the peaks of upper limb joint kinetics to compare the energy flow during the serve between injured and non-injured tennis players. Their results showed that ball velocity increased and upper limb joint kinetics decreased with the quality of energy flow from the trunk to the hand + racket segment. Injured players showed a lower quality of energy flow through the upper limb kinetic chain, a lower ball velocity, and higher rates of energy absorbed by the shoulder and elbow compared with non-injured players. Consequently, it appears that the alterations of energy flow from the trunk to the racket can play a predictive role in both serve performance and injury [4].

1.5 The Effects of the Stance Technique on Serve Biomechanics

The goal of the preparation phase for the server, during which they get their body and legs into position, is to use ground reaction forces in order to generate the power required for the service motion. Tennis players can generally use two stance techniques: some bring the back foot up to the front foot during the ball toss, prior to the swing (Murray, Tsonga, Del Potro); while others leave the rear foot back until leg extension begins (Federer, Djokovic). The first is known as the "foot-up" technique, while the second is called the "foot-back" technique. During the 2007 French Open, the distribution of the two stance techniques was analyzed [33]. Results showed that 72.4% of players used the foot-up technique. However, when we look at technique selection according to game style, we notice that this percentage changes considerably (Table 1.4). Close to 50% of players who serve and volley regularly or occasionally (doubles players or attacking players) use the foot-back stance when serving, compared with only one player in six among those who never move to the net after their serve (Table 1.4). What are the advantages and disadvantages of each stance technique?

1.5.1 Effect of the Stance Technique on Ball Velocity

A recent study has shown that when expert players use the foot-up technique, they generate on average higher ball velocities (173.2 km/h vs. 166.3 km/h with the foot-back technique) [34]. This represents a mean difference of 7 km/h in favor of the foot-up technique. How can we explain this result? It is known that the larger the base of support, the more balanced the player is. That is what happens with the foot-back technique which gives the player good stability. By contrast, with the foot-up technique, as both feet get closer until they touch one another and the server moves forward and pushes off the ground to hit the ball, the base of support narrows, which means the player becomes less balanced. The body of the server starts rotating forward. As the result of the blocking of a body part in motion (in this instance, the feet), an amount of body rotation is produced (as is also the case during a trip or somersault). That amount of forward body rotation (known as "angular momentum" in biomechanics) is greater with the foot-up technique than with the foot-back technique. And we know that the greater the amount of forward body rotation, the higher the ball velocity [15]. That is why the foot-up stance allows players to serve a little harder.

1.5.2 Effect of the Stance Technique on Ball Impact Height

Another major advantage of the foot-up technique is that it produces higher upward ground reaction forces compared with the foot-back technique (2.1 times the body weight vs. 1.5 times the body weight, respectively) [35, 36]. Consequently, the foot-up technique allows players to impact the ball higher compared with the foot-back technique. A mean difference of 11 cm was recorded between the two stance techniques (2.65 m with the foot-up technique vs. 2.54 m with the foot-back technique) in expert tennis players [35]. As we know, the higher the ball impact, the greater the net clearance, the higher the chances of increasing first and second serve percentages, and the more chances you have of achieving short and cross-court angles. It has been shown that increasing the height of ball impact from 2.60 to 2.70 m allowed players to reach zones 25–30 cm shorter in the service box.

Table 1.4 Distribution of techniques according to game style among players at the French Open, adapted from Renoult [33]

Serve stance	Attacking game style, %	Baseline game style, %
Foot-up	54.3	82.7
Foot-back	45.7	17.3

1.5.3 Effect of the Stance Technique on Running Time to the Net During the Serve and Volley

A scientific study has focused on the influence of stance techniques on the running time of expert tennis players (male and female) to the net during the serve and volley [34]. Results showed that players using the foot-back technique were able to reach the service line faster than those using the foot-up technique (1.49 s vs. 1.56 s, respectively). Even though the difference of 70 ms between the two techniques may appear insignificant at first sight, in reality it makes quite a difference in relation to one of the biggest challenges of serve-and-volley play. Indeed, serve-and-volley players look to run as quickly as possible in order to play the volley in good conditions; this can be achieved by getting as close as possible to the net. For instance, in the case of a return of serve hit at 140 km/h, a 70 ms time difference means that the serve and volleyer can get approximately 2.4 m closer to the net, thus greatly enhancing the likelihood of a successful first volley. How is it possible to explain such a difference between the two stance techniques? According to the results of this study, the loss of time recorded with the foot-up technique happens mostly during the landing phase. The duration of the first foot-floor contact after the serve is extended by 20 ms on average with the foot-up technique.

Because players push more upward when using the foot-up technique, they need more time to recover balance during the landing phase before running to the net. Another factor explains the shorter running time to the net with the foot-back technique, and that is the forward impulse. With the foot-back technique, players cover a greater distance inside the court during the serve (60 cm compared with 46 cm with the foot-up technique) because they are able to generate larger propulsive forces to the net (0.20 times the body weight vs. 0.16 times the body weight with the foot-up technique) [35, 36].

1.5.4 Effect of the Stance Technique on Upper Limb Joint Loadings and Risks of Chronic Injuries

Some scientists studied the loadings (forces and torques) that are placed on the shoulder joint during the serving motion depending on the stance technique used in order to determine if one technique was more traumatic than the other. No noticeable difference in joint loading was observed between the foot-back and the foot-up techniques [25].

1.6 Biomechanical Differences Between the Type of Spins

1.6.1 Kinematic Differences Between the Type of Spins: Flat, Slice, and Kick Serves

The spin is particularly important in tennis success. The direction of ball spin for the flat and slice serves is similar, while the kick serve is different since it is hit with more topspin than the other serves [37]. There is a negative relationship between speed and spin. Indeed, when ball spin rate increases, ball velocity decreases (Table 1.5).

Racket velocity during the serve is influenced by the type of spins [24, 39, 40]. Significant differences in the direction of the racket velocity vector between serves have been demonstrated (Table 1.6): the kick serve had the largest lateral and smallest forward racket velocity components, while the flat serve had the smallest vertical component. The slice serve had lateral velocity, like the kick, and large forward velocity, like the flat [40].

Reid et al. [24, Sheets et al. [40], and Abrams et al. [41] investigated tennis players' kinematics

Table 1.5 Ball velocity versus spin trade-off in the serve from high-performance players [38]

	Flat serve	Slice serve	Kick serve
Ball velocity (km/h)	190	170	150
Spin rate (rpm)	1200	2200	3200

1 Biomechanics of the Tennis Serve

Table 1.6 Racket kinematics for the flat and kick serves

Racket kinematics	References	Flat serve	Kick serve
Absolute maximal velocity (km/h)	[24]	156 ± 11	145 ± 10
	[39]	140 ± 8	135 ± 9
Maximal horizontal velocity (km/h)	[24]	146 ± 12	126 ± 10
	[39]	123 ± 11	115 ± 14
Maximal vertical velocity (km/h)	[24]	108 ± 11	100 ± 10
	[39]	60 ± 17	68 ± 14
Right lateral velocity (km/h)	[24]	5 ± 20	37 ± 8
	[39]	21 ± 15	59 ± 10

Table 1.7 Racket lateral flexion angle at impact across ages and type of serves [38]

	Flat serve	Slice serve	Kick serve
Adults	15°	30°	40°
14–15 years	20°	30°	40°
11–12 years	20°	30°	25°

Table 1.8 Racket face twist (pronation) angle at impact across ages and types of serves [38]

	Flat serve	Slice serve	Kick serve
Adults	5°	30°	20°
14–15 years	10°	20°	15°
11–12 years	10°	10°	10°

1.6.2 Kinetic Differences Between the Type of Spins and Injury Risks

The kick serve is frequently linked with shoulder and lower limb pain and injuries in tennis. Reid et al. [24] observed comparable shoulder joint loadings between the flat and kick serves in 12 high-performance male players. However, a more recent study in seven collegiate tennis players reported larger posteriorly directed shoulder forces in the kick serve [41]. Moreover, the kick serve had a higher force magnitude at the back than the flat and slice serves. Force and torque magnitudes at the elbow and wrist were not significantly different between the serves [41]. According to those results, one may consider that the kick serve induces the greatest amount of loadings on the back and shoulder and thus may pose the greatest risk for injury. Moreover, the combination of the posteromedial contact point and the increased vertical and lateral linear velocities of the racket during the kick serve contributes to increased stress loadings on the back (ligaments, disks, and vertebrae of the spinal column) and activity levels of trunk muscles as previously reported [42]. Conversely, the slice serve demonstrated lower overall joint loadings [41]. Consequently, it should be considered as the most "physiologic" of the serve types and may be the first serve type to introduce when attempting to return to play, especially when recovering from injury [41].

during the flat and kick serves. They showed similar shoulder joint kinematics between the flat and kick serves, but Sheets et al. [40] reported differences in velocity components at the wrist and elbow. Velocity components at the wrist and elbow were smaller in the lateral direction during the flat serve than during the kick and had larger downward velocities. Moreover, a more vigorous lower limb drive for the kick serve has been observed since the peak vertical velocity of the rear hip in the kick serve (2.3 ± 0.3 m/s) was significantly higher than in the flat serve (2.1 ± 0.3 m/s) [24]. By using a more dynamic vertical leg drives, players can maximize the "up and out" racket trajectory and the spin rate transferred to the ball at impact. Moreover, the body position at ball impact is significantly different between the flat and kick serves [40]. Indeed, the racket in the kick serve was positioned 9 cm more posterior and 21 cm more medial than the shoulder compared with the flat. This position could increase the risk of shoulder and back injuries associated with the kick serve. The combination of racket angle at impact and racket trajectory with reference to the ball allows the players to produce various spins on the ball. Racket lateral flexion angle and racket face twist angle are influenced by the type of spin and players' age (Tables 1.7 and 1.8) [38].

1.7 Influence of Fatigue on Serve Biomechanics

The typical average tennis match duration is between 1 and 2 h, but in some cases, this duration can be prolonged (from 3 to 6 h) [43, 44].

In Grand Slam tournaments, the mean duration of five-set matches is between 137 and 154 min, according to the court surface [45]. Tennis match play is defined by intermittent exercise: short bouts of high intensity (<10 s) are interrupted by short active recovery bouts (10–20 s) and passive recovery periods of longer duration (90–120 s). Throughout an extreme five-set tennis match, players can hit more than 1000 ground strokes and 400 serves [44] leading to muscular fatigue, which is considered both as a cause of performance impairment and an injury risk factor [46]. The influence of muscular fatigue on serve ball velocity during tennis is unclear since previous studies have reported conflicting results. Indeed, it has been shown that serve ball velocity did not change between the beginning and the end of 2 h 30 and 4-h tennis matches [47, 48], while it has been reported that a 2-h tennis match or training session decreased serve accuracy (from −12% to −30%), ball speed (−4.5%), and increased percentage of errors [49–51]. Moreover, the effects of tennis fatigue on muscle capacities have been previously analyzed [50, 52]. Electromyographic activity (EMG) and force measured during isometric maximal voluntary contraction decreased in knee extensors, in plantar flexors during a 3-h tennis match [52], and in pectoralis major and flexor carpi radialis during a 40-min tennis exercise composed by four series of 12 repetitions of one serve followed by eight forehand strokes [50]. However, this last result was measured during "artificial" fatigue protocol that may fail to reflect fatigue level obtained for prolonged tennis match [46]. Indeed, one of the limitations in these previous studies [49–51] is that the duration of tennis exercise ranged from 40 to 120 min, and the total number of serves was limited to 100 or fewer. Yet, it is essential that scientific researches reflect the true competition situation to accurately understand the fatigue effects on tennis performance and muscular activity [46]. Consequently, a recent study has quantified kinematic, kinetic, and performance changes that occurred in the serve throughout a 3-h real tennis match play in male advanced tennis players [53]. Their results showed that a 3-h tennis match induces decrease in mean power frequency values for several upper limb muscles (biceps brachii, anterior deltoid, pectoralis major, middle trapezius, triceps brachii, and infraspinatus) that is an indicator of local muscular fatigue. Moreover, decreases in serve ball velocity (−6.4 km/h, −3.9%) and ball impact height (−4 cm) were reported after the match. Between the beginning and the end of the match, the results show significant decreases in maximal angular velocity of shoulder internal rotation (−7.5%), elbow extension (−6.0%), wrist flexion (−13.8%), pelvis longitudinal rotation (−4.7%), trunk transversal rotation (−5.1%), and trunk sagittal rotation (−6.0%) (Fig. 1.1). With fatigue, the majority of the upper limb joint kinetics decreased between the beginning and the end of the match (Fig. 1.2). Conversely, no change in timing of maximal angular velocities was observed throughout the match. This consistency suggests that advanced tennis players are able to use a robust segmental coordination, which allows them to maintain the temporal pattern of their serve technique, in spite of the muscular fatigue development.

1.8 The Effect of Repetitive Serving on Shoulder Range of Motion

Objective measurement of range of motion (ROM) of the shoulder joint is important for tennis performance as well as rehabilitation and prevention of shoulder injury [54]. Chandler et al. [55] were the first to compare active internal and external rotation ROM for the shoulder with 90° of abduction in junior elite tennis players. They found significantly less mean internal rotation range in the dominant arm compared with the non-dominant arm (−11°) [55]. Conversely, greater external rotation was reported on the dominant shoulder compared with the non-dominant one (13°). Similar results in later studies have been found [56, 57]. Kibler et al. [58] analyzed the chronic effect of tennis play on shoulder range of motion, and they reported that dominant internal rotation of the shoulder decreased and the difference between the

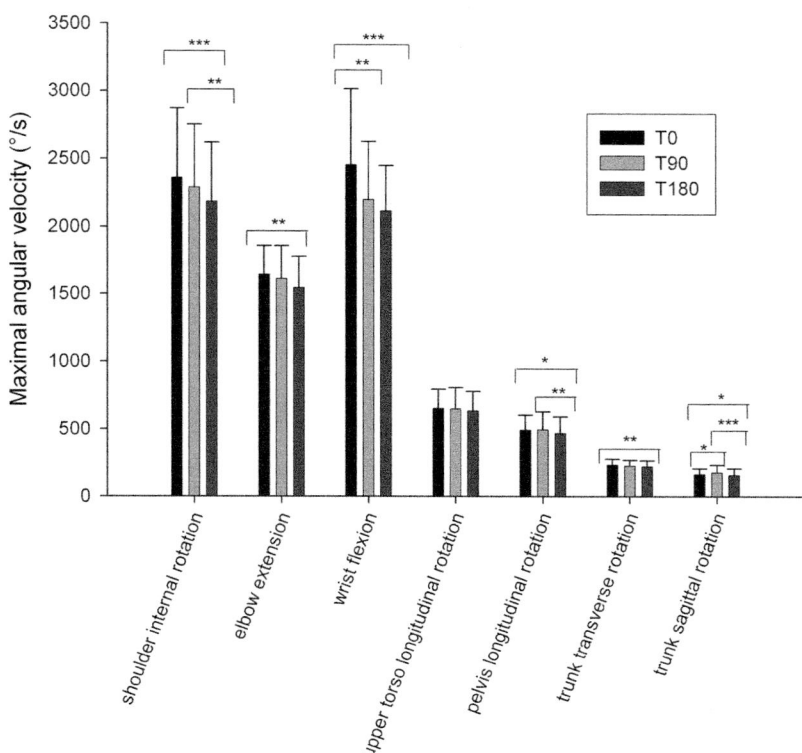

Fig. 1.1 Upper body maximal angular velocities before (T0), at mid-match (T90) and immediately after the match (T180). Values are mean ± SD. ***$p < 0.001$; **$p < 0.01$; *$p < 0.05$ [53]

dominant and non-dominant internal rotation increased with both age and years of tournament play. This deficit in shoulder internal rotation ROM of approximately 10° between dominant and non-dominant arm is currently considered as a physiological adaptation that occurs normally in tennis players [59]. Wilk et al. [60] introduced the concept of shoulder total rotation ROM. It involves adding the internal and external rotation ROM at 90° of abduction together [60]. In elite junior tennis players, significantly less dominant shoulder total rotation ROM was identified (149.1° vs. 158.2°) [57]. Pathologic shoulder internal rotation is identified when there is a loss of shoulder internal rotation greater than 18°–20° associated with a corresponding loss of total ROM greater than 5° when compared bilaterally [61]. Indeed, recent findings support that a loss of total shoulder ROM is predictive of future shoulder injury in professional overhead throwing athletes [62]. In baseball, it has been shown that pitchers whose total ROM comparison was greater than 5° exhibited a 2.5 times greater risk of sustaining a shoulder injury [62]. In tennis, a statistically significant correlation was observed between dominant shoulder internal rotation deficits and shoulder pain [63]. Moreover, a significant relationship between serve velocity and increased dominant shoulder internal rotation at 0° of abduction has been found in expert tennis players [64].

Determining the acute effect of a prolonged tennis match on shoulder ROM may be insightful for understanding shoulder injury potential and serve performance. As a consequence, two studies analyzed the acute effect of prolonged tennis match play on shoulder ROM [65, 66]. In the study of Martin et al. [65], shoulder passive internal and external rotation ROM were measured on 8 male advanced tennis players before, every 30 min during and just after a 3-h tennis match during which players hit approximately 250 serves and 547 ground strokes. In the study of Moore-Reed et al. [66], shoulder passive internal and external rotation ROM were evaluated in 79 professional female tennis players at three

Fig. 1.2 Maximal values of upper limb joint forces and torques before (T0), at mid-match (T90) and immediately after the match (T180). Values are mean ± SD.
***$p < 0.001$; **$p < 0.01$; *$p < 0.05$ [53]

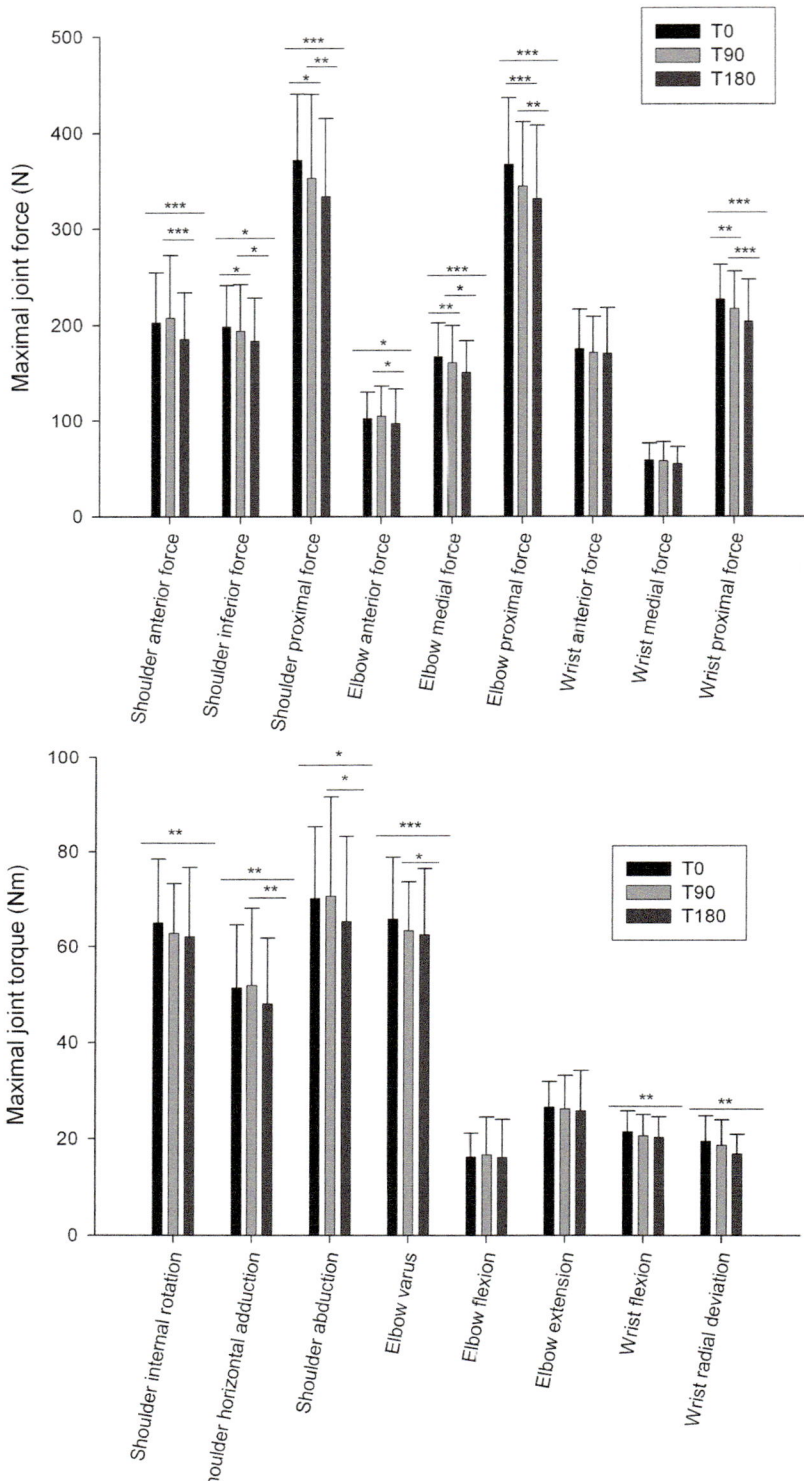

different time points (TP): baseline before match play (TP1), immediately after match play (TP2), and 24 h after baseline (TP3). Both studies demonstrated significant decreases in shoulder internal rotation and total ROM between the beginning and the end of the match (Figs. 1.3 and 1.4). Moreover, shoulder internal ROM continued to decrease 24 h after the acute match exposure [66]. No statistically significant difference was observed for shoulder external rotation after the match.

According to Manske et al. [61], pathologic shoulder internal rotation is identified when there is a loss of shoulder internal rotation greater than 18°–20°, with a corresponding loss of total ROM greater than 5° when compared bilaterally. A nonacceptable level of shoulder internal rotation deficit is defined as (1) more than 20° loss of shoulder internal rotation or (2) greater than a 10% loss of the total ROM [32]. In the study of Martin et al. [65], the mean loss of shoulder internal rotation reached 20.8° and the mean loss of total ROM approximated 25° (i.e., 15%) after the match. Although this study did not compare dominant and non-dominant shoulders, the results show that a prolonged tennis match play can bring the dominant shoulder to a risky situation when compared with the beginning of the match. The decreases in shoulder internal rotation and total ROM measured could be the result of repetitive eccentric contractions [67] caused by the numerous powerful serves hit by the players during the match. Repetitive eccentric contractions can cause posterior muscle-tendon unit and capsular tightness that has been shown to create abnormal shoulder biomechanics [68]. Indeed, it has been reported that posterior capsule tightness of the shoulder causes subsequent anterior and superior translations of the humeral head [69]. As a consequence, this phenomenon could reduce subacromial space and lead to soft tissue impingement. Moreover, Muraki et al. [70] reported increased peak subacromial pressure and increased contact area on the coracoacromial ligament in the follow-through position of overhead throwing after modifying the posteroinferior shoulder capsule. Further support for posterior shoulder tightness as a risk factor of shoulder injuries comes from Wilk et al. [62] and Vad et al. [63], who observed decreased shoulder internal rotation in baseball and tennis players with shoulder impingement symptoms. Consequently, one may argue that shoulder ROM changes caused by a prolonged

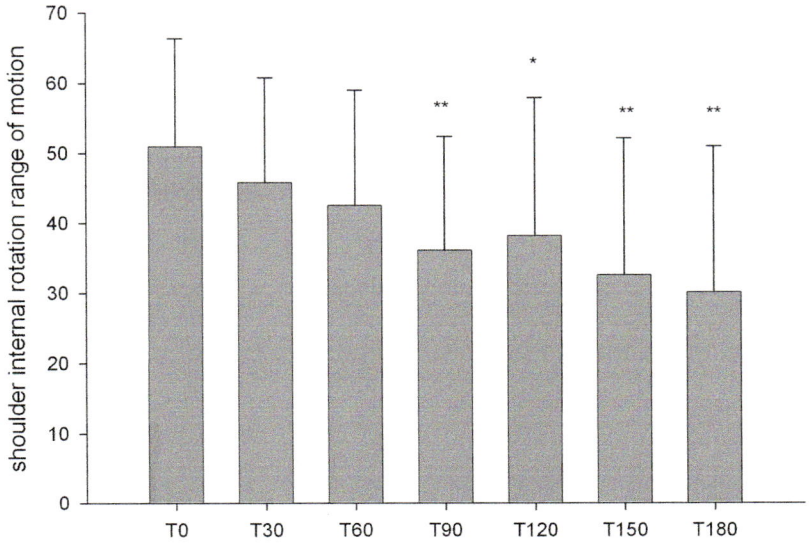

Fig. 1.3 Shoulder internal range of motion before (T0), during (T30, T60, T90, T120, and T150), and immediately after the match (T180). Values are means 6 SD. *$p < 0.05$; **$p < 0.01$ (significantly different from T0) [65]

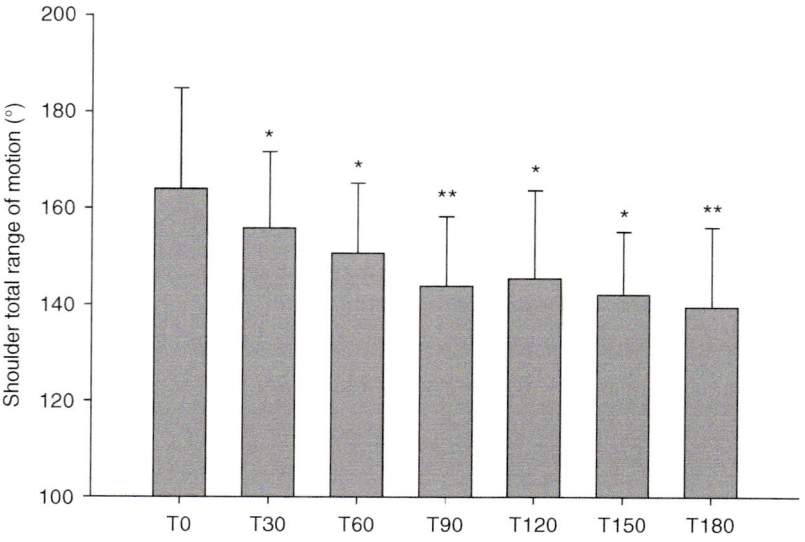

Fig. 1.4 Shoulder total range of motion before (T0), during (T30, T60, T90, T120, and T150), and immediately after the match (T180). Values are means 6 SD. $*p < 0.05$; $**p < 0.01$ (significantly different from T0) [65]

tennis match could increase the risk of shoulder injuries. Moreover, shoulder internal ROM continued to decrease 24 h after the acute match exposure [66]. This phenomenon is problematic for tennis players who regularly play one or two matches per day during tournaments. One may hypothesize that many tennis players play one tennis match after another, while their shoulder ROM does not return to baseline. Although an acute decrease in shoulder ROM may be a normal physiological response [71], tennis players may be more vulnerable to shoulder injury if they continue to play with decreased shoulder internal rotation and total ROM. Consequently, it appears necessary to restore the tennis player's normal shoulder ROM before having to play the next match. Throughout a prolonged tennis match (especially during a "best of 5 sets" format used in men's tennis during Grand Slam tournaments), tennis players could take advantage of changing ends for practicing cross-body stretches and pendulum exercises to limit loss of shoulder ROM. After the match, stretching (cross-body and sleeper stretches) [68], joint mobilization, ice, and instrument-assisted soft tissue mobilization [72] are recommended for tennis players because these techniques have been studied and found to be beneficial for increasing shoulder ROM.

References

1. Johnson C, McHugh M, Wood T, Kibler B. Performance demands of professional male tennis players. Br J Sports Med. 2006;40:696–9.
2. Roetert EP, Kovacs M. Tennis anatomy. Champaign, IL: Human Kinetics; 2011.
3. Hjelm N, Werner S, Renstrom P. Injury risk factors in junior tennis players: a prospective 2-year study. Scand J Med Sci Sports. 2012;22:40–8.
4. Martin C, Bideau B, Bideau N, Nicolas G, Delamarche P, Kulpa R. Energy flow analysis during the tennis serve: comparison between injured and noninjured tennis players. Am J Sports Med. 2014;42:2751–60. https://doi.org/10.1177/0363546514547173.
5. Abrams G, Sheets A, Andriacchi T, Safran M. Review of tennis serve motion analysis and the biomechanics of three serve types with implications for injury. Sports Biomech. 2011;10:378–90.
6. Jayanthi N, Sallay P, Hunker P, Przybylski M. Skill-level related injuries in recreational competition tennis players. J Med Sci Tennis. 2005;40:12–5.
7. Pluim B, Staal J, Windler G, Jayanthi N. Tennis injuries: occurrence, aetiology and prevention. Br J Sports Med. 2006;40:464–8.
8. Fleisig G, Nicholls R, Elliott B, Escamilia R. Kinematics used by world class tennis players to produce high-velocity serves. Sports Biomech. 2003;2:51–64.
9. Elliott B, Marshall N, Noffal G. Contributions of upper limb segment rotations during the power serve in tennis. J Appl Biomech. 1995;11:433–42.
10. Gordon B, Dapena J. Contributions of joint rotations to racquet speed in the tennis serve. J Sports Sci. 2006;24:31–49.
11. Sprigings E, Marshall R, Elliott B, Jennings L. A three-dimensional kinematic method for deter-

mining the effectiveness of arm segment rotations in producing racquet-head speed. J Biomech. 1994;27:245–54.
12. Tanabe S, Ito A. A three-dimensional analysis of the contributions of upper limb joint movements to horizontal racket head velocity at ball impact during tennis serving. Sports Biomech. 2007;6:418–33.
13. Wagner H, Pfustersched J, Tilp M, Landlinger J, von Duvillard S, Muller E. Upper-body kinematics in team-handball throw, tennis serve, and volleyball spike. Scand J Med Sci Sports. 2012;24(2):345–54.
14. Bahamonde R. Changes in angular momentum during the tennis serve. J Sports Sci. 2000;18:579–92.
15. Martin C, Kulpa R, Delamarche P, Bideau B. Professional tennis players' serve: correlation between segmental angular momentums and ball velocity. Sports Biomech. 2013;12:2–14. https://doi.org/10.1080/14763141.2012.734321.
16. Elliott B, Fleisig G, Nicholls R, Escamilia R. Technique effects on upper limb loading in the tennis serve. J Sci Med Sport. 2003;6:76–87.
17. Davis J, Limpisvasti O, Fluhme D, Mohr K, Yocum L, Elattrache N, Jobe F. The effect of pitching biomechanics on the upper extremity in youth and adolescent baseball pitchers. Am J Sports Med. 2009;37:1484–91.
18. Aguinaldo A, Buttermore J, Chambers H. Effects of upper trunk rotation on shoulder joint torque among baseball pitchers of various levels. J Appl Biomech. 2007;23:42–51.
19. Martin C, Bideau B, Ropars M, Delamarche P, Kulpa R. Upper limb joint kinetic analysis during tennis serve: assessment of competitive level on efficiency and injury risks. Scand J Med Sci Sports. 2014;24:60–75. https://doi.org/10.1111/sms.12043.
20. Kibler WB. Biomechanical analysis of the shoulder during tennis activities. Clin Sports Med. 1995;14:79–85.
21. Lintner D, Noonan T, Kibler W. Injury patterns and biomechanics of the athlete's shoulder. Clin Sports Med. 2008;27:527–51.
22. Kannus P. Etiology and pathophysiology of chronic tendon disorders in sports. Scand J Med Sci Sports. 1997;7:78–85.
23. Reid M, Elliott B, Alderson J. Shoulder joint kinetics of the elite wheelchair tennis serve. Br J Sports Med. 2007;41:739–44. https://doi.org/10.1136/bjsm.2007.036145.
24. Reid M, Elliott B, Alderson J. Shoulder joint loading in the high performance flat and kick tennis serves. Br J Sports Med. 2007;41(12):884–9.
25. Reid M, Elliott B, Alderson J. Lower-limb coordination and shoulder joint mechanics in the tennis serve. Med Sci Sports Exerc. 2008;40:308–15.
26. Marx R, Sperling J, Cordasco F. Overuse injuries of the upper extremity in tennis players. Clin Sports Med. 2001;20:439–51.
27. Fortenbaugh D, Fleisig G, Andrews J. Baseball pitching biomechanics in relation to injury risk and performance. Sports Health. 2009;1:314–20.
28. Kibler W, Thomas S. Pathomechanics of the throwing shoulder. Sports Med Arthrosc Rev. 2012;20:22–9.
29. Girard O, Micallef J, Millet G. Influence of restricted knee motion during the flat first serve in tennis. J Strength Cond Res. 2007;21:950–7.
30. Martin C, Kulpa R, Ropars M, Delamarche P, Bideau B. Identification of temporal pathomechanical factors during the tennis serve. Med Sci Sports Exerc. 2013;45:2113–9. https://doi.org/10.1249/MSS.0b013e318299ae3b.
31. Mihata T, McGarry M, Kinoshita M, Lee T. Excessive glenohumeral horizontal abduction as occurs during the late cocking phase of the throwing motion can be critical for internal impingement. Am J Sports Med. 2010;38:369–74.
32. Burkhart S, Morgan C, Kibler W. The disabled throwing shoulder: spectrum of pathology. Part I: pathoanatomy and biomechanics. Arthroscopy. 2003;19:404–20.
33. Renoult M. Les positions de départ au service et le relais d'appuis. Lett Club Fédéral Enseign Prof Tennis. 2007;2007:2–3.
34. Martin C, Bideau B, Nicolas G, Delamarche P, Kulpa R. How does the tennis serve technique influence the serve-and-volley? J Sports Sci. 2012;30:1149–56.
35. Elliott B, Wood G. The biomechanics of foot-up and foot-back tennis service techniques. Aust J Sports Sci. 1983;3:3–6.
36. Bahamonde R, Knudson D. Ground reaction forces and two types of stances and tennis serves. Med Sci Sports Exerc. 2001;33:102.
37. Sakurai S, Reid M, Elliott B. Ball spin in the tennis serve: spin rate and axis of rotation. Sports Biomech Int Soc Biomech Sports. 2013;12:23–9. https://doi.org/10.1080/14763141.2012.671355.
38. Elliott B, Reid M, Crespo M. Technique development in tennis stroke production. London: International Tennis Federation; 2009. p. 71–88.
39. Chow JW, Carlton LG, Lim Y-T, Chae W-S, Shim J-H, Kuenster AF, Kokubun K. Comparing the pre- and post-impact ball and racquet kinematics of elite tennis players' first and second serves: a preliminary study. J Sports Sci. 2003;21:529–37. https://doi.org/10.1080/0264041031000101908.
40. Sheets A, Abrams G, Corazza S, Safran M, Andriacchi T. Kinematics differences between the flat, kick and slice serves measured using a markerless motion capture method. Ann Biomed Eng. 2011;39:3011–20.
41. Abrams G, Harris A, Andriacchi T, Safran M. Biomechanical analysis of three tennis serve types using a markerless system. Br J Sports Med. 2013;48:339–42.
42. Chow JW, Shim JH, Lim YT. Lower trunk muscle activity during the tennis serve. J Sci Med Sport Sports Med Aust. 2003;6:512–8.
43. Kovacs MS. Applied physiology of tennis performance. Br J Sports Med. 2006;40:381–6. https://doi.org/10.1136/bjsm.2005.023309.

44. Reid M, Duffield R. The development of fatigue during match-play tennis. Br J Sports Med. 2014;48:i7–i11. https://doi.org/10.1136/bjsports-2013-093196.
45. Morante SM, Brotherhood JR. Match characteristics of professional singles tennis. J Med Sci Tennis. 2005;13:12–3.
46. Hornery D, Farrow D, Mujika I, Young W. Fatigue in tennis. Mechanisms of fatigue and effect on performance. Sports Med. 2007;37:199–212.
47. Girard O, Millet G, Micallef J. La vitesse du service et les forces de réaction du sol sont-elles modifiées suite à une session de tennis prolongée? ITF Coach Sport Sci Rev. 2012;20:18–20.
48. Gescheit DT, Cormack SJ, Reid M, Duffield R. Consecutive days of prolonged tennis matchplay: performance, physical, and perceptual responses in trained players. Int J Sports Physiol Perform. 2015. https://doi.org/10.1123/ijspp.2014-0329.
49. Hornery DJ, Farrow D, Mujika I. An integrated physiological and performance profile of professional tennis. Br J Sports Med. 2007;41:531–6. https://doi.org/10.1136/bjsm.2006.031351.
50. Rota S, Morel B, Saboul D, Rogowski I, Hautier C. Influence of fatigue on upper limb muscle activity and performance in tennis. J Electromyogr Kinesiol. 2014;24:90–7. https://doi.org/10.1016/j.jelekin.2013.10.007.
51. Vergauwen L, Brouns F, Hespel P. Carbohydrate supplementation improves stroke performance in tennis. Med Sci Sports Exerc. 1998;30:1289–95.
52. Girard O, Racinais S, Micallef J-P, Millet GP. Spinal modulations accompany peripheral fatigue during prolonged tennis playing. Scand J Med Sci Sports. 2011;21:455–64. https://doi.org/10.1111/j.1600-0838.2009.01032.x.
53. Martin C, Bideau B, Delamarche P, Kulpa R. Influence of a Prolonged Tennis Match Play on Serve Biomechanics. PLoS One. 2016;11:e0159979. https://doi.org/10.1371/journal.pone.0159979.
54. Ellenbecker TS, Roetert EP, Piorkowski PA, Schulz DA. Glenohumeral joint internal and external rotation range of motion in elite junior tennis players. J Orthop Sports Phys Ther. 1996;24:336–41. https://doi.org/10.2519/jospt.1996.24.6.336.
55. Chandler TJ, Kibler WB, Uhl TL, Wooten B, Kiser A, Stone E. Flexibility comparisons of junior elite tennis players to other athletes. Am J Sports Med. 1990;18:134–6.
56. Ellenbecker T. Shoulder internal and external rotation strength and range of motion of highly skilled junior tennis players. Isokinet Exerc Sci Ther. 1992;2:1–8.
57. Ellenbecker TS, Roetert EP, Bailie DS, Davies GJ, Brown SW. Glenohumeral joint total rotation range of motion in elite tennis players and baseball pitchers. Med Sci Sports Exerc. 2002;34:2052–6. https://doi.org/10.1249/01.MSS.0000039301.69917.0C.
58. Kibler B, Chandler T, Livingston B, Roetert E. Shoulder range of motion in elite tennis players. Effect of age and years of tournament play. Am J Sports Med. 1996;24:279–85.
59. Ellenbecker TS, Roetert EP, Safran M. Shoulder injuries in tennis. In: Wilk KE, Reinold MM, Andrews JR, editors. Athletes Shoulder. 2nd ed. Philadelphia, PA: Churchill Livingstone; 2009. p. 429–44.
60. Wilk K, Meister K, Andrews J. Current concepts in the rehabilitation of the overhead throwing athlete. Am J Sports Med. 2002;30:136–51.
61. Manske R, Wilk KE, Davies G, Ellenbecker T, Reinold M. Glenohumeral motion deficits: friend or foe? Int J Sports Phys Ther. 2013;8:537–53.
62. Wilk K, Macrina L, Fleisig G, Porterfield R, Simpson C, Harker P, Paparesta N, Andrews J. Correlation of glenohumeral internal rotation deficit and total rotational motion to shoulder injuries in professional baseball pitchers. Am J Sports Med. 2011;39:329–35.
63. Vad V, Gebeh A, Dines D, Altchek D, Norris B. Hip and shoulder internal rotation range of motion deficits in professional tennis players. J Sci Med Sport. 2003;6:71–5.
64. Cohen D, Mont M, Campbell K, Vogelstein B, Loewy J. Upper extremity physical factors affecting tennis serve velocity. Am J Sports Med. 1994;22:746–50.
65. Martin C, Kulpa R, Ezanno F, Delamarche P, Bideau B. Influence of playing a prolonged tennis match on shoulder internal range of motion. Am J Sports Med. 2016;44(8):2147–51. https://doi.org/10.1177/0363546516645542.
66. Moore-Reed SD, Kibler WB, Myers NL, Smith BJ. Acute changes in passive glenohumeral rotation following tennis play exposure in elite female players. Int J Sports Phys Ther. 2016;11:230–6.
67. Proske U, Morgan DL. Muscle damage from eccentric exercise: mechanism, mechanical signs, adaptation and clinical applications. J Physiol. 2001;537:333–45.
68. Manske RC, Meschke M, Porter A, Smith B, Reiman M. A randomized controlled single-blinded comparison of stretching versus stretching and joint mobilization for posterior shoulder tightness measured by internal rotation motion loss. Sports Health. 2010;2:94–100. https://doi.org/10.1177/1941738109347775.
69. Harryman DT, Sidles JA, Clark JM, McQuade KJ, Gibb TD, Matsen FA. Translation of the humeral head on the glenoid with passive glenohumeral motion. J Bone Joint Surg Am. 1990;72:1334–43.
70. Muraki T, Yamamoto N, Zhac KD, Sperling JW, Steinmann SP, Cofield RH, An K-N. Effect of posteroinferior capsule tightness on contact pressure and area beneath the coracoacromial arch during pitching motion. Am J Sports Med. 2010;38:600–7. https://doi.org/10.1177/0363546509350074.
71. Reinold M, Wilk K, Macrina L, Sheheane C, Dun S, Fleisig G, Crenshaw K, Andrews J. Changes in shoulder and elbow passive range of motion after pitching in professional baseball players. Am J Sports Med. 2008;36:523–7.
72. Laudner K, Compton BD, McLoda TA, Walters CM. Acute effects of instrument assisted soft tissue mobilization for improving posterior shoulder range of motion in collegiate baseball players. Int J Sports Phys Ther. 2014;9:1–7.

Biomechanics of Groundstrokes and Volleys

Bruce Elliott, Machar Reid, and David Whiteside

2.1 Groundstrokes

2.1.1 Introduction

How prevalent are groundstrokes in match play and how important are they to tennis success? Hawk-Eye, a technical development that was introduced to assist in officiating the game, has provided a unique opportunity to fully appreciate the structure of the professional game. Data from this source should benefit coaching and help improve performance and reduce the risk of injury. Figure 2.1 provides Hawk-Eye data captured at the 2012–2015 Australian Open tournaments. It is clear that groundstrokes provide the cornerstone for Grand Slam tennis with marginally more shots played on the forehand ($\approx$38%) than the backhand ($\approx$35%). In absolute terms, women hit 1–3 more groundstrokes per game than men, suggesting that they need to be conditioned for higher hitting volumes. However, from a cumulative standpoint, during the first week of the Australian Open, the average man hits almost 800 more shots during the competition than his female counterpart. In light of this, it could be argued that men are more predisposed to mechanical related groundstroke injuries than women, simply due to the sheer volume of balls they hit during competition (Table 2.1).

Therefore while the serve is considered the most important stroke in tennis and when joint forces and moments, together with muscle activation are considered, loads the body more than any other stroke [1], the more frequently played groundstrokes are arguably the key to tennis success. Notational analysis of Grand Slam tournaments has shown that groundstrokes are 1.75 times more prevalent than the serve [2]. Also, while mean service velocity for professionals is typically 185 km/h and 155 km/h for male and female players, respectively (a differential of 15–20% that remarkably seems to hold across all performance levels), the typical velocity of female groundstrokes (~105 km/h), while lower than that recorded for the male counterparts (~110 km/h) from a practical perspective, is a closer velocity differential (~5%) than observed for the serve [2]. Although the forehand is associated with a greater number of points won [3] and is generally hit with higher ball velocity than its backhand counterpart [4], it is the evolution of the backhand from using one (1H) to two hands (2H) that represents one of the biggest mechanical changes in the game over recent times. Having said that, research has produced inconclusive

B. Elliott (✉)
The University of Western Australia,
Perth, WA, Australia
e-mail: Bruce.Elliott@uwa.edu.au

M. Reid
Tennis Australia and International Tennis Federation,
London, UK
e-mail: mreid@tennis.com.au

D. Whiteside
New York Yankees, New York, NY, USA
e-mail: dwhiteside@yankees.comtennis.com.au

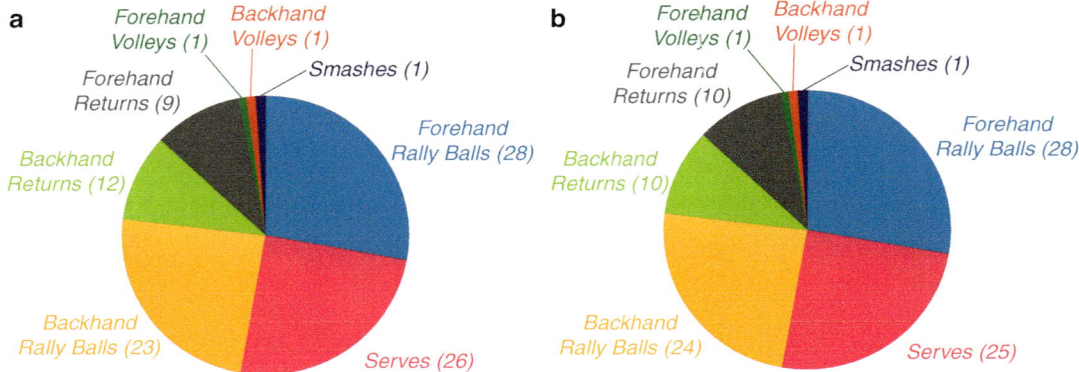

Fig. 2.1 Breakdown of stroke types per 100 shots at the Australian Open (**a**, males; **b**, females). Data captured by Hawk-Eye between 2012 and 2015

Table 2.1 Women's and men's mean player (±SD) cumulative shots played across the first four rounds of the 2015 Australian Open

Stroke	Women: mean (SD)	Men: mean (SD)
First serves	278 (48)	433 (78)
Second serves	99 (19)	154 (34)
Forehand returns	145 (27)	203 (44)
Backhand returns	164 (38)	271 (28)
Forehand groundstrokes	412 (99)	631 (196)
Backhand groundstrokes	359 (67)	516 (196)
Forehand volleys	16 (5)	30 (10)
Backhand volleys	14 (7)	28 (11)
Smashes	9 (5)	16 (6)
Shots	1496 (205)	2282 (507)

results when comparing these two backhand approaches for racket velocity [5, 6], ball velocity [7] and accuracy [8].

This predominance of groundstrokes in match play stresses the need for correct technique to be learned at an early age, as half of the injuries to paediatric tennis players have been reported to be located in the upper limb [9]. The biomechanical basis of these strokes is therefore equally important, irrespective of sex, if a player is to attain optimal performance and stay injury-free. From a biomechanical perspective, while accuracy is dictated by racket orientation and trajectory at impact, ball velocity is primarily governed by two primary factors:

- The *velocity of the incoming ball*
- *Racket velocity* (remember, velocity is just speed with direction, or alternatively if you talk about racket speed or resultant velocity, you are referring to the combination of racket horizontal, lateral and vertical velocities)

Approximately 25% of hitting velocity is dictated by the horizontal velocity of the incoming ball. This velocity, while it is in part beyond your control, is influenced by court surface (consider the velocity of the ball from the grass at Wimbledon compared with the clay of Roland Garros). However, 75% of the velocity of your groundstroke is determined by your racket velocity at impact [10]. Although the importance of racket velocity is therefore obvious, one may also ask how important racket design and string composition are to groundstroke success. The larger sweet spot (larger hitting area where optimal rebound velocity and lesser impact forces are recorded compared with impacts recorded near the periphery of the strings) and improved string design of modern rackets have enabled players to swing more vigorously and hit the ball consistently with more power. Cross [11], in modelling the contribution of various mechanical factors to hitting velocity, emphasized the importance of racket movement by showing that a 20% increase in racket velocity elicited an approximate 20% increase in that of the ball, yet a similar percentage improvement in racket and string design only yielded a 6% gain.

Groundstroke mechanics are therefore integrally linked with the development of racket velocity, trajectory and orientation for impact, over a variety of tactical situations.

The following chapter should be read in conjunction with the ITF publications *Biomechanics of Advanced Tennis* [12] and *Technique Development in Tennis Stroke Production* [13], together with *Tennis Science: Optimizing Performance on the Court* [14], for a complete understanding of the concepts presented.

2.1.2 Stroke Variability

The variability of body movements creating a consistent positioning of the racket for impact from varying joint movements, under similar and different tactical situations, underpins stroke production.

Biomechanics is often accused of trying to create a one-style-fits-all approach to stroke production, where all mechanical factors from player to player are the same. Nothing could be further from the truth, as while there are certain mechanical factors that are relatively invariant (e.g. the angle of the racket at impact), many others vary for an individual player and with the morphology of one player compared with another. From a morphological perspective, consider the stroke mechanics (and tactics) used by two top ATP players: the 1.75 m (5 ft 9 in.) David Ferrer compared with the 1.96 m (6 ft 5 in.) Milos Raonic. However, once players have decided on 'game plans' based on their morphology among other factors, stable racket positioning and velocity at impact across a multitude of tactical situations are achieved via controlled but inherently variable movements. This movement variability is an essential feature of human motor behaviour, affording the necessary flexibility and adaptability required for skilled performance [15].

In other words, we are not talking about variations in stroke mechanics between Djokovic and Federer or between Williams and Kerber, but rather variations across multiple forehands hit by Djokovic. As alluded to above, Djokovic's racket orientation at impact will be relatively constant, yet how the racket gets there is variable. More specifically, science has shown that forehand shots are characterized by:

- Relatively constant rotations about the shoulder joint
- Variable velocity and acceleration profiles at the elbow and wrist, even for a similar tactically based stroke [16]

The only way to concertedly integrate such a concept into the development of a player's stroke mechanics is to challenge the player with precise target hitting in a variety of tactical situations (e.g. deep balls, short balls, those fed with a variety of spins). Indeed, German tennis scientist Richard Schonborn emphasized that it is through the linking of these two factors, target hitting and variable tactical situations, that functional variability is systematically honed. As part of this, he stressed the importance of target hitting, in that it allows the success of each shot to be evaluated by the brain—a prerequisite in the continual refinement of stroke production. Here, he advocated the use of blocks of three shots to five different targets to achieve highly refined strokes. In this context, it is important to note that while the focus is on harnessing variability to improve stroke performance, it is done through a combination of variable and serial practice schedules.

Clinician's Corner
1. Once the rudimentary mechanics of stroke production are achieved, it is imperative to emphasize variable practice that provides for self-evaluation of stroke success (feedback on outcomes) to refine the development of stroke mechanics.
2. From a loading perspective, overuse injuries are the result of repetitive micro-trauma to the tendons, bones and joints [17]. It has been proposed that movement variability acts to distribute loads and thwart repetitive uniform

loading [18–20], which may help to avert overuse injuries.
3. Equally pertinent for the practitioner is the evidence revealing that hitting loads increase as players progress deeper into the tournament. Put simply, the number of shots a player hits in the fourth round is significantly greater than what is required of them in their two opening rounds. With that in mind, sufficient recovery during Grand Slam competition should not only focus on helping a player back up their performance from the previous round but actually withstand greater workloads, particularly on groundstrokes. Practically, this might involve progressively increasing a player's groundstroke hitting load during a 2-week training block to simulate competition. With effective playing time (i.e. the proportion of total match duration spent in point play) also having been shown to increase as the tournament progresses, there is a logical expectation for fatigue to become a bigger issue in later rounds. With fatigue having been proposed as a reason for the emergence of upper extremity pain in overhead movements [21–24], this may emphasize the importance of sufficient physical preparation for averting the development of pain.
4. Research has also shown that it is beneficial to train on different surfaces [25], as the magnitude of knee flexion is reduced on impact in running forehands played on clay courts as compared with a cushioned acrylic surface. Players adapted to the characteristics of the surface, and this adaptation favours sliding on the low-friction surface (clay). Greater flexion contributes to reducing the load transmitted to the lower limb during braking on the harder surface—*practising on various surfaces teaches the body to adapt.*

2.1.3 Cueing, Footwork and Stance

Mechanics involved in early stroke preparation are the basis upon which the following phases are built.

Where players look in preparation for and during the early phases of a stroke can be considered to encompass their approach to **cueing**. For the purposes of this chapter, this sits separate to the role of vision (and head position) during racket-ball impact. Consequently, cueing can be thought of as the gaze or visual search approach adopted by players from the moment when the ball bounces on the other side of the net to the point at which it lands on their side of the court.

A player's gaze traverses objects and locations, constantly fluctuating between periods of stability and rapid movement. A more stable gaze gives the brain time to process information. When objects are stationary or moving within small visual angles for >100 ms [26], fixations and pursuit tracking (a more stable gaze) predominate. Depending on the situation in which players find themselves during game play, it is possible that this type of gaze behaviour can contribute to the way players process information. For example, when players are going toe-to-toe cross-court (hitting successive cross-court balls back and forth), it stands to reason that pursuit tracking is involved. Indeed, in these situations, as well as other rally-based scenarios, players tend to be in what is called the *object recognition phase*. This means that they likely have the time to focus or cue in on the stroke kinematics of the opponent, as well as his/her court position. Depending on the speed with which shots are hit, it may also be that smooth pursuit tracking is suitable for players to process what's coming and to begin to prepare a response. However, more commonly, when the ball travels quickly, saccades—which are rapid eye movements from one tracked location to another—are required. The average player/person can 'saccade' three times per second, ranging from 60 to 100 ms, which limits the extent to which conscious information processing is possible. In essence, this means that when tracking oncoming ball trajectories, players employ saccades to forecast or get ahead of the ball's flight so that pursuit tracking (which can consciously pick up changes in ball flight) can be re-engaged.

The **footwork** that players use to get to and then recover from each and every shot could form the basis of its own book chapter, if not book! So, rather than attempt to cover all manner of movement nuance here, and in so doing belittle the very importance of such an integral part of the game, we will highlight the key aspects of moving to and from groundstrokes. Given that we're discussing the way in which the feet are interacting with the court to produce force, it's intuitive to also introduce the role of the stance in stroke production.

It's not uncommon to hear experts refer to one player as having good **balance** and another as being poorly balanced. When pressed to expand, a player's ability to be stable, maintain their base, be strong with their legs, or hold position is often then woven into the conversation. Balance, when described in this way, almost takes on an intangible or ephemeral entity. In essence, however, experts are simply describing the known relationship between a player's centre of gravity (COG) and base of support. In standing or stationary positions, balance is static; while when moving, as is typically the case in tennis, it is termed dynamic. Players continuously refine this relationship between their COG and base of support to place themselves at mechanical advantage during both movement and stroke production. On a practical level, this is most evident in the initiation of movement and use of different stances upon arriving at the ball, as discussed below.

When preparing to move, players initially assume a balanced ready position (static), but this posture is temporary, such that a dynamic response to the opponent and/or ball is possible [27]. These ready positions are invariably linked to the use of the split step. The split step is a combined anticipatory-movement response by players that involves coordinating the ground contact and orientation of the outside foot (one furthest from where the ball is being directed) and inside foot (one closest to where the ball is being directed) to ensure the fastest possible transition to the ball. Expertise-based differences in the temporal characteristics of the split step have been observed [27], while from a mechanical point of view, it eccentrically stretches and stores elastic energy in the quadriceps and gastrocnemius muscle groups to aid a player's first step [12].

2.1.3.1 Arriving and Adopting the Appropriate Stance

As players approach the ball and/or the ball approaches players, a variety of decisions are contemplated—what shot to play, where to hit, and so on. As part of that process, players decide upon the stance most appropriate for the situation. In so doing, they consider the time pressure that they're under, as well as their strategic intent—both of which ultimately impact stroke mechanics.

While it is true that players can orientate their feet anywhere in the 360 degree space that surrounds them, it is more common for a player's feet to be displaced somewhere in the 135 degree arcs to the right or left (Fig. 2.2). The four common stances that feature within these arcs, namely, are:

- Open stance, where both feet are parallel to the baseline or at 0° (a)
- Semi-open stance, where the inside or front foot is displaced 30–45° forward (b)
- Square stance, where the inside or front foot is displaced perpendicular to the baseline or is rotated 90° forward (c)
- Closed stance, where the inside or front foot crosses perpendicular to the baseline or is rotated 110–135° forward (d)

While the effect of stance on stroke velocity has revealed mixed results in the literature, researchers have revealed certain links to joint loading (see Clinician's Corner). In generalizing

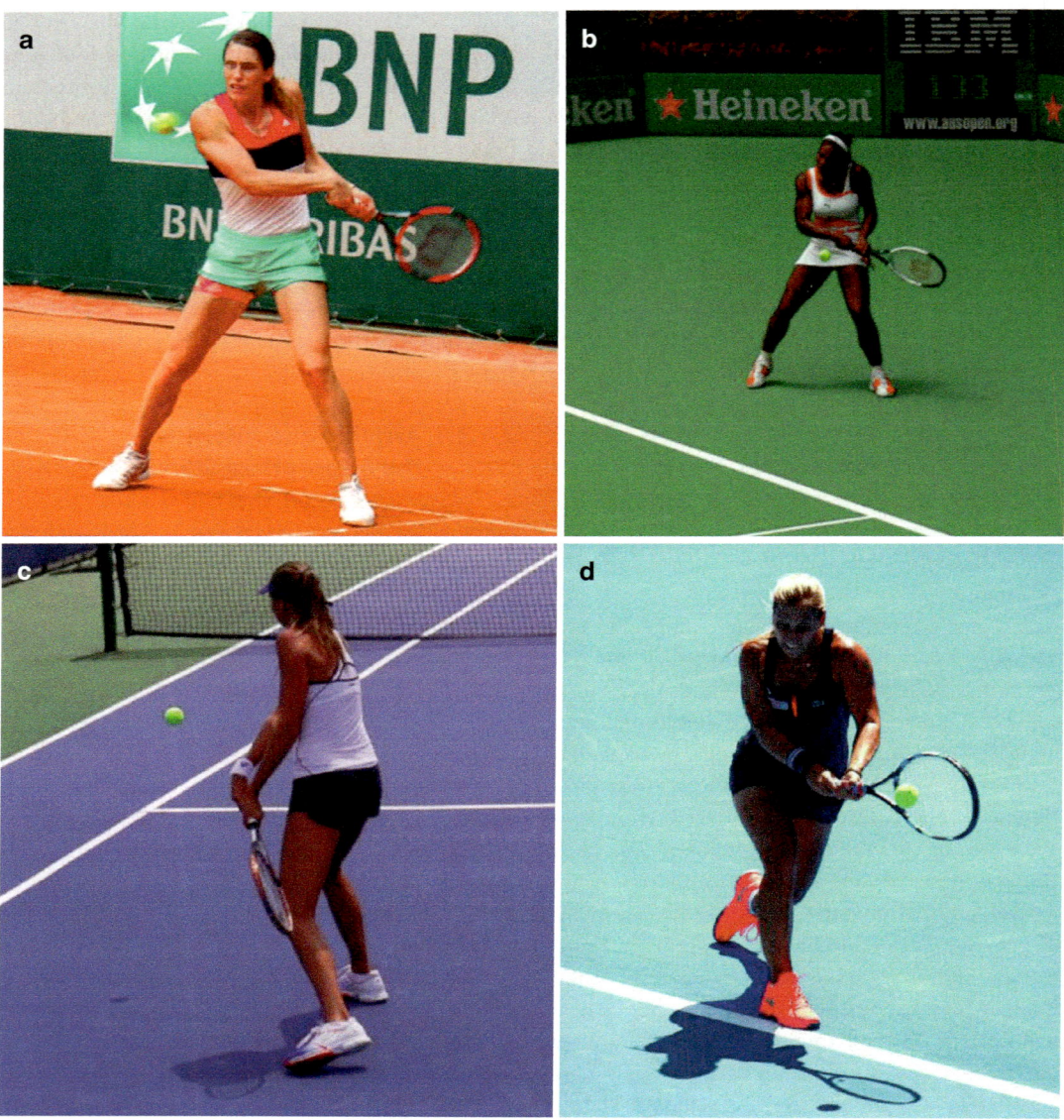

Fig. 2.2 Stances (**a**, open; **b**, semi-open; **c**, square; **d**, closed)

to practice, one can consider the open stance and square stance to exist at opposing ends of a time/space pressure continuum (high, open; low, square) and the semi-open stance to reside somewhere in between (Fig. 2.3). The closed stance is something of a special case, often called upon in extremes (i.e. end-range recovery or very low bouncing balls).

Roger Federer	Open *	Square	Closed
Clay court	77%	13%	10%
Grass court	72%	19%	9%

Alejandro Falla	Open *	Square	Closed
Clay court	72%	12%	18%
Grass court	34%	41%	25%

Maria Sharapova	Open *	Square	Closed
Clay court	66%	25%	9%
Hard court	62%	27%	11%

Sam Stosur	Open *	Square	Closed
Clay court	68%	23%	9%
Hard court	74%	17%	9%

Fig. 2.3 Case studies of professional players illustrating the effect of court surface on stance type [28]

Clinician's Corner
1. Triolet et al. [29] have reported that anticipation informs player responses in only 6.1–13.4% of tennis situations, which tend to those situations when opponents are at notable tactical advantage. This highlights the importance of tactical context in developing these types of skills, especially among advanced players.
2. The stances adopted by players are thought to have implications for joint loading. While Knudson and Blackwell [30] revealed the open and square stance forehand to share similar trunk muscle activity, square stance forehands have been noted to produce higher upper limb joint torques (shoulder internal rotation and wrist flexion) than open stance forehands [31].
3. Stance was also implicated in the variable lumbar loading patterns observed in the study of Campbell et al. [1], where the open stance forehand generated significantly greater anterior force than open and square stance backhands. The forehand, hit with both open and square stances, also featured larger right lateral flexion moments than the backhands, independent of stance used.

2.1.4 Grips

How a player holds the racket is at the heart of stroke mechanics.

It stands to reason that the manner in which players hold their rackets will influence stroke production, from both racket velocity and injury standpoints. Logically, it then follows that there is a range of acceptable grips for each of the game's strokes. Significantly, research has been able to illustrate the effect of different grips on aspects of the skill performance-injury paradigm.

For example, on the forehand, eastern but more commonly semi-western and western grips are used by top players. In comparing the racket velocity profiles of forehands played with western versus eastern forehand grips, Elliott et al. [32] highlighted the different functional roles of ulnar, radial and palmar wrist flexion depending on grip position. Interestingly, the way that the wrist flexes—in accordance with grip—to assist the development of racket velocity has also been shown to relate to types of wrist injuries that players sustain. That is, Tagliafico et al. [33] investigated the site of wrist injury, as a function of forehand grip among 370 non-professional players and linked radial-side and ulnar-side injuries to the use of the eastern and western forehand grips, respectively. In a similar vein, albeit through visual inspection rather than 3D measurement, Eng and Hagler [34] have identified the bottom hand and top hand in the 2H backhand to assume three and six different grip positions, respectively, among a sample of 174 top 100 male and female professionals. The authors related grip selection to the precision or power prerogative of players, with men more likely to use power grips (i.e. where the thumb of the top hand is placed in the plane of its palm above the fingers) than women. However, in so doing, they were unable to discount the effect of the grip length (i.e. males, with larger hand sizes, ran out of space on the grip to adopt precision grips) on the orientation of the hands, meaning that it may also influence grip selection. King et al. [35] used computer simulation to relate impact position and grip tightness in the 1HB. They showed that off-centre impacts increased wrist extensor torque. Altering grip tightness had no significant effect on central impacts. However, there was a 20% increase in wrist extensor torque when central and off-centre impacts were compared with a 'normal' grip. Consequently off-centre impacts may be a contributing factor for tennis elbow, with a tight grip aggravating the effect due to high eccentric wrist extensor torque.

Wei et al. [36] also investigated the proliferation of vibrations through the forearms of experienced and recreational players when hitting 1HBs. Despite experiencing significantly greater racket vibrations at impact, experienced players were far more adept at attenuating these vibrations to protect the hitting arm. Specifically, only 11.8% (7.4 g) of the initial racket vibration was transferred to experienced players' elbow, compared with 38.2% (13.3 g) in recreational players. Consistent with previous research, it was determined that this was a product of recreational players maintaining a firm grip after ball impact, which acted to create a stiffer ball-racket system. This evidence points to more protective mechanics in experienced players, thereby underlining the importance of grip technique in preventing injury.

Clinician's Corner
1. Knudson [37], through the findings of case study analyses, recommended that players at risk of tennis elbow pain should reduce the force (firmness) of their grips at impact in the forehand.
2. The use of western and semi-western forehand grips, coupled with an increased intensity of play, has been implicated in the presentation of stress fractures in the second and, to a lesser extent, the third metacarpal of the racket-hand of adolescent tennis players [38].
3. Rossi et al. [39] simulated the effect of three different grip sizes on the grip forces and wrist joint moments of intermediate and advanced players' hitting forehands under different fatigued and non-fatigued conditions. Results revealed the prominent activation of the wrist extensor muscles during the forehand shot but the potential for extensor tendon loading (and any associated lateral epicondylitis) to be reduced with the selection of an optimal grip size.

2.1.5 Backswing

This phase of stroke production involves increasing the distance the racket has to accelerate under control for impact, enabling muscles involved in the movement to be put on stretch, while positioning the racket for the required tactical situation.

It is certainly possible to accelerate the racket rapidly over a short distance, as in tactical situations where backswing length is reduced in order to 'take' the return early and thus reduce the time afforded to an opponent. However, efficient stroke production is typically characterized by a controlled and yet extended backswing. Wu et al. [40] demonstrated the importance of a sufficiently long backswing in that this reduced upper limb loading at least for the 1HB stroke. In groundstrokes this is characterized by rotation of the shoulders (the alignment between the two shoulder joints) more than the hips (the line joining the two hip joints) creating what is referred to as a separation angle (Fig. 2.4). Creating this angle is integrally involved in the stretch phase of the *stretch-shorten cycle*, where elastic energy is stored, as the associated muscles contract eccentrically. Some of this stored energy is then used to assist in building rotational velocity for impact.

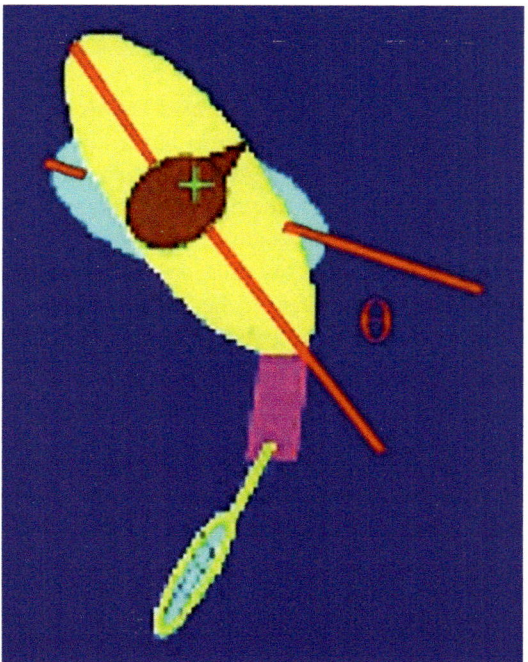

Fig. 2.4 Separation angle is the difference in shoulder and hip alignments—shown here for a forehand

Table 2.2 Backswing positions in tennis groundstrokes

Alignment[a]	Forehand (°)	Backhand (°)	
		One-handed	Two-handed
Shoulders	110	120	80
Hips	90	90	70
Separation angle	20	30	20
Racket[b]	210	250	200

[a]Alignment with the shoulders or hips parallel with the baseline equates to zero degrees
[b]The racket pointed at 90° to the baseline toward your opponent equates to 0°

Absolute positions at the completion of the forehand and backhand backswings are recorded in Table 2.2 [5, 32, 41, 42].

The level of trunk rotations is similar for forehand and 1HB groundstrokes; however, they are reduced in the 2HB, where both hands are on the racket. These rotations are affected by tactical situation, particularly if the ball is to be directed across the court compared with down-the-line. Elliott and Christmass [41] further reported increased shoulder rotation for shoulder compared with hip-height impacts in the 1H slice backhand, showing that stroke selection and tactics are integrally related.

The 20–30° of trunk twist (separation angle—see Fig. 2.5a–c) is similar for all groundstrokes. However, there is a tendency for females to have ≈10% more separation than males, which may be related to the ≈20% less trunk rotational strength recorded for females on the backhand side [7, 43, 44]. For these mechanics to function effectively, it is important for spinal mobility to be addressed, as the lower lumbar region approaches end range of motion in both groundstrokes [1].

Trunk rotation also plays a role in racket displacement, which is highest in the 1HB and similar in the other groundstrokes. In general, it is always good to have the upper arm and shoulders in line in the forehand (i.e. for the upper arm not to pass beyond the line of the shoulders), such as is evident in Fig. 2.5a, to reduce shoulder loading. Unfortunately, in the serve, internal impingement at the shoulder may be unavoidable due to the nature of the overhead movement [45].

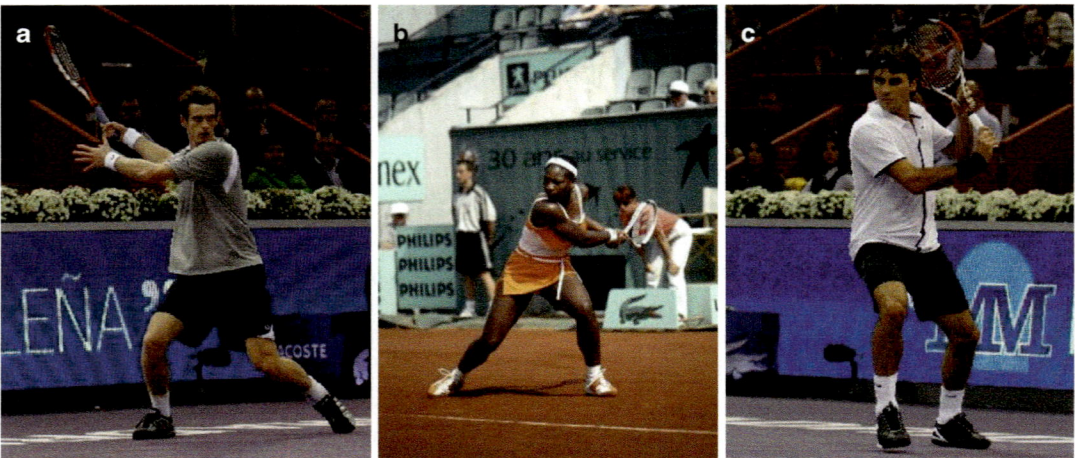

Fig. 2.5 Backswing positions for forehand (**a**—Murray) and two- (**b**—Williams) and one-handed backhands (**c**—Federer; slice stroke)

Clinician's Corner

1. Adolescent players with a history of recurrent lower back pain rotated beyond their lumbar end range during groundstrokes compared with those who were injury-free [1], emphasizing the need for good technique linked to appropriate physical preparation.
2. Groundstrokes are less injurious than the serve (in an acute sense) due to mechanics, intensity and more variable movement.
3. The amount of force required to swing a racket is directly related to its inertial characteristics. In this regard, high twist weight (that is the amount of mass distributed away from the midline of the racket, e.g. on the sides of the head) has been shown to increase shoulder and elbow loading in the serve [46, 47]. It is therefore logical to assume that upper limb joint loading will increase in line with increases in racket moment of inertia for groundstrokes.

2.1.6 Forward Swing: Generation of Racket Velocity

The summation of the drive from the lower limbs and then the rotations of the trunk and segments of the upper limb (upper arm, forearm and hand) must be coordinated if optimal racket speed (horizontal, vertical and lateral velocities) is to be created for impact.

2.1.6.1 Lower Limb Drive and Trunk

The right lower limb, for a right-handed player, is responsible for 'firing' the kinetic chain in the forehand. Specifically, it is the right hip that extends to initiate forward hip rotation (Fig. 2.6a, b; [48]. While left hip (rear leg) extension was observable in the 1HB, it was larger in the 2H stroke that was characterized by higher pelvis rotation [6, 42]. This suggests a certain analogy between the roles of the lower limbs in trunk rotation in the 2HB and forehand stroke.

The energy flow from the legs through the trunk typically follows the sequence for the forehand stroke:

- Force initially from back foot (R)
- R-knee extension (Fig. 2.6a, b)

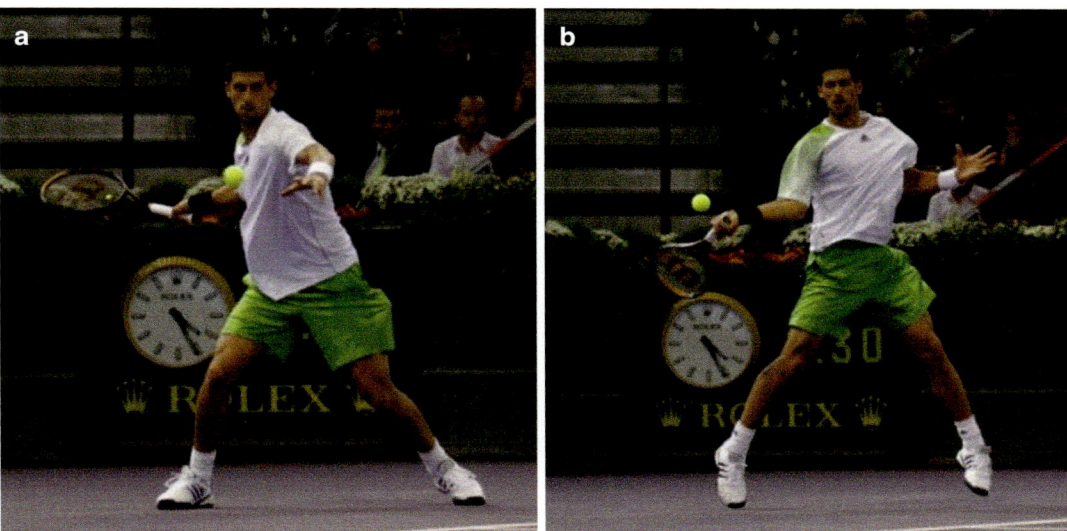

Fig. 2.6 Lower limb drive and trunk rotations in the early forward swing phase of a Djokovic forehand

- R-hip extension important for pelvic rotation (Fig. 2.6a, b)
- Flow from R-gluteal area diagonally across the body to left shoulder region

There are also indications that tennis players are at risk for femoroacetabular impingement syndrome (FAI). Several high-profile players such as Lleyton Hewitt, David Nalbandian and Tommy Haas have reportedly missed tennis due to this condition in recent times. Additionally, a study of 148 adolescent players revealed 62% exhibited hips at risk for femoroacetabular impingement [49]. It has been proposed that prolonged participation in sports that require demanding hip motion during childhood may provoke the bony adaptations that characterize this condition [50, 51]. While this remains unexplored in tennis junior populations, the notion of tennis-specific morphological changes is already well established in the upper extremity [52] and, therefore, appears a plausible scenario at the hip. Ultimately, FAI-related pain is incited by end-range internal rotation and/or flexion at the hip—a posture that is part of the follow-through in the serve (Fig. 2.7a) and backhand (Fig. 2.7b) and unconventional end-range shots (Fig. 2.7c, d).

Trunk rotation has been directly linked with racket forward velocity (Fig. 2.8) in both groundstrokes, irrespective of stance or playing level [7, 53]. Hip (pelvic) rotation, which is evident in all groundstrokes, is particularly important in the 2HB. Research has shown that rotations were twice as high in the 2H stroke (9.4 versus 5 rad/s) when compared with the 1H stroke [6, 7]. The 1H and 2H backhands therefore involve different strategies to develop horizontal racket velocity. The 2H stroke relies more on trunk rotation (shoulder alignment rotates beyond the hip alignment at impact [54]), whereas the 1H backhand relies more on linear movement [41, 55], created by greater rotations of the segments of the hitting limb [42]. Female players have also been shown to rotate their shoulder alignment more than males in the backswing and subsequently increase the level of forward rotation by approximately 10% [54]. It is evident from the vigour of trunk rotation that scapulothoracic movement plays an integral role in the link between the trunk and the racket-limb.

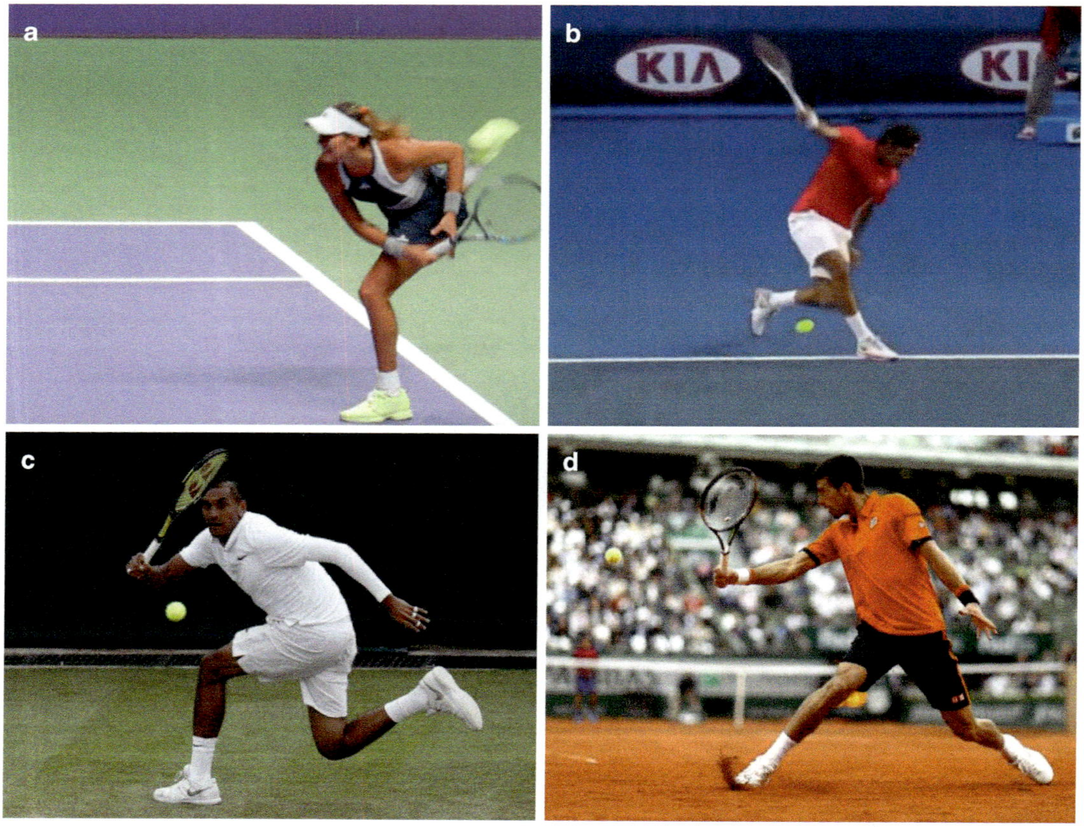

Fig. 2.7 At-risk hip postures during stroke production

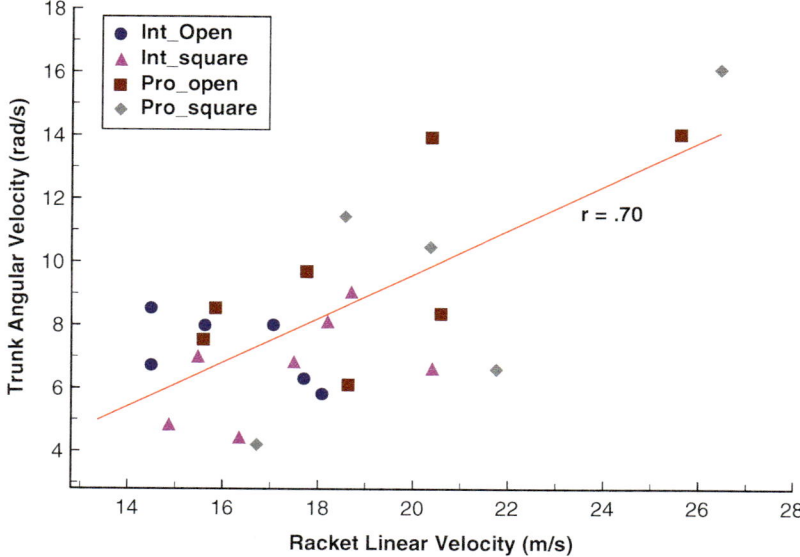

Fig. 2.8 Relationship between trunk rotational and racket velocities in the forehand [53]

It appears trunk rotation is almost linearly linked to velocity development in the forehand, where a doubling of ball velocity was accompanied by a doubling of the trunk rotational velocity [56]. Male, collegiate players increased their trunk rotation velocity when they were asked to increase ball velocity from slow to medium and then fast forehand groundstrokes. Landlinger et al. [57] further illustrated the importance of the trunk in the forehand when they compared high-performance juniors (≈16 years of age) with ATP ranked male players (≈23 years of age). The 2 m/s higher racket velocity for the senior players could be attributed primarily to the level of trunk rotation. When one considers the mechanics of the swing in the generation of racket velocity for impact, it is evident that you can approach this situation in one of two ways.

Velocity of a segment endpoint (e.g. point of impact on the racket or wrist joint) = angular velocity of segment (ω) multiplied by length of the segment – radius of rotation) (l)

Conceptually increasing velocity requires that you either increase the radius of rotation (l) or increase the rate of rotation (ω), *and in the 2H stroke, you have little choice but to adopt the latter.*

It is evident from the vigour of this rotation that scapulothoracic movement plays an integral role in the link between the trunk and the racket-limb. The need for scapula stabilization has been clearly established, if one wants an effective and injury-free approach to stroke production [58].

2.1.6.2 The Kinetic or Kinematic Chain

The theory behind this concept is discussed in another section of this book, so we will present its practical application to groundstrokes. Figure 2.7a–c visualizes how the kinetic chain unfolds in groundstroke production, while we expand on the individual joint contributions to racket velocity at impact below (see [59] for actual forehand contributions):

- Racket-shoulder: It is evident that the lower limb drive and trunk rotation move this shoulder in the direction of the hit and hence add linear velocity (in the direction of the target) to the racket in both single-handed groundstrokes (Fig. 2.9a2, b2), more than is the case in the 2H stroke (Fig. 2.9c2).
- Upper arm horizontal movement at the shoulder: Fig. 2.9a2–3, b1–2 and c1–2 shows how the upper arm flexes horizontally to contribute to impact racket velocity in both groundstrokes. In the 2H stroke, the dominant side plays the role of stabilizing the non-dominant extremity that is an important contributor to horizontal racket velocity [54, 60].
- Forearm pronation and extension at the elbow: Only play a minor role in generating racket velocity. The pronation angle of the forearm changes in the forehand; however this is caused by shoulder internal rotation, while grip and type of stroke will dictate the contribution to racket velocity from elbow extension. Elbow extension again plays a minor role in both backhand strokes.
- Upper arm internal rotation at the shoulder in the forehand (Fig. 2.9a2–3): This varies depending on the velocity of the incoming ball and the direction of the player's response. It is greater when generating power, particularly in directing the ball cross-court, than when absorbing and responding to the powerful stroke of an opponent. Remember, you will almost always have internal rotation, as a key and observable movement characteristic of the follow-through. Bahamonde and Knudson [31] highlighted shoulder joint internal rotation torque occurred very late in the forehand forward swing, just before impact. Obviously shoulder internal rotation does not play the same role for the backhand groundstroke; however, the role of external rotation and horizontal abduction in the dominant arm during the 1HB is evidenced through muscular activity [61].
- Hand flexion: This movement plays an important role on groundstrokes with levels of radial and palmar velocity varying depending on grip and the spin placed on the ball (forehand: Fig. 2.9a2–3). The wrist angle typically decreased from the position observed in the backswing to the late forward swing phase of

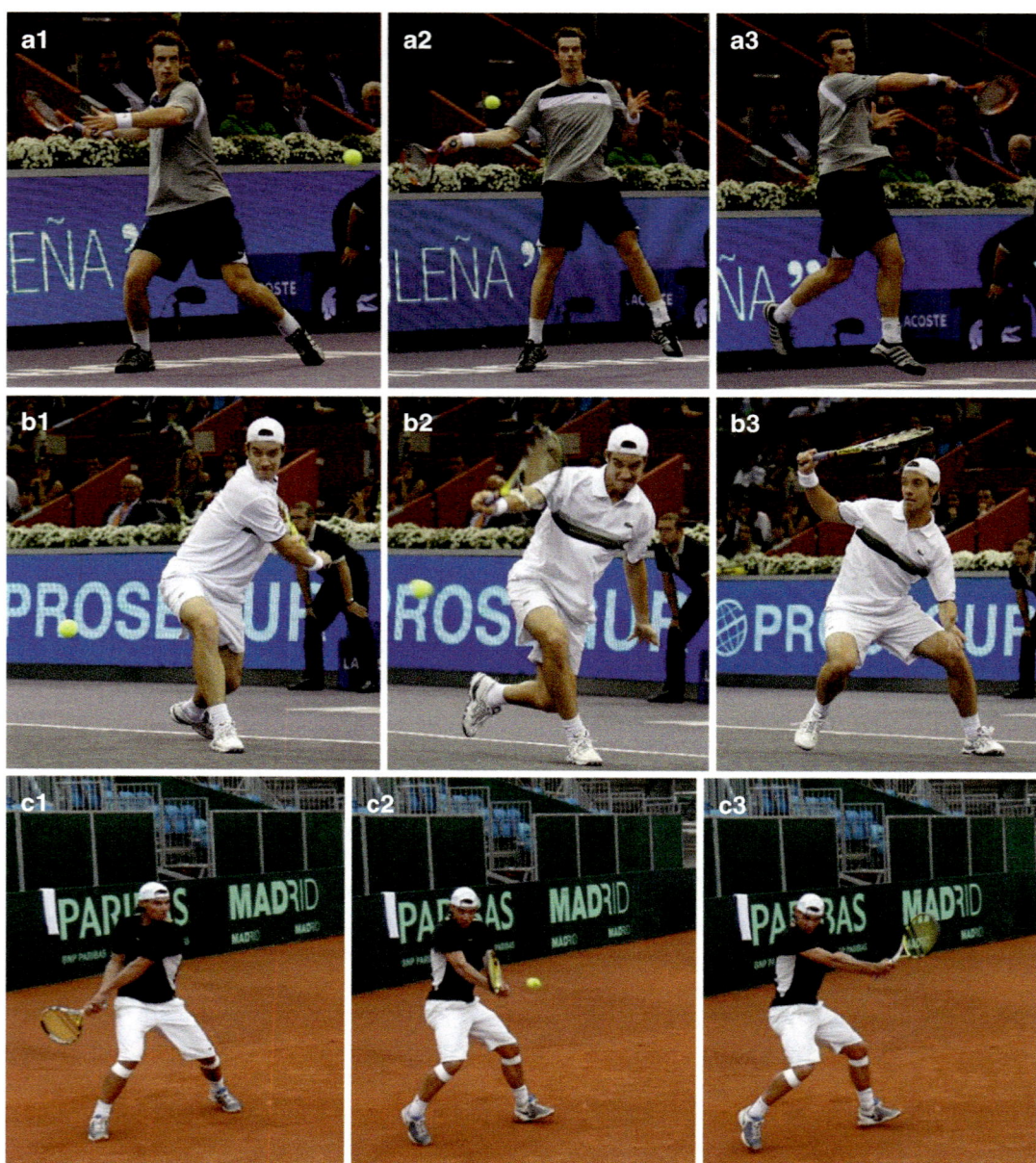

Fig. 2.9 Kinetic chain sequencing in the forehand (**a**), 1H (**b**) and 2H backhands (**c**)

the stroke, as the racket trailed the forward moving limb [62] (Fig. 2.9a2). Wrist flexion, in the forehand, then occurred to increase the speed of the racket (vertical, lateral and horizontal velocities) for impact (Fig. 2.9a2–3). Seeley et al. [56] reported increased hand flexion velocity in the forehand drive (low velocity, 460°/s; medium velocity, 780°/s; and high velocity, 1070°/s) accompanying increases in ball velocity from low to medium to high. They showed that an increase in hand rotational velocity was required to double ball velocity, although this should not be interpreted as requiring more muscle action about the wrist, as higher rotational velocities up the kinetic chain may have contributed to a *whip-*

like response with the hand (inertial transfer of energy). While the wrist joint is hyperextended at the completion of the backswing (≈160°), it is often still hyperextended (to a lesser extent) at impact, showing that flexion has occurred during the forward swing, as mentioned above [62]. The direction of forces about the wrist at impact is determined by the grip used [33], and there was effective hand movement (flexion/radial or ulnar flexion) irrespective of stance in the forehand drive [31].

- In a similar manner, the hand plays an important role in the 1HB with the hand again playing an integral role in the stroke, as the last segment in the kinetic chain [63] (Fig. 2.9b1–2). In the 2H stroke, wrist flexion is observed from Fig. 2.9c1–2. However, a player may adopt a different mechanical approach to that used in the 1H action, to produce varying racket velocity and trajectory. With both hands on the racket, it is possible to create a force couple, where the hands work independently to angle the racket forward in a 'push-pull' scenario, as shown in Fig. 2.10, while in hitting topspin the hands may move in a more up-down action.

- As you can see, all strokes are the product of the coordinated action of several body parts. While we have explored each of those contributors in isolation, their presentation during stroke production is clearly not independent. In this regard, evidence has been presented to demonstrate that the energy flow through the kinetic chain of the serve is more efficient in uninjured tennis players, compared with injured players [64]. A holistic view of stroke production is, therefore, just as critical to injury prevention as servicing the sum of its individual parts.

Clinician's Corner
1. Lower limb (knee joint) flexes more on a hard compared with clay surface in the running forehand, to accommodate court hardness and reduce the force transmitted to the body [25].
2. The upper limb will be additionally loaded, to achieve the same outcome, if the trunk is not actively involved in the kinetic chain.
3. More emphasis is needed on lumbar spine for training in the 2H stroke, as more axial rotation and lateral flexion were found in this stroke [65].
4. The tennis forehand may contribute to scapular dyskinesis, mainly due to the greater amplitude in scapulothoracic anterior tilt and internal rotation during the follow-through [58], thus emphasizing the need for scapula stabilization.
5. When groups with pain and no pain in the lumbar region were compared for groundstrokes, it was evident that active extension, right rotation and left lateral flexion ranges were significantly greater in the no pain group [1]. This increased range caused the pain group to typically position their lower lumbar spine closer to end of range for left lateral flexion (Fig. 2.11) and extension.

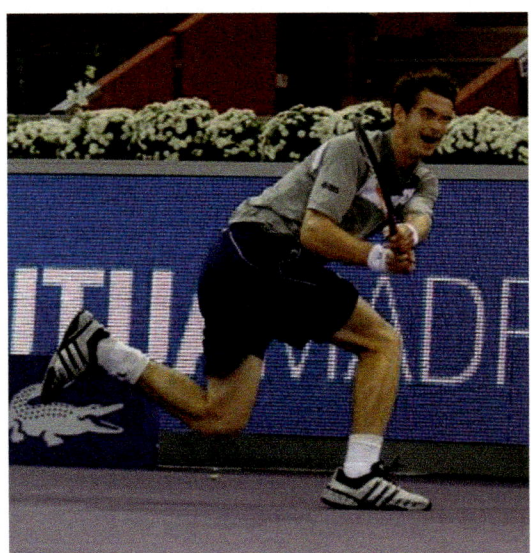

Fig. 2.10 Murray backhand showing the ability to create a force couple with the hands

6. Strengthening the muscles associated with wrist flexion was beneficial to energy efficiency in groundstrokes [66].
7. Players using a 2HB should learn the 1H slice early in the development process.

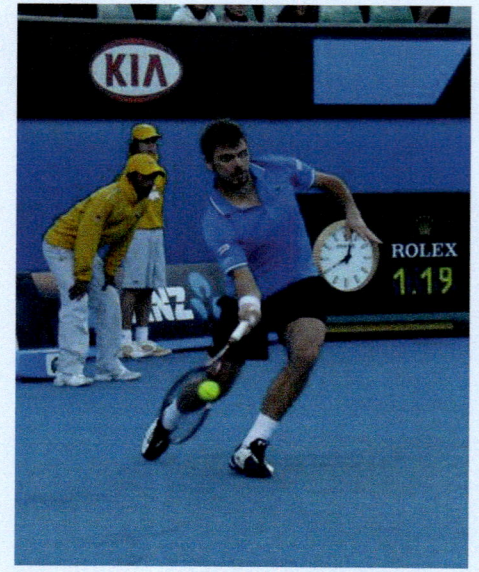

Fig. 2.11 Trunk lateral flexion in the forehand

2.1.7 Forward Swing: Racket Trajectory and Spin

Weight or heaviness of a groundstroke (the appropriate mix of spin and velocity) is the result of racket mechanics about impact.

The ability to create topspin on the ball, or hit a 'heavy' ball (a combination of spin and velocity), requires a low-to-high racket trajectory (Fig. 2.12a–c) in combination with an almost vertical racket-head at impact, whereas the backspin shot requires the reverse profile. That is, while forward velocity is highest, the vertical component of the velocity is higher in topspin (upward) and backspin (downward) when compared with flat hits [5, 59, 62]. However, the racket does not follow a single trajectory, as shown in Table 2.3. It appears that a player develops one trajectory up until just before impact and then increases this to the required level once impact is assured.

Blackwell and Knudson [67] showed that high-performance players, when compared with intermediate-level players, were able to hit a forehand with higher speed (resultant velocity), approached impact with a steeper racket trajectory (28° vs 23° to the horizontal, respectively) and aligned the racket-face differently immediately before impact (closed by 4° vs open by 3° to the horizontal, respectively) when asked to hit a topspin stroke. Intermediate players often use a flatter trajectory to impact ($\approx 20°$) compared with more advanced players ($\geq 30°$) when attempting a topspin stroke. The range of acceptability typically quoted for the racket at impact is from vertical (i.e. cross strings aligned with the vertical) to a tilt forward by 5° (closed) in topspin strokes (Fig. 2.12c) and from vertical to tilted back by 10° (open) for the slice backhand. Rogowski et al. [68] reported that with young players the vertical racket velocity in topspin compared with flat forehands was created at impact by radial deviation more than shoulder abduction, stressing the need for full body movements in creating the appropriate racket trajectories.

Nadal is certainly the king when it comes to hitting a heavy ball with spin rates of 4000 rpm recorded on his forehand topspin stroke. Compare this value with rotations reported for Agassi of 2000 rpm—another hard hitter of the ball—and you can see why the weight on Nadal's stroke is so difficult to counter.

During heavy topspin, the ball has as much energy in its rotation, as it does in its forward movement. This is why on returning a 'heavy' topspin with a 1HB stroke, it is so much easier to hit with backspin (the ball is rotating in the same direction) rather than topspin, where you must reverse the direction of the incoming ball [69].

The spin imparted to the ball certainly influences its bounce from the court, although this does not always match the results one finds in a laboratory, where for the same approach angle, a ball with topspin will bounce lower than one with backspin. How can this be so, as any player will tell you that the ball with topspin 'jumps'

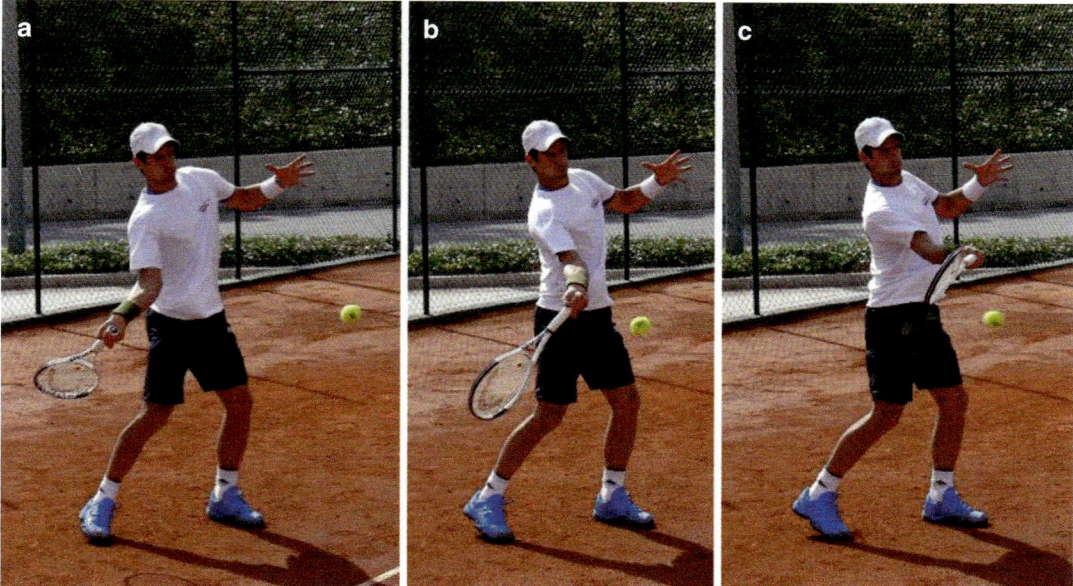

Fig. 2.12 An upward and forward trajectory of the racket is required to develop power and spin

Table 2.3 Pre- and post-impact racket trajectories for groundstrokes

Stroke	Forehand [59]		Backhand [5, 41]	
	Pre-impact	Post-impact	Pre-impact	Post-impact
Flat	20°	40°		
Topspin	40°	50°	20°	45°
Topspin lob	50°	75°		

viciously, while one hit with backspin appears to 'shoot through', as shown in Fig. 2.13a, b?

2.1.8 Impact

The racket mechanics at impact are the sole determinant of ball velocity and flight.

The mechanics of the total body are all important at impact if one is to achieve the appropriate racket velocity and trajectory. Mean forehand resultant racket velocity (combination of vertical, horizontal and lateral velocities) for high-performance players, which is in the order of 22 m/s [72], and loading [30, 31] were not significantly different when players used an open or square stance.

2.1.8.1 The Head

Because of its weight, the head is a key feature at impact, particularly with younger players, irrespective of groundstroke. A characteristic of many ($\approx$15%) elite players is that they 'fix' (***complete fixation***) their head for impact and hold this position into the follow-through [70, 71]. Figure 2.14a of Federer clearly shows this characteristic. The majority of professionals though demonstrate ***partial head fixation***. Remember, when gazing into the impact zone and holding the head still—you do not actually see impact. To this end, Ferrer (b) holds this head position for impact but quickly moves his head/eyes to follow the ball following impact, in what can be considered a sign of a player that uses partial fixation. Developing players often do not fix the head and eyes (***no fixation***), and this is one of the reasons they lack consistency in their stroke production (Fig. 2.14c).

2.1.8.2 Trunk

The mechanical similarities between the open and square stance forehand techniques at impact would appear consistent and at odds, respectively, with the teachings of many coaching professionals [72]. In the forehand the shoulders rotate more than the hips during the forward

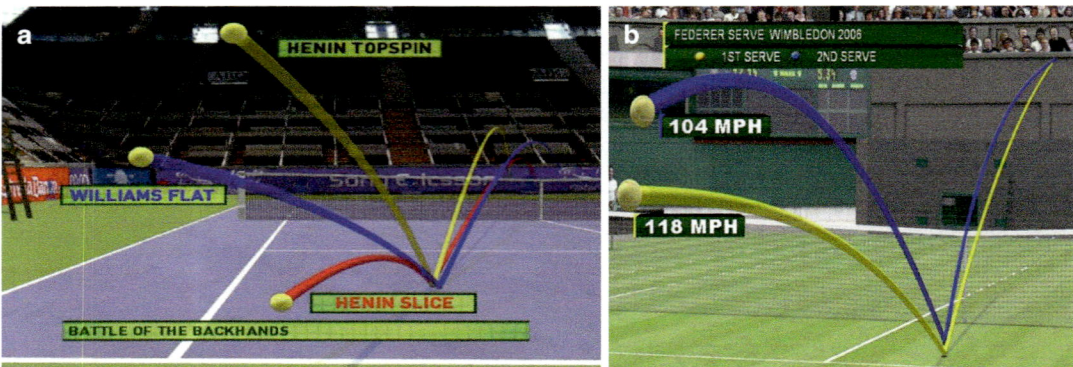

Fig. 2.13 Bounces for balls with a variety of spins in groundstrokes (**a**) and the serve (**b**). In a match environment, sliced shots bounce lower (**a**) because they have a reduced angle of approach (red curve). This contrasts with topspin strokes, which bounce higher owing to their greater angle of approach (compare the yellow and red trajectories). The same effect can be seen when comparing trajectories for the first and second serves, whereby the second serve (blue) is hit with more forward rotation landing with a higher trajectory and therefore bounces (kicks) higher off the court (**b**)

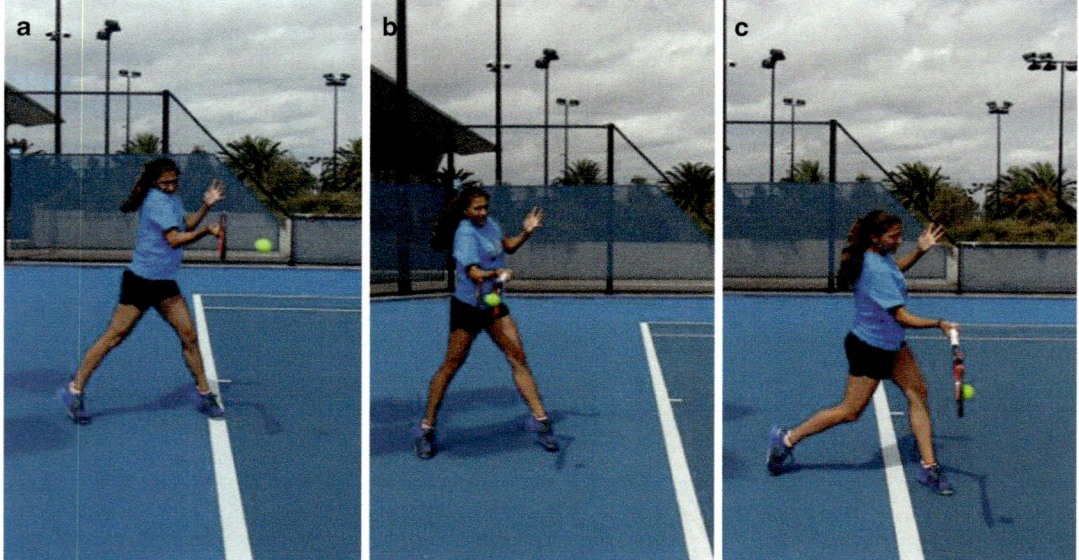

Fig. 2.14 Head positions at impact (**a**, full fixation; **b**, partial fixation; **c**, no fixation)

swing, so that by impact they are almost parallel to the net (Fig. 2.12b; [62]). While this characteristic will vary depending on the intended direction of the shot, the trunk rotational velocity recorded a similar level for open and square stances at impact [72].

A more varied trunk alignment can be found with the backhand stroke, where style and tactical situation dictate impact positions. Hip rotation commences trunk involvement, and a similar range of movement ($\approx 30°$ to $35°$) was exhibited in both backhand styles. Shoulder alignment rotation occurred with players using the 2H stroke rotating further to impact ($\approx 65°$) compared with the 1H action ($\approx 50°$). They were therefore more parallel to the baseline in the 2H compared with the 1HB (Fig. 2.9b2, c2 [5]).

2.1.8.3 Elbow/Wrist Joint

While grip type plays a large role in the impact height, hand force at impact does not significantly affect the coefficient of restitution of the ball in the flat forehand drive [37]. However it does influence elbow angle at impact with players using a western grip for the forehand typically having a more flexed elbow at impact, whereas those using an eastern grip were more extended [62]. Hitting positions were also dependent on type of backhand wherein the elbow was more flexed and the wrist joint more extended in the 2H [5], compared with 1H strokes. Players whose bottom hand is a more western grip in the 2HB will typically use an 'in-out swing', whereas those who adopt a more 'balanced' grip structure (eastern grips) will follow a more 'out-in swing path'. Elbow extension leads to a relatively straight but not fully extended upper limb at impact for backspin ($\approx 170°$) and topspin ($\approx 165°$) 1HB and is more flexed in the 2H stroke ($\approx 130°$) [5, 41, 73] (Fig. 2.9b2, c2).

Although the wrist joint flexes during the forehand forward swing, it is still hyperextended at impact, particularly when hitting down-the-line (Fig. 2.12b, c [62]). This angle will, of course, be partly determined by the direction of the stroke. In the 1HB, the hand was involved in the transfer of momentum from the forearm (kinetic chain) and thus was integral to the generation of racket velocity for impact [54, 55].

The impact position relative to the body is similar for one-handed groundstrokes on both sides of the body, with the ball impacted forward (≈ 0.65 m) and lateral to the body (≈ 0.70 m). The 2HB was hit closer (≈ 0.45 m), but at a similar distance laterally from the body (≈ 0.70 m) to the 1H stroke [5]. Impact height will vary depending on grip and stance; however, it has been shown that skilled players adjust the position of the racket to meet varying tactical situations, at least in part, by modification of lower limb movement [74]. Although with consideration to the section on variability above, King et al. [69] observed that for similar ball-racket impact conditions, there were comparable angle-time relationships at the wrist and elbow joints but with major kinematic differences evident at the shoulder joint in the 1H topspin and backspin strokes.

Clinician's Corner
1. Forearm muscle loading in the 1HB provides some insight into the development of 'tennis elbow'. Intermediate players with tennis elbow eccentrically contracted the wrist extensor muscles at impact, and novices have also been shown to generate less force yet load the extensor musculature eccentrically at impact. In a similar manner, different levels of wrist rotation were also recorded at impact, with better players forcibly extending through impact, while novice players were only marginally extending [75, 76].
2. Giangarra et al. [77] reported that the decreased occurrence of lateral epicondylitis in players using a 2HB compared with the 1H stroke may be more related to poor technique rather than decreased wrist extensor activity.
3. By not fully extending the elbow at impact, the upper limb is not 'locked', so as to avoid undue stress on the elbow region.

2.1.8.4 Timing and Disguise

One of the advantages of the 2H stroke compared with its 1H counterpart, at least for the backhand, is the ability to use disguise to confuse your opponent. How often have you approached the net only to have your opponent use their 2HB to 'flick' the ball over your head with a topspin lob? While racket velocity profiles have been reported as similar at impact for 1H and 2H strokes, maximum accelerations have been recorded closer to impact in the 2H style (Fig. 2.15 [5]). This ability to make what may be considered a very late tactical decision is an advantage for the stroke, notwithstanding that much of the swing time of the 1H stroke sees the racket behind the body.

2.1.9 Follow-Through and Recovery

This permits optimal racket mechanics for impact, allows fast moving parts of the body to 'slow under control' and involves movements that position the player for the next stroke.

Figure 2.16 shows David Ferrer executing his forehand follow-through, an integral part of all groundstrokes, where his shoulder abduction angle is ≈90° and his elbow is typically pointing in the direction of the shot.

The backhand stroke, irrespective of style, displays a full follow-through (Fig. 2.17a, b). Notice the position of the head and the role of the left arm in both strokes. In the 2H stroke, this arm is used to help 'hit through the line of impact', while in the 1H stroke, it balances the forward movement of the racket, even for intermediate players.

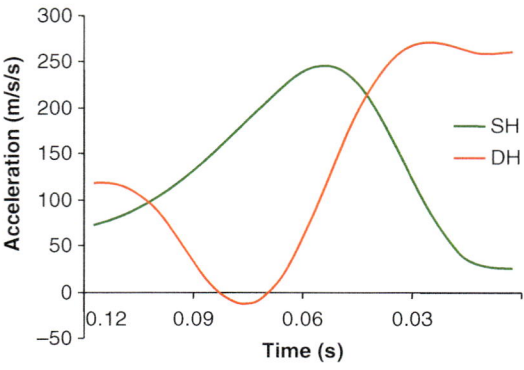

Fig. 2.15 Racket acceleration profiles in the backhand stroke (SH, 1H, and DH, 2H), where time 0 = impact [5]

Clinician's Corner
1. A full follow-through is needed in all groundstrokes to ensure optimal performance at impact and to slow the racket under eccentric muscle control.
2. The high levels of internal rotation in the forehand, either just before or after impact, mean that the external rotators, at the shoulder, must be trained *eccentrically* to protect the shoulder region from injury (as with the serve).

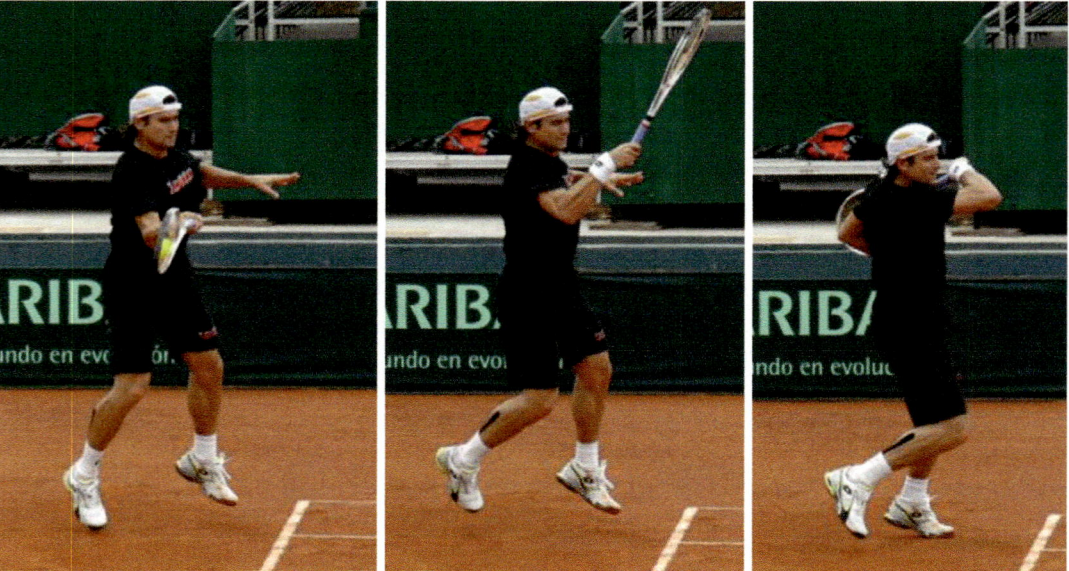

Fig. 2.16 Ferrer's forehand showing a complete follow-through

2 Biomechanics of Groundstrokes and Volleys

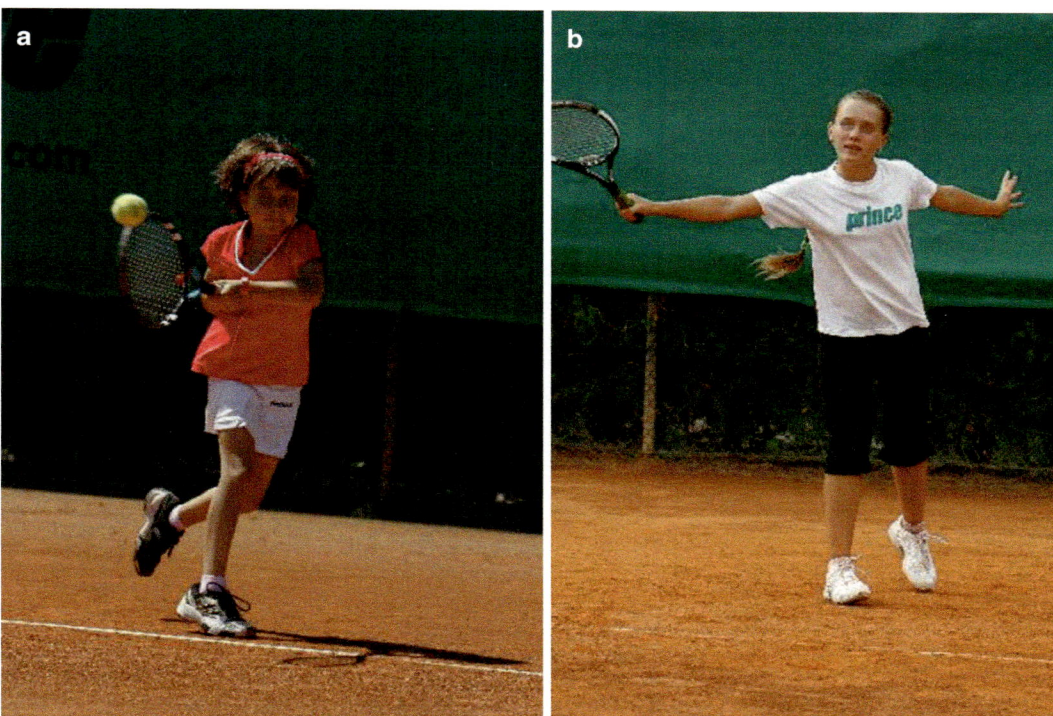

Fig. 2.17 Follow-throughs for the 2H and 1H backhands for junior players

2.2 Volleys

2.2.1 Introduction

Contemporary tactics are typically built around groundstrokes and the serve, with the volley now only playing an integral role in doubles tennis. For instance, volleys only account for 2% of total shots played in both men's and women's professional tennis (Fig. 2.1 and Table 2.1). While this number is very small, it was evident men hit almost double the number of volleys to women when the first four rounds of the Australian Open in 2015 were analyzed (58 vs 30).

Although it should be stated that doubles tennis is the cornerstone of most recreational programs, so the volley is an important stroke in tennis generally. Anecdotally, while it is rare for the volley to feature prominently in most development approaches, it is still a shot that if mastered may enhance one's chance of success. The lesser number of repetitions during play and reduced emphasis on velocity generation also mean that mechanical loading and the associated possibility of injury are not a major concern in most instances, at least at the professional level.

The complexity of the transition to the net and volley has meant that few scientific papers provide data to assist in providing guidance with respect to this stroke. While the drive-volley is played from an elevated return and does not require the same preparation as occurs with the serve-volley or approach shot-volley scenarios. For that reason the following section will deal primarily with these two latter situations.

Volley mechanics are integrally linked with the appropriate positioning and movement of the

racket for impact in a variety of tactical situations (drive, conventional and drop-volleys).

2.2.2 Preparation

Mechanical aspects need to be linked with the movement and orientation of the body and racket commensurate with tactical considerations.

The primary mechanical consideration following a serve or approach shot is to adopt a balanced pose that is tactically appropriate. In groundstrokes where approximately 75% of the ball velocity was generated from the racket, in the volley, which does not need to be hit with as high a velocity as a groundstroke, more of the ball velocity can be 'taken' from the incoming ball.

> **Clinician's Corner**
> 1. A 'split step' is the cornerstone of dynamic balance needed for a volley. The dynamic balance created by this movement enhances volley performance while reducing the chance of lower limb injuries compared with a rushed or unbalanced pose.
> 2. Research has shown that movement improves by 10–20% if elastic energy stored during the 'split step' is tactically used to advantage with minimal pause between the stretch and shorten phases of the quadriceps *stretch-shorten cycle* [78, 79].

The cornerstone to this balanced position is the 'split step'. While this movement permits the player to adopt a balanced but not stable position for the volley, it also places the quadriceps muscle group on stretch. The energy stored during the eccentric contraction of this muscle group may then be partially returned to assist subsequent movement to the ball. The very quick action involved in the volley to intercept the return inevitably means that there is little pause between the stretch and shorten phases of quadriceps contraction and therefore a maximal level of stored energy is returned to assist movement to the ball.

2.2.3 Backswing

Mechanical considerations will vary in line with the tactical situation.

Studies by Chow et al. [80, 81] for varying ball speed and impact positions reported players initiated racket movement earlier, as the speed on the incoming ball increased. Skilled players completed a volley—from initial racket movement to impact—in less than 400 ms; however slower-approaching balls afforded players 800 ms, which explains why drive-volleys may be played with a greater backswing, in a similar manner to that seen in a groundstroke. During this preparation phase, relatively low muscular activity was recorded in the arm and shoulder muscles, although the muscles of the lower trunk were active, in preparing for the forward movement of the body to the ball.

Racket movement, shoulder alignment turn and back foot pivot all occurred in one synchronous action for both forehand and 1HB volleys, both at the service line and net [82]. Shoulder alignment rotations for volleys at the service line and net were greater for 1HB ($\approx 80°$ and 95°, respectively), compared with forehand volleys ($\approx 55°$ and $\approx 60°$, respectively). A larger shoulder rotation occurred in all 1HB volleys compared with forehand volleys, irrespective of court location, as the racket had to be moved to the opposite side of the body. These rotations meant that immediately prior to forward movement, the racket was in a position behind the line of the hitting shoulder for volleys from the service line but not necessarily for those played at the net. The elbow angle was significantly larger in forehand service-line volleys compared with those at the net ($\approx 145°$ and $\approx 130°$, respectively), whereas 1HB values were similar at both court locations ($\approx 140°$), which suggests the racket moves through a larger arc in preparation for the forehand volley at the service line.

2.2.4 Forward Swing to Impact

Mechanics *of forward movement of the body (momentum) and racket must be linked.*

The body needs to create forward momentum for impact; however, there was no sequential pattern to suggest that a summation of segment velocities, as in the kinetic chain, took place as movement tended to occur at different joints at the same time. That is, the forward swing was characterized by a velocity-accuracy trade-off, whereby tasks, such as a volley that requires precise racket orientation, are summed at a similar point in time.

Trunk rotation and lower limb drive increased the linear velocity of the shoulder until just prior to impact. At impact while the front leg was on the ground in the fast ball condition studied by Chow et al. [80, 81], when time permitted the contralateral leg landed on the ground simultaneously with impact. In match conditions it would be logical to assume that this dynamic approach to volleying is linked with the tactical situation. Low-impact positions therefore require greater stability than higher impacts and may require this front foot to be on the court for impact.

The racket moved on a downward path between the backswing position and impact for all volleys, irrespective of court location, a desirable trajectory to achieve backspin on the ball [82]. Trunk rotation, lower limb drive and upper limb movements then all contributed to the impact racket velocity ($\approx$13 m/s). The best players, ranked on their ability to play forehand volleys, all achieved higher upper limb segment velocities compared with the lesser level volleyers and maintained an almost straight line between the long axis of the racket and the hand through impact.

The closing velocity of the racket and ball was approximately 30 m/s ($\approx$65 mph), well below the theoretical value of 45 m/s proposed for groundstroke situations, where if the ball was travelling slower, the racket would be swung faster. However, there was $\approx$20% increase in the velocity of the ball after impact (accepting a change in direction), far less than typically occurs for groundstrokes [62].

2.2.5 Follow-Through and Recovery

Mechanical considerations are integrally linked with preparation for the next stroke.

The post-impact racket velocity was reduced by $\approx$50% by impact, as the racket pushed through the line of impact [82]. Racket linked with body movement then occurred as the player prepares for the next stroke.

Clinician's Corner

1. Upper limb loading is not typically an issue with volleying, although it should be stressed that more off-centre impacts occur in this stroke, so good technique should be stressed to optimize performance and reduce any possibility of injury.

Conclusion

External load, irrespective of whether hitting groundstrokes or volleys, can be thought of as a combination of:

- Movement load: the nature of player's movement on court
- Hitting load: the volume of balls they hit and the intensity at which they do so

While these factors are always present, it is evident that technique also plays a part in enhancing performance and reducing load and thus the likelihood of injury. It is the job of the coach and support staff to sufficiently prepare players for competition and keep them healthy. Thus, they need to establish a balanced training regime that provides enough load to elicit improvements in performance, without exceeding a load threshold that places the athlete at a significant risk of injury. This chapter has presented the mechanical factors that should be considered in preparing a player's groundstrokes and volleys for match play. In other words, how can we sufficiently prepare a player for competition that requires so many groundstrokes, if we don't know the mechanical structure of these strokes? Hopefully this chapter has provided a mechanical background to stroke production for the coach and player alike.

References

1. Campbell A, Straker L, Whiteside D, O'Sullivan P, Elliott B, Reid M. Lumbar mechanics in tennis groundstrokes: Differences in elite adolescent players with and without low back pain. J Appl Biomech. 2016;32:32–9.
2. Reid M, Morgan S, Whiteside D. Matchplay characteristics of Grand Slam tennis: implications for training and conditioning. J Sports Sci. 2016;34(19):1791–8.
3. Cam I, Turhan B, Onag Z. The analysis of the last shots of top-level tennis players in open tennis tournaments. Turk J Sport Exerc. 2013;15(1):54–7.
4. Landlinger J, Stöggl T, Lindinger S, Wagner H, Müller E. Differences in ball speed and accuracy of tennis groundstrokes between elite and high-performance players. Eur J Sport Sci. 2012;12(4):301–8.
5. Reid M, Elliott B. The one- and two-handed backhands in tennis. Sports Biomech. 2002;1:47–68.
6. Akutagawa S, Kojima T. Trunk rotation torques through the hip joints during the one- and two-handed backhand strokes. J Sports Sci. 2005;23(8):781–93.
7. Fanchiang H, Finch A, Ariel G. Effects of one and two handed tennis backhands hit with varied power levels on torso rotation. XXXI international symposium on biomechanics in sport, Taiwan; 2013. p. 7–11.
8. Muhamad T, Rashid A, Razak M, Salamuddin N. A comparative study of backhand strokes in tennis among national tennis players in Malaysia. Proc Soc Behav Sci. 2011;15:3495–9.
9. Kibler B, Safran M. Tennis Injuries. Med Sport Sci. 2005;48:120–37.
10. Brody H. Bounce of a tennis ball. J Sci Med Sport. 2003;6(1):113–9.
11. Cross R. Customising a tennis racquet by adding weights. Sports Eng. 2001;4:1–14.
12. Elliott B, Reid M, Crespo M, editors. Biomechanics of advanced tennis. Valencia, Spain: ITF Ltd.; 2003.
13. Elliott B, Reid M, Crespo M, editors. Technique development in tennis stroke production. Valencia, Spain: ITF Ltd.; 2009.
14. Reid M, Elliott B, Crespo M, editors. Tennis science: optimizing performance on the court. London: Ivy Press; 2015.
15. Davids K, Glazier P, Araújoe D, Bartlett R. Movement systems as dynamical systems: the functional role of variability and its implications for sports medicine. Sports Med. 2003;33(4):245–60.
16. Knudson D. Intra-subject variability of upper extremity kinematics in the tennis forehand drive. Int J Sports Biomech. 1990;6:415–21.
17. Matava M. Stop sports injuries: overuse injuries [Pamphlet]. Rosemont, IL: American Orthopedic Society for Sports Medicine; 2010.
18. Hamill J, van Emmerik RE, Heiderscheit BC, Li L. A dynamical systems approach to lower extremity running injuries. Clin Biomech. 1999;14(5):297–308.
19. Heiderscheit BC. Variability of Stride Characteristics and Joint Coordination among Individuals. J Appl Biomech. 2002;18:110–21.
20. James CR, Dufek JS, Bates BT. Effects of injury proneness and task difficulty on joint kinetic variability. Med Sci Sports Exerc. 2000;32(11):1833–44.
21. Fortenbaugh D, Fleisig G, Andrews J. Baseball pitching biomechanics in relation to injury risk and performance. Sports Health. 2009;1(4):314–20.
22. Grantham W, Byram I, Meadows M, Ahmad C. The impact of fatigue on the kinematics of collegiate baseball pitchers. Orthop J Sports Med. 2014;2(6):2325967114537032.
23. Lyman S, Fleisig G, Waterbor J, et al. Longitudinal study of elbow and shoulder pain in youth baseball pitchers. Med Sci Sport Exerc. 2001;33(11):1803–10.
24. Olsen SJ, Fleisig G, Dun S, Loftice J, Andrews J. Risk factors for shoulder and elbow injuries in adolescent baseball pitchers. Am J Sports Med. 2006;34(6):905–12.
25. Damm L, Low D, Richardson A, Clarke J, Carré M, Dixon S. The effects of surface traction characteristics on frictional demand and kinematics in tennis. Sports Biomech. 2013;12(4):389–402.
26. Carl JR, Gellman RS. Human smooth pursuit: stimulus-dependent responses. J Neurophysiol. 1987;57(5):1446–63.
27. Avilès C, Benguigui N, Beaudoin E, Godart F. Developing early perception and getting ready for action on the return of serve. ITF Coaching Sport Sci Rev. 2002;28:6–8.
28. Reid M, Elliott B, Crespo M. Mechanics and learning practices associated with the tennis forehand: a review. J Sports Sci Med. 2013;12(2):225–31.
29. Triolet C, Benguigui N, Le Runigo C, Williams AM. Quantifying the nature of anticipation in professional tennis. J Sports Sci. 2013;31(8):820–30.
30. Knudson D, Blackwell J. Trunk muscle activation in open and square stance tennis forehands. Int J Sports Med. 2000;21:321–4.
31. Bahamonde R, Knudson D. Kinetics of the upper extremity in the open and square stance tennis forehand. J Sci Med Sport. 2003;6(1):88–101.
32. Elliott B, Takahashi K, Noffal G. The influence of grip position on upper limb contributions to racket head velocity in a tennis forehand. J Appl Biomech. 1997;13(2):182–96.
33. Tagliafico A, Ameri P, Michaud J, Derchi L, Sormani M, Martinoli C. Wrist injuries in nonprofessional tennis players: relationships with different grips. Am J Sports Med. 2009;37(4):760–7.
34. Eng D, Hagler D. A novel analysis of grip variations on the two-handed backhand. ITF Coaching Sport Sci Rev. 2014;62:14–6.
35. King M, Kentel B, Mitchell S. The effects of ball impact location and grip tightness on the arm, racquet and ball for one-handed tennis backhand groundstroke. J Biomech. 2012;45(6):1048–52.
36. Wei SH, Chiang JY, Shiang TY, Chang HY. Comparison of shock transmission and forearm

electromyography between experienced and recreational tennis players during backhand strokes. Clin J Sport Med. 2006;16(2):129–35.
37. Knudson D. Hand forces and impact effectiveness in the tennis forehand. J Hum Mov Stud. 1989;17(1):1–7.
38. Balius R, Pedret C, Estruch A, Hernández G, Ruiz-Cotorro Á, Mota J. Stress fractures of the metacarpal bones in adolescent tennis players. A case series. Am J Sports Med. 2010;38(6):1215–20.
39. Rossi J, Vigouroux L, Barla C, Berton E. Potential effects of racket grip size on lateral epicondilalgy risks. Scand J Med Sci Sports. 2014;24(6):e462–70.
40. Wu S, Gross M, Prentice W, Yu B. Comparison of ball-and-racquet impact force between two tennis backhand stroke techniques. J Orthop Sports Phys Ther. 2001;31(5):247–54.
41. Elliott B, Christmass M. A comparison of the high and low backspin backhand drives in tennis using different grips. J Sports Sci. 1995;13(2):141–51.
42. Kawasaki S, Imai S, Inaoka H, Masuda T, Okawa A, Shinomiya K. The lower lumbar spine movement and the axial rotational movement of a body during one-handed and double-handed backhand stroke in tennis. Int J Sports Med. 2005;26(8):617–21.
43. Ellenbecker T, Roetert P. An isokinetic profile of trunk rotation strength in elite tennis players. Med Sci Sports Exerc. 2004;36(11):1959–63.
44. Kibele A, Classen C, Triebfuerst K. Standardized testing of forehand and backhand groundstrokes in tennis through a bird's eye perspective. ITF Coaching Sport Sci Rev. 2009;49:14–6.
45. Charbonnier C, Chagué S, Kolo FC, Lädermann A. Shoulder motion during tennis serve: dynamic and radiological evaluation based on motion capture and magnetic resonance imaging. Int J Comput Assist Radiol Surg. 2015;10(8):1289–97.
46. Creveaux T, Dumas R, Hautier C, Macé P, Chèze L, Rogowski I. Joint kinetics to assess the influence of the racket on a tennis player's shoulder. J Sports Sci Med. 2013;12(2):259–66.
47. Rogowski I, Creveaux T, Chèze L, Macé P, Dumas R. Effects of the racket polar moment of inertia on dominant upper limb joint moments during tennis serve. PLoS One. 2014;9(8):1–8.
48. Iino Y, Kojima T. Torque acting on the pelvis about its superior-inferior axis through the hip joint during a tennis forehand stroke. J Hum Mov Stud. 2001;40:269–90.
49. Cotorro AR, Philippon M, Briggs K, Boykin R, Dominguez D. Hip screening in elite youth tennis players. Br J Sports Med. 2014;48(7):582.
50. Philippon MJ, Ho CP, Briggs KK, Stull J, LaPrade RF. Prevalence of increased alpha angles as a measure of cam-type femoro-acetabular impingement in youth ice hockey players. Am J Sports Med. 2013;41(6):1357–62.
51. Siebenrock KA, Kaschka I, Frauchiger L, Werlen S, Schwab JM. Prevalence of cam-type deformity and hip pain in elite ice hockey players before and after the end of growth. Am J Sports Med. 2013;41(10):2308–13.
52. Ireland A, Maden-Wilkinson T, McPhee J, Cooke K, Narici M, Degens H, Rittweger J. Upper limb muscle–bone asymmetries and bone adaptation in elite youth tennis players. Med Sci Sports Exerc. 2013;45(9):1749–58.
53. Bahamonde R. Producing an explosive forehand and backhand. In: Elliott B, Gibson B, Knudson D, editors. Proceedings of the XVII international symposium on biomechanics. Perth, Australia: Edith Cowan University; 1999.
54. Stepien A, Bober T, Zawadzki J. The kinematics of trunk and upper extremities in one-handed and two-handed backhand stroke. J Hum Kinet. 2011;30:37–47.
55. Wang L, Lin H. Momentum transfer of upper extremity in tennis one-handed backhand drive. J Mech Med Biol. 2005;5(2):231–41.
56. Seeley M, Funk M, Denning W, Hager R, Hopkins T. Tennis forehand kinematics change as post-impact ball speed is altered. Sports Biomech. 2011;10(4):415–26.
57. Landlinger J, Lindinger S, Stoggl T, Wagner H, Muller E. Key factors and timing patterns in the tennis forehand of different skill levels. J Sports Sci Med. 2010;9(4):643–51.
58. Rogowski I, Creveaux T, Cheze L, Dumas R. Scapulothoracic kinematics during tennis forehand drive. Sports Biomech. 2014;13(2):166–75.
59. Takahashi K, Elliott B, Noffal G. The role of the upper limb segment rotations in the development of spin in the tennis forehand. Aust J Sci Med Sport. 1996;28(4):106–13.
60. Huang Y, Tang W, Wang S. Intermuscular coordination analysis of skilled double-handed backhand and single-handed forehand players. XX international society of biomechanics congress, Cleveland, USA; 2005.
61. Ryu K, McCormick F, Jobe F, Moynes D, Antonell D. An electromyographic analysis of shoulder function in tennis players. Am J Sports Med. 1988;16:481–5.
62. Elliott B, Marsh T, Overheu P. A biomechanical comparison of the multi-segment and single unit topspin forehand drives in tennis. Int J Sport Biomech. 1989;5(3):350–64.
63. Wang L, Lin H, Lo K, Hsieh Y, Su F. Comparison of segmental linear and angular momentum transfers in two-handed backhand stroke stances for different skill level tennis players. J Sci Med Sport. 2010;13(4):452–9.
64. Martin C, Bideau B, Bideau N, Nicolas G, Delamarche P, Kulpa R. Energy flow analysis during the tennis serve comparison between injured and non-insured tennis players. Am J Sports Med. 2014;42(11):2751–60.
65. Ray J. The biomechanical analysis of the one-handed and two-handed backhand in tennis. XIII international symposium on biomechanics in sport, Thunder Bay, Canada; 1995. p. 18–22.

66. Yue Z, Kleinoder H, Mester J. Power and energy analysis of tennis forehand. In: 6th annual congress of the European College of Sports Sciences, Cologne, Germany; 1994. p. 1305.
67. Blackwell J, Knudson D. Vertical plane margins in the topspin forehand of intermediate tennis players. Med Sport. 2005;9(3):83–6.
68. Rogowski I, Rouffet D, Lambalot F, Brosseau O, Hautier C. Trunk and upper limb muscle activation during flat and topspin forehand drives in young tennis players. J Appl Biomech. 2011;27:15–21.
69. King M, Glynn J, Mitchell S. Subject-specific computer simulation model for determining elbow loading in one-handed tennis backhand groundstroke. Sports Biomech. 2011;10(4):391–406.
70. Lafont D. Towards a new hitting model in tennis. Int J Perform Anal Sport. 2007;7(3):106–16.
71. Lafont D. Gaze control during the hitting phase in tennis: a preliminary study. Int J Perform Anal Sport. 2008;8(1):85–100.
72. Knudson W, Bahamonde R. Trunk and racket kinematics at impact in the open and square stance tennis forehand. Biol Sport. 1999;16(1):3–10.
73. Elliott B, Marsh A, Overheu P. The topspin backhand drive: a biomechanical analysis. J Hum Mov Stud. 1989;16:1–16.
74. Nesbit S, Serrano M, Elzinga M. The role of knee positioning and range-of-motion on the closed-stance forehand tennis swing. J Sports Sci Med. 2008;7:114–24.
75. Kentel B, King M, Mitchell S. Evaluation of a subject-specific, torque-driven computer simulation model of one-handed tennis backhand ground strokes. J Appl Biomech. 2011;27:345–54.
76. Reik S, Chapman A, Milner T. A simulation of muscle force and internal kinematics of extensor carpi radialis brevis during backhand tennis stroke: implications for injury. Clin Biomech. 1999;14:477–83.
77. Giangarra C, Conroy B, Jobe F, Pink M, Perry J. Electromyographic and cinematographic analysis of elbow function in tennis players using single- and double-handed backhand strokes. Am J Sports Med. 1993;21(3):394–9.
78. Wilson G, Elliott B, Wood G. The effect of imposing a delay during a stretch-shorten cycle movement. Med Sci Sport Exerc. 1991;23:364–70.
79. Walshe A, Wilson G, Ettema G. Stretch-shorten cycle compared with isometric preload contributions to enhanced muscular performance. J Appl Physiol. 1998;84:97–106.
80. Chow J, Carlton L, Chae W, Lim J, Kuenster A. Muscle activation during the tennis volley. Med Sci Sports Exerc. 1999;31(6):846–54.
81. Chow J, Carlton L, Woen-Sik C, Jae-Ho S, Young-Tae L, Kuenster A. Movement characteristics of the tennis volley. Med Sci Sports Exerc. 1999;31(6):855–63.
82. Elliott B, Overheu P, Marsh A. The service line and net volley in tennis: a cinematographic analysis. Aust J Sci Med Sport. 1988;20(2):10–8.

Epidemiology of Tennis Injuries

Babette M. Pluim and Gary Windler

3.1 Introduction

Tennis is one of the most popular sports worldwide based on the level of participation. It is played at various levels of skill (beginner, intermediate, advanced, elite, and professional) among both sexes and all ages, from early childhood to octogenarians and beyond. Both the singles and doubles format are popular at all levels of play. Tennis is not a clock-based sport, but is rather scoring based. As a result, duration of matches varies considerably. The sport is played on a variety of court surfaces, both indoors and outdoors, and in a broad range of environmental conditions. Although the basic equipment, consisting of racquets, strings, balls, and net, generally conform to standards imposed by the governing bodies within the sport and followed by equipment manufacturers, there remains considerable variation in racquets and strings which may influence injury patterns.

Epidemiological studies on tennis injuries can play an important part in the development of injury prevention strategies. Tennis epidemiologists, however, must take into account the many factors mentioned above, including age, sex, skill level, surface, equipment, etc. in interpretation of injury data and in designing meaningful studies. Retrospective studies often fail to adequately account for many of these variables generally making them of more limited value than prospective designs.

3.2 Evolution of Tennis

The sport of tennis has been significantly impacted by advancements in equipment technology. This applies primarily to the racquet and strings. The most apparent change came about in the 1980s with the replacement of the wood racquet, initially with various metal designs and ultimately with composite materials used almost exclusively today. The racquet material affects its stiffness which ultimately affects the force transmission to the upper extremity. Perhaps an even more drastic result of the material change was a reduction in the overall weight of the racquet by approximately 20–30%, which has allowed for increased swing (racquet head) speed. This, along with advancements in string technology material and design, has resulted in a game driven today by more power and spin than at any time in the past. This, in turn, directly impacts the style of play, the length of rallies, biomechanical loads, and other important aspects of the game that relate to injuries.

B. M. Pluim (✉)
Royal Netherlands Lawn Tennis Association (KNLTB), Amersfoort, The Netherlands
e-mail: b.pluim@knltb.nl

G. Windler
ATP World Tour, Ponte Vedra Beach, FL, USA

South Carolina Sports Medicine & Orthopaedic Center, P.A., Charleston, SC, USA
e-mail: gwindler@atpworldtour.com

Equipment changes have directly and indirectly impacted stroke mechanics as well. Major changes have included the advent of the two-handed (double-handed) backhand which is the predominant backhand in professional tennis today. Other significant changes have included the shift to the semi-western and more extreme western grip from the more traditional continental and eastern forehand grips, and the implementation of the open stance forehand and backhand. Presumably, the biomechanical alterations resulting from the changes in stroke technique have affected injury patterns seen in today's game.

In addition, as in most other sports and particularly at the professional level, tennis has experienced an improvement in the general level of fitness of the players [1]. Much of that can be attributed to the increase in knowledge in the fields of strength and conditioning, nutrition, and hydration. Players generally spend more time doing off-court fitness training now than in the past. Many professional players today travel with their own physiotherapists and fitness trainers, a distinct change from years past. The impact of improved strength, flexibility, and endurance on injury risk has been studied in many sports, including tennis, and continues to be an area of intense study.

Another interesting trend evolving in the game is a relatively recent shift in the age of the top players in professional tennis. At the time of the writing of this chapter, the top five male players in the world were all over the age of 30. Additionally, 43 of the top 100 professional tennis players on the ATP World Tour were 30 years of age or greater. This appears to indicate an extended longevity in the careers of professional tennis players. Though there are likely many factors contributing to this trend, it suggests that there may be a decrease in the incidence of career-ending injuries. This in turn could be related to better fitness, optimization of players' tournament schedule allowing better recovery, or perhaps better treatment of serious injuries.

Thus, based upon the multifaceted and continued evolution of the game, it should be recognized that generally, more recent tennis injury studies are most relevant to today's game.

3.3 Incidence of Injuries

Determination of injury incidence by epidemiological methods requires the recording of both the number of new injuries and the number of individuals within the population being studied. A "definition of injury" must be included in any study on injury incidence. Injuries can be defined by players simply reporting or seeking or receiving treatment for a musculoskeletal complaint [2–6]. Others prefer to utilize "time loss from tennis" as the defining measure of injury. Several studies have also reported on retirements from matches due to injury as a measure of injury incidence [7–10]. It is crucial that injury definition is examined carefully when trying to compare incidence of injury across studies.

In a consensus statement on epidemiological studies in tennis for the International Tennis Federation, Pluim et al. [11] recommended the following: "Any physical or psychological complaint or manifestation sustained by a player that results from a tennis match or tennis training irrespective of the need for medical attention or time loss from tennis activities." It must be recognized that this was proposed as a definition for "medical condition" with the intent of using the definition to study both injury and illness related to the sport of tennis.

Another important consideration when examining injury rates in sports is defining the underlying time frame. Injury incidence in tennis has been studied and calculated using various time parameters including number of injuries per hours of play [5, 12], per set [4], per match [3], per tournament [10, 13], per season, and per year.

A meta-analysis conducted by Pluim, et al. included 28 descriptive epidemiological studies across all age groups and skill levels dating back as far as 1976 [14]. This review found an injury incidence ranging from 0.05 to 2.9 injuries per player per year and 0.04 to 3.0 injuries per 1000 hours played. The definition of injury varied considerably however among all studies.

Collegiate tennis is an ideal population for tennis injury studies as college teams typically have a team doctor and physiotherapist/athletic trainer to oversee and document all aspects of injuries. Lynall et al. [15] showed that injury rates in NCAA men's and women's tennis were similar overall (4.9/1000 Athletic Exposures) and that injury rates were higher during match play than during practice.

Several studies have examined the incidence of injury in junior players [12, 13, 16]. Although injury incidence generally is not markedly dissimilar from that seen in studies of adults, variation in definition of injury and overall study design makes it difficult to draw valid conclusions based on comparison of the studies in juniors.

3.4 Injury Trends by Region and Body Part

Examination of tennis injury studies of differing designs focusing on different populations using varying injury definitions is quite difficult. However, some general injury trends can be noted.

The greatest number of injuries is seen in the lower extremities, followed by the upper extremities and finally the trunk [14, 15]. Acute injuries more commonly occur in the lower extremities, while chronic injuries are seen more commonly in the upper extremities and trunk.

Ankle sprains and thigh strains are two of the most common acute injuries, while low back pain, rotator cuff conditions, and elbow epicondylitis commonly account for chronic symptoms.

3.5 Common Upper Extremity Injuries

As expected shoulder injuries in tennis occur predominantly in the dominant shoulder. As in other overhead sports, the repetitive overhead motion on the serve likely plays an important role in the pathomechanics of the shoulder. Much less common are injuries to the nondominant shoulder which, when it does occur, may be related to the two-hand backhand or the repetitive overhead motion of the service toss.

Most injuries to the shoulder are overuse in nature. These include rotator cuff and long-head biceps tendinosis and tears, anterior and internal impingement, labral tears, and both acromioclavicular and glenohumeral osteoarthritis. Acute tears of the rotator cuff, particularly the supraspinatus and infraspinatus tendon and less often the subscapularis, may be seen but are generally attritional in nature. Instability patterns are more common in junior players, while glenohumeral osteoarthritis is common in older players who have played tennis for many years [17].

As has been reported in other overhead sports including baseball and volleyball, infraspinatus atrophy is not uncommon. Young et al. [18] reported a 52% incidence of visual infraspinatus muscle atrophy in the dominant shoulder found at pre-participation physicals among 125 professional female players examined. Ellenbecker et al. [19] have found a slightly higher rate of infraspinatus atrophy in male professional tennis players (60.1%) which was positively correlated with external rotation weakness measured with a handheld dynamometer.

Elbow injuries also occur primarily in the dominant elbow. Lateral epicondylitis ("tennis elbow") is very common in the recreational player and is most often associated with eccentric load on the one-handed backhand stroke. Medial epicondylitis ("golfer's elbow") is more commonly seen in advanced players and is typically associated with the serve and forehand. Factors such as stroke technique, racquet characteristics, string material and tension, and grip size have all been implicated as contributing factors to tendinosis on both the medial and lateral side of the elbow.

Although tears of the ulnar collateral ligament of the elbow do occur in tennis players, they are less frequent than in throwers, especially baseball pitchers. Similarly, ulnar nerve problems including neuritis and symptomatic subluxation are less common than in throwers. Triceps tendinosis and posterior elbow osteophytes and loose bodies may be seen, usually in more advanced players and wheelchair tennis players.

Unlike shoulder and elbow problems, wrist injuries are common in both the dominant and nondominant extremities. This is due to use of the nondominant arm in stabilizing and in some cases being the primary force generator during the two-hand backhand. Tendinopathy of both the flexor and extensor tendons at the wrist is a common cause of wrist discomfort. Structural injuries are more common on the ulnar side of the wrist and typically involve tears of either the triangular fibrocartilage complex (TFCC) or the extensor carpi ulnaris (ECU) tendon or subsheath. Tagliafico et al. [20] found that in nonprofessional players, radial-sided injuries were associated with the eastern grip, while ulnar-sided injuries were more frequently associated with the western and semi-western grips. This most probably accounts for the preponderance of ulnar-sided injuries as the semi-western grip is the predominant grip in the game today. As a whole, wrist injuries appear to be on the rise in tennis over the past two decades [21]. This may be related to the shift to the two-hand backhand and western and semi-western grips along with the more extreme ranges of motion utilized to impart maximum spin on the ball on both the forehand and backhand strokes.

Hand and finger injuries are generally not very common, although falls onto the outstretched hand can result in finger, hand, wrist, or elbow injuries. More commonly, the hand and fingers are affected by pressure- and abrasion-related skin conditions such as blisters and calluses. Factors such as grip size and material, grip technique, and a rapid increase in the volume of play may be etiological factors.

3.6 Common Lower Extremity Injuries

As is the case in many sports, hip and groin injuries in tennis represent a spectrum of conditions which may be present alone or in combination. These include adductor, abductor and hip flexor muscle strains, athletic pubalgia, osteitis pubis, and acetabular labral tears usually in conjunction with femoroacetabular impingement (FAI). The start-stop nature of the game, including frequent changes of direction, does provide a mechanism for eccentric overload of the lower extremity musculature, including the hip. However, as clinicians have developed a better understanding of these conditions, it is becoming clear that many injuries that in past years were reported as primary hip muscle strains more likely were manifestations of FAI. The incidence of FAI with and without associated labral tearing in tennis has not yet been clearly elucidated. The apparent increase in hip injuries in general and FAI in particular seen in professional tennis may be related to the more common use of the open stance forehand and backhand in today's game although this association is not clear.

Similar to other sports that require explosive movement and direction change, quadriceps, hamstring, and adductor strains are common in tennis at all levels, primarily the result of eccentric overload.

The knee is a frequently injured joint in tennis. Patellar tendinosis (jumper's knee) is perhaps the most common knee pathology at the professional level. The injury is typically related to repetitive eccentric overload. Quadriceps tendinosis, though also seen in tennis, is significantly less common.

The incidence of meniscal tears in tennis is not known; however, the torsional nature of the forehand and backhand ground strokes likely contributes to the forces exerted on the meniscus. As expected reparable tears are more typically seen in younger players, while degenerative tears are more common in seniors.

Medial collateral ligament injuries are the most common ligament injury about the knee in tennis. Anterior cruciate ligament and lateral collateral injuries are seen less frequently. Posterior cruciate ligament and both posteromedial and posterolateral corner injuries are uncommon.

Muscle strains in the lower leg are quite common as a result of the repetitive start-stop pattern of movement. The medial head of the gastrocnemius is frequently involved, with this condition termed "tennis leg." Achilles tendinopathy and insertional Achilles pathology are also quite common. While Achilles tendon ruptures, both complete and partial, can occur, they are much less frequent and are more typically seen in middle-aged players.

Ankle sprains are the most common acute injury in the lower extremity. They usually occur either while planting the foot in preparation for a change of direction or catching of the foot on the surface during lateral movement. As in many other sports, the lateral ligament complex is most frequently injured as a result of an inversion-plantarflexion mechanism.

Both anterior and posterior impingements of the ankle occur in tennis, primarily at the more elite level of play. Plantar fasciitis is a relatively common problem and presumably court surface plays an important role in its pathogenesis.

As in the hand, blisters and calluses on the foot may be seen frequently in tennis. They are generally related to shoe and sock wear. Similarly, subungual hematoma in the toe (tennis toe) is often related to shoe and sock wear.

3.7 Fractures

As a noncontact sport, tennis players are at much lower risk for acute fractures than participants in contact sports such as American football, rugby, soccer, wrestling, etc. Acute fractures in tennis, though rare, can occur anywhere in the upper extremity and typically result from a fall onto an outstretched hand or arm. Similarly, falls can also result in acute lower extremity fractures as well. Osteoporosis and balance problems, both seen most commonly in seniors, are risk factors. Thus it would appear that senior tennis players are most at risk for fracture in the tennis-playing population.

Due to the repetitive nature of the sport, stress fractures do occur in tennis. As in most sports, they are more common in the lower extremities. A study by Maquirriain et al. [22] of elite players 13–35 years of age showed the tarsal navicular, metatarsals, and pars interarticularis (L5) as the most common sites for stress fracture. Other lower extremity locations include the tibia and fibula. In the upper extremity, stress fractures have been reported in the lunate, metacarpals, and ulna. In addition, stress reactions of the humerus have been described in competitive players [23, 24].

3.8 Injuries on the ATP World Tour

Data collected at the professional level often provides important epidemiological information on sport-specific injuries. It must be recognized that injuries at the highest level may be unique in some ways and therefore cannot necessarily be directly extrapolated to other populations within the sport. Nevertheless, this data can still provide important insights into the various aspects of the injuries that may affect participants.

The ATP World Tour is the organization representing players and tournaments in men's professional tennis worldwide. As the Tour is an individual rather than team sport and is played all over the world, both provision of medical care and comprehensive and accurate injury data collection are very challenging.

Staff and consultants of the ATP World Tour working closely with their counterparts in the Women's Tennis Association (WTA) developed an electronic Internet-based sport-specific healthcare documentation system. The system was designed to fulfill three primary objectives: (1) provide the necessary clinical information to optimize continuing care of players' injuries and illnesses at tournaments, (2) fulfill the required standards of medical-legal documentation, and (3) develop a clinical database for epidemiological analysis and focused injury studies.

Clinical evaluation, diagnosis, and data input on the ATP World Tour are performed by the Tour physiotherapists and tournament physicians. An injury is defined as any musculoskeletal complaint for which a player seeks evaluation and/or treatment from the physiotherapist or physician. Time loss from tennis is not a criterion for a musculoskeletal complaint to be considered and recorded as an injury.

Implementation of the system began in mid-year of the 2011 professional tennis season. Full season data has therefore been collected over a 5-year period (2012–2016). Review of the injury data showed relatively consistent results since 2013. The number of recorded injuries in 2012 was significantly lower than in subsequent years. This was likely related to the learning curve associated with use of the new system by the physiotherapists and tournament physicians. Therefore, data collected over the 4 years including 2013–2016 is felt to represent the most accurate injury data available for the ATP World Tour identifying consistent injury frequencies with only 1–3% year-to-year variation during this time period.

The spine, inclusive of cervical, thoracic, and lumbar regions, was the most common area of injury when the data was broken out by anatomical areas. This was followed in order by the foot/ankle, thigh, shoulder, knee, hip, elbow, wrist, and lower leg. Less commonly injured areas included the hand, abdominal, and rib (see Chap. 25 for Hip Injury information and Chap. 8 for Spinal Injury information).

The most common diagnosis in each anatomical area of injury was identified for years 2014–2016. This data is summarized in Table 3.1. Of interest is the change in the most frequent injury location in the thigh from hamstring in 2013 to adductor in 2014, to quadriceps in 2015. Medial epicondylitis was the most common diagnosis at the elbow, with an approximate 3:1 ratio as compared to lateral epicondylitis. This differs from the recreational tennis population where lateral epicondylitis is significantly more common. Also of interest is the finding of femoroacetabular impingement (FAI) as the most common hip diagnosis. The relatively high incidence of this condition in other sports such as soccer, basketball, and ice hockey has been recognized. Although the true incidence in tennis is not yet known, this early data on professional tennis players suggests it is not uncommon.

As has been noted earlier, the spine is the anatomical area accounting for the most injuries on the ATP World Tour. When broken down further, the lumbar spine is the most frequently injured region followed by the cervical spine, thoracic spine, and finally sacroiliac joint (Chap. 31).

Table 3.1 Most common diagnoses per anatomical area (2014-2016)

Region	Most common diagnosis (%) of region category
Abdominal	Rectus abdominis strain
Rib	Costovertebral dysfunction
Blister	Foot blister
Hand	Hand abrasion
Foot/ankle	Anterior talofibular ligament sprain
Thigh	Hamstring 2013/adductor 2014/quadriceps 2015
Elbow	Medial epicondylitis
Shoulder	Rotator cuff tendonitis/impingement
Wrist	Extensor tenosynovitis 2013/2014 /sprain 2015
Knee	Patellar tendinopathy
Hip	Femoroacetabular impingement
Spine	Facet syndrome

Although this initial 4-year injury data compiled by the ATP World Tour does add important epidemiologic information to our knowledge of tennis injuries at the professional level, one must recognize some important limitations of the data collection. Unlike many other international professional sports in which the athletes' medical care is provided by a small group of team physicians and physiotherapists or athletic trainers, professional tennis players on the ATP World Tour are cared for by several ATP physiotherapists and different tournament doctors at each of the over 60 tournaments. As a result, players are evaluated and data input by 100–200 different healthcare providers annually. Further, many diagnoses are made only on a clinical basis and not always confirmed by imaging or surgical findings. These factors surely influence the accuracy and consistency of the data to some extent.

3.9 Court Surface: How Does It Affect Injuries?

Tennis is played on a variety of surfaces at the professional, collegiate, junior, and recreational levels. There are many different court surfaces available. At the professional level, they include the broad categories "hard", "clay", and grass. Hard courts are made from a variety of different composite layers. The hard court surfaces vary significantly, especially between indoor and outdoor courts. Clay courts are typically made from either crushed brick or crushed stone. A recent study by Pluim et al. [25] showed that there was no significant difference in the overall prevalence of injury on clay, hard court, sand-fill artificial grass, and red-sand-fill artificial grass, but that there was a higher prevalence of lower limb overuse injuries when playing on hard court compared to the other court surfaces. Also, players who played on multiple surfaces had a higher injury prevalence, particularly of overuse injuries, than those who primarily played on one court surface.

The speed of the court, a function of the interaction between the ball and the court surface, can be controlled for all three surfaces. For hard courts this is accomplished primarily by the formulation of the paint applied to the surface. The rougher the surface paint, the slower the court due to the increased coefficient of friction. Clay surface speed depends somewhat on the composition of the crushed brick or stone, but to an even greater extent on the moisture level of the surface. This is directly related to both environmental conditions and maintenance watering practices. Greater moisture slows down court speed. Grass court speed depends on the type of grass and length at which it is maintained. During the course of a tournament, the grass typically degrades with play, changing both the surface contour and speed. Typically, grass is the fastest court surface, while clay is the slowest.

Court speed may affect injury incidence and patterns in several ways. Rally length is typically longer on slower courts as it is more difficult for a player to end the point with an offensive shot or service winner. Increased rally length increases time exposure to injury and muscle fatigue. It also increases the number of changes of direction by each player. In addition, court speed affects the ball speed at contact with the racquet which ultimately affects force transmission to the racquet arm.

The height of the ball bounce varies considerably depending on the surface with grass providing the lowest bounce. Low balls generally require increased knee flexion, hip flexion, and/or flexion at the lumbar spine in order for the player to get down to the level of the ball effectively. On the other hand, returning high bouncing shots requires hitting forehands and backhands with the hitting arm in more abduction and forward flexion, respectively, in order to get the racquet up to the level of the ball.

The shoe–surface interaction changes considerably between surfaces. This is most apparent in the players' choice of different outsole patterns based on the court surface in order to achieve optimal footing. The varying shoe–surface interactions allow for differing lower extremity mechanics on each type of court. As an example, the consistency and coefficient of friction of the clay surface allow the players to slide into shots. This technique can also be used on hard and grass courts, but to a much lesser extent. Similarly, hard courts typically provide the most friction between the shoe and the surface maximizing the ability to change direction. However, this increased shoe–surface friction may also promote injuries, such as ankle sprains, if the movements are not properly coordinated.

Injury incidence and patterns may be affected by court surface characteristics in other ways as well. As an example, players tend to use the kick serve more on clay due to the effectiveness with which the spin of the ball reacts to the surface. On the other hand, the flat serve is typically used more often on grass due to the court's speed and tendency to keep the ball low. The biomechanical differences between these two serves may have implications with regard to injuries to the upper extremity and trunk.

Finally, falls onto the court may result in upper or lower extremity injuries due to the impact of the fall. By the nature of their mechanical properties, grass courts typically cushion this impact more than clay or hard courts, likely reducing the risk of injury in a fall to some degree.

Although court surface clearly has many potential effects on the incidence, type, and severity of injury, little information exists in the literature at this time documenting differences in injury rates and patterns on the various surfaces. While it is relatively easy to study acute injuries related to playing surface, it is more difficult to investigate the epidemiological relationship of overuse injuries to court type. This is due primarily to the insidious nature of the onset of symptoms typically seen in overuse injuries. As overuse injuries are very common in tennis, this is an area that is extremely important and will require very thoughtful investigation.

Conclusions

The health benefits of tennis as a lifelong sport have been well described. However, despite the fact that it is a noncontact sport, injuries are not uncommon. Overuse injuries are more common in the upper extremities, while acute injuries are more common in the lower extremities with ankle sprains being the most common. The lumbar spine is a frequent source of injury.

Multiple factors including stroke technique, equipment (racquets and strings), court surface, fitness, and volume of play are just some of the many factors which may play a role in the precipitation of injury.

Further studies are necessary to better understand the epidemiological aspects of tennis injuries. It is important that researchers utilize a similar definition of "injury" so that study results may be effectively compared. Injury data from the WTA is collected in a similar fashion using the same injury documentation system as the ATP World Tour. This represents a great opportunity going forward to examine similarities and differences between injuries in men and women at the highest level of tennis.

Further studies looking at volume of play would seem to be particularly important. Very few studies have examined the impact of training and competition loads on the incidence and pattern of injuries. Looking at serve counts, a concept similar to pitch counts in baseball, as a means to reduce injuries is also an exciting area of research.

Prospective, well-designed studies looking at incidence of injuries, injury patterns, injury severity, and risk factors are needed. Information obtained from such studies can then be used to develop effective injury prevention strategies and programs in tennis.

References

1. Gale-Watts AS, Nevill AM. From endurance to power athletes: the changing shape of successful male professional tennis players. Eur J Sport Sci. 2016;16(8):948–54.
2. Gaw CE, Chounthirath T, Smith GA. Tennis-related injuries treated in United States emergency departments, 1990 to 2011. Clin J Sport Med. 2014;24(3):226–32.
3. Sell K, Hainline B, Yorio M, Kovacs M. Injury trend analysis from the US Open Tennis Championships between 1994 and 2009. Br J Sports Med. 2014;48(7):546–51.
4. McCurdie I, Smith S, Bell PH, Batt ME. Tennis injury data from The Championships, Wimbledon, from 2003 to 2012. Br J Sports Med. 2017;51(7):607–11.
5. Gescheit DT, Cormack SJ, Duffield R, Kovalchik S, Wood TO, Omizzolo M, Reid M. Injury epidemiology of tennis players at the 2011–2016 Australian Open Grand Slam. Br J Sports Med. 2017 pii: bjsports-2016-097283. https://doi.org/10.1136/bjsports-2016-097283.
6. Correia JP. Injury surveillance at 23 International Tennis Federation Junior and Pro Circuit tournaments between 2011 and 2015. Br J Sports Med. 2016;50:1556. https://doi.org/10.1136/bjsports-2016-096255.
7. Okholm Kryger K, Dor F, Guillaume M, Haida A, Noirez P, Montalvan B, Toussaint JF. Medical reasons behind player departures from male and female professional tennis competitions. Am J Sports Med. 2015;43:34–40.
8. Hartwell MJ, Fong SM, Colvin AC. Withdrawals and retirements in professional tennis players. Sports Health. 2017;9(2):154–61.
9. Breznik K, Batagelj V. Retired matches among male professional tennis players. J Sports Sci Med. 2012;11:270–8.
10. Maquirriain J, Baglione R. Epidemiology of tennis injuries: an eight-year review of Davis Cup retirements. Eur J Sport Sci. 2016;16(2):266–70.
11. Pluim BM, Fuller CW, Batt ME, Chase L, Hainline B, Miller S, Montalvan B, Renström P, Stroia KA, Weber K, Wood TO. Consensus statement on epidemiological studies of medical conditions in tennis, April 2009. Br J Sports Med. 2009;43(12):893–7.
12. Pluim BM, Loeffen FG, Clarsen B, Bahr R, Verhagen EA. A one-season prospective study of injuries and illness in elite junior tennis. Scand J Med Sci Sports. 2016;26:564–71.
13. Silva RT, Takahashi R, Berra B, Cohen M, Matsumoto MH. Medical assistance at the Brazilian juniors tennis circuit—a one-year prospective study. J Sci Med Sport. 2003;6(1):14–8.
14. Pluim BM, Staal JB, Windler GE, Jayanthi N. Tennis injuries: occurrence, aetiology, and prevention. Br J Sports Med. 2006;40(5):415–23.
15. Lynall RC, Kerr ZY, Djoko A, Pluim BM, Hainline B, Dompier TP. Epidemiology of National Collegiate

Athletic Association men's and women's tennis injuries, 2009/2010–2014/2015. Br J Sports Med. 2016;50(19):1211–6.
16. Hjelm N, Werner S, Renstrom P. Injury profile in junior tennis players: a prospective two year study. Knee Surg Sports Traumatol Arthrosc. 2010;18(6):845–50.
17. Maquirriain J, Ghisi JP, Amato S. Is tennis a predisposing factor for degenerative shoulder disease? A controlled study in former elite players. Br J Sports Med. 2006;40:447–50.
18. Young SW, Dakic J, Stroia K, Nguyen ML, Harris AH, Safran MR. High incidence of infraspinatus muscle atrophy in elite professional female tennis players. Am J Sports Med. 2015;43(8):1989–93.
19. Ellenbecker TS, Dines D, Renstrom P, Windler G. Visual observation of apparent infraspinatus muscle atrophy in professional male tennis players. J Orthop Sports Phys Ther. 2018;48(1):A38.
20. Tagliafico AS, Ameri P, Michaud J, Derchi LE, Sormani MP, Martinoli C. Wrist injuries in nonprofessional tennis players: relationships with different grips. Am J Sports Med. 2009;37(4):760–7.
21. Stuelcken M, Mellifont D, Gorman A, Sayers M. Wrist injuries in tennis players: a narrative review. Sports Med. 2017;47(5):857–68.
22. Maquirriain J, Ghisi JP. The incidence and distribution of stress fractures in elite tennis players. Br J Sports Med. 2006;40(5):454–9.
23. Silva RT, Hartmann LG, Laurino CF. Stress reaction of the humerus in tennis players. Br J Sports Med. 2007;41(11):824–6.
24. Hoy G, Wood T, Phillips N, Connell D, Hughes DC. When physiology becomes pathology: the role of magnetic resonance imaging in evaluating bone marrow oedema in the humerus in elite tennis players with an upper limb pain syndrome. Br J Sports Med. 2006;40(8):710–3.
25. Pluim BM, Clarsen B, Verhagen E. Injury rates in recreational tennis players do not differ between different playing surfaces. Br J Sports Med. 2018;52:611–5. pii: bjsports-2016-097050. https://doi.org/10.1136/bjsports-2016-097050.

Pathophysiology of Tennis Injuries: The Kinetic Chain

Natalie L. Myers and W. Ben Kibler

4.1 Introduction

The tennis serve is a complex dynamic activity involving the entire body. Serving results in repetitive high velocity, high load, and large range of motion demands on all parts of the body. Understanding the normal mechanics that produce function and the pathomechanics associated with dysfunction will enable clinicians to optimize performance and minimize injury risk. This chapter describes the kinetic chain mechanics in function and dysfunction and suggests implications for clinical evaluation and rehabilitation.

4.2 Kinetic Chain Mechanics in the Serve: What Makes the Ball Go

The serving motion is developed and regulated through a sequentially coordinated and task-specific kinetic chain of force development and a sequentially activated kinematic chain of body positions and motions [1]. The kinematics of the tennis serve have been well described and may be broken down into phases [2–4]. These descriptions show how muscles can move the individual segments and show the temporal sequence of the motions. The kinetics are not as well described but are important due to the forces and motions that are developed. These forces and motions are applied to all the body segments to allow their summation, regulation, and transfer throughout the segments, resulting in performance of the task of throwing or hitting the ball. The term, kinetic chain, is used to collectively describe both of these mechanical linkages.

An effective kinetic chain is characterized by three components [4]: (1) optimized anatomy in all segments; (2) optimized physiology (muscle flexibility and strength and well-developed, efficient, task-specific motor patterns for muscle activation); and (3) optimized mechanics (sequential generation of forces appropriately distributed across motions that result in the desired athletic function).

The kinetic chain has several functions:

1. Using integrated programs of muscle activation to temporarily link multiple body segments into one functional segment (e.g., the back leg in cocking stance and push-off and the arm in long-axis rotation prior to ball impact) to decrease the degrees of freedom (DOFs) in the entire motion [2, 5, 6]
2. Providing a stable proximal base for distal arm mobility

N. L. Myers (✉)
Department of Health & Human Performance,
Texas State University, San Marcos, TX, USA
e-mail: natalie.myers@txstate.edu

W. B. Kibler
Shoulder Center of Kentucky, Lexington Clinic Orthopedics, Lexington, KY, USA

3. Maximizing force development in the large muscles of the core and transferring it to the hand [2, 7, 8]
4. Producing interactive moments at the distal joints that develop more force and energy than the joint itself could develop and decrease the magnitude of the applied loads at the distal joint [9–14];
5. Producing torques that decrease deceleration forces [12–16]

Several studies have clearly established the basic role of the kinetic chain in tennis [7, 17–21]. Each body part has specific roles in the entire motion [2]. The feet are contact points with the ground and allow maximum ground reaction force for proximal stability and force generation. The legs and core are the mass for the stable base and the engine for the largest amount of force generation. The shoulder is the funnel for force regulation and transmission and the fulcrum for stability during the rapid motion of the arm. The arm and hand is the rapidly moving delivery mechanism of the force to racquet.

To achieve its role in kinetic chain function, the shoulder must develop precise ball-and-socket kinematics to create maximum concavity compression [22] that optimizes functional stability throughout the entire range of rapid motion. Requirements for functional stability include optimum alignment of the humerus and glenoid with ±30° angulation [16], co-contraction and compression force couples of the rotator cuff and shoulder muscles [23, 24], a stable scapular base [25], adequate balanced rotational range of motion [26–28], and labral integrity to act as a washer, allowing best fit of the humerus into the glenoid [29].

Tasks performed in tennis occur as a result of the summation of speed principle, which states that in order to maximize the speed at the distal end of a linked system, the movement should start with the proximal segments (the hips and core) and progress to the distal segments. (shoulder, elbow, and wrist) [12]. Each segment in this link system can influence motions of its adjacent segments. For example, during a baseball pitch, stability of the back and stride legs allows rotation of the trunk, which, in turn, allows for maximal throwing arm external rotation. The stable lower extremity serves as a platform for trunk and upper extremity motion, where the amount of trunk rotation is proportionate to the amount of arm motion, which can occur. Variations in motor control and physical fitness components, such as strength, flexibility, and muscle endurance, can affect the efficiency and effectiveness of all segments of the linked system [5, 6, 30].

Efficient mechanics can be improved by decreasing the possible DOFs throughout the entire motion [5, 6, 31, 32]. There are 244 possible DOFs in the body from the foot to the hand. Most models of maximum efficiency in body motions find that limiting DOFs to approximately 6–8 maximizes the total force output and minimizes effort and load [32]. DOFs can be limited by coordinated muscle activation coupling, called integrative complexes, which constrain and couple positions and motions so that several segments move as one [31]. The few independent DOFs are called nodes and represent key positions and motions in the overhead tasks [2]. These key positions are thought to be correlated with the optimum force development and minimal applied loads and are considered the most efficient method of coordinating kinetic chain activation. The tennis serve motion can be evaluated by analyzing a set of nine nodes or positions and motions; these nodes are an extension of those presented by Lintner et al. [2] and Kibler et al. [33] and have been refined by the Shoulder Center of Kentucky and the Women's Tennis Association (WTA) (Table 4.1).

The analysis includes optimal foot placement, adequate knee flexion in cocking progressing to knee extension at ball impact, hip counter rotation away from the court into cocking, back hip tilt downward in cocking, lack of front hip forward lean in cocking, coupled hip/trunk rotation with a separation of approximately 30°, trunk rotation, and coupled arm motion in the scapular plane [19, 20, 34–40]. The majority of the nodes have been shown to have above substantial interobserver reliability [41, 42]. These nodes can be evaluated by visual observation or by

Table 4.1 The observational tennis serve analysis tool

Node	Efficient mechanics (normal mechanics)	Inefficient mechanics (pathomechanics)
Foot position	Good: back foot stays behind front foot	Bad: back foot stays in front of front foot
Knee position	Good: substantial knee bend (both knees to bend >15°)	Bad: none to minimal knee bend (both knees bend ≤15°)
Counterhip rotation	Good: the hip on back side is rotating away from the net	Bad: the hip on back side is not rotating away from the net
Posterior hip tilt and loading	Good: the hip on back side is dropping toward the ground, and the back leg is loaded	Bad: the hip on back side is not dropping toward the ground, and the back leg is not loaded
Front hip lean	Good: the hip on front side is not leaning forward toward the net	Bad: the hip on front side is leaning forward toward the net
X-angle	Good: x-angle describes the relationship between the shoulders and the hips and should be approximately equal to 30°	Shoulders don't rotate behind the hips Bad: the x-angle is >30° Bad: the x-angle is <30°
Trunk rotation	Good: trunk rotation around a vertical axis	Bad: no trunk rotation around a vertical axis
Arm position	Good: the shoulder in line with the plane of the scapula	Bad: hypercocking—shoulder behind of the plane of the scapula hypococking—shoulder in front of plane of the scapula
Composite motion of kinetic chain	Good: used knee flexion and back leg drive to maximize ground reaction forces that push the body upward from the cocking position into ball impact (push-through motion)	Bad: use the trunk muscles to pull the trunk and arm from cocking into ball impact (pull-through motion)

Note: Evaluate nodes 1–8 at maximum knee bend. Composite motion of kinetic chain should be evaluated throughout the entire motion
Copyright © WTA Tour Inc., The Shoulder Center of Kentucky. All Rights Reserved

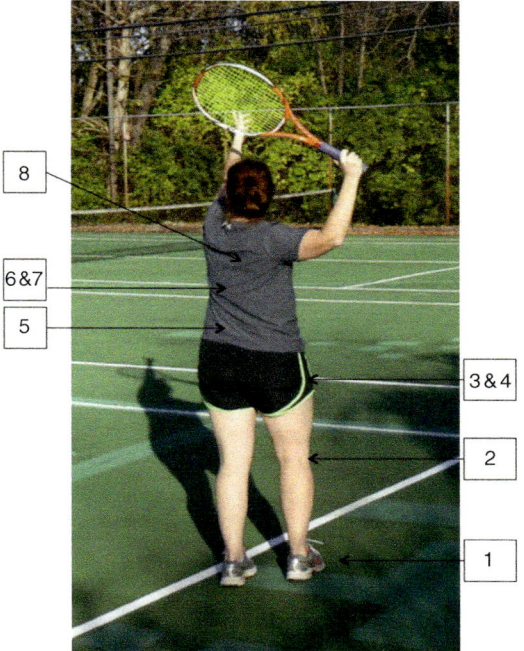

Fig. 4.1 Improper tennis serve nodes suggested to negatively affect function. The number sequence correlates with the inefficient mechanics description in Table 4.1. There is minimal foot loading, minimal knee flexion, no hip rotation or tilting, no trunk rotation, and an x-angle of 0°

video recording and analysis. An example of tennis-specific pathomechanics is illustrated in Fig. 4.1 with detailed descriptions of the deleterious motions listed in Table 4.2.

4.3 Pathomechanics in the Serve Motion: What Happens When the Ball Doesn't Go

Tennis players with a painful shoulder have been shown to have a multitude of possible causative factors contributing to the presenting complaints of pain and decreased function, either by causing the anatomic injury or increasing the dysfunction from the injury. There may be alterations in anatomy, physiology, and/or biomechanics. They can combine to produce an alteration in the normal mechanics, resulting in pathomechanics that may create decreased efficiency in the kinetic chain, impaired performance, increased injury risk, or

Table 4.2 Tennis nodes and possible consequences (Adapted from Kibler et al. Mechanics and Pathomechanics in the Overhead Athlete. *Clin. Sports Med.* 2013;32(4): 637–651)

Nodes	Result of inefficient mechanics	Musculoskeletal areas to be evaluated
Node 1: foot position	Increased load on the trunk or shoulder	Hip and/or trunk flexibility and strength
Node 2: knee position	Increased load on anterior shoulder and medial elbow	Hip and knee strength
Node 3: Counterhip rotation	Increased load on shoulder and trunk; inability to push through increasing load on abdominals	Hip and trunk flexion flexibility and strength
Node 4: posterior hip tilt and loading	Increased load on the shoulder and trunk; inability to push through increasing load on abdominals	Hip and trunk flexion flexibility and strength
Node 5: front hip lean	Increased load on the shoulder and trunk; inability to push-through increasing load on abdominals	Hip and trunk flexion flexibility and strength
Node 6: x-angle	Increased load on abdominals and "slow arm"; increased load on anterior shoulder	Hip, trunk, and shoulder flexibility
Node 7: trunk rotation	Increased load on abdominals and "slow arm"; increased load on anterior shoulder	Hip, trunk, and shoulder flexibility
Node 8: arm position	Increased load on anterior shoulder	Scapular and shoulder strength and flexibility
Node 9: kinetic chain	Inability to generate maximal energy and force	Postural control, flexibility, and strength

actual injury [12, 19, 20]. These pathomechanics contribute to the disabled throwing shoulder (DTS) [43], a general term that describes the limitations of function that exist in symptomatic overhead athletes in that they cannot optimally perform the task of throwing or hitting the ball. In a large percentage of cases, DTS is the result of a cascade to injury [43], a process in which the body's response to the inherent demand of hitting results in a series of alterations throughout the kinetic chain that can affect the optimal function of all segments in the chain.

In a closed system, such as the kinetic chain, alteration in one area creates changes throughout the entire system [29]. This is known as the catch-up phenomenon, where the changes in the interactive moments alter the forces in the distal segments [12, 44]. The increased forces place extra stress on the distal segments, which often results in the sensation of pain or actual anatomic injury [20].

The legs and core connect the body to the ground, producing the ground reaction force that is important for force development, create the proximal base of stability required for distal mobility, and generate more than 50% of the kinetic energy and force delivered to the hand [7, 44]. Alterations creating pathomechanics in this area are seen in up to 50% of DTS patients [1].

Foot position is important in the tennis serve. Research has shown no major mechanical differences between the "foot-back" and "foot-up" positions. However, the "foot-forward" position, in which the back foot is advanced forward of the front foot, limits hip rotation and optimal cocking, which may increase loads on the trunk and shoulder.

Alteration of knee flexion has also been associated with increased stresses in the arm. Tennis players who did not have adequate bend in the knees, breaking the kinetic chain and decreasing the contribution by the hip and trunk, had 23–27% increased loads in horizontal adduction and rotation at the shoulder and valgus load at the elbow [19]. Quadriceps inflexibility and decreased eccentric strength may also alter knee motion.

Weakness or tightness at the hip can also affect other segments. Decreased hip flexibility in rotation or strength in abduction (positive Trendelenburg) was seen in 49% of athletes with arthroscopically proved posterior-superior labral tears [45]. Vad and colleagues [46] reported a 33% increase of low back pain in professional golfers with tight hip muscles. Altered hip and trunk motion was found to increase shoulder loads [47]. The musculoskeletal alterations could potentially be due to tissue maladaptations from repetitively imposed loads [48]. Strength imbalances around the hip and lumbar spine have been demonstrated by many studies, suggesting that these deficits may play a role in the dysfunction of the kinetic chain [49, 50]. These alterations can also alter the three nodes around the hip. Weak or tight hip muscles can alter the amount of back hip loading and the degree of hip counter rotation and increase the amount of front hip loading and lean.

Scapular dyskinesis may also be seen in athletes who present with the DTS. Dyskinesis represents an alteration of static scapular position or dynamic scapular motion in coordination with arm motion. The altered position and motions create a loss of control of retraction and posterior tilt, resulting in protraction, anterior tilt, and excessive internal rotation. Alteration of scapular retraction control can also affect coupled arm/scapular motion, increasing posterior joint loads.

Alterations in glenohumeral rotation are consistently found in overhead athletes with DTS and are the factors most highly associated with shoulder pain and injury [1, 51, 52]. They create multiple problems in and around the throwing shoulder, including scapular dyskinesis due to windup of the tight posterior structures [25], impingement due to anterior superior humeral head translation in follow-through [26, 53], and posterior-superior humeral head translation in cocking and anterior superior translation in flexion, which increase labral shear [27, 43]. Increased evidence suggests that both glenohumeral internal rotation deficit (GIRD) and total range of motion deficit (TROMD) may create the pathomechanics [51, 52].

Also multiple muscles around the shoulder have been found to develop tightness as a result of the overhead motion. The most commonly affected muscles are the pectoralis minor, subscapularis, and latissimus dorsi. The pathophysiology is believed to result from chronic tensile overload or from a muscle adaptive response [54]. The tight pectoralis minor creates a tendency for scapular anterior tilt and acromial downward tilt, decreasing the arm's ability to cock or reach maximal abduction [55–57]. The tight subscapularis decreases arm external rotation, limiting arm cocking. The tight latissimus dorsi limits overhead positioning and cocking.

The ultimate pathomechanical factor in the DTS is loss of optimal concavity-compression and functional glenohumeral stability. This can result from a combination of misalignment of the humerus on the glenoid [58], alteration of muscle force couples, scapular dyskinesis [59, 60], GIRD/TROMD [26, 27], rotator cuff disease [1], and/or labral injury [1]. Consequently, these factors may contribute to the loss of velocity and accuracy in the overhead athlete while presenting clinically with symptoms of pain, clicking, sliding, weakness, and injury.

4.4 Clinical Implications

The body works as a unit to achieve optimum overhead throwing function and can fail as a unit in altered performance or the DTS. Therefore, the evaluation of tennis players with DTS needs to be comprehensive and can involve evaluation of the pertinent normal mechanics, evaluation of possible pathomechanics, identification of physiologic and biomechanical factors contributing to the pathomechanics, and the kinetic chain examination as well as identification of all pathoanatomic factors that may exist in the shoulder. Similarly, treatment should include optimization of the pathoanatomy as well as restoration of the pathophysiology and pathomechanics [1].

The observational tennis serve analysis (OTSA) was developed by the Women's Tennis Association (WTA) and the Shoulder Center of Kentucky (SCKY) as a method for assessing serve mechanics by direct observation and/or video analysis. Specific methods for evaluation and criteria for determining presence (yes) or absence (no) of the nodes have been developed for tennis and are summarized in Table 4.1. This examination can identify anatomic areas and mechanical motions that may be contributing to the symptoms and suggest areas for more detailed evaluation. The eight nodes can be demonstrated to be present (1) or absent (0). One more point is awarded for displaying the biomechanically efficient "push-through" motion compared to the inefficient "pull through" motion, creating a score from 0 to 9. It can be used as part of the comprehensive evaluation for tennis players who either desire to improve their performance or who have an injury. The evaluation can highlight areas of the kinetic chain that demonstrate mechanical deficits. Further clinical evaluation may identify musculoskeletal factors that can create the mechanical deficits.

The kinetic chain evaluations can be organized into three components, the leg/hip/core, the scapula, and the shoulder. The shoulder examination should be comprehensive, emphasizing evaluation of the anatomy (labrum, biceps, and/or rotator cuff internal derangement), physiology (muscle weakness/imbalance and flexibility), and mechanics (scapular dyskinesis, GIRD, and TROMD). Treatment should also involve a comprehensive approach, including restoration of all kinetic chain deficits, altered mechanics, and functional joint stability. Rehabilitation should address all the physiologic and mechanical factors [1, 61–63]. These include restoration of hip range of motion and leg strength, core stability and strength, scapular control, shoulder muscle flexibility and strength, and glenohumeral rotation. Surgery should address repairing joint structures to optimize the capability for functional stability [1].

Conclusion

Optimal performance of the tennis requires precise mechanics that involve coordinated kinetic and kinematic chains to develop, transfer, and regulate the forces the body needs to withstand the inherent demands of the serve and to allow optimal performance. These chains have been evaluated, and the basic components, called nodes, have been identified.

Impaired performance and/or injury, the DTS, is associated with alterations in the mechanics that are called pathomechanics. They can occur at multiple locations throughout the kinetic chain. They must be evaluated and treated as part of the overall problem.

Observational analysis of the mechanics and pathomechanics using the observational tennis serve analysis tool can be useful in highlighting areas of alteration that can be evaluated for anatomic injury or altered physiology. The comprehensive kinetic chain examination can evaluate sites of kinetic chain breakage, and a detailed shoulder examination can assess joint internal derangement of altered physiology that may contribute to the pathomechanics.

Treatment of the DTS should be comprehensive, directed toward restoring physiology and mechanics and optimizing anatomy. This maximizes the body's ability to develop normal mechanics to accomplish the overhead throwing task.

References

1. Kibler WB, Kuhn JE, Wilk K, et al. The disabled throwing shoulder: spectrum of pathology-10-year update. Arthroscopy. 2013;29(1):141–161.e126.
2. Lintner D, Noonan TJ, Kibler WB. Injury patterns and biomechanics of the athlete's shoulder. Clin Sports Med. 2008;27(4):527–51.
3. Kovacs M, Ellenbecker T. An 8-stage model for evaluating the tennis serve: implications for performance enhancement and injury prevention. Sports Health. 2011;3(6):504–13.
4. Sciascia A, Thigpen C, Namdari S, Baldwin K. Kinetic chain abnormalities in the athletic shoulder. Sports Med Arthrosc. 2012;20(1):16–21.
5. Davids K, Glazier P, Arajuo D, Bartlett R. Movement systems as dynamic systems, the functional role of variability and its implications for sports medicine. Sports Med. 2003;33(4):245–60.
6. Sporns O, Edelman GM. Solving Bernstein's problem: a proposal for the development of coordinated movement by selection. Child Dev. 1993;64(4):960–81.
7. Elliott BC, Marshall RN, Noffal GJ. Contributions of upper limb segment rotations during the power serve in tennis. J Appl Biomech. 1995;11:433–42.
8. Toyoshima S, Miyashita M. Force-velocity relation in throwing. Res Q. 1973;44(1):86–95.
9. Hirashima M, Yamane K, Nakamura Y, Ohtsuki T. Kinetic chain of overarm throwing in terms of joint rotations revealed by induced acceleration analysis. J Biomech. 2008;41(13):2874–83.
10. Hirashima M, Kadota H, Sakurai S, Kudo K, Ohtsuki T. Sequential muscle activity and its functional role in the upper extremity and trunk during overarm throwing. J Sports Sci. 2002;20(4):301–10.

11. Hirashima M, Kudo K, Watarai K, Ohtsuki T. Control of 3D limb dynamics in unconstrained overarm throws of different speeds performed by skilled baseball players. J Neurophysiol. 2007;97(1):680–91.
12. Putnam CA. Sequential motions of body segments in striking and throwing skills: description and explanations. J Biomech. 1993;26:125–35.
13. Fleisig GS, Andrews JR, Dillman CJ, Escamilla RF. Kinetics of baseball pitching with implications about injury mechanisms. Am J Sports Med. 1995;23(2):233–9.
14. Fleisig GS, Barrentine SW, Escamilla RF, Andrews JR. Biomechanics of overhand throwing with implications for injuries. Sports Med. 1996;21:421–37.
15. Young JL, Herring SA, Press JM, Casazza BA. The influence of the spine on the shoulder in the throwing athlete. J Back Musculoskelet Rehabil. 1996;7:5–17.
16. Nieminen H, Niemi J, Takala EP, Viikari-Juntura E. Load-sharing patterns in the shoulder during isometric flexion tasks. J Biomech. 1995;28(5):555–66.
17. Fleisig G, Nicholls R, Elliott B, Escamilla R. Kinematics used by world class tennis players to produce high-velocity serves. Sports Biomech. 2003;2(1):51–64.
18. Marshall RN, Elliott BC. Long-axis rotation: the missing link in proximal-to-distal segmental sequencing. J Sports Sci. 2000;18(4):247–54.
19. Elliott B, Fleisig G, Nicholls R, Escamilia R. Technique effects on upper limb loading in the tennis serve. J Sci Med Sport. 2003;6(1):76–87.
20. Martin C, Kulpa R, Ropars M, Delamarche P, Bideau B. Identification of temporal pathomechanical factors during the tennis serve. Med Sci Sports Exerc. 2013;45(11):2113–9.
21. Martin C, Bideau B, Bideau N, Nicolas G, Delamarche P, Kulpa R. Energy flow analysis during the tennis serve: comparison between injured and noninjured tennis players. Am J Sports Med. 2014;42:2751.
22. Lippitt SB, Vanderhooft JE, Harris SL, Sidles JA, Harryman DT, Matsen FA. Glenohumeral stability from concavity-compression: a quantitative analysis. J Shoulder Elbow Surg. 1993;2(1):27–35.
23. DiGiovine NM, Jobe FW, Pink M, Perry J. An electromyographic analysis of the upper extremity in pitching. J Shoulder Elbow Surg. 1992;1(1):15–25.
24. Speer K, Garrett W. Muscular control of motion and stability about the pectoral girdle. The shoulder: a balance of mobility and stability. Rosemont, IL: AAOS; 1994. p. 159–73.
25. Kibler WB. The role of the scapula in athletic shoulder function. Am J Sports Med. 1998;26(2):325–37.
26. Harryman DT, Sidles JA, Clark JM, McQuade KJ, Gibb TD, Matsen FA. Translation of the humeral head on the glenoid with passive glenohumeral motion. J Bone Joint Surg. 1990;72-A(9):1334–43.
27. Grossman MG, Tibone JE, McGarry MH, Schneider DJ, Veneziani S, Lee TQ. A cadaveric model of the throwing shoulder: a possible etiology of superior labrum anterior-to-posterior lesions. J Bone Joint Surg Am. 2005;87(4):824–31.
28. Wilk KE, Meister K, Andrews JR. Current concepts in the rehabilitation of the overhead throwing athlete. Am J Sports Med. 2002;30(1):136–51.
29. Veeger HE, van der Helm FC. Shoulder function: the perfect compromise between mobility and stability. J Biomech. 2007;40(10):2119–29.
30. Kibler WB, Press J, Sciascia A. The role of core stability in athletic function. Sports Med. 2006;36(3):189–98.
31. Glazier PS, Davids K. Constraints on the complete optimization of human motion. Sports Med. 2009;39(1):15–28.
32. Bernstein NA. The co-ordination and regulation of movements. Oxford: Pergamon Press; 1967.
33. Kibler WB, Wilkes T, Sciascia A. Mechanics and pathomechanics in the overhead athlete. Clin Sports Med. 2013;32(4):637–51.
34. Elliott B, Wood G. The biomechanics of the foot-up and foot-back tennis service techniques. Aust J Sports Sci. 1983;3(2):3–6.
35. Bahamonde RE. Changes in angular momentum during the tennis serve. J Sports Sci. 2000;18(8):579–92.
36. Campbell A, Straker L, O'Sullivan P, Elliott B, Reid M. Lumbar loading in the elite adolescent tennis serve: link to low back pain. Med Sci Sports Exerc. 2013;45(8):1562–8.
37. Reid M, Elliott B, Alderson J. Shoulder joint loading in the high performance flat and kick tennis serves. Br J Sports Med. 2007;41(12):884–9. Discussion 889.
38. Whiteside D, Elliott B, Lay B, Reid M. The effect of age on discrete kinematics of the elite female tennis serve. J Appl Biomech. 2013;29(5):573–82.
39. Martin C, Bideau B, Ropars M, Delamarche P, Kulpa R. Upper limb joint kinetic analysis during tennis serve: assessment of competitive level on efficiency and injury risks. Scand J Med Sci Sports. 2014;24(4):700–7.
40. Girard O, Micallef JP, Millet GP. Influence of restricted knee motion during the flat first serve in tennis. J Strength Cond Res. 2007;21(3):950–7.
41. Myers NL, Kibler WB, Lamborn L, Smith BJ, English RA, Jacobs C, Uhl TL. Reliability and validity of a biomechanically based analysis method for the tennis serve. Int J Sports Phys Ther. 2017;12(3):437.
42. Myers NL, Kibler WB, Capilouto GJ, Westgate P, English RA, Uhl TL. Reliabiity of an observational method used to asses tennis serve mechanics in a group of novice raters. J Med Sci Tennis. 2017;22(3):6–12.
43. Burkhart SS, Morgan CD, Kibler WB. The disabled throwing shoulder: spectrum of pathology Part I: pathoanatomy and biomechanics. Arthroscopy. 2003;19(4):404–20.
44. Kibler WB. Biomechanical analysis of the shoulder during tennis activities. Clin Sports Med. 1995;14:79–85.

45. Burkhart SS, Morgan CD, Kibler WB. Shoulder injuries in overhead athletes, the "dead arm" revisited. Clin Sports Med. 2000;19(1):125–58.
46. Vad VB, Bhat AL, Basrai D, Gebeh A, Aspergren DD, Andrews JR. Low back pain in professional golfers: the role of associated hip and low back range-of-motion deficits. Am J Sports Med. 2004;32(2):494–7.
47. Robb AJ, Fleisig G, Wilk K, Macrina L, Bolt B, Pajaczkowski J. Passive ranges of motion of the hips and their relationship with pitching biomechanics and ball velocity in professional baseball pitchers. Am J Sports Med. 2010;38(12):2487–93.
48. Kibler WB, McMullen J. Scapular dyskinesis and its relation to shoulder pain. J Am Acad Orthop Surg. 2003;11:142–51.
49. Nadler SF, Malanga GA, Feinberg JH, Prybicien M, Stitik TP, DePrince M. Relationship between hip muscle imbalance and occurrence of low back pain in collegiate athletes: a prospective study. Am J Phys Med Rehabil. 2001;80(8):572–7.
50. Nadler SF, Malanga GA, Bartoli LA, Feinberg JH, Prybicien M, Deprince M. Hip muscle imbalance and low back pain in athletes: influence of core strengthening. Med Sci Sports Exerc. 2002;34(1):9–16.
51. Wilk KE, Macrina LC, Fleisig GS, et al. Correlation of glenohumeral internal rotation deficit and total rotational motion to shoulder injuries in professional baseball pitchers. Am J Sports Med. 2011;39(2):329–35.
52. Kibler WB, Sciascia A, Thomas SJ. Glenohumeral internal rotation deficit: pathogenesis and response to acute throwing. Sports Med Arthrosc. 2012;20(1):34–8.
53. Silliman JF, Hawkins RJ. Classification and physical diagnosis of instability of the shoulder. Clin Orthop Relat Res. 1993;291:7–19.
54. Butterfield TA. Eccentric exercise in vivo: strain-induced muscle damage and adaptation in a stable system. Exerc Sport Sci Rev. 2010;38(2):51–60.
55. Lukasiewicz A, McClure P, Michener L, Pratt N, Sennett B. Comparison of 3-dimensional scapular position and orientation between subjects with and without shoulder impingement. J Orthop Sports Phys Ther. 1999;29(10):574–83. discussion 584–576.
56. Borstad JD, Ludewig PM. The effect of long versus short pectoralis minor resting length on scapular kinematics in healthy individuals. J Orthop Sports Phys Ther. 2005;35(4):227–38.
57. Kebaetse M, McClure P, Pratt N. Thoracic position effect on shoulder range of motion, strength, and three-dimensional scapular kinetics. Arch Phys Med Rehabil. 1999;80:945–50.
58. Mihata T, McGarry MH, Kinoshita M, Lee TQ. Excessive glenohumeral horizontal abduction as occurs during the late cocking phase of the throwing motion can be critical for internal impingement. Am J Sports Med. 2010;38(2):369–74.
59. Weiser WM, Lee TQ, McMaster WC, McMahon PJ. Effects of simulated scapular protraction on anterior glenohumeral stability. Am J Sports Med. 1999;27(6):801–5.
60. Mihata T, Jun BJ, Bui CN, et al. Effect of scapular orientation on shoulder internal impingement in a cadaveric model of the cocking phase of throwing. J Bone Joint Surg. 2012;94(17):1576–83.
61. McMullen J, Uhl TL. A kinetic chain approach for shoulder rehabilitation. J Athl Train. 2000;35(3):329–37.
62. Wilk KE, Macrina LC, Arrigo C. Passive range of motion characteristics in the overhead baseball pitcher and their implications for rehabilitation. Clin Orthop Relat Res. 2012;470(6):1586–94.
63. Ellenbecker TS, Cools A. Rehabilitation of shoulder impingement syndrome and rotator cuff injuries: an evidence-based review. Br J Sports Med. 2010;44(5):319–27.

Tennis Equipment and Technique Interactions on Risk of Overuse Injuries

5

Tom Allen, Sharon Dixon, Marcus Dunn, and Duane Knudson

5.1 Introduction

Tennis is a popular sport played throughout the world. Sports with repetitive movements like tennis can create sport-specific anthropometric, strength, and flexibility imbalances in athletes that may be related to risk of injury [1]. In a review of 28 epidemiological studies published between 1966 and 2005, Pluim et al. [2] identified that reported incidences of tennis injury ranged between 0.04 and 3.0 injuries/1000 player-hours. The majority of tennis injuries reported at the upper extremity were characterised as chronic/overuse injuries, whereas injuries experienced at the lower extremity were characterised as acute injuries [2]. Consequently, many advanced tennis players invest considerable effort in physical training to increase the neuromuscular and skeletal system's strength to withstand the rigours of the sport. Another area where athletes may be able to mediate the risk of injury in competitive tennis play may be in the selection of equipment used in training and competition.

This chapter focuses on biomechanics and engineering research on tennis equipment and its likely effects on the risk of overuse injuries in the sport since overuse injuries are common in elite adult [3–5] and junior players [6]. The effect of changes in tennis equipment on injury risk can be difficult to predict given that player stroke and court movement biomechanics interact with equipment [7–9] and the large variation in movements and hand loading in the sport [10–12]. This chapter first summarises the interaction of the player with the racquet, strings, and ball system in tennis strokes. The chapter concludes describing the research on the interaction of the player, shoes, and court surface in court movements common in the sport. Biomechanical testing of player interactions with tennis equipment provides initial evidence about the potential effects of that equipment on risk of overuse injuries. Prospective studies, however, are needed to verify if the hypothesised benefits of most adjustments of tennis equipment on injury risk are correct.

5.2 Player-Racquet Interactions

A challenge facing engineers in designing new tennis racquets to influence performance or injury risk is the interaction of the design with the biomechanics of the player and the context of the sport. In the late twentieth century, lighter and larger head racquets increased the speed of

T. Allen
Manchester Metropolitan University, Manchester, UK

S. Dixon
University of Exeter, Exeter, UK

M. Dunn
Sheffield Hallam University, Sheffield, UK

D. Knudson (✉)
Texas State University, San Marcos, TX, USA
e-mail: dknudson@txstate.edu

strokes and the sport. The lighter frames, larger power regions on the face, and increased resistance to off-centre impacts allowed players to adapt stroke technique with more open-stance and extreme topspin groundstrokes. Initial concerns about greater use of open-stance strokes were fueled by new case studies of upper extremity stress fractures in tennis players. Fortunately, an epidemic of upper extremity injuries did not happen, and several studies reported similar stroke kinematics, kinetics, and muscle actions between open- and square-stance forehands [13–15]. A variety of research methods are necessary for engineers to validate the hypothesised benefits of new racquet designs interacting with the biomechanical characteristics of players and the evolving nature of the sport of tennis.

5.2.1 Racquet Frame

Previous reviews have focused on the relationship between racquet design and player performance (e.g. [7, 8]), but there is limited research into how tennis equipment may affect overuse injury risk. A first step is to quantify the number of strokes a player will typically perform during a match. Quantifying ball and racquet speeds during strokes, and associated forces, can inform the design of laboratory tests and help further our understanding of the cumulative effect repetitive impact may have on the player. The effect of racquet design on stroke speed, ball/string bed impact forces and loads, and vibrations transmitted to the player can then be investigated. Impact-induced translation and rotation of the racquet can force eccentric stretching of muscle and are the likely mechanism of overuse injury, rather than frame vibrations which are quickly damped out.

Lane et al. [16] categorised ball impacts in ATP 250 tour events—on hard courts between 2011 and 2013—reporting around 200 serves and 600 other strokes per match. Serves are often the focus of racquet testing and modelling, with the assumption that the ball is impacted perpendicular to the string bed with negligible velocity before it is struck [8]. Lane and colleagues reported ball speeds of around 40–50 m/s for serves in agreement with recent work [17], indicating impulses between the ball and string bed in the region of 2–3 N s (estimated from change in ball momentum), and time-averaged forces of 400–700 N assuming contact times of 4–6 ms [18–20]. Racquet velocity—normal to the face at the impact point with the ball—has been reported in the region 24–34 m/s for serves [21, 22]. Whilst measuring temporal forces between the ball and string bed is challenging, finite element simulations have produced results in broad agreement with the above predictions from ball speeds for serves, as shown in Fig. 5.1 [23].

Impact forces will be dependent on stroke parameters, such as the impact velocity and region of ball contact [11, 24, 25], and frame properties such as mass and stiffness (Fig. 5.1). There are three 'sweet spots' and contact positions that can affect ball speed and how the racquet recoils and vibrates post-impact [8], which may influence how loads are transmitted to the player and how the stroke 'feels'. The 'Power Zone' provides the highest ball speed; its location changes with the inertial properties of the racquet and stroke parameters [26]. Impact at the centre of percussion of an unconstrained racquet is said to result in no reaction at the handle, but the concept does not account for the player's grip and is, therefore, irrelevant to actual strokes [27]. Elite players 'aim' to hit the ball towards the centre of the string bed at the node for groundstrokes [28, 29] to minimise frame vibrations, which are influenced by racquet design and their grip.

A number of authors have investigated how a tennis racquet vibrates (e.g. [1, 30–36]). When comparing a handheld to a freely suspended racquet in a modal test, the frequency of the lowest bending mode is slightly reduced, the node point in the handle is closer to the butt and the vibrations damp out sooner. Increasing grip tightness further reduces the vibration frequency of the handheld racquet whilst increasing damping. The frequency of the lowest bending mode of a racquet reduces further during tennis strokes than when handheld in a modal test. Adding mass to the handle of a freely suspended racquet—as a simple representation of player grip—reduces vibration frequency [30, 35], but the amount

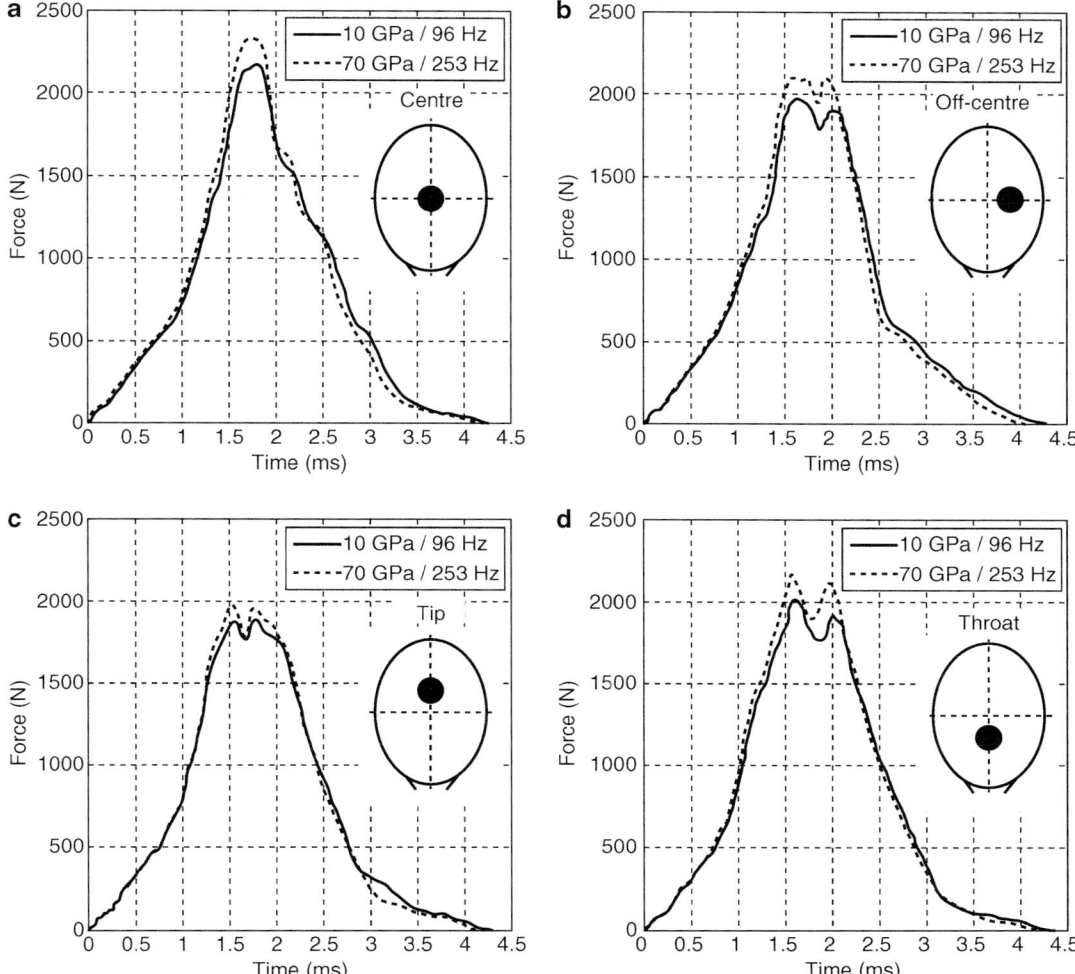

Fig. 5.1 Resultant force plots obtained from a finite element model for a ball impacting perpendicular to a stationary unconstrained racquet at 40 m/s, (**a**) centre, (**b**) off-centre, (**c**) tip, and (**d**) throat [23]

required to match the lowest bending mode to the value corresponding to a tennis stroke is lower than that of a hand [33].

Miller [37] hypothesised that modern frame designs may have led to an increase in overuse injuries, such as 'tennis elbow', but there is little direct evidence of this hypothesis. There is evidence that modern frames can be swung faster due to their lower swing moment of inertia (swing weight) [22, 37–40], which may reduce stroke accuracy and increase any vibrations and loads transmitted to the player. Larger hitting areas [41] allow the ball to be struck further 'off-centre', with impacts away from the longitudinal axis (off-axis) increasing any torque applied to the player. Despite having wider heads, modern frames don't have a higher polar moment of inertia as they are lighter [41], which means they offer similar resistance to torque from off-axis impacts. King et al. [42] reported increased racquet rotation about the longitudinal axis and forced wrist flexion/extension when the ball was struck off-axis during one-handed backhands. High stiffness combined with low mass also means modern racquets vibrate at a higher frequency [41] when the ball is struck away from the node. Vethecan and Subic [36] concluded that racquet vibrations can be attenuated with an appropriately positioned frame damper, although their findings were based on a model which did not account for the player's hand.

Clearly, understanding the effect of frame design on overuse injuries is a challenging topic due to the complex interaction with the player. Increasing frame mass or stiffness, or moving the balance point closer to the tip, will increase 'collision efficiency', resulting in higher ball speed and spin for the same impact conditions [24]. Cross [35] investigated how frame parameters affect forces applied to the hand, modelling the racquet as an unconstrained flexible beam with a distributed mass at the handle to represent player grip. He predicted hand forces to reduce as the mass and stiffness of the frame increased and as the balance point moved closer to the tip, based on the assumption that the player would keep ball serve speed constant utilising higher collision efficiency to swing the racquet slower. Elite players may actually utilise developments in frame design to increase ball speed and spin, and further work is required to fully understand the complex relationship between racquet parameters, swing mechanics, and injury risks.

The best evidence on the effect of racquet design interacting with players to influence risk of injury are prospective studies, but very few of these are conducted and published. Modern technology has been applied to frame design in an attempt to reduce overuse injury risks, or decrease symptoms. HEAD developed 'intelligence' racquets, utilising piezoelectric fibres and built-in electronics to capture frame deformation energy to be used to actively damp subsequent frame vibrations [43, 44]. Early work testing frames with *intelligence* technology on players experiencing tennis elbow appeared to decrease their symptoms [45], whilst a more recent 'double-blind' study reported decreased symptoms compared to regular racquets [46]. Production and sale of these frames were discontinued, possibly due to their high cost and sales, and consumers may be more influenced by manufacturers' claims related to benefits to performance than injury prevention than scientific evidence.

The effect of frame design on overuse injuries is complex, and further work is required before it is fully understood. Future work should look further to characterise the number of strokes a player will typically perform, alongside the resultant velocity between ball and racquet, impact location on the string bed and acceleration of their upper limb. Modern technology—such as sensors (e.g. Babolat Connect and Pay) and camera and image analysis systems (e.g. [38, 47])—combined with the introduction of player analysis technology (PAT) [48] should help with gathering and processing of this information. Experimental protocols and models—with appropriate constraint at the handle (e.g. [35, 49]) and representative impact conditions—can then be developed specifically for investigating how 'shock' and frame vibrations are transmitted to the player. Any potential benefits of frame design identified from these experiments or models should be tested in prospective studies.

5.2.2 Strings

The elasticity of tennis strings has a dramatic influence on the speed and spin created at impact with the ball, but a smaller effect on the impulsive and vibrational loads transmitted to the racquet and player. Decreasing string bed stiffness—via reductions in string material stiffness, stringing tension, the number of strings 'open string bed pattern' or increasing the size of the racquet head—will increase out-of-plane deformation, marginally reducing impact force and slightly increasing contact time and perpendicular ball velocity. Finite element simulations have shown peak impact force to reduce with the Young's modulus (stiffness) of the strings [50], and spring damper models have predicted increases in ball velocity with reductions in string bed stiffness [51]. Laboratory experiments have shown lower stringing tension [51, 52] and more open string patterns [53, 54] to marginally increase perpendicular ball velocity.

Tennis players can expect peak impact accelerations or force transmitted to the hand or elbow to be reduced 5–20% by reducing string tension from typically recommended high to low values [55–57]. String dampers can influence the vibration of the string bed and the sound and 'feel' of ball impact, but they do not change how the frame vibrates or the loads transmitted to the player [34, 58–61]. Whilst players feel differences between string types, differences in peak forces are smaller with only minor reductions in peak impact force for gut and nylon strings compared to polyester and Kevlar strings [56]. Tennis players with elbow pain should be encouraged to string their racquets at a lower tension. Prospective studies are needed to determine if these mechanical effects on peak impact forces can reduce symptoms or reduce risk of future elbow pain.

5.2.3 Ball

Until fairly recently, tennis players only had a choice of a few brands of pressurised tennis balls, colours, and a pressure-less ball. Now players have choices of various felt density, practice/regular/premium, foam, developmental, and the larger type 3 tennis ball. The International Tennis Federation (ITF) rigorously tests balls for meeting the rules of the game. Whilst players can intuitively sense apparent differences in the speed, bounce, and feel of strokes with different balls, there is limited systematic research on potential injury risk with different balls. Player perceptions of comfort and speed of strokes with different balls largely overlap [62]. Two examples are summarised in this section, the larger (type 3) and developmental balls.

Near the turn of the twenty-first century, advances in racquets had increased the speeds of shots and the game. For example, larger and lighter racquets meant players used more open-stance strokes with more sequential coordination [14]. About this time the ITF approved the type 3 ball that was 6% larger in diameter, but with a thinner rubber core to maintain the same mass as a regular tennis ball. The greater frontal area of the ball slowed it down in flight, and some players worried it felt different and might pose a greater risk of overuse injury. The United States Tennis Association (USTA) funded several studies to explore the potential injury risk of play with the type 3 ball.

Three studies of the immediate effects of the type 3 ball on court motion, muscle activation, player movement, and racquet acceleration at impact supported the hypothesis that this new ball posed no different risk of upper extremity overuse injuries than regular balls. The dynamic nature of tennis means that there is large variability in stroke positions on court, peak racquet acceleration, and muscle activation and no systematic difference across regular and type 3 balls [63]. Follow-up studies of more controlled conditions of the serve [64] and reacting to volleys [65] confirmed these results. Whilst there have been no prospective studies, the type 3 ball does not appear to pose any greater risk of injury given its use over time, although lack of player interest in this ball has dramatically decreased its use.

Recently the ITF, USTA, and other professional organisations have promoted the use of the developmental tennis balls and racquets for children learning the sport. Using a smaller racquet on a small court, along with three stages of balls makes logical sense to help children learn the sport. A lower and slower bounce of stage 1 (red, ages 5–8), stage 2 (orange, ages 8–10), and stage 3 (green, ages 9 and older) does significantly improve the immediate match-play statistics of young players, making them more successful and similar to adults [66, 67]. It is, however, unclear if these immediate effects translate into long-term improvements in rate of development and ultimate level of skill or performance. There have been no retrospective or prospective studies comparing long-term tennis performance between children learning the sport with traditional and developmental equipment. It is possible that the interaction of the player and equipment confounds potential benefits. For example, a player with an aggressive temperament with faster initial stroke success could develop high-risk tactical play that ultimately limits the development of defensive skills needed for advanced play.

5.3 Player-Surface Interactions

A defining characteristic of tennis is that it is played on different court surfaces [68]. Grand Slam tournaments, i.e. Wimbledon, Roland Garros, Australian Open, and US Open, are played on grass, clay, and acrylic court surfaces. The physical properties of these court surfaces, e.g. friction and energy restitution, vary greatly and must meet standards published by the ITF to ensure consistency between competitions and safety of use. The ITF has implemented a court pace rating protocol (ITF CS 01/02) [69], based on friction and energy restitution of ball-surface interactions, to characterise the 'speed' of court surfaces, e.g. slow, medium, or fast. Whilst ball-surface interactions are well understood, current knowledge of player-surface interaction with different court surfaces is limited [37]. The tennis shoe provides an important link between the player and court: player-surface interaction is a dynamic quantity dependent on loading conditions at the shoe-surface interface. The biomechanics of player-shoe-surface interaction during tennis-specific movements are, therefore, important considerations when optimising performance and minimising injury risk.

5.3.1 Player Injury Profile

The incidence of reported tennis injuries varies greatly; injury incidence variation has primarily been attributed to different reporting methods [2]. Indeed, the normalisation of injury incidence to factors such as exposure time is considered inappropriate [2] because factors such as rally duration are affected by court surface [70, 71]. However, when compared to other sports, tennis has a unique 'injury profile' [2]. Pluim et al. [2] highlighted that the lower extremities now comprise the most frequently injured sites in tennis (31.1–67.0%), followed by the upper extremities (20.0–48.6%) and trunk (3.0–22.0%). Further, a chronological progression from predominantly upper extremity injuries (three studies between 1976 and 1989) to lower extremity injuries (ten studies between 1986 and 2005) was demonstrated [2], whilst the nature of lower extremity injuries was predominantly acute injuries, in contrast to chronic, upper extremity injuries.

A review of 408 tennis injuries between 2009 and 2015, incurred during practice and match play, reaffirmed the lower extremity as the most frequently injured site in tennis [4]. Specifically, 47.0% and 52.4% of men's and women's tennis injuries involved the lower extremity, followed by the trunk (16.6% and 17.6%, respectively) and the shoulder and clavicle (14.4% and 11.9%, respectively). Both men and women reported similar diagnosis-specific injury rates at similar injury sites, with the most prevalent tennis injury being lateral ankle ligament complex sprains (7.7% and 9.7% for men and women, respectively) [4]. Further, the most prevalent severe injury site (defined as more than 3 weeks of time lost or season ending injuries) involved the ankle and foot (20.0% and 30.8% for men and women, respectively). Potential injury causes were suggested as high acceleration movement, play on different court surfaces and high-load, frontal plane movements. However, court surface effects could not be explored due to survey limitations [72]. An evolving tennis injury profile, whereby acute, lower extremity injuries frequently involving the foot and ankle, is evident. The increased athleticism of 'modern era' tennis movement and different court surface characteristics have been identified as contributory factors in tennis injury [73, 74]. However, current injury reporting mechanisms have not allowed the exploration of factors such as player movement and surface type.

Movement demands of match-play tennis affect injury rate. During tennis match play, injury rates have been reported as 2.3 and 1.8 times higher than during practice (men and women, respectively) [4]. Whilst injury rates reflect increased intensity of match play over practice, court surface—as an environmental factor of match play—has also been demonstrated to influence the injury profile of tennis players [74]. For match-play tennis, player injury rates are linked to match retirement; match retirements are only recorded in the event of player injury or illness [75]. Breznik and Batageli [76] quantified match retirements for 420,489 matches (comprising 17,553 ATP ranked players) between 1968 and 2010. Over time and for all court surfaces, the proportion of match retirements has increased, with match retirement rate for matches played after 2002 twice that of matches played prior to 1990 (3.0% vs. 1.5%, respectively) [76]. Further, for Grand Slam tournaments, match retirement rates for clay and hard court surfaces (2.8% and 2.6%, respectively) were significantly higher than retirement rates for matches played on grass (1.6%). Breznik and Batageli [76] concluded that clay and hard court surfaces were the most likely surfaces to result in match-play retirement. The authors noted limitations to their approach when explaining injury related to court surface. For example, rally duration, a central characteristic of match-play intensity [72], could not be assessed. Further, tournament quality was inversely related to match retirement rate, indicating that match retirement comprised of other factors than injury.

For grass and clay court surfaces, match-play retirement rate due to injury opposed previous reports of match-play injury treatment rate. In a 3-year study examining injury treatment, Bastholt [77] reported that most injury treatments were required for match play on grass court surfaces. Further, injury treatments on clay court surfaces were required less often than on hard court surfaces. However, grass court surfaces are not played on as frequently as clay and hard court surfaces. Of matches analysed by Breznik and Batageli [76], 51.4% and 42.6% were played on clay and hard court surfaces, respectively; only 6.0% of matches were played on grass court surfaces.

The inverse relationship between match retirement and tournament quality might explain disparity between match retirement and injury treatment rate. In a 10-year review of injuries sustained at Wimbledon (2002–2012), most presented injuries were pre-existing or recurrent injuries and were predominantly acute, muscle, and ligament injuries [5]. Whilst findings could not support nor refute the notion of the faster, grass court surface as a contributory factor in treated injuries, it was noted that professional players must transition for play on all three court surfaces within very short time frames [5]. The high-quality, prestige and perceived importance of Grand Slam tournaments such as Wimbledon—which would comprise most grass court match play for most professional players—might explain low retirement rates [76] but high injury treatment rates [78]. Modern professional tennis challenges players to adapt movement for court-specific performance, without sustaining injury [5]. Therefore, to understand the biomechanics of injury related to court surface, movement demands of match-play tennis on different court surfaces must be assessed.

5.3.2 Player Movement

Player movement differs between court surfaces. Notational analyses highlight that rallies at Roland Garros were longer and consisted of more baseline play than rallies at the US and Australian Opens [70]. Similarly, rallies at the US and Australian Opens were longer and consisted of more baseline play than rallies at Wimbledon. Recently, rally duration between court surfaces has become more similar [71]. Between 1997 and 1999, average rally duration at Roland Garros was 3.5 s longer than at Wimbledon; in 2007 this had shortened to 2.2 s (longer rallies at Wimbledon) [71]. It was suggested that rally duration changes reflected the use of larger, slower type 3 tennis balls (reducing service dominance) as well as improved player fitness and technical ability [71]. Whilst useful for characterisation, notational analyses cannot quantify the precise movement demands of players and, as such, are limited when understanding player-surface interaction.

An experimental analysis of simulated matches revealed that players travelled 25% further for points played on clay surfaces (11.6 ± 1.5 m) when compared to points played on acrylic surfaces (9.3 ± 1.8 m) [77]. Court surface effects at the point level correspond to match level distances, where players travelled 21% further on clay (1447 ± 143 m) than on acrylic surfaces (1199 ± 168 m). However, again the volume and variability of Grand Slam matches—which can exceed 5 h in duration—have clear implications for the validity of experimentally derived player movement data, particularly when injury rates between practice and match-play tennis are considered [4]. It is therefore imperative that player movement, to inform player-surface interaction research, is characterised during match-play tennis, as experimental characterisations often fail to fully capture the movement demands of match play [79].

5.3.3 Player Movement During Match Play

Spatial representations of player position data (e.g. Fig. 5.2) can provide useful visualisations of match-play tennis. However, much information, regarding the intensity and variation of movement, is omitted [79]. Using data provided by HawkEye, Reid et al. [80] presented a gender comparison of player movement during rallies (102 males and 95 females) at Australian Open tournaments between 2012 and 2014. Reid et al. [80] reported differences for distance travelled during men's (2110 ± 839 m) and women's (1232 ± 440 m) matches, although travel differences largely reflected match format (i.e. three and five sets for women and men, respectively). Other distance metrics, such as distance travelled per set or per point, did not reveal gender differences. However, mean in-point movement speed during men's games (3.7 m/s) was greater than during women's games (3.4 m/s), indicating a higher intensity of movement within the men's game, despite similar movement frequencies [80].

Reid et al. [80] noted that both male and female players travelled further during points won (~10.5 m) compared to points lost (~8.8 m). The necessity to travel greater distances to win points reflects previous analyses of match play on acrylic surfaces. Using the SAGIT (two overhead cameras) tracking system [81], Martinez-Gallego et al. [82] quantified player movement during eight matches of the 2011 Valencia Open. Per game, the median distance travelled by game winners was 84.2 m, compared to 80.2 m travelled by game losers [82]. Game winners, however, travelled at lower speeds than game losers (median speed, 1.3 m/s and 1.4 m/s, respectively). Game winners dictated game pace, forcing losers to adopt defensive movement strategies (i.e. high acceleration movement) in defensive court areas (e.g. >1.5 m behind baseline) [82]. The external pace of match play highlights limitations of experimentally characterising tennis movement [79].

Player movement speeds are characterised by non-normal distributions, reflecting the variety of movement that comprises match-play tennis [80, 82]. However, no information regarding movement direction was provided. Tennis-specific movements, such as lateral and turning movements, have been identified as potential tennis injury mechanisms [74]. Therefore, it is imperative to assess the magnitude, direction, and frequency of tennis movement at the rally level [82], to allow the integration of match-play tennis movement and biomechanical player-surface interaction research.

In unpublished work, Dunn [83] developed a portable, single-camera tracking system to measure player movement and step strategy during match-play tennis. To demonstrate the system's application, match-play movements of a player (2011 ATP rank 3), during 20 rallies of a semi-

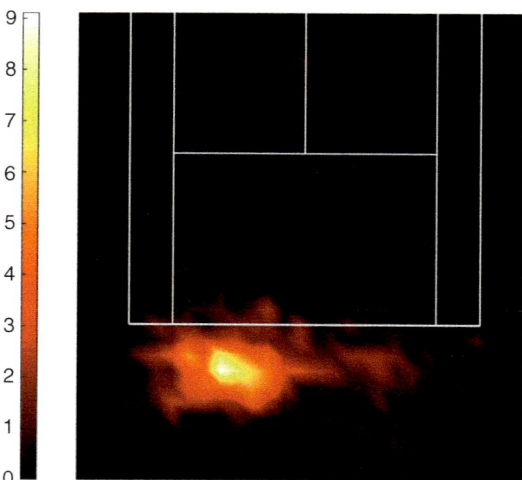

Fig. 5.2 Heat map illustrating player-court occupancy (colour bar indicates duration in seconds) during match-play tennis rallies (n = 20) [83]

final match at the 2011 ATP World Tour Finals, were quantified. Rallies were between 6 and 28 s in duration and comprised of between two and ten strokes. Per rally, the player travelled 32.9 ± SD15.6 m, which comprised of 25.3 ± 12.4 m and 20.1 ± 10.4 m in baseline and centreline directions, respectively [83]. Further, mean baseline direction movements were faster (1.9 m/s) than centreline movements (1.4 m/s), whilst 95% of movements were below 4.1 m/s (resultant direction). Finally, median speed (resultant direction) was 1.4 m/s [82], reflecting previous analyses of match play on acrylic surfaces [82].

Whilst rallies were nearly twice the duration of previously reported rallies [70, 84] and unlikely to be match representative [83], analyses provide insight into rally level movement strategies that characterise top ranked match-play tennis. For example, the analysed player won 60% of rallies and the match, despite occupying defensive court areas for 30.8% of the rallies [83]. When assessing elite tennis player (ATP rank, 5–113) court occupancy, MartÍnez-Gallego et al. [82] reported that match winners and losers occupy defensive court areas for 10.3% and 14.2% of rallies, respectively. Exploiting movement strategies traditionally considered to be defensive to win points might characterise top-ranked match-play tennis movement. This highlights the necessity of integrating match-play movement analysis with player-surface interaction research.

Match-play analyses of player movement on other court surfaces are limited. In an analysis of player movement on clay, Pereira et al. [85] used bespoke, dual-camera tracking software [86] to quantify match-play movements of eight players (644 rallies) at the 2012 Brazil F24 Futures tournament. Players travelled 3160.0 ± 880.1 m during rallies per match, comprising of 1702.4 ± 448.2 m and 1457.6 ± 678.1 m in first and second sets, respectively [85]. Match and set travel was markedly greater than match-play assessments of acrylic surfaces; Reid et al. [80] reported that players travelled 2110 ± 839 m and 572 ± 152 m per match and set, respectively. Further, per game, Pereira et al. [85] reported that players travelled 117.7 ± 94.4 m and 102.9 ± 92.6 m (first and second sets, respectively) markedly higher than game travel on acrylic (e.g. median distance, 82.2 m [82]). However, player mean travel per rally was 5.8 ± 7.2 m and 5.3 ± 6.6 m (first and second sets, respectively) [85], markedly shorter than rally travel on acrylic surfaces (e.g. 10.3 m) [80]. Disproportionately short travel during rallies suggests a high proportion of low return rallies (e.g. ace or return of serve not defended). Indeed, Pereira et al. [85] noted that disparity reflected player ability and match duration; however, experimental evidence [77] supports the notion that players travel greater distances during match play on clay surfaces.

Analyses of player movement during match-play tennis are limited. During match-play, player movement has been reported at match [80, 85], set [80, 85], game [82, 85], and rally [80, 83] levels for clay and acrylic court surfaces. To the authors' knowledge, no research has quantified player movement during match play on grass court surfaces. This might reflect the small proportion (6%) of competitive matches played on grass [76]. However, evidence indicates that players travel considerably further during match play on clay surfaces than on acrylic surfaces, reflecting longer rally durations on clay [70, 71]. During match-play rallies, tennis players walk, jog, run, and sprint [86]. High acceleration movement [4] and extreme, side-to-side turning and lunging movements [74] have been indicated as potential tennis injury mechanisms. Therefore, an integrated approach to player-surface interaction must consider locomotor requirements of tennis-specific movements observed during match play, to inform biomechanical research of potential injury mechanisms.

5.3.4 Player Step Strategy During Match Play

At the 2011 Roland Garros Qualifying Tournament, Dunn et al. [87] manually characterised step length and step frequency for forehand groundstrokes. A gender comparison of 40 match-play rallies revealed that women adopted higher step frequencies than men (6.9 and 5.3 Hz, respectively); however, forehand groundstroke step lengths did not reveal gender differences (1.0 and 0.9 m for men and women, respectively). Further analysis of men's rally movements indicated trends towards higher frequencies of large (>4.5 m [72]) baseline directed movements, when compared to women's rallies. Aggressive, baseline rallying on clay surfaces has been identified as a potential tennis injury mechanism [74]. Whilst movement data were limited by sample size, different step frequencies might be indicative of different step strategies to performing tennis-specific movements on clay court surfaces.

As noted previously (Sect. 5.3.3), Dunn [83] developed a single-camera tracking system to measure tennis player movement and step strategy. In addition to tracking player location, a view- and gait-independent algorithm automatically identified foot contacts during 20 match-play rallies to derive step length and step time data [83]. Analysis revealed that match-play step strategy comprised of 38.1 ± 20.8 steps, with step lengths and frequencies of 0.87 ± 0.39 m and 3.4 ± 6.5 Hz, respectively [83]. Large variation in step frequency highlights step strategy consisting of tennis-specific movements, e.g. side steps, skip steps, shuffle steps, and lunges [86]. Further, positively skewed step length data (e.g. Fig. 5.3) reflect that most rally movements were comprised of short step lengths.

The integrated measurement of player step and movement strategy allows player movement data (e.g. player location or preceding movement velocity [83]), for specific step parameters during match play to be identified. Figure 5.3 illustrates player location for step lengths ≥1.12 m (fourth quartile step length data), which are indicative of high loads, inducing high utilised friction coefficients at the shoe-surface interface (e.g. Sect. 5.3.5). Step lengths ≥1.12 m were predominantly observed behind the baseline, aligned with both the deuce and advantage court singles sideline. This reflects the lateral extremes of player movement (e.g. baseline lunging and turning manoeuvres). High acceleration whole-body court movement [4] and extreme, side-to-side turning and lunging [74], characteristic of movements that yield large step lengths (e.g. Fig. 5.4), have been identified as potential tennis injury mechanisms. Therefore, quantifying the location,

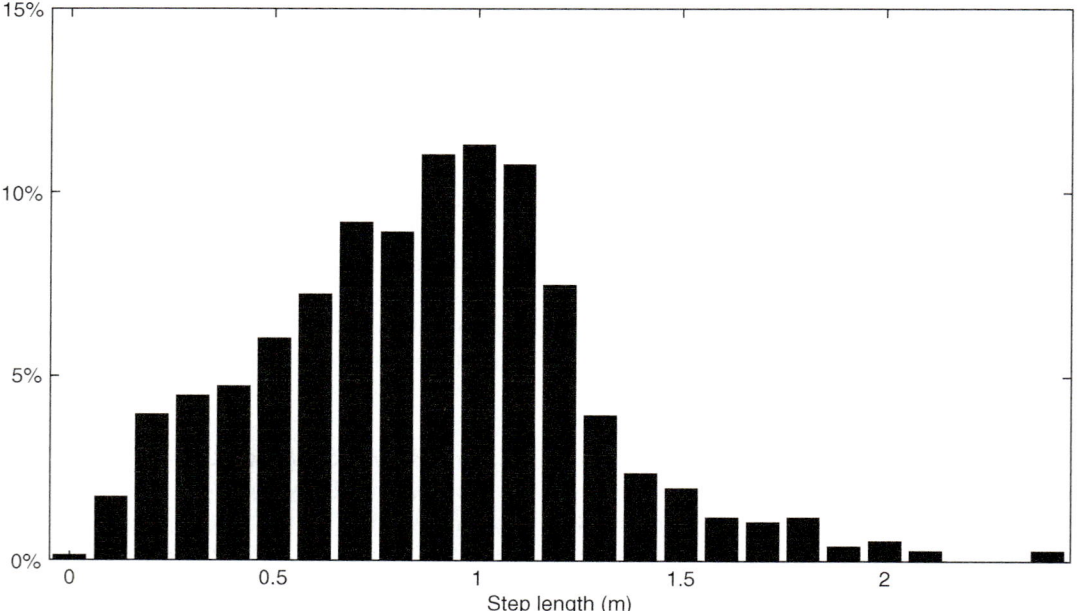

Fig. 5.3 Distribution of step length during match-play tennis rallies ($n = 20$) [83]

magnitude, and frequency of key, tennis step strategy, as well as corresponding player movement data during match-play, can directly inform future biomechanical research into potential injury mechanisms in tennis.

5.3.5 Player-Shoe-Surface Biomechanics

The variations observed in global movement patterns between court surfaces and the resulting differences in overall workload are likely to contribute to the differences in injury risk between court types. In addition to differences in overall movement patterns and workload, the specific loads experienced by structures of the lower limb for each step during interaction with the ground will influence the risk of specific injuries. Interest in the loads experienced for different tennis court surfaces has led to several studies of the influence of court surface on lower limb biomechanics for tennis-specific movements. The comparison of surfaces with different mechanical characteristics can reveal the relative role of specific design features on player biomechanics, informing the design of safer, high performance surfaces.

The two main surface types that have been studied in terms of biomechanical response and links with injury risk are acrylic hard courts and traditional red clay courts. These surface types are distinctly different in terms of their hardness and friction properties. Acrylic hard courts comprise of an asphalt or concrete base overlaid with a rubber shock-absorbing layer coated with acrylic/polyurethane paint. Acrylic hard courts provide the stiffest surface yielding a high ball-bounce and the highest player-surface frictional coefficient as a result of the rough paint finish. 'Clay' consists of crushed stone layers topped with fine gritty clay. Differences in injury incidence suggested by previous studies are therefore likely to be the result of variations in mechanical characteristics of the surfaces, primarily differences in surface friction and/or hardness. It is challenging to isolate the influence of friction and hardness, since both are likely to change to

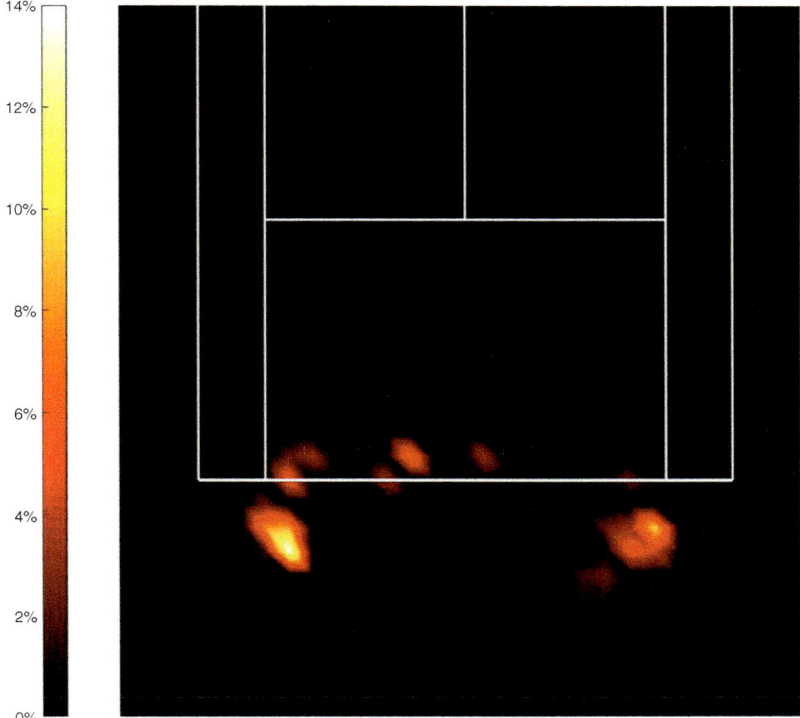

Fig. 5.4 Player-court location map (accumulated into 50 cm² bins) for step lengths ≥1.12 m (colour bar indicates frequency) for 20 match-play tennis rallies [83]

some extent when comparing surfaces and vary over time and wear. Comparisons have typically focused on one or other of these characteristics, where the difference between compared surfaces has been predominately in hardness or friction.

The influence of surface hardness on lower limb biomechanics and associated loading has most typically been assessed using a force plate placed beneath the surface. These devices provide the magnitude, direction, and point of application of the resultant force vector, known as the ground reaction force (GRF). The peak rate at which the vertical force is applied, or the peak rate of loading, is the maximum steepness of the vertical force curve during the ascending impact phase (Fig. 5.5), occurring during the first 50 ms of ground contact. This loading rate has been suggested to be a reliable indicator of the loading associated with the shoe-surface interaction for different shoes [87, 88] and surfaces [89] which differ in terms of mechanical cushioning characteristics. As an example, the peak loading rates for young adults running at a relaxed pace over a force plate have been reported in the range 30–40 bodyweights per second (BW/s) [90]. During the foot plant of the more dynamic sport-specific

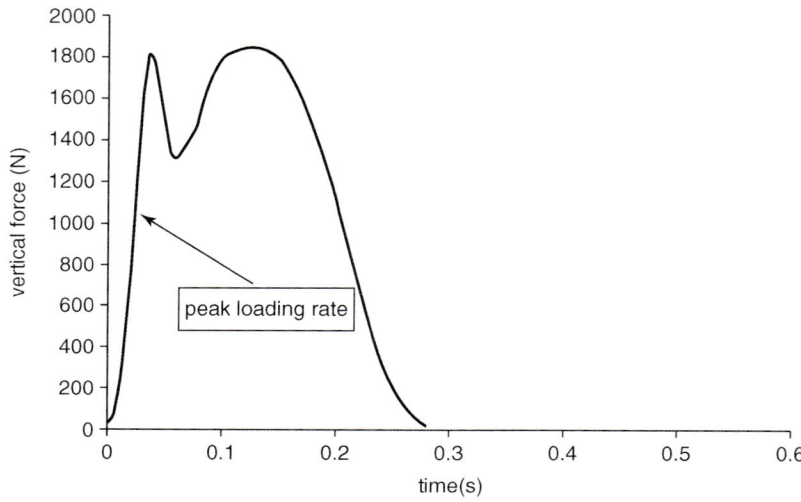
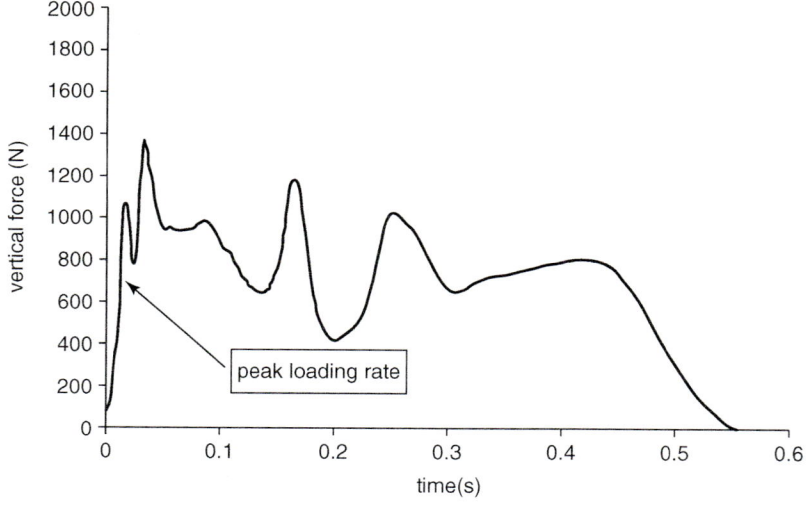

Fig. 5.5 Typical vertical ground reaction force for (top) running and (bottom) tennis running forehand, identifying the peak loading rate (peak steepness of the curve)

movement of a tennis running forehand, peak rate of loading was reported to be in the region of 360 BW/s [74], highlighting the relatively large magnitude of loading during foot-ground contact during dynamic tennis movements. The performance of this tennis-specific movement on surfaces with increased levels of cushioning resulted in significant reductions in the peak loading rate [91], suggesting that the loads experienced by the structures of the lower limb are reduced when playing on courts that possess greater mechanical cushioning.

The application of force plates to quantify levels of cushioning has generally been restricted to measurements taken within a laboratory environment, rather than in the applied setting of tennis courts. The use of pressure insoles placed within footwear has enabled the collection of loading in a more applied setting. Pressure insole data provide the distribution of vertical load across the foot plantar surface. Applications of this technology in tennis have identified different loading patterns for different court surfaces. For example, a greater load was measured under the hallux (big toe) and lesser toes for hard courts compared with clay [74]. Greater loads, however, were observed for clay courts than for hard courts under the medial and lateral midfoot. This change in distribution of loading under the foot plantar surface was suggested to be a result of the different movement strategies for the distinct surface types—hard courts were associated with an aggressive front-foot landing style compared with more defensive responses and deep baseline play on clay. The movement pattern on clay includes more side-to-side steps exerting pressure through the midfoot, suggesting that, rather than different cushioning of tennis courts simply directly influencing load, the resulting differences in style of play also contribute to the loading and subsequent risk of injury. This highlights the importance of combining the approaches for quantifying global player movement and step strategies (see Sects. 5.3.2–5.3.4) with detailed biomechanical analysis of specific tennis movements, to fully characterise player-surface interactions. In addition, clay and hard court surfaces differ not only in their hardness, and ability to provide cushioning, but also in the level of friction at the shoe-surface interface.

Friction is dependent on the interaction between two surfaces, in this case the shoe and surface. The peak horizontal force measured using a force plate can be used to indicate the shear requirements of a surface for different movements. In addition, the ratio of vertical to horizontal ground reaction force can provide a utilised coefficient of friction. Sliding (kinetic) friction is usually around 30% lower than static friction. Stucke and colleagues [92] reported how the utilised coefficient of friction altered with tennis court surface, with acceleration from rest on a hard court resulting in a coefficient of friction of 0.8 compared with a value of 0.65 on a cinder surface. This comparison of surfaces with different resistance to sliding also demonstrated differences in movement patterns, or kinematics. For a stopping movement, it was reported that the knee joint continues to flex when stopping on a hard court, with relatively high friction. This movement was suggested to contribute to reducing the load experienced by the knee joint compared with that would be experienced if the knee were kept relatively straight [92]. When performing the same task on cinder, with low friction, a fixed knee flexion angle was observed, and braking was achieved by sliding occurring between the shoe and surface interfaces. This study of the influence of shoe-surface friction on player biomechanics was performed using a controlled design, where players performed the stopping and accelerating movements in a controlled, repeatable manner. Results suggested that players adjust to shoe-surface combinations with lower mechanical coefficient of friction by applying a lower horizontal ground reaction force component, resulting in a lower utilised coefficient of friction. However, recent comparison of hard court and clay surfaces during a simulated forehand movement has revealed that the relationship between shoe-surface friction and adaptation of lower limb biomechanics may be more complex than initially thought [93]. For this tennis-specific movement, a greater horizontal force was observed on clay than on a hard court surface, leading to a greater utilised coefficient of friction for the clay surface. The authors suggested that players adapt to clay by applying high horizontal force to facilitate sliding on this type of surface. This example highlights the importance of considering how players respond to shoe-surface combinations for movements that are specific to tennis and that the comparison of shoe-surface combinations under conditions that are too controlled may not provide valid results regarding player biomechanics and resulting injury risk.

As previously highlighted, observed changes in the distribution of plantar pressures attributed to differences in playing surface hardness may also be influenced by differences in shoe-surface friction. A study by Damm and colleagues [94] compared in-shoe pressures for a controlled jumping movement and two standardised tennis movements, performed on court surfaces to simulate tennis playing conditions. These authors reported lower pressures on clay compared to hard court, with longer step duration and a greater number of unloading episodes on clay. Mechanical characterisation of the court surfaces indicated that they differed primarily in their friction characteristics, resulting in the observed differences during player interaction being attributed primarily to variations in friction rather than hardness of the court surfaces. The higher pressures on a hard court were suggested to support an association with increased levels of overuse injuries. Lower pressures and a longer braking step on clay were suggested to facilitate sliding by preventing sticking, with unloading episodes also suggested to be part of the strategy to slide on clay.

Whilst force plate and pressure insole data provide us with detail regarding external loading for different tennis court surface types, these measurements do not provide information on the loading experienced directly by specific lower limb structures. An estimation of differences in internal loading can be obtained using joint moments, providing a measure of the net rotational effect of all forces acting about a joint. Although generally limited to studies performed in a laboratory environment, the comparison of joint moments for clay versus hard court surfaces has revealed greater knee moments on hard courts, suggesting greater loads are experienced by structures controlling knee movement [95]. Continued use of these approaches to develop models to estimate loading at frequently injured sites, such as the lateral ankle ligaments, will increase understanding of the role surface properties may play in influencing injury risk.

It has typically been assumed that changes in ground reaction force, in-shoe pressure and/or movement patterns indicate changes in internal loading and thus injury risk. In support of the use of these biomechanical measures to detect injury risk, it has been suggested that evidence from studies with three different designs—those focused on 'sports surfaces and injury', 'sports surfaces and biomechanics', and 'injury and biomechanics'—be combined [96]. Adopting this approach has allowed links to be developed to support biomechanical mechanisms for surface-related knee and ankle injuries. For example, lateral ankle ligament sprains are common in tennis [61]. Although detailed data for injury site are not available across court types, acrylic hard courts are typically associated with a greater coefficient of friction and associated with shorter stopping times and less likelihood of sliding [95]. Hard court surfaces have also been associated with greater lateral pressures during turning, suggesting the subtalar joint is in a more inverted orientation [74]. Greater inversion places the lateral ligaments under increased load and increases the likelihood of failure of these structures. Thus, the detection of greater lateral concentration of pressure may be used as an indicator of risk of ankle inversion injury for different surface types. Whilst this argument appears logical, prospective studies which integrate the mechanical characterisation of surfaces, identification of differences in player movement strategies during match play, and measurement of lower limb biomechanics are required, alongside the monitoring of injury rates. Taking this approach will increase our confidence in the use of biomechanical measures to identify potential differences in injury risk.

The main focus of biomechanical studies of player-shoe-surface interaction in tennis has been on the manipulation of the surface. Since footwear is also a component of the player-shoe-surface interaction, consideration of the potential role of footwear on injury risk is also important. A study of tennis player satisfaction with footwear identified that the majority of players found tennis footwear comfortable, with only 9% reporting that their footwear was uncomfortable [97]. A study of ten different types of tennis shoe during a sideways cutting movement on a consistent surface reported that the only variables influenced by footwear were the contact time and the peak subtalar joint inversion [98]. A positive correlation between contact time and peak inversion led the authors to conclude footwear that provided inversion control also increased player performance (in terms of time taken for changing direction). Thus footwear appears to be an important consideration when a specific playing surface has been identified. However, compared with the large differences between court surface, footwear has been found to have a relatively small effect. Damm and colleagues compared two footwear types (clay court and acrylic hard court shoes, Fig. 5.6) for clay and hard court playing surfaces [94]. It was found that the difference in footwear worn had a negligible influence on lower limb biomechanics compared with the effect of surface. It is suggested that the change from hard court to clay is so extreme that injury risk on clay will be governed predominantly by the surface characteristics. For hard court surfaces, there is some evidence that footwear design can influence biomechanics, particularly during turning, but marked differences in design characteristics may be required to achieve these differences. An example of this is provided by the development of a tennis shoe designed to facilitate sliding on hard court surfaces [99]. Investigators reported that the introduction of a plastic plate to the shoe outsole design to allow sliding on hard courts resulted in players being able to perform changes of direction using a sliding technique on a hard court surface and that this technique was associated with an improvement in performance time. Future manipulations of footwear design may therefore facilitate larger differences in lower limb biomechanics, and thus injury risk, than have been reported to date.

5.4 Chapter Summary

The relationship between equipment and injury risk in tennis is complex, mainly due to the interaction with the player and the evolving nature of the sport. Impulsive forces from ball/racquet impact during strokes can lead to overuse injuries to the upper extremity, whereas player-surface interactions often lead to acute injuries to the lower limbs. These lower limb injuries are more common, and a range of tennis surfaces adds complexity when investigating how shoe design may influence player-surface interactions. Modern technology—such as cameras and movement and pressure sensors—can play an important role by assisting with data collection on court, ideally in elite match play. Data collected from actual tennis movements can help inform the development of appropriate laboratory tests concerning athlete and equipment, predictive models, and universal testing standards. Any potential benefits identified through changes to equipment should be validated with prospective studies.

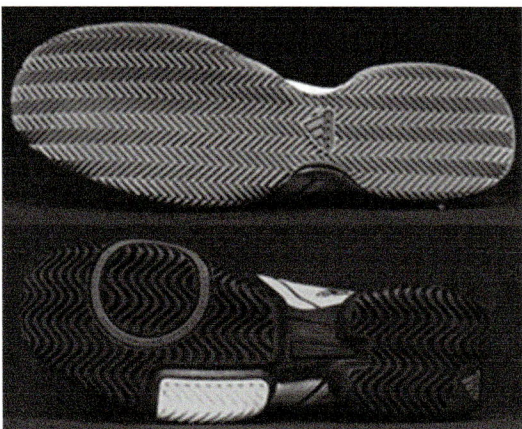

Fig. 5.6 Example tennis shoe soles, showing a clay court outsole (top) and a hard court outsole

References

1. Rogowski I, Creveaux T, Triquigeneaux S, et al. Tennis racquet vibrations and shock transmission to the wrist during forehand drive. PLoS ONE. 2015;10(7):e0132925. https://doi.org/10.1371/journal.pone.0132925.
2. Pluim B, Staal J, Windler G, et al. Tennis injuries: occurrence, aetiology, and prevention. Br J Sports Med. 2006;40:415–23. https://doi.org/10.1136/bjsm.2005.023184.
3. Sell K, Hainline B, Yorio M, et al. Injury trend analysis from the US Open tennis championships between 1994 and 2009. Br J Sports Med. 2014;48:546–51. https://doi.org/10.1136/bjsm-2012-091175.
4. Lynall RC, Kerr ZY, Djoko A, et al. Epidemiology of National Collegiate Athletic Association men's and women's tennis injuries, 2009/2010–2014/2015. Br J Sports Med. Online First. 2015. https://doi.org/10.1136/bjsports-2015-095360.
5. McCurdie I, Smith S, Bell PH, et al. Tennis injury data from The Championships Wimbledon, from 2003 to 2012. Br J Sports Med. Online First. 2015. https://doi.org/10.1136/bjsports-2015-095552.
6. Pluim BM, Loeffen FGJ, Clarsen B, et al. A one-season prospective study of injuries and illness in elite junior tennis. Scand J Med Sci Sports. 2016;26:564–72. https://doi.org/10.1111/sms.12471.
7. Knudson D, Allen T, Choppin S. Interaction of tennis racquet design and biomechanical factors. In: Hong Y, editor. Routledge handbook of ergonomics in sport and exercise. London: Routledge; 2014. p. 423–39.
8. Allen T, Choppin S, Knudson D. A review of tennis racquet performance parameters. Sports Eng. 2016;19:1–11. https://doi.org/10.1007/s12283-014-0167-x.
9. Knudson D. Biomechanical aspects of the tennis racquet. In: Hong Y, Bartlett R, editors. Routledge handbook of biomechanics and human movement science. London: Routledge; 2008. p. 248–60.
10. Knudson D. Intra-subject variability of upper extremity angular kinematics in the tennis forehand drive. Int J Sport Biomech. 1990;6:415–21.
11. Knudson D. Factors affecting force loading in the tennis forehand. J Sports Med Phys Fit. 1991;31:527–31.
12. Plagenhoef S. Tennis racquet testing. In: Terauds J, editor. Biomechanics in sports. Del Mar, CA: Research Center for Sports; 1982. p. 411–21.
13. Bahamonde R, Knudson D. Kinetics of the upper extremity in the open and square stance tennis forehand. J Sci Med Sport. 2003;6:88–101.
14. Knudson D, Bahamonde R. Trunk and racquet kinematics at impact in the open and square stance tennis forehand. Biol Sport. 1999;16:3–10.
15. Knudson D, Blackwell J. Trunk muscle activation in open stance and square stance tennis forehands. Int J Sports Med. 2000;21:321–4.
16. Lane B, Sherratt P, Xiao H, et al. Characterisation of ball impact conditions in professional tennis: matches played on hard court. Proc Inst Mech Eng P J Sports Eng Technol. 2015. https://doi.org/10.1177/1754337115617580.
17. Mecheri S, Rioult F, Mantel B, et al. The serve impact in tennis: first large-scale study of big Hawk-Eye data. Stat Anal Data Mining. 2016;9(5):310–25. https://doi.org/10.1002/sam.11316.
18. Brody H. Physics of the tennis racquet. Am J Phys. 1979;47:482–7. https://doi.org/10.1119/1.11787.
19. Brody H, Cross R, Lindsey C. The physics and technology of tennis. CA: Racquet Tech Pub; 2002.
20. Cross R, Lindsey C. Technical tennis. CA: Racquet Tech Pub; 2005.
21. Elliott B, Marshall R, Noffal G. Contributions of upper limb segment rotations during the power serve in tennis. J Appl Biomech. 1995;11:433–42.
22. Mitchell S, Jones R, King M. Head speed vs. racquet inertia in the tennis serve. Sports Eng. 2000;3:99–110. https://doi.org/10.1046/j.1460-2687.2000.00051.x.
23. Allen T. Finite element model of a tennis ball impact with a racquet. Doctoral dissertation, Sheffield Hallam University, 2009.
24. Allen T, Haake S, Goodwill S. Effect of tennis racquet parameters on a simulated groundstroke. J Sports Sci. 2011;29(3):311–25. https://doi.org/10.1080/02640414.2010.526131.
25. Hennig E. Influence of racquet properties on injuries and performance in tennis. Exerc Sport Sci Rev. 2007;35:62–6.
26. Choppin S. An investigation into the power point in tennis. Sports Eng. 2013;16:173–80. https://doi.org/10.1007/s12283-013-0122-2.
27. Cross R. Center of percussion of hand-held implements. Am J Phys. 2004;72:622–30. https://doi.org/10.1119/1.1634965.
28. Choppin S, Goodwill S, Haake S. Impact characteristics of the ball and racquet during play at the Wimbledon qualifying tournament. Sport Eng. 2011;13:163–70. https://doi.org/10.1007/s12283-011-0062-7.
29. Hatze H. Impact probability distribution, sweet spot, and the concept of an effective power region in tennis racquets. J Appl Biomech. 1994;10:43–50.
30. Caross R. The sweet spots of a tennis racquet. Sports Eng. 1998;1:63–78. https://doi.org/10.1046/j.1460-2687.1999.00011.x.
31. Cross R. Factors affecting the vibration of tennis racquets. Sports Eng. 2015;18:135–47. https://doi.org/10.1007/s12283-015-0173-7.
32. Creveaux T, Sevrez V, Coste B, et al. Methodological contribution to study the vibratory behaviour of tennis racquets following real forehand drive impact. Comput Methods Biomech Biomed Eng. 2014;17:150–1. https://doi.org/10.1080/10255842.2014.931610.
33. Banwell G, Roberts J, Halkon B, et al. Understanding the dynamic behaviour of a tennis racquet under play

34. Brody H. Vibration damping of tennis racquets. Int J Sport Biomech. 1989;5:451–6.
35. Cross R. Impact forces and torques transmitted to the hand by tennis racquets. Sports Technol. 2010;3(2):102–11. https://doi.org/10.1080/19346182.2010.538398.
36. Vethecan JK, Subic AJ. Vibration attenuation of tennis racquets using tuned vibration absorbers. Sports Eng. 2002;5:155–64. https://doi.org/10.1046/j.1460-2687.2002.00105.x.
37. Miller S. Modern tennis racquets, balls, and surfaces. Br J Sports Med. 2006;40:401–5. https://doi.org/10.1136/bjsm.2005.023283.
38. Whiteside D, Elliott B, Lay B, et al. The effect of racquet swing weight on serve kinematics in elite adolescent female tennis players. J Sci Med Sport. 2013;17:124–8. https://doi.org/10.1016/j.jsams.2013.03.001.
39. Schorah D, Choppin S, James D. Effects of moment of inertia on restricted motion swing speed. Sports Biomech. 2015;14:157–67. https://doi.org/10.1080/14763141.2015.1027949.
40. Cross R, Bower R. Effects of swing-weight on swing speed and racquet power. J Sports Sci. 2006;24:23–30. https://doi.org/10.1080/02640410500127876.
41. Haake S, Allen T, Choppin S, et al. The evolution of the tennis racquet and its effect on serve speed. In: Miller S, Capel-Davies J, editors. Tennis science and technology, vol. 3. London: International Tennis Federation; 2007. p. 257–71.
42. King M, Hau A, Blenkinsop G. The effect of ball impact location on racquet and forearm joint angle changes for one-handed tennis backhand groundstrokes. J Sports Sci. 2016:1–8. https://doi.org/10.1080/02640414.2016.1211308.
43. Lammer H. Racquet with self-powered piezoelectric damping system. U.S. Patent 6,974,397, 13 Dec 2005
44. Lammer H. Racquet with self-powered piezoelectric damping system. U.S. Patent 7,160,286, 9 Jan 2007
45. Kotze J, Lammer H, Cottey R, et al. The effects of active piezo fibre racquets on tennis elbow. In: Miller S, editor. Tennis science and technology 2. London: International Tennis Federation; 2003. p. 55–60.
46. Cottey R, Kotze J, Lammer H, et al. An extended study investigating the effects of tennis racquets with active damping technology on the symptoms of tennis elbow. In: Moritz E, Haake S, editors. Engineering of sport 6. New York: Springer; 2006. p. 391–6.
47. Elliott N, Choppin S, Goodwill S, et al. Markerless tracking of tennis racquet motion using a camera. Procedia Eng. 2014;72:344–9. https://doi.org/10.1016/j.proeng.2014.06.060.
48. ITF. 2016 ITF rules of tennis, 2016. http://www.itftennis.com/officiating/rulebooks/rules-of-tennis.aspx. Accessed 22 June 2016
49. Choppin S, Goodwill S, Haake S. Investigations into the effect of grip tightness on off-centre forehand strikes in tennis. Proc Inst Mech Eng P J Sport Eng Technol. 2010;224(4):249–57. https://doi.org/10.1243/17543371JSET75.
50. Allen T, Haake S, Goodwill S. Comparison of a finite element model of a tennis racquet to experimental data. Sports Eng. 2009;12:87–98. https://doi.org/10.1007/s12283-009-0032-5.
51. Goodwill SR, Haake SJ. Spring damper model of an impact between a tennis ball and racquet. Proc Inst Mech Eng C J Mech Eng Sci. 2001;215:1331–41.
52. Haake SJ, Carré M, Goodwill SR. The dynamic impact characteristics of tennis balls with tennis racquets. J Sport Sci. 2003;21:839–50.
53. Nicolaides A, Elliott N, Kelley J, et al. Effect of string bed pattern on ball spin generation from a tennis racquet. Sports Eng. 2013;16:181–8.
54. Washida Y, Elliott N, Allen T. Measurement of main strings movement and its effect on tennis ball spin. Procedia Eng. 2014;72:557–62. https://doi.org/10.1016/j.proeng.2014.06.097.
55. Kawazoe Y. Effects of string pre-tension on impact between ball and racquet in tennis. Ther Appl Mech. 1994;43:223–32.
56. Cross R, Lindsay C, Andruczyk D. Laboratory testing of tennis strings. Sports Eng. 2000;4:219–30.
57. Mohandhas BR, Makaram N, Drew TS, et al. Racquet string tension directly affects force experienced at the elbow: implications for the development of lateral epicondylitis in tennis players. Shoulder Elbow. 2016;8(3):184–91. https://doi.org/10.1177/1758573216640201.
58. Stroede CL, Noble L, Walker HS. The effect of tennis racquet string vibration dampers on racquet handle vibrations and discomfort following impacts. J Sport Sci. 1999;17:379–85. https://doi.org/10.1080/026404199365894.
59. Li FX, Fewtrell D, Jenkins M. String vibration dampers do not reduce racquet frame vibration transfer to the forearm. J Sport Sci. 2004;22:1041–52. https://doi.org/10.1080/02640410410001729982.
60. Wilson JF, Davis JS. Tennis racquet shock mitigation experiments. J Biomech Eng. 1995;117:479–84. https://doi.org/10.1115/1.2794211.
61. Mohr S, Cottey R, Lau D, et al. Dynamics of a stringbed damper on tennis racquets. In: The engineering of sport 7. Paris: Springer; 2008. p. 179–89.
62. Baszczynski P, Chevrel-Fraux C, Flcheux C, et al. Settings adjustment for string tension and mass of a tennis racquet depending on ball characteristics: laboratory and field testing. Procedia Eng. 2016;147:472–7. https://doi.org/10.1016/j.proeng.2016.06.343.
63. Knudson D, Blackwell J. Effect of type 3 ball on upper extremity EMG and acceleration in the tennis forehand. In: Blackwell JR, editor. Proceedings of oral sessions: XIX international symposium on biomechanics in sports. San Francisco, CA: University of San Francisco; 2001. p. 32–4.

64. Blackwell J, Knudson D. Effect of the type 3 (oversize) tennis ball on serve performance and upper extremity muscle activity. Sports Biomech. 2002;1:187–92.
65. Andrew DPS, Chow JW, Knudson D, et al. Effect of ball size on player reaction and racquet acceleration during the tennis volley. J Sci Med Sport. 2003;6:102–12.
66. Buszard T, Farrow D, Reid M, et al. Modifying equipment in early skill development: a tennis perspective. Res Quart Exerc Sport. 2014;85:218–25. https://doi.org/10.1080/02701367.2014.893054.
67. Buszard T, Reid M, Masters RSW, et al. Scaling the equipment and play area in children's sport to improve motor skill acquisition: a systematic review. Sports Med. 2016;46:829–43. https://doi.org/10.1007/s40279-015-0452-2.
68. International Tennis Federation. International Tennis Federation, 2015. http://www.itftennis.com/about/organisation/history.aspx. Accessed 20 Nov.
69. International Tennis Federation Technical Department. International Tennis Federation Technical Department, 2016. http://www.itftennis.com/technical/home.aspx. Accessed 20 Nov.
70. O'Donoghue P, Ingram B. A notational analysis of elite tennis strategy. J Sports Sci. 2001;19:107–15. https://doi.org/10.1080/026404101300036299.
71. Brown E, O'Donoghue PG. Gender and surface effect on elite tennis strategy. ITF Coach Sport Sci Rev. 2008;46(12):9–12.
72. Kerr ZY, Dompier TP, Snook EM, et al. National collegiate athletic association injury surveillance system: review of methods for 2004–2005 through 2013–2014 data collection. J Athl Train. 2014;49:552–60. https://doi.org/10.4085/1062-6050-49.3.58.
73. Fernandez J, Mendez-Villanueva A, Pluim BM. Intensity of tennis match play. Br J Sports Med. 2006;40:387–91. https://doi.org/10.1136/bjsm.2005.023168.
74. Girard O, Eicher F, Fourchet F, et al. Effects of the playing surface on plantar pressures and potential injuries in tennis. Br J Sports Med. 2007;41:733–8. https://doi.org/10.1136/bjsm.2007.036707.
75. Dragoo JL, Braun HJ. The effect of playing surface on injury rate. Sports Med. 2010;40:981–90. https://doi.org/10.2165/11535910-000000000-00000.
76. Breznik K, Batagelj V. Retired matches among male professional tennis players. J Sports Sci Med. 2012;11:270–8.
77. Murias JM, Lanatta D, Arcuri CR, et al. Metabolic and functional responses playing tennis on different surfaces. J Strength Cond Res. 2007;21:112–7.
78. Bastholt P. Professional tennis (ATP tour) and number of medical treatments in relation to type of surface. Med Sci Tennis. 2000;5:2.
79. Reid M, Duffield R. The development of fatigue during match-play tennis. Br J Sports Med. 2014;48:i7–i11. https://doi.org/10.1136/bjsports-2013-093196.
80. Reid M, Morgan S, Whiteside D. Match play characteristics of Grand Slam tennis: implications for training and conditioning. J Sports Sci. 2016;34:1791–8. https://doi.org/10.1080/02640414.2016.1139161.
81. Perš J, Bon M, Kovačič S, et al. Observation and analysis of large-scale human motion. Hum Mov Sci. 2002;21:295–311. https://doi.org/10.1016/S0167-9457(02)00096-9.
82. Martínez-Gallego R, Guzmán JF, James N, et al. Movement characteristics of elite tennis players on hard courts with respect to the direction of ground strokes. J Sports Sci Med. 2013;12:275–81.
83. Dunn MD. Video-based step measurement in sport and daily living. Ph.D. Thesis, Sheffield Hallam University, 2014.
84. Fernandez-Fernandez J, Sanz-Rivas D, Fernandez-Garcia B, et al. Match activity and physiological load during a clay-court tennis tournament in elite female players. J Sports Sci. 2008;26:1589–95. https://doi.org/10.1080/02640410802287089.
85. Pereira TJC, Nakamura FY, Jesus MTD, et al. Analysis of the distances covered and technical actions performed by professional tennis players during official matches. J Sports Sci. 2016:1–8. https://doi.org/10.1080/02640414.2016.1165858.
86. Hughes M, Meyer R. Movement pattern in elite men's singles tennis. Int J Perform Anal Sport. 2005;5:110–34.
87. Dunn M, Goodwill S, Wheat J, et al. Assessing tennis player interactions with tennis courts. In: Vilas-Boas JP, Machado L, Kim W, Veloso AP, editors. Biomechanics in sports 29. Portugal: University of Porto; 2011. p. 859–62.
88. Clarke TE, Frederick EC, Cooper LB. Effects of cushioning upon ground reaction forces in running. Int J Sports Med. 1983;4:247–51.
89. Stiles VH, Dixon SJ. Biomechanical response to systematic changes in impact interface cushioning properties while performing a tennis specific movement. J Sports Sci. 2007;25:1229–39.
90. Lilley K, Dixon S, Stiles V. A biomechanical comparison of the running gait of mature and young females. Gait Posture. 2011;33:496–500.
91. Stiles VH, Dixon SJ. The influence of different playing surfaces on the biomechanics of a tennis running forehand foot plant. J Appl Biomech. 2006;22:14–24.
92. Stucke H, Baudzus W, Baumann W. On friction characteristics of playing surfaces. In: Frederick FC, editor. Sports shoes and playing surfaces. Champaign, IL: Human Kinetics; 1984. p. 87–97.
93. Damm L, Low D, Richardson A, Clarke J, Carré M, Dixon S. The effects of surface traction characteristics on frictional demand and kinematics in tennis. Sports Biomech. 2013;12:389–402. https://doi.org/10.1080/14763141.2013.784799.
94. Damm L, Starbuck C, Stocker N, Clarke J, Carré M, Dixon S. Shoe-surface friction in tennis: influ-

ence on plantar pressure and implications for injury. Footwear Sci. 2014;6:155–64. https://doi.org/10.1080/19424280.2014.891659.
95. Dixon S, Damm L, Starbuck C, Clarke J, Carré M. Understanding player response to changes in shoe-surface friction during tennis-specific movements. In Proceedings of the world congress of biomechanics, Boston, 2014.
96. Stiles V, Dixon S. Sports surfaces, biomechanics and injury. In: Dixon S, Fleming P, James I, Carre M, editors. The science and engineering of sport surfaces. Oxon: Routledge; 2015. p. 70–97.
97. Llana S, Brizuela G, Alcántara E, Martínez A, García A. Study of comfort associated with tennis footwear. In: Riehle HJ, Vieten M, editors. 16th International symposium on biomechanics in sports. Konstanz: University of Konstanz; 1998. p. 1124–7.
98. Llana-Belloch S, Brizuela G, Pérez-Soriano P, García-Belenguer A, Crespo M. Supination control increases performance in sideward cutting movements in tennis. Sports Biomech. 2013;12:38–47. https://doi.org/10.1080/14763141.2013.765906.
99. Pavailler S, Horvais N. Sliding allows faster repositioning during tennis specific movements on hard court. Procedia Eng. 2014;72:859–64. https://doi.org/10.1016/j.proeng.2014.06.157.

Part II

Player Evaluation

Evaluation of the Shoulder and Elbow in the Elite Tennis Player

David Dines, Todd S. Ellenbecker, and Jonathan Berkowitz

6.1 Introduction

The evaluation of the shoulder and elbow in the elite tennis player is of extreme importance to determine the ultimate cause of the injury/pathology and prepares the foundation for the development of evidence-based rehabilitation and treatment programs. The high interplay and close association of the shoulder, scapulothoracic, and elbow articulations in the upper extremity kinetic chain make a thorough evaluation of all three regions of paramount importance regardless of the specific area of injury in the elite tennis player. The purpose of this chapter is to overview key evaluation methods for the shoulder and elbow of particular relevance to the elite tennis player to provide this foundation. Reference to descriptive findings contained in Chap. 10 will also be provided to highlight specific anatomic adaptations and musculoskeletal strength and range of motion profiling inherent in elite-level players.

D. Dines (✉)
Hospital for Special Surgery, New York, NY, USA

ATP World Tour, Ponte Vedra Beach, FL, USA

T. S. Ellenbecker
ATP World Tour and Rehab Plus Sports Therapy, Scottsdale, AZ, USA
e-mail: tellenbecker@atpworldtour.com

J. Berkowitz
Southern California Orthopedic Institute, Van Nuys, CA, USA

6.2 Shoulder Examination

While it is beyond the scope of this chapter to review all aspects of the clinical examination, the reader is referred to specific texts that have more complete descriptions of all aspects of the clinical shoulder exam [1, 2]. Key components of the exam will be covered below.

6.2.1 Observation and Posture

Evaluation of posture for the patient with shoulder dysfunction begins with shoulder heights evaluated in the standing position, as well as use of the hands-on-hips position to evaluate the prominence of the scapula against the thoracic wall. Typically, the dominant shoulder is significantly lower than the nondominant shoulder in neutral, non-stressed standing postures, particularly in unilaterally dominant athletes like tennis players [3] (Fig. 6.1). The dominant shoulder is visibly lower in male ATP professional tennis players 82% of the time [4]. Although the exact reason for this phenomenon is unclear, theories include increased mass in the dominant arm, leading the dominant shoulder to be lower secondary to the increased weight of the arm, as well as elongation of the periscapular musculature on the dominant or preferred side secondary to eccentric loading.

In the standing position, the clinician can observe the patient for symmetrical muscle

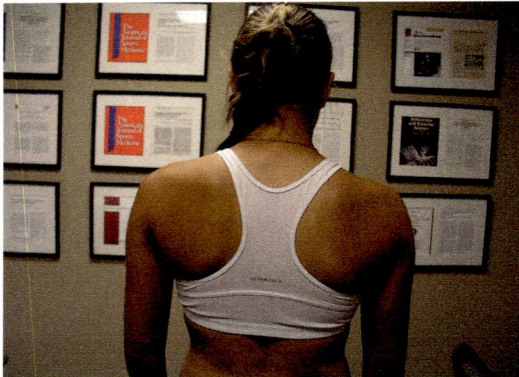

Fig. 6.1 Unilaterally dominant right handed athlete from posterior view showing the variation in shoulder heights

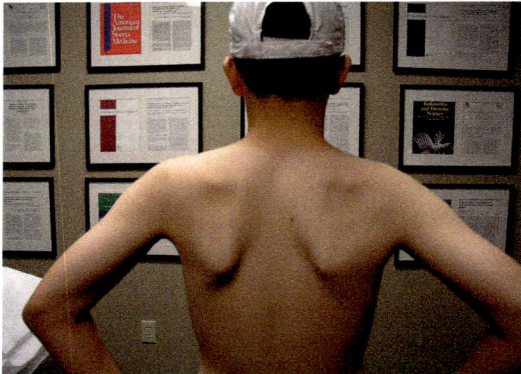

Fig. 6.2 Hands-on-hips position posterior view showing atrophy in the infraspinous fossa and scapular prominence

development and, more specifically, focal areas of muscle atrophy. One of the positions recommended, in addition to observing the patient with the arms at the sides in a comfortable standing posture, is the hands-on-hips position, which simply places the patient's shoulders in approximately 45°–50° of abduction with slight IR. The hands are placed on the iliac crests of the hips such that the thumbs are pointed posteriorly (Fig. 6.2). Placement of the hands on the hips allows the patient to relax the arms and often enables the clinician to observe focal pockets of atrophy along the scapular border, as well as more commonly over the infraspinous fossa of the scapula. Observable unilateral atrophy of the infraspinatus on the dominant extremity as compared to the nondominant extremity has been reported to be found in 73% of male professional ATP tennis players (Ellenbecker Chap. 10). Young et al. [5] reported this finding on the dominant arm in 52% of female professional tennis players on the WTA tour.

Thorough visual inspection using this position can often identify excessive scalloping over the infraspinous fossa, which may be present in patients with rotator cuff dysfunction, as well as in patients with severe atrophy who may have suprascapular nerve involvement. Impingement of the suprascapular nerve can occur at the suprascapular notch and the spinoglenoid notch and from paralabral cyst formation commonly found in patients with superior labral lesions [6]. Further diagnostic testing of the patient with extreme wasting of the infraspinatus muscle is warranted to rule out suprascapular nerve involvement.

6.2.2 Scapular Evaluation

While scapular movement and biomechanics are very technical and complex, clinical evaluation of the scapulothoracic joint is an integral part of the complete evaluation of the patient with shoulder dysfunction. It is important to note that several movements and translations occur in the scapulothoracic joint during arm elevation. These include scapular upward and downward rotation, IR and ER, and anterior and posterior sagittal plane tilting. In addition to those three rotational movements, two translations occur, superior and inferior translation, as well as protraction and retraction [7]. It is important to point out that with normal healthy arm elevation, scapular upward rotation, posterior tilting, and ER occur [8].

Kibler and associates [9] have outlined three primary scapular dysfunctions. This classification system consists of three primary scapular conditions and is named for the portion of the scapula that is most pronounced or most prominently visible when viewed during the clinical examination and can be used during the evaluation of the elite tennis player with shoulder and elbow pathology. The scapular examination recommended by Kibler includes visual inspection of the patient from a posterior view in resting stance, again in the hands-on-hips position (hands placed upon the hips such that the thumbs are pointing backward on the iliac crests), and during active movements bilaterally in the sagittal, scapular, and frontal planes [9]. These scapular dysfunctions are termed inferior angle, medial border, and superior.

Several key issues are important to point out regarding the use of visual scapular evaluation methods. It is important to use multiple repetitions and multiple planes of movement to allow the evaluator to assess the effects of fatigue and several planes of elevation and their effect on the patient's ability to dynamically control and stabilize the scapula [1, 9, 10]. Additionally, the use of an external load may be necessary to further provoke and load the extremity to elicit scapular dysfunction especially in athletes with subtle presentations of shoulder pathology, particularly in elite-level tennis players [11–13]. Scapular disassociation away from the thorax often is most pronounced during the slow eccentric lowering of the extremities from overhead elevation rather than during the concentric phase of arm elevation, so the examiner should be sure to closely observe the scapula during all phases of movement (Fig. 6.3). Finally, scapular dysfunction does not always present according to the previously outlined clear patterns of dysfunction, and often multiple patterns of dysfunction can occur simultaneously due to the complex movement patterns of the human scapula [9, 14].

Kibler [14] has described the scapular assistance test (SAT). This test (Fig. 6.4) involves the assistance of the scapular through the examiner's hands applied to the inferior medial aspect of the scapula and the second hand at the superior base of the scapula to provide an upward rotation assistance type motion while the patient actively elevates the arm in either the scapular plane or sagittal plane. A negation of symptoms or increased ease in arm elevation during the application of this pressure as compared to the response of the patient doing the movement independently without the assistance of the examiner determines a positive or negative test.

One final scapular test or sign that can be used during evaluation of the shoulder is the flip sign. Kelley et al. [15] originally described this test which consists of resisted ER at the side by the examiner with close visual monitoring to the medial border of the scapula during the ER resistance applied by the examiner (Fig. 6.5). A positive flip sign is present when the medial border of the scapula "flips" away from the thorax and becomes more prominent. This indicates a loss of scapular stability and would direct the clinician to further evaluate the scapula and integrate exercise progressions aimed at the serratus anterior and trapezius force couple to stabilize the scapula [15].

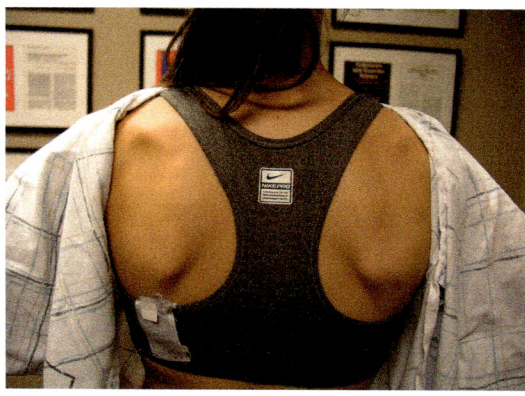

Fig. 6.3 Kibler type I inferior angle scapular dysfunction

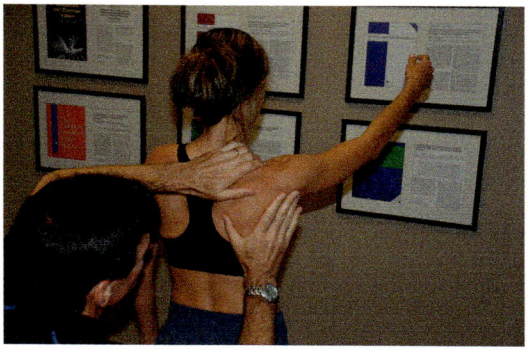

Fig. 6.4 Kibler scapular assistance test

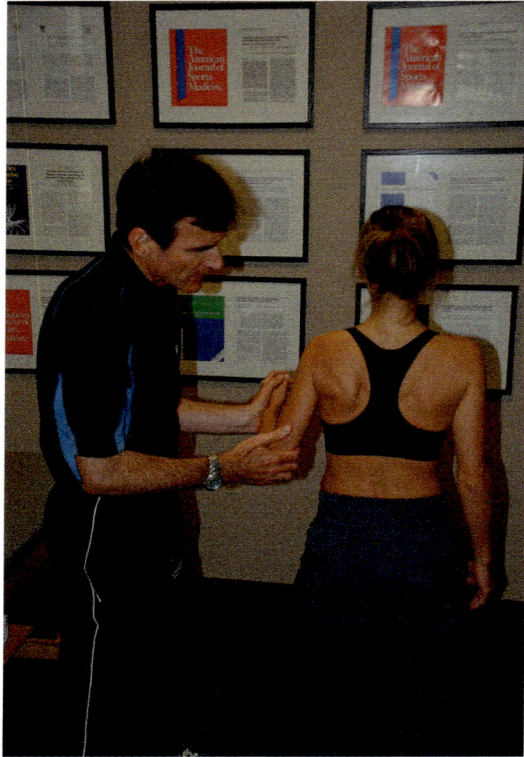

Fig. 6.5 Flip sign showing prominence of the scapula with external rotation manual muscle testing

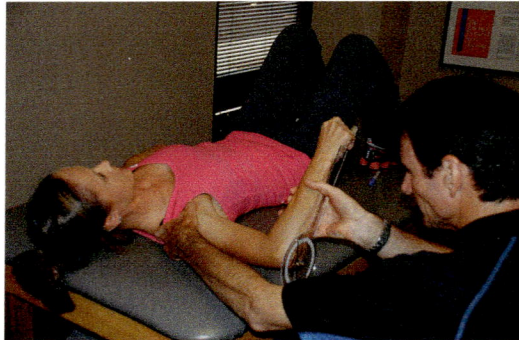

Fig. 6.6 Assessment of glenohumeral joint internal rotation range of motion with scapular stabilization

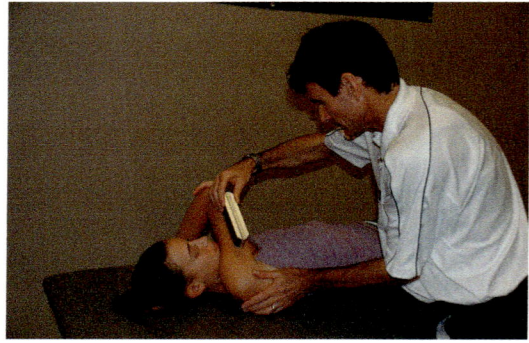

Fig. 6.7 Crossarm horizontal adduction measurement technique for the glenohumeral joint

6.2.3 Glenohumeral Joint Range of Motion Measurement

A detailed, isolated assessment of GH joint ROM is a key ingredient to a thorough evaluation of the patient with shoulder dysfunction. Measurement of several cardinal movements of the shoulder is important; however GH joint IR and ER have significant clinical importance and will be discussed in greater length and detail here. Selective loss of IR ROM on the dominant extremity has been consistently reported in patient populations as well as in overhead athletes such as elite tennis players [16–18], professional and youth baseball pitchers [17, 19–21], and softball players [21]. A goniometric method using scapular stabilization by the examiner (Fig. 6.6) to minimize the scapulothoracic contribution and or substitution is recommended by Ellenbecker and other authors to better isolate and represent GH rotational motion [1, 22, 23]. Additional ROM measures specifically recommended for the overhead athlete include horizontal (crossarm) adduction. This measure also assesses the status of the posterior shoulder and includes not only the posterior capsule but also the posterior muscle-tendon units as well [24–26]. Laudner et al. [26] and Shanley et al. [21] have published studies quantifying crossarm adduction ROM in overhead athletes. Both studies recommend the use of a supine technique where scapular stabilization is provided by the clinician's hand along the lateral aspect of the scapula providing a retraction containment type force (Fig. 6.7) while the arm is guided without overpressure into horizontal crossarm adduction.

6.3 Manual Muscle Testing (MMT)

While it is beyond the scope of this monograph to completely review all aspects of MMT, this section will cover several studies which have objectively identified positions for testing muscles in the shoulder complex, with particular emphasis on the rotator cuff [27]. The reader is referred to more detailed texts dedicated to MMT for comprehensive descriptions and theory on the technique itself [28, 29].

Kelley et al. [27] found the optimal muscle testing position for the supraspinatus to be at 90° of elevation, with the patient in a seated position. The scapular plane position was used (in this research this represented 45° of horizontal adduction from the coronal plane) with ER of the humerus such that the forearm was placed in neutral and the thumb was pointing upward toward the ceiling. This position was termed the full can testing position. Another frequently used test position to assess the strength of the supraspinatus muscle-tendon unit is the empty can test. This test position has been advocated by Jobe et al. [30] and has been found to have high levels of supraspinatus muscular activation using indwelling EMG [31]. Chalmers et al. [32] recently advocated a testing position called the "champagne toast" to better isolate supraspinatus function. This test showed higher EMG of the supraspinatus and decreased activation levels of the deltoid and recommended this position for clinical use.

Kelly et al. [27] reported the optimal position to test for infraspinatus strength is with the patient in a seated position, with 0° of GH joint elevation and in 45° of IR from neutral as pictured (Fig. 6.8).

An alternative position for testing the infraspinatus has been recommended by Jenp et al. [33]. They recommend testing the infraspinatus in 90° of elevation in the sagittal plane, with the arm in half-maximal ER.

Kelly et al. [27] did not specifically report on the teres minor muscle; however the use of the Patte test to best isolate the teres minor has been recommended by both Walch et al. [34] and Leroux et al. [35]. The position of the GH joint for the Patte test to isolate the teres minor has been reported as 90° of GH joint abduction in the scapular plane and 90° of ER (Fig. 6.9) [36]. Additionally, Kurokawa et al. [37] have recently delineated the muscular activity of external rotation strength testing in neutral and 90° of abduction concluding that greater infraspinatus activation is present with testing in neutral (arm at side) and greater teres minor activation is present with ER testing in 90° of abduction.

Kelley et al. [27] reported the optimal position for subscapularis muscular activation to be in the Gerber lift-off position (Fig. 6.10). This is consistent with Gerber [38] but in contrast to Stefko

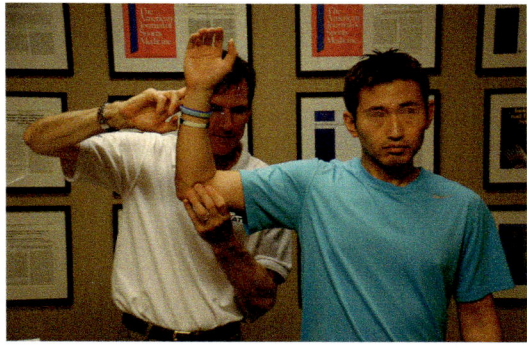

Fig. 6.9 Manual muscle test used to assess external rotation strength in 90° of abduction in the coronal plane

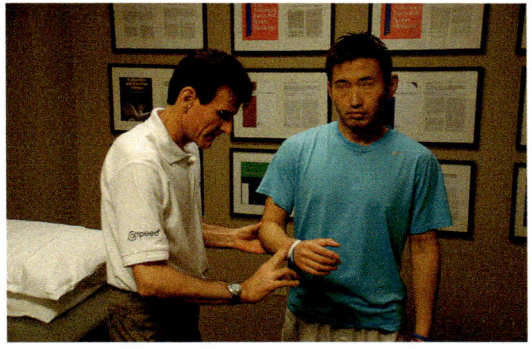

Fig. 6.8 External rotation manual muscle testing for assessing the strength of the infraspinatus

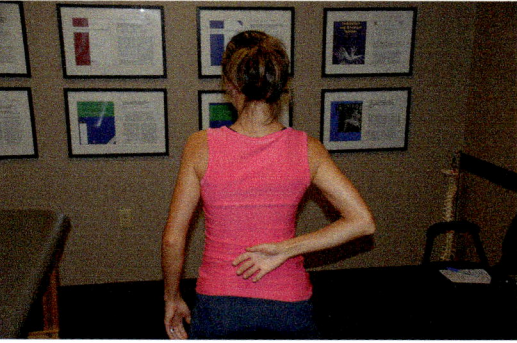

Fig. 6.10 Gerber lift-off test to assess strength and integrity of the subscapularis

et al. [39] who found the highest isolated muscular activity with the dorsal aspect of the hand placed up near the inferior border of the ipsilateral scapula.

6.4 Shoulder Special Tests

Discussion of several types of manual orthopedic tests is warranted as their inclusion in the comprehensive examination sequence gives the clinician the ability to determine the underlying cause or causes of shoulder dysfunction. Tests discussed in this chapter will include impingement, instability, rotator cuff, and labral tests.

6.4.1 Impingement Tests

Tests to identify GH impingement primarily involve the re-creation of subacromial shoulder pain using maneuvers that are known to reproduce and mimic functional positions in which significant subacromial compression is present. These motions involve forcible forward flexion (Neer impingement sign) [40] (Fig. 6.11), forced IR in the scapular plane (Hawkins impingement sign) [41] (Fig. 6.12), forced IR in the sagittal plane (coracoid impingement test) [42] (Fig. 6.13), and crossarm adduction impingement tests (Fig. 6.14) [2]. These tests all involve passive movement of the GH joint. The Yocum's impingement test involves the active combination of elevation with IR and can provide a valuable understanding of the patient's ability to control superior humeral head translation during active arm elevation in a compromised position [43] (Fig. 6.15). Valadie et al. [44] have provided objective evidence of the degree of encroachment and compression of the rotator cuff tendons against the coracoacromial arch during several impingement tests.

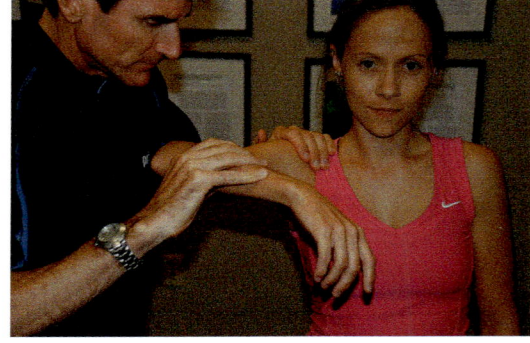

Fig. 6.12 Hawkins impingement test

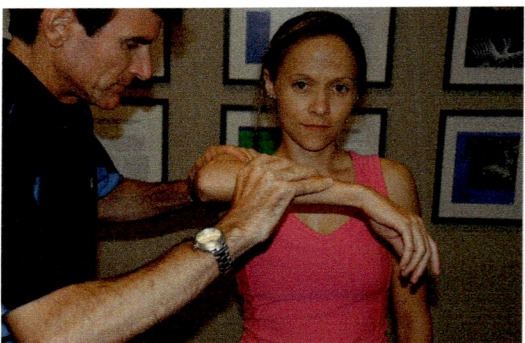

Fig. 6.13 Coracoid impingement test

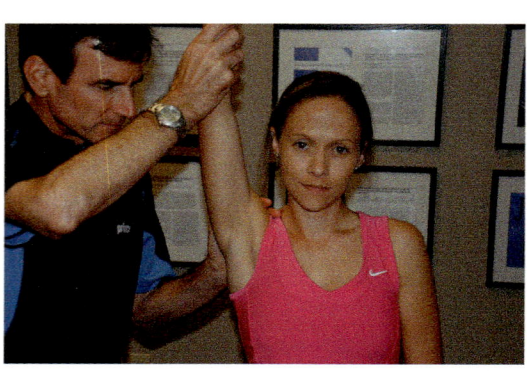

Fig. 6.11 Neer "forward flexion" impingement test

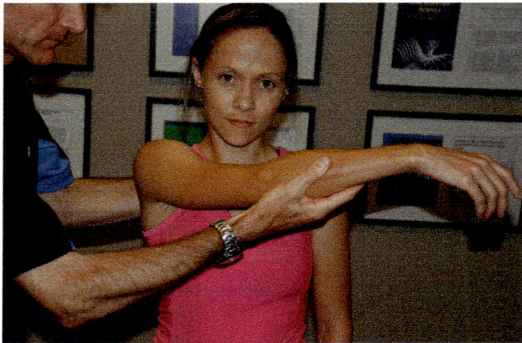

Fig. 6.14 Crossarm adduction impingement test

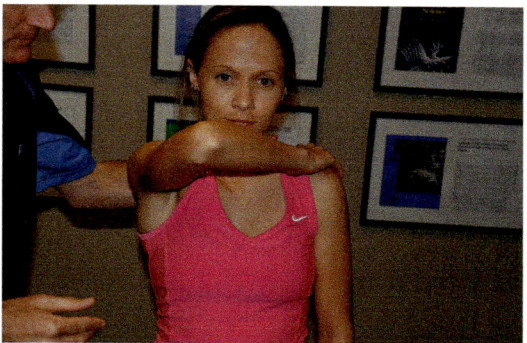

Fig. 6.15 Yocum's impingement test

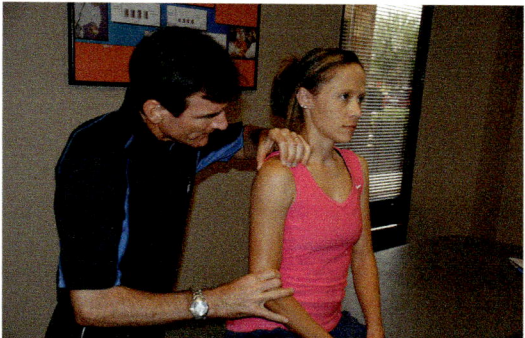

Fig. 6.16 MDI sulcus test

6.4.2 Instability Tests

Another major type of clinical test that must be included during the examination of the shoulder is instability testing. There are two main types of instability tests that are used and recommended. These are humeral head translation tests and provocation tests. Each type is presented in this section.

6.4.3 Humeral Head Translation Tests

Several authors believe that the most important tests used to identify shoulder joint instability are humeral head translation tests [45, 46]. These tests attempt to document the amount of movement of the humeral head relative to the glenoid through the use of carefully applied directional stresses to the proximal humerus. There are three main directions of humeral head translation testing, anterior, posterior, and inferior. Inferior humeral head translation testing is also referred to as multidirectional instability or MDI [45].

6.4.4 Multidirectional Instability Sulcus Tests (MDI Sulcus Sign)

One key test used to evaluate the stability of the shoulder is the MDI sulcus test (Fig. 6.16). This test is the primary test used to identify the patient with MDI of the GH joint. Excessive translation in the inferior direction during this test most often indicates a forthcoming pattern of excessive translation in an anterior or posterior direction or in both anterior and posterior directions [45]. This test, when performed in the neutral adducted position, directly assesses the integrity of the superior GH ligament and the coracohumeral ligament [47]. These ligaments are the primary stabilizing structures against inferior humeral head translation in the adducted GH position [48]. To perform this test, it is recommended that the patient be examined in the seated position with the arms in neutral adduction and resting gently in the patient's lap. The examiner grasps the distal aspect of the humerus using a firm but unassuming grip with one hand, while several brief, relatively rapid downward pulls are exerted to the humerus in an inferior (vertical) direction (Fig. 6.16). A visible "sulcus sign" (tethering of the skin between the lateral acromion and the humerus from the increase in inferior translation of the humeral head and the widening subacromial space) is usually present in patients with MDI [49].

6.4.5 Anterior and Posterior Translation (Drawer) Tests

Gerber and Ganz [46] and McFarland et al. [45] believe that testing for anterior and posterior shoulder laxity is best performed with the patient in the supine position because of greater inherent relaxation of the patient. This test allows the patient's extremity to be tested in multiple positions of GH joint abduction, thus selectively stressing specific portions of the GH joint anterior capsule and capsular ligaments. It is important to note that the direction of translation must be along the line of the GH joint, with an anteromedial and posterolateral direction used because of the 30° version of the glenoid [50]. This is accomplished by ensuring that the examiner places the patient's GH joint in the scapular plane as pictured (see Fig. 6.17). Testing for anterior translation is performed in the range between 0° and 30° of abduction, between 30° and 60° of abduction, and at 90° of abduction to test the integrity of the superior, middle, and inferior GH ligaments, respectively [48, 49]. Posterior translation testing typically is performed at 90° of abduction because no distinct thickenings of the capsule are noted, with the exception of the posterior band of the inferior GH ligament complex [48]. Grading (assessing the translation) for this test is performed using the classification of Altchek and Dines [51]. This classification system defines grade I translation as humeral translation within the glenoid without edge loading or translation of the humerus over the glenoid rim. Grade II represents translation of the humeral head up over the glenoid rim with spontaneous return on removal of the stress. The presence of grade II translation in an anterior or posterior direction without symptoms does not indicate instability but instead merely represents laxity of the GH joint. Unilateral increases in GH translation in the presence of shoulder pain and disability can ultimately lead to the diagnosis of GH joint instability [1, 52]. Grade III translation, which is not seen clinically in orthopedic and sports physical therapy, involves translation of the humeral head over the glenoid rim without relocation upon removal of stress.

6.4.6 Subluxation/Relocation Test

One final instability test to be discussed in this section is the subluxation relocation test. This test may be one of the most important tests used to identify subtle anterior instability in the overhead-throwing athlete or the individual with symptoms in overhead positions. The subluxation relocation test is a subtle form of provocation test that does not measure actual humeral head translation. Originally described by Jobe [30], the subluxation/relocation test is designed to identify subtle anterior instability of the GH joint. Fowler described the diagnostic quandary of microinstability (subtle anterior instability) versus rotator cuff injury or both in swimmers and advocated the use of this important test to assist in the diagnosis. The subluxation/relocation test is performed with the patient's shoulder held and stabilized in the patient's maximal end range of ER at 90° of abduction in the coronal plane. The examiner then provides a mild anterior subluxation force (Fig. 6.18a) being sure to exert the subluxation force to the proximal humerus to create anterior translational stress or loading. The patient is then asked if this subluxation force reproduces his or her symptoms. Reproduction of patient symptoms of anterior or posterior shoulder pain with subluxation leads the examiner to reposition his hand on the anterior aspect of the patient's shoulder and perform a posterior-lateral directed force, using a soft, cupped hand to minimize anterior shoulder pain from the hand-shoulder (e.g., examiner-patient) interface (see Fig. 6.18b). Failure to reproduce the patient's symptoms with end-range ER and 90° of abduction leads the examiner to reattempt the subluxation maneuver with 110° and 120° of abduction. Reproduction of anterior or posterior shoulder pain with the subluxation portion of this test, with subsequent diminution or disappearance of anterior or posterior shoulder pain with the relocation maneuver, constitutes a positive test. Production of apprehension with any position of abduction during the anteriorly directed subluxation force phase of testing would indicate

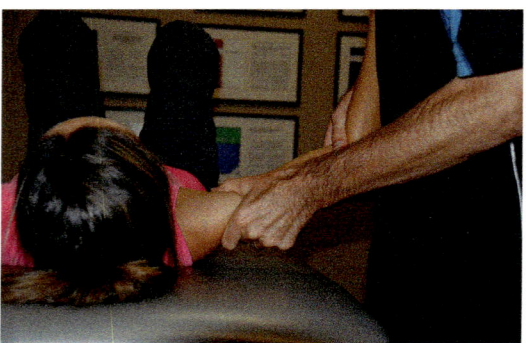

Fig. 6.17 Supine anterior humeral head translation test

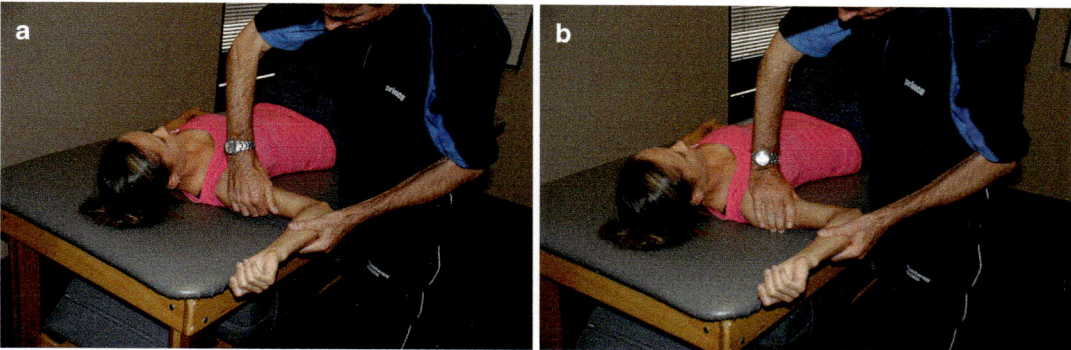

Fig. 6.18 (**a**) Subluxation relocation test (subluxation). (**b**) Relocation

occult anterior instability. The primary ramifications of a positive test would indicate subtle anterior instability and secondary GH joint impingement (anterior pain) or posterior or internal impingement in the presence of posterior pain with this maneuver.

6.4.7 Beighton Hypermobility Index

The Beighton hypermobility scale or index was originally introduced by Carter and Wilkinson [53] and modified by Beighton and Horan [54]. This scale is comprised of nine individual tests each assessed bilaterally (except for trunk flexion) which are used to assess the generalized hypermobility of the individual. These tests include passive hyperextension of the fifth MCP joint, passive thumb opposition to the forearm, bilateral elbow and knee hyperextension, and standing trunk flexion with knees fully extended. Several authors have documented the psychometric properties of the Beighton scale with reliability estimates ranging from 0.74 to 0.84 [55]. Several cutoff criteria have been used to determine how many of the individual tests must be positive to rate an individual as hypermobile with no overwhelming consensus [56].

6.4.8 Rotator Cuff Testing

Several clinical tests are presently recommended for use to assess the integrity of the rotator cuff muscle-tendon unit. These include tests that assess strength of the rotator cuff (covered previously in Sect. 6.3) as well as tests to provoke symptoms and pain reproduction.

6.4.9 Empty Can Test

In addition to using the empty or full can test to solely assess muscle strength of the rotator cuff, Itoi et al. [57] tested the effectiveness of both the full can and empty can test to predict the presence of a rotator cuff tear. Their results showed that greater predictive values were present when weakness was encountered during the use of both the full can and empty can tests as compared to when pain was encountered during testing. There was no significant difference in the ability of these two tests to predict a full-thickness rotator cuff tear, and the author concluded that both test positions could be used for supraspinatus testing. A recent study has introduced the champagne toast test for the supraspinatus [32]. This test was found with EMG to better isolate the supraspinatus and is performed similar to a manual muscle test in a position simulating that used when "toasting" with a glass of champagne [32].

6.4.10 Subscapularis Tests

Three tests are commonly used to assess the integrity of the subscapularis muscle-tendon unit. These include the Gerber lift-off position (Fig. 6.10), Napoleon or belly-press test (Fig. 6.19), and the bear hugger sign (Fig. 6.20) [58]. Recent research has assessed the effects of subscapularis muscular activation in each of

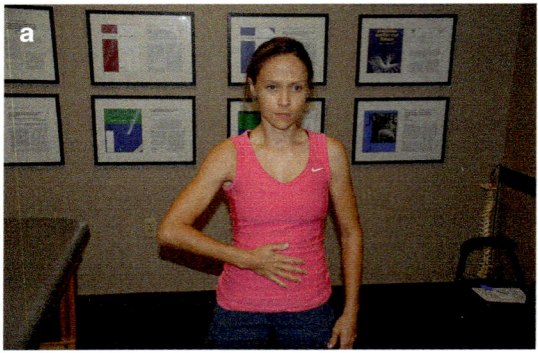 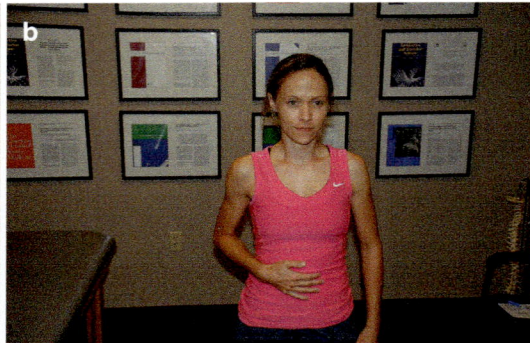

Fig. 6.19 Belly-press or Napoleon sign for subscapularis testing (Negative Test on Left, positive test sign on right with wrist flexed)

these three clinical tests as well as slight variations (+/) 10° positional changes to the reference positions described in the literature. This study concluded that all three tests (Gerber lift-off/ Napoleon and bear hugger) isolate the subscapularis and are recommended for use to evaluate the integrity of the subscapularis muscle-tendon unit.

6.4.11 Labral Testing

Many clinical examination maneuvers have been published in the literature to assess the integrity of the glenoid labrum. Both general labral tests that can be used to identify labral pathology in any region of the labrum as well as site-specific (i.e., superior labrum) tests will be described. It is beyond the scope of this chapter to describe a generous number of labral tests, and for that the reader is referred to texts that cover labral testing in a more complete fashion as well as contain diagnostic accuracy information for each test [1, 2, 59], Hegedus et al. [60], Hegedus[61], Cook et al. [62], and Michener et al. [63].

Many general labral tests such as the clunk test, circumduction test (Fig. 6.21), and compression rotation test utilize a long-axis compression exerted through the humerus to scour the glenoid and to attempt to trap the torn or detached labral fragment between the humeral head and the glenoid, much like a mortar and pestle-type mechanism [64–67]. The circumduction and clunk tests

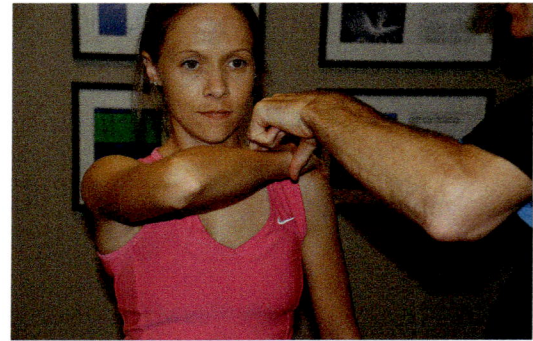

Fig. 6.20 Bear hugger sign for subscapularis testing

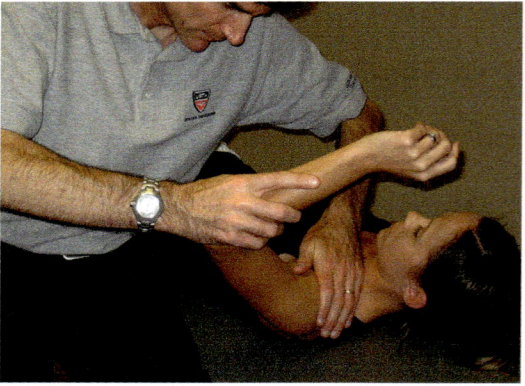

Fig. 6.21 Circumduction test

literally scour the perimeter of the glenoid trying to trap the labral tear with the compression and rotation performed by the examiner during the test. One key clinical application with these tests is the frequent finding of crepitus and grating during the movements as well as increases in humeral head translation that can create "noise" from the joint. These tests typically when positive will recreate the pain experienced by the patient. Noise generation or a feeling of traversing across the glenoid rim does not indicate a torn labrum and can fool an inexperienced clinician during the interpretation of the exam findings.

Of all the clinical tests in the orthopedic and sports medicine literature today, there are likely more clinical tests described for identifying superior labral lesions than for any other structure in the shoulder. Tests that specifically utilize muscular tension exerted in the bicep long head to tension the superior labrum include the O'Brien active compression test (Fig. 6.22a, b), the Mimori test, speeds test [1, 68], and the biceps load test. These tests all place or develop a traction-type force through and active contraction of the bicep muscle by the patient resisted by the examiner [1, 69]. Additional tests for the glenoid labrum utilize the combined position of abduction and external rotation to create or mimic the peel-back mechanism of the cocking position of the throwing motion. These tests include the ER supination test, dynamic labral shear tests [70] (Fig. 6.23), and the crank test. One additional test called the anterior slide test [63, 71] utilizes internal rotation rather than external rotation in the hands-on-hips position to provoke the labrum through an anteriorly and superiorly directed movement by the examiner. A positive anterior slide test (reproduction of pain and/or a click or pop) and a combined finding of a clinical history of popping catching and clicking have been found to have moderate diagnostic utility for type II–IV labral lesions [63].

6.5 Examination of the Elbow

Stability of the elbow joint is a function of joint congruity, capsuloligamentous integrity, and balanced arm and forearm musculature. Between 20° and 120° of elbow flexion, stability is maintained by soft-tissue restraints of which the medial collateral ligament (UCL) is the most important [72, 73]. In the kinetic chain, the elbow functions as a link between the body and racquet, allowing for the transfer of considerable kinetic energy [74].

High-speed video analysis studies have demonstrated that during a serve in tennis the elbow moves from 116° to 20° of flexion within 0.21 s, with an angular velocity of 982°/s for elbow extension [75]. Clearly, the elbow must absorb extreme forces during tennis activity. The decreased internal shoulder rotation found in many overhead athletes often results in compensatory increased internal rotation forces in the elbow joint.

The "valgus extension overload" syndrome in overhead athletes results from high valgus forces combined with rapid extension of the elbow. The medial elbow experiences significant tensile force,

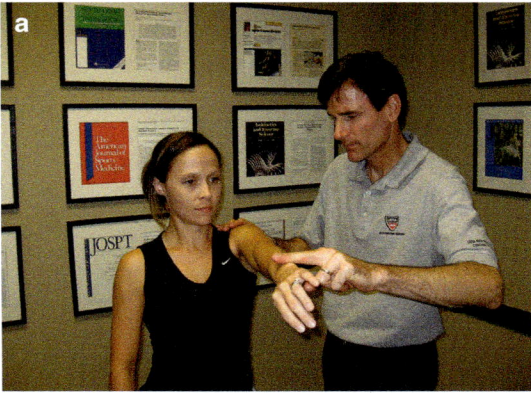
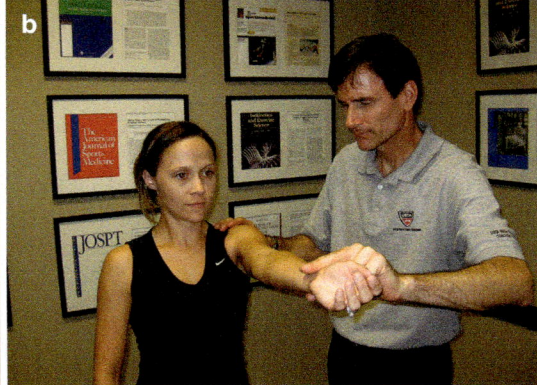

Fig. 6.22 O'Brien active compression test. (**a**) Pronated, internal rotation initial test position; (**b**) supinated external rotation second test position

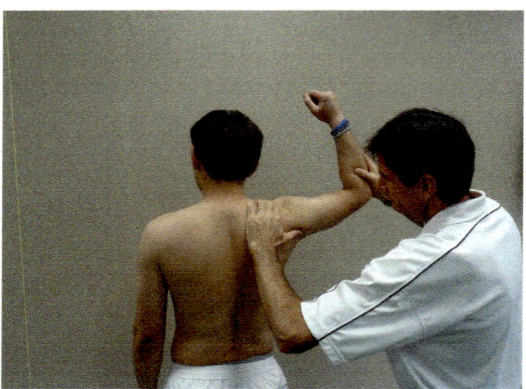

Fig. 6.23 Dynamic labral shear test for SLAP lesions

while the lateral elbow is under compressive force load and the posterior compartment is sustaining shear force loads.

In addition to the effects of "valgus extension overload" from serving, tennis players are also vulnerable to great stress on the medial and lateral musculo-ligamentous structures during ground strokes, especially on the lateral side in "one-handed" backhands [74].

In the physical examination of the elbow in tennis players, the examining practitioner must take into account the high loads which are placed across the elbow joint during this sport. A systemic anatomic approach can aid in the diagnosis of the myriad of musculoskeletal injuries in the elbow of elite tennis players.

6.6 Proximal Upper Extremity Examination

An assessment of the cervical spine should be performed in the evaluation of any upper extremity injury in order to rule out any cervical radiculitis symptoms which can mimic primary elbow dysfunction in some cases. Palpation, cervical range of motion (ROM), and a Spurling's Test should be performed. Resting posture and any asymmetry or deformity should be included in the observation portion of the exam.

Since thoracic outlet syndrome can present as vague arm and elbow pain, an Adson's test can be performed to rule it out [76]. The patient's neck is extended and rotated away from the examined side, and the elbow is held in extension while the radial pulse is palpated. The shoulder is abducted, extended, and externally rotated while the patient opens and closes their fist. A positive result is considered if there is an absent or decreased palpable pulse strength.

6.7 Shoulder

The shoulder girdle should be assessed as per discussed in the beginning of this chapter.

6.8 Clinical Examination of the Elbow

Normal carrying angle of 11–14° of valgus in men and 13–16° in women should be seen. Larger carrying angles can be seen in skeletally immature athletes due to medial epicondylar hypertrophy. Assessment of normal active and passive ROM should reveal 0–140° flexion with 80° of pronation and supination. Loss of motion compared to the contralateral limb could be a result of contraction, swelling/effusion, loose bodies, or impingement. It should be noted which motion is painful or blocked and at what point in the normal motion arc the symptom occurs. Osteophytes in the coronoid fossa can present as a block during flexion ROM, and similarly, olecranon fossa osteophytes can result in blocks during extension ROM. If encountered at the terminal arc of motion, suspect osteophytes. If encountered at mid-arc, the block to ROM may be from an osteochondral lesion. While extension is normally decreased after elbow injuries, in overhead athletes loss of terminal extension may be from a developmental flexion contracture.

6.8.1 Lateral Elbow

Bony landmarks such as the radial head, lateral epicondyle, and tip of the olecranon should be palpated. Any joint effusion can be felt in between the triangle formed by these bony landmarks, which is known as the "soft spot." Palpation of the radial head should be performed in active and passive supination and pronation, checking for any subluxation or frank dislocation. Additionally, any tenderness or clicking in the radiocapitellar joint should be noted. Inflamed bursa, loose bodies, or articular radiocapitellar lesions can cause pain in the lateral elbow during passive ROM testing.

In some cases, long-term load transmission and subsequent degeneration of the articular surface may lead to osteochondritis dissecans (OCD) of the capitellum. OCD of the capitellum will often present as tenderness over the radiocapitellar joint and is commonly associated with a loss of 15°–20° of extension. The "active radiocapitellar compression test," which can be positive for OCD lesions, elicits pain in the lateral compartment of the elbow when the patient pronates and supinates the forearm with the elbow axially loaded in extension [77].

Inflamed plicae can be a cause of snapping or catching symptoms accompanied by lateral elbow pain [78]. A palpable snap can be encountered during provocative testing and is considered a positive test. An anterior radiocapitellar plica can be painful during passive elbow flexion with the forearm pronated and under a valgus load. A posterior plica is painful in an extended elbow with the forearm supinated under a valgus load [79].

Although rarely encountered in elite tennis players, up to 50% of those who play recreational tennis regularly will develop lateral elbow tendinopathy classically referred to as "tennis elbow." This syndrome can cause pain with wrist extension, pain while gripping, and even decreased grip strength [80]. Tenderness can be elicited anterior and distal to the lateral epicondyle at the origin of extensor carpi radialis brevis. The Cozen test can diagnose for lateral epicondylitis and is performed by reproducing pain in an extended elbow during passive wrist flexion and resisted wrist extension.

6.8.2 Medial Elbow

The only bony prominence on the medial side is the medial epicondyle. The flexor/pronator mass and UCL attach at this site. During repetitive overhead activity and groundstrokes, this tendinous insertion is subject to recurring and significant tensile loading. This often results in flexor-pronator strains and micro-tearing (golfer's elbow). In addition to producing active pronation and wrist extension, the flexor/pronator mass acts as a dynamic stabilizer of medial aspect of the elbow. It reduces the tension on the ulnar collateral ligament during high torque activity [81].

The UCL bears the brunt of the intense valgus force through the tennis player's elbow. Tenderness can be elicited anywhere along the course of its anterior oblique ligament (AOL) component which courses from the inferior medial epicondyle to the sublime tubercle which lies on the medial side of the coronoid process of the proximal ulna. The anterior oblique ligament (AOL) is the main static stabilizer of the MCL complex from 20° to 120° of flexion. The posterior oblique ligament originates deep to the AOL and fans out to its insertion on the medial ulnar sigmoid notch [82].

Athletes with a UCL injury will often experience tenderness localized approximately 2 cm distal to the medial epicondyle or more commonly in the acute setting at the medial joint line. The absence of pain with resisted wrist flexion and the location of pain slightly posterior to the common flexor-pronator origin can help differentiate medial epicondylitis from UCL injury. Yet, it is important to note that these two pathologic processes may coexist in the same injured elbow [82–84].

The diagnosis of a UCL injury is made by evaluation of the functional integrity of the ligament complex. There have been several provocative tests described over the years that evaluate each portion of the UCL complex. Classically, UCL ligament evaluation is carried out by providing a valgus stress to a well-stabilized humerus with the elbow in approximately 20°–30° of flexion (Fig. 6.24). This degree of flexion brings the olecranon out of the posterior fossa and limits the osseous contribution to medial elbow stability. This test has been found to stress the anterior band of the AOL. A positive test is manifested by increased medial joint space widening compared to the contralateral elbow and pain provocation [82–85].

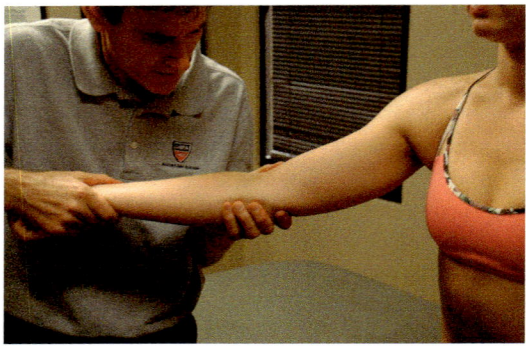

Fig. 6.24 UCL ligament is evaluated by providing a valgus stress to a well-stabilized humerus with the elbow in approximately 20°–30° of flexion

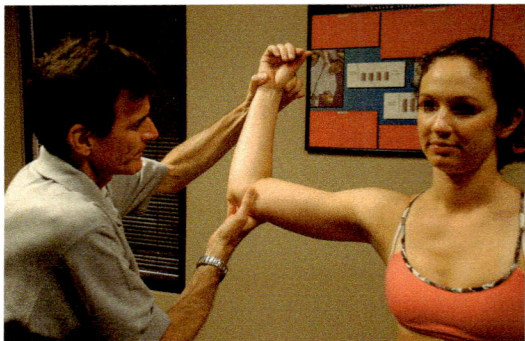

Fig. 6.26 The "moving valgus stress test" more accurately assesses UCL continuity or injury

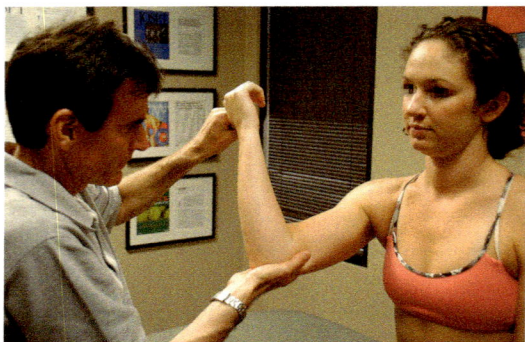

Fig. 6.25 The "milking maneuver" demonstrated here tests the posterior band of the AOL

Testing the posterior band of the AOL can be performed by administering the "milking maneuver." In this test the patient brings the affected elbow into flexion beyond 90° and uses the opposite hand to grasp the thumb and apply a valgus moment to the elbow [84, 85]. The UCL is palpated by the physician to evaluate tenderness and joint space widening, which, when present, confers a positive test (Fig. 6.25). The contralateral arm should also be examined for comparison. Modifications to this test have been proposed that decrease the amount of flexion such that the coronoid does not engage the anterior fossa and contribute additional osseous stability.

The "moving valgus stress test" was described by O'Driscoll and Lawton in 2005 [86] and provides a dynamic assessment of UCL insufficiency. To perform the moving valgus stress test, the examiner applies and maintains a constant moderate valgus torque to the fully flexed elbow and then quickly extends the elbow. Medial elbow pain reproduced during an arc of motion from 70° to 120° of flexion denotes a positive test (Fig. 6.26). In their study of 21 patients, the authors found the test to be 100% sensitive and 75% specific when compared to surgical inspection.

Ulnar nerve pathology is frequently encountered in tennis players with medial elbow pain. It should be palpated along its course from its emergence at the medial intermuscular septum, into the cubital tunnel, and then as it courses between the two heads of the flexor carpi ulnaris. The recurrent forces and impact encountered by the nerve due to its proximity to the elbow joint can cause neuritis. As a result of increased medial elbow laxity due to an injured MCL, the ulnar nerve can be stretched and damaged. Pressure over the ulnar nerve while the elbow is maximally flexed replicates this pain. Gross dislocation can be assessed by visual inspection as the patient actively flexes and extends the elbow. Hypermobility can also be assessed by having the patient maximally flex the elbow with the forearm supinated, the examiner's finger placed on the medial epicondyle, and the arm brought into extension. If the nerve is trapped anterior to the examiner's finger, it is considered to be dislocating [87].

6.8.3 Posterior Elbow

Palpation of the triceps tendon and tip of the olecranon should reveal any triceps tendinopathy. In order to best palpate the posterolateral or posteromedial olecranon, flex the elbow 20°–30° to relax the triceps. Olecranon bursitis will present as posterior elbow swelling, bogginess, and erythema. The long, lateral, and medial heads of the triceps should be palpated individually at their convergence point to assess for tendinopathy or injury.

The "snapping triceps syndrome" can be encountered as well. This clinical entity occurs when the distal band of the medial triceps tendon subluxes over the medial epicondyle. If it occurs concurrent with ulnar nerve instability, two separate snaps may be palpated during elbow flexion. This has been reported in tennis players [88].

In younger players, repetitive acceleration and deceleration of the upper extremity can result in stress fractures of the ulna. This injury should be considered in situations where there is pain in forced extension in serving especially in younger athletes and tenderness to palpation on the olecranon distal to the tip. These injuries can be quite subtle, and in cases where stress fracture is considered, proper imaging including X-rays and bone scans should be carried out [89].

The valgus extension overload (VEO) mechanism described above also causes a shear force between the medial portion of the tip of the olecranon and the olecranon fossa. Under supraphysiologic stress, the posteromedial elbow undergoes chondrolysis, loose body formation, and reactive osteophyte formation [90, 91]. Clinically, there is a resulting loss of extension, crepitus, and discomfort. Assessment of VEO syndrome can be performed by repeatedly bringing the elbow from near full extension (20° flexion) into a fully extended position. While performing this motion, the examiner palpates the posteromedial olecranon for tenderness. Next, the test is repeated with a valgus force applied, to see if the posteromedial pain is from VEO itself or if there is any additional associated instability [91].

6.8.4 Anterior Elbow

Biceps tendinosis or frank rupture is the most important diagnosis to consider when evaluating the anterior elbow. Distal biceps rupture is clearly a very rare phenomenon; however in cases of acute trauma with pain and deformity, it must be considered. The "reverse 'Popeye' sign," or proximal retraction of the biceps muscle belly, can be seen on visual inspection often associated with acute ecchymosis. Strength testing will reveal decreased supination strength. The hook test can be used to evaluate for the presence of an intact distal biceps tendon. With the patient's shoulder abducted and elbow flexed to 90°, the examiner hooks an index finger laterally under the tendon as the patient attempts active supination. A positive test is one in which no tendon can be felt [92].

More commonly, these athletes will present with distal biceps tendinitis or an inflamed distal biceps bursa. They may present with localized pain at tendon insertion into the radial tuberosity or a painful clicking sensation with active forearm rotation and flexion.

Conclusion

Care for the injured shoulder and elbow in elite overhand tennis athletes requires a comprehensive history and physical examination as well as appropriate diagnostic imaging and testing. The anatomic diagnostic approach to examination including the cervical spine, shoulder, elbow, and wrist described in this chapter allows for a thorough evaluation of all causes of elbow pathology which might affect the injured athlete. With this information, proper treatment plans can be undertaken to get the player back to the competition safely and expeditiously.

References

1. Ellenbecker TS. Clinical examination of the shoulder. St Louis, MO: Elsevier Saunders; 2004.
2. Ellenbecker TS, Wilk KE. Sport therapy for the shoulder. Champaign, IL: Human Kinetics Publishers; 2017.
3. Priest JD, Nagel DA. Tennis shoulder. Am J Sports Med. 1976;4(1):28–42.
4. Ellenbecker TS. Chap. 10 Musculoskeletal screening for the elite and developing tennis player. In: DiGiacomo G, Ellenbecker T, Kibler WB, editors. Tennis medicine. Cham: Springer; 2018.
5. Young SW, Dakic J, Stroia K, Nguyen ML, Harris AH, Safran MR. High incidence of infraspinatus

muscle atrophy in elite professional female tennis players. Am J Sports Med. 2015;43(8):1989–93.
6. Piatt BE, Hawkins RJ, Fritz RC, Ho CP, Wolf E, Schickendantz M. Clinical evaluation and treatment of spinoglenoid notch ganglion cysts. J Shoulder Elb Surg. 2002;11:600–4.
7. Kibler WB. Role of the scapula in the overhead throwing motion. Contemp Orthop. 1991;22:525.
8. Bourne DA, Choo AM, Regan WD, MacIntyre DL, Oxland TR. Three-dimensional rotation of the scapula during functional movements: an in-vivo study in healthy volunteers. J Shoulder Elb Surg. 2007;16(2):150–62.
9. Kibler WB, Uhl TL, Maddux JW, Brooks PV, Zeller B, McMullen J. Qualitative clinical evaluation of scapular dysfunction: a reliability study. J Shoulder Elb Surg. 2002;11:550–6.
10. Ellenbecker TS, Kibler WB, Bailie DS, Caplinger R, Davies GJ, Riemann BL. Reliability of scapular evaluation in professional baseball players. Clin Orthop Relat Res. 2012;470:1540–4.
11. McClure PW, Tate AR, Kareha S, Irwin D, Zlupko E. A clinical method for identifying scapular dyskinesis, Part 1: Reliability. J Athl Train. 2009;44:160–4.
12. Tate AR, McClure P, Kareha S, Irwin D, Barbe MF. A clinical method for identifying scapular dyskinesis, Part 2: Validity. J Athl Train. 2009;44:165–73.
13. Tate AR, McClure P, Kareha S, Irwin D, Barbe MF. A clinical method for identifying scapular dyskinesis, Part 1. J Athl Train. 2009;44:165–73.
14. Kibler WB. The role of the scapula in athletic shoulder function. Am J Sports Med. 1998;26:325–37.
15. Kelley MJ, Kane TE, Leggin BG. Spinal accessory nerve palsy: associated signs and symptoms. J Orthop Sports Phys Ther. 2008;38(2):78–86.
16. Ellenbecker TS. Shoulder internal and external rotation strength and range of motion of highly skilled junior tennis players. Isokinet Exerc Sci. 1992;2:1–8.
17. Ellenbecker TS, Roetert EP, Bailie DS, Davies GJ, Brown SW. Glenohumeral joint total rotation range of motion in elite tennis players and baseball pitchers. Med Sci Sports Exerc. 2002;34(12):2052–6.
18. Chandler TJ, Kibler WB, Uhl TL, Wooten B, Kiser A, Stone E. Flexibility comparisons of elite junior tennis players to other athletes. Am J Sports Med. 1990;18:134–6.
19. Wilk KE, Macrina LC, Arrigo C. Passive range of motion characteristics in the overhead baseball pitcher and their implications for rehabilitation. Clin Orthop Relat Res. 2012;470:1586–94.
20. Wilk KE, Macrina LC, Fleisig GS, Porterfield R, Simpson CD II, Harker P, Paparesta N, Andrews JR. Correlation of glenohumeral internal rotation deficit and total rotational motion to shoulder injuries in professional baseball pitchers. Am J Sports Med. 2011;39:329–35.
21. Shanley E, Rauh MJ, Michener LA, Ellenbecker TS, Garrison JC, Thigpen CA. Shoulder range of motion measures as risk factors for shoulder and elbow injuries in high school softball and baseball players. Am J Sports Med. 2011;39:1997–2006.
22. Ellenbecker TS, Roetert EP, Piorkowski P. Shoulder internal and external rotation range of motion of elite junior tennis players: a comparison of two protocols (abstract). J Orthop Sports Phys Ther. 1993;17:A65.
23. Wilk KE, Reinold MM, Macrina LC, Porterfield R, Devine KM, Suarez K, Andrews JR. Glenohumeral internal rotation measurements differ depending on stabilization techniques. Sports Health. 2009;1(2):131–6.
24. Tyler TF, Roy T, Nicholas SJ, Gleim GW. Reliability and validity of a new method of measuring posterior shoulder tightness. J Orthop Sports Phys Ther. 1999;29(5):262–74.
25. Tyler TF, Nicholas SJ, Lee SJ, Mullaney M, McHugh MP. Correction of posterior shoulder tightness is associated with symptom resolution in patients with internal impingement. Am J Sports Med. 2010;38(1):114–9.
26. Laudner KG, Stanek JM, Meister K. Assessing posterior shoulder contracture: the reliability and validity of measuring glenohumeral joint horizontal adduction. J Athl Train. 2006;41(4):375–80.
27. Kelly BT, Kadrmas WH, Speer KP. The manual muscle examination for rotator cuff strength. An electromyographic investigation. Am J Sports Med. 1996;24:581–8.
28. Daniels L, Worthingham C. Muscle testing: techniques of manual examination. 4th ed. Philadelphia, PA: WB Saunders; 1980.
29. Kendall FD, McCreary EK. Muscle testing and function. 3rd ed. Baltimore, MD: Williams and Wilkins; 1983.
30. Jobe FW, Bradley JP. The diagnosis and nonoperative treatment of shoulder injuries in athletes. Clin Sports Med. 1989;8:419–37.
31. Malanga GA, Jemp YN, Growney E, An K. EMG analysis of shoulder positioning in testing and strengthening the supraspinatus. Med Sci Sports Exerc. 1996;28:661–4.
32. Chalmers PN, Cvetanovich GL, Kupfer N, Wimmer MA, Verma NN, Cole BJ, Romeo AA, Nicholson GP. The champagne toast position isolates the supraspinatus better than the Jobe test: an electromyographic study of shoulder physical examination tests. J Shoulder Elb Surg. 2016;25(2):322–9.
33. Jenp YN, Malanga BA, Gowney ES, An KN. Activation of the rotator cuff in generating isometric shoulder rotation torque. Am J Sports Med. 1996;24:477–85.
34. Walch F, Boulahia A, Calderone S, Robinson AH. The 'dropping' and 'hornblower's' signs in evaluation of rotator cuff tears. J Bone Joint Surg Br. 1998;80(4):624–8.
35. Leroux JL, Codine P, Thomas E, Pocholle M, Mailhe D, Flotman F. Isokinetic evaluation of rotational strength in normal shoulders and shoulders with impingement syndrome. Clin Orthop. 1994;304:108–15.

36. Patte D, Goutallier D, Monpierre H, Debeyre J. Over-extension lesions. Rev Chir Orthop. 1988;74:314–8.
37. Kurokawa D, Sano H, Nagamoto H, Omi R, Shinozaki N, Watanuki S, Kishimoto KN, Yamamoto N, Hiraoka K, Tashiro M, Itoi E. Muscle activity pattern of the shoulder external rotators differs in adduction an abduction: an analysis using positron emission tomography. J Shoulder Elb Surg. 2014;23:658–64.
38. Gerber C, Krushell RJ. Isolated rupture of the tendon of the subscapularis muscle. Clinical features in 16 cases. J Bone Joint Surg Br. 1991;73:389–94.
39. Stefko JM, Jobe FW, Vander Wilde RS, Carden E, Pink M. Electromyographic and nerve block analysis of the subscapularis liftoff test. J Shoulder Elb Surg. 1997;6:347–55.
40. Neer CS, Welsh RP. The shoulder in sports. Orthop Clin North Am. 1977;8:583–91.
41. Hawkins RJ, Kennedy JC. Impingement syndrome in athletes. Am J Sports Med. 1980;8:151–8.
42. Davies GJ, DeCarlo MS. Examination of the shoulder complex, Current concepts in rehabilitation of the shoulder. La Crosse, WI: Sports Physical Therapy Association; 1995.
43. Yocum LA. Assessing the shoulder. Clin Sports Med. 1983;2:281–9.
44. Valadie AL III, Jobe CM, Pink MM, Ekman EF, Jobe FW. Anatomy of provocative tests for impingement syndrome of the shoulder. J Shoulder Elb Surg. 2000;9(1):36–46.
45. McFarland EG, Torpey BM, Carl LA. Evaluation of shoulder laxity. Sports Med. 1996;22:264–72.
46. Gerber C, Ganz R. Clinical assessment of instability of the shoulder with special reference to anterior and posterior drawer tests. J Bone Joint Surg Br. 1984;66(4):551–6.
47. Pagnani MJ, Warren RF. Stabilizers of the glenohumeral joint. J Shoulder Elb Surg. 1994;3:73–90.
48. O'Brien SJ, Neves MC, Arnvoczky SP, et al. The anatomy and histology of the inferior glenohumeral ligament complex of the shoulder. Am J Sports Med. 1990;18:449–56.
49. Hawkins RJ, Mohtadi NGH. Clinical evaluation of shoulder instability. Clin J Sports Med. 1991;1:59–64.
50. Saha AK. Mechanism of shoulder movements and a plea for the recognition of "zero position" of the glenohumeral joint. Clin Orthop. 1983;(173):3–10.
51. Altchek DW, Dines DW. The surgical treatment of anterior instability: selective capsular repair. Oper Tech Sports Med. 1993;1:285–92.
52. Hawkins RJ, Schulte JP, Janda DH, Huckell GH. Translation of the glenohumeral joint with the patient under anesthesia. J Shoulder Elb Surg. 1996;5:286–92.
53. Carter C, Wilkinson J. Persistent joint laxity and congenital dislocation of the hip. J Bone Joint Surg Br. 1964;46:40–5.
54. Beighton P, Horan F. Orthopaedic aspects of the Ehlers-Danlos syndrome. J Bone Joint Surg Br. 1969;51(3):444–53.
55. Juul-Kristensen B, Rogind H, Jensen DV, Remvig L. Inter-examiner reproducibility of tests and critera for generalized joint hypermobility and benign joint hypermobility syndrome. Rheumatology (Oxford). 2007;46(12):1835–41.
56. Cameron KL, Duffey ML, DeBerardino TM, Stoneman PD, Jones CJ, Owens BD. Association of generalized joint hypermobility with a history of glenohumeral joint instability. J Athl Train. 2010;45(3):253–8.
57. Itoi E, Kido T, Sano A, Urayama M, Sato K. Which is more useful, the "full can test" or the "empty can test" in detecting the torn supraspinatus tendon? Am J Sports Med. 1999;27(1):65–8.
58. Pennock AT, Pennington WW, Torry MR, Decker MJ, Vaishnav SB, Provencher MT, Millet PJ, Hackett TR. The influence of arm and shoulder position on the bear-hug, belly-press, and lift-off tests: an electromyographic study. Am J Sports Med. 2011;39:2338–46.
59. Pandya NK, Colton A, Webner D, Sennett B, Huffman GR. Physical examination and magnetic resonance imaging in the diagnosis of superior labrum anterior-posterior lesions of the shoulder: a sensitivity analysis. Arthroscopy. 2008;24(3):311–7.
60. Hegedus EJ, Goode A, Campbell S, et al. Physical examination tests of the shoulder: a systematic review with meta-analysis of individual tests. Br J Sports Med. 2008;42:80–92.
61. Hegedus EJ. Which physical examination tests provide clinicians with the most value when examining the shoulder ? Update of a systematic review with meta-analysis of individual tests. Br J Sports Med. 2012. https://doi.org/10.1136/bjsports-2012-091066.
62. Cook C, Beaty S, Kissenberth MJ, Siffri P, Pill SG, Hawkins RJ. Diagnostic accuracy of five orthopedic clinical tests for diagnosis of superior labrum anterior posterior (SLAP) lesions. J Shoulder Elb Surg. 2012;21(1):13–22.
63. Michener LA, Doukas WC, Murphy KP, Walsworth MK. Diagnostic accuracy of history and physical examination of superior labrum anterior-posterior lesions. J Athl Train. 2011;46(6):343–8.
64. Andrews JR, Gillogly S. Physical examination of the shoulder in throwing athletes. In: Zarins B, Andrews JR, Carson WG, editors. Injuries to the throwing arm. Philadelphia, PA: WB Saunders; 1985.
65. Ellenbecker TS. Etiology and evaluation of rotator cuff pathologic conditions and rehabilitation. In: Donatelli RA, editor. Physical therapy of the shoulder. 4th ed. Philadelphia, PA: Churchill Livingstone; 2004. p. 337–58.
66. Liu SH, Henry MH, Nuccion S. A prospective evaluation of a new physical examination in predicting glenoid labrum tears. Am J Sports Med. 1996;24(6):721–5.
67. Stetson WB, Templin K. The crank test, the O'Brien test, and routine magnetic resonance imaging scans in the diagnosis of labral tears. Am J Sports Med. 2002;30(6):806–9.

68. O'Brien SJ, Pagnani MJ, Fealy S, McGlynn SR, Wilson JB. The active compression test: a new and effective test for diagnosing labral tears and acromioclavicular joint abnormality. Am J Sports Med. 1998;26(5):610–3.
69. Magee DJ. Orthopaedic physical assessment. 3rd ed. Philadelphia, PA: WB Saunders; 1997.
70. Kibler BW, Sciascia AD, Hester P, Dome D, Jacobs C. Clinical utility of traditional and new tests in the diagnosis of biceps tendon injuries and superior labrum anterior and posterior lesions in the shoulder. Am J Sports Med. 2009;37(9):1840–7.
71. Kibler WB. Specificity and sensitivity of the anterior slide test in throwing athletes with superior glenoid labral tears. Arthroscopy. 1995;11(3):296–300.
72. Morrey BF, Tanaka S, An KN. Valgus stability of the elbow: a definition of primary and secondary constraints. Clin Orthop Relat Res. 1991;(265):187–95.
73. Regan WD, Korinek S, Morrey BF, An KN. Biomechanical study of ligaments around the elbow joint. Clin Orthop Relat Res. 1991;(271):170–9.
74. Kibler WB. Clinical biomechanics of the elbow in tennis: implications for evaluation and diagnosis. Med Sci Sports Exerc. 1994;26:1203–6.
75. Elliott B, Fleisig G, Nicholls R, Escamilia R. Technique effects on upper limb loading in the tennis serve. J Sci Med Sport. 2003;6(1):76–87.
76. Strukel RJ, Garrick JG. Thoracic outlet compression in athletes. Am J Sports Med. 2016;6(2):35–9.
77. Churchill RW, Munoz J, Ahmad CS. Osteochondritis dissecans of the elbow. Curr Rev Musculoskelet Med. 2016;9(2):232–9.
78. Antuna SA, O'Driscoll SW. Snapping plicae associated with radiocapitellar chondromalacia. Arthroscopy. 2001;17(5):491–5.
79. Kim DH, Gambardella RA, Elattrache NS, Yocum LA, Jobe FW. Arthroscopic treatment of posterolateral elbow impingement from lateral synovial plicae in throwing athletes and golfers. Am J Sports Med. 2006;34(3):438–44.
80. Nirschl RP. Elbow tendinosis/tennis elbow. Clin Sports Med. 1992;11:851–70.
81. Hamilton CD, Glousman RE, Jobe FW, et al. Dynamic stability of the elbow: electromyographic analysis of the flexor pronator group and the extensor group in pitchers with valgus instability. J Shoulder Elb Surg. 1996;5:347–54.
82. Bruce JR, Andrews JR. Ulnar collateral ligament injuries in the throwing athlete. J Am Acad Orthop Surg. 2014;22(5):315–25.
83. Dines J, Altchek D, Dines DM. Medial collateral ligament reconstruction of elbow; current concepts in surgical technique. J Shoulder Elb Surg. 2010;19:110–7.
84. Safran M, Ahmad C, Elattrache N. Ulnar collateral ligament of the elbow. Arthroscopy. 2005;21(11):1381–95.
85. Cain EL Jr, Dugas J, Wolf R, Andrews J. Elbow injuries in the throwing athletes; a current review. Am J Sports Med. 2005;33(2):231–9.
86. O'Driscoll SW, Lawton RL, Smith AM. The "moving valgus stress test" for medial collateral ligament tears of the elbow. Am J Sports Med. 2005;33(2):231–9.
87. Calfee RP, et al. Clinical assessment of the ulnar nerve at the elbow: reliability of instability testing and the association of hypermobility with clinical symptoms. J Bone Joint Surg Am. 2010;92(17):2801–8.
88. Lasecki M, et al. The snapping elbow syndrome as a reason for chronic elbow neuralgia in a tennis player - MR, US and sonoelastography evaluation. Pol J Radiol. 2014;79:467–71.
89. Brucker J, Sahu N, Sandella B. Olecranon stress injury in an adolescent overhand pitcher: a case report and analysis of the literature. Sports Health. 2015;7(4):308–11.
90. Park JY, Yoo HY, Chung SW, Lee SJ, Kim NR, Ki SY, Oh KS. Valgus extension overload syndrome in adolescent baseball players: clinical characteristics and surgical outcomes. J Shoulder Elb Surg. 2016;25(12):2048–56.
91. Paulino FE, Villacis DC, Ahmad CS. Valgus extension overload in baseball players. Am J Orthop (Belle Mead NJ). 2016;45(3):144–51.
92. O'Driscoll S, Goncalves L, Dietz P. The Hook test for distal biceps tendon avulsion. Am J Sports Med. 2007;35(11):1865–9.

Physical Evaluation of the Hip

Paul K. Herickhoff and Marc R. Safran

7.1 Introduction

Tennis players subject their bodies to extreme forces; the hip joint may experience forces up to five times body weight during activities such as running, jumping, and twisting [1]. One to 27% of injuries in high-level tennis players originate in the hip, pelvis, and groin [2]. Furthermore, alteration of biomechanics from any pathologic process in the hip places the tennis player at increased risk of injury to the shoulder and upper extremity by disturbing the kinetic chain [1]. This is critical, as proper hip function is critical to performance in tennis (Kibler, Presented at 2016 STMS meeting).

A detailed history and physical examination is essential to the diagnosis and treatment of hip pathology. The differential diagnosis of the painful hip is extensive and includes intra-articular and extra-articular pathology and pain referred from other locations (Table 7.1). Because radiographic abnormalities are found in up to 60% of asymptomatic patients [4] and labral tears are found in as many as 90% of magnetic resonance imaging (MRI) studies of asymptomatic volunteers [5], these studies should be utilized for confirmation of the diagnosis after completion of the physical exam and to rule out other pathology. The purpose of this chapter is to describe the history and physical examination of the hip in the tennis player.

7.2 History

Evaluation of hip pain in the tennis player begins with a careful history. The patient should relate the onset and duration of symptoms, the presence or absence of trauma (including the mechanism of injury), and if there have been any changes to their training, the surface area being played on, or mechanics. The location and character of the pain should be discerned, as well as exacerbating and alleviating factors. "Which tennis motions make the hip pain worse?" and "When does the pain occur?" (before, during, or after the match, does it improve after warming up), "Is it worse or better on any particular playing surface," are valuable questions in determining how the athlete is affected [3].

It is important to ask what prior treatments have been attempted, such as rest, ice, physical therapy, orthotics, oral medication, injections, or

P. K. Herickhoff
Orthopaedic Surgery, Penn State Sports Medicine,
Pennsylvania State University,
State College, PA, USA

Orthopaedic Sports Medicine, Stanford University,
Redwood City, CA, USA
e-mail: pherickhoff@pennstatehealth.psu.edu

M. R. Safran (✉)
Orthopaedic Sports Medicine, Stanford University,
Redwood City, CA, USA

Department of Orthopaedic Surgery,
Stanford University, Redwood City, CA, USA
e-mail: msafran@stanford.edu

Table 7.1 Common sources of hip pain in tennis players [3]

Intra-articular	Femoroacetabular impingement Labral tears Chondral damage Loose bodies Ligamentum teres tears Hip dysplasia Hip instability
Extra-articular	Pubic symphysis dysfunction Osteitis pubis Athletic pubalgia/sports hernia/core muscle injury Inguinal or femoral hernia Iliopsoas tendonitis, strain, and tendinopathy Internal snapping hip syndrome External snapping hip syndrome Greater trochanteric pain syndrome (including trochanteric bursitis, as well as gluteus medius and minimus strain, tendinopathy, and tears) Piriformis syndrome Hamstring strain and tendinopathy
Referred	Abdominal muscle strain Abdominal—gastrointestinal Pelvis—genitourinary Lumbar spine (disc herniation or degeneration, facet arthropathy, pars injuries)

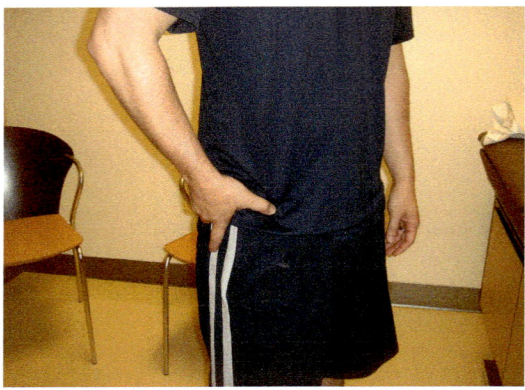

Fig. 7.1 The C-sign. Patients with intra-articular hip pain may grasp their lateral hip, forming the shape of a "C" with the thumb and fingers. They note that the pain is deep inside, where their thumb and fingers would meet

surgeries. If injections were performed, the exact location of the injection and amount and duration or relief should be recorded by either asking the patient or reviewing outside medical records. If prior surgery was performed, obtaining the outside physician's operative note and arthroscopic pictures is extremely helpful. The physician should also inquire about previous hip injuries or problems at a younger age, recalling that developmental dysplasia of the hip typically presents in infants, Legg-Calve-Perthes disease in elementary and middle-school aged children, and slipped capital femoral epiphysis (SCFE) in adolescents. A social history of steroid use, alcohol abuse, or deep sea diving may suggest avascular necrosis as the underlying cause [6].

The location and description of the pain can be helpful in determining its point of origin. Intra-articular pain typically localizes to the groin or inguinal region but may be referred to the medial thigh or lateral hip. The C-sign is noted when the patient grabs his or her hip with the thumb in the inguinal region and the long finger posterolaterally and states that the pain is at the junction of the fingers (Fig. 7.1). Pain with the hip in a flexed position such as squatting, sitting, or driving for long periods of time or arising from a seated position is often due to intra-articular pain generators. Pain resulting from twisting or pivoting on the affected hip also suggests an intra-articular source [3].

Extra-articular or referred pain will have varying complaints. Pain in the lower abdomen or adductor tubercle may indicate pubic symphysis dysfunction, athletic pubalgia/core muscle injury/sports hernia, osteitis pubis, or inguinal hernia, while pain in the lateral hip suggests trochanteric bursitis or gluteus medius syndrome. Pain in the buttocks or thigh may be coming from the proximal hamstrings, piriformis, or ischiofemoral impingement or referred from the lumbar spine. Neurologic complaints of numbness, weakness, back pain, or symptoms worsening with coughing or sneezing most likely result from lumbar spine pathology.

Mechanical symptoms may be intra- or extra-articular in origin. Chondral flaps and labral tears within the joint can cause painful catching or clicking in the hip, but are not visible and rarely audible. Audible popping felt in the groin while bringing the hip from flexion to extension is caused by the iliopsoas tendon sliding over the iliopectineal eminence or femoral head, known as internal snapping of the hip. External snapping of the hip, on the other hand, results from a tight iliotibial band sliding over the greater trochanter, is visible and palpable in the lateral hip, and will often be accompanied by the patient complaining that "my hip joint is dislocating."

Traumatic posterior hip dislocation from playing tennis, to our knowledge, has not been reported in the literature, though the senior author has seen a tennis player who sustained a posterior hip subluxation playing tennis. Atraumatic microinstability of the hip, however, may be a source of hip pain and results from repetitive microtrauma, ligamentous laxity, hip dysplasia, or a combination of the above factors [7]. Microinstability is more common in females than males, and patients may complain of a sensation of instability in the hip. Particular hip positions or movements which cause the hip to feel unstable should be recorded, and any personal or family history of ligamentous laxity or Marfan or Ehlers-Danlos syndrome must be noted as well [8].

7.3 Physical Examination

The key to the physical examination is to determine if the pain originates from intra-articular or extra-articular pathology and to confirm the pain is not referred from the spine, gastrointestinal or genitourinary systems, or lower abdomen. Intra-articular pathologies tend to be aggravated by passive motion of the hip joint, while extra-articular causes are often painful to palpation or manual strength testing [3]. Both hips should be inspected, palpated, measured for range of motion and strength, and subjected to provocative tests in five different positions. The senior author and others have found the most efficient order of exam begins in the standing position followed by seated, supine, and lateral and ends with prone examinations [9].

First observe the patient during the history part of the evaluation. Are they slouched to prevent flexion of the hip, or are they listing to stay off the buttock on one side? Are they constantly moving side to side?

7.3.1 Standing Examination

Begin by asking the patient to stand with their back facing toward the examiner. Observe the patient arising from the seated position, making note of over-reliance on the arms to push up out of the chair and if the patient splints or compensates for the affected hip. With the feet (with shoes off) shoulder width apart, palpate the iliac crests to assess for leg length discrepancy. In patients with equal leg lengths, the height of the iliac crests will be the same. When the iliac crests are at different heights, a leg length discrepancy exists. Incremental wooden blocks placed under the short side heel will aid in orthotic considerations for patients whose leg lengths are unequal [9].

Hip abductor strength is measured with the Trendelenburg test (Fig. 7.2). While palpating the iliac crests and posterior superior iliac spines, the patient is asked to sequentially lift each knee. The iliac crest will rise up in patients with normal hip abductor strength. If the iliac crest does not rise, or if the athlete shifts their upper body toward the standing leg, the hip abductors are weak [10].

Gait evaluation involves observation of the patient walking from the front and the back. Key points of gait evaluation include foot rotation (internal/external progression angle), pelvic rotation, stance phase, hip motion, and stride length. The foot progression angle will detect osseous or static rotatory malalignment. A pelvic wink is the result of excessive rotation toward the affected hip to obtain terminal hip extension. Pelvis wink during gait may be the result of intra-articular hip pathology, abnormal femoral version, and ligamentous laxity of the hip. An antalgic gait is characterized by a shortened stance phase on the painful side limiting the duration of weight bearing [9].

7.3.2 Seated Examination

Inspect the patient in a seated position for abnormal posture. Patients with piriformis syndrome may lean away from the affected hip, while patients with femoroacetabular impingement (FAI) slouch

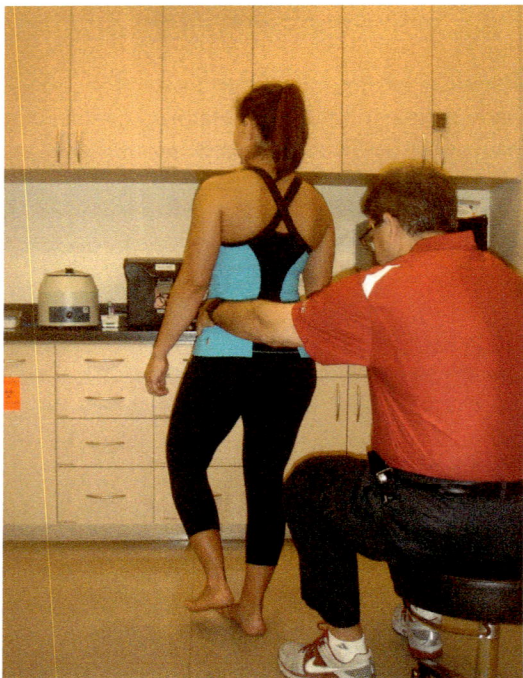

Fig. 7.2 Trendelenburg sign and leg length discrepancy. Evaluating the patient from the back, standing on both legs, the examiner evaluates the iliac crest heights for determination of leg length discrepancy. Next, the athlete lifts one knee while the examiner still has their hands on the iliac crests and posterior iliac spines. The iliac crest on the side the leg is lifted should rise up, indicative of good strength on the contralateral hip abductors. If it does not raise or if the athlete shifts their upper body toward the standing leg, then there is hip abductor weakness [3]

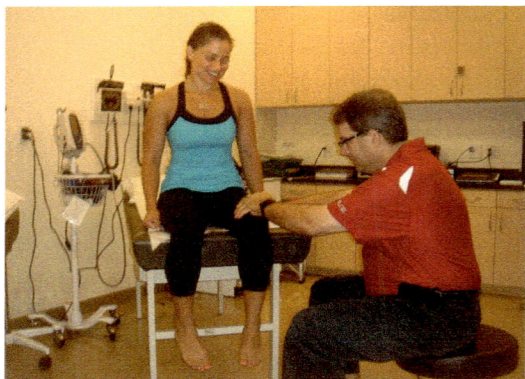

Fig. 7.3 Iliopsoas strength test—resisted hip flexion while seated is useful to evaluate the iliopsoas for weakness as well as pain

to reduce hip flexion. A neurovascular examination should be performed, including pulses, deep tendon reflexes, sensation and manual motor testing, and seated straight leg raise test. The strength of the iliopsoas is assessed by having the patient raise the knee off the table (Fig. 7.3). Pain with resisted hip flexion suggests tendonitis or bursitis of the iliopsoas. Passive hip ROM in internal rotation (IR) and external rotation (ER) should be recorded in the seated position—as the ischium is stable, reducing compensatory motion [3].

7.3.3 Supine Examination

Inspect the anterior hip, inguinal region, and pubic symphysis, and palpate the inguinal canal, pubic bone, pubic symphysis, rectus abdominis, and adductor longus. Tenderness at the superficial inguinal ring with swelling that becomes more prominent with Valsalva maneuvers is indicative of an inguinal hernia. Osteitis pubis presents with tenderness over the pubic bone and pain with a pelvic compression test, performed by pushing the anterior superior iliac spines toward the midline (this can also be done in the lateral position). The pubic symphysis stress test creates a shear force at the pubic symphysis by grabbing the superior border of the pubic bone on one side, the inferior border of the pubic bone on the contralateral side, and pressing the two hands together. A positive test recreates the patient's pain at the pubic symphysis. Hesselbach's test (Fig. 7.4) is performed by palpating the edge of the rectus abdominis insertion into the pubis while the patient performs a sit up. Exacerbation of the patient's symptoms with this maneuver is consistent with athletic pubalgia/core muscle injury/sports hernia. Tenderness over the adductor longus which worsens with resisted hip adduction at 0° or 90° of hip flexion indicates tendinopathy or tearing of the adductor longus [3].

Range of motion of the hip is measured in flexion, extension, adduction, abduction, and internal and external rotation with the hip flexed to 90° and in neutral flexion-extension are recorded, and it should be noted if the patient experiences discomfort at the end range of motion. Normal range of motion values is listed

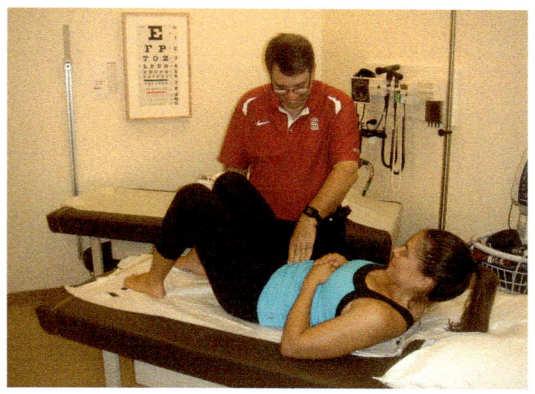

Fig. 7.4 Hesselbach's test. This test is performed by palpating the edge of the rectus abdominis insertion while the patient performs a sit up. Exacerbation of the patient's symptoms with this maneuver is consistent with athletic pubalgia/core muscle injury/sports hernia

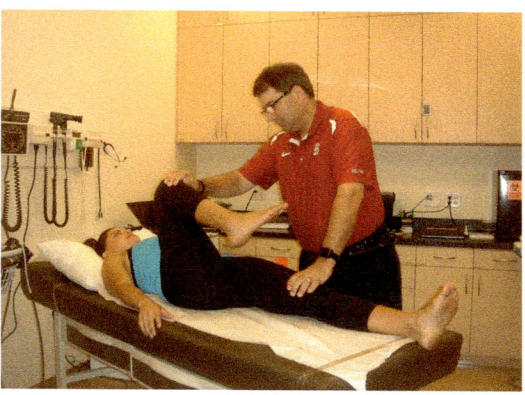

Fig. 7.5 Thomas test. This test evaluates for hip flexion contracture. The patient pulls the knee of one leg up to his/her chest. If there is no flexion contracture, the contralateral extended hip and extremity will be flat on the examination table. Care is taken to be sure the lumbar spine is flat against the examination table during this test and can be assessed by the examiner placing their hand underneath the athlete's lower back

Table 7.2 Normal range of motion values of the hip [3]

Flexion	110°–120°
Extension	10°–15°
Abduction in extension	30°–50°
Adduction in extension	30°
External rotation in flexion	40°–60°
Internal rotation in flexion	30°–40°

in Table 7.2. Groin pain at maximal hip flexion which improves with hip abduction may indicate FAI secondary to a low-lying anterior inferior iliac spine (AIIS), while obligate abduction and external rotation while the hip is being flexed is known as Drehmann's sign, seen in patients with SCFE. Hamstring tightness is assessed by flexing the hip to 90° and passively extending the knee from 90° of flexion until muscle tightness resistance is felt. This is the popliteal angle, and an angle greater than 60° is considered tight in general, though less degrees may also be indicative of tightness for some patients, and thus, contralateral hamstring tightness should be measured as well.

The Thomas test (Fig. 7.5) is utilized to evaluate for hip flexion contracture, which may be found in association with abdominal muscle strains. The flexion/adduction/internal rotation (FADIR) test, also known at the impingement test (Fig. 7.6), is very sensitive for intra-articular hip pathology, but is not specific for FAI. The

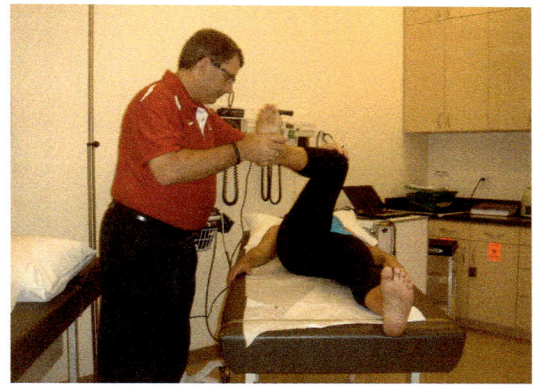

Fig. 7.6 Flexion/adduction/internal rotation (FADIR) or "impingement" test. The hip is flexed to 90°, adducted, and internally rotated. This test is sensitive to intra-articular pathology, but is not pathognomonic for femoroacetabular impingement

dynamic labral stress test, or scour maneuver (Fig. 7.7), pinches the labrum between the femoral neck and acetabulum and may indicate a symptomatic labral tear if it reproduces the patient's pain. The Stinchfield test (Fig. 7.8) is performed by having the patient perform a resisted straight leg raise and may be positive with either intra-articular (labral tear) or extra-articular pathology, such as rectus femoris or iliopsoas strains or tendonitis. The foveal distraction

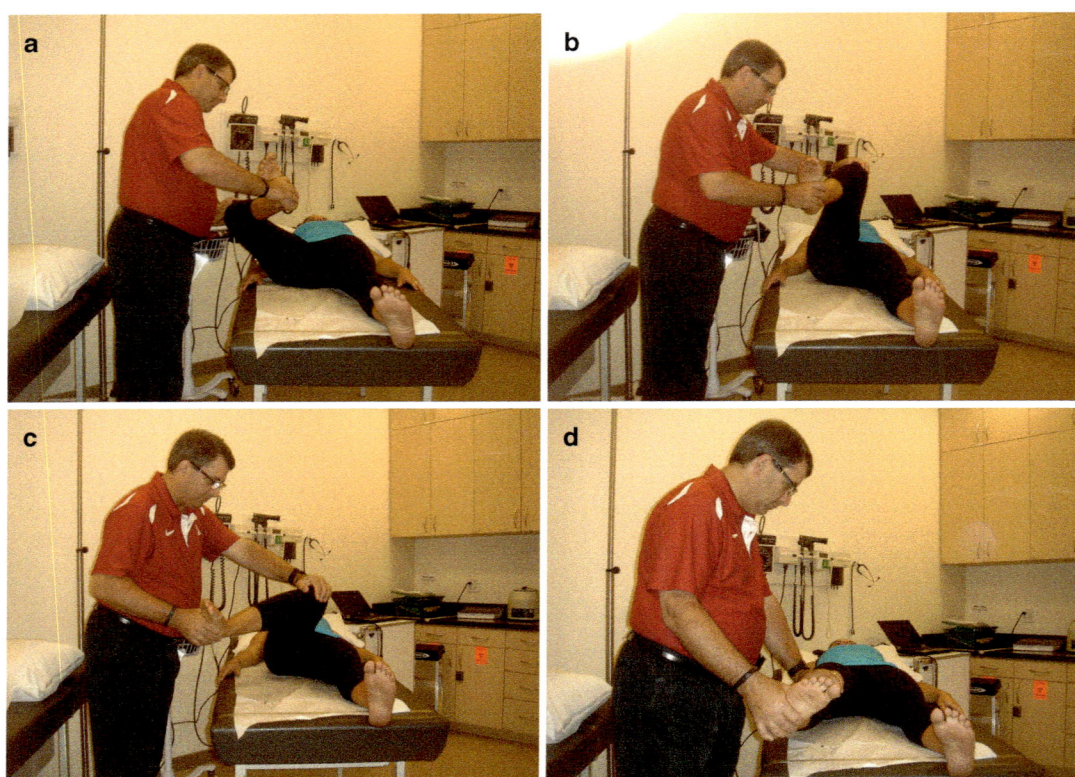

Fig. 7.7 Labral stress test or scour maneuver. The patient's hip is flexed, abducted, and externally rotated to start (**a**). The hip is then adducted and internally rotated (**b**) while extending the hip (**c** and **d**). The hip is then passively ranged from flexion through a wide arc of abduction and external rotation toward hip extension

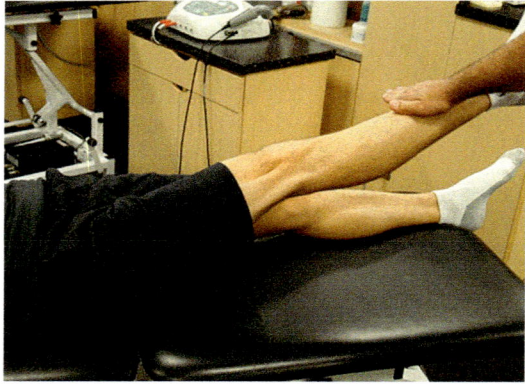

Fig. 7.8 Stinchfield test. This test is performed with a straight leg raise against resistance. Pain while performing this test may indicate either intra-articular hip pathology or hip flexor inflammation or injury

test is performed by placing axial traction on the leg with the hip in 30° of abduction, which reduces intra-articular pressure. Relief of pain during this maneuver also indicates in intra-articular source of hip pain.

The Patrick test (Fig. 7.9) and Gaenslen's test (Fig. 7.10) are used to evaluate the sacroiliac joint. The Byrd test (Fig. 7.11) attempts to reproduce internal snapping of the hip by having the patient actively flex and externally rotate the hip, followed by abduction and then extending and internally rotating the hip as the hip is adducted to the starting position. The examiner should palpate the groin during this maneuver to feel for popping or clicking of the iliopsoas in the front of the hip, though the snap is usually audible.

The logroll test is a sensitive test for intra-articular pain in patients with acute hip injuries. A modified logroll test evaluates for hip instability. With the patient relaxed, the external rotation position of the foot is noted. The foot is passively

7 Physical Evaluation of the Hip

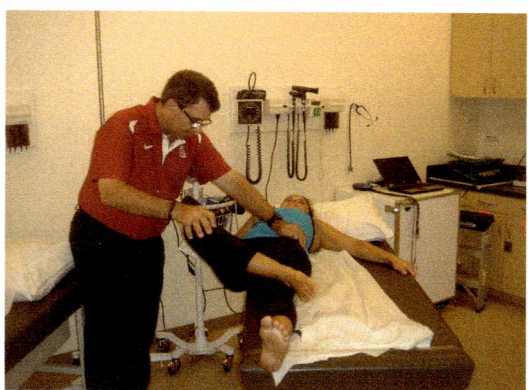

Fig. 7.9 FABER test/Patrick's test. In this test, the patient's buttock is off the edge of the table, and then the ipsilateral leg is brought into a "figure-of-4" position (flexion, abduction, and external rotation—FABER). While stabilizing the contralateral anterior superior iliac spine with one hand, the examiner applies a downward force to the knee with the other hand. Posterior pain is often elicited as a result of sacroiliac pathology, while anterior pain may be the result of pubic symphysis pain or anterior labral damage

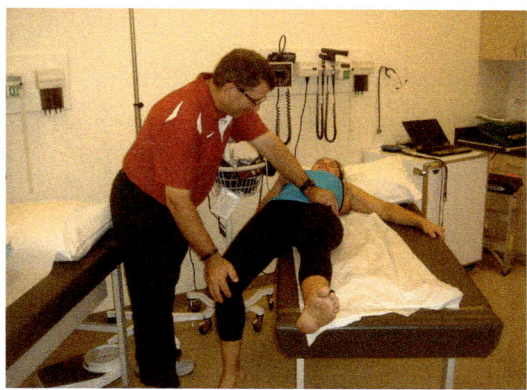

Fig. 7.10 Gaenslen's test. The patient lies supine with the buttock off the edge of the table. The ipsilateral leg is then extended toward the floor. This maneuver stresses the sacroiliac joint and is positive if the patient experiences posterior hip pain on the provoked side

internally rotated then released to fall back into external rotation. Anterior hip pain and external rotation of the foot past 75° suggests iliofemoral ligament laxity which may be consistent with anterior microinstability of the hip. The hyperextension-external rotation test (Fig. 7.12) also evaluates for anterior instability of the hip. During this test, the patient lies supine with the pelvis at the end of the examination table with the legs dangling free. The hip not being examined is flexed and held by the patient stabilizing the pelvis, while the contralateral hip is externally rotated in hyperextension. Anterior groin pain may indicate and anterior labrum tear and/or anterior microinstability [3].

7.3.4 Lateral Examination

Palpation of the trochanteric bursa, gluteus medius, and piriformis is performed in the lateral position. Ober's test (Fig. 7.13) evaluates for contracture of the iliotibial band. External snapping hip syndrome should be investigated by having the patient simulate pedaling a bicycle with their upper leg. A positive test reproduces snapping of the iliotibial band over the greater trochanter. Instability testing in the lateral position as described by Guanche (Fig. 7.14) involves applying an anterior force to the posterior greater trochanter with the hip in an extended, abducted, and externally rotated position [11]. Anterior hip pain indicates a positive test.

7.3.5 Prone Examination

Hip instability may also be tested in the prone position, as described by Domb (Fig. 7.15). With the hip in external rotation, an anteriorly directed force is applied to the posterior greater trochanter. A positive test results in anterior hip pain [11].

Internal and external rotation of the hip should be measured in the prone position with the knee flexed to 90°. Craig's test is performed by internally rotating the foot until the trochanter is felt most prominently laterally. Femoral version may then be estimated by noting the angle between the axis of the tibia and an imaginary vertical line, which normally is between 10° and 20°. Ely's test assesses for rectus femoris contracture by maximally flexing the knee in the prone position. A negative test demonstrates full flexion of the knee to the thigh with no movement in the

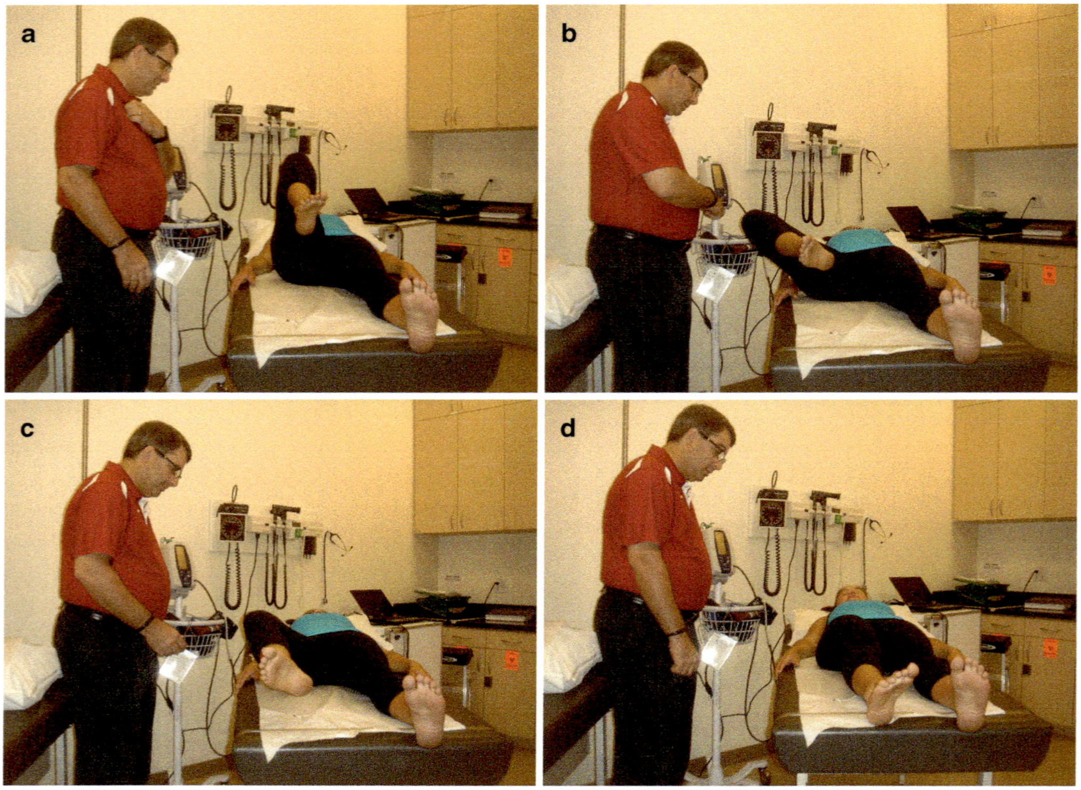

Fig. 7.11 Byrd test. While the examiner palpates the groin, the patient actively brings the hip into (**a**) flexion, then (**b**) abducts, and (**c**) externally rotates while (**d**) extending the hip. This test is used to detect popping of the iliopsoas tendon over the iliopectineal eminence or femoral head, known as internal snapping of the hip

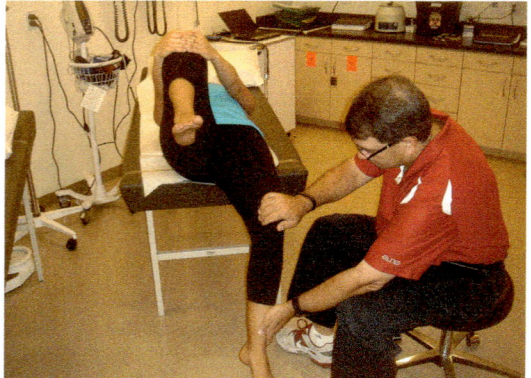

Fig. 7.12 Hyperextension-external rotation test. The patient lies supine with the pelvis at the end of the examination table, and the lower extremities are dangling free. The hip not being examined is flexed and held by the patient while the other extremity is externally rotated while in hyperextension. Anterior hip pain may be the result of an anterior labral tear and/or anterior microinstability

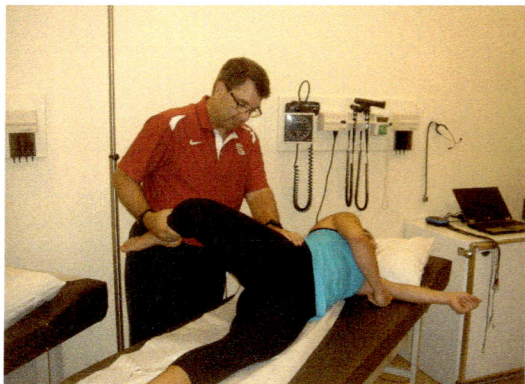

Fig. 7.13 Ober test. This test is for hip abductor tightness or iliotibial band contracture. With the patient in the lateral decubitus position, the hip and knee are first flexed, then the hip abducted, then extended, and let fall into adduction. Inability of the knee to drop below neutral indicates tightness of the iliotibial band

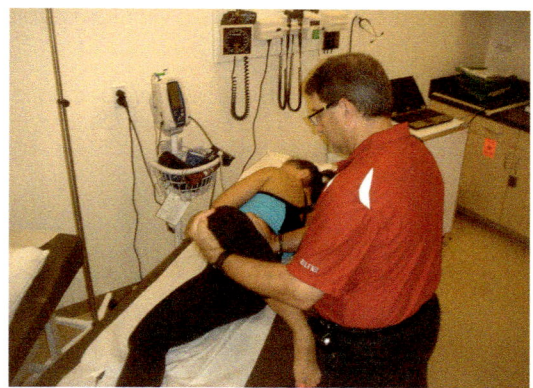

Fig. 7.14 Abduction-extension-external rotation test. In this test, the patient's hip is held in abduction, extension, and external rotation, and then an anteriorly directed force is applied to the greater trochanter. Pain in the groin or anterior hip indicates anterior labral tear and/or anterior microinstability

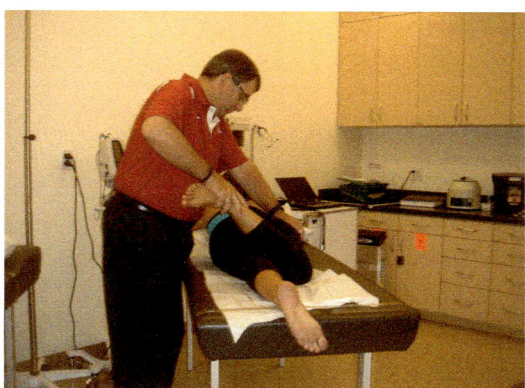

Fig. 7.15 Prone instability test. With the patient prone, and the hip externally rotated, an anterior force is directed against the posterior aspect of the greater trochanter. Pain in the anterior hip indicates anterior labral tear and/or anterior microinstability

pelvis. Any limitation of knee flexion or elevation of the buttocks from the table is a positive test for rectus femoris contracture [12].

Palpating the gluteus maximus with the index finger of one hand and the hamstring muscle belly with the index finger of the other hand while asking the patient to raise his or her flexed knee off the table will allow differentiation of which muscle fires first to extend the hip. Normally, the gluteus maximus will fire first, known as gluteal dominance. If the hamstrings contract before the gluteus maximus, the patient is hamstring dominant. Hamstring-dominant patients will benefit from referral to a physical therapist for neuromuscular reeducation to achieve gluteal dominance. Finally, tenderness over the ischial tuberosity or pain with resisted hamstring firing may be found in patients with proximal hamstring tendinopathy or tearing.

7.4 Summary

Hip pain in the tennis player comprises an extensive differential diagnosis. The deep location of the hip joint, its thick soft tissue envelope, and the potential for referred pain patterns highlight the importance of performing a comprehensive history and physical examination. Proper execution of the history and physical examination techniques detailed in this chapter, in combination with confirmatory imaging and diagnostic injection tests, allows the physician to formulate the correct diagnosis and initiate appropriate treatment.

References

1. Dines JS, Williams PN, Dodson CC, Ellenbecker TS, Altchek DW, Windler G, Dines DM. Tennis injuries: epidemiology, pathophysiology, and treatment. J Am Acad Orthop Surg. 2015;23(3):181–9.
2. Abrams GD, Renstrom P, Safran MR. Epidemiology of musculoskeletal injury in the tennis player. Br J Sports Med. 2012;46(7):492–8. https://doi.org/10.1136/bjsports-2012-091164.
3. Safran M. Evaluation of the painful hip in tennis players. Aspetar Sports Med J. 2014;3:516–25.
4. Jung KA, Restrepo C, Hellman M, AbdelSalam H, Morrison W, Parvizi J, Morrison W. The prevalence of cam-type femoroacetabular deformity in asymptomatic adults. J Bone Joint Surg Br. 2011;93-B(10):1303–7. https://doi.org/10.1302/0301-620X.93B10.26433.
5. Schmitz MR, Campbell SE, Fajardo RS, Kadrmas WR. Identification of acetabular labral pathological changes in asymptomatic volunteers using optimized, noncontrast 1.5-T magnetic resonance imaging. Am J Sports Med. 2012;40(6):1337–41. https://doi.org/10.1177/0363546512439991.
6. Safran MR. Evaluation of the hip: history, physical examination, and imaging. Oper Tech Sports Med. 2005;13(1):2–12. https://doi.org/10.1053/j.otsm.2004.09.006.

7. Shu B, Safran MR. Hip instability: anatomic and clinical considerations of traumatic and atraumatic instability. Clin Sports Med. 2011;30(2):349–67. https://doi.org/10.1016/j.csm.2010.12.008.
8. Kalisvaart MM, Safran MR. Hip instability treated with arthroscopic capsular plication. Knee Surg Sports Traumatol Arthrosc. 2016;25:24–30. https://doi.org/10.1007/s00167-016-4377-6.
9. Martin HD, Shears SA, Palmer IJ. Evaluation of the hip. Sports Med Arthrosc Rev. 2010;18(2):63–75. https://doi.org/10.1097/JSA.0b013e3181dc578a.
10. Trendelenburg F. Trendelenburg's test: 1895. Clin Orthop Relat Res. 1998;(355):3–7. http://www.ncbi.nlm.nih.gov/pubmed/9917586
11. Domb BG, Brooks AG, Guanche C. Physical examination of the hip. In: Hip and pelvis injuries in sports medicine. Philadelphia: Lippincott Williams and Wilkins; 2010. p. 62–70.
12. Braly BA, Beall DP, Martin HD. Clinical examination of the athletic hip. Clin Sports Med. 2006;25(2):199–210. https://doi.org/10.1016/j.csm.2005.12.001.

Spine Injuries in Tennis

8

Stephan N. Salzmann, Javier Maquirriain, Jennifer Shue, and Federico P. Girardi

8.1 Introduction

Tennis is a popular sport played by more than 75 million individuals around the world [1]. It attracts people from all age groups and is played at both recreational and professional levels [2]. Health benefits associated with tennis include improved aerobic fitness, lower risk for cardiovascular disease, and favorable effects on bone health [3]. Multiple studies have shown that the bone mineral density (BMD) of the dominant (playing) arm of tennis players was significantly higher in comparison to the nondominant arm [3–5]. More interestingly, an increased bone mass was also observed in the lumbar spine of tennis players. Thereby tennis might have a beneficial effect on bone mass not only in the humerus but also in the lumbar spine [3, 6, 7].

S. N. Salzmann · J. Shue · F. P. Girardi (✉)
Department of Orthopedic Surgery, Spine and Scoliosis Service, Hospital for Special Surgery, Weill Cornell Medical College, New York, NY, USA
e-mail: GirardiF@hss.edu

J. Maquirriain
Centro Nacional de Alto Rendimiento Deportivo (CeNARD, Secretaría de Deporte, Ministerio de Desarrollo Social de la Nación),
Buenos Aires, Argentina

Consejo Nacional de Investigaciones Científicas y Técnicas (CONICET), Ministerio de Ciencia y Tecnología e Innovación Productiva,
Buenos Aires, Argentina

Asociación Argentina de Tenis,
Buenos Aires, Argentina

However, as with any other sport, tennis players are at risk for injury [8]. In general, tennis is a low-risk sport. Since it is a noncontact sport, the injury incidence is lower in comparison to contact team sports and described in the literature ranging from 0.04 to 3.0 per 1000 h of play [1, 8]. Impact-related injuries are relatively rare in tennis. Although many common tennis injuries, such as a sprained ankle, also occur in other related sports, tennis has its own unique injury profile. A predominance of lower extremity injuries followed by upper extremity injuries and trunk injuries have been described [1, 8, 9].

Low back pain is very common among tennis players. The repetitive nature of tennis in conjunction with the extreme motion and the speed of trunk movement puts the lower back at risk for injury [10]. Studies have shown that most recurrent injuries in tennis occur in the lumbar spine [2]. In addition, more than one third of professional tennis players missed at least one tournament due to low back pain [11]. The aim of this chapter is to provide a general overview of spine injuries in tennis with a focus on commonly described pathologies in the lumbar spine of tennis players including facet joint arthropathy, disc degeneration, disc herniation, and pars injuries [12, 13].

8.2 Anatomy and Biomechanics

The spinal column is composed of multiple functional units lying on each other. Each unit consists of an anterior and posterior segment.

The function of the anterior segment, which includes the vertebral bodies and intervertebral disc, is mainly weight bearing. The posterior segment protects the spinal cord and directs the permitted vertebral movement by the orientation of the facets [14].

The intervertebral disc consists of an outer annulus fibrosus and an inner nucleus pulposus that functions as a shock absorbing fluid system. Compressive loads are transferred from one spinal level to the next via the disc. Adapting to this increased weight-bearing stresses, the caudal vertebral bodies and intervertebral discs are bigger in size when compared to more cephalad levels. The fluid content of the intervertebral disc decreases as we age. As a result, compressive loads might cause stress on primary non-weight-bearing structures [11, 14].

The facet joints determine the direction of motion permitted. In contrast to other parts of the spinal column, the orientation of the facets is more sagittal in the lumbar spine. This orientation permits flexion and extension while constricting lateral flexion and rotation [11, 14].

Numerous ligaments (ligamentum flavum, interspinous, supraspinous, anterior, and posterior longitudinal ligaments) support the spinal column in its function and prevent extreme motion. The anterior and posterior longitudinal ligaments extend along the vertebral column and strengthen the annulus fibrosus of the disc. To comprehend certain disc pathologies, it is important to note that the posterior longitudinal ligament narrows caudally in the lumbar spine. Consequently, the annulus is less reinforced in the lower lumbar region, which is already prone to biomechanical overstress [14].

Several muscles are involved in lumbar trunk motion. They can be divided into an anterior and posterior group. The anterior muscles primarily involved in lumbar motion are the abdominal muscles. The posterior muscles consist of a superficial, middle, and deep layer. The superficial layer, also known as the erector spinae, includes the medial spinalis, the intermediate longissimus, and the lateral iliocostalis. The middle muscle layer consists of the multifidus, while the deep layer includes the interspinalis, intertransversarii, and rotators [11, 14].

8.3 Tennis-Specific Movements

Comparable to many other racket sports, the four main strokes in tennis include the serve, the forehand groundstroke, the backhand groundstroke, and the volley. All of these strokes as well as the simple movement to pick up the ball put the spine at potential risk for injury, especially if these movements are not performed correctly. The serve is a complex movement including an initial hyperextension and rotation of the spine followed by a forceful flexion and derotation. It is the stroke causing the greatest stress on the lower back. Also the two-handed backhand is considered to put the lumbar spine at an increased risk for injury, since a higher degree of rotation is necessary to perform the movement in comparison with the one-handed variant [11, 14].

8.4 Effect of Tennis on the Spine During Growth

Besides the positive effects of sports on the musculoskeletal system during adolescence, there are some concerns that certain athletic activities might increase the risk for spinal deformities, especially if performed competitively [15]. Many experts consider asymmetric sports like tennis as a risk factor for the development of scoliosis in adolescents. A recent study compared the prevalence of spinal deformities in adolescent competitive tennis players with non-tennis players of the same age. Interestingly, this study showed no correlation between tennis and spinal deformities in adolescents. The authors concluded that tennis does not appear to be dangerous for the spine during growth. Therefore parents and physicians should not prevent children and adolescents from playing tennis [16].

8.5 Lumbar Strain

Acute strains in the lumbar region are probably among the most common back injuries in tennis players. The erector spinae and multifidus are at risk due to repetitive muscle contraction during extension and rotation of the trunk. Factors leading to a lumbar strain might include a change in training intensity/frequency or the use of a different tennis technique. In the majority of cases, the only symptom is local tenderness over the paraspinal muscles. The treatment is conservative and includes rest, ice, and anti-inflammatory drugs. This is followed by a gradual return to activity. Imaging is not necessary for this type of diagnosis. However, persistent pain, worsening of pain with extension, or existence of any neurological symptoms are cause for concern for a more serious etiology that may require further diagnostic workup [14, 17]. Besides the back muscles, the abdominal muscles are at risk for acute muscle strain secondary to repetitive rotation and trunk flexion in tennis [14, 18, 19].

8.6 Facet Joint Arthropathy

Facet joint changes are a common pain generator in athletes. Possible pain-promoting mechanisms include joint capsule stretching, trapped synovial villi between articular surfaces, nerve impingement by osteophytes, and release of inflammatory mediators [12, 20]. Imaging studies in tennis players revealed facet joint arthropathy as the most frequently encountered lumbar spine pathology. The incidence of facet joint arthropathy in tennis players was significantly higher in comparison to the general population suggesting premature facet joint degeneration in these athletes. A possible explanation for this finding might be the frequent and repetitive axial rotation of the lumbar spine in this sport. Especially during the serve and the double-handed groundstrokes, increased forces on the facets can occur. The most affected levels are typically L4/L5 and L5/S1 [12, 13]. Under physiologic conditions the facets are not supposed to approximate in a weight-bearing manner. However, approximation of the facets might occur as a result of lumbar degenerative disc changes. Degenerative disc disease and facet joint arthropathy are traditionally believed to occur in sequence. Interestingly, this typical sequential pattern does not always apply in tennis, since many patients with facet joint changes were shown to have normal intervertebral discs.

Symptoms of facet joint arthropathy include pain in the lower back which may radiate into the buttocks. The neurologic exam is usually normal. Sometimes a convex spinal curvature on the side of pain can be noticed. Diagnostic imaging is essential since degenerative disc pathologies often coexist [12–14]. Identifying the facet joint as the primary pain generator is challenging. For this reason controlled local anesthetic blocks of the facet joint and its nerve supply are often used to diagnose patients with facet joint pain. The management is primarily conservative and includes drug therapy, chiropractic treatment, or physical therapy. If conservative management fails, interventional techniques and surgery can be considered. For long-term improvement, radiofrequency neurotomy and facet joint nerve blocks may be beneficial [20, 21].

8.7 Lumbar Degenerative Disc Disease

The etiology of lumbar degenerative disc disease is multifactorial. The degenerative process is influenced by age, environmental factors, and genetic predisposition. Physical loading has only a modest effect on disc degeneration in the general population. In contrast, athletes are exposed to high repetitive physical forces on the spine for a longer duration, which might explain the higher prevalence of lumbar degenerative disc disease compared to nonathletes [22, 23]. The clinical presentation of patients with lumbar disc disease can vary and may include pain, radicular symptoms, and weakness. Position and movement often influence the symptoms. In general, extension relieves discogenic back pain, whereas flexion exacerbates it [23]. The initial imaging should consist of plain radiographs in two planes. Plain radiographs not only help to rule out other pathologies (deformity, fracture, metastatic cancer) but may reveal typical degenerative changes including disc space narrowing, end-plate sclerosis, osteophytes, and vacuum phenomenon in the disc. In addition, MRI is a sensitive imaging modality for disc pathologies. With its use, the hydration of the disc, bulging of the annulus, and associated vertebral end plate (Modic) changes can be assessed. In order to identify a specific disc as the primary pain generator, a discography can be performed as a confirmation study. Its use, however, remains controversial [22–24]. The most common localization of lumbar degenerative disc disease is the L5/S1 level followed by L4/L5 [12, 13]. In comparison to sports with high axial loading (e.g., weight lifting), multilevel disease and advanced degenerative changes are less common in tennis [12]. Conservative treatment including physical therapy and nonsteroidal anti-inflammatory drugs remains the initial treatment of choice for discogenic pain [24]. In patients with progressively symptomatic disc degeneration and failed conservative treatment, surgical intervention can be considered. For a long time, surgical treatment was limited to fusion of the affected level. Lumbar spinal fusion can be performed by a variety of approaches and is still considered the gold standard of surgical treatment for degenerative disc disease. However, there are several potential shortcomings of lumbar fusion including failure to achieve a solid fusion mass (pseudarthrosis), adjacent segment degeneration, and bone donor site complications. Theoretically, lumbar total disc replacement overcomes all these shortcomings and maintains motion at the operated level (Fig. 8.1) [25]. Studies of lumbar total disc replacement in high performance individuals such as athletes and military personnel showed highly satisfactory results [26, 27]. Nonetheless, concerns regarding possible late complications and implant durability in athletic individuals remain [25].

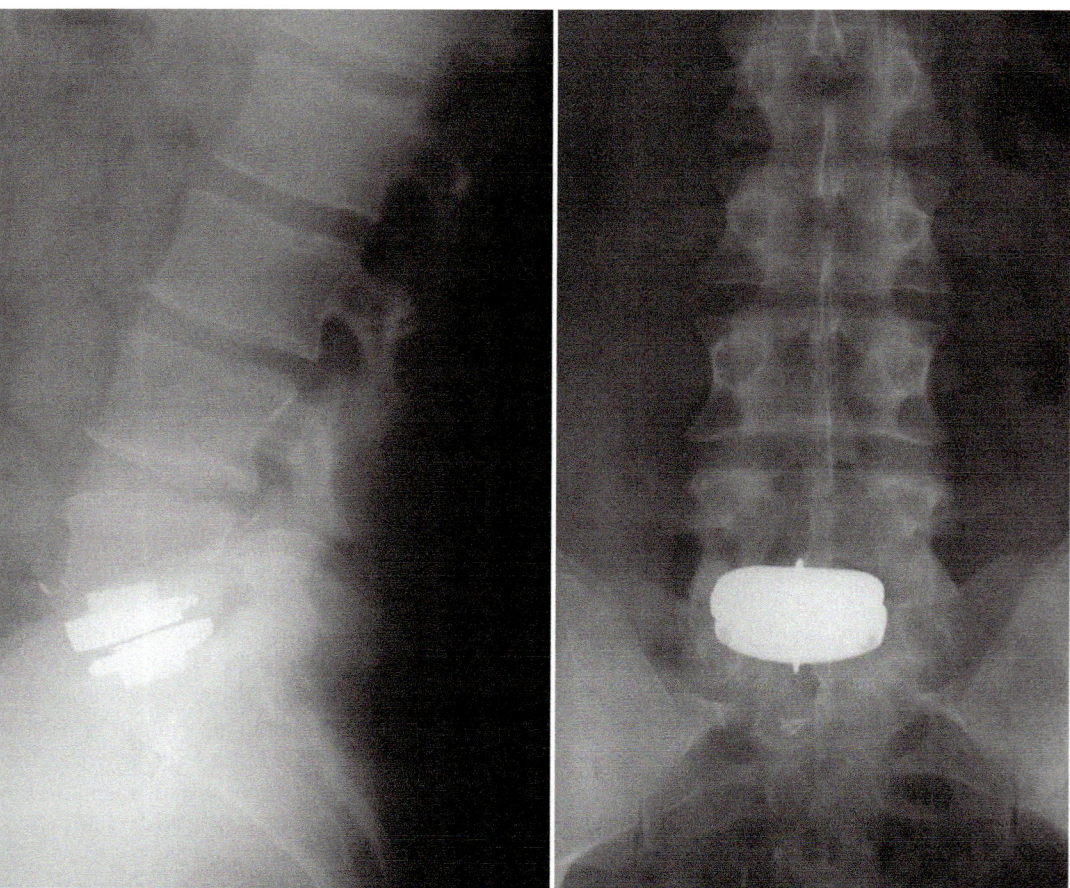

Fig. 8.1 Lateral and anteroposterior radiographs of a lumbar total disc replacement

8.8 Herniated Nucleus Pulposus (HNP)

Lumbar disc herniation is a common condition in athletes, especially in tennis players. Microtrauma to the lumbar disc from repetitive hyperextension and rotation (especially during the serve and the two-handed ground strokes) might be a possible cause for the high incidence of disc herniation in tennis players. Symptoms of an acute lumbar disc herniation may vary from back pain only, leg pain only, or a combination of back and leg symptoms.

The degree of radiating pain in association with numbness and weakness is determined by the anatomic location of the disc herniation. In the setting of large central disc herniations with a severely compromised spinal canal, bowel and bladder symptoms may occur [14]. From a diagnostic standpoint, plain radiographs are of limited value, since they are often normal or show only a mild reduction in disc space height. MRI is considered the gold standard imaging modality (Fig. 8.2). It is important to correlate the MRI findings with the clinical symptoms, since disc herniations are also

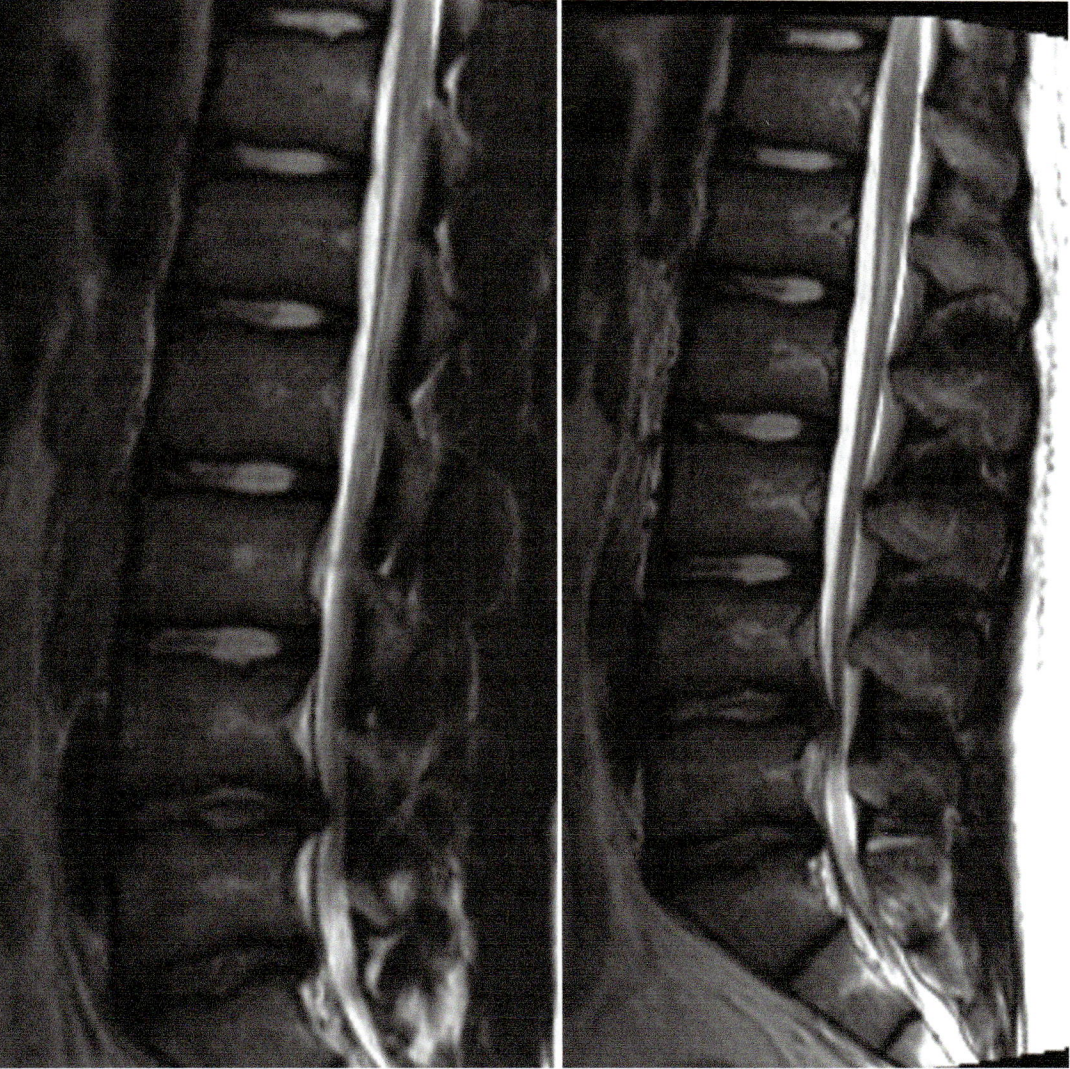

Fig. 8.2 HNP of the lower lumbar spine shown on MRI

commonly found in asymptomatic nonathletes. Nonoperative treatment includes physical therapy with lumbar extension and core strengthening exercises. Additional pain relief can often be achieved with epidural steroid injections as an alternative to surgery [17, 22]. Failed conservative treatment and existence of neurological deficits are indications for surgery. Standard discectomy and microdiscectomy are two available treatment options. The standard discectomy involves a laminotomy, removal of the disc fragment, incision of the annulus fibrosus, and removal of central and lateral portions of the nucleus. The use of an operating microscope in the setting of a microdiscectomy enables the surgeon to perform a smaller incision with the potential benefits of less scarring and less muscle denervation [17, 28].

8.9 Spondylolysis

Spondylolysis is defined as a defect in the pars interarticularis of a vertebra. Compared to the general population, the prevalence of spondylolysis is much higher in athletes, especially in disciplines requiring repetitive lumbar hyperextension like in tennis. Spondylolysis is often found in younger athletes, since the pars interarticularis is still immature and vulnerable to repeated stress from hyperextension. The most common location for pars injuries is the L5 level, followed by L4. Patients typically complain of local lumbar pain which worsens with extension. Initial workup includes anteroposterior and lateral radiographs. Additionally a fracture through the pars interarticularis is sometimes visible as the "Scotty dog sign" on oblique radiographs. Nonetheless, the use of oblique radiographs for the diagnosis of spondylolysis remains controversial. A CT scan is considered the best modality to accurately diagnose a pars defect. However, it is often not possible to differentiate between active and inactive lesions, and therefore a SPECT is sometimes used in combination with CT. Some authors recommend the use of MRI as a first-line diagnostic tool to diagnose juvenile spondylolysis. Primary treatment of pars defects is conservative (rest, activity modification, and bracing). The majority of cases show good results without surgery. If conservative treatment fails, several surgical options are available including decompression, fusion with or without instrumentation, and direct pars repair. The decision is dependent on the type of pars defect (unilateral, bilateral, complex), and existence of neurologic signs or instability [17, 22, 29].

8.10 Spondylolisthesis

Bilateral pars fractures or defects may result in slipping of one vertebral body relative to an adjacent level. This condition is known as spondylolisthesis. The grading is based on the degree of transition (width of the vertebral body): Grade I <25%, Grade II 26–50%, Grade III 51–75%, Grade IV 76–100%, and Grade V >100% (spondyloptosis). A different and simplified grading system differentiates between stable (<50% translation) and unstable (>50% translation) cases. Depending on the severity of the slip, symptoms resulting from central and foraminal stenosis can occur. Similar to spondylolysis the initial treatment is conservative. Surgery should be considered for patients with failed conservative treatment, traumatic cases, or higher-grade spondylolisthesis (Fig. 8.3) [17, 30].

8.11 Return to Play

Currently there is no consensus regarding the time to return to play after a lumbar spine injury and surgery in tennis players. However, general recommendations for returning to play include that the individual should be pain-free after an adequate time for recovery (rehabilitation program following surgery), have preoperative range of motion and full strength, and not show any signs of neurologic injury [17, 22].

8.12 Prevention

There is limited data on measures proven to prevent spine injuries in tennis [8]. However, there is consensus on several recommendations.

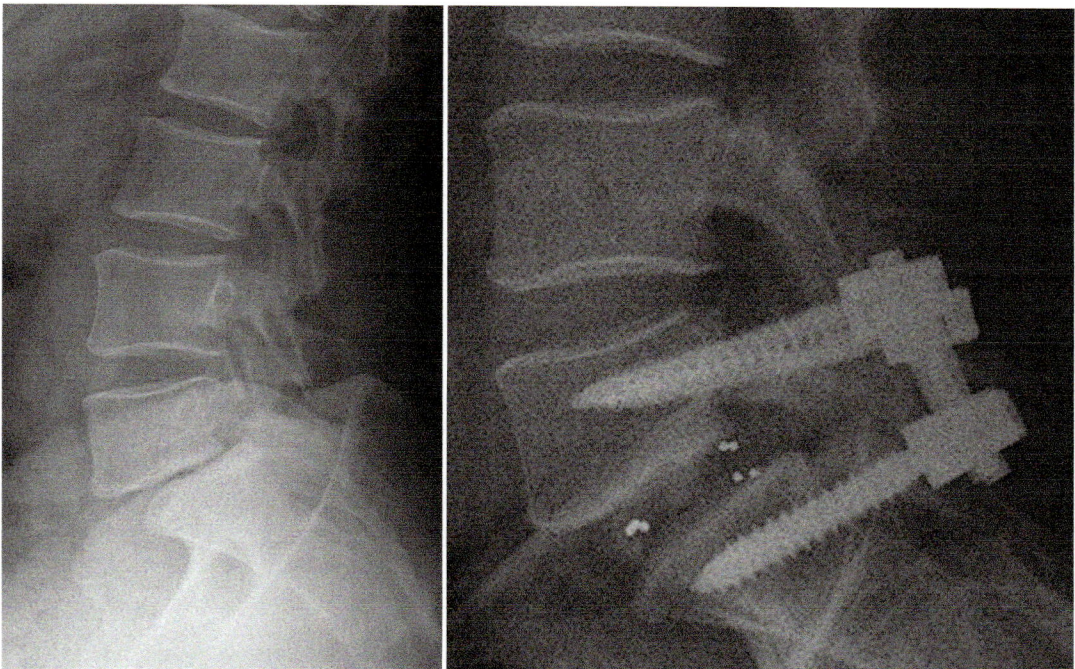

Fig. 8.3 Pre- and postoperative images of a spondylolisthesis L5/S1

Establishing basic fitness with strong core muscles (abdominal and back muscles) is essential. Warming up before a game can reduce the likelihood of muscle strains and spasms. Learning the right technique with a professional coach is a good way not only to improve the play but also in preventing spine injuries. Since the serve is considered the most dangerous stroke in tennis, a different movement such as a slice serve rather than a topspin serve could be considered to reduce the stress on the lower back from hyperextension. Also learning a one-handed backhand might reduce rotational stress on the lumbar spine. Proper tennis equipment (especially the right racket and tennis shoes) is important to prevent injuries. Indirect stress to the spine could be a result of altered biomechanics of the swing due to inadequate equipment [31, 32]. Although a recent study showed that the overall injury rates do not differ between different playing surfaces, it is generally believed that playing on high shock-absorbing and low-friction surfaces such as clay courts might reduce the risk for injury [33].

8.13 Summary

Spine injuries in tennis players are very common. The underlying injury mechanisms are complex and multifactorial in nature. Training, adequate technique, and proper equipment are paramount to preventing long-lasting injuries. The majority of tennis players with a spine injury do not require surgical intervention since resolution of symptoms can often be accomplished with conservative management.

References

1. Changstrom B, Jayanthi N. Clinical evaluation of the adult recreational tennis player. Curr Sports Med Rep. 2016;15:437–45.
2. Hjelm N, Werner S, Renstrom P. Injury profile in junior tennis players: a prospective two year study. Knee Surg Sport Traumatol Arthrosc. 2010;18:845–50.
3. Pluim BM, Staal JB, Marks BL, Miller S, Miley D. Health benefits of tennis. Br J Sports Med. 2007;41:760–8.
4. Haapasalo H, Kannus P, Sievanen H, Pasanen M, Uusi-Rasi K, Heinonen A, Oja P, Vuori I. Effect of

long-term unilateral activity on bone mineral density of female junior tennis players. J Bone Miner Res. 1998;13:310–9.
5. Haapasalo H, Sievanen H, Kannus P, Heinonen A, Oja P, Vuori I. Dimensions and estimated mechanical characteristics of the humerus after long-term tennis loading. J Bone Miner Res. 1996;11:864–72.
6. Etherington J, Harris PA, Nandra D, Hart DJ, Wolman RL, Doyle DV, Spector TD. The effect of weight-bearing exercise on bone mineral density: a study of female ex-elite athletes and the general population. J Bone Miner Res. 1996;11:1333–8.
7. Jacobson PC, Beaver W, Grubb SA, Taft TN, Talmage RV. Bone density in women: college athletes and older athletic women. J Orthop Res. 1984;2:328–32.
8. Pluim BM, Staal JB, Windler GE, Jayanthi N. Tennis injuries: occurrence, aetiology, and prevention. Br J Sports Med. 2006;40:415–23.
9. Pluim BM, Loeffen FGJ, Clarsen B, Bahr R, Verhagen EALM. A one-season prospective study of injuries and illness in elite junior tennis. Scand J Med Sci Sports. 2016;26:564–71.
10. Donatelli R, Dimond D, Holland M. Sport-specific biomechanics of spinal injuries in the athlete (throwing athletes, rotational sports, and contact-collision sports). Clin Sports Med. 2012;31:381–96.
11. Marks MR, Haas SS, Wiesel SW. Low back pain in the competitive tennis player. Clin Sports Med. 1988;7:277–87.
12. Alyas F, Turner M, Connell D. MRI findings in the lumbar spines of asymptomatic, adolescent, elite tennis players. Br J Sports Med. 2007;41:836–41; discussion 841.
13. Rajeswaran G, Turner M, Gissane C, Healy JC. MRI findings in the lumbar spines of asymptomatic elite junior tennis players. Skelet Radiol. 2014;43:925–32.
14. Hainline B. Low back injury. Clin Sports Med. 1995;14:241–65.
15. Tanchev PI, Dzherov AD, Parushev AD, Dikov DM, Todorov MB. Scoliosis in rhythmic gymnasts. Spine (Phila Pa 1976). 2000;25:1367–72.
16. Zaina F, Donzelli S, Lusini M, Fusco C, Minnella S, Negrini S. Tennis is not dangerous for the spine during growth: results of a cross-sectional study. Eur Spine J. 2016;25:2938–44.
17. Huang P, Anissipour A, McGee W, Lemak L. Return-to-play recommendations after cervical, thoracic, and lumbar spine injuries: a comprehensive review. Sports Health. 2016;8:19–25.
18. Maquirriain J, Ghisi JP, Kokalj AM. Rectus abdominis muscle strains in tennis players. Br J Sports Med. 2007;41:842–8.
19. Maquirriain J, Ghisi JP. Uncommon abdominal muscle injury in a tennis player: internal oblique strain. Br J Sports Med. 2006;40:462–3.
20. Manchikanti L, Kaye AD, Boswell MV, et al. A systematic review and best evidence synthesis of effectiveness of therapeutic facet joint interventions in managing chronic spinal pain. Pain Physician. 2015;18(4):E535–82.
21. Manchikanti L, Hirsch JA, Falco FJE, Boswell MV. Management of lumbar zygapophysial (facet) joint pain. World J Orthop. 2016;7:315–37.
22. Burgmeier RJ, Hsu WK. Spine surgery in athletes with low back pain-considerations for management and treatment. Asian J Sports Med. 2014. https://doi.org/10.5812/asjsm.24284.
23. Taher F, Essig D, Lebl DR, Hughes AP, Sama AA, Cammisa FP, Girardi FP. Lumbar degenerative disc disease: current and future concepts of diagnosis and management. Adv Orthop. 2012;2012:970752.
24. Madigan L, Vaccaro AR, Spector LR, Milam RA. Management of symptomatic lumbar degenerative disk disease. J Am Acad Orthop Surg. 2009;17:102–11.
25. Salzmann SN, Plais N, Shue J, Girardi FP. Lumbar disc replacement surgery—successes and obstacles to widespread adoption. Curr Rev Musculoskelet Med. 2017. https://doi.org/10.1007/s12178-017-9397-4.
26. Tumialán LM, Ponton RP, Garvin A, Gluf WM. Arthroplasty in the military: a preliminary experience with ProDisc-C and ProDisc-L. Neurosurg Focus. 2010;28:E18.
27. Siepe CJ, Wiechert K, Khattab MF, Korge A, Mayer HM. Total lumbar disc replacement in athletes: clinical results, return to sport and athletic performance. Eur Spine J. 2007;16:1001–13.
28. Porchet F, Bartanusz V, Kleinstueck FS, Lattig F, Jeszenszky D, Grob D, Mannion AF. Microdiscectomy compared with standard discectomy: an old problem revisited with new outcome measures within the framework of a spine surgical registry. Eur Spine J. 2009;18:360–6.
29. Li Y, Hresko MT. Lumbar spine surgery in athletes: outcomes and return-to-play criteria. Clin Sports Med. 2012;31:487–98.
30. Maquirriain J. Low back pain in the young tennis player. ASPETAR Sport Med J. 2014;3:508–14.
31. From Backhand to Backache. http://www.thespinehealthinstitute.com/news-room/health-blog/from-backhand-to-backache-5-ways-to-keep-tennis-from-troubling-your-spine.
32. Tennis and Back Pain. http://www.spine-health.com/conditions/sports-and-spine-injuries/tennis-and-back-pain.
33. Pluim BM, Clarsen B, Verhagen E. Injury rates in recreational tennis players do not differ between different playing surfaces. Br J Sports Med. 2017. https://doi.org/10.1136/bjsports-2016-097050.

Imaging of the Shoulder, Hip and Pelvis

9

Giuseppe Monetti, Gianluca Rampino, Giuseppe Rusignuolo, and Serena Tripoli

9.1 Imaging of the Shoulder

The tennis player's shoulder joint is subject to severe and repetitive stress. The forceful and explosive movements of the sport, especially serve and smash shots, place a heavy strain on musculotendinous and capsuloligamentous structures. Moreover, the fast and forceful movements required to wield increasingly light racquets—the result of continuous advances in materials research—also involve severe impacts on soft tissues.

A variety of diagnostic imaging techniques are employed to assess the injuries sustained by tennis players. They include plain radiography, computed tomography (CT), and dynamic ultrasound (US), the latter offering the additional valuable tools of power and colour Doppler and elastography. Yet, magnetic resonance imaging (MRI) remains the gold standard method to assess most of these lesions. High-field magnets provide a wide range of sequences that are suitable to assess changes in tendons, ligaments, cancellous bone, and cartilage. In addition, MR arthrography with injection of an intra-articular contrast agent supplies highly detailed morphological images of capsuloligamentous and fibro-cartilage structures. Notably, last-generation low-field magnets enable patients to be examined both lying down and standing, which is especially useful when dynamic evaluation is required.

Damage to the long head of the biceps tendon (LHBT), in the form of reactive tenosynovitis or of trauma involving its proximal insertion into the glenoid labrum, is by far the most common injury sustained by tennis players. The rotator cuff tendons are also frequently injured due to repetitive shoulder rotation. Partial- and full-thickness tears result in microinstability and eventually in severe impingement, most often posterosuperior impingement.

The most common conditions affecting tennis players are listed below.

9.1.1 Tenosynovitis of the Long Head of Biceps Tendon

Tenosynovitis of the extra-articular LBHT portion, which is covered by a synovial sheath, is a highly frequent painful condition among tennis players.

G. Monetti (✉)
Dipartimento di Diagnostica per Immagini, Ospedale Privato Accreditato Nigrisoli,
Bologna, Italy
e-mail: info@muskultrasound.it

G. Rampino
Unità operativa di Diagnostica per Immagini Friuli Coram, Udine, Italy

G. Rusignuolo
Struttura Complessa di Radiologia Azienda Ospedaliera Santa Maria di Terni, Terni, Italy

S. Tripoli
Centro di Diagnostica Sportiva D-Lab, Bologna, Italy

US is the imaging method of choice to assess it, especially because colour and power Doppler provide optimal evaluation of the inflammatory processes affecting the richly vascularized and innervated tendon sheath. US accurately detects the involvement of the synovial sheath through the presence of fluid and enables its examination under relaxation and contraction, providing clear evidence of any change in the myotendinous junction or of tendon instability in the bicipital groove (Fig. 9.1). The more severe injuries involve detachment of the tendon from the muscle component, accompanied by proximal tendon retraction and formation of a large haematoma; in such patients, valuable follow-up information is provided by elastography, which affords accurate assessment of the elasticity of musculotendinous components. US, together with MRI, also provides optimal follow-up imaging after tenodesis, clearly depicting the healing process of the tendon after bone fixation (Fig. 9.2a, b).

9.1.2 Superior Labral Tear from Anterior to Posterior (SLAP) Lesions

The LHBT inserts proximally at the level of the supraglenoid tubercle, where it attaches to the labrum anteriorly and posterosuperiorly. The repetitive stress borne by the tendon, especially in serve and smash shots, may induce fraying of the fibrocartilage labrum; moreover, the traction exerted by the robust tendon may eventually give rise to partial or complete labral tears.

MRI is the diagnostic method of choice to assess this condition: by providing accurate anatomical and topographic information, it clearly depicts any pathological changes. However, since standard MRI does not employ contrast media, MR arthrography is more suitable to diagnose SLAP lesions, since injection of ca. 15 cc of contrast agent into the joint distends the capsule and demonstrates any fissures in the labrum (Fig. 9.3a).

Upright MRI is a highly advanced technique that provides excellent images. Application of mechanical traction (2–4 kg) on the arm highlights any pathological labral detachment (Fig. 9.3b). A key advantage of the method, besides the fact that it obviates the use of intra-articular contrast agents, is that it provides dynamic, real-time images that enable optimal functional evaluation of the region. It should however be noted that this type of examination may be hampered by anatomical variants, whose common presence may result in misdiagnosis.

9.1.3 Rotator Cuff

The rotator cuff tendons are involved in all movements made by tennis players and are subject to severe strain. The tendon most commonly affected is the supraspinatus, at the level of the critical area on the lateral side of the joint.

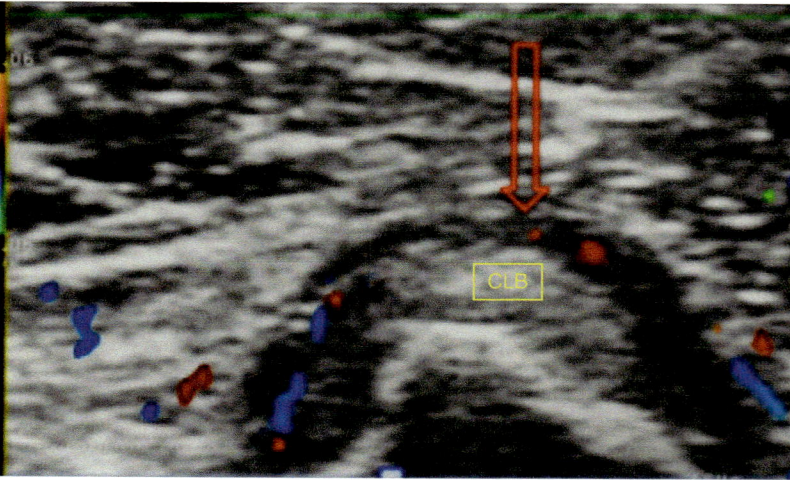

Fig. 9.1 Dynamic US scan through the axial plane: subluxation of the long head of biceps tendon at the level of the lesser tuberosity associated with severe tenosynovitis

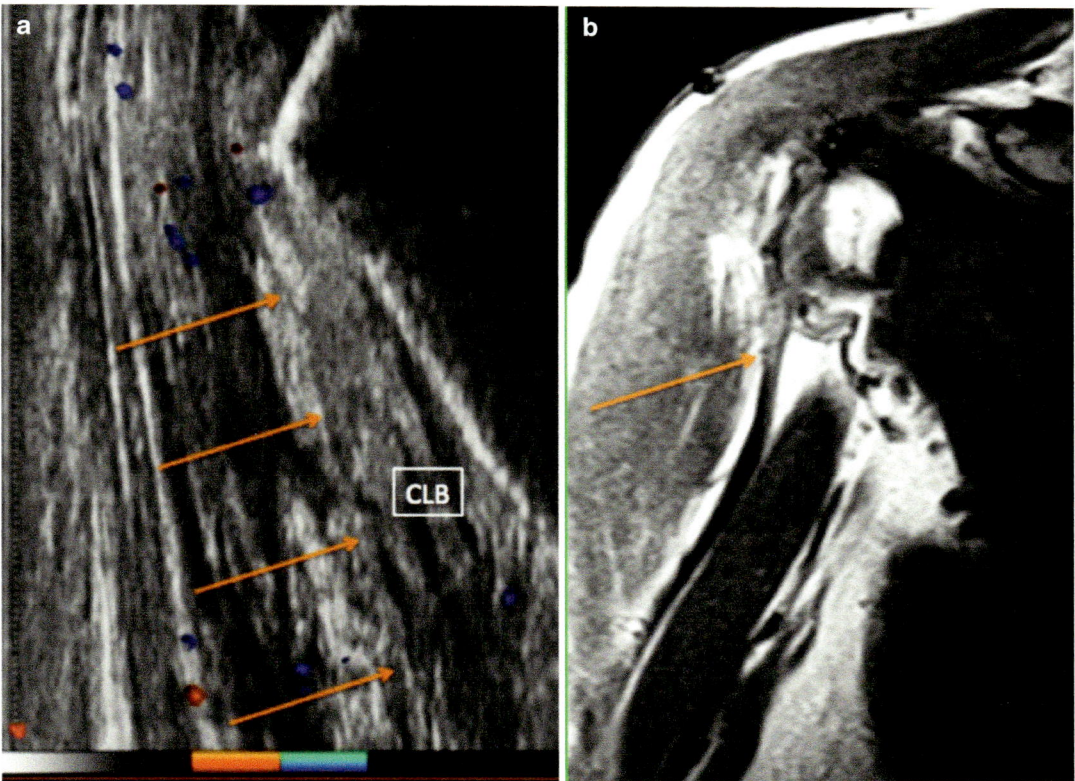

Fig. 9.2 Follow-up scans of long head of biceps tenodesis as assessed by US (**a**) and MRI (**b**). The tendon has been attached at the level of the proximal third of the humerus

Rotator cuff tendon lesions are first examined with dynamic US. In patients where the findings are difficult to interpret, valuable information can be obtained from high-contrast MRI sequences. The advent of dynamic MRI has greatly improved the diagnostic potential of the method. Dynamic MRI provides extremely accurate images, especially in those cases where US and standard MRI do not supply conclusive diagnostic information despite strong clinical evidence of tendon injury. Scans acquired with the shoulder in abduction and dynamic external rotation clearly demonstrate even small lesions that are undetectable both by US and by standard MRI (Fig. 9.4a, b).

9.1.4 Posterosuperior Impingement

Posterosuperior or internal impingement is due to entrapment of the articular portion of the supraspinatus and infraspinatus between the humeral head and the glenoid during shoulder abduction and external rotation. In professional athletes repeated entrapment gives rise to tendon wear that may eventually lead to high-grade tears.

In such cases US provides useful diagnostic information on the articular portion of the tendon, but cannot exclude a possible, concomitant SLAP lesion. The diagnostic technique of choice to assess these conditions is therefore MRI, which provides wide panoramic views. In particular, dynamic MRI can demonstrate the impingement during abduction and external rotation as the tendon glides between the humeral head and the glenoid (Fig. 9.5a, b).

Dynamic MRI also provides excellent information to assess humeral head engagement due to anterior shoulder dislocation. In these patients a very posterior Hill-Sachs lesion may involve engagement of the head at the level of the posterosuperior glenoid rim during abduction and external rotation (Fig. 9.6a, b).

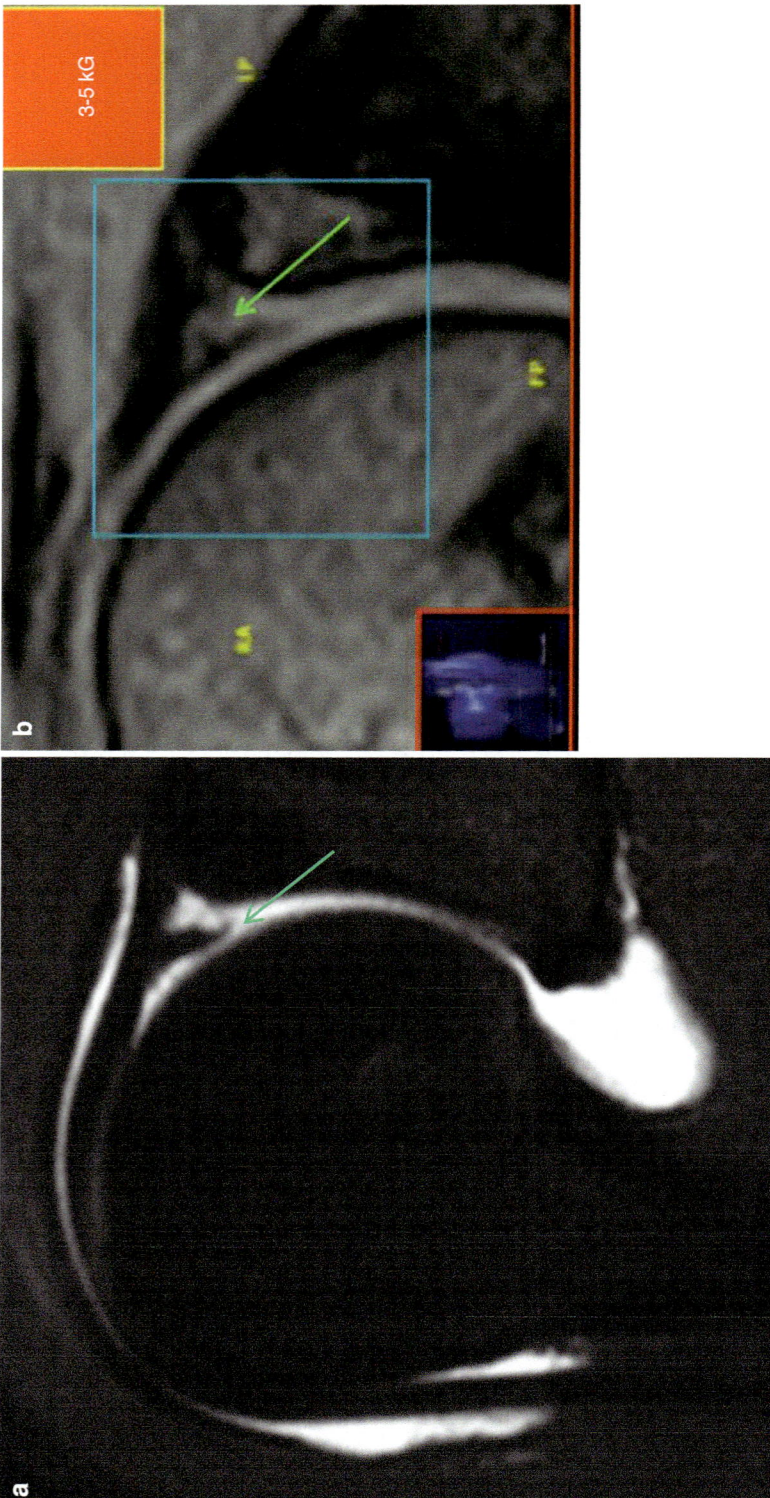

Fig. 9.3 Fissures in the labrum (**a**) and labral detachment (**b**) Type III SLAP lesion diagnosed by dynamic upright MRI with 5 kg traction

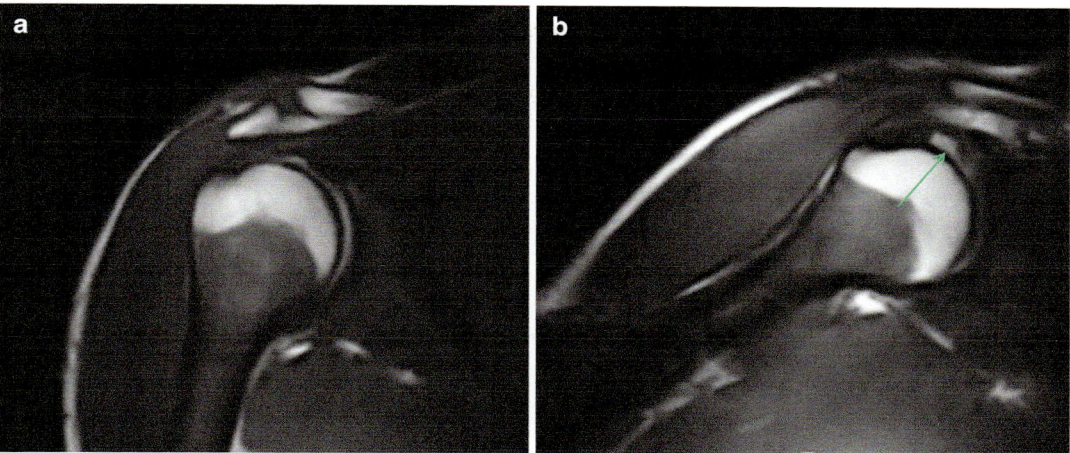

Fig. 9.4 Dynamic MRI. At rest (**a**) the rotator cuff lesion is undetectable, whereas the tear is demonstrated by the dynamic scan acquired with the shoulder in forced adduction and internal rotation (**b**)

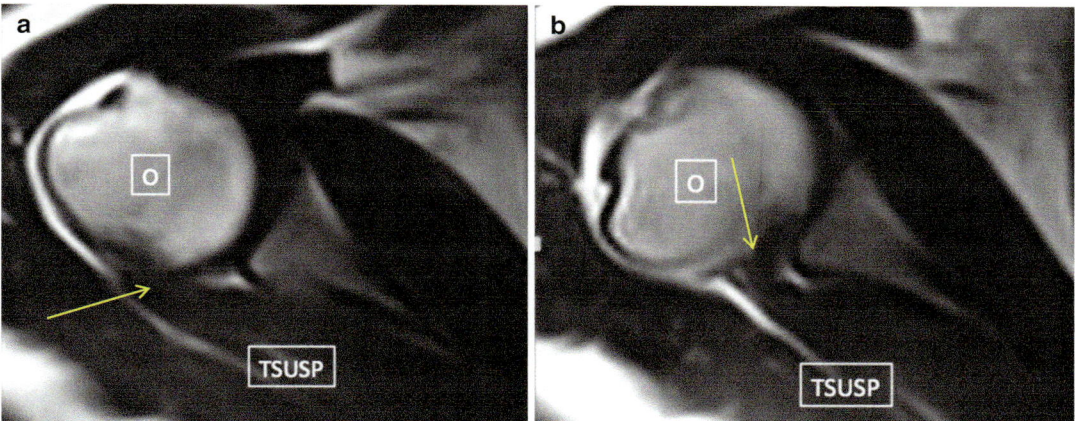

Fig. 9.5 Clear posterosuperior impingement (**a**), where abduction and external rotation (**b**) allow visualization of the impingement with entrapment of the infraspinatus tendon between the glenoid and the humeral head

Dynamic US, MR arthrography, and dynamic upright MRI are the methods of choice to assess the conditions discussed above, which are the most common problems affecting tennis players. Plain X-rays and 3D CT reconstructions can also be employed in patients whose condition is complicated by a bone fracture in the same area.

9.2 Imaging of the Hip and Pelvis

The different surfaces of tennis courts have different effects on the lower limbs; they involve different impacts on anatomical structures and induce discrete lesions. The softer clay courts are associated with muscle distraction and avulsion of the tendons of insertion, most often of the adductors, as players slide through the court, typically as they respond to angled shots. In contrast, the harder surfaces of concrete and synthetic courts, which are characterized by greater vibration and limited lateral mobility, are more often associated with injury to capsuloligamentous structures.

The conditions affecting tennis players, especially those involved in competitions, are predominantly trochanteric or iliopsoas bursitis, impingement of the tensor fasciae latae and gluteus medius in the peritrochanteric region, and

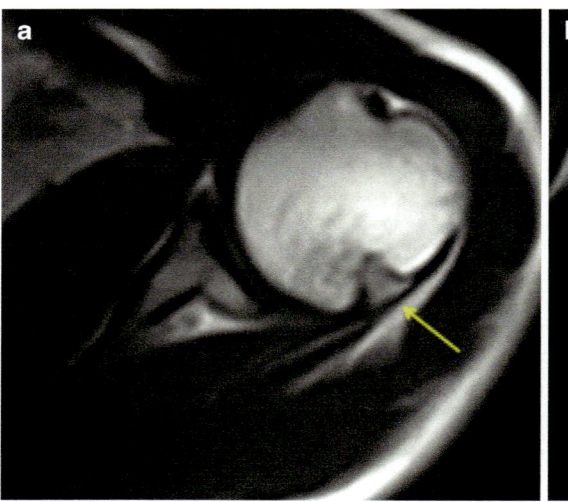

Fig. 9.6 Sequelae of anterior shoulder dislocation. The dynamic MRI scan, acquired in maximum external rotation, demonstrates the engagement of the humeral head fracture with the posterosuperior glenoid labrum (**a**) and infraspinatus impingement (**b**)

femoroacetabular impingement (of the cam or pincer type), which is becoming increasingly common.

The diagnostic imaging methods of choice to assess these injuries include dynamic US, especially in patients with bursitis or inflammation of the myotendinous junction, MR arthrography, and, recently, dynamic upright MRI.

The major pathological conditions affecting tennis players are listed and discussed below.

9.2.1 Bursitis

The portion of the hip bursa that is most often affected by inflammation is the peritrochanteric region, where the bursa tends to become inflamed during the typical lateral movements involved in the sport. The bursitis is sometimes accompanied by impingement of the tensor fasciae latae and gluteus medius, which often gives rise to external snapping hip syndrome.

Snapping hip may be caused by inflammation and distension of the peritrochanteric bursa, bony changes, or intratendinous calcifications. The imaging method of choice to assess these conditions is dynamic US, which can demonstrate the snapping event, depict the actual impingement, and, in the dynamic scanning phase, detect any tendon injury (Fig. 9.7a–c).

Inflammation in the iliopsoas bursa gives rise to internal snapping hip syndrome, which is often due to impingement of the tendon of the iliopsoas muscle at the level of the iliopubic eminence, resulting in bursitis or intratendinous changes. Given the considerable depth of this bursa, US is not very informative, whereas standard and dynamic upright MRI scans, acquired where needed with internal and external rotation, provide highly accurate findings (Fig. 9.8a, b).

9.2.2 Inguinal and Sports Hernia

In tennis players, internal/external rotation and adduction/abduction of the hip may give rise to hernias. They are either inguinal hernias or sports hernias, the latter due to laxity of the aponeurotic wall that is found between adjacent muscles at this site.

The technique of choice to diagnose this condition is US, in particular power Doppler and elastography, because it makes it possible to acquire dynamic scans during a Valsalva manoeuvre (Fig. 9.9).

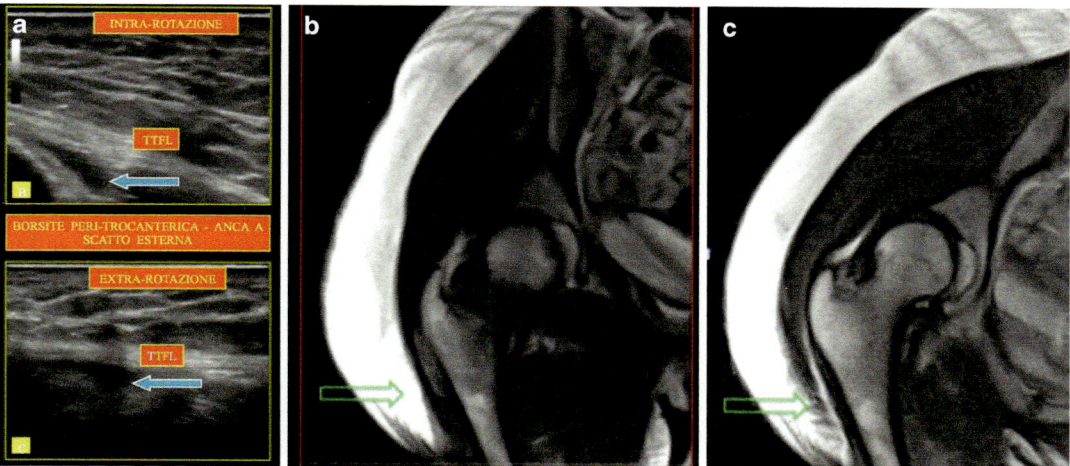

Fig. 9.7 (**a–c**) Peritrochanteric bursitis inducing external snapping hip demonstrated by dynamic US and dynamic upright MRI

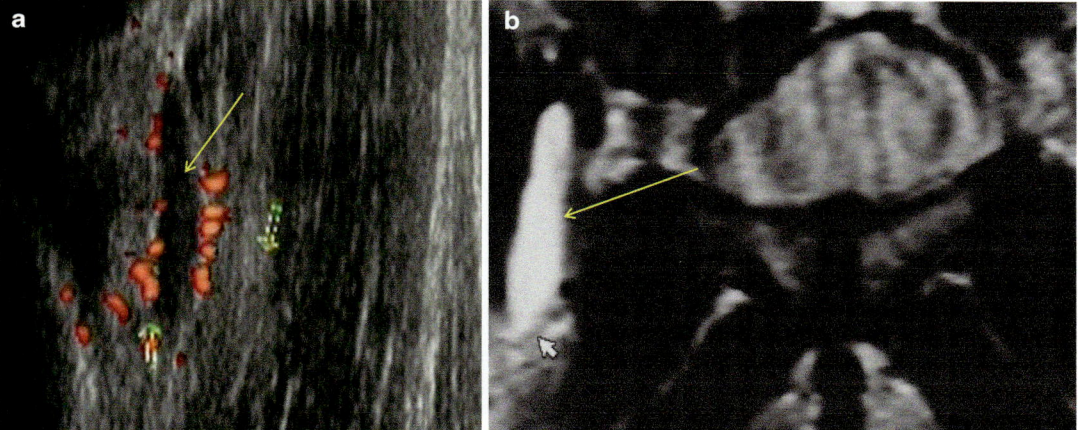

Fig. 9.8 Internal snapping hip due to iliopsoas bursitis depicted by US (**a**) and MRI (**b**)

9.2.3 Muscle Lesions

The most commonly injured pelvic muscles in tennis players are the adductors, especially the adductor longus, the rectus femoris, and the iliopsoas muscle. Involvement of the posterior ischiocrural muscles is less common (Figs. 9.10, 9.11, and 9.12).

The method of choice to depict these lesions is dynamic elastography, especially where the more superficial muscles are involved. The diagnosis of pelvic adductor injury is best made on standard MRI and upright MR scans taken with weight bearing (each leg and both legs). X-rays, including pelvic views, may also provide useful diagnostic information.

9.2.4 Femoroacetabular Impingement

Femoroacetabular impingement may be of cam or pincer type. Young, especially male, athletes suffer predominantly from the cam type, where deformation of the femoral neck close to the junction with the head, on the anterolateral side,

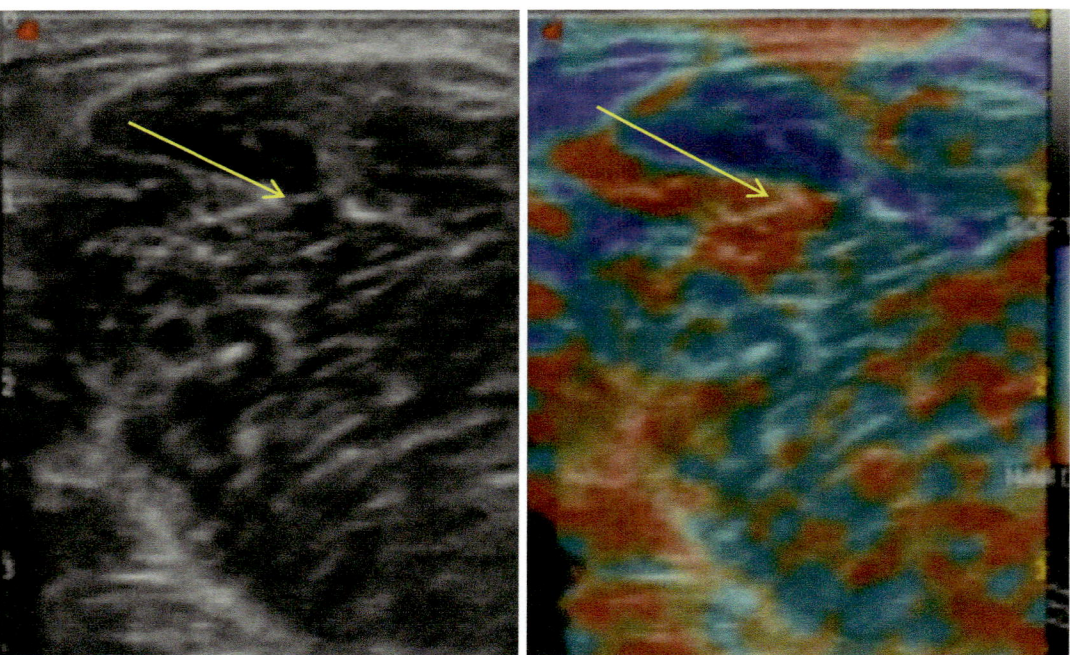

Fig. 9.9 Dynamic elastography: scan showing a sports hernia

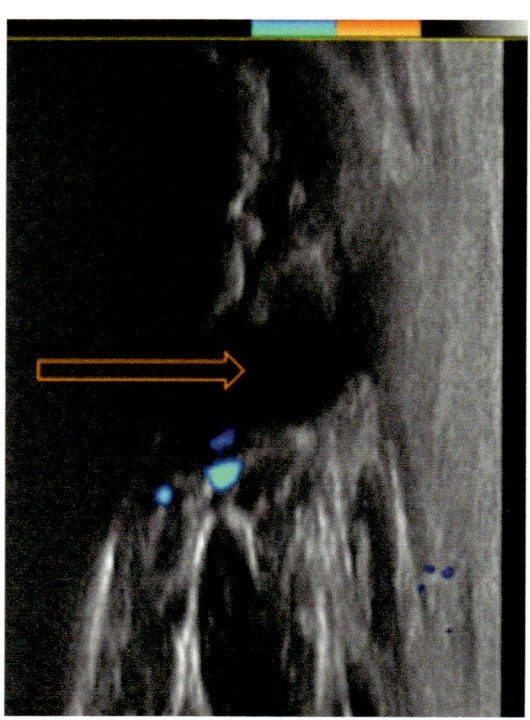

Fig. 9.10 Acute, full-thickness tear of the insertion of the tendon of the long adductor muscle depicted by dynamic US with the hip in passive contraction

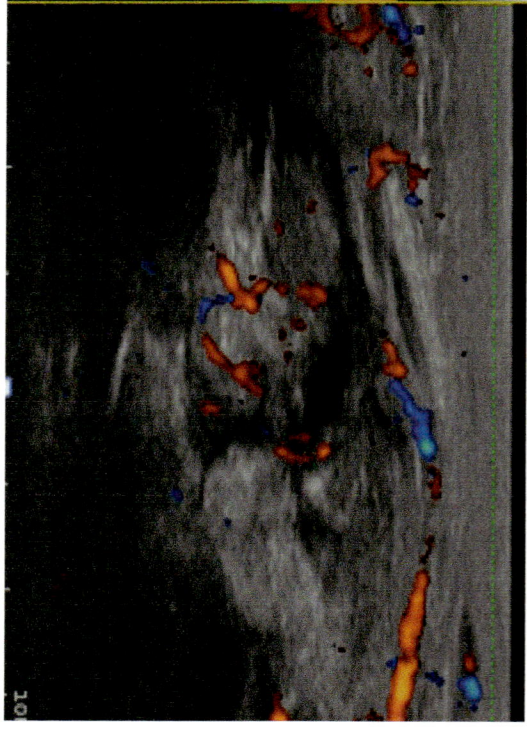

Fig. 9.11 High-grade partial rupture of the myotendinous junction of the tendon of the long adductor muscle depicted by dynamic US. Inflammation is clearly demonstrated by colour Doppler

9 Imaging of the Shoulder, Hip and Pelvis

the femoral head and the anterosuperior labrum as the patient performs internal/external rotation and adduction/abduction movements (Fig. 9.13a, b). The less common pincer type is assessed in the same way. The methods of choice are dynamic elastography and MRI, especially dynamic and upright MRI. Plain X-rays and CT with 3D reconstructions (where needed) are further valuable diagnostic tools.

9.2.5 Piriformis Syndrome

Intense physical and athletic activity, as in the case of professional tennis players, may affect the piriformis, resulting in muscle hypertrophy or oedema. The sciatic nerve, which traverses the muscle belly, may undergo compression mimicking lumbar pain and sciatica.

US is not the method of choice to diagnose this condition, given the wide and flat shape of the piriformis and the availability of only axial and sagittal views. MRI in the coronal plane is more informative, since its panoramic views enable comparison with the contralateral muscle, thus providing at least morphological data, i.e. hypotrophy or hypertrophy due to muscle stress or trauma. Currently, the method of choice to assess piriformis syndrome is dynamic upright MRI with muscle contraction and relaxation, especially through the sagittal plane. In these patients we have often detected a significant involvement of the quadratus femoris muscle, whose contraction directly compresses the sciatic nerve, giving rise to neurological pain (Fig. 9.14a, b).

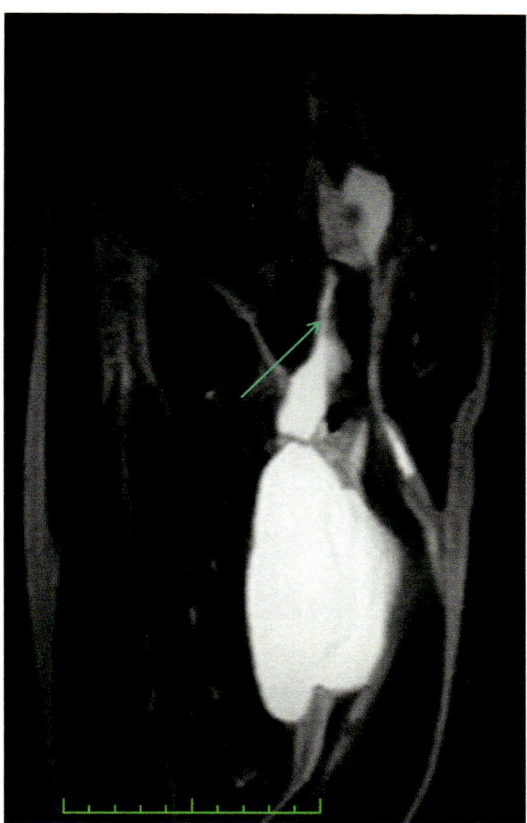

Fig. 9.12 Dynamic upright MRI. Full rupture of the ischiocrural muscle tendons of insertion

gives rise to impingement with the anterosuperior portion of the labrum during internal and external rotation of the leg.

Besides standard MRI, the imaging method of choice for this condition is dynamic upright MRI, which depicts the actual impingement between

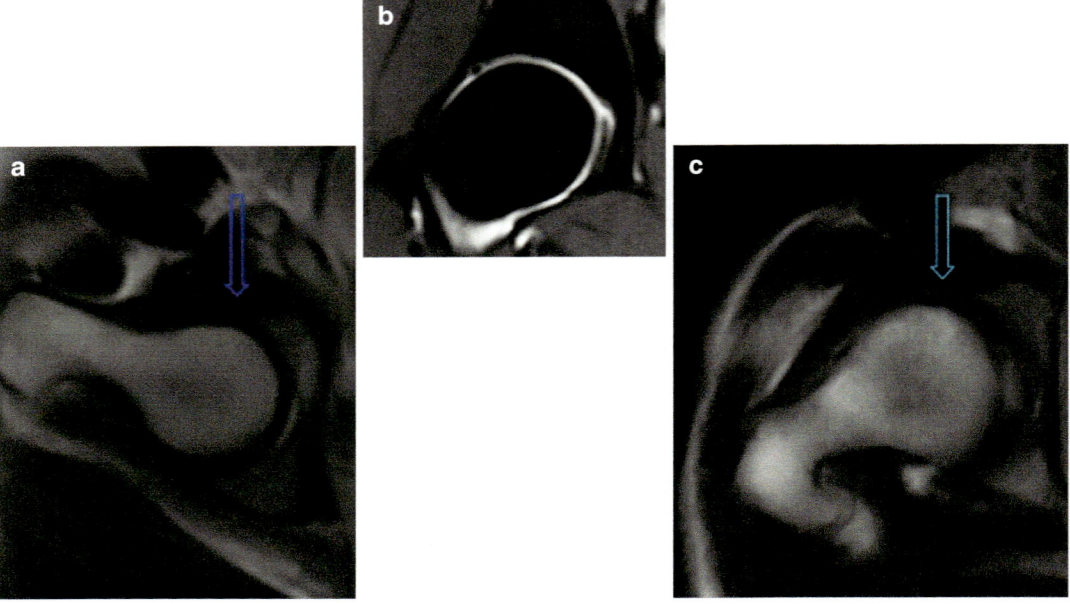

Fig. 9.13 Dynamic upright MRI. The scans acquired with internal (**a**) and external rotation (**b**) show clearly the cam type femoroacetabular impingement. (**c**) MR arthrography: rupture of the anterosuperior portion of the labrum

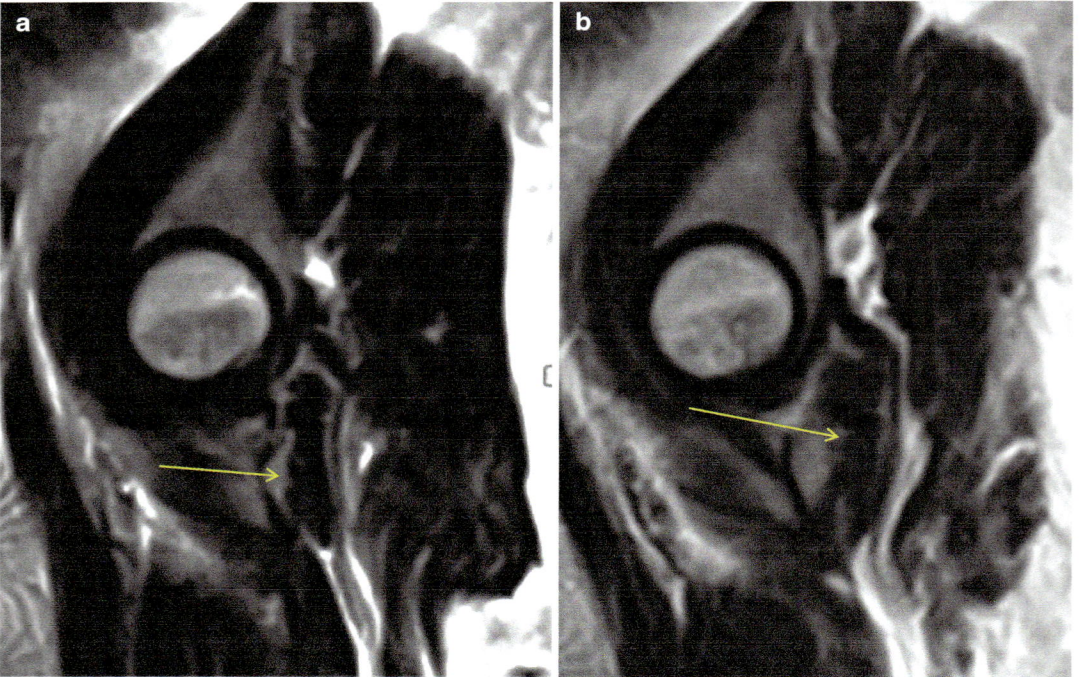

Fig. 9.14 (**a**, **b**) Upright MRI. Impingement of the quadratus femoris and the sciatic nerve during muscle contraction

Suggested Reading

Ahuja A, Antonio GF, Griffith JF, et al. Diagnostic and surgical imaging anatomy ultrasound. Salt Lake City, UT: Amirsys; 2007.

Baert AL, Sartor K. Paediatric musculoskeletal disease with an emphasis on ultrasound. In: Wilson D, Editor. Berlin: Springer. p. 2005.

Baert AL, Knauth M, Sartor K. High resolution sonography of the peripheral nervous system. In: Peer S, Bodner G, Editors. 2nd revised edition. Springer: Berlin; 2008

Barbolini G, Monetti G. L'esame ecografico dell'anca del neonato e del lattante. In: Ziviello M, editor. Ecotomografia, vol. 2. Napoli: Idelson.

Basford JR, Jenkyn TR, An KN, Ehman RL, Heers G, Kaufman KR. Evaluation of healthy and diseased muscle with magnetic resonance elastography. Arch Phys Med Rehabil. 2002;83(11):1530–6.

Bianchi S, Martinoli C. Ultrasound of the musculoskeletal system. Berlin: Springer; 2007.

Bradley M, O'Donnell P. Atlas of musculoskeletal ultrasound anatomy. London: Greenwich Medical Media; 2002.

Callaghan MJ, McCarthy CJ, Al-Omar A, Oldham JA. The reproducibility of multi-joint isokinetic and isometric assessments in a healty and patient population. Clin Biomech (Bristol, Avon). 2000;15:678.

Chevrot A. Imagerie des tendons, ligaments et muscles periphetiques. Paris: Masson; 1993.

Chhem RK, Cardinal E. Guidelines and gamuts in muscloscheletal ultrasound. New York: Wiley-Liss; 1999.

Cohen M. Echoanatomie des ischio-jambiers. Gel Contact. 2002;9:4–8.

Couture A, Baud C, Ferran SL, Veyrac C. Ecographie de la hanche chez l'enfant. Montpellier: Axone; 1988.

De Marchi A, Pozza S, Faletti C. Atlante di Ecografia Muscolotendinea Tecnica Anatomia Quadri Patologici. Torino: Utet; 2007.

Di Giacomo G, et al. Atlas of functional shoulder anatomy. Milan: Springer; 2008.

Downey DB, Fenster A. Three-dimensional ultrasound: a maturing technology. Ultrasound Q. 1998;14:25.

Downey DB, Fenster A, Williams JC. Clinical utility of three-dimensional ultrasound. Radiographics. 2000. https://doi.org/10.1148/radiographics.20.2.g00mc19559.

Dresner MA, Rose GH, Rossman PJ, et al. Magnetic resonance elastography of skeletal muscle. J Magn Reson Imaging. 2001;13:269.

Fenster A, Downey DB. 3D ultrasound imaging: a review. IEEE Eng Med Biol. 1996;15:41.

Fornage BD. Ultrasonography of muscles and tendons. Examination technique and atlas of normal anatomy of the extremities. New York: Springer; 1988.

Fukashiro S, Itoh M, Ichinose Y, et al. Ultrasonography gives directly but noninvasively elastic characteristic of human tendon in vivo. Eur J Appl Physiol Occup Physiol. 1995;71:555.

Garfinkel S, Cafarelli E. Relative changes in maximal force, EMG, and muscle crosssectional area after isometric training. Med Sci Sports Exerc. 1992;24:1220–7.

Graf R. Fundamentals of sonographic diagnosis of infant hip dyspasia. J Pediatr Orthop. 1984;4:735–40.

Harcker HT. Screening newborns for developmental dysplasia of the hip: the role of sonography. AJR Am J Roentgenol. 1994;162:395–7.

Heers G, Jenkyn T, Dresner MA, et al. Measurement of muscle activity with magnetic resonance elastography. Clin Biomech (Bristol, Avon). 2003;18(6):537–42.

Jenkyn TR, Ehman RL, An KN. Noninvasive muscle tension measurement using the novel technique of magnetic resonance elastography (MRE). J Biomech. 2003;36:1917.

Khurana A, Dahiya N. 3D-4D ultrasound: a text and atlas. Kent, UK: Anshan-Jaypee; 2004.

Manaster DJ, et al. Diagnostic and surgical imaging anatomy musculoskeletal. Salt Lake City, UT: Amirsys; 2006.

Manduca A, Oliphant TE, Dresner MA, et al. Magnetic resonance elastography: non invasive mapping of tissue elasticity. Med Image Anal. 2001;5:237.

Martin BJ, Park H-S. Analysis of tonic vibration reflex: influence of vibration variables on motor unit synchronization and fatigue. Eur J Phys. 1997;75(6):504–11.

Martino F, Monetti G. Semeiotica ecografica delle malattie reumatiche. Padova: Piccin editore; 1993.

Martino F, Silvestri E, Grassi W, Garlaschi G. Ecografia dell'Apparato Osteoarticolare, Anatomia, Semeiotica e Quadri Patologici. New York: Springer; 2006.

McNally EG. Practical musculoskeletal ultrasound. Philadelphia: Elsevier; 2005.

Monetti G. Ecografia muscolare. In: Neurosonologia. III Meeting SINS, Torino; 1986.

Monetti G. Ecografia muscolo-tendinea e dei tessuti molli. Milano: Solei ed; 1989.

Monetti G. Ecografia osteo-articolare e muscolo-tendinea. Napoli: Gnocchi Editore; 1994a.

Monetti G. Muscoli e tendini. In: Bazzocchi M, editor. Napoli: Gnocchi Ed; 1994b.

Monetti G. L'impiego degli ultrasuoni nella diagnostica della patologia neuromuscolare. Ultrasonica. 1998

Monetti G. Ecografia muscolo-scheletrica imaging integrato. Napoli: Idelson Gnocchi; 2000.

Monetti G. Elastographie Muscolaire et Tendineuse – Atti Convegno Hitachi Maggio. Paris; 2009a.

Monetti G. Musculo-skeletal elastosonography – Atti 18th annual conference- Musoc 22–24 octobre 2009b, Buenos Aires.

Monetti G. Ecografia muscolo-scheletrica, Tecnica, anatomica ed imaging integrato, vol. 1. Bologna: Timeo Editore; 2009c.

Monetti G. Muskuloskeletal ultrasound, Technique, anatomy and integrated imaging, vol. 1. Bologna, Italy: Timeo Publisher; 2009d.

Monetti G. Ecografia muscolo-scheletrica, Patologia ed imaging integrato di muscoli, tendini e tecniche speciali, vol. 2. Bologna: Timeo Editore; 2010a.

Monetti G. Ecografia muscolo-scheletrica, Patologia ed imaging integrato delle articolazioni, vol. 3. Bologna: Timeo Editore; 2010b.

Monetti G. L'Elastographie en Ecographie de l' appareil locomoteur – Actualites en ecographie de l'appareil locomoteur. Paris: J.L. Brasseur – Sauramps Medical; 2012.

Monetti G, Minafra P. Trattato di Ecografia Clinica CA.A. V.V.C. Ed. Edison Gnocchi; 2006.

Monetti G, Minafra P. The muskuloskeletal elastography. Medix Supplement; 2007. p. 43–5.

Monetti G, Minafra P. La Elastosonografia come Indagine Funzionale nella Patologia Muscolo-Tendinea Atti 43° Nazionale SIRM- 23-27 maggio, Roma; 2008.

Monetti G, Minafra P. Ultrasound elastography. Musculoskeletal ultrasound, Anatomy, technique and integrated imaging, vol. 1. Bologna, Italy: Timeo Editore; 2010.

Monetti G, et al. Valore della ecotomografia nello studio della patologia muscolo tendinea. In: Landscape. 1986;1:11.

Monetti G, Minafra P, Pruna R, Till L. Sonoelastography main applications: muskuloskeletal system. Pavia, Italy: EdiMes; 2012.

Monetti G, et al. La spalla. Rome: Verducci Editore; 2014.

Monetti G, et al. Small-parts in pediatria. In: La ecotomografia nella diagnostica per immagini. Atti Convegno R.E., 83-6, 28 Settembre 1985.

Morel-Lavallee M. Décollements traumatiques de la peau et des couches sous-jacentes. Arch Gen Med. 1863;1:20–38, 172–200, 300–32.

Moritani T, De Vries H. Neural factors versus hypertrophy in the time course of muscle strength gain. Am J Physical Med. 1979;58(3):115–30.

Muthupillai R, Lomas DJ, Rossman PJ, et al. Magnetic resonance elastography by direct visualization of propagating acousticstrain waves. Science. 1995;269:1854.

O'Neill J. Musculoskeletal ultrasound anatomy and technique. New York: Springer; 2008.

Ophir J, Céspedes I, Ponnekanti H, Yazdi Y, Li X. A quantitative method for imaging the elasticity of biological tissue. Ultrason Imaging. 1991;13(2):111–34.

Parker KJ, Huang SR, Musulin RA, Lerner RM. Tissue response to mechanical vibration for "Sonoelasticity imaging". Ultrason Med Biol. 1990;16:241.

Pecina M. Tunnel syndromes. Boca Raton: CRC Press; 1991.

Peetrons P, Chhem R. Atlas D'Echographie du Systeme Locomoteur. Tome 1: Le membre superieur. Tome 2: Le membre inferieur. Sauramps Medical; 2000.

Pesavento A, Lorenz A, Siebers S, Ermert H. New real-time strain imaging concept using diagnostic ultrasound. Phys Med Biol. 2000;45:1423.

Porcellini G, et al. La spalla. Patologia, tecnica chirurgica e riabilitazione. 1st ed. Rome: Verducci Editore; 2003.

Porcellini G, et al. La spalla. Patologia, tecnica chirurgica e riabilitazione. 2nd ed. Rome: Verducci Editore; 2014.

Prior BM, Foley JM, Javaraman RC, Meyer RA. Pixel T2 distribution in functional magnetic resonance images of muscle. J Appl Physiol. 1999;87:2107.

Psenner K, Ortore PG, Fodor G. L'ecografia nella displasia dell'anca del neonato, da G. Monetti, Ecografia muscolo-tendinea e dei tessuti molli. SOLEI Ed.; 1989.

Segal RL. Using imaging to assess normal and adaptive muscle function. Phys Ther. 2007;87:704.

Shina T, Nitta N, et al. Real time tissue elasticity imaging using combined autocorrelation method. J Med Ultrasound. 1999;29:119–28.

Smirniotou A, Katsikas C, Paradisis G, Argeitaki P, Zacharogiannis E, Tziortzis S. Strength-power parameters as predictors of sprinting performance. J Sports Med Phys Fitness. 2008;48(4):447–54.

Stoller DW. Stoller's atlas of orthopaedics and sports medicine. Philadelphia, PA: Wolters Kluwer-Lippicott Williams & Wilkins; 2008.

Thompson JC. Atlante di anatomia ortopedica di Netter. Ed. In: Masson; 2004.

Tomà P, Rossi UG. Pediatric ultrasound. II. Other applications. Eur Radiol. 2001;11:2369–98.

Torvinen S, Kannus P, Sievanen H, Jarvinen M, Oja P, Vuori I. Effect of vibration exposure muscular performance and body balance. Randomized cross-over study. Clin Physiol Funct Imaging. 2002;22(2):145–52.

Van Holsbeeck, Introcaso J.H., Musculoskeletal ultrasound. Mosby Year Book, St. Louis, MO 1991.

Van Holsbeeck MT, Introcaso JH. Musculoskeletal ultrasound. 2nd ed. Philadelphia, PA: Mosby; 2001.

Musculoskeletal Screening for the Elite and Developing Tennis Player

Todd S. Ellenbecker

10.1 Introduction

The use of musculoskeletal testing in sports medicine is a widespread practice, typically with a dual goal of injury prevention and performance enhancement. Knowledge regarding sport-specific normative results of musculoskeletal tests is important for the optimal interpretation of test findings in individual populations of athletes. Sport-specific descriptive data aids in the interpretation of these tests and helps to define characteristic adaptations inherent in certain homogenous athletic populations. The purpose of this chapter is to present the current methods and descriptive findings of a tennis-specific musculoskeletal screening examination used for elite junior and professional tennis players.

Prior research has identified shoulder and hip range of motion (ROM) and muscular strength patterns in elite juniors [1–6] and adult [7] tennis players. Similar studies can also be found for high-level baseball players [8–12] and in other overhead athletes [13, 14]. Musculoskeletal profiling research is also available for the lower extremity in tennis and soccer players [15–17]. These studies have most often utilized a single means of testing (i.e., isokinetic strength, goniometric range of motion, etc.).

Injuries in elite tennis players involve virtually all anatomical regions of the body, with acute injuries more common in the lower extremities and chronic overuse injuries more common in the upper extremity and trunk. Repetitive forces and loads are imparted through the sequential segmental rotational loading of the entire kinetic chain during performance of the primary tennis strokes (serve, forehand, backhand) [15–25]. Therefore, a musculoskeletal screening examination to identify subtle muscular weakness, muscular imbalance, and both flexibility and range of motion deficits using a series of tests throughout the entire body (rather than just a single joint or a small series of joints) is appropriate for the elite tennis player.

10.2 Historical Perspective of Musculoskeletal Screening for Elite Tennis Players

In 2003, the United States Tennis Association (USTA) Sport Science Committee originally developed a musculoskeletal evaluation for elite junior tennis players called the High Performance Profile (HPP). It consisted of ten evidence-based tests for the upper body, lower body, and core musculature, specific to the demands and adaptations reported in the litera-

T. S. Ellenbecker
ATP World Tour and Rehab Plus Sports Therapy, Scottsdale, AZ, USA
e-mail: tellenbecker@atpworldtour.com

ture for elite-level tennis players. These tests were designed to assess the entire kinetic chain and be readily performed by physical therapists, athletic trainers, and physicians. The committee reevaluated the HPP in 2012 and updated the profile changing several tests based on an initial review of the data from the HPP and reflecting several changes in emphasis specifically adding tests for hip rotation range of motion and hip and core stabilization testing. Table 10.1 lists the original and updated tests for the USTA HPP. Clinicians continue to utilize the updated battery of musculoskeletal tests for elite junior tennis players.

In 2006, ATP Medical Services initiated the Performance and Injury Prevention Screening (PIPS) program. The USTA HPP formed the initial platform for the screening program. Several tests were added by the ATP Medical Services Committee to provide further descriptive information on professional-level male players. Testing considerations for the ATP program included the ability to perform the entire screening within 30 min with portable equipment and within the confines of an athletic training room at professional tennis tournaments. As the ATP PIPS program was developed primarily as a player service, the tests selected to be included generally allowed for implementation of corrective exercises to address any deficiencies found in the individual tests (Fig. 10.1). Additionally, tests selected could not be too fatiguing or induce pain or significant post-examination soreness which might affect players' performance as it was being performed during participation in the tournament. Table 10.2 lists the tests and measures carried out in the ATP Performance and Injury Prevention Screening (PIPS) program.

Table 10.1 USTA High Performance Profile Tests. Original (2003) and updated (2012)

HPP original tests	HPP updated tests
Scapular stabilization test	Scapular stabilization test
External rotation manual muscle test	External rotation manual muscle test
Grip strength	Shoulder internal and external rotation ROM
Shoulder internal and external rotation ROM	One-leg stability test
One-leg stability test	Drop vertical jump test
Hip external rotation test (Patrick's)	Prone hip IR and ER ROM
Thomas (hip flexor) test	Thomas (hip flexor) test
Hamstring SLR test	Hamstring SLR test
Quadriceps prone flexibility test	Quadriceps prone flexibility test
Abdominal bracing core stab test	Plank (prone and side) tests

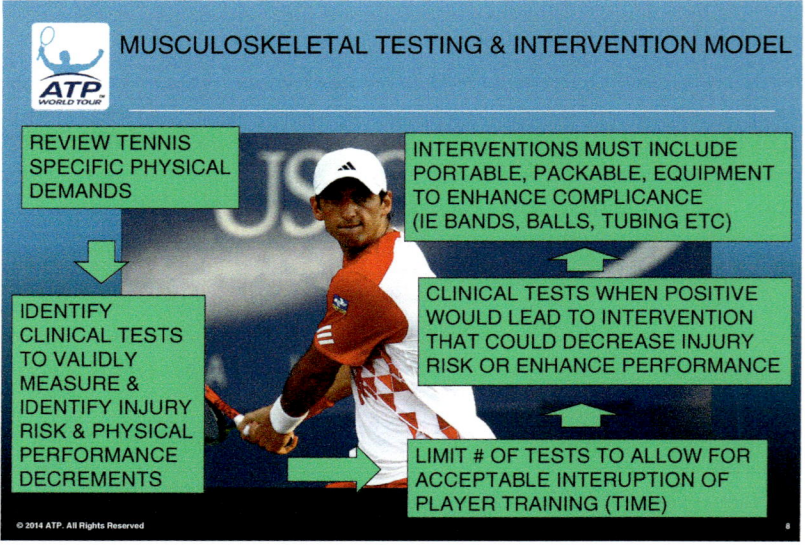

Fig. 10.1 ATP musculoskeletal screening and intervention model (Figure 1)

Table 10.2 The ATP Performance and Injury Prevention Screening program tests

Posture/shoulder heights
Visual observation of infraspinatus atrophy
Scapular dyskinesis test[a]
External rotation strength with handheld dynamometer (neutral and 90° of abduction)
Supraspinatus strength with handheld dynamometer
Glenohumeral joint internal and external rotation range of motion (90° ABD)[a]
Glenohumeral joint cross-arm adduction range of motion
Elbow extension range of motion
Forearm pronation/supination range of motion
Grip strength[a]
Hamstring straight leg raise flexibility[a]
Prone knee flexion range of motion[a]
Prone hip internal and external rotation range of motion
Thomas test[a]
Ankle dorsiflexion range of motion
One-leg stability test[a]
Abdominal bracing core stability test[a]
Plank test
Bridging test
Rotary stability test

[a]Denotes original test from USTA high-performance profile (HPP)

10.3 Overview of Key Tests Used in Musculoskeletal Screening of Elite Tennis Players

For the purposes of this chapter, a brief review of each of the key screening tests will be undertaken citing both a methodological description and scientific rationale for these tests.

10.3.1 Upper Extremity Tests

10.3.1.1 Range of Motion

Passive Glenohumeral Joint Rotation

Glenohumeral joint range of motion (ROM) is measured with the player in a supine position and with the shoulder abducted 90° in the coronal plane using a universal goniometer. The player's elbow is maintained in 90° of elbow flexion, while passive external (ER) and internal (IR) rotation ROM were measured, while the exam-

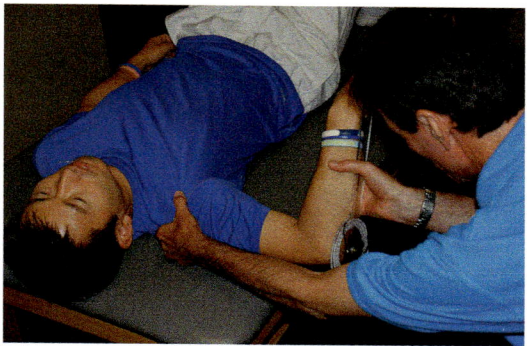

Fig. 10.2 Shoulder internal rotation range of motion measurement using a goniometer with technique for scapular stabilization used during testing

iner's hand stabilizes the scapula so that scapulothoracic movement is prevented [2, 3, 26] (Fig. 10.2). End range of motion is determined by the weight of the limb and gravity, with no overpressure exerted by the examiner. Total rotation ROM is obtained by adding the IR and ER measures together. It is important that these tests be performed bilaterally, to allow for comparison to the non-dominant extremity. The test-retest reliability of this range of motion technique for shoulder internal rotation in 90° of abduction with scapular stabilization has been studied by Wilk et al. [26] with intraclass correlation coefficients reported as 0.62 for intra-rater reliability and 0.43 for inter-rater reliability.

Shoulder Cross-Arm (Horizontal) Adduction

The test is performed with the player in the supine position using a digital inclinometer. The player's shoulder is passively brought to 90° of shoulder flexion in the sagittal plane, with the examiner stabilizing the lateral border of the scapula and with the examiner's other hand against the lateral border prior to the initiation of the cross body movement. No overpressure is applied to the horizontal adduction motion, with the extremity's weight against gravity used to determine the end point. Bilateral measurement of this movement pattern is recorded using the value generated from the digital inclinometer relative to the vertical (neutral) starting position (Fig. 10.3).

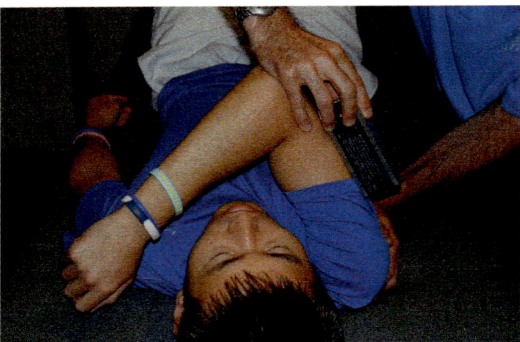

Fig. 10.3 Shoulder cross-arm adduction testing performed with an inclinometer with scapular stabilization

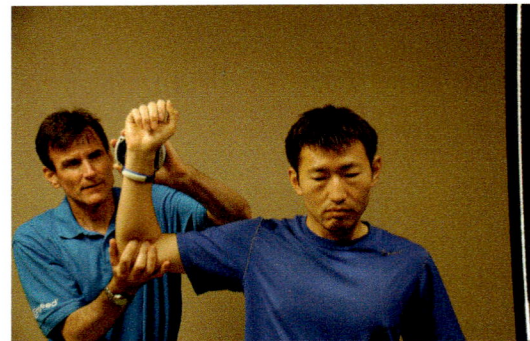

Fig. 10.4 Shoulder external rotation manual muscle test with handheld dynamometer with 90° of glenohumeral joint abduction

Elbow and Wrist ROM

With the player in a seated position, elbow extension ROM is measured using a universal goniometer bilaterally. The shoulder is placed in 90° of flexion, with the forearm supinated during measurement. The goniometer is aligned along the lateral aspect of the elbow, using consistent landmarks [27]. Players actively extend their elbow to end ROM. Active forearm pronation and supination are also measured, with the player in the seated position and the elbow flexed to 90° with the arm at the side. The goniometer axis is placed in line with the third metacarpal of the hand, and the degrees of pronation and supination motion from neutral are recorded [27]. Additionally, flexion and extension of the wrist are measured with the elbow extended fully and the forearm in pronation (palm-down position). The goniometer is used and aligned with the lateral aspect of the ulna (proximal arm) and the fifth metacarpal (distal arm) to perform this measurement.

10.3.1.2 Strength and Stability

Shoulder ER Strength

Players are tested using a Lafayette (Lafayette Instrument Company, Lafayette, IN, USA) handheld dynamometer (HHD) in a seated position, with the shoulder abducted 90° in the coronal plane (Fig. 10.4). The best of two maximal contractions are recorded in kilograms. The HHD is placed on the dorsal aspect of the forearm, immediately proximal to the ulnar styloid process. The elbow remains flexed 90° during testing. This

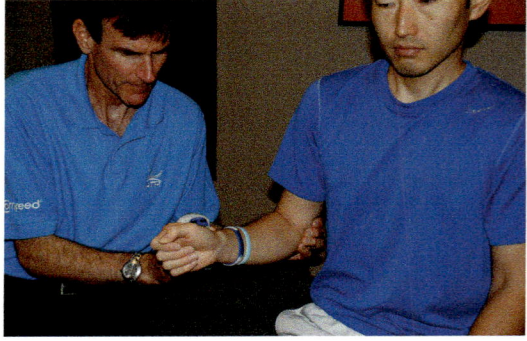

Fig. 10.5 Shoulder external rotation manual muscle test with handheld dynamometer with the shoulder in neutral (ab/adduction) at the side

primarily tests the strength of the teres minor. Kurokawa et al. [28] tested muscle activity in both the 90° abducted and neutral (at side) positions and reported significantly more teres minor activity versus infraspinatus activity in the 90° abducted position when assessing shoulder external rotation strength. Muscle strength testing with the arm in 0° of abduction (neutral at side) produced greater infraspinatus activity and a lower teres minor/infraspinatus ratio than testing external rotation strength at 90° of abduction.

Therefore, shoulder external rotation strength is also tested with the arm by the side to assess the strength of the infraspinatus [28, 29], as injury to the suprascapular nerve has been reported in overhead athletes [30–33] (Fig. 10.5). An upright-seated position is used, with the elbow flexed 90° and the shoulder in

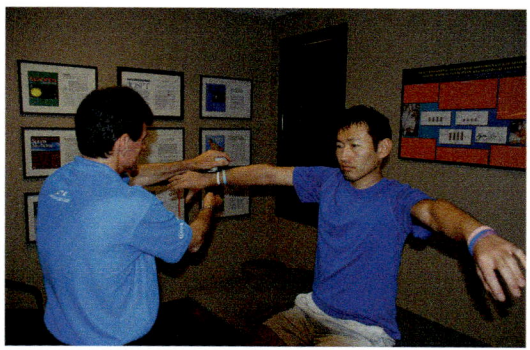

Fig. 10.6 Empty can test position used to test for supraspinatus strength with a handheld dynamometer

resting adduction positioning. The player is instructed to maximally externally rotate the shoulder with the HHD positioned just proximal to the ulnar styloid process above the wrist. The best of two maximal contractions is recorded in kilograms.

Supraspinatus Strength

Testing utilizes the empty can position (scapular plane abduction with internal rotation) [32, 33] in the seated position. The shoulder is maintained in 90° of elevation during testing, with the HHD placed just proximal to the ulnar styloid process (Fig. 10.6). The best of two maximal contractions is recorded bilaterally in kilograms.

Grip Strength

A Jamar handgrip dynamometer is used, with the player in a standing position. The elbow is maintained in an extended position, with no contact of the dynamometer with the player's body during testing. The best of two maximal effort trials is recorded bilaterally in kilograms.

Scapular Evaluation

Using a 1 kg (2.2 pound) weight, players are visually observed from behind during 4–5 repetitions of simultaneous bilateral shoulder overhead forward flexion, scapular plane abduction, and coronal plane abduction performed in the standing position (Fig. 10.7). Using the classification proposed and researched by Kibler [34, 35], each scapula is independently evaluated.

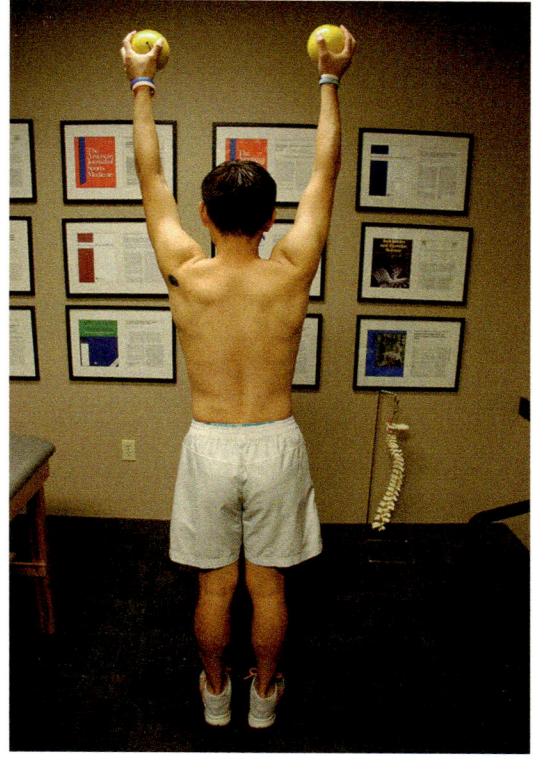

Fig. 10.7 Test for scapular stabilization using a 2 pound weight with self-directed elevation in the scapular plane

Scapular dyskinesis is considered to be present if abnormal motion or positioning of the scapular relative to the thorax is identified [34]. A yes/no determination is used. Test-retest reliability of the Kibler system of scapular dysfunction has been studied, with coefficient of agreements reported as 79% (Kappa 0.40) for the yes/no classification [34].

10.3.1.3 Posture

Shoulder Heights

Shoulder heights are assessed individually by both examiners with the player in a resting standing position, with the arms hanging freely by the sides, and with examiners positioned behind the player. The assessment of shoulder height is determined by visual inspection and documented as dominant shoulder higher, dominant shoulder lower, or shoulder heights equal bilaterally by each examiner.

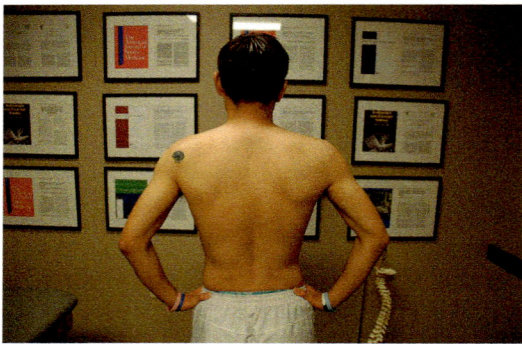

Fig. 10.8 Visual observation of infraspinatus atrophy using the hands on hip position

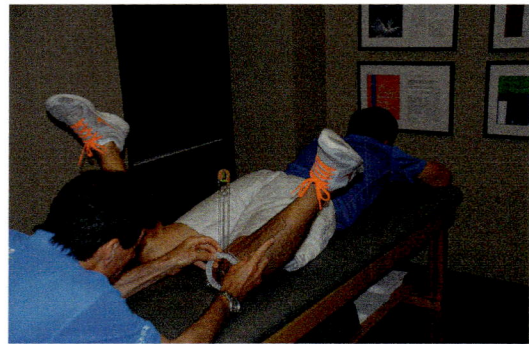

Fig. 10.9 Prone hip internal rotation range of motion measurement method

Visual Observation of Infraspinatus Atrophy

The player is instructed to place their hands on their hips with their thumbs pointing posteriorly, placing the shoulder in slight internal rotation and slight scapular protraction and upward rotation (Fig. 10.8). Visual inspection and, when necessary, palpation of the infraspinatus fossa of both shoulders are performed independently by both examiners and recorded as yes/no (yes atrophy or no atrophy) of the infraspinatus muscle bilaterally.

10.3.2 Lower Extremity Tests

10.3.2.1 Range of Motion

Hip Rotation

Hip rotation ROM is measured with the player in the prone position, with the knees flexed 90°. Hip IR is measured by having the subject actively internally rotate both hips simultaneously, to minimize trunk and body rotation (Fig. 10.9). A goniometer is used with the axis of rotation along the femur, with one arm placed along the tibia and the other remaining vertical [4]. Hip ER is measured one extremity at a time, with the examiner's hand placed on the ipsilateral pelvis to stabilize and minimize motion/rotation during measurement. Similar goniometer landmarks are again used for hip ER. Hip total rotation is obtained by summing the IR and ER measurements.

Thomas Test

This well-known and widely used flexibility test for the hip flexors is performed with the player in a supine position on a plinth. The description of this test is well referenced elsewhere [35]. A positive test indicating tightness of the hip flexors is determined when the femur does not achieve a position parallel to the ground (hip flexor tightness) (Fig. 10.10). Additionally, rectus femoris tightness is determined when the knee cannot be passively flexed to 90° without concomitant flexion of the femur [7]. Each extremity is assessed independently.

Prone Knee Flexion

Players are tested in a prone position and asked to actively flex their knee, moving their heel to their buttock. A goniometer is placed along the lateral aspect of the femur and fibula to measure knee flexion [3]. Testing of bilateral extremities is performed and compared.

Hamstring Flexibility

Multiple methods of assessing the flexibility of the hamstrings are reported in the literature and are used in the screening of elite tennis players. One method, the straight leg raise (SLR) test, is performed by measuring passive hip flexion ROM with the knee extended and recording the angle of the thigh relative to the trunk using a goniometer [35]. Another method involves the active extension of the knee from a 90/90 position and measures the angle from vertical of the tibia [35]. Both tests involve a neutral extended

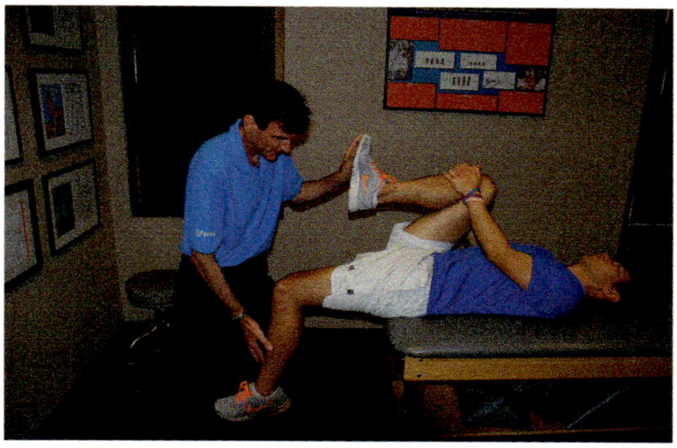

Fig. 10.10 Thomas test used to assess flexibility of the hip flexors

position of the contralateral extremity. We use the passive straight leg raise test to measure each extremity independently.

Ankle Dorsiflexion

The measurement of active ankle dorsiflexion range of motion is performed with the player in a supine position on a treatment table with the knee in extension. The goniometer is aligned with the lateral aspect of the lower leg (fibula) and the lateral border of the foot. Each extremity is assessed independently. Following the recording of the values for ankle dorsiflexion with knee extension which represent gastrocnemius flexibility, the player is placed in the prone position to assess ankle dorsiflexion with 90° of knee flexion, using identical landmarks for goniometer placement. Ankle dorsiflexion with knee flexion represents soleus flexibility. Both measurements are used to assess ankle joint ROM and posterior calf muscle flexibility, as well as prescreen the player prior to performance of the one-leg stability test. Significant limitations in ankle dorsiflexion identified with isolated testing assist with interpretation of hip and core deviations or alterations during the one-leg squat test. Players with limited ankle dorsiflexion range of motion are tested with and without a towel roll under the heel, to minimize the effect of limited ankle movement on subsequent hip and core stability tests.

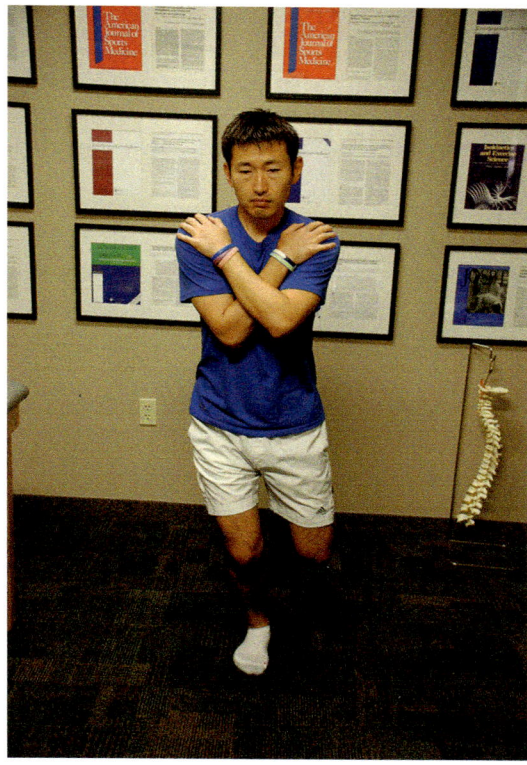

Fig. 10.11 One-leg stability test used to test for hip and core stabilization

10.3.2.2 Lower Extremity Strength and Core Stability Tests

One-Leg Stability Test

The one-leg stability test measures the player's ability to stand on one leg (Fig. 10.11) and perform a 1/3 (30°–45° of knee flexion) squat while maintaining proper balance and trunk and lower extremity alignment [36, 37]. Several repetitions are viewed by both examiners from in front of the player, with particular attention focused on the following three abnormal movement patterns:

1. Trendelenburg sign (contralateral hip drop)
2. Knee valgus angulation during descent
3. Excessive forward lean of the trunk

The presence of any one or combination of these three abnormal movement patterns results in a failed test. The test is performed bilaterally, with the arms of the player crossed over their chest. Test-retest reliability of the single-leg stability test has been reported for both inter- and intra-rater applications, with coefficients of agreement reported as 73–87% and kappa coefficients of 0.60–0.80.

Abdominal Bracing Test

The original core stability test recommended by the USTA Sport Science Committee consists of abdominal bracing during a series of independent leg extensions from the initial position of 90° of hip and knee flexion [38]. A blood pressure cuff is placed in the lumbar region of the player, with initial inflation of the cuff to 40 mmHg during contraction of the abdominal musculature to produce a posterior tilt of the pelvis into the cuff. The player is then instructed to alternatively lower one leg at a time to a position of hip and knee extension approximately 6 in. off the supporting surface (Fig. 10.12a, b). To pass the test, the player has to maintain the pressure in the cuff at or above 40 mmHg for ten repetitions with each leg. Inability to perform ten repetitions with each leg results in a "failed" test [36, 38].

Plank Tests (Prone and Unilateral Side Support)

The plank tests involve a sustained hold in prone and right and left side-lying positions, while maintaining optimal body alignment and postural control [36, 38]. Each of the positions must be maintained for 30 s to pass the test (Figs. 10.13 and 10.14).

Bridging

A modification of the bridge test is utilized to evaluate posterior chain core stability and strength. Players are tested in the supine position. Their arms are crossed over their chests to eliminate upper extremity utilization during testing. They are asked to perform a bridge by extending their hips and trunk and raising their buttocks from the supportive surface until a straight alignment is achieved. From that position they are then instructed to engage their core and gluteal musculature, prior to extending one of the knees such that the leg is extended outward, forming a straight line from the shoulders through the hip and knee (Fig. 10.15). Players are required to limit any trunk and pelvic rotation during the unilateral support phase of the bridge. The procedure is repeated multiple times with each leg to ensure that the player is able to support his hip and core during alternating periods of unilateral support. To pass the test, the player has to

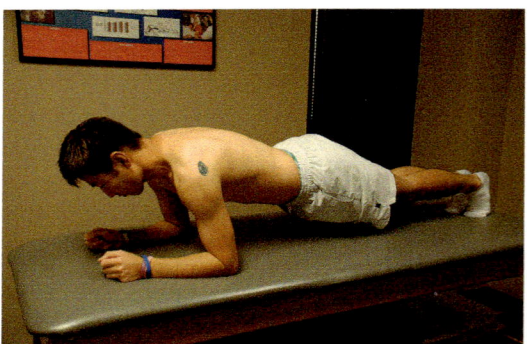

Fig. 10.13 Prone plank position

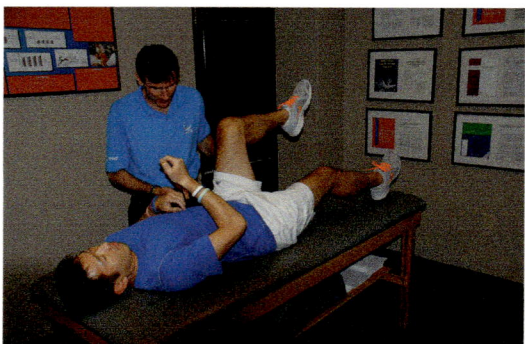

Fig. 10.12 Abdominal bracing test with unilateral leg lowering using a blood pressure cuff in the lumbar region

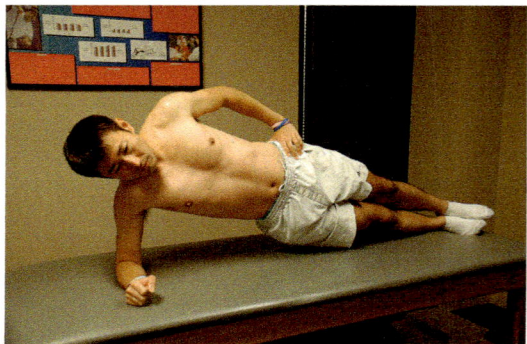

Fig. 10.14 Side plank position

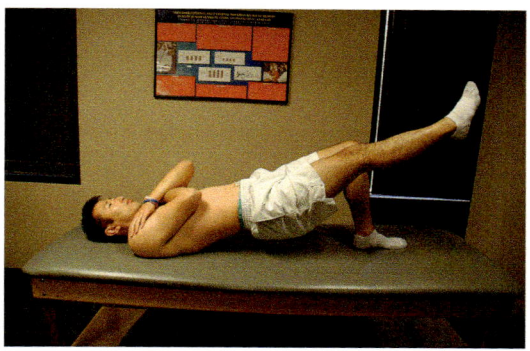

Fig. 10.15 Bridging test with unilateral knee extension

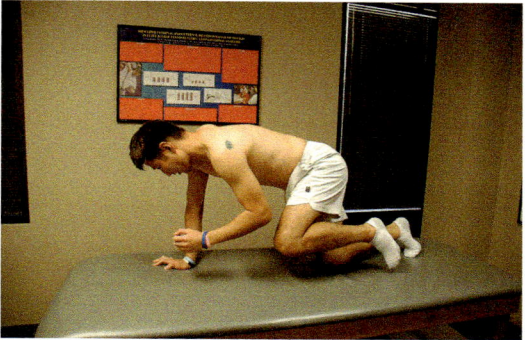

Fig. 10.16 Rotary stability test with ipsilateral arm/leg movement

exhibit complete control, with no loss of alignment or rotational movement of the hips and pelvis during the test.

Rotary Stability Test
This test, a component of the functional movement screen (FMS), is performed with the player in the quadruped position [39]. The player is instructed to alternatively extend diagonal extremity pairs (left arm/right leg then right arm/left leg) while maintaining a neutral spinal alignment with minimal trunk motion during the movements. Multiple repetitions are performed. Inability to maintain alignment constitutes a failed test. A more advanced version of this test is also recommended for application for elite-level tennis players. This test is called the ipsilateral arm/leg extension rotary stability test. This test is identical to the contralateral version but, as the name implies, involves successive repetitions of ipsilateral arm and leg extension (Fig. 10.16).

10.4 Interpretation/Application of Musculoskeletal Test Findings for Elite Tennis Players

To facilitate the interpretation of musculoskeletal evaluation of elite tennis players, this portion of the chapter will be dedicated to the discussion and presentation of descriptive data from two primary populations of elite players. One sample for presentation comes from a 10-year period of testing of 232 male professional players who were tested as part of the ATP PIPS program. The second data set comes from screening of elite male and female tennis players ($n = 299$). All players were currently training and/or competing and were free from injuries that prohibited their full participation in their competition or training activities at the time of testing. Table 10.3A, B list the demographic parameters and characteristics of each testing group.

Table 10.3A displays the demographics of the 232 professional players tested in the ATP Performance and Injury Prevention Program from 2006 to 2015. The average age of the players tested was 25.6 ± 3.85 years. The median ATP World Tour singles ranking was 140 and doubles ranking 120. A majority of players were right-handed (86.2%), and, for the purposes of this article and our analysis, all data was processed using the dominant and non-dominant classification rather than left or right. Two-handed backhands were used by 74% of the players in this sample reflecting the predominance of the two-handed backhand in the modern game. The forehand grip used by the players was 70.2% semi-Western, 15.3% Western, and 3% Eastern.

Table 10.3B displays the demographics of the 299 elite junior tennis players. To be considered elite, players were training year round in tennis and competing in tournaments leading to the achievement of rankings in local, sectional, national, and international standings. Two-handed backhands were used by 75% of elite male junior players and 97% of elite female junior players. Additionally, the Beighton Hypermobility Index was positive in 25% of elite male junior players

Table 10.3 Player demographics from ATP World Tour professional male players (A) and elite junior male and female players (B)

(A) ATP World Tour professional male tennis player demographics ($n = 232$)			
Variable	Mean	Standard deviation	Frequency
Player age (years)	25.6	(3.85)	–
Player weight (kg)	79.8	(6.73)	–
Arm dominance (right)			86.2%
Two-handed backhand			74%
(B) Elite male and female junior tennis players ($n = 299$)			
Variable	Males (mean ± sd)	Females (mean ± sd)	
Age (years)	17.2 (3.2)	16.5 (3.5)	
Height (in.)	69.9 (4.0)	66.6 (3.9)	
Weight (lbs)	150.1 (31.3)	128.9 (25.7)	
Years of tennis play	8.3 (3.4)	6.9 (3.7)	
Number of tournaments/year	16.8 (7.8)	16.7 (8.3)	
Two-handed backhand	75%	97%	
Right-handed players	90%	94%	
Beighton Hypermobility Index (+)	25%	62%	

and 62% of elite female junior players in this testing sample.

Although many players were screened multiple times, the results presented in this article contain the musculoskeletal screening data only from the player's initial screening in the program. It is recommended that players follow up after initial screenings for an ongoing assessment of their strength, range of motion, and overall musculoskeletal health at regular time intervals, which was routinely followed for a large proportion of the players in these two samples; however, follow-up data is not presented in this chapter. Players received an evidence-based exercise program to address key areas of deficiency identified during the musculoskeletal screening protocol.

10.5 Descriptive Musculoskeletal Findings in Elite Tennis Players

The remainder of this chapter will discuss the findings from the two samples of musculoskeletal screenings performed on ATP professional players and elite juniors. While it is beyond the scope of this chapter to discuss all results in detail, tables with complete data are included to provide a descriptive profile from these populations.

10.5.1 Upper Extremity Testing

Posture: Evaluation of posture showed that professional male players presented with their dominant shoulder lower than the contralateral shoulder 82.7% of the time. Players' non-dominant shoulder was lower only 4.4% of the time, while shoulder heights appeared level 12.9% of the time. Visual atrophy of the infraspinatus muscle was apparent in the dominant shoulder 73% of the time and present 5% of the time in the non-dominant shoulder.

Scapular Testing: Scapular dyskinesis was identified in 52% of the dominant shoulders and 38% of the non-dominant shoulders of the male professional tennis players. For the elite junior players, female players had visually observed scapular dyskinesis 75% of the time on the dominant arm and 56% in the non-dominant extremity. For the male elite junior players, slightly lower values of 65% for the dominant extremity and 48% on the non-dominant extremity were observed and recorded.

Upper Extremity Range of Motion and Strength: Tables 10.4 and 10.5 display the results of the upper extremity range of motion and strength testing from the ATP male professional players and the elite junior players, respectively.

Players had an average of 4.58° more dominant shoulder glenohumeral external rotation

Table 10.4 Upper extremity range of motion and strength test results in ATP professional male tennis players

Test	Dominant Mean (sd)	Non-dominant Mean (sd)	Difference (Dom − Ndom) Mean (sd)
Shoulder ER at 90	100.4 (8.2)	95.8 (10.9)	4.58 (10.3)
Shoulder IR at 90	39.8 (8.0)	49.9 (7.4)	−10.09 (8.8)
Total rotation ROM	140.1 (10.4)	146.4 (9.6)	−6.28 (9.0)
Cross-arm adduction	34.4 (6.4)	42.3 (7.4)	−7.86 (6.6)
Elbow extension	−2.9 (6.9)	4.3 (6.1)	−7.29 (6.4)
Forearm pronation	69.9 (7.0)	71.9 (7.9)	−2.03 (7.5)
Forearm supination	80.0 (14.2)	87.8 (14.0)	−7.26 (8.6)
Shoulder ER (neutral)	13.6 (3.0)	15.6 (2.4)	−2.03 (2.7)
Shoulder ER (neutral) Force/BW ratio	17.1%	19.5%	–
Shoulder ER (90 ABD)	15.2 (3.0)	14.6 (2.7)	0.58 (2.01)
Shoulder ER (90 ABD) Force/BW ratio	19%	18.3%	–
Supraspinatus	11.1 (2.4)	11.4 (2.2)	−0.38 (1.8)
Supraspinatus Force/BW ratio	13.8%	14.3%	–
Grip strength	56.8 (9.6)	50.9 (8.7)	5.9 (8.0)

Note: All measures for range of motion expressed in degrees. All strength measures expressed in kilograms. Force/BW ratios are in kilograms of force relative to body weight in kilograms

Table 10.5 Upper extremity variables in elite junior tennis players

Variable	Males (mean ± sd)			Females (mean ± sd)		
	Dominant	Non-dominant	(Diff)	Dominant	Non-dominant	(Diff)
Shoulder IR	39.4 (9.5)	52.2 (9.7)	−12.8	41.5 (7.9)	53.1 (7.0)	−11.6
Shoulder ER	103.2 (9.3)	99.1 (9.8)	4.1	105.6 (7.5)	101.3 (7.9)	4.3
Total rotation	142.6 (11.2)	151.2 (10.5)	−8.6	147.2 (9.2)	154.4 (8.9)	−7.2
Elbow extension	−0.86 (6.8)	+2.75 (5.8)	3.61	+2.89 (6.4)	+5.91 (6.6)	2.9
Wrist flexion	68.2 (9.3)	73.1 (8.7)	−4.9	73.0 (9.0)	75.2 (7.2)	−2.2
Wrist extension	70.2 (11.0)	75.4 (9.8)	−5.2	73.1 (7.5)	77.4 (7.8)	−4.3
Empty can (kg)	8.3 (2.6)	8.3 (2.4)	0.0	6.9 (2.5)	6.9 (2.2)	0.0
Supraspinatus Force/BW ratio	12.2%	12.2%		11.8%	11.8%	
ER 90 abduction (kg)	11.5 (3.7)	11.5 (3.7)	0.0	10.4 (3.0)	9.9 (2.3)	0.5
Shoulder ER (90 ABD) Force/BW ratio	16.9%	16.9%		17.9%	17.0%	
Grip strength (kg)	45.3 (13.2)	39.6 (12.0)	5.7	31.8 (9.1)	27.1 (8.3)	4.7
Scapular dyskinesis	65%	48%	17%	75%	56%	14%

Notes: All measures in degrees except for strength testing (empty can/supraspinatus), ER at 90° of abduction, and grip strength which are in kilograms
**Scapular dyskinesis expressed as number of positive findings for each extremity in percent

measured at 90° of abduction, while internal rotation was 10.0° less on average when compared to the non-dominant extremity. This resulted in an overall decrease in total rotation range of motion of the dominant shoulder of 6.2°. Similar findings were identified in the elite junior test results with dominant shoulder external rotation being approximately 4° greater than the non-dominant, with 11°–12° less dominant arm internal rotation measured in both male and female junior players compared to their non-dominant extremity. This resulted in a decrease in dominant arm total rotation range of motion similar to the professional male players of 7°–8°. Also identified in the professional male tennis players was a loss of a mean of 7.8° of dominant arm horizontal adduction ROM compared to the non-dominant side as measured with an inclinometer.

This data has ramifications for the prescription of shoulder stretching programs to treat and prevent shoulder injury. Normal uninjured players from our two samples had between 6° and 8° of total rotation ROM loss on the dominant extrem-

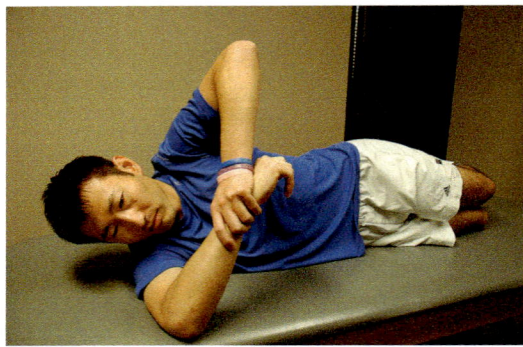

Fig. 10.17 Sleeper Stretch performed to improve internal rotation range of motion

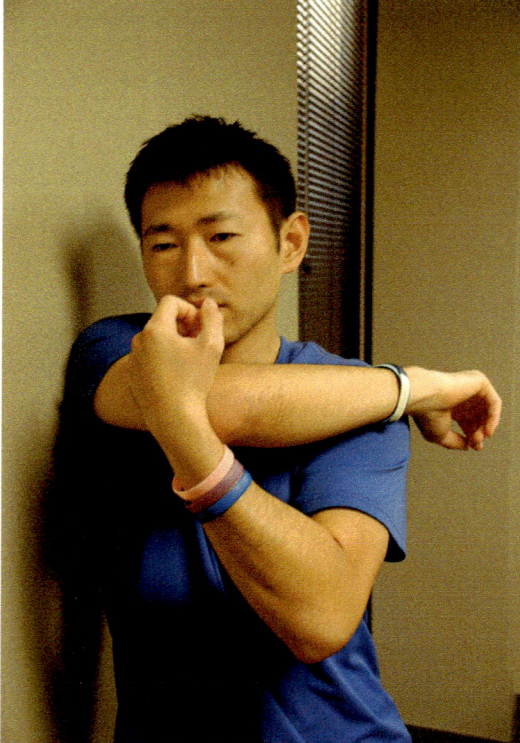

Fig. 10.18 Cross arm stretch performed against a wall to enhance scapular stabilization and improve stretching of the posterior shoulder

ity when compared bilaterally. This range (6°–8°) is used as a criterion or cutoff whereby players with more ROM loss are given sleeper stretches and cross-arm stretches (Figs. 10.17 and 10.18) to address internal rotation range of motion loss [40–43]. Players with less than 6°–8° of ROM loss are still instructed on these important stretches to maintain their current ROM values and profile, but players with more ROM loss are prescribed with these exercises with the goal of normalizing their ROM patterning on the dominant extremity.

Results for elbow and forearm ROM are also displayed in Tables 10.4 and 10.5. Professional male players had an average of 7.2° less elbow extension on the dominant arm as compared to the non-dominant arm. Forearm pronation was found to be 2° less while supination averaged 7.6° less in the dominant forearm. Elite juniors showed only 2°–3° less dominant arm elbow extension range of motion compared to the non-dominant extremity with the female players showing hyperextension values on both the dominant and non-dominant extremities. This is consistent with the finding of a positive Beighton hypermobility being documented in 62% of the female players and only 25% of the male elite junior players. Wrist range of motion was measured only in the elite junior tennis players and ranged between 4° and 5° of ROM loss in wrist extension and flexion on the dominant extremity in both male and female players.

Shoulder ER and supraspinatus strength results are displayed in Tables 10.4 and 10.5 as well. For the male professional players, shoulder external rotation strength measured in 0° of abduction (neutral) was 2.0 kg weaker in the dominant extremity as compared to the non-dominant extremity. Testing in this position is most representative of infraspinatus strength [28]. Values obtained for shoulder external rotation at 90° of abduction were essentially equal bilaterally (0.58 kg difference between extremities) as was supraspinatus strength in the empty can position (0.3 kg bilateral difference). To allow for more generalized application of ER and supraspinatus strength data, measures are expressed relative to body weight as "force/body weight" ratios in Tables 10.4 and 10.5 as well. Ratios of 13–15% of body weight for ER measured in neutral were found along with ratios of 18–19% for ER at 90° of abduction for professional male tennis players. Supraspinatus torque-to-body weight ratios were 14% for this population as well.

Table 10.6 Lower extremity range of motion test results in ATP professional male tennis players

Test	Dominant Mean (sd)	Non-dominant Mean (sd)	Difference (Dom − Ndom) Mean (sd)
Prone hip ER	35.9 (7.4)	35.3 (7.5)	0.53 (5.5)
Prone hip IR	32.9 (9.0)	32.0 (8.6)	0.95 (6.4)
Hip total rotation	68.8 (11.5)	67.4 (12.0)	1.41 (7.2)
Prone knee flexion	128.0 (6.0)	126.4 (5.9)	1.58 (12.4)
Straight leg raise	80.7 (9.0)	81.1 (9.2)	−0.46 (3.8)
Ankle dorsiflexion (G)	8.5 (4.3)	9.2 (4.1)	−0.63 (3.2)
Ankle dorsiflexion (S)	14.6 (4.7)	13.3 (4.3)	1.34 (3.9)
Thomas test (+)	60.8%	58.1%	2.7%
One-leg stability (+)	54.5%	49.0%	5.5%

Note: All measures in degrees. Percent positive (failed) tests for Thomas and one-leg stability tests reported

Table 10.7 Lower extremity variables in elite junior tennis players

Variable	Males (mean ± sd)			Females (mean ± sd)		
	Dominant	Non-dominant	(Diff)	Dominant	Non-dominant	(Diff)
Prone hip IR	35.9 (9.3)	34.1 (8.8)	1.8	45.3 (9.9)	43.3 (9.4)	2.0
Prone hip ER	36.8 (9.7)	36.7 (8.8)	0.1	34.7 (6.8)	35.3 (6.6)	−0.6
Hip total rotation	72.9 (13.6)	70.7 (13.6)	2.2	80.2 (12.3)	78.8 (11.7)	1.4
Prone knee flexion	132.7 (8.9)	131.5 (9.6)	1.2	133.1 (7.9)	132.3 (7.9)	0.8
Thomas test (+)	45%	45%	0.0	50%	50%	0.0
One-leg stability (+)	56%	65%	−9%	65%	68%	3.0

Note: All measures in degrees. Percent positive (failed) tests for Thomas and one-leg stability tests reported

In the elite junior players, only ER at 90 abduction and empty can testing were performed. For male and female junior players, the testing identified no difference between the dominant and non-dominant side with the use of a handheld dynamometer for both ER at 90 and the empty can test. One exception was in the female players where a 0.5 kg increase in dominant arm ER strength was measured. Force-to-body weight values calculated from this data show 16–17% ER ratios at 90 abduction and 11–12% ratios for the empty can supraspinatus test for males and female players.

For the professional male tennis players, grip strength was stronger on the dominant extremity by a mean of 5.9 kg. Differences of 4–5 kg with the dominant arm being stronger were also measured in the elite junior players.

10.5.2 Lower Extremity and Core Testing

Tables 10.6 and 10.7 present the lower extremity range of motion data from both populations of elite tennis players. In contrast to upper extremity shoulder range of motion, goniometrically measured prone hip rotation measurements generated from these two samples show essentially symmetrical IR, ER, and total rotation values bilaterally. Prone knee flexion representing quadriceps flexibility, SLR hamstring measurements, and ankle dorsiflexion measures were within 1–2° when compared between the dominant and non-dominant sides. Tightness of the hip flexors measured via a positive Thomas test was recorded in 60.8% for the professional male players on the dominant limb, and in 58.1% of the non-dominant limbs, and in 45–55% of the elite male and female junior players as well.

To assess lower extremity hip and core strength, the one-leg stability test was used. Failure of the one-leg stability test occurred in 54.5% of players on the dominant limb, and 49% on the non-dominant limb in the ATP male players, and in a slightly higher percentage of elite female and male players (55–65%).

Another test used to measure core stability was the abdominal bracing test. To pass this test, ten repetitions of reciprocal leg lowering had to be performed while maintaining abdominal bracing against a blood pressure cuff. In the sample of male professional players, 64% of the players performed ten repetitions on this test, with only 4.6% being unable to perform even one repetition with abdominal control. In the elite junior players, the core stability test was failed by 61% of the male players and 56% of the female players.

Additional testing was performed in the testing cohort of professional male players. The bridging test was passed by 73.5% of the players. The rotary stability test (contralateral arm and leg extension) was passed successfully by 90% of players and has been replaced by the ipsilateral arm and leg extension rotary stability test which is more challenging. Data on this test are not yet available for reporting due to the recent addition of this test to the protocol. The prone and side-lying plank test was passed by 98.6% of the players tested in the program.

10.6 Summary

This chapter provides an overview and description of a musculoskeletal testing program that has been used on both professional and elite junior tennis players. The objective musculoskeletal descriptive results from this testing battery are presented to provide a descriptive profile of the musculoskeletal adaptations that can be expected in healthy elite-level tennis players. Knowledge of the typical findings and results of the tests presented in this chapter can assist individuals providing musculoskeletal screening for elite-level tennis players. The tennis players in these cohorts had an extensive competitive tennis and training history and present with significant sport-specific musculoskeletal findings. Knowledge of the expected results and descriptive profile in this population will assist clinicians in the evaluation and interpretation of findings of musculoskeletal testing in elite-level tennis players.

References

1. Ellenbecker TS. Shoulder internal and external rotation strength and range of motion in highly skilled tennis players. Isokinet Exerc Sci. 1992;2:1–8.
2. Ellenbecker TS, Roetert EP, Piorkowski PA. Shoulder internal and external rotation range of motion of elite junior tennis players: a comparison of two protocols. J Orthop Sports Phys Ther. 1993;17:65.
3. Ellenbecker TS, Roetert EP, Bailie DS, Davies GJ, Brown SW. Glenohumeral joint total rotation range of motion in elite tennis players and baseball pitchers. Med Sci Sports Exerc. 2002;34:2052–6.
4. Ellenbecker TS, Ellenbecker GA, Roetert EP, Silva RT, Keuter G, Sperling F. Descriptive profile of hip rotation range of motion in elite tennis players and professional baseball pitchers. Am J Sports Med. 2007;35:1371–6.
5. Ellenbecker TS, Roetert EP. Age specific isokinetic glenohumeral internal and external rotation strength in elite junior tennis players. J Sci Med Sport. 2003;6(1):63–70.
6. Roetert EP, Ellenbecker TS, Brown SW. Shoulder internal and external rotation range of motion in nationally ranked junior tennis players: a longitudinal analysis. J Strength Cond Res. 2000;14(2):140–3.
7. Ellenbecker TS. A total arm strength isokinetic profile of highly skilled tennis players. Isokinet Exerc Sci. 1991;1:9–21.
8. Wilk KE, Andrews JR, Arrigo CA, Keirns MA, Erber DJ. The strength characteristics of internal and external rotator muscles in professional baseball pitchers. Am J Sports Med. 1993;21:61–6.
9. Wilk KE, Macrina LC, Fleisig GS, Porterfield R, Simpson CD, Harker P, Paparesta N, Andrews JR. Correlation of glenohumeral internal rotation deficit and total rotational motion to shoulder injuries in professional baseball pitchers. Am J Sports Med. 2011;39:329–35.
10. Shanley E, Rauh MJ, Michener LA, Ellenbecker TS, Garrison JC, Thigpen CA. Shoulder range of motion measures as risk factors for shoulder and elbow injuries in high school softball and baseball players. Am J Sports Med. 2011;39:1997–2006.
11. Ellenbecker TS, Mattalino AJ. Concentric isokinetic shoulder internal and external rotation strength in professional baseball pitchers. J Orthop Sports Phys Ther. 1999;25:323–8.
12. Robb AJ, Fleisig G, Wilk KE, Macrina L, Bolt B, Pajaczkowski J. Passive ranges of motion of the hips and their relationship with pitching biomechanics and ball velocity in professional baseball pitchers. Am J Sports Med. 2010;38:2487–93.
13. Stickley CD, Hetzler RK, Freemyer BG, Kimura IF. Isokinetic peak torque ratios and shoulder injury history in adolescent female volleyball athletes. J Athl Train. 2008;43(6):571–7.

14. Reeser JC, Joy EA, Porucznik CA, Berg RL, Colliver EB, Willick SE. Risk factors for volleyball related shoulder pain and dysfunction. PM R. 2010;2:27–36.
15. Ellenbecker TS, Roetert EP, Sueyoshi T, Riewald S. A descriptive profile of age-specific knee extension flexion strength in elite junior tennis players. Br J Sports Med. 2007;41:728–32.
16. Chiala TA, Maschi RA, Stuhr RM, Rogers JR, Sheridan MA, Callahan LR, Hannifan JA. A musculoskeletal profile of elite female soccer players. HSS J. 2009;5(2):186–95.
17. Paul DJ, Nassis P. Testing strength and power in soccer players: the application of conventional and traditional methods of assessment. J Strength Cond Res. 2015;29(6):1748–58.
18. Kovacs M, Ellenbecker TS, Kibler WB, Roetert EP, Lubbers P. Injury trends in American competitive junior tennis players. J Sci Med Tennis. 2014;19:19–24.
19. Pluim BM, Staal JB, Windler GE, et al. Tennis injuries: occurrence, aetiology, and prevention. Br J Sports Med. 2006;40:415–23.
20. Ellenbecker TS, Pluim B, Vivier S, Sniteman C. Common injuries in tennis players: exercises to address muscular imbalances and reduce injury risk. J Strength Cond. 2009;31(4):50–8.
21. Kibler WB, McQueen C, Uhl T. Fitness evaluation and fitness findings in competitive junior tennis players. Clin Sports Med. 1988;7:403–16.
22. Kryger KO, Dor F, Guillaume M, Haida A, Noirez P, Montalvan B, Toussaint JF. Medical reasons behind player departures from male and female professional tennis competitions. Am J Sports Med. 2015;43(1):34–40.
23. Reece LA, Fricker PA, Maguire KA. Injuries to elite young tennis players at the Australian Institute of Sports. Aust J Sci Med Sport. 1986;18:11–5.
24. Jayanthi NA, O'Boyle J, Durazo-Arvizu RA. Risk factors for medical withdrawals in United States Tennis Association Junior National Tennis Tournaments: a descriptive epidemiologic study. Sports Health. 2009;1:231–5.
25. Hjelm N, Werner S, Renstrom P. Injury profile in junior tennis players: a prospective two year study. Knee Surg Sports Traumatol Arthrosc. 2010;18:845–50.
26. Wilk KE, Reinold MM, Macrina LC, Porterfield R, Devine KM, Suarez K, Andrews JR. Glenohumeral internal rotation measurements differ depending on stabilization techniques. Sports Health. 2009;1(2):131–6.
27. Norkin CC, White DJ. Measurement of joint motion: a guide to goniometry. 2nd ed. Philadelphia: FA Davis; 1995.
28. Kurokawa D, Sano H, Nagamoto H, Omi R, Shinozaki N, Watanuki S, Kishimoto KN, Yamamoto N, Hiraoka K, Tashiro M, Itoi E. Muscle activity pattern of the shoulder external rotators differs in adduction an abduction: an analysis using positron emission tomography. J Shoulder Elb Surg. 2014;23:658–64.
29. Kelly BT, Kadrmas WH, Speer KP. The manual muscle examination for rotator cuff strength. An electromyographic investigation. Am J Sports Med. 1996;24:581–8.
30. Lajtai G, Pfirrmann CWA, Aizetmuller G, Pirkl C, Gerber C, Jost B. The shoulders of professional beach volleyball players. Am J Sports Med. 2009;37(7):1375–82.
31. Cummins CA, Messer TM, Schafer MF. Infraspinatus muscle atrophy in professional baseball players. Am J Sports Med. 2004;32:116–20.
32. Safran M. Nerve injury about the shoulder in athletes, Part 1. Am J Sports Med. 2004;32(3):803–19.
33. Jobe FW, Bradley JP. The diagnosis and nonoperative treatment of shoulder injuries in athletes. Clin Sports Med. 1989;8:419–37.
34. Kibler WB, Uhl TL, Maddux JW, Brooks PV, Zeller B, McMullen J. Qualitative clinical evaluation of scapular dysfunction: a reliability study. J Shoulder Elb Surg. 2002;11:550–6.
35. Ellenbecker TS, Kibler WB, Bailie DS, Caplinger R, Davies GJ, Riemann BL. Reliability of scapular evaluation in professional baseball players. Clin Orthop Relat Res. 2012;470:1540–4.
36. Reiman MP, Manske RC. Functional testing in human performance. Champaign, IL: Human Kinetics Publishers; 2009.
37. Crossley KM, Zhang WJ, Schache AG, Bryant A, Cowan SM. Performance on the single-leg squat task indicates hip abductor muscle function. Am J Sports Med. 2011;39(4):866–73.
38. Hoogenboom BJ, Bennett JL, Clark M. Establishing core stability in rehabilitation. In: Hoogenboom BJ, Voight ML, Prentice WE, editors. Musculoskeletal interventions. 3rd ed. New York: McGraw Hill.
39. Cook G, Burton L, Hoogenboom BJ, Voight M. Functional movement screening: the use of fundamental movements as an assessment of function – Part 2. Int J Sports Phys Ther. 2014;9(4):549–63.
40. Kibler WB, Chandler TJ, Livingston BP, Roetert EP. Shoulder range of motion in elite tennis players: effect of age and years of tournament play. Am J Sports Med. 1996;24:279–85.
41. Laudner KG, Sipes RC, Wilson JT. The acute effects of sleeper stretch on shoulder range of motion. J Athl Train. 2008;43(4):359–63.
42. Moore SD, Laudner KG, McLoda TA, Shaffer MA. The immediate effects of muscle energy technique on posterior shoulder tightness: a randomized controlled trial. J Orthop Sports Phys Ther. 2011;41(6):400–7.
43. Wilk KE, Macrina LC, Arrigo C. Passive range of motion characteristics in the overhead baseball pitcher and their implications for rehabilitation. Clin Orthop Relat Res. 2012;470(6):1586–94.

The Preparticipation Physical: The WTA Experience and Findings

11

Walter C. Taylor, Brian Adams, Kathy Martin, Susie Parker-Simmons, Marc Safron, Belinda Herde, and Kathleen Stroia

11.1 Introduction

The Women's Tennis Association (WTA) requires that players have a periodic health evaluation (PHE) every 2 years similar to that proposed by the International Olympic Committee (IOC) in 2009 [1]. This is performed predominately by the team of WTA medical advisors at two large tournaments in March, which is toward the beginning of the new season. The medical advisors conducting the WTA physicals include a primary care sports medicine physician (family medicine), orthopedic surgeon, dermatologist, registered sports dietician, and a mental health counselor. The physicals are performed on site at the tournament and are supported by several of the Primary Health Care Providers (PHCPs), who are licensed physical therapists and certified athletic trainers (or the international equivalent specializing in sports medicine). For players who are not present or playing in the two tournaments where the medical advisors are present, the player may have the evaluation performed by a tournament physician or their private physician. Ultimately the medical advisors review all of these completed physical evaluation forms to ensure adequate completion of the form and to review and make additional recommendations for the player based on the data present in the form and the recommendations of the completing provider(s).

The reasons for performing these physicals are the same as those outlined by other organizations such as the Preparticipation Physical Evaluation Monograph [2], the NCAA [3], and the International Olympic Committee (IOC) [1]. The primary objective of the PPE is to detect conditions that predispose athletes to serious injury, illness, or sudden death. A recent joint consensus statement regarding the preparticipation evaluation

W. C. Taylor (✉)
Department of Family Medicine, Mayo Clinic College of Medicine, Jacksonville, FL, USA

Women's Tennis Association, St. Petersburg, FL, USA
e-mail: WTaylor@wtatennis.com

B. Adams
Department of Dermatology, University of Cincinnati College of Medicine, Cincinnati, OH, USA

VAMC, Cincinnati, OH, USA

K. Martin · B. Herde
Women's Tennis Association, St. Petersburg, FL, USA

S. Parker-Simmons
Womens Tennis Association and United States Olympic Committee, St. Petersburg, FL, USA

United States Olympic Committee, Colorado Springs, CO, USA

M. Safron
Women's Tennis Association, St. Petersburg, FL, USA

Division of Sports Medicine, Department of Orthopedic Surgery, Stanford University, Stanford, CA, USA

K. Stroia
Sport Sciences & Medicine and Transitions, Women's Tennis Association, St. Petersburg, FL, USA

(PPE) by the ACSM and FIMS discussed that there are many variations of the PPE between different countries [4]. In the end, this group recommended a human-centered design for PPE which includes electronic collection of data and storage in order to better understand the value of the PPE and to drive evidence-based decisions as to what pieces of information are most pertinent to the athlete and sports medicine healthcare provider. They also determined that the PPE is not just a screen for cardiac disease that places the athlete at risk for sudden cardiac death/arrest. The PPE allows for the provider to counsel the athlete on the risk of sport, injury prevention, and other social, medical, and behavioral risk factors. The WTA PHE is modeled after this human-/athlete-centered design.

Matheson et al. [5] reviewed data from the PPE on 1693 collegiate athletes that was collected utilizing an electronic version of the PPE. They showed that 11% of athletes present for their PPE with ongoing issues from a prior injury. The premise is that by identifying these athletes early enough, programs can be designed to either obtain further investigations to better determine the cause of ongoing symptoms and to rehabilitate the injury to the point where symptoms are resolved or greatly improved and to reduce the risk of aggravation or recurrence of the injury. The idea is that athletes with a prior injury that is not completely resolved are at greater risk for reinjury [1]. The WTA philosophy is based on this idea that identifying persistent symptoms related to injury, illness, and emotional or dietary issues in our players allows for the opportunity to improve those issues to improve player health, well-being longitudinally, and in turn sport performance.

Other specific goals of the WTA PHE are to counsel the player on a variety of issues regarding prevention of injury and illness, emotional health, and nutrition. Since players travel to different cities throughout the world to play in tournaments, it is helpful to have baseline medical information, as each tournament has a different tournament physician(s). These physicians have access to the player's medical record for the duration of that tournament. They are able to review the player's past medical history, surgeries, medications, allergies, and any very serious medical conditions (termed red alerts). The WTA PHCPs are full-time employees or independent contractors of the WTA, and each travels to multiple tournaments per year. Since there is a different tournament physician(s) at each tournament, the PHCPs really allow for continuity of care. They have continuous access to the player's electronic medical record (EMR). It is most helpful for the PHCPs to know what medical issues each player has, so they can work as a medical team with the tournament physician(s) to provide the player(s) with optimal care during the tournament. Because they are familiar with the player's medical history, the PHCPs frequently bring the tournament physicians up to date on the player's history and ongoing issues when the physician is evaluating the player for a new or ongoing health condition.

The WTA medical advisors make recommendations for preventative programs utilizing a holistic approach including medical, musculoskeletal, and dermatological and skin cancer prevention, emotional health, and nutrition for health and performance. Having access to the data from the physical examinations allows the medical advisors and the PHCPs to design and monitor these recommendations on a longitudinal basis.

The WTA periodic health evaluation is a comprehensive evaluation that includes the following components: general medical, psychological (emotional health), nutrition, dermatologic, orthopedic, and a tennis-specific screen (TSS), which is a functional screen. Players complete the medical history portion of the form, and then a physical examination is performed. The healthcare provider completing each section records their findings and recommendations, which are discussed with the player at that time. After the player completes all the different stations/sections, they discuss the recommendations with Kathleen Stroia, Senior Vice President of Sport Sciences & Medicine and Transitions, and develop a plan for follow-up of the recommendations. In this chapter we review the various components of the WTA periodic health evaluation.

11.2 General Medical Examination

The general medical examination is performed as noted to identify any medical conditions that would affect the player's ability to safely

Table 11.1 Components of the WTA medical history periodic health evaluation

Medications/supplements
Immunizations
General medical concerns
Cardiac symptoms and family history
Pulmonary—those with asthma
Menstrual and female health questions
Fatigue
Heat illness
Allergic disorders
Concussion
Gastrointestinal disorders
Family medical history
Past surgical history

Table 11.2 The 14-element AHA recommendations for preparticipation cardiovascular screening

Medical history
  Personal history
  1. Chest pain/discomfort/tightness/pressure related to exertion
  2. Unexplained syncope/near-syncope
  3. Excessive and unexplained dyspnea/fatigue or palpitations, associated with exercise
  4. Prior recognition of a heart murmur
  5. Elevated systemic blood pressure
  6. Prior restriction from participation in sports
  7. Prior testing for the heart, ordered by a physician
  Family history
  8. Premature death (sudden and unexpected or otherwise) before age 50 years old attributable to heart disease in ≥1 relative
  9. Disability from heart disease in a close relative <50 years old
  10. Hypertrophic or dilated cardiomyopathy, long QT syndrome or other channelopathies, Marfan's syndrome, or clinically significant arrhythmia and specific knowledge of genetic cardiac conditions in family members

Physical examination
  11. Heart murmur
  12. Femoral pulses to exclude coarctation of the aorta
  13. Physical stigmata of Marfan's syndrome
  14. Brachial artery blood pressure in sitting position

(Reprinted with permission, Circulation. 2014;130: 1303–34, @2014 American Heart Association, Inc.)

participate on the WTA Tour. While the primary goal of the evaluation is to identify players at risk for sudden cardiac death, there are many other aspects to the physical. The medical evaluation includes the player's personal and family medical history. The history components are listed in Table 11.1. For the cardiac history, the questions for athletic preparticipation cardiac screening as recommended by the American Heart Association are included in Table 11.2 [6]. The physical examination of the cardiovascular system is completed in accordance with the AHA recommendations.

Since 2014, the WTA has recommended that all players have a screening ECG in order to complement the cardiac history and physical examination. The ECG is recommended every 2 years until the age of 20. The sports medicine community has yet to reach a consensus on the utilization of the screening ECG for young athletes across all levels of competition. However, after review of the medical literature, and due to the elite, professional level of its athletes, the WTA medical advisors determined it was prudent to add this test to aid in screening for underlying cardiac disease that would place the player at significant risk for sudden cardiac death or arrest. This was based on the findings of Corrado et al. [7] and Baggish et al. [8] and the recommendation of the European Society of Cardiology [9], the IOC [1], and the FIFA [10]. It is also consistent with the cardiovascular screening protocol used by major professional sports teams in North America [11]. More recently, the AMSSM Position Statement on Cardiovascular Preparticipation Screening in Athletes indicated that the group could not recommend for or against the use of the ECG in assessing risk for sudden cardiac death or arrest in the athlete [12]. However, they did indicate that it is reasonable to leave this decision up to the individual team physician or athletic organization. In a joint statement, the American Heart Association and the American College of Cardiology recommended against the use of ECG screening of large populations of young athletes and nonathletes to attempt to detect underlying cardiovascular disease [6]. However, this statement does state that ECG screening—in combination with a clinical history and physical examination—may be considered in small cohorts of young healthy persons in order to identify or raise suspicion of underlying cardiovascular diseases, if one understands the known and anticipated limitations of the 12-lead ECG. Considering the above studies and recommendations, the WTA has committed to the addition of the 12-lead ECG, combined with the 14-point AHA history and physical examination recommendations, to screen WTA players for underlying cardiovascular disease that may place them at risk for sudden cardiac arrest or death.

The electronic medical record (EMR) used by the WTA allows the medical advisors to identify subpopulations of players with certain medical conditions. The EMR allows the medical advisors to perform quality improvement projects as part of a population health approach to a cohort of athletes. For example, as part of a quality improvement project in 2016, during the physical examinations, all players identified as having asthma completed an asthma control test form [13, 14], and then the medical advisor discussed an individualized asthma action plan [15]. Since players are traveling and playing globally, it is key that prior to long durations away from home, they are aware of when they need refills of their medications and when their medications will expire. They are counseled to be proactive to make sure they travel with enough medication to get them through these long durations away from their home or training base.

The PHE allows the medical advisors to provide individual counseling and recommendations to each player on various topics. An example of several topics in which the player may be counseled is listed in Table 11.3. The medical advisor may recommend that a player who has a specific medical concern be evaluated further. The WTA also recommends that players have annual laboratory studies as listed in Table 11.4. These are recommended but not required.

11.3 Dermatologic

All players complete a dermatologic history which includes any ongoing or prior skin disorders; personal or family history of skin cancer; abnormal nevi, greater than 50 nevi; and toenail conditions. Players are asked how many days a week do they apply and then reapply sunscreen and what SPF of sunscreen they use.

A full-skin examination is then performed by a dermatologist during the team-based physicals. If a player does not have their physical performed during the team-based physical examinations,

Table 11.3 Topics for player counseling

Medications—if athletes need a therapeutic use exception
Supplements in compliance with the tennis antidoping program
Iron deficiency
Asthma
Mitigating fatigue
Bone health
Menstrual concerns
Players follow up plans for any ongoing medical issues
Laboratory work

Table 11.4 Components of the WTA musculoskeletal examination

Spine
  Presence of scoliosis, kyphosis, lordosis
  Range of motion of cervical, thoracic, lumbar spine
  Neurologic
    Strength of lower extremity
    Deep tendon reflexes
Shoulder
  Inspection
    Presence of scapular winging
    Infraspinatus atrophy
    Swelling
  Tenderness to palpation
  Range of motion
    Abduction
    Forward flexion
    Internal rotation at 90° abduction in degrees
    External rotation at 90° abduction in degrees
    External rotation in adduction
  Strength testing of above range of motion
  Special tests
    Apprehension/relocation test
    O'Brien's test
    Sulcus sign
    Hawkins impingement test
    Adson's test
Elbow
  Inspection
    Swelling, effusion, deformity
  Range of motion
    Flexion
    Extension
    Pronation
    Supination
  Special tests
    Moving valgus stress test
    Milking maneuver
    Ulnar nerve position

Table 11.4 (continued)

- Tinel's cubital tunnel
- Wrist/hand
  - Inspection
  - Range of motion
    - Wrist
      - Flexion
      - Extension
      - Radial deviation
      - Ulnar deviation
    - Fingers
      - Flexion
      - Extension
  - TFCC compression rest
  - Watson's test
  - Subluxation extensor carpi ulnaris tendon
  - Laxity of ulnar collateral ligament 1st MCP joint
  - Grip strength
- Hip
  - Inspection
  - Range of motion
    - Flexion
    - Abduction
    - Adduction
    - Extension
    - External rotation (90° flexion of hip) in degrees
    - External rotation (prone) in degrees
    - Internal rotation (90° flexion of hip) in degrees
    - Internal rotation (prone) in degrees
  - Special tests
    - FABER test
    - FADIR test
    - Scour test
    - Adductor flexibility
    - Evidence of leg length discrepancy
    - Hamstring flexibility
    - Thomas test
    - Test for snapping hip
    - Hamstring vs. gluteal dominance for hip extension in prone position
    - Resisted sit-up test
- Knee
  - Inspection
    - Effusion
    - Deformity
    - Atrophy of quadriceps
  - Palpation for tenderness or crepitus
  - Range of motion
    - Flexion
    - Extension
  - Ligament testing
    - Lachman test
    - Anterior drawer test
    - Posterior drawer test

Table 11.4 (continued)

- Valgus stress test for medial collateral ligament laxity
- Varus stress test for lateral collateral ligament laxity
- McMurray's test
- Patellar mobility testing
  - Apprehension
  - Abnormal lateral tracking
- Ankle
  - Inspection
  - Range of motion
    - Dorsiflexion
    - Plantar flexion
    - Inversion
    - Eversion
  - Ligament tests
    - Anterior drawer test
    - Eversion stress test
    - Syndesmosis external rotation stress test
    - Subtalar joint motion
  - Special tests
    - Peroneal subluxation
    - Posterior impingement test
- Foot
  - Type: Normal, pronation, supination
  - Navicular drop test
  - Standing rotation test: neutral, flexible, rigid
  - First metatarsal mobility test
  - Deformity
  - Range of motion of toes
  - Palpation for tenderness
- Gait: Note any abnormality

this section is completed by a primary care sports physician or a tournament physician. Recommendations are then made for the player for any ongoing treatment or evaluation of any concerning dermatologic lesions or conditions. For further information regarding skin disorders in elite tennis players, refer to Chap. 37.

11.4 Emotional Health and Safety Section

The WTA recognizes the importance of mental health in the overall health, well-being, and peak competitive participation of its players. The psychological health of athletes impacts upon athletic performance and prevalence rates of injury and illness and is a contributing factor to premature dropout from sport [16–18]. It is also understood that athletes experience mental illnesses at similar rates to nonathletes, estimated at a rate of 20–25% over their lifetime [17–20]. It has been proposed that the intense physical and mental demands placed upon elite athletes and the personality traits associated with being an elite athlete (such as perfectionism) predispose them to *higher* rates of some psychiatric disorders [19, 21–23]. Furthermore, the inherent injury risks associated with professional and elite sports are also a significant stress factor for athletes; injuries are predictive of and/or may expose psychological concerns in athletes [24]. There is also evidence that mood and anxiety disorders affect young females at higher rates than young males [18]. The average age of a WTA player ranked in the top 225 is 24 (data accurate as of Monday, 6 February, 2017). This age coincides with the age at which there are increased rates of mental illnesses in the population (aged 15–25), which are at rates up to *twice* the incidence as older adults (aged over 50) [18, 25].

In addition to psychological stressors, it is important to screen the athlete for non-accidental violence (harassment and abuse) concerns. These issues are prevalent in society, and unfortunately, athletes are not immune and are possibly at *higher* risk. It is also recognized that non-accidental violence is a causative factor in many psychological concerns [26–29].

It is also recognized that many athletes do *not* actively seek professional psychological support, despite their rates of psychological injury. There are many reasons for this: the stigma associated with getting help, which is prevalent in many cultures; a fear of being seen to be "weak" in an athletic culture which values "mental toughness"; denial of psychological distress by athletes; lack of available expert counseling or psychological resources; lack of organizational support for psychological help-seeking behaviors; inattention of medical and allied practitioners to nonphysiological causes of performance deficits, injuries, and illnesses; and simply not being asked if they need help [17, 18, 27, 28, 30–35].

The WTA screen consists of three sections:

1. *Safety and Emotional Health*
   This is derived from recommended sports psychological screening tools [2, 25, 36], known prevalence of psychiatric illnesses in athletes [19, 23, 33], best practices in psychosocial screening for adolescents and young adults [37], and recommended questions relating to non-accidental violence [26–28]. Specifically, athletes are asked about:
   - Sleep: Sleep disturbances can be symptomatic of a psychological concern or may be a clinical disorder [38, 39]. They are common in athletes and negatively impact athletic performance [39, 40]. WTA players are subjected to extensive long-distance travel and thus are also susceptible to jet lag, which is also known to negatively impact athletic performance [41, 42]. A positive answer here allows for further evaluation to identify underlying causes and possible solutions.
   - Substance use and/or dependence: WTA players are obliged to follow the Tennis Anti-Doping Program rules (http://www.itftennis.com/antidoping). It is recognized that athletes may struggle with substance use, especially alcohol and prescription medicines, which may subsequently cause psychiatric or physical health issues [17, 19, 25, 43].
   - Participation in high-risk or self-harming behaviors: Life stressors, including harassment and abuse, and psychological issues such as depression and anxiety disorders are associated with higher risks of deliberate self-harm (DSH). Being female also increases the risk [44, 45]. Contrary to popular opinion, DSH is a sign of both seeking attention and help *and* of psychological distress [45], and is *not* necessarily suicidal in intent [46]. DSH includes behaviors such as self-cutting, burning, and other self-induced bodily injuries and ingesting substances above prescribed doses or other harmful items [46]. There is a lack of research about the prevalence in sports.
   - Suicide attempts and/or ideation: It is known that suicide is a leading cause of death in young people, with a significantly higher

prevalence in young men [47, 48]. Persons committing suicide frequently meet criteria for a clinical mental illness [38, 49] and/or maybe victims of interpersonal violence [28, 37]. It is imperative that the psychological screening of WTA players includes questions regarding suicide. Athletes at risk can be identified early so that effective interventions can be applied [47].

- Relationship safety: According to international best practices, questions about non-accidental violence, including psychological, physical, and sexual abuse, are included [27–29, 50]. It is clear that there is an association between these practices and poor mental and physical health outcomes for athletes, which include asset depreciation due to dropout from sport [28, 50]. It is vital that these topics are not "taboo" and that WTA athletes know they have access to expert, confidential help.
- Use of any type of psychological or counseling services, including WTA Athlete Assistance, and if the player found these helpful: This may indicate a proactive approach to mental wellness and/or a willingness to engage in help-seeking behavior and/or a history of mental health concerns. This information is important to guide the Athlete Assistance team about player readiness to receive psychological help and to inform psychological recommendations.

Other areas of the physical also contain psychologically related sections. These are reviewed in conjunction with the above and with the other practitioners. Specifically:

- Medical red alert section, which has a checkbox list which includes depression, recurring anxiety and fatigue, hair loss, headaches, and gastrointestinal issues, any of which may be symptomatic of psychological issues or clinical psychiatric disorders [17, 18, 38].
- Reproductive history, which allows identification of any player with history of amenorrhea, which can be related to reduced energy intake which may in turn be associated with disordered eating or a clinical eating disorder.

Questions relating to safe sex practices may also indicate risk-taking behavior which may have psychosocial antecedents [51–53].
- Sport Concussion Assessment Tool (SCAT3). A history of concussion is known to be associated with higher incidence of cognitive and memory impairment and psychological issues in athletes [54, 55].
- Body composition may indicate tendencies for body dysmorphia and faulty thinking associated with issues related to disordered eating and eating disorder pathology [51–53].
- Additional questions or information may be gathered if any of the above sections indicate further follow-up. For example, a player reporting sleep difficulties will be asked to complete the WTA Sleep Questionnaire. A player with ongoing fatigue will complete the WTA Performance and Fatigue Questionnaire. Then appropriate management plans can be activated.

2. *Sport Performance*
   This section gathers information relating to the Player Support Team (PST):
   - The PST occupy positions of trust and authority with the player. It is important to establish if the PST are qualified, ethical, and helpful, as these factors are correlated with improved athletic performance and with reduced risk of harm from non-accidental violence [28, 50].

3. *Summary and Recommendations*
   This is the "plan of action" discussed with the player. It includes a variety of options:
   - General education about Athlete Assistance resources, including a free website and 24/7 counseling.
   - Provision of relevant information and resources, such as hard copies of education materials, Physically Speaking and Athlete Assistance topics, and/or email of further education resources. Physically Speaking and Athlete Assistance topics are documents by the WTA medical advisors and other healthcare professionals on various patient education topics specific for WTA players.
   - Option to assist player to access psychologists and/or psychiatrists with appropriate

- experience and expertise to assist her to manage the psychological issue when she is at home and when traveling to tournaments.
- Option to meet with Athlete Assistance personnel for more in-depth interview of psychological concerns and subsequently devise a psychological plan of care.
- Other follow-ups, for example, the option to provide team consultation between player and the WTA's Athlete Assistance, medical advisors, and sports dietician for management of athlete triad concerns or to provide team consultation with player and her PST members, such as her psychologist or coach and Athlete Assistance personnel.
- Encourage and reinforce players in their use of effective psychological strategies where applicable, to help them maintain mental health and manage the complexities of life as a professional athlete.

The WTA physical includes psychological health and safety as an integral aspect of athlete health and performance; it helps destigmatize psychological concerns, to reframe them in a performance context and to optimize athlete well-being [34].

11.5 Nutrition

The aim of an athlete's diet is to provide adequate energy and nutrients for training and competition, sustain optimal health and function, support growth and development, enhance adaptation and recovery, achieve and maintain an ideal physique, and adopt lifelong healthy eating behaviors [56]. An inadequate diet, however, can lead to fatigue, slow recovery, inadequate concentration, poor motivation, and reduced competitive performance. It may also increase the risk of illness, injury, and poor decision-making [57]. Dietary assessment is the first stage in assisting a tennis player optimizes their nutrition-related factors of health and sporting performance.

The dietary assessment portion of the Women's Tennis Association (WTA) preparticipation physical is performed by the WTA sport dieticians. It creates the basis of nutrition evaluation and intervention of each player in the areas of health and athletic performance. This screening then forms the foundation of nutrition monitoring, treatment, and education throughout the annual year.

The dietary assessment section of the preparticipation physical includes the collection of social, cultural, medical, and psychological influences on food choices. It also includes gathering medical, biochemical, training, and anthropometric data. Below is a list of information collected in the dietary assessment portion of the WTA preparticipation physical.

1. Medical history as it related to nutrition
   - For example, food intolerances, abnormal blood work, abnormality in menstrual cycle, illness, etc.
2. Body composition
   - Objective anthropometric data
   - Subjective assessment of body composition
   - Methods they adopt to obtain the ideal body composition
3. Training diet
   - Through completing an athlete food frequency form and 24-h record
4. Hydration
   - History of heat stress and muscle cramping
   - Strategies adopted to prevent dehydration
5. Competition diet
   - Pre-event meal strategies
   - Event fueling methods adopted to delay the onset of fatigue and dehydration
   - Recovery strategies to ensure readiness to compete and/or train
6. Supplements
   - What brand and type of supplements are used by the player
   - Which supplements (if any) are recommended for the athlete to optimize her health and performance
7. Dietician contact details
   - Contact details of the sport dietician they work with in their country of origin

Upon conclusion of the consultation, the WTA sport dietician provides the player with the outcomes of the dietary assessment, individual-specific goals, and a plan. In addition, this information is shared with the WTA medical advisory team, who then collectively establishes goals and a structural framework that helps optimize the player's health and tennis performance.

11.6 Orthopedic

As these women are professional athletes that participate in a physically demanding sport, the musculoskeletal examination is a key component of the preparticipation physical examination for WTA players. The orthopedic examination is a complete examination from the neck to the feet, though special focus is paid to certain areas, as this is a unilateral arm-dominant (or asymmetric) sport. In tennis, as in other sports, physical adaptations occur in the growing athlete, as well as in the adult player. These adaptations may be advantageous to the player, but excessive adaptations may become maladaptations, resulting in altered joint mechanics, pain, and injury, as frequently seen in the dominant shoulder. Significant stresses are applied throughout the body, and areas are susceptible to acute injuries, as well as overuse injury.

The purpose of the orthopedic PPE, then, is to identify areas of players at risk of injury, to provide them with counseling about risk of injury, to provide a rehabilitation program to correct the maladaptation or imbalance, and to help reduce the risk of injury. Additionally, a database of normative values in players can help future players reduce risk of injury. The data collected has led to identification of the prevalence of suprascapular nerve dysfunction in female tennis players [58] and the prevalence of internal snapping hip in WTA players [59], as well as identifying associations of physical exam findings with injury, such as iliopsoas weakness in those with the a history of abdominal muscle strains [59].

The preparticipation orthopedic history also provides information about prior musculoskeletal injury, whether symptoms are recurrent, ongoing, or resolved. This allows extra focus during the PPE to assure the injury is resolved and/or what may be necessary to treat it or prevent recurrence. Further, players playing with an injury may compensate for the injury, putting other musculoskeletal structures at risk for breakdown/injury.

A general screening of joint range of motion and strength is carried out. Any prior history of injury limiting play or practice, area of prior surgery, or current pain or dysfunction is examined in full detail. Additionally, limitations in motion or strength are further evaluated with special tests of the given area or joint. Finally, areas of common maladaptation or particular overuse in tennis players are examined in greater detail—the shoulders, low back, wrists, knees, and ankles.

The examination begins with the athlete standing in front of the examiner. Neck range of motion is assessed in all planes—flexion, extension, rotation, and bending. This is followed by assessing shoulder range of motion and strength, in addition to testing the rotator cuff and evaluating for SLAP lesions and instability signs and AC joint pain. Shoulder range of motion, particularly internal and external rotation in 90° of abduction with scapula stabilized, is measured with an electronic goniometer. Special attention is paid to making sure the player does not have glenohumeral rotational deficit (GIRD) or scapular dyskinesis. Both of these are common in the overhead athlete, including tennis players, and are associated with shoulder pain and dysfunction and injury, but correctible with appropriate rehabilitation. As return to play at the same or higher level after shoulder surgery is not as consistent or predictable as one would like [60], this is a critical part of the examination, where the PPE may make a huge impact on preventing injury or the need for surgery.

Next, elbow, wrist, and hand/finger range of motion and strength are evaluated. Tests for wrist tenderness, as well as TFCC integrity and ECU stability, are carried out. Scapular muscle stabilizing function is evaluated for symmetry and stability in forward elevation and abduction. Back motion is assessed in all planes, and their lower extremity alignment is evaluated while standing in front of the examiner. Single-leg stance for hip abductor weakness is also evaluated from behind the player, usually right after scapular motion is assessed. The athlete then will do a squat and duck walk for loaded knee flexion and meniscus function. Gait, including toe to toe and heel to heel, is studied, as is heel raise. Assessment for flat feet is also carried out while the athlete is walking, barefoot.

The athlete then lays supine on the examination table. Shoulder apprehension and relocation tests are performed, as are supine core tests. A detailed knee examination is accomplished—assessing for patellar mobility and tenderness, effusion, ligamentous integrity, and hamstring tightness. Quadriceps muscular bulk, symmetry, and tone are recorded. A detailed hip examination is also performed for range of motion (flexion, as well as internal and external rotation in 90° of flexion), impingement and scour maneuvers, snapping iliopsoas tests, and lateral knee joint line to table distance. If needed, Patrick's and Gaenslen's tests are performed to assess for SI joint dysfunction. If there is any suspicion for IT band problems at the knee, a Noble test is executed. The player's adductor muscles are tested in flexion and extension. The player then does a resisted sit-up, evaluating for athletic pubalgia/core muscle injury.

The patient is then placed in the lateral decubitus position assessing for IT band tightness, trochanteric bursal or gluteus medius tenderness, and hip stability. The athlete is then rotated prone to measure hip internal and external rotation in the neutral flexion-extension position (with an electronic goniometer) and to evaluate for gluteus dominance in hip extension. Finally, the player is brought supine at the end of the examination table to evaluate for hip instability and iliopsoas tightness.

The patient then is seated on the examination table where iliopsoas strength (and any pain with resisted strength testing) is evaluated. Hip internal and external rotation is measured in this position, as the pelvis is stable against the examination table, making the goniometric measurement more accurate, since potential pelvic motion is eliminated. Ankle range of motion, both tibiotalar and subtalar, is tested to assure there is adequate ankle dorsiflexion, which can be associated with a number of lower extremity problem, and subtalar motion, which may be the cause of recurrent ankle sprains. Ankle strength testing is also carried out, focusing particularly on inversion and eversion strength, as inversion weakness has been associated with shin splints and eversion weakness may be a sign of inadequately treated ankle sprain. Ankle stability tests, particularly the anterior drawer test, are performed, while the player is seated. Toes are also evaluated for a myriad of potential foot issues, dermatologic, as well as structural, like hammer and claw toes and bunions.

The physical exam findings that may put the player at risk of injury/reinjury, whether due to current or past injury or surgery, or are the result of adaptations, even if asymptomatic, are discussed with the athlete. The information is passed on to the PHCPs who provide a rehabilitation program to eliminate these muscular weaknesses, imbalances, or inflexibilities. The PHCPs also provide recommendations on activities to avoid if an athlete's musculoskeletal anatomy when combined with the particular activity puts them at risk of injury. For example, a player with the anatomy of hip femoroacetabular impingement, though not having any hip pain or symptoms, will be advised against performing deep squats and recommended to maintain gluteal strength.

11.7 Tennis-Specific Screen

Musculoskeletal screening aims to prevent injury by identifying risk and to ultimately improve performance through development of a sport-specific profile and exercise interventions [61]. The WTA developed the tennis-specific screen (TSS) in an attempt to identify muscle weakness and imbalances and flexibility or range of movement deficits that may contribute to injury risk or reduce performance. Injuries may occur throughout the body in tennis, and specific movement patterns in multiple directions are required with integration of body segments to use the kinetic chain [62]. Therefore the screen requires multiple body area assessment and must be specific to tennis. The TSS was developed utilizing the following criteria: 1. previous injury trends and musculoskeletal assessment findings from the WTA Annual Physical Examinations; 2. the main actions of tennis and sport specificity [61]; 3. utilizing musculoskeletal examination tests which are often used in the daily assessment of athletes and require minimal equipment to accommodate the nature of international traveling tennis; 4. preference for reliable and valid tests; and 5. based on other tennis screening protocols within the literature, such as the USTA High Performance Profile [63]. When possible the TSS utilized dichotomous tests with a yes or no outcome as these have been found to be more clinically useful at predicting subsequent injury risk [64]. The ten screening tests comprising the TSS involve tests throughout the body and are listed below:

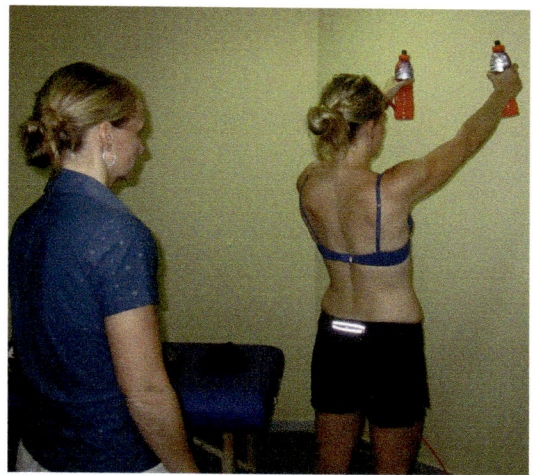

Fig. 11.1 Scapula stabilization test. The subject raises their arms overhead in flexion, and the examiner observes for evidence of scapular dyskinesis

1. Scapula stabilization test
   - Test: Active shoulder forward flexion and abduction are repeated with a 2 kg weight five times in each direction to detect presence or absence of scapula dyskinesis (Fig. 11.1). Scapula dyskinesis was classified as winging of medial or inferior scapula border or lack of smooth and coordinated movement [65].
   - Evidence: Observation is a reliable method for assessing scapula function with elevation [66–68] and found to be a reliable method [65]. Poor scapula control has been associated with upper extremity injury, with scapula muscular endurance and strength deficits being associated with lateral epicondylalgia [69, 70] and a correlation of shoulder symptoms with dyskinesis [68]. Altered elbow kinematics was also seen in throwing athletes associated with fatigue of scapula stabilizers [71]. A stable scapula base appears important to upper extremity function in the overhead athlete; therefore identifying scapula dyskinesis may reduce shoulder injury risk.
2. Shoulder strength test
   - Test: Manual muscle test of shoulder external rotation and internal rotation in 90/90 position of abduction/elbow flexion. Standing position chosen for functionality to tennis. Dynamometer is used if available or the oxford scale.
   - Evidence: Rotator cuff weakness has been proposed to contribute to shoulder injury [72], and external rotation weakness is associated with throwing injury and surgery [73]. Muscle imbalance in the dominant arm has been found in both overhead athletes [74, 75] and elite junior tennis players [76, 77]. Inter-rater reliability has been established ([78–80] and using a handheld dynamometer appears the most reliable method for isometric strength of the rotator cuff [81]. External rotation to internal rotation ratio in the dominant arm has been described at between 65% and 70% [63], while an internal rotation: external rotation ratio of greater than 1.5:1 is likely to lead to shoulder injury in baseball [82].
3. Single-leg squat
   - Test: Athlete places hands across the chest and lowers as far as able keeping the heel on ground and maintaining upright body (Fig. 11.2). Test classified as stable or unstable. Unstable, subclassified by presence of hip adduction, internal rotation or foot pronation, pelvic drop, loss of balance, or forward lean, is reported.
   - Evidence: Single-leg squat may correlate with hip muscle dysfunction and has good reliability and is shown to be valid [83].

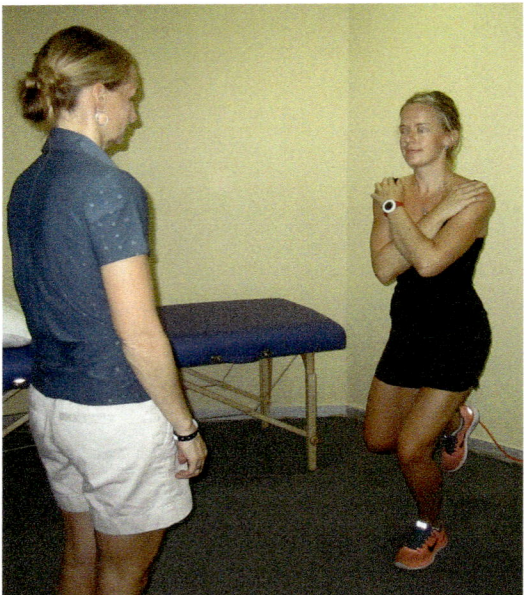

Fig. 11.2 Single-leg squat test. Athlete places hands across the chest and lowers as far as able keeping the heel on ground and maintaining upright body. Test classified as stable or unstable. Unstable, subclassified by the presence of hip adduction, internal rotation or foot pronation, pelvic drop, loss of balance, or forward lean, is reported

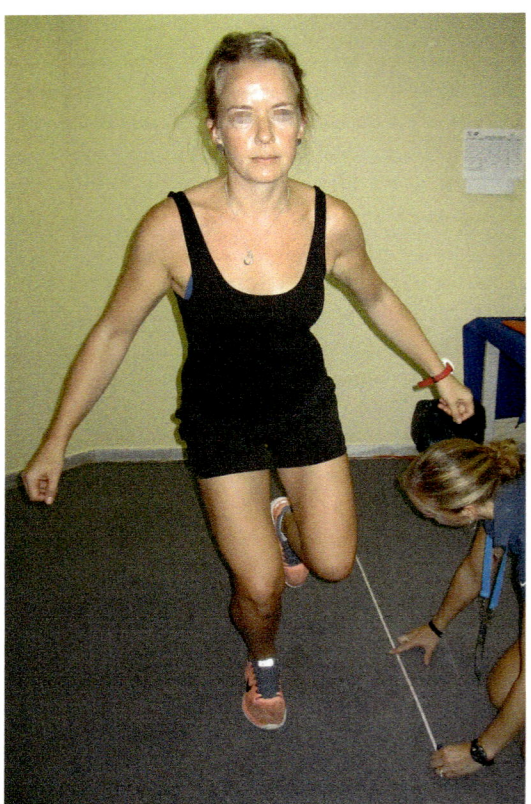

Fig. 11.3 Multidirectional hop test. This test is performed with one practice hop and best of two hops for distance in anterior, lateral, and medial directions controlling the landing for 5 s. The figure demonstrates measurement of a subject performing an anterior hop

Weakness of hip stabilizing muscles may cause lower extremity injuries [84] and lead to poor lower limb biomechanics while running [85].

4. Multidirectional hop test
   - Test: Multidirectional hop test is performed with one practice hop and best of two hops for distance in anterior, lateral, and medial directions controlling the landing for 5 s (Fig. 11.3).
   - Evidence: Assessment of unilateral leg power, coordination, leg dominance, and muscle imbalances may be detected through hop tests [86], and there is a reported four-time increase in foot or ankle injury with a greater than 10% side-to-side difference in single-leg hop test [87] (Brumitt et al. 2013). Several different types of hop tests have been found to be valid and reliable post-ACL reconsruction [88, 89].
5. Dorsiflexion lunge test
   - Test: Dorsiflexion (DF) lunge test (knee to wall). Active ankle dorsiflexion measured on tape is measured in centimeters by furthest distance able to dorsiflex ankle while touching the knee to the wall (Fig. 11.4).
   - Evidence: Reduced DF is recognized as a risk factor for lower extremity injury [90–92]. Weight-bearing tests of DF have high intra-rater [93–95] and inter-rater reliability [94, 96, 97]. Validity for lunge test is supported [97]. Lunge test with tape measure is more reliable than goniometer and inclinometer [98].
6. Thoracic rotation
   - Test: Thoracic rotation test is performed in sitting with hands across the chest and rolled towel between knees to stabilize position (Fig. 11.5). A goniometer measures

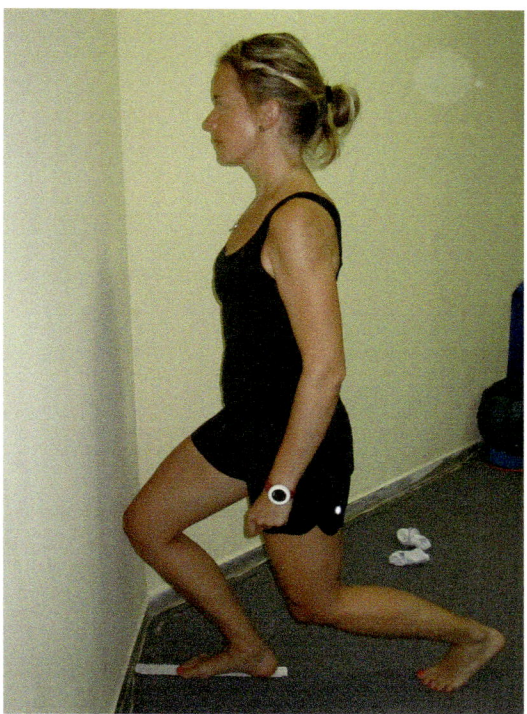

Fig. 11.4 Dorsiflexion (DF) lunge test (knee to wall). Active ankle dorsiflexion measured on tape measured in centimeters by furthest distance able to dorsiflex ankle while touching the knee to the wall

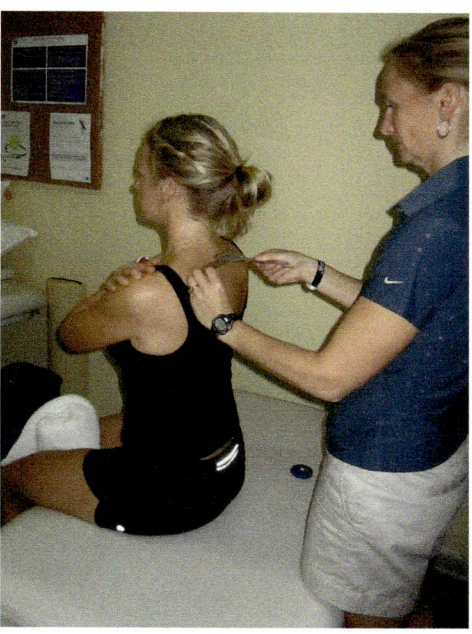

Fig. 11.5 Thoracic rotation test is performed in sitting with hands across the chest and rolled towel between knees to stabilize position. A goniometer measures angle of active rotation measured between T1 and T2 spinous processes with one arm perpendicular and one parallel to line of scapula

angle of active rotation measured between T1 and T2 spinous processes with one arm perpendicular and one parallel to line of scapula.
- Evidence: Tennis involves large rotary component; therefore it is necessary to quantify thoracic range of motion [99]. Good inter-rater reliability was found with thoracic rotation test [99].

7. Hip mobility
   - Test: Modified Thomas test (Fig. 11.6) is performed on edge of plinth stabilizing pelvis in neutral position and measuring angle of hip extension with an inclinometer at a level midpoint of the thigh.
   - Evidence: An association between abdominal strains and the presence of hip flexion contracture or positive Thomas test was found in WTA female tennis players [59]. When pelvic tilt is controlled, the Thomas test appears to be a valid test in evaluating hip extension angle [100]. Variable reporting of reliability in the literature exists, with poor reliability [101] and high inter- and intra-rater reliability with inclinometer and goniometer reported [102, 103].
   - Test: Hip external rotation (ER) and internal rotation (IR) passively assessed with an inclinometer placed proximal to lateral malleolus and medial malleolus, respectively. Athlete sits upright with both fists placed between knees to keep thighs parallel.
   - Evidence: Normal hip motion is an essential component for proper kinematics in the overhead athlete. A bilateral difference in total hip rotation arc of greater than 10° has a significant association with thigh injury in professional female WTA players [104]. In other overhead athletes,

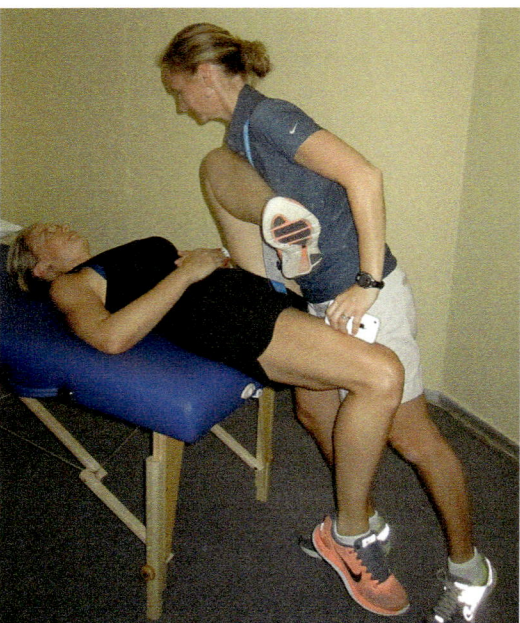

Fig. 11.6 Modified Thomas test is performed on edge of plinth stabilizing pelvis in neutral position and measuring angle of hip extension with an inclinometer at a level midpoint of the thigh

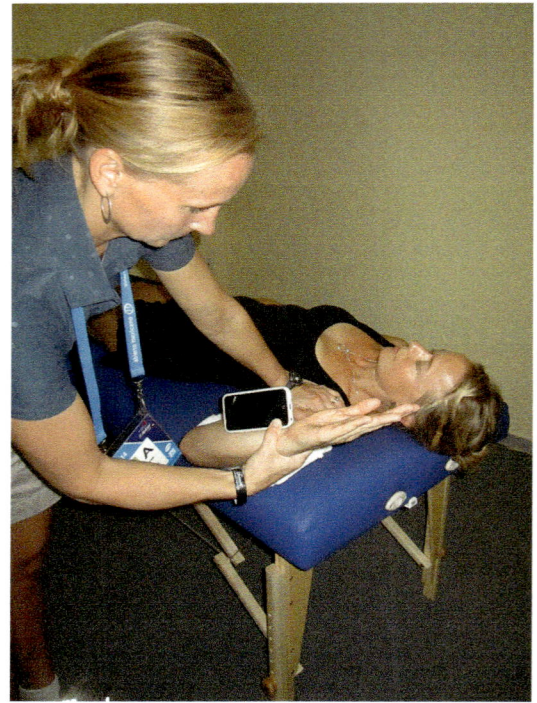

Fig. 11.7 Passive glenohumeral joint external rotation (ER) is shown in this figure. This is assessed in supine position with the shoulder in 90° of abduction and 90° of elbow flexion with an inclinometer. Internal rotation in this position is also assessed but not shown

a correlation between reduced hip internal rotation and total arc of motion with hip, hamstring, and groin injuries in baseball has been reported [105]. Hip rotation mobility is reliable [106, 107] and no difference in reproducibility reported between prone, supine, and seated positions [108].

8. Shoulder mobility
   - Test: Passive glenohumeral joint internal (IR) and external rotation (ER) (Fig. 11.7) is assessed in supine position with the shoulder in 90° of abduction and 90° of elbow flexion with an inclinometer.
   - Evidence: A loss of glenohumeral joint IR and/or total glenohumeral joint range of motion has been associated with both shoulder injury in overhead athletes [109–111] and altered joint kinematics [112]. In the dominant shoulder, both reductions in IR and total range of movement have been found following acute exposure to tennis play [113]; therefore identification of athletes for motion alterations is important to implement intervention strategies. Reliability of assessment has been reviewed in varying positions [114] and intra-rater reliability established with this particular method of measurement [113].
9. Hamstring length/SLR
   - Test: The straight leg raise test was chosen to assess hamstring length for its ease in application and potential combined ability to detect neurodynamic restriction [115].
   - Evidence: Reduced length reported to be associated with increased injury risk [116]. High reliability is reported in literature [103, 117, 118].
10. Core stabilization test
    - Test: Modified Closed Kinetic Chain Upper Extremity Stability test (CKCUES

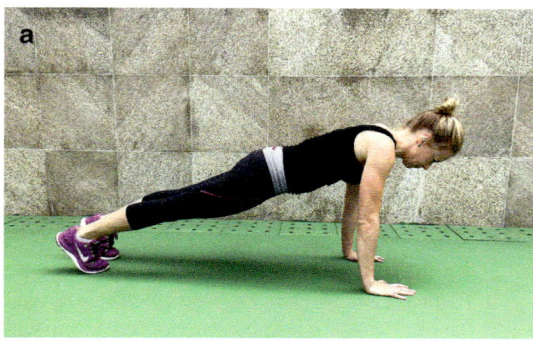 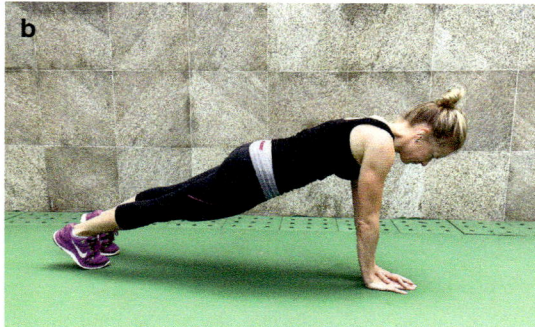

Fig. 11.8 Core stability test. (**a**) Starting position in push-up position with hands 30 in. apart. (**b**) Hands alternate touching the other hand. Measure number of hand touches in 15 s

test) is performed in the push-up position with hands 30 in. apart on tape and feet hip width apart. In 15 s, maximal alternate hand touch is completed aiming to maintain trunk and scapula control (Fig. 11.8).

- Evidence: Preseason performance of CKCUES test significantly correlated with shoulder injury [119] correlates to rotator cuff strength [120]. CKCUES test is reliable [121, 122] and reported to be clinically useful [123].

The TSS is a method of assessment that may be used preseasonally or regularly throughout the season to monitor athletes and identify any areas of weakness to ensure deficits can be addressed to prevent injury and optimize performance. The test aims to assess the whole body, as there is integration from multiple segments in the kinetic chain to produce powerful strokes. A breakage in one of these segments may lead to compensatory actions and/or overload to more distal segments [62]. The TSS aims to identify potential musculoskeletal deficiencies and address these deficits to be with a focus of treatment and physical training.

11.8 Check Out and Follow-Up

Once the player has completed all the examination/evaluation stations during their WTA physical examination, they present their file to the WTA's Senior Vice President, Sport Sciences & Medicine and Transitions, to review all the recommendations made by the various WTA medical advisors from each station. The player identifies if they want help from the WTA medical staff to arrange for any further education, monitoring, and treatment that was suggested. Any player that needs follow-up of some issue or condition is added to a database that is used by the WTA PHCP's to monitor any recommendations that have been made. This helps to improve player compliance with the medical plan that was suggested at the time of their physical. The PHCP's follow up and document in the database and the player's WTA EMR if the player has completed the recommended suggestions.

References

1. Ljungqvist A, Jenoure P, Engebretsen L, Alonso JM, Bahr R, Clough A, DeBondt G, Dvorak J, Maloley R, Matheson G, Meeuwisse W, Meijboom E, Mountjoy M, Pelliccia A, Schwellnus M, Sprumont D, Schamasch P, Gauthier JB, Dubi C, Stupp H, Thill C. The International Olympic Committee (IOC) consensus statement on periodic health evaluation of Elite Athletes March 2009. Br J Sports Med. 2009;43(9):631–43.
2. American Academy of Family Physicians, American Academy of Pediatrics, American College of Sports Medicine, American Medical Society for Sports Medicine, American Orthopedic Society for Sports Medicine & American Osteopathic Academy of Sports Medicine. Preparticipation physical evaluation. 4th ed. Elk Grove Village, IL: American Academy of Pediatrics; 2010.

3. Hainline B, Drezner J, Baggish A, Harmon FG, Emery MS, Myeburg RJ, Sanchez E, Molossi S, Parsons JT, Thompson PD. Interassociation consensus statement on cardiovascular care of college student-athletes. Br J Sports Med. 2016;51(2):74–85.
4. Roberts WO, Löllgen H, Matheson GO, Royalty AB, Meeuwisse WH, Levine B, Hutchinson MR, Coleman N, Benjamin H, Spataro A, Debruyne A, Bachl N, Pigozzi F. Advancing the preparticipation physical evaluation: an ACSM and FIMS Joint Consensus Statement. Clin J Sports Med. 2014;24(6):442–7.
5. Matheson GO, Anerson S, Robell K. Injuries and illnesses in the preparticipation evaluation data of 1693 college student-athletes. Am J Sports Med. 2015;43(6):1518–25.
6. Maron BJ, Friedman RA, Kligfield P, Levine BD, Viskin S, Chaitman BR, Okin PM, Saul JP, Salberg L, Van Hare GF, Soliman EZ, Chen J, Matherne GP, Bolling SF, Mitten MJ, Caplan A, Balady GJ, Thompson PD, American Heart Association Council on Clinical Cardiology; Advocacy Coordinating Committee; Council on Cardiovascular Disease in the Young; Council on Cardiovascular Surgery and Anesthesia; Council on Epidemiology and Prevention; Council on Functional Genomics and Translational Biology; & Council on Quality of Care and Outcomes Research, and American College of Cardiology. Assessment of the 12-lead electrocardiogram as a screening test for detection of cardiovascular disease in healthy general populations of young people (12-25 years of age): a scientific statement from the American Heart Association and the American College of Cardiology. J Am Coll Cardiol. 2014;64(14):1479–514.
7. Corrado D, Basso C, Pavei A, Michieli P, Schiavon M, Thiene G. Trends in sudden cardiovascular death in young competitive athletes after implementation of a preparticipation screening program. J Am Med Assoc. 2006;296(13):1593–601.
8. Baggish AL, Hutter AM, Wang F, Yared K, Weiner RB, Kupperman E, Picard MH, Wood MJ. Cardiovascular screening in college athletes with and without electrocardiography: a cross-sectional study. Ann Intern Med. 2010;152(5):269–75.
9. Corrado D, Pelliccia A, Bjørnstad HH, Vanhees L, Biffi A, Borjesson M, Panhuyzen-Goedkoop N, Deligiannis A, Solberg E, Dugmore D, Mellwig KP, Assanelli D, Delise P, van-Buuren F, Anastasakis A, Heidbuchel H, Hoffmann E, Fagard R, Priori SG, Basso C, Arbustini E, Blomstrom-Lundqvist C, McKenna WJ, Thiene G. Cardiovascular preparticipation screening of young competitive athletes for prevention of sudden death: proposal for a Common European Protocol. Consensus Statement of the Study Group of Sports Cardiology Exercise Physiology and the Working Group of Myocardial and Pericardial Diseases of the European Society of Cardiology. Eur Heart J. 2005;26(5):516–24.
10. Dvorak J, Grimm K, Schmied C, Junge A. Development and implementation of a standardized precompetition medical assessment of international elite football players – 2006 FIFA World Cup Germany. Clin J Sport Med. 2009;19(4):316–21.
11. Harris KM, Sponsel A, Hutter AM, Maron BJ. Brief communication: cardiovascular screening practices of major North American professional sports teams. Ann Intern Med. 2006;145(7):507–11.
12. Drezner JA, O'Connor FG, Harmon KG, Fields KB, Asplund CA, Asif IM, Price DE, Dimeff RJ, Bernhardt DT, Roberts WO. AMSSM position statement on cardiovascular preparticipation screening in athletes: current evidence, knowledge gaps, recommendations and future directions. Clin J Sport Med. 2016;26(5):347–61.
13. Nathan RA, Sorkness CA, Kosinski M, Schatz M, Li JT, Marcus P, Murray JJ, Pendergraft TB. Development of the asthma control test: a survey for assessing asthma control. J Allergy Clin Immunol. 2004;113(1):59–65.
14. Schatz M, Sorkness CA, Li JT, Marcus P, Murray JJ, Nathan RA, Kosinski M, Pendergraft TB, Jhingran P. Asthma control test: reliability, validity, and responsiveness in patients not previously followed by asthma specialists. J Allergy Clin Immunol. 2006;117(3):549–56.
15. American Lung Association. Asthma Action Plan, viewed 31 December 2016. http://www.lung.org/assets/documents/asthma/asthma-action-plan.pdf.
16. American College of Sports Medicine (ACSM), American Academy of Family Physicians (AAFP), American Academy of Orthopaedic Surgeons (AAOS), American Medical Society for Sports Medicine (AMSSM), American Orthopaedic Society for Sports Medicine (AOSSSM), & American Osteopathic Academy of Sports Medicine (AOASM). Psychological issues related to injury in athletes and the team physician: a consensus statement. Med Sci Sports Exerc. 2006;38(11):2030–4.
17. Markser V. Sport psychiatry and psychotherapy. Mental strains and disorders in professional sports. Challenges and answer to societal changes. Eur Arch Psychiatry Clin Neurosci. 2011;261(Suppl 2):S182–5.
18. Neal TL, Diamond AB, Goldman S, Klossner D, Morse ED, Pajak DE, Putukian M, Quandt EF, Sullivan JP, Wallack C, Welzant V. Inter-association recommendations for developing a plan to recognize and refer student-athletes with psychological concerns at the collegiate level: an executive summary of a consensus statement. J Athl Train. 2013;48(5):716–20.
19. Rice SM, Purcell R, de Silva S, Mawren D, McGorry PD, Parker AG. The mental health of elite athletes: a narrative systematic review. Sports Med. 2016;46(9):1333–53.
20. Stull T. The psychiatrist perspective. In: Brown GT, editor. Mind, body, sport. Understanding and sup-

21. Gulliver A, Griffiths KM, Mackinnon A, Batterham PJ, Stanimirovic R. The mental health of elite Australian athletes. J Sci Med Sport. 2015;18(3):255–61.
22. Hughes L, Leavey G. Setting the bar: athletes and vulnerability to mental illness. Br J Psychiatry. 2012;200(2):95–6.
23. Stillman MA, Brown T, Ritvo EC, Glick ID. Sport psychiatry and psychotherapeutic intervention, circa 2016. Int Rev Psychiatry. 2016;28(6):614–22.
24. Putukian M. The psychological response to injury in student athletes: a narrative review with a focus on mental health. Br J Sports Med. 2016;50(3):145–8.
25. National Collegiate Athletics Association (NCAA), NCAA Sport Sciences Institute. Mental health best practices. Inter-association consensus document: best practices for understanding and supporting student-athlete mental wellness, viewed on 31 Dec 2016. 2016. http://www.ncaa.org/sport-science-institute/mental-health.
26. Brown LK, Puster KL, Vazquez EA, Hunter HL, Lescano CM. Screening practices for adolescent dating violence. J Interpers Violence. 2007;22(4):456–64.
27. Marks S, Mountjoy M, Marcus M. Sexual harassment and abuse in sport: the role of the team doctor. Br J Sports Med. 2012;46(13):905–8.
28. Mountjoy M, Brackenridge C, Arrington M, Blauwet C, Carska-Sheppard A, Fasting K, Kirby S, Leahy T, Marks S, Martin K, Starr K, Tiivas A, Budgett R. International Olympic Committee consensus statement: harassment and abuse (non-accidental violence) in sport. Br J Sports Med. 2016;50(17):1019–29.
29. National Collegiate Athletics Association (NCAA), NCAA Sport Sciences Institute. Addressing sexual assault and interpersonal violence, viewed on 31 Dec 2016. 2014. http://www.ncaa.org/sites/default/files/Sexual-Violence-Prevention.pdf.
30. Carr C, Davidson J. The psychologist perspective. In: Brown GT, editor. Mind body, sport. Understanding and supporting student athlete mental wellness. Indianapolis: National Collegiate Athletic Association; 2014.
31. Chew K, Thompson R. Potential barriers to accessing mental health services. In: Brown GT, editor. Mind body, sport. Understanding and supporting student athlete mental wellness. Indianapolis: National Collegiate Athletic Association; 2014.
32. Gulliver A, Griffiths KM, Christensen H. Barriers and facilitators to mental health help-seeking for young elite athletes: a qualitative study. BMC Psychiatry. 2012;12:157–70.
33. Prinz B, Dvorak J, Junge A. Symptoms and risk factors of depression during and after the football career of elite female players. BMJ Open Sport Exerc Med. 2016;2(1):e000124.
34. Stillman MA, Ritvo EC, Glick ID. Psychotherapeutic treatment of athletes and their significant others. In: Reardon CL, Baron SH, editors. Clinical sports psychiatry: an international perspective. Hoboken, NJ: Wiley; 2013.
35. Trojian T. Depression is under-recognised in the sport setting: time for primary care sports medicine to be proactive and screen widely for depression symptoms. Br J Sports Med. 2016;50(3):137–9.
36. Conley KM, Bolin DJ, Carek PJ, Konin JG, Neal TL, Violette D. National Athletic Trainers' association position statement: preparticipation physical examinations and disqualifying conditions. J Athl Train. 2014;49(1):102–20.
37. Klein DA, Goldenring JM, Adelman WP. HEEADSSS 3.0 The psychosocial interview for adolescents updated for a new century fueled by media. Contemp Pediatr. 2014;31:16–28.
38. American Psychiatric Association (APA). Diagnostic and statistical manual of mental disorders, 5th Edition: DSM-5. Arlington, VA: American Psychiatric Association; 2013.
39. Juliff LE, Halson SL, Peiffer JJ. Understanding sleep disturbance in athletes prior to important competitions. J Sci Med Sport. 2015;18(1):13–8.
40. Sargent C, Lastella M, Halson SH, Roach GD. Impact of training schedules on sleep and fatigue in elite athletes. Chronobiol Int. 2014;31(10):1160–8.
41. Fowler PM, Duffield R, Lu D, Hickmans JA, Scott TJ. Effects of long-haul transmeridian travel on subjective jet-lag and self-reported sleep and upper respiratory symptoms in professional rugby league players. Int J Sports Physiol Perform. 2016;11(7):876–84.
42. Kraemer WJ, Hooper DR, Kupchak BR, Saenz C, Brown LE, Vingren JL, Luk HY, DuPont WH, Szivak TK, Flanagan SD, Caldwell LK, Eklund D, Lee EC, Häkkinen K, Volek JS, Fleck SJ, Maresh CM. The effects of a roundtrip trans-American jet travel on physiological stress, neuromuscular performance, and recovery. J Appl Physiol. 2016;121(2):438–48.
43. McDuff DR, Baron D. Substance use in athletics: a sports psychiatry perspective. Clin Sports Med. 2005;24(4):885–97.
44. Chang EC, Lee J, Wright KM, Najarian AS-M, Yu T, Chang OD, Hirsch JK. Examining sexual assault victimization and loneliness as risk factors associated with nonlethal self-harm behaviors in female college students: is it important to control for concomitant suicidal behaviors (and vice versa)? J Interpers Violence. 2016. https://doi.org/10.1177/0886260516675920.
45. Madge N, Hawton K, McMahon EM, Corcoran P, De Leo D, de Wilde EJ, Fekete S, van Heeringen K, Ystgaard M, Arensman E. Psychological characteristics, stressful life events and deliberate self-harm: findings from the Child & Adolescent Self-Harm in Europe (CASE) study. Eur Child Adolesc Psychiatry. 2011;20(10):499–508.

46. Carter G, Page A, Large M, Hetrick S, Milner AJ, Bendit N, Walton C, Draper B, Hazell P, Fortune S, Burns J, Patton G, Lawrence G, Dadd L, Robinson J, Christensen H. Royal Australian and New Zealand College of Psychiatrists Clinical Practice Guideline for the management of deliberate self-harm. Aust N Z J Psychiatry. 2016;50(10):939–1000.
47. Rao AD, Asif IM, Drezner JA, Toresdahl BG, Harmon KG. Suicide in National Collegiate Athletic Association (NCAA) athletes: a 9-year analysis of the NCAA resolutions database. Sports Health. 2015;7(5):452–7.
48. Rao AL, Hong ES. Understanding depression and suicide in college athletes: emerging concepts and future directions. Br J Sports Med. 2016;50(3):136–7.
49. Mann JJ, Apter A, Bertolote J, Beautrais A, Currier D, Haas A, Hegerl U, Malone K, Marusic A, Mehlum L, Patton G, Phillips M, Rutz W, Rihmer Z, Schmidtke A, Shaffer D, Silverman M, Takahashi Y, Varnik A, Wasserman D, Yip P, Hendin H. Suicide prevention strategies: a systematic review. J Am Med Assoc. 2005;294(16):2064–74.
50. Brackenridge C, Fasting K, Kirby S, Leahy T. Protecting children from violence in sport: a review from industrialized countries. Florence, Italy: UNICEF Innocenti Research Centre; 2010.
51. de Souza MJ, Nattiv A, Joy E, Misra M, Williams NI, Mallinson RJ, Gibbs JC, Olmsted M, Goolsby M, Matheson G, Expert Panel. 2014 female athlete triad coalition consensus statement on treatment and return to play of the female athlete triad: 1st International Conference held in San Francisco, California, May 2012 and 2nd International conference held in Indianapolis, Indiana, May 2013. Br J Sports Med. 2014;48(4):289.
52. Joy E, Kussman A, Nattiv A. Update on eating disorders in athletes: a comprehensive narrative review with a focus on clinical assessment and management. Br J Sports Med. 2016;50(3):154–62.
53. Mountjoy M, Sundgot-Borgen J, Burke L, Carter S, Constantini N, Lebrun C, Meyer N, Sherman R, Steffen K, Budgett R, Ljungqvist A. The IOC consensus statement: beyond the female athlete triad—relative energy deficiency in sport (RED-S). Br J Sports Med. 2014;48(7):491–7.
54. Ip A. Concussion and mental health: a concise review. Univ B C Med J. 2016;8(1):44–5.
55. McCrory P, Meeuwisse WH, Aubry M, Cantu B, Dvorák J, Echemendia RJ, Engebretsen L, Johnston K, Kutcher JS, Raftery M, Sills A, Benson BW, Davis GA, Ellenbogen RG, Guskiewicz K, Herring SA, Iverson GL, Jordan BD, Kissick J, McCrea M, McIntosh AS, Maddocks D, Makdissi M, Purcell L, Putukian M, Schneider K, Tator CH, Turner M. Consensus statement on concussion in sport: the 4th international conference on concussion in sport held in Zurich, November 2012. Br J Sports Med. 2013;47(5):250–8.
56. Burke L. Practical sports nutrition. South Australia: Human Kinetics; 2007.
57. Burke L, Deakin V. Clinical sports nutrition. 5th ed. Australia: McGraw-Hill Education Pty Ltd; 2015.
58. Young SW, Dakic J, Stroia K, Nguyen ML, Harris AHS, Safran MR. High incidence of infraspinatus atrophy in elite professional female tennis players. Am J Sports Med. 2015;43(8):1989–93.
59. Young SW, Dakic J, Stroia K, Nguyen ML, Harris AH, Safran MR. Hip range of motion and association with injury in female professional tennis players. Am J Sports Med. 2014;42(11):2654–8.
60. Young SW, Dakic J, Stroia K, Nguyen ML, Harris AHS, Safran MR. Arthroscopic shoulder surgery in female professional tennis players: ability and timing to return to play. Clin J Sports Med. 2016;27:357. https://doi.org/10.1097/JSM.0000000000000361.
61. Murphy DF, Connolly DA, Beynnon BD. Risk factors for lower extremity injury: a review of the literature. Br J Sports Med. 2003;37(1):13–29.
62. Kibler WB, Press J, Sciascia AD. The role of core stability in athletic function. Sports Med. 2006;36(3):189–98.
63. Ellenbecker T. Musculoskeletal examination of elite junior tennis players. Aspetar Sports Med J. 2014;3:548–56.
64. Bahr R. Why screening tests to predict injury do not work-and probably never will…: a critical review. Br J Sports Med. 2016;50(13):776–80.
65. Kibler WB, Uhl TL, Maddux JW, Brooks PV, Zeller B, McMullen J. Qualitative clinical evaluation of scapular dysfunction: a reliability study. J Shoulder Elb Surg. 2002;11(6):550–6.
66. McClure P, Tate A, Kareha S, Irwin D, Zlupko E. A clinical method for identifying scapular dyskinesis, part 1: Reliability. J Athl Train. 2009;44(2):160–4.
67. Tate AR, McClure P, Kareha S, Irwin D. Effect of the scapula reposition test on shoulder impingement symptoms and elevation strength in overhead athletes. J Orthop Sports Phys Ther. 2008;38(1):4–11.
68. Uhl TL, Kibler WB, Gecewich B, Tripp BL. Evaluation of clinical assessment methods for scapular dyskinesis. Arthroscopy. 2009;25(11):1240–8.
69. Day JM, Bush H, Nitz AJ, Uhl TL. Scapular muscle performance in individuals with lateral epicondylalgia. J Orthop Sports Phys Ther. 2015;45(5):414–24.
70. Lucado AM, Kolber MJ, Cheng MS, Echternach JL Sr. Upper extremity strength characteristics in female recreational tennis players with and without lateral epicondylalgia. J Orthop Sports Phys Ther. 2012;42(12):1025–31.
71. Hidetomo S, Swanik KA, Huxel KC, Kelly JD IV, Swanik CB. Alterations in upper extremity motion after scapular-muscle fatigue. J Sport Rehabil. 2006;15:71–88.
72. Wilk KE, Obma P, Simpson CD, Cain EL, Dugas JR, Andrews JR. Shoulder injuries in the overhead athlete. J Orthop Sports Phys Ther. 2009a;39(2):38–54.
73. Byram IR, Bushnell BD, Dugger K, Charron K, Harrell FE Jr, Noonan TJ. Preseason shoulder strength measurements in professional baseball

pitchers: identifying players at risk for injury. Am J Sports Med. 2010;38(7):1375–82.
74. Dehnavi H, Daneshmandi H, Glosalari M, Shahrokhi H. A comparison of internal/external rotation strength and range of motion in the shoulder joint between zurkhaneh athletes and non-athletes. Am J Sports Sci. 2013;1(3):39–43.
75. Yildiz Y. Shoulder terminal range eccentric antagonist/concentric agonist strength ratios in overhead athletes. Scand J Med Sci Sports. 2006;16(3):174–80.
76. Ellenbecker TS, Roetert EP. Age specific isokinetic glenohumeral internal and external rotation strength in elite junior tennis players. J Sci Med Sport. 2003;6(1):63–70.
77. Saccol MF. Shoulder functional ratio in elite junior tennis players. Phys Ther Sport. 2010;11(1):8–11.
78. Ellenbecker TS, Davies GJ. The application of isokinetics in testing and rehabilitation of the shoulder complex. J Athl Train. 2000;35(3):338–50.
79. Hurd WJ, Kaufman KR. Glenohumeral rotational motion and strength and baseball pitching biomechanics. J Athl Train. 2012;47(3):247–56.
80. Cools AM, De Wilde L, Van Tongel A, Ceyssens C, Ryckewaert R, Cambier DC. Measuring shoulder external and internal rotation strength and range of motion: comprehensive intra-rater and inter-rater reliability study of several testing protocols. J Shoulder Elbow Surg. 2014;23(10):1454–61.
81. Hayes K, Walton JR, Szomor ZL, Murrell GA. Reliability of 3 methods for assessing shoulder strength. J Shoulder Elb Surg. 2002;11(1):33–9.
82. Whiteley R, Oceguera MV, Valencia EB, Mitchell T. Adaptations at the shoulder of the throwing athlete and implications for the clinician. Tech Should Elbow Surg. 2012;13(1):36–44.
83. Crossley KM, Zhang WJ, Schache AG, Bryant A, Cowan SM. Performance on the single-leg squat task indicates hip abductor muscle function. Am J Sports Med. 2011;39(4):866–73.
84. Leetun DT, Ireland ML, Willson JD, Ballantyne BT, Davis IM. Core stability measures as risk factors for lower extremity injury in athletes. Med Sci Sports Exerc. 2004;36(6):926–34.
85. Ferber R, Hreljac A, Kendall KD. Suspected mechanisms in the cause of overuse running injuries: a clinical review. Sports Health. 2009;1(3):242–6.
86. Hewit JK, Cronin JB, Hume PA. Asymmetry in multi-directional jumping tasks. Phys Ther Sport. 2012;13(4):238–42.
87. Brumitt J, Heiderscheit BC, Manske RC, Niemuth PE, Rauh MJ. Lower extremity functional tests and risk of injury in division iii collegiate athletes. Int J Sports Phys Ther. 2013;8(3):216–27.
88. Reid A, Birmingham TB, Stratford PW, Alcock GK, Giffin JR. Hop testing provides a reliable and valid outcome measure during rehabilitation after anterior cruciate ligament reconstruction. Phys Ther. 2007;87(3):337–49.
89. Gustavsson A, Neeter C, Thomee P, Silbernagel KG, Augustsson J, Thomee R, Karlsson J. A test battery for evaluating hop performance in patients with an ACL injury and patients who have undergone ACL reconstruction. Knee Surg Sports Traumatol Arthrosc. 2006;14(8):778–88.
90. Hadzic V, Sattler T, Topole E, Jarnovic Z, Burger H, Dervisevic E. Risk factors for ankle sprain in volleyball players: a preliminary analysis. Isokinet Exerc Sci. 2009;17(3):155–60.
91. Pope R, Herbert R, Kirwan J. Effects of ankle dorsiflexion range and pre-exercise calf muscle stretching on injury risk in army recruits. Aust J Physiother. 1998;44(3):165–72.
92. Willems TM, Witvrouw E, Delbaere K, Mahieu N, De Bourdeaudhuij I, De Clercq D. Intrinsic risk factors for inversion ankle sprains in male subjects: a prospective study. Am J Sports Med. 2005;33(3):415–23.
93. Collins N, Teys P, Vicenzino B. The initial effects of a Mulligan's mobilization with movement technique on dorsiflexion and pain in subacute ankle sprains. Man Ther. 2004;9(2):77–82.
94. Venturini C, Ituassu NT, Teixeira LM, Deus CVO. Intrarater and interrater reliability of two methods for measuring the active range of motion for ankle dorsiflexion in healthy subjects. Rev Bras Fisioter. 2006;10(4):377–81.
95. Vicenzino B, Prangley I, Martin D. The initial effect of two Mulligan mobilisation with movement treatment techniques on ankle dorsi-flexion. In A sports medicine odyssey—challenges, controversies and change: proceedings of the Australian Conference of Science and Medicine in Sport, 23–27 October, Perth, Australia, Sports Medicine Australia; 2001.
96. Bennell KL, Talbot RC, Wajswelner H, Techovanich W, Kelly D, Hall AJ. Intra-rater and inter-rater reliability of a weight-bearing lunge measure of ankle dorsiflexion. Aust J Physiother. 1998;44(3):175–80.
97. Chisolm MD, Birmingham TB, Brown J, MacDermid J, Chesworth BM. Reliability and validity of a weight-bearing measure of ankle dorsiflexion range of motion. Physiother Can. 2012;64(4):347–55.
98. Konor MM, Morton S, Eckerson JM, Grindstaff TL. Reliability of three measures of ankle dorsiflexion range of motion. Int J Sports Phys Ther. 2012;7(3):279–87.
99. Johnson KD, Kim KM, Yu BK, Saliba SA, Grindstaff TL. Reliability of thoracic spine rotation range-of-motion measurements in healthy adults. J Athl Train. 2012;47(1):52–60.
100. Vigotsky AD, Lehman GJ, Beardsley C, Contreeras B, Chung B, Feser EH. The modified Thomas test is not a valid measure of hip extension unless pelvic tilt is controlled. PeerJ. 2016;4:e2325.
101. Peeler J, Anderson JE. Reliability of the Thomas test for assessing range of motion about the hip. Phys Ther Sport. 2007;8(1):14–21.
102. Clapis PA, Davis SM, Davis RO. Reliability of inclinometer and goniometric measurements of hip extension flexibility using the modified Thomas test. Physiother Theory Pract. 2007;24(2):135–41.

103. Gabbe BJ, Bennell KL, Wajswelner H, Finch CF. Reliability of common lower extremity musculoskeletal screening tests. Phys Ther Sport. 2004;5(2):90–7.
104. Dakic J, Gosling C, Smith B. Hip and shoulder rotation range of motion and shoulder strength ratios and association with injury in professional female tennis players. J Sci Med Sport. 2017;20(Suppl 1):e58–9.
105. Li X, Ma R, Zhou H, Thompson M, Dawson C, Nguyen J, Coleman S. Evaluation of hip internal and external rotation range of motion as an injury risk factor for hip, abdominal and groin injuries in professional baseball players. Orthop Rev. 2015;7(4):111–5.
106. Ellison JB, Rose SJ, Sahrmann S. Patterns of hip rotation range of motion: a comparison between healthy subjects and patients with low back pain. Phys Ther. 1990;70(9):537–41.
107. Van Dillen LR, Bloom NJ, Gombatto SP, Susco TM. Hip rotation range of motion in people with and without low back pain who participate in rotation related sports. Phys Ther Sport. 2008;9(2):72–81.
108. Kouyoumdjian P, Coulomb R, Sanchez T, Asencio G. Clinical evaluation of hip joint rotation range of motion in adults. Orthop Traumatol Surg Res. 2012;98(1):17–23.
109. Clarsen B, Bahr R, Andersson SH, Munk R, Myklebust G. Reduced glenohumeral rotation, external rotation weakness and scapular dyskinesis are risk factors for shoulder injuries among elite male handball players: a prospective cohort study. Br J Sports Med. 2014;48(17):1327–33.
110. Myers JB, Laudner KG, Pasquale MR, Bradley JP, Lephart SM. Glenohumeral range of motion deficits and posterior shoulder tightness in throwers with pathologic internal impingement. Am J Sports Med. 2006;34(3):385–91.
111. Wilk KE, Macrina LC, Fleisig GS, Porterfield R, Simpson CD II, Harker P, Paparesta N, Andrews JR. Correlation of glenohumeral internal rotation deficit and total rotational motion to shoulder injuries in professional baseball pitchers. Am J Sports Med. 2011;39(2):329–35.
112. Borich MR, Bright JM, Lorello DJ, Cieminski CJ, Buisman T, Ludewig PM. Scapular angular positioning at end range internal rotation in cases of glenohumeral internal rotation deficit. J Orthop Sports Phys Ther. 2006;36(12):926–34.
113. Moore-Reed SD, Kibler WB, Myers NL, Smith BJ. Acute changes in passive glenohumeral rotation following tennis play exposure in elite female players. Int J Sports Phys Ther. 2016;11(2):230–6.
114. Wilk KE, Reinold MM, Macrina LC, Porterfield R, Devine KM, Suarez K, Andrews JR. Glenohumeral internal rotation measurements differ depending on stabilization techniques. Sports Health. 2009b;1(2):131–6.
115. Butler DS. Mobilisation of the nervous system. Melbourne: Churchill Livingstone; 1994.
116. Freckleton G, Pizzari T. Risk factors for hamstring muscle strain injury in sport: a systematic review and meta-analysis. Br J Sports Med. 2013;47(6):351–8.
117. Carregaro RL, Silva LCCB, Gil Coury HJC. Comparison between two clinical tests for the evaluation of posterior thigh muscles flexibility. Braz J Phys Ther. 2007;11(2):125–30.
118. Hsieh CY, Walker JM, Gillis K. Straight leg raising test: comparison of three instruments. Phys Ther. 1983;63(9):1429–33.
119. Pontillo M, Spinelli BA, Sennett BJ. Prediction of in-season shoulder injury from preseason testing in division I collegiate football players. Sports Health. 2014;6(6):497–503.
120. Pontillo M, Horneff JG, Huffman GR, Sennett BJ. The relationship between upper extremity strength, functional testing, and self-reported disability in collegiate athletes. J Orthop Sports Phys Ther. 2010;40(1):A108.
121. Goldbeck TG, Davies GJ. Test-retest reliability of the closed kinetic chain upper extremity stability test: a clinical field test. J Sport Rehabil. 2000;9:35–45.
122. Tucci HT, Martins J, de Carvalho Sposito G, Ferreira Camarini PM, de Oliveira AS. Closed kinetic chain upper extremity stability test (CKCUES test): a reliability study in persons with and without shoulder impingement syndrome. BMC Musculoskelet Disord. 2014;15(1):1–9.
123. Roush JR, Kitamura J, Waits MC. Reference values for the closed kinetic chain upper extremity stability test (CKCUEST) for collegiate baseball players. N Am J Sports Phys Ther. 2007;2(3):159–63.

Assessment of Physical Performance for Individualized Training Prescription in Tennis

12

Alexander Ferrauti, Alexander Ulbricht, and Jaime Fernandez-Fernandez

12.1 Introduction

Tennis requires a complex interaction of technical, tactical, psychological, and several physical components (i.e., strength, agility) and metabolic pathways (i.e., aerobic and anaerobic) [1] (Fig. 12.1). In order to achieve an optimum cost-benefit ratio of training input, goals and contents during physical conditioning must be defined according to the specific workload and the most important limiting performance factors in tennis but also closely corresponding to the individual needs (strengths and weaknesses) of each athlete. The dominance of the technical and tactical requirements for tennis performance can be figured out by an upper position in a hierarchical model of performance-limiting aspects (Fig. 12.1). The weekly training volume has to be adjusted correspondingly, and the respective volume for physical conditioning remains comparably low. Therefore, on an elite performance level, it becomes of predominant importance that physical training has to be combined with technical and tactical training on-court and during off-court sessions that should meet precisely the individual requirements which have to be regularly assessed by physical performance tests [2–5].

Testing procedures [e.g., [6]] as well as complex test batteries [e.g., [7]] are described in the tennis-specific literature, and all measurements (i.e., laboratory as well as field-based tests) have to consider the specific criteria of proper testing, which are validity, reliability, and objectivity [4, 8, 9]. While laboratory tests are used to evaluate basic performance characteristics in standardized conditions, field-based methods are better suited to the demands of complex intermittent sports like tennis, since the variability in energy system, muscle group, and skill incorporated in their performance is difficult to replicate in the laboratory [6, 10]. Field tests seem to be more ecologically valid, and usually they allow the testing of large numbers of subjects simultaneously [11, 12]. However, the testing surroundings in the laboratory often show a higher standardization and reproducibility, and, therefore, coaches and scientists have to decide between a comparably higher validity and a lower but acceptable reliability (e.g., specific field tests), compared to a lower validity and a correspondingly higher reliability (e.g., laboratory tests) [6].

The development and application of physical performance tests in tennis should be integrated into a complex scientific approach, which can be used to construct a long-term sport-specific

A. Ferrauti (✉) · A. Ulbricht
Faculty of Sport Science, Department of Training Science, Ruhr-Universität Bochum,
Bochum, Germany
e-mail: alexander.ferrauti@rub.de;
alexander.ulbricht@rub.de

J. Fernandez-Fernandez
Faculty of Physical Activity and Sports Sciences,
University of León, León, Spain
e-mail: jaime.fernandez@unileon.es

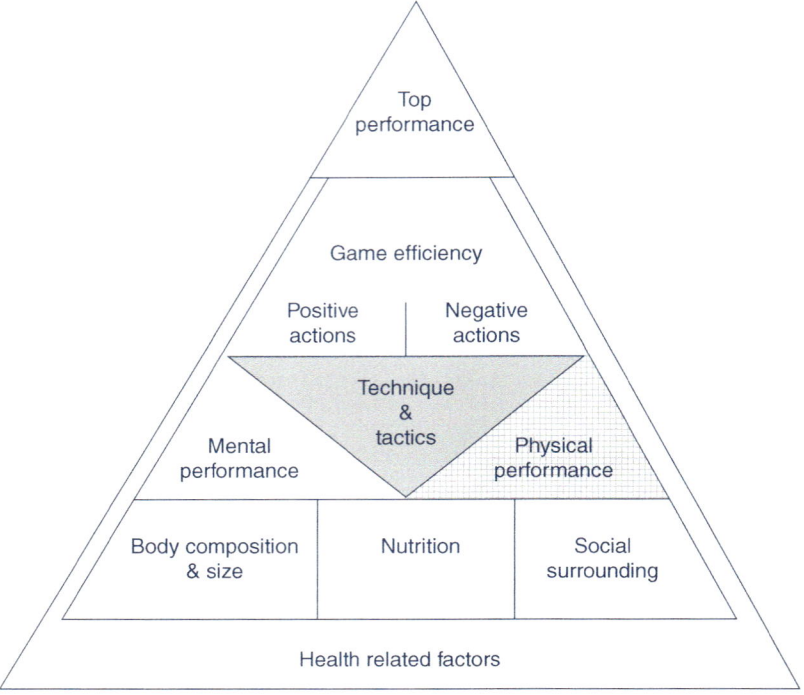

Fig. 12.1 Hierarchical model of performance limiting aspects in tennis [2]

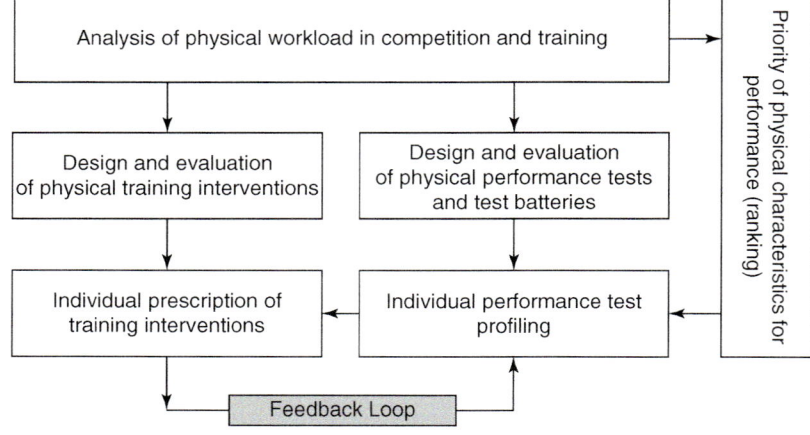

Fig. 12.2 Schematic representation of the sport specific training optimization model [3]

and individual training optimization model (Fig. 12.2). A major first step in this model is the knowledge of the workload profile during competition, which could be defined as the description of the athletes' external demands (i.e., running distances and directions) combined with physiological internal demands (i.e., heart rate (HR), sources of muscular energy). Thus, data obtained during tennis competition can be used as external criteria for the validation of tennis-specific tests and for the design of specific training interventions [1, 13–17].

Once a physical test or a test battery is standardized with representative data samples (e.g., different levels of performance, age, and sex groups), a statistical multiple regression approach can be applied using the national or international ranking position as external criteria to identify the most sensitive physical characteristics of performance [18–20]. This systematic approach is directly related to the specificity training principle, which states that to target these performance characteristics or components, and elicit specific adaptations, training must be focused on the desired elements of performance [4]. At the final stage of the schematic representation of the sport-specific training optimization model (Fig. 12.2), tennis players have to regularly complete a test battery, which allows an individual performance profiling and an individual prescription of training. This important last step has to include several pieces of information: the individual strengths and weaknesses compared to the (biological) age-related norm values, the individual anthropometrics and in youth players the estimated prospective body size, and the actual and prospective individual tactical playing style [7, 21]. Finally, this process has to be repeated in a regular feedback loop while adapting training interventions to obtain changes in physical performance (Fig. 12.2).

The present chapter first gives an overview about the different testing protocols related to tennis, mainly published by national tennis federations [7, 22, 23], trying to cover the tennis-specific physical qualities (Sect. 12.2). As selection criteria for the testing procedures, mainly tennis-specific field tests were initially selected, followed by intermittent sports-related tests, while laboratory tests are only complemented if necessary. Since some of the different physical qualities allow a less specific approach for physical testing (e.g., general endurance as well as strength and power), some basic tests are also included. The second part of the chapter includes some reference values for specific tests in different sex and age groups of elite youth tennis players in the German Tennis Federation and statistically analyzes the most important physical characteristics of top-ranked youth tennis players (Sect. 12.3). Finally, an individual approach for an evidence- and guideline-based individual training prescription is presented. This very important step from diagnostics to training prescription is a great challenge for coaches and yet not well prepared in literature (Sect. 12.4).

12.2 Physical Performance Testing in Tennis

12.2.1 Aerobic Endurance Tests

A look into the tennis literature concerning endurance testing provides an extreme variability of procedures, ranging from non-specific laboratory to more or less specific (semi-specific) and tennis-specific field tests [24]. Incremental exercise tests in the laboratory are generally accepted as a measure of aerobic power, and although they can be conducted on a variety of ergometers, a motorized treadmill is recommended for testing tennis players [24]. A wide range of test protocols with different characteristics (i.e., incremental stage durations and intensities, rest intervals, number of stages) are described elsewhere [25]. The determination of the $VO_{2\,max}$ and blood lactate-related thresholds are commonly used as general aerobic fitness markers of athletes [10, 26]. It is generally accepted that these unidirectional continuous running patterns are of limited validity compared to the tennis-specific demands. The constancy of laboratory conditions and the availability of motivation-independent submaximal markers (e.g. ventilatory or blood lactate thresholds) on the other hand give more reliable information compared to field tests.

As an interesting alternative, laboratory-based incremental treadmill test protocols can also be transferred to field conditions [26], allowing groups of players (e.g., all players of a national or regional squad) to run simultaneously (e.g., on a 400 m track divided into sections) and follow an acoustic signal. For practical reasons (e.g., club level; no technical or physiological measurements available), the Cooper 12-min run test could be useful [27], although tests of this category are characterized by a lower reproducibility because of tactical and motivational aspects [26]. Other protocols such as the Montréal track test or the Vameval test were originally devised for running on a track following acoustic signals, providing an indirect estimation of maximum oxygen uptake (VO_{2max}) [28, 29]. However, the lack of specificity of continuous running as mode of assessment is not reflective of the intermittent nature of tennis.

During the last two decades, several discontinuous incremental field tests based on shuttle runs have been developed, in order to improve the specificity of assessment modes. Their aim is to establish maximal aerobic levels under acoustically controlled conditions for distance covered and running velocity [30–33]. These tests are validated by VO_2 measurements, and the estimated VO_{2max} can be predicted by gender- and age-related equations. Since tests include accelerations, decelerations, and changes of direction, they can be categorized as semi-specific. The 20-m multistage shuttle test (MSST) (i.e., "multistage fitness test," "beep test," or Léger test) consists of 20-m shuttle runs performed at increasing speeds, until exhaustion [30, 31], and has become a standard field test, being part of the regular test battery of different national tennis federations (United States Tennis Association (USTA), Tennis Australia) [22, 34]. However, based on the demands of intermittent sports [35], the relevance of these tests has been questioned, leading to the development of more valid and reliable sport-specific tests like the Yo-Yo intermittent recovery (IR) and the 30–15 intermittent fitness tests (30–15IFT) [32, 33]. The Yo-Yo IR tests consist of 2 × 20-m shuttle runs at increasing speeds, interspersed with a 10-s period of active recovery (controlled by audio signals). Level 1 (Yo-Yo IR1) starts at a lower speed, with increases in speed being more moderate than for level 2 (Yo-Yo IR2) test (IR1, 10 km/h; IR2, 13 km/h). In the 30–15IFT [33], subjects run 40-m shuttles for 30 s at a given velocity interspersed with 15 s of active recovery; running velocity for the work bouts is progressively increased with each run (0.5 km/h).

In tennis, the use of these semi-specific field tests (MSST, Yo-YoIR, 30–15IFT) seems to be a good recommendation although it has to be pointed out that in all presented tests, the respective running distances, movement characteristics, and muscle groups involved still offer considerable differences compared to the tennis-specific workload profile. To the best of our knowledge, there is almost no scientific information regarding their use in tennis-specific settings and just some normative values for the MSST offered from national tennis federations [22, 34]. To close the remaining gap, tennis researchers endeavor to develop more specific protocols (Figs. 12.3 and 12.4), mainly based on the use of the tennis court dimensions and combining specific footwork and strokes. In this regard, different protocols have been published with an acceptable accuracy under standardized conditions [6, 10, 36–41]. Weber and Hollmann [38] were the first authors describing an incremental on-court exercise test for assessing aerobic power in tennis players. The standardization of the test was conducted using a ball-feeding machine projecting balls alternatively to the right and the left corners of the baseline, adjusting the intensity controlling the ball frequency [38]. Following this approach, several similar test protocols were developed, all of them using a ball-feeding machine [36, 37, 40–42] (Fig. 12.3).

To further enhance reproducibility and practicability (i.e., no expensive equipment required),

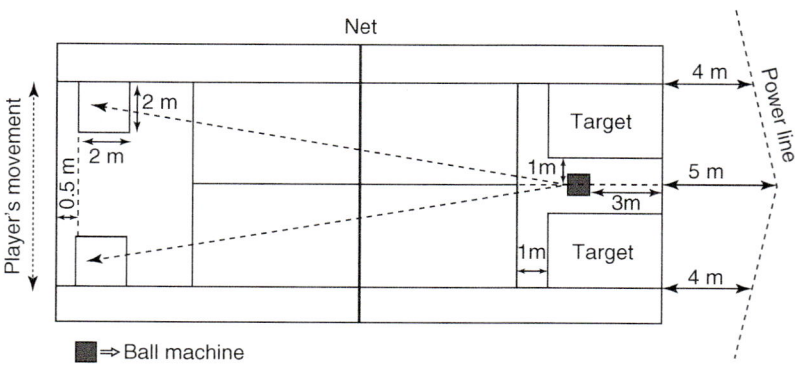

Fig. 12.3 Schematic setting for a tennis-specific endurance field test [36–38]

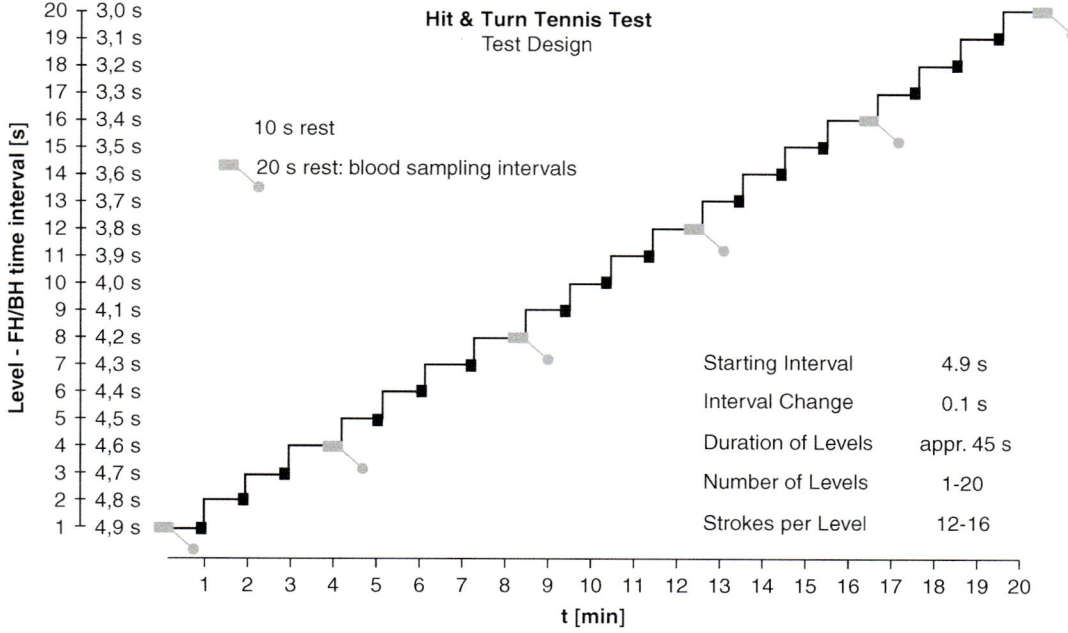

Fig. 12.4 Progressive test design with beep time intervals [6]

two tests have been published during the last decade (e.g., the Girard Test and the Hit & Turn Tennis Test from Ferrauti et al.) [6, 10, 43]. These protocols follow an incremental protocol to exhaustion, combining tennis footwork and stroke simulation with movement velocities and directions controlled by visual or acoustic feedback [6, 10]. Test stages are of 40–50 s in duration and interspersed by 10–20 s of rest (Fig. 12.4), with some differences in the protocols. In the Girard Test, running direction, movement technique, and stroke position are more variable and partly uncertain than during the Hit & Turn test. This ensures a closer approach to real tennis but complicates test preparation and execution. In both cases it should be emphasized that stroke quality is far removed from reality and individual differences exist. This has to be considered, since it was shown that the upper limb work contributes considerably to the overall energetic demand in tennis [44]. Regarding the practical use of these tests, the Hit & Turn test already offers age- and sex-related normative values (see Tables 12.1 and 12.2) [7].

12.2.2 Anaerobic Endurance Tests

Since the direct measurement of the anaerobic pathway is difficult, several indirect methods of measuring anaerobic ATP turnover have been developed under laboratory conditions [3]. Because of its practicability, in most sports, peak power output is determined during the 30-s Wingate test [45]. Regarding its use in tennis, the validity of a cycling test should be questioned [46]. The use of power output measurements with non-motorized treadmills could be a future option for intermittent sports [47] including single or multiple sprint protocols [48].

Classical anaerobic field tests include the step-running test or the measure of maximal lactate production during one all-out sprint over an established distance (e.g., 80, 100, or 200 m) [49, 50]. However, a more specific approach for anaerobic testing consists in the measurement of repeated sprint ability (RSA) [51–53]. RSA is usually determined by using running protocols with several repeated short sprints (e.g., 6–10 × 4–6 s or 20–40 m) interspersed with brief

Table 12.1 Norm values (mean and SD) for physical qualities in male and female junior tennis players [7]

			Chronological age					Biological age (years from peak height velocity)				
Girls	**Measurements**		Under 12 (n = 194)	Under 14 (n = 485)	Under 16 (n = 300)	Under 18 (n = 148)		−1.5 to 0 yrs (n = 178)	0–1.5 yrs (n = 385)	1.5–3 yrs (n = 347)	3–4.5 yrs (n = 197)	
Anthropometry	PHV	[years]	−0.6 ± 0.6	0.9 ± 0.7	2.4 ± 0.5	3.8 ± 0.5		−0.6 ± 0.4	0.7 ± 0.4	2.1 ± 0.4	3.6 ± 0.4	
	Height	[cm]	150.3 ± 7.2	160.6 ± 7.0	167.8 ± 6.2	171.5 ± 6.4		148.9 ± 4.6	159.3 ± 4.7	166.9 ± 5.1	172.5 ± 5.9	
	Weight	[kg]	39.6 ± 6.5	48.6 ± 7.5	58.3 ± 6.6	64.2 ± 6.2		37.9 ± 4.4	47.4 ± 5.6	56.8 ± 5.3	64.5 ± 5.9	
	BMI	[kg/m²]	17.4 ± 1.8	18.8 ± 1.9	20.6 ± 2.1	21.8 ± 1.6		17.1 ± 1.6	18.6 ± 1.7	20.4 ± 1.7	21.7 ± 1.5	
Strength and power	Grip strength[a]	[kg]	21.8 ± 4.5	27.8 ± 5.3	33.7 ± 4.7	37.1 ± 6.4		20.9 ± 3.6	27.0 ± 4.4	33.1 ± 4.5	36.8 ± 5.9	
	CMJ	[cm]	28.1 ± 4.5	29.7 ± 3.6	31.6 ± 3.7	32.0 ± 4.0		28.4 ± 4.0	29.4 ± 3.6	30.9 ± 3.8	32.1 ± 3.9	
	Medicine ball[b]	[cm]	511.5 ± 94.7	620.5 ± 101.8	735.4 ± 113.7	829.3 ± 129.0		503.0 ± 87.1	607.2 ± 91.3	709.1 ± 105.1	828.6 ± 117.7	
	Service velocity	[km/h]	112.8 ± 12.3	129.8 ± 12.0	144.2 ± 12.2	153.5 ± 8.5		112.2 ± 11.0	128.0 ± 11.1	140.8 ± 11.6	153.5 ± 8.6	
Speed and agility	10 m	[s]	2.04 ± 0.09	1.98 ± 0.10	1.94 ± 0.09	1.93 ± 0.10		2.02 ± 0.12	2.00 ± 0.09	1.95 ± 0.10	1.93 ± 0.09	
	20 m	[s]	3.62 ± 0.14	3.49 ± 0.14	3.40 ± 0.12	3.37 ± 0.15		3.60 ± 0.16	3.52 ± 0.14	3.42 ± 0.13	3.37 ± 0.13	
	Shuttle sprint FH	[s]	3.05 ± 0.14	2.95 ± 0.14	2.86 ± 0.15	2.83 ± 0.14		3.04 ± 0.13	2.95 ± 0.13	2.89 ± 0.15	2.82 ± 0.16	
	Shuttle sprint BH	[s]	3.16 ± 0.14	3.08 ± 0.14	3.01 ± 0.14	2.97 ± 0.12		3.16 ± 0.15	3.07 ± 0.14	3.04 ± 0.15	2.98 ± 0.13	
Endurance	Hit & Turn test	[level]	11.7 ± 2.1	13.1 ± 1.9	14.2 ± 1.9	14.7 ± 1.9		11.9 ± 2.2	13.0 ± 2.0	13.8 ± 1.8	14.8 ± 1.8	
Boys	**Measurements**		Under 12 (n = 281)	Under 14 (n = 699)	Under 16 (n = 482)	Under 18 (n = 289)		−3.0 to −1.5 yrs (n = 381)	−1.5 to 0 yrs (n = 515)	0–1.5 yrs (n = 354)	1.5–3 yrs (n = 341)	
Anthropometry	PHV	[years]	−2.3 ± 0.5	−0.9 ± 0.8	1.1 ± 0.8	2.8 ± 0.7		−2.1 ± 0.4	−0.9 ± 0.4	0.7 ± 0.4	2.2 ± 0.5	
	Height	[cm]	149.7 ± 7.0	160.8 ± 8.8	175.2 ± 7.9	181.8 ± 5.7		150.0 ± 5.2	161.3 ± 5.6	173.8 ± 5.3	180.8 ± 5.4	
	Weight	[kg]	38.9 ± 5.4	47.3 ± 8.3	61.9 ± 9.1	72.1 ± 7.5		38.6 ± 4.2	47.4 ± 5.3	59.9 ± 6.3	69.7 ± 6.4	
	BMI	[kg/m²]	17.3 ± 1.5	18.1 ± 1.8	20.1 ± 1.8	21.8 ± 1.7		17.2 ± 1.4	18.2 ± 1.5	19.8 ± 1.7	21.3 ± 1.7	
Strength and power	Grip strength[a]	[kg]	22.4 ± 4.0	28.7 ± 6.7	41.1 ± 8.9	50.1 ± 7.2		22.7 ± 3.8	28.7 ± 5.2	38.6 ± 6.9	48.4 ± 7.0	
	CMJ	[cm]	28.9 ± 4.1	31.2 ± 4.1	36.3 ± 4.5	40.2 ± 4.2		29.3 ± 3.9	31.3 ± 4.2	35.2 ± 4.5	39.0 ± 4.1	
	Medicine ball[b]	[cm]	525.4 ± 84.1	649.0 ± 124.7	893.9 ± 164.1	1087.4 ± 165.6		530.6 ± 84.6	655.5 ± 99.1	851.0 ± 129.4	1027.4 ± 157.4	
	Service velocity	[km/h]	121.3 ± 10.5	138.8 ± 12.9	162.5 ± 13.1	178.0 ± 10.8		123.7 ± 10.5	139.6 ± 10.8	158.5 ± 11.0	174.1 ± 10.2	

Speed and agility	10 m	[s]	2.04 ± 0.10	1.96 ± 0.12	1.85 ± 0.10	1.77 ± 0.08	2.02 ± 0.14	1.96 ± 0.09	1.88 ± 0.09	1.79 ± 0.08
	20 m	[s]	3.60 ± 0.16	3.46 ± 0.16	3.24 ± 0.16	3.08 ± 0.12	3.57 ± 0.16	3.46 ± 0.16	3.29 ± 0.16	3.12 ± 0.12
	Shuttle sprint FH	[s]	3.00 ± 0.15	2.89 ± 0.14	2.72 ± 0.14	2.63 ± 0.11	2.98 ± 0.14	2.87 ± 0.13	2.74 ± 0.15	2.65 ± 0.11
	Shuttle sprint BH	[s]	3.13 ± 0.15	3.01 ± 0.15	2.88 ± 0.15	2.78 ± 0.12	3.09 ± 0.16	3.00 ± 0.15	2.89 ± 0.15	2.81 ± 0.12
Endurance	Hit & Turn test	[level]	12.5 ± 2.0	14.5 ± 2.0	16.6 ± 1.9	17.9 ± 1.7	13.1 ± 2.2	14.5 ± 2.0	16.3 ± 1.9	17.6 ± 1.8

BH backhand, *CMJ* countermovement jump, *FH* forehand, *PHV* years to/from peak height velocity, *U12–U18* under 12 to under 18, *yrs* years

[a]Dominant hand
[b]Overhead medicine ball throw

Table 12.2 Percentile table for male elite junior tennis players aged 15.0–15.5 years old ($n = 54$)

		Anthropometry			Strength					Speed and jumping				Tennis-specific sprint		Upper-body power			Serve velocity	Endurance
					Grip strength						Linear sprint					Medicine ball throw				Hit & Turn test
		Height [cm]	BM [kg]	BMI [kg/m²]	dh [kg]	ndh [kg]	Push-ups [n]	Sit-ups [n]	CMJ [cm]		10 m [s]	20 m [s]	FH [s]	BH [s]		OH [cm]	FH [cm]	BH [cm]	[km/h]	level max
Mean ± SD		177.4 ± 6.5	65.5 ± 7.3	20.8 ± 1.7	42.8 ± 8.3	37.6 ± 7.8	24.2 ± 15.4	31.4 ± 14.7	37.5 ± 3.6		1.84 ± 0.07	3.19 ± 0.13	2.72 ± 0.12	2.88 ± 0.13		924.4 ± 126.3	1227.9 ± 127.3	1169.9 ± 132.1	168.5 ± 9.44	17.0 ± 1.5
Percentiles	10	168.4	53.9	18.6	31	27	14	13	33.5		1.94	3.35	2.88	3.05		782	1050	963	155.5	15.0
	20	171.3	61.0	19.0	35	29	16	19	34.6		1.90	3.31	2.82	3.01		822	1112	1080	159.0	15.9
	30	172.9	63.2	19.8	38	33	18	23	35.0		1.88	3.28	2.79	2.95		856	1166	1107	163.7	16.0
	40	175.6	63.9	20.4	40	36	21	26	35.7		1.86	3.24	2.75	2.92		897	1214	1120	168.4	16.4
	50	177.5	65.5	21.0	42	38	22	31	36.9		1.85	3.22	2.72	2.88		905	1220	1170	169.3	17.0
	60	179.0	67.0	21.3	45	39	24	36	38.6		1.84	3.15	2.69	2.85		944	1250	1194	170.6	17.2
	70	181.1	68.9	21.6	47	41	25	41	39.1		1.79	3.12	2.65	2.80		980	1280	1227	172.6	17.8
	80	184.0	70.9	21.9	52	45	28	48	40.0		1.76	3.09	2.60	2.77		1048	1328	1319	177.7	18.1
	90	185.4	74.7	23.2	54	49	30	50	43.3		1.72	3.01	2.57	2.70		1099	1399	1360	181.6	19.0

dh dominant hand, *ndh* non-dominant hand, *BM* body mass, *BMI* body mass index, *CMJ* counter movement jump, *FH* forehand, *BH* backhand

recovery periods (e.g., 10–30 s) [35, 52]. Since multiple metabolic and neuromuscular factors (i.e., PCr availability, anaerobic glycolytic flow) are responsible for RSA, a clear classification of RSA as an anaerobic field test is questioned [52]. Assessments of RSA generally provide two performance indices: (a) the overall test performance (e.g., total sprint time or work [s], mean sprint time [s], best sprint time [s]) and (b) percentage decrement scores [35]. Some protocols calculate a fatigue index (i.e., change from the first to the last or from the best to the worst sprint); however, the percentage decrement score (i.e., [[mean sprint time/best sprint time] × 100] − 100) is a more valid and reliable measure of fatigue for RSA [51].

In tennis, the use of RSA tests is scarce, with just some information about different protocols and normative values. Tennis Australia recommend 10 × 20 m with 20 s rest, with two performance scores: the real accumulated sprint time in seconds and the percent decrement score [34]. Fernandez-Fernandez et al. [54] conducted a more tennis-specific test, including 10 × ~20-m shuttle sprints, with mean time and percent decrement as the main performance measures.

Some aspects should be highlighted about RSA testing, as athletes usually develop pacing strategies throughout the test and therefore, potentially do not exert a maximal effort [11]. Moreover, the performance score selection seems to be difficult, with the total accumulated sprint time being more reliable than the decrement scores [55]. Since the total accumulated sprint time is almost perfectly correlated with the best sprint time [56], a simple 20 m sprint may be enough, being more practical and less demanding for the athletes. More research is needed to clarify this issue.

12.2.3 Strength and Power Tests

The modern game of tennis has evolved to a current fast-paced, explosive sport based on strength and power [1, 57, 58]. Maximal strength is defined as the result of force-producing muscles performing maximally, either in isometric or dynamic patterns during a single voluntary effort of a defined task [59]. Power production is the product of force and velocity and is probably the most important factor in determining success in many sports. Thus, the "ability to generate force (strength)" is an integral part of power production and therefore may be a key component in determining athletic success [60]. Moreover, strength and power can represent specific or independent qualities of neuromuscular performance and therefore can be assessed and trained independently [61].

Dynamic strength can be assessed in a variety of ways using an assortment of testing equipment (i.e., free weights or fixed resistance machines). Traditionally, performance-related changes in maximal voluntary dynamic strength capabilities have been assessed using one-repetition maximum (1RM, the maximal amount of weight that can be lifted in one repetition) test protocols. The use of free weights is usually the most accurate way in determining functional strength in a sport-specific context [62], as the athlete has a greater freedom of movement. The rationale for maximal tests is that an increase in maximal strength is usually connected with an improvement in relative strength and therefore with improvement of power abilities [50]. For example, in female tennis players, ball velocities of the serve and forehand and backhand strokes have been moderately correlated to 1RM military press, but not to bench press performance [20]. This relationship between maximal strength and performance is also supported by jump test results, as well as sprint times over 10–30 m in other intermittent sports [11, 62, 63]. However, such procedures may not be easy to control, as athletes need to be proficient in the movement patterns and able to handle maximal loads. Moreover, determining 1RM values for large groups is very time-consuming and has been suggested to expose those being tested to increased injury risk. Other measures such as the 3RM, 5RM, 10RM, and the maximum number of repetitions that can be performed at a fixed resistance can also be determined, although it is important to take into account the body mass or using different formulas depending on the sport (i.e., Wilks formula) [64].

Thus, the use of single set tests in which 1RM values are predicted based on the number of repetitions performed with a submaximal weight has been recommended [65]. In tennis, the use of these measurements is scarce, with just some information about different protocols as well as normative values extracted from some national tennis federations [7, 34].

In tennis, more field-based power-related measurements should be included in the testing procedures, taking into account that power is generally tested using isoinertial protocols with resistance loads [66]. Squat jumps and countermovement jumps are commonly used for the lower body, while bench throws or bench pulls, with varying inertial loads, are used for the upper body [60]. Assessments typically employ apparatuses such as a Smith machine, with power encoders used to quantify mechanical power output (in Newtons). The load at which peak power output is achieved (P_{max}) has been used as a performance measure in different intermittent sports, such as rugby or American football [66], highlighting the need of tennis-specific research on this topic.

A typical test which is used in most of the scientific research is the vertical jump (i.e., countermovement jump (CMJ)). The rationale of its use is based on the biomechanical similarities to various acceleration- and game-related dynamic movements, and that is a common action in several sports [58]. Furthermore, the strong correlations observed between sprint times (e.g., 10- and 20-m sprints) and vertical jumps (e.g., power during CMJ and drop jumps) in previous research [20, 67] underline the importance of muscle strength and power in the lower extremities to produce explosive actions in tennis players. In terms of practicability, vertical jumps are usually conducted in the field using contact mats to obtain basic measurements like contact and flying times. Regarding the CMJ, its relationship with tennis-specific performance (i.e., serve velocity, ground strokes) has been shown to be moderate [22], if not insignificant [68], questioning if vertical jump performance reflects lower limb activity during tennis stroke production.

Regarding upper-body power, medicine ball tests (i.e., overhead throw) seem to be useful for tennis players, as they show high external validity, because they involve the coordination of body segments (i.e., kinetic chain) and allow generation, summation, transfer, and regulation of forces from the lower body to the upper body, which is similar to tennis strokes [68]. Moreover, previous research showed significant correlations between ball toss and strength (i.e., isokinetic trunk rotation; individual values of velocity at 30% of 1RM bench press) [69, 70], as well as serve velocity [71], suggesting that these tests are fundamental indicators of whole-body explosive power regardless of throwing technique [70]. Thus, the use of vertical jump tests and medicine ball throws has been part of the regular testing of tennis players in different national tennis associations [7, 34] (Tables 12.1 and 12.2).

Since sport-specific technical skills are predominant factors (e.g., stroke skills) in tennis, the most appropriate tests seem to be those measuring serve and groundstrokes velocities [72]. In this regard the tennis serve velocity test appears to show high external validity in terms of its relationship with tennis functional performance, as it is a basic action relying on multiple body segments to produce power through properly timed rotations and complex coordinated muscular activations [67]. Moreover, it has been considered the most stable and predictable measure of on-court tennis performance [56], with recent data showing medium to large correlations with individual rankings in male and female players (i.e., from U14 to U18) [7, 71]. Previous research also showed reliable and valid tests aiming to assess performance of groundstrokes in low- to intermediate-level tennis players [70]. Figure 12.5 shows the representation of a serve performance test [72–74]. Serve velocity is measured with a radar gun positioned behind the server. The highest speed recorded is used for analysis [72, 73]. Serve accuracy is determined by counting the number of times the ball landed within the designated target perimeter. Participants serve from the deuce court and are instructed to "serve first serves flat and down the T" (center line). Shots landing within target areas are ranked according

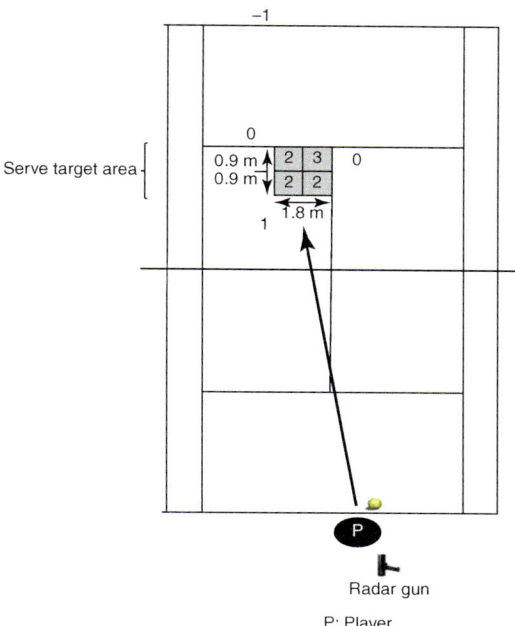

Fig. 12.5 A schematic representation of the serve performance test (right handed players) and an example for target area dimensions

to a 3, 2, 1, scoring system. Balls landing outside the perimeter of the target areas (i.e., errors) received a score of 0. A total score is recorded for each trial.

12.2.4 Speed and Agility Tests

In tennis, speed comprises the ability to move at high velocity in a variety of directions, and often not in a straight line. Players need to be exceptional movers in a linear direction (i.e., acceleration) but also laterally and multidirectionally. Speed has been defined as the rate of change of distance with respect to time, whereas acceleration is the rate of change in speed with respect to time [59]. Due to the constant changes of direction, players are not able to achieve maximal running speeds (i.e., obtained between 30 and 60 m in a straight-line sprint). Therefore, acceleration and deceleration seem to be fundamental for tennis players.

Because of its good reproducibility, the 20 m sprint test, with splits at 5 and 10 m, is used as a general measure of linear acceleration and speed [59]. In tennis, although the distances of 5 and 10 m are most specific to those covered in any one effort during a match, the evaluation of speed over 20 m can be also informative [34] (Tables 12.1 and 12.2). These tests are usually included in the regular testing of national federations [7, 34], using electronic timing gates, as they offer higher degrees of accuracy and reliability than stopwatch-recorded times.

Besides linear acceleration tests, several agility tests are recommended in literature. "Agility" is defined as a rapid whole-body movement with change of velocity or direction in response to a stimulus [75]. Previous research showed that straight-line sprinting and change of direction tests typically show a limited statistical relationship [76], suggesting that acceleration, maximum speed, and change of direction are distinct and partly separate abilities [75]. A wide variety of tests that measure change of direction ability is employed in different sports and could be used in tennis, like the "5–0–5 test," in which the player turns once to sprint 5 m back to the start line, or the "Illinois agility test," which features multiple slalom cuts through cones and 180° turns [75, 77]. Both tests show positive correlations with acceleration measurements [77]. Due to the complexity of tennis in terms of movement, there are just a few studies analyzing speed and agility components in tennis players. Change of direction tests have been modified to incorporate a simple reaction component to the movement task, so that the movement is executed in response to an external cue. The time recorded by the athlete on tests of this type represents a combination of both reaction time and the time taken to complete the movement task [74]. Cooke et al. [78] designed a test using an electronic timing system with programmable light stimuli in which the athlete had to move as quickly as possible from the baseline to three different gates in reaction to light signals (Fig. 12.6). A contact mat acted as a switch turning on the light on a random gate. On reaching the gate, the player was instructed to step over a line marker placed 30 cm beyond the gate and then return to the contact mat and repeat for a total of three gates. Ulbricht et al. [7]

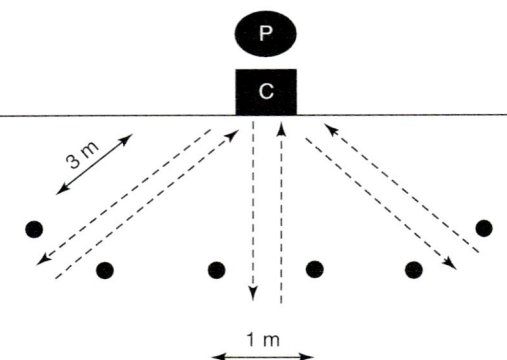

Fig. 12.6 Planned and reactive agility test setup [78]. Light cells, P: player; C: contact mat

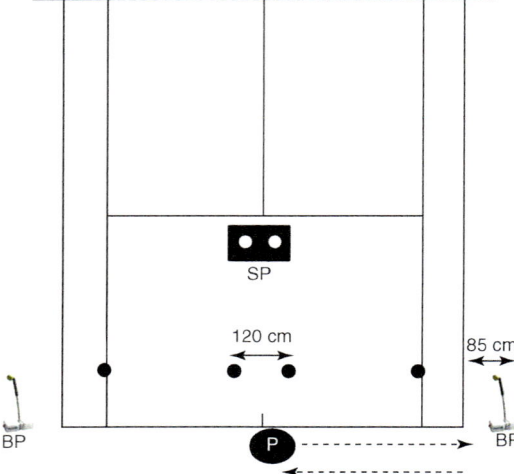

Fig. 12.7 Tennis specific sprint test [7]. Light cells; P: player; SP: signal panel; BP: ball pendulum

designed a tennis-specific sprint test (Fig. 12.7) with the use of a twofold signal panel with two light-emitting diodes (right-left). The player stands with his racket in a frontal position in the middle of the baseline. By activating one diode of the signal panel, the time is initiated, and players turn and run in a straight line to the prescribed corner, perform a stroke simulation against a ball pendulum, and return to the initial position. Each player performs two maximal repetitions to each side, interspersed with 90-s rest of passive recovery, and the fastest time (total time and split times for direction change in the forehand and backhand corners) achieved is recorded [7].

12.2.5 Musculoskeletal Tests

General musculoskeletal assessment protocols comprise static measurements and clinical examinations of joint integrity (e.g., hip and shoulder), ROM (e.g., passive assessment), together with muscular strength patterns [79]. These assessments are widespread practice with the dual goal of injury prevention and performance enhancement. In general, tests of ROM and muscle flexibility are recommended to identify players at risk of muscle strain injury [79]. Since injuries in tennis can involve all the areas of the body, the application and use of a comprehensive musculoskeletal examination using a series of tests throughout the entire body are recommended [15, 80]. Among the most used testing protocols, we can find shoulder and hip ROMs, aiming to measure passive glenohumeral rotation as well as passive hip extension and passive hip internal/external rotation. An inclinometer (e.g., ISOMED, Portland, Oregon) with a telescopic arm is normally used as the key measure for all ROMs, with methods well described in previous literature [81–83]. Although results can be different depending on the measures, population analyzed, level of play, or history of pain, specific alterations in the different joints analyzed can be identified. The USTA Sport Science Committee developed a test battery ("high-performance profile") which is recommended for use by competitive players [84], comprising ten tests, which have been shown to be valid and reliable in athletes (i.e., shoulder internal and external range of motion at 90° abduction, straight leg raise test) [85–88] (Fig. 12.8).

In recent years, movement-based protocols have become more popular, together with the use of standard musculoskeletal assessments. The Functional Movement Screen (FMS) is a relatively new tool that attempts to address multiple movement factors, with the goal of predicting general risk of musculoskeletal conditions and injuries [89, 90]. The FMS consists of seven fundamental movement component tests (i.e., deep squat, in-line lunge, hurdle step) that are scored on a scale of 0–3, with the sum creating a composite score ranging from 0 to 21 points. Based on recent research

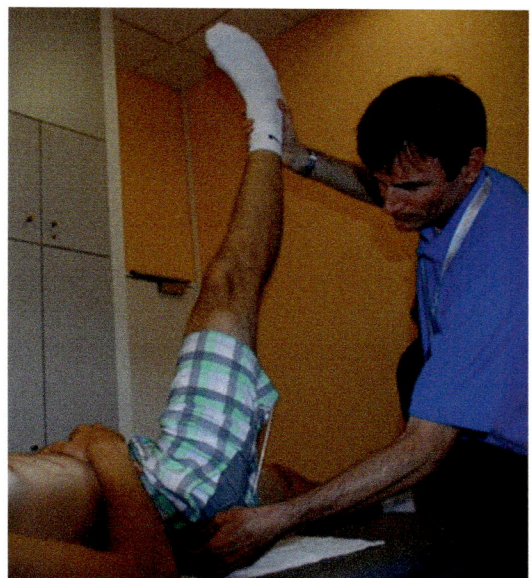

Fig. 12.8 Example of the straight leg raise test (photo courtesy of Todd S. Ellenbecker)

[91–93], FMS is found to show good reliability and appears to be a valid method to detect deficits in gross movement quality and identify movement asymmetries. However, to date, FMS normative values are only related to active populations or high school athletes [94]. Results suggest that the FMS may be useful for recognizing deficiency in certain movements. However, this data suggests that it should not be used for overall prediction of injury in high school athletes throughout the course of a season. This could help coaches interpret the raw data collected during testing, and, therefore, future research is recommended to further refine and validate the FMT as a screening tool that can be used in multiple sporting settings, including tennis.

12.3 Sex- and Age-Related Fitness Characteristics and Their Impact on Tennis Performance

Norm values and percentile tables for junior tennis players which have been generated and used to assess a given performance are commonly based on chronological age [95, 96]. However, since there is a large variation in physical, emotional, and cognitive development of athletes in adolescence (i.e., fundamental changes in biological characteristics especially at the age of 12–15 years) [97], it seems that chronological age is not the only indicator on which to base athletes training programs or evaluate physical performance. A practical approach to design optimal individual training programs which are related to certain periods of trainability during the process of maturation is the use of an athletes' peak height velocity (PHV) as a reference point [98]. The PHV is the fastest rate of growth during the adolescent growth spurt and can be a useful reference point providing valuable information about an individual's stage of maturation, enhancing the efficiency of development training, competition, and recovery programs [99]. Established profiles just based on the chronological age do not consider the individual stage of maturation, thus obviously representing a weakness in the testing procedures. Table 12.1 presents reference values for boys and girls of different age groups from the "German Physical Condition Tennis Test," a biannual nationwide physical testing established in 2009 [7]. Based on the results, it is possible to create percentile tables (examples shown in Table 12.2 for male tennis players) that take chronological and biological age in consideration and enable the identification of weaknesses in different parameters and allow to design efficient physical training programs.

Knowledge about the impact of fitness characteristics on tennis performance is important for talent detection but also to define the priority of training goals during the individual physical training prescription (Fig. 12.1). One statistical approach for that is to test how close different physical characteristics are related to the players' competitive level (i.e., national or international ranking lists). The huge database including male and female junior players (aged 11–16 years), all nationally ranked in the German Tennis Federation, is perfectly designed for that statistical correlation (Table 12.3) [18].

The results show that the serve velocity ($r = -0.43$ to 0.64 for females [♀]; $r = -0.33$ to

Table 12.3 Correlation coefficients between anthropometric and fitness characteristics and the ranking position in males and females of different age groups (Correlation coefficients >0.3 are highlighted in red)

		Male players			Female players		
		U12	U14	U16	U12	U14	U16
		n = 122	n = 254	n = 165	n = 82	n = 177	n = 97
Chronological age (years)	r	−0.17	−0.40	−0.42	−0.29	−0.34	−0.28
	P	0.06	0.00	0.00	0.00	0.00	0.01
APHV	r	−0.05	−0.30	−0.33	−0.19	−0.29	−0.31
	P	0.59	0.00	0.00	0.10	0.00	0.00
Height (cm)	r	−0.06	−0.29	−0.27	−0.17	−0.18	−0.15
	P	0.53	0.00	0.00	0.13	0.01	0.15
Weight (kg)	r	−0.07	−0.23	−0.34	−0.17	−0.17	−0.30
	P	0.44	0.00	0.00	0.13	0.03	0.00
Grip strength dh (kg)	r	−0.23	−0.29	−0.38	−0.21	−0.19	−0.30
	P	0.02	0.00	0.00	0.06	0.01	0.00
CMJ (cm)	r	0.02	−0.17	−0.01	0.00	0.01	0.16
	P	0.86	0.01	0.87	0.98	0.87	0.13
10-m sprint (s)	r	0.14	0.23	0.13	−0.06	0.15	−0.06
	P	0.13	0.00	0.12	0.58	0.05	0.56
20-m sprint (s)	r	0.16	0.31	0.23	−0.05	0.19	0.00
	P	0.08	0.00	0.00	0.67	0.01	0.97
TSS forehand (s)	r	0.00	0.17	0.16	0.01	0.16	−0.10
	P	1.00	0.01	0.04	0.91	0.03	0.37
TSS backhand (s)	r	0.18	0.26	0.21	0.14	0.28	0.12
	P	0.04	0.00	0.01	0.21	0.00	0.24
MBT over-head (cm)	r	−0.17	−0.33	−0.37	−0.26	−0.35	−0.36
	P	0.07	0.00	0.00	0.02	0.00	0.00
MBT forehand (cm)	r	−0.20	−0.42	−0.43	−0.15	−0.47	−0.38
	P	0.03	0.00	0.00	0.20	0.00	0.00
MBT backhand (cm)	r	−0.24	−0.40	−0.45	−0.17	−0.49	−0.45
	P	0.01	0.00	0.00	0.13	0.00	0.00
Serve velocity (km/h)	r	−0.33	−0.48	−0.49	−0.43	−0.61	−0.64
	P	0.00	0.00	0.00	0.00	0.00	0.00
Hit and turn test (level)	r	−0.19	−0.39	−0.30	0.04	−0.20	−0.46
	P	0.04	0.00	0.00	0.71	0.01	0.00

APHV estimated age at peak height velocity, *BMI* body mass index, *CMJ* counter movement jump, *TSS* tennis-specific sprint test, *MBT* medicine ball throws, *dh* dominant hand

0.49 for males [♂]) and the upper-body power (e.g., medicine ball throw $r = -0.26$ to -0.49 ♀; $r = -0.20$ to -0.49 ♂) are significantly and closely correlated with the tennis ranking in both female and male tennis players compared to other physical performance characteristics. On a second level, also significantly correlated, we found the specific endurance performance (Hit & Turn Tennis Test), while speed, agility, and jumping performance was of less importance (Table 12.3). These results underline the importance of physical fitness but also show that in elite junior players fitness is not the most important factor that leads to a successful tennis player (Fig. 12.1). According to our findings, upper-body strength/power (i.e., MBT and serve velocity) and tennis-specific endurance (i.e., Hit & Turn Tennis Test) seem to be important physical components in adolescent tennis players. Therefore, we would recommend using these tests in the framework of physical testing and talent identification programs. A stronger focus should be given to training interventions aimed at increasing upper-body power and stroke velocity (Fig. 12.11).

12.4 Evidence- and Guideline-Based Individual Training Prescription

Regular fitness testing provides a useful frame for the development of an individualized database and a more efficient training prescription. Results obtained from sex- and age-related norm values will give coaches and physical trainers an individual follow-up and the possibility to observe the development of physical qualities. An individual report (including the percentile rank relative to the chronological and biological age) should be provided for each player and discussed with their coaching staff and parents. In addition to this information, specific individualized training program recommendations have to be designed. The following two case studies will illustrate that procedure.

Player A (Fig. 12.9) is a right-handed male player at age 15.2 years old; he passed his age at peak height velocity at 13.5 years (average for males is 13.8 years). Body height and body mass as well as the body mass index clearly show that this player belongs to the heavier and taller boys and, thus, to the higher percentiles compared to the biological and chronological norm values. Interestingly, there is a significant body mass increase in the last 2 years, from 48.5 to 72.4 kg, which leads to an increase of the body mass index (BMI) from 18.0 to 22.0. Regarding the physical performance, the results clearly show very high scores in most of the power as well as the speed and jumping categories. We assume that the increase in body mass is mainly induced by an increase in muscle mass, which is illustrated by a continuous increase in the strength and power qualities analyzed (i.e., grip strength and medicine ball throws) and, finally, in the transfer of dynamic power into tennis-specific skill performance, with an increase in the serve velocity from 140 to 180 km/h in the last 2 years.

Analyzing speed and jumping performance, results show that player A has a really good base for tennis, reaching the highest percentile in all jumping tests as well as in the linear sprint test (20 m). However, the transfer of speed qualities into tennis-specific movements seems to be not perfectly adjusted, with the player showing average percentiles in agility sprint tests (e.g., 50–60), especially when running to the forehand corner. It is reasonable to assume that specific running velocity (i.e., short runs with changes of direction) is one of the determining factors in tennis performance.

Finally, in the endurance performance, player A shows a major weakness compared with his peers, with his individually results categorized in the lower third of his reference group. It can be speculated that the player's body composition (relatively high body weight and muscle mass) and muscle fiber profile (perhaps a huge amount of fast twitch fibers) has a negative impact on endurance capacity. In this regard, as a training recommendation, the focus will be on endurance training, especially during the preseason cycle, with 3–4-week training blocks. These training blocks might include a combination of high-intensity and repeated sprint-based training as it has been shown that this might be an appropriate tool to optimize the development of cardiorespiratory fitness in competitive tennis players. A positive effect on the change of direction would also be expected, as during acceleration and deceleration movements, the involvement of specific muscles (e.g., biceps femoris, rectus femoris, hip adductors, iliopsoas) could lead players to positive changes in specific coordination and agility.

Player B is a male player aged 13.1 years old (Fig. 12.10). However, the age of peak height velocity for player B was estimated to be at an age of 15.3 years. This means that, from a biological point view, player B is almost 2 years behind his peers (player A). The anthropometric data show that player B belongs to the smallest and lightest percentile of his chronological age group, which means he is a "late" mature compared with his peers. There are substantial differences between percentiles based on chronological or biological age (Tables 12.1). For example, while player B shows poor upper-body power performance when he is analyzed from a chronological point of view

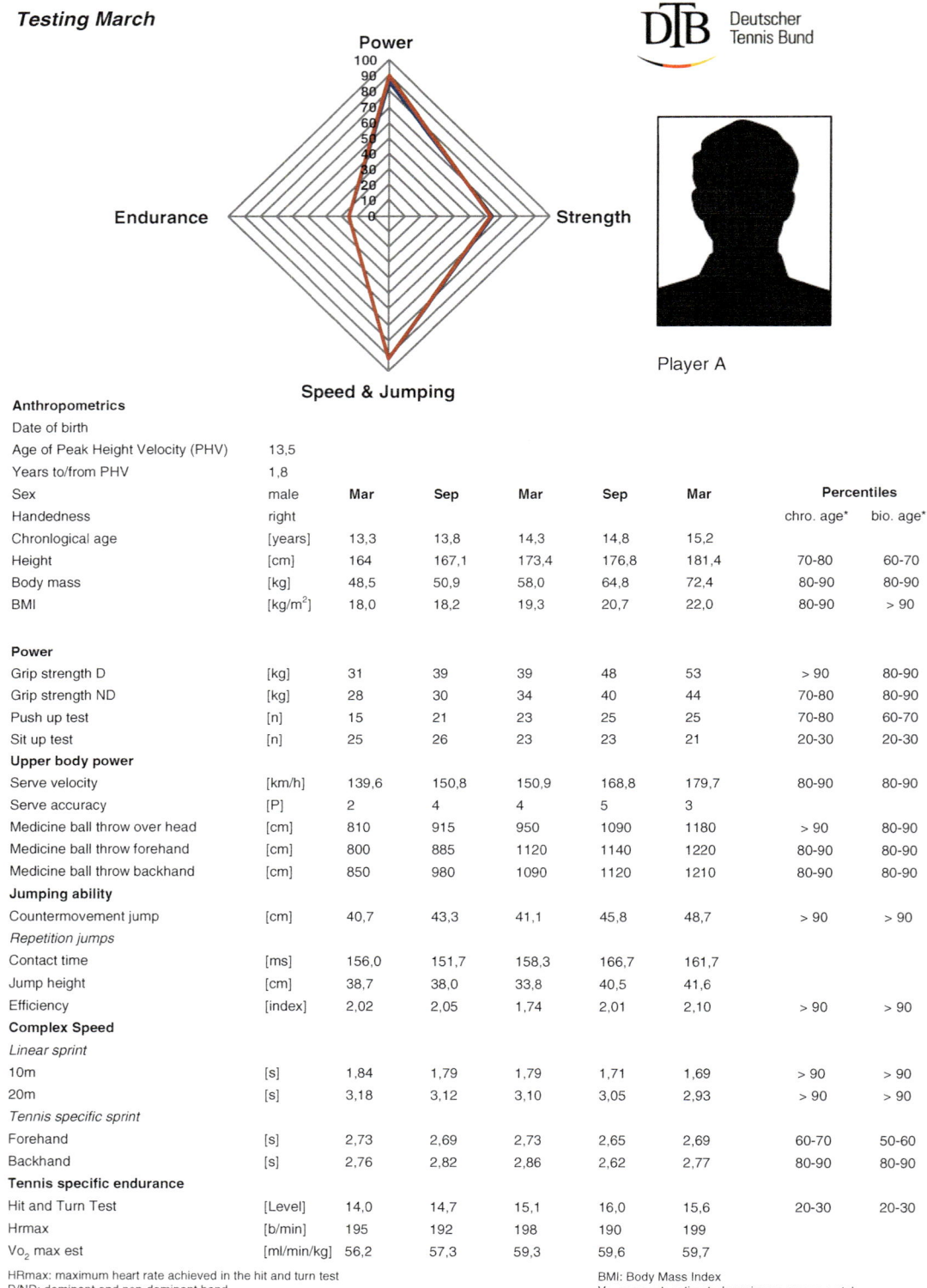

Anthropometrics		Mar	Sep	Mar	Sep	Mar	Percentiles	
Date of birth							chro. age*	bio. age**
Age of Peak Height Velocity (PHV)	13,5							
Years to/from PHV	1,8							
Sex	male							
Handedness	right							
Chronlogical age	[years]	13,3	13,8	14,3	14,8	15,2		
Height	[cm]	164	167,1	173,4	176,8	181,4	70-80	60-70
Body mass	[kg]	48,5	50,9	58,0	64,8	72,4	80-90	80-90
BMI	[kg/m^2]	18,0	18,2	19,3	20,7	22,0	80-90	> 90
Power								
Grip strength D	[kg]	31	39	39	48	53	> 90	80-90
Grip strength ND	[kg]	28	30	34	40	44	70-80	80-90
Push up test	[n]	15	21	23	25	25	70-80	60-70
Sit up test	[n]	25	26	23	23	21	20-30	20-30
Upper body power								
Serve velocity	[km/h]	139,6	150,8	150,9	168,8	179,7	80-90	80-90
Serve accuracy	[P]	2	4	4	5	3		
Medicine ball throw over head	[cm]	810	915	950	1090	1180	> 90	80-90
Medicine ball throw forehand	[cm]	800	885	1120	1140	1220	80-90	80-90
Medicine ball throw backhand	[cm]	850	980	1090	1120	1210	80-90	80-90
Jumping ability								
Countermovement jump	[cm]	40,7	43,3	41,1	45,8	48,7	> 90	> 90
Repetition jumps								
Contact time	[ms]	156,0	151,7	158,3	166,7	161,7		
Jump height	[cm]	38,7	38,0	33,8	40,5	41,6		
Efficiency	[index]	2,02	2,05	1,74	2,01	2,10	> 90	> 90
Complex Speed								
Linear sprint								
10m	[s]	1,84	1,79	1,79	1,71	1,69	> 90	> 90
20m	[s]	3,18	3,12	3,10	3,05	2,93	> 90	> 90
Tennis specific sprint								
Forehand	[s]	2,73	2,69	2,73	2,65	2,69	60-70	50-60
Backhand	[s]	2,76	2,82	2,86	2,62	2,77	80-90	80-90
Tennis specific endurance								
Hit and Turn Test	[Level]	14,0	14,7	15,1	16,0	15,6	20-30	20-30
Hrmax	[b/min]	195	192	198	190	199		
Vo$_2$ max est	[ml/min/kg]	56,2	57,3	59,3	59,6	59,7		

HRmax: maximum heart rate achieved in the hit and turn test
D/ND: dominant and non-dominant hand
*Percentiles based on chronological age

BMI: Body Mass Index
Vo$_2$ max est: estimated maximum oxygen uptake
**Percentiles based on biological maturation (PHV)

Fig. 12.9 Individual performance profile of player A including the percentiles referring to his biological (red line in the spider net diagram) and chronological age reference (blue line)

12 Assessment of Physical Performance for Individualized Training Prescription in Tennis

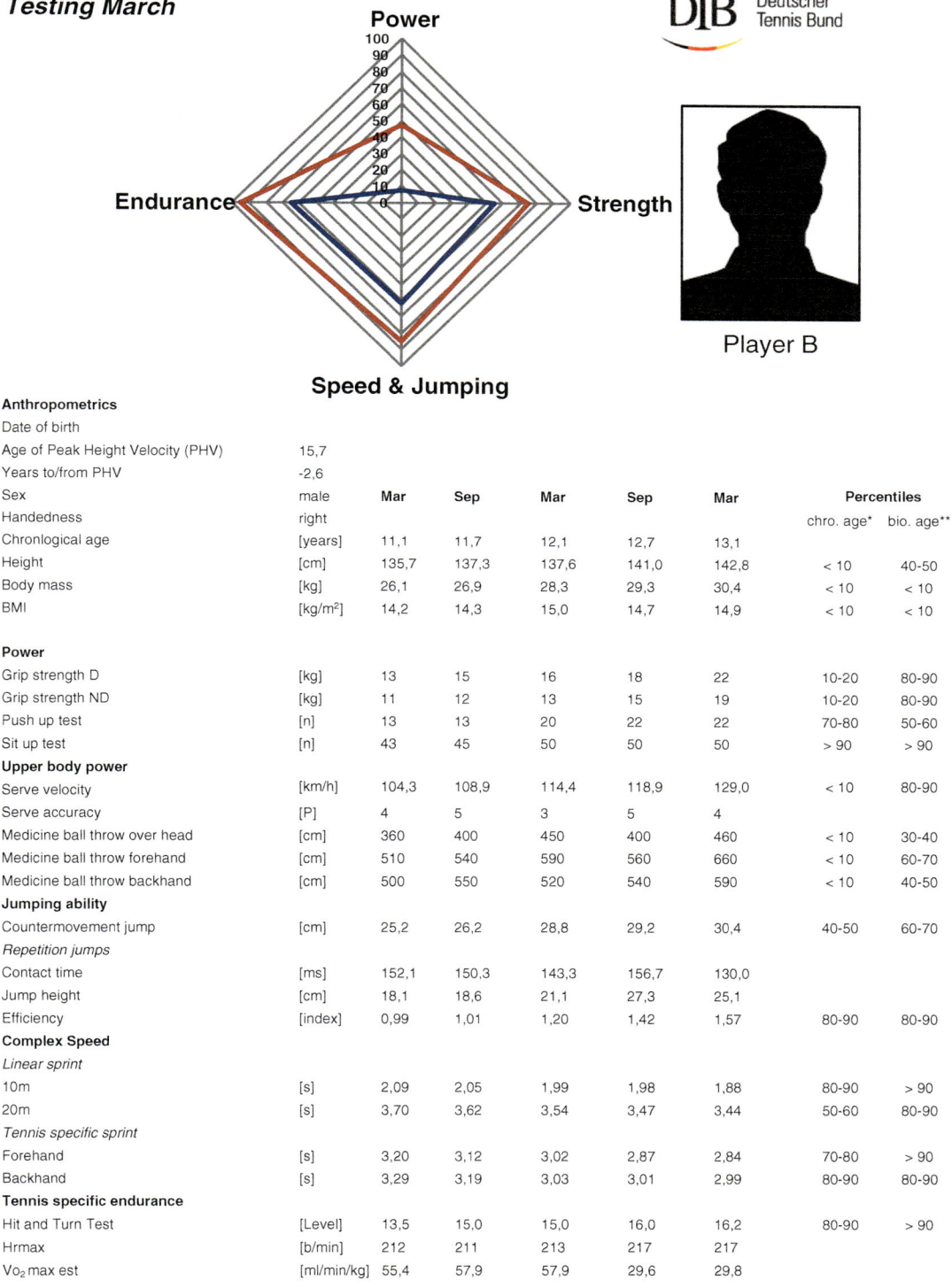

Testing March — Player B

Anthropometrics		Mar	Sep	Mar	Sep	Mar	Percentiles	
Date of birth							chro. age*	bio. age**
Age of Peak Height Velocity (PHV)		15,7						
Years to/from PHV		-2,6						
Sex	male							
Handedness	right							
Chronological age	[years]	11,1	11,7	12,1	12,7	13,1		
Height	[cm]	135,7	137,3	137,6	141,0	142,8	< 10	40-50
Body mass	[kg]	26,1	26,9	28,3	29,3	30,4	< 10	< 10
BMI	[kg/m²]	14,2	14,3	15,0	14,7	14,9	< 10	< 10
Power								
Grip strength D	[kg]	13	15	16	18	22	10-20	80-90
Grip strength ND	[kg]	11	12	13	15	19	10-20	80-90
Push up test	[n]	13	13	20	22	22	70-80	50-60
Sit up test	[n]	43	45	50	50	50	> 90	> 90
Upper body power								
Serve velocity	[km/h]	104,3	108,9	114,4	118,9	129,0	< 10	80-90
Serve accuracy	[P]	4	5	3	5	4		
Medicine ball throw over head	[cm]	360	400	450	400	460	< 10	30-40
Medicine ball throw forehand	[cm]	510	540	590	560	660	< 10	60-70
Medicine ball throw backhand	[cm]	500	550	520	540	590	< 10	40-50
Jumping ability								
Countermovement jump	[cm]	25,2	26,2	28,8	29,2	30,4	40-50	60-70
Repetition jumps								
Contact time	[ms]	152,1	150,3	143,3	156,7	130,0		
Jump height	[cm]	18,1	18,6	21,1	27,3	25,1		
Efficiency	[index]	0,99	1,01	1,20	1,42	1,57	80-90	80-90
Complex Speed								
Linear sprint								
10m	[s]	2,09	2,05	1,99	1,98	1,88	80-90	> 90
20m	[s]	3,70	3,62	3,54	3,47	3,44	50-60	80-90
Tennis specific sprint								
Forehand	[s]	3,20	3,12	3,02	2,87	2,84	70-80	> 90
Backhand	[s]	3,29	3,19	3,03	3,01	2,99	80-90	80-90
Tennis specific endurance								
Hit and Turn Test	[Level]	13,5	15,0	15,0	16,0	16,2	80-90	> 90
Hrmax	[b/min]	212	211	213	217	217		
Vo₂ max est	[ml/min/kg]	55,4	57,9	57,9	29,6	29,8		

Fig. 12.10 Individual performance profile of player B including the percentiles referring to his biological (red line in the spider net diagram) and chronological age reference (blue line)

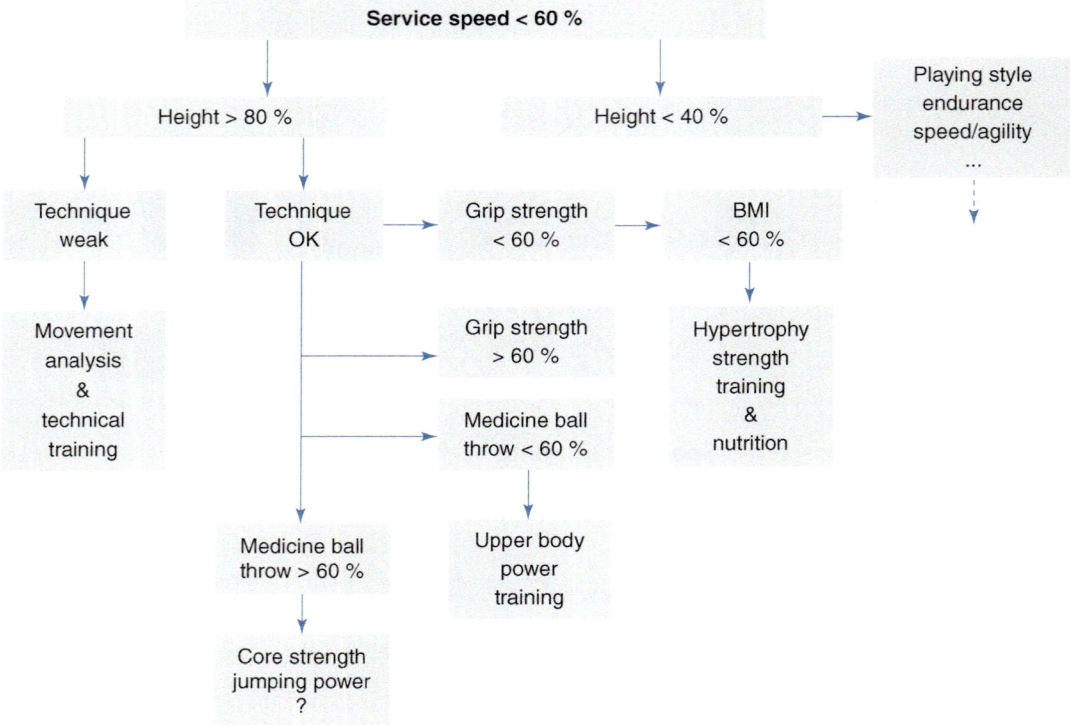

Fig. 12.11 A multivariate guideline flowchart for discussion and prescription of the athletes individual training focus. An example for the improvement of the serve velocity

(i.e., percentile 10–20), he seems to be average (i.e., percentile 40–50) when he is analyzed from a biological point of view. If we just use results based on the chronological age percentiles, it would probably lead to an inaccurate interpretation of the results. Moreover, the setup for an optimal training program could be disturbed. Therefore, we highly recommend the additional use of References normative data and percentiles which consider an individual's stage of maturation.

Both case studies show that interpretation and individual prescription of training programs is not easy and a great challenge for coaches. To avoid that physical testing is not the endpoint—what we often see—but an important starting point for individual training optimization (Fig. 12.2), evidence-based guidelines and flowcharts have to be developed for tennis coaches to facilitate the individual database construction of training programs.

As serve velocity and upper-body power were identified as important limiting aspects for the complex tennis performance, Fig. 12.11 shows an example for these flowcharts related to diagnostic of a poor serve velocity, which was defined to be lower than the 60th age-related percentile. On a first view, coaches and parents should realize the actual body height and prognostic final body height. Depending on these factors, players who are currently below the average body height and whose prognostic final body height is also clearly below the average should align their playing style accordingly and focus on other aspects of physical training (i.e., endurance, agility, and speed) rather than to invest too many resources in the improvement of serve velocity. For those players who fulfill the anthropometrical requirements (i.e., body height percentile >80) but do not achieve the appropriate serve velocity (i.e., serve velocity percentile <60%), a comprehensive technique analysis of the tennis serve should be carried out to identify possible weaknesses regarding technical elements. Whenever the serve technique is found to be impeccable, further test results can provide information regarding the subsequent training programs and following analysis. Therefore, a player with accurate technique and a basic body strength and body mass index around or below average (i.e., grip strength and BMI percentile <60%) could benefit from hypertrophy strength training and an according nutrition. On the other hand, an upper-body power training would be appropriate for players who reveal an according weakness (i.e., medicine ball throw percentile <60%). To further optimize the athletic training interventions, a great future task for sports science and sports coaches will be the development of evidence-based training programs.

12.5 Summary

Assessment of physical performance in tennis provides a framework for the development of an individualized database and a more efficient program of the physical fitness training, especially in junior players. Several testing protocols for different physical qualities are presented. With the results obtained from these testing protocols and the respective normative values, coaches and physical trainers can develop individual profiles of the players, based on age and sex group percentiles, with their respective strengths and weaknesses. This would lead to a more efficient design of physical training programs, saving time for the tennis-specific training. Examples for a guideline-based flowchart for making individual training decisions more evidence based are given. This very important step from diagnostics to training prescription is a great challenge for coaches and yet not well prepared in literature.

References

1. Fernandez-Fernandez J, Sanz-Rivas D, Mendez-Villanueva A. A review of the activity profile and physiological demands of tennis match play. Strength Cond. 2009;31(4):15.
2. Ferrauti A, Maier P, Weber K. Handbuch für Tennistraining, Leistung – Athletik - Gesundheit. Aachen: Meyer & Meyer; 2014.
3. Fernandez-Fernandez J, Ulbricht A, Ferrauti A. Fitness testing of tennis players: how valuable is it? Br J Sports Med. 2014;48:i22–31.
4. Reilly T, Morris T, Whyte G. The specificity of training prescription and physiological assessment: a review. J Sports Sci. 2009;27(6):575–89.
5. MacDougall JD, Wenger HA, Green HJ. Physiological testing of the high-performance athlete. Champaign: Human Kinetics; 1991.
6. Ferrauti A, Kinner V, Fernandez-Fernandez J. The Hit & Turn Tennis Test: an acoustically controlled endurance test for tennis players. J Sports Sci. 2011;29(5):485–94.
7. Ulbricht A, Fernandez-Fernandez J, Ferrauti A. Conception for Fitness Testing and individualized training programs in the German Tennis Federation. Sports Orthopaed Traumatol. 2013;29:180–92.
8. Bangsbo J. The physiology of soccer with special reference to intense intermittent exercise. Acta Physiol Scand Suppl. 1994;619:1.
9. Hoff J. Training and testing physical capacities for elite soccer players. J Sports Sci. 2005;23(6):573–82.
10. Girard O, Chevalier R, Leveque F, Micallef JP, Millet GP. Specific incremental field test for aerobic fitness in tennis. Br J Sports Med. 2006;40(9):791–6.
11. Svensson M, Drust B. Testing soccer players. J Sports Sci. 2005;23(6):601–18.
12. Alricsson M, Harms-Ringdahl K, Werner S. Reliability of sports related functional tests with emphasis on speed and agility in young athletes. Scand J Med Sci Sports. 2001;11(4):229–32.
13. Bangsbo J, Mohr M, Poulsen A, Krustrup P. Training and testing the elite athlete. J Exerc Sci Fit. 2006;4(1):1–13.
14. Stolen T, Chamari K, Castagna C, Wisloff U. Physiology of soccer: an update. Sports Med. 2005;35(6):501–36.
15. Kovacs MS. Tennis physiology: training the competitive athlete. Sports Med. 2007;37(3):189–98.
16. Signorile J, Sandler D, Smith W, Perry AC. Correlation analyses and regression modeling between isokinetic testing and on-court performance in competitive adolescent tennis players. J Strength Cond Res. 2005;19(3):519–26.
17. Gabbett TJ. Science of rugby league football: a review. J Sports Sci. 2005;23(9):961–76.
18. Ulbricht A, Fernandez-Fernandez J, Villanueva A, Ferrauti A. Impact of physical fitness characteristics on tennis performance in elite junior tennis players. J Strength Cond Res. 2016;30(4):989–98.
19. Girard O, Millet GP. Physical determinants of tennis performance in competitive teenage players. J Strength Cond Res. 2009;23(6):1867–72.
20. Kraemer WJ, Hakkinen K, Triplett-Mcbride NT, Fry AC, Koziris LP, Ratamess NA, Bauer JE, Vlek JS, McConnel T, Newton RU, Gordon SE, Cummings

D, Hauth J, Pullo F, Lynch JM, Fleck SJ, Mazzetti SA, Knuttgen HG. Physiological changes with periodized resistance training in women tennis players. Med Sci Sports Exerc. 2003;35(1):157–68.
21. Ulbricht A, Fernandez-Fernandez J, Villanueva A, Ferrauti A. The relative age effect and physical fitness characteristics in German male tennis players. J Sports Sci Med. 2015;14:634–42.
22. Roetert P, Ellenbecker TS. Complete conditioning for tennis. Champaign: Human Kinetics; 2007.
23. Buckeridge A, Farrow D, Gastin P, McGrath M, Morrow P, Quinn A, Young W. Protocols for the physiological assessment of high-performance tennis players. Physiological Tests for Elite Athletes Australian Sports Commission. Champaign: Human Kinetics; 2000.
24. Reid M, Quinn A, Crespo M. Strength and conditioning for tennis. London: International Tennis Federation; 2003.
25. Bourdon P. Blood lactate thresholds: concepts and applications. In: Gore CJ, Tanner RK, editors. Physiological tests for elite athletes. 2nd ed. Champaign: Human Kinetics; 2013. p. 77–102.
26. Ferrauti A, Weber K, Wright PR. Endurance: basic, semi-specific and tennis specific. In: Reid M, Quinn A, Crespo M, editors. Strength and conditioning for tennis. London: ITF; 2003. p. 93–112.
27. Maksud MG, Coutts KD. Application of the Cooper twelve-minute run-walk test to young males. Res Q Am Assoc Health. 1971;42(1):54–9.
28. Leger L, Boucher R. An indirect continuous running multistage field test: the Universite de Montreal track test. Can J Appl Sport Sci. 1980;5(2):77–84.
29. Chtara M, Chamari K, Chaouachi M, Chaouachi A, Koubaa D, Feki Y, Millet GP, Amri M. Effects of intra-session concurrent endurance and strength training sequence on aerobic performance and capacity. Br J Sports Med. 2005;39(8):555–60.
30. Léger LA, Lambert J. A maximal multistage 20 m shuttle run test to predict VO2 max. Eur J Appl Physiol Occup Physiol. 1982;49(1):1–12.
31. Leger L, Mercier D, Gadoury C, Lambert J. The multistage 20 metre shuttle run test for aerobic fitness. J Sports Sci. 1988;6(2):93–101.
32. Bangsbo J, Iaia FM, Krustrup P. The Yo-Yo intermittent recovery test: a useful tool for evaluation of physical performance in intermittent sports. Sports Med. 2008;38(1):37–51.
33. Buchheit M. The 30-15 intermittent fitness test: accuracy for individualizing interval training of young intermittent sport players. J Strength Cond Res. 2008;22(2):365–74.
34. Reid M, Sibte N, Clark S, Whiteside D. Tennis players. In: Gore CJ, Tanner RK, editors. Physiological tests for elite athletes. 2nd ed. Champaign: Human Kinetics; 2013. p. 449–61.
35. Spencer M, Bishop D, Dawson B, Goodman C. Physiological and metabolic responses of repeated-sprint activities: specific to field-based team sports. Sports Med. 2005;35(12):1025–44.
36. Smekal G, Pokan R, von Duvillard SP, Baron R, Tschan H, Bachl N. Comparison of laboratory and "on-court" endurance testing in tennis. Int J Sports Med. 2000;21(4):242–9.
37. Baiget E, Fernández-Fernández J, Iglesias X, Vallejo L, Rodriguez FA. On-court endurance and performance testing in competitive male tennis players. J Strength Cond Res. 2014;28(1):256–64.
38. Weber K, Hollmann W. Neue Methoden zur Diagnostik und Trainingssteuerung der tennisspezifischen Ausdauerleistungsfähigkeit. In: Gabler H, editor. Talentsuche und Talentförderung im Tennis. Ahrensberg: Czwalina; 1984. p. 186–209.
39. Weber K. Der Tennisport aus internistisch-sportmedizinisher Sicht. Schriften der Deutschen Sporthoschule Köln. St. Augustin: Academia; 1987.
40. Vergauwen L, Spaepen AJ, Lefevre J, Hespel P. Evaluation of stroke performance in tennis. Med Sci Sports Exerc. 1998;30(8):1281–8.
41. Davey PR, Thorpe RD, Williams C. Fatigue decreases skilled tennis performance. J Sports Sci. 2002;20(4):311–8.
42. Brechbuhl C, Girard O, Millet GP, Schmitt L. Technical alterations during an incremental field test in elite male tennis players. Med Sci Sports Exerc. 2017;49(9):1917–26.
43. Urso R, Okuno N, Gomes R, Bertuzzi R. Validity and reliability evidences of the Hit & Turn Tennis Test. Sci Sports. 2013;29(4):e47–53.
44. Fernandez-Fernandez J, Kinner V, Ferrauti A. The physiological demands of hitting and running in tennis on different surfaces. J Strength Cond Res. 2010;24(12):3255–64.
45. Inbar O, Bar-Or O, Skinner JS. The Wingate anaerobic test. Champaign: Human Kinetics; 1996.
46. Kovacs MS, Pritchett R, Wickwire PJ, Green JM. Physical performance changes after unsupervised training during the autumn/spring semester break in competitive tennis players. Br J Sports Med. 2007;41(11):705–10.
47. Lakomy HKA. The use of a non-motorised treadmill for analysing sprint performance. Ergonomics. 1987;30:627–37.
48. Ratel S, Williams C, Oliver J, Armstrong N. Effects of age and recovery duration on performance during multiple treadmill sprints. Int J Sports Med. 2006;27(01):1–8.
49. Spriet LL, Howlett RA, Heigenhauser GJ. An enzymatic approach to lactate production in human skeletal muscle during exercise. Med Sci Sport Exerc. 2000;32(4):756–63.
50. Bleicher A, Mader A, Mester J. Zur Interpretation von Laktatleistungskurven – experimentelle Ergebnisse mit computergestützten Nachberechnungen. Spektrum der Sportwissenschaften. 1998;10:92–104.
51. Dawson B. Repeated-sprint ability: where are we? Int J Sports Physiol Perform. 2012;7(3):285–9.
52. Girard O, Mendez-Villanueva A, Bishop D. Repeated-sprint ability - Part I: Factors contributing to fatigue. Sports Med. 2011;41(8):673–94.

53. Bishop D, Girard O, Mendez-Villanueva A. Repeated-sprint ability - Part II: Recommendations for training. Sports Med. 2011;41(9):741–56.
54. Fernandez-Fernandez J, Zimek R, Wiewelhove T, Ferrauti A. High-intensity interval training vs. repeated-sprint training in tennis. J Strength Cond Res. 2012;26(1):53–62.
55. Buchheit M. Repeated-sprint performance in team sport players: associations with measures of aerobic fitness, metabolic control and locomotor function. Int J Sports Med. 2012;33(3):230–9.
56. Kovacs MS, Ellenbecker TS. A performance evaluation of the tennis serve: implications for strength, speed, power, and flexibility training. Strength Cond J. 2011;33(4):22.
57. Reid M, Schneiker K. Strength and conditioning in tennis: current research and practice. J Sci Med Sport. 2008;11(3):248–56.
58. Cronin JB, Henderson ME. Maximal strength and power assessment in novice weight trainers. J Strength Cond Res. 2004;18(1):48–52.
59. Cronin JB, Hansen KT. Strength and power predictors of sports speed. J Strength Cond Res. 2005;19(2):349–57.
60. Cormie P, McGuigan MR, Newton RU. Developing maximal neuromuscular power. Sports Med. 2011;41(1):17–38.
61. Wisløff U, Castagna C, Helgerud J, Jones R. Strong correlation of maximal squat strength with sprint performance and vertical jump height in elite soccer players. Br J Sports Med. 2004;38(3):285–8.
62. Baker D, Nance S. The relation between running speed and measures of strength and power in professional rugby league players. J Strength Cond Res. 1999;13(3):230–5.
63. Brown L, Weir J. Accurate assessment of muscular strength and power, ASEP procedures recommendation. J Exerc Physiol. 2001;4(3):1–21.
64. Reynolds JM, Gordon TJ, Robergs RA. Prediction of one repetition maximum strength from multiple repetition maximum testing and anthropometry. J Strength Cond Res. 2006;20(3):584–92.
65. Cronin J, Sleivert G. Challenges in understanding the influence of maximal power training on improving athletic performance. Sports Med. 2005;35(3):213–34.
66. Girard O, Micallef JP, Millet GP. Lower-limb activity during the power serve in tennis: effects of performance level. Med Sci Sports Exerc. 2005;37(6):1021–9.
67. Elliott B. Biomechanics and tennis. Br J Sports Med. 2006;40(5):392–6.
68. Roetert E, Piorkowski P, Woods R, Brown SW. Establishing percentiles for junior tennis players based on physical fitness testing results. Clin Sport Med. 1995;14(1):1.
69. Ellenbecker TS, Roetert EP. An isokinetic profile of trunk rotation strength in elite tennis players. Med Sci Sports Exerc. 2004;36(11):1959–63.
70. Ikeda Y, Kijima K, Kawabata K, Fuchimoto T, Ito A. Relationship between side medicine-ball throw performance and physical ability for male and female athletes. Eur J Appl Physiol. 2007;99(1):47–55.
71. Ulbricht A, Ferrauti A, Pfannkoch P, Gewehr J, Fernandez-Fernandez J. Impact of physical performance on tennis ranking in juniors-results from nationwide German tennis test (abstract). In: Cable T, George K, editors. 16th Annual Congress of the European College of Sports Science, Liverpool; 2011.
72. Hornery DJ, Farrow D, Mujika I, Young WB. Caffeine, carbohydrate, and cooling use during prolonged simulated tennis. Int J Sports Physiol Perform. 2007;2(4):423.
73. Fernandez-Fernandez J, Ellenbecker T, Sanz-Rivas D, Ulbricht A, Ferrauti A. Effects of a 6-week Junior Tennis Conditioning Program on Service Velocity. J Sports Sci Med. 2013;12(2):232–9.
74. Ferrauti A, Bastiaens K. Short-term effects of light and heavy load interventions on service velocity and precision in elite young tennis players. Br J Sports Med. 2007;41(11):750–3.
75. Sheppard J, Young W. Agility literature review: classifications, training and testing. J Sports Sci. 2006;24(9):919–32.
76. Little T, Williams AG. Specificity of acceleration, maximum speed, and agility in professional soccer players. J Strength Cond Res. 2005;19(1):76–8.
77. Stewart PF, Turner AN, Miller SC. Reliability, factorial validity, and interrelationships of five commonly used change of direction speed tests. Scand J Med Sci Sports. 2014;24(3):500–6.
78. Cooke K, Quinn A, Sibte N. Testing speed and agility in elite tennis players. Strength Cond J. 2011;33(4):69–72.
79. Ellenbecker T, De Carlo M, DeRosa C. Effective functional progressions in sport rehabilitation. Champaign: Human Kinetics; 2009.
80. Pluim BM, Staal JB, Windler GE, Jayanthi N. Tennis injuries: occurrence, aetiology, and prevention. Br J Sports Med. 2006;40(5):415–23.
81. Cools AM, De Wilde L, Van Tongel A, Ceyssens C, Ryckewaert R, Cambier DC. Measuring shoulder external and internal rotation strength and range of motion: comprehensive intra-rater and inter-rater reliability study of several testing protocols. J Shoulder Elb Surg. 2014;23:1454–61.
82. Almeida GPL, de Souza VL, Sano SS, Saccol MF, Cohen M. Comparison of hip rotation range of motion in judo athletes with and without history of low back pain. Man Ther. 2012;17:231–5.
83. Cejudo A, Sainz de Baranda P, Ayala F, Santonja F. Test-retest reliability of seven common clinical tests for assessing lower extremity muscle flexibility in futsal and handball players. Phys Ther Sport. 2015;16:107–12.
84. Ellenbecker TS. Musculoskeletal examination of elite junior tennis players. Sports Med J. 2014;3:548–56.

85. Kibler WB, Uhl TL, Maddux JW, Brooks PV, Zeller B, McMullen J. Qualitative clinical evaluation of scapular dysfunction: a reliability study. J Shoulder Elb Surg. 2002;11(6):550–6.
86. Ellenbecker TS. Physical examination of the shoulder. Philadelphia: Saunders; 2004.
87. Peeler J, Anderson J. Reliability of the Thomas test for assessing range of motion about the hip. Phys Ther Sport. 2007;8(1):14–21.
88. Magee DJ. Orthopaedic physical assessment. Amsterdam: Elsevier; 2008.
89. Cook G, Burton L, Hoogenboom B. Pre-participation screening: the use of fundamental movements as an assessment of function–Part 1. N Am J Sports Phys Ther. 2006;1(2):62.
90. Minick KI, Kiesel KB, Burton L, Taylor A, Plisky P, Butler RJ. Interrater reliability of the functional movement screen. J Strength Cond Res. 2010;24(2):479–86.
91. Gribble PA, Brigle J, Pietrosimone BG, Pfile KR, Webster KA. Intrarater reliability of the functional movement screen. J Strength Cond Res. 2013;27(4):978–81.
92. Elias JE. The inter-rater reliability of the functional movement screen within an athletic population using untrained raters. J Strength Cond Res. 2015;30(9):1533–4287.
93. Smith CA, Chimera NJ, Wright NJ, Warren M. Interrater and intrarater reliability of the functional movement screen. J Strength Cond Res. 2013;27(4):982–7.
94. Bardenett SM, Micca JJ, DeNoyelles JT, Miller SD, Jenk DT, Brooks GS. Functional movement screen normative values and validity in high school athletes: can the FMS be used as a predictor of injury? Int J Sports Phys Ther. 2015;10(3):303–8.
95. Birrer R, Levine R, Gallippi L, Tischler H. The correlation of performance variables in preadolescent tennis players. J Sports Med Phys Fitness. 1986;26(2):137–9.
96. Kibler WB, McQueen C, Uhl T. Fitness evaluations and fitness findings in competitive junior tennis players. Clin Sports Med. 1988;7:403–16.
97. Roetert EP, Garrett GE, Brown SW, Camaione D. Performance profiles of nationally ranked junior tennis players. J Strength Cond Res. 1992;6(4):225–31.
98. Malina RM, Bouchard C, Bar-Or O. Growth, maturation and physical activity. Champaign: Human Kinetics; 2004.
99. Ford P, De Ste Croix M, Lloyd R, Meyers R, Moosavi M, Oliver J, Till K, Williams C. The long term athlete development model: physiological evidence and application. J Sports Sci. 2011;29(4):389–402.

Part III

Shoulder Injuries

Diagnosis and Management of Partial- and Full-Thickness Rotator Cuff Tears in Tennis Players

Christopher L. Camp, David M. Dare, and David W. Altchek

13.1 Introduction

Tennis continues to be one of the most popular sports in the world, and as interest grows, our understanding of the physiologic demands of the sport also increases. During the course of a standard tennis match, players are required to repetitively exert themselves in short, but explosive, bursts of energy several hundred times [1]. This is especially true during the serve, but all types of strokes place very unique demands on the upper extremity [2–4]. To better understand the physiologic processes occurring during the serve, it has been broken down into five distinct phases: (1) windup, (2) early cocking, (3) late cocking, (4) acceleration, and (5) follow-through [4, 5]. In order to successfully execute these phases, energy must be transferred efficiently and effectively along the entire kinetic chain of motion. Although the greatest stress to the shoulder occurs during the cocking and acceleration phases, disruption of the kinetic chain at any point in the process can place the shoulder at risk for injury [6].

Accordingly, shoulder injuries are common in tennis players of all skill levels. While lower extremity injuries tend to occur in an acute fashion, shoulder and other upper extremity injuries are generally the result of chronic attrition and over exertion. Ultimately, upper extremity injuries represent 20–49% of all musculoskeletal injuries in tennis players, and they occur in players of all ages and experience levels [7–9]. Although the most common upper extremity injury reported by tennis players is lateral epicondylitis, up to 24% of juniors and 50% of middle age players experience shoulder pain [10]. While the most common shoulder pathology in younger players is generally related to subtle instability, rotator cuff injuries are more common in older tennis athletes [11]. Internal impingement and scapular dyskinesia are also common findings in this group [5, 6, 10, 12].

Rotator cuff tears in tennis players represent a unique challenge to practitioners, as the physiologic demands of these overhead athletes are quite different from those of the normal population, and rotator cuff injuries commonly coexist with other pathologic processes such as internal impingement, scapular dyskinesia, superior labral injury, biceps tendonitis, chondral injury, and even arthritis [5, 6, 12, 13]. When treating these patients, it is critical that these potential concomitant processes are identified and addressed. Generally speaking, a comprehensive course of nonoperative treatment is the preferred management for rotator cuff injuries in overhead athletes, and indications for surgical intervention remain controversial. Nonoperative management generally includes a period of activity

C. L. Camp (✉)
Sports Medicine Center, Mayo Clinic,
Rochester, MN, USA
e-mail: camp.christopher@mayo.edu

D. M. Dare · D. W. Altchek
Sports and Shoulder Service, Hospital for Special Surgery, New York, NY, USA

modification, anti-inflammatory medications, and a comprehensive regimen of physical therapy targeted at optimizing the entire kinetic chain. When these measures fail to provide sufficient relief, surgical intervention is considered, and this typically exists in the form of tear debridement, intra-substance repair, or formal repair of the tendon back to the humeral head [13].

13.2 Etiology and Tear Types

The vast majority of rotator cuff injuries occurring in tennis players are the result of chronic degeneration and overuse, and this is true for both partial- and full-thickness tears. Partial tears can occur on the articular side, remain intra-tendinous, or develop on the bursal (subacromial) side. Although most rotator cuff injuries in tennis players are the result of chronic, repetitive overuse, acute injuries are certainly possible. The spectrum of rotator cuff pathology in tennis players generally spans four main groups: (1) small partial articular-sided tears often associated with internal impingement in younger adult tennis athletes; (2) chronic tendinosis, intra-substance tears, or bursal-sided tears secondary to overuse in middle-aged players; (3) acute, potentially full-thickness, injuries in middle-aged players; and finally, (4) degenerative full-thickness tears in the older tennis population.

13.2.1 Partial Articular-Sided Tears

Partial articular-sided tears are likely a result of eccentric tensile stress, internal impingement, or a combination of both. The tensile stress theory is supported by a number of biomechanical studies that have demonstrated tremendous repetitive eccentric loads transmitted through the rotator cuff during the follow-though portion of overhead activity [3, 14, 15]. The more recent prevailing theory is that of internal impingement, where the posterior portion of the supraspinatus and anterior portion of the infraspinatus are compressed between the greater tuberosity of the humerus and the superior glenoid and labrum when the arm is in the overhead position (90° abduction and 90° external rotation) [16]. Also seen in throwing athletes, repetitive overhead activity can lead to posterior capsular contracture, which causes the humeral head to migrate superiorly on the glenoid during the overhead motion increasing the risk for internal impingement [16]. It is worth noting that many authors have suggested that partial articular-sided rotator cuff tears in the setting of internal impingement can commonly be found in asymptomatic overhead athletes [17, 18]. The specific factors or qualities that cause some of these patients to develop symptomology while others remain pain free are not yet fully elucidated.

13.2.2 Intra-tendinous Tears

A robust body of basic science research has demonstrated that the tendinous portion of the rotator cuff is actually composed of five different histologic layers [19–23]. Each of these layers experiences shear stresses in distinct ways during rotator cuff contraction. Accordingly, intra-tendinous delamination often accompanies rotator cuff injuries [16, 19, 24, 25]. Generally, this delamination is seen in the setting of articular-sided, bursal-sided, or full-thickness tears; however, it can occur in isolation.

13.2.3 Partial Bursal-Sided Tears

Although it is believed that most tears in overhead athletes begin on the articular side and propagate through the five histologic layers toward the bursal side, isolated tears of the bursal side of the rotator cuff commonly occur. These can be a result of chronic overuse and degeneration and/or subacromial impingement (also known as secondary, outlet, or external impingement).

13.2.4 Full-Thickness Tears

Chronic, full-thickness tears in overhead athletes are generally thought to begin as articular-sided tears that fully propagate through the tendon to the bursal side. The time it takes for this process to occur is unknown, and it likely varies significantly depending upon the individual patient, physiologic demand, and quality of the tendon and surrounding structures. Acute, traumatic, full-thickness tears can occur de novo or in the setting of previous chronic partial tears. These acute injuries are generally identified by the patient's history when they describe an acute onset of pain and dysfunction following a single serve or stroke.

13.3 Diagnosis

13.3.1 Clinical Presentation

Rotator cuff tears in tennis players can present in a multitude of ways; however, the most common symptoms include pain, weakness, shoulder fatigue, and decreased motion. More subtle, sport-specific symptoms may include decreased playing endurance, reduce service speed, and loss of ball control. Other important factors to elucidate are chronicity, presence of night pain, quality of symptoms, worsening and mitigating factors, presence of mechanical symptoms, history of prior treatment, associated neurologic symptoms, and status of the cervical spine.

It is also critical to determine the location of pain and the precise motions that bring it out. For instance, patients who notice posterior shoulder pain during their backhand may have isolated (or predominant) infraspinatus and/or teres minor injury. Those with lateral or superior shoulder pain when trying to elevate the arm overhead are more likely to have sustained injury to the supraspinatus. Patients with isolated anterior shoulder pain and weakness during their forehand may have subscapularis deficiency. Other common shoulder pathologies that should be ruled out include shoulder instability, superior labral injury, biceps tendonitis or instability, and acromioclavicular joint arthrosis to name a few.

13.3.2 Physical Examination

A comprehensive physical exam should be performed on all patients with special attention paid to tests specific to rotator cuff pathology. The exam actually begins as soon as the patient walks into the office or training room. One can glean a great deal of information by observing how the patient carries the arm while walking, doffing a jacket, etc. The formal examination of the shoulder should include assessment of the cervical spine, neurologic evaluation, vascular exam, inspection of the shoulder and peri-scapular musculature, measurement of range of motion (ROM), strength assessment, and special tests as indicated.

13.3.2.1 Cervical Spine Exam

Prior to investigating the shoulder, the cervical spine can be evaluated. This is accomplished by assessing motion, areas of tenderness to palpation, presence of neurologic deficits, and the Sperling's test. If any of these components is positive, it is critical that they be correlated with the patient's history and symptoms. If any of these maneuvers recreates the patient's symptoms, further investigation into the cervical spine is warranted. It is not uncommon that patients will have some pain or restriction related to the cervical spine that co-exists with rotator cuff disease. In these situations, each problem should be addressed accordingly.

13.3.2.2 Inspection

It is critical that the entire shoulder and scapula be visualized during the shoulder exam. Standing behind the patient, the surgeon can look for atrophy of the supraspinatus, infraspinatus, or any of the other peri-scapular musculature. Isolated atrophy of supraspinatus is often indicative of fatty degeneration following supraspinatus tear. Isolated atrophy of both the supraspinatus and infraspinatus may indicate a two-tendon tear or compression of the suprascapular nerve at the level at the suprascapular notch. Isolated infraspinatus atrophy may occur secondary to an isolated tendon tear, or it commonly is the result of a spinoglenoid notch cyst compressing the suprascapular nerve distal to its innervation of the supraspinatus.

Following static inspection, it is helpful to observe the patient elevate the arms overhead. At this time, special attention should be paid to the scapula. Not uncommonly, patients with rotator cuff injuries will demonstrate scapular hiking (either to avoid impingement or to increase the motion that is limited by weakness) or winging. When there is concern for winging (either medial or lateral), this is often made more apparent by having the patient repeatedly elevate and lower their arms or perform a modified push-up against a wall or table.

13.3.2.3 Range of Motion

ROM should be assessed for both arms in multiple planes including forward flexion, elevation in the scapular plane, abduction, and internal rotation (IR)/external rotation (ER) at the side and with the arm abducted 90°. Where active motion is limited, passive motion should be assessed. In all planes, the injured arm is compared to the non-injured side. Decreased elevation is often secondary to supraspinatus injury, and decreased active external rotation (ER) may suggest injury to the supraspinatus. Increased external rotation can occur in the setting of subscapularis deficiency.

13.3.2.4 Strength

Similar to ROM, strength should be assessed in all planes of motion. Patients with supraspinatus injury will typically have pain and weakness with resisted elevation in the scapular plane. Injury to the infraspinatus may cause ER weakness with the arm at the side, and teres minor dysfunction leads to ER weakness with the arm abducted to 90°. Decreased internal rotation strength is often secondary to subscapularis injury.

13.3.2.5 Special Tests

A multitude of special tests have been described for evaluation of the rotator cuff [26]. For the supraspinatus, the most common tests include neer impingement sign (pain with passive elevation), Jobe's test (pain with resisted elevation in scapular plane), Hawkins test (pain with forceful internal rotation of the abducted arm), and the drop sign (pain when lowering the arm or inability to maintain arm position after passive elevation).

The infraspinatus is best evaluated by assessing ER strength and ER lag. The most common special tests for the subscapularis include IR lag sign, the lift-off test (inability to lift the hand off back or maintain the hand in lifted position), belly press test (inability to bring elbow forward while pressing on the belly), and the bear hug test (in ability to keep the hand against contralateral chest during resistance). The significance of internal impingement is assessed by evaluating for a posterior impingement sign [27]. This test is positive when the patient's pain is recreated when the arm is placed in 90° abduction, 10° forward flexion, and maximal external rotation.

13.3.3 Imaging Studies

13.3.3.1 Plain Radiographs

Standard X-rays, including anteroposterior (AP), axillary, and scapular Y views, are often unrevealing; however they should be assessed for the presence of arthritic changes, superior humeral head migration, cystic changes at the insertional footprint of the cuff, and altered acromial morphology [28, 29].

13.3.3.2 Magnetic Resonance Imaging

Magnetic resonance imaging (MRI) has become the standard imaging modality for diagnosing soft tissue pathology in the shoulder (Fig. 13.1). The diagnostic accuracy is generally enhanced by the addition of intra-articular contrast [30–32]. This is particularly true for partial articular-sided tears where the addition of contrast has resulted in a 91% diagnostic accuracy with 84% sensitivity and 96% specificity [33]. In patients with suspected internal impingement or tears isolated to the articular side, MRI of the shoulder in the abducted and externally rotated position may improve diagnostic accuracy [32, 34]. MRI also has the added benefit of permitting evaluation of the quality of rotator cuff musculature, degree of retraction, and dimensions of the tear [35]. It is also beneficial in assessing surrounding structures such as the biceps tendon and labrum, and it

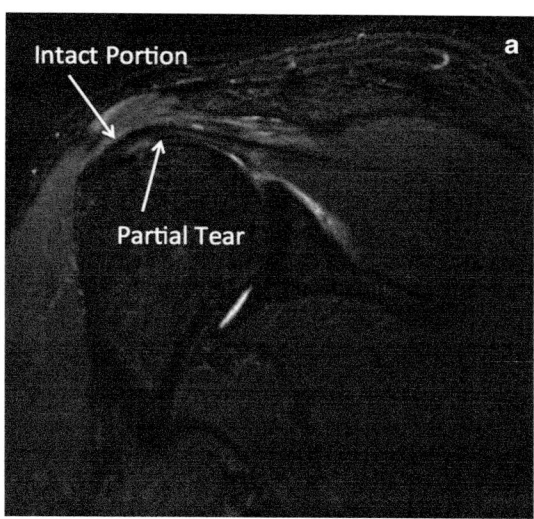
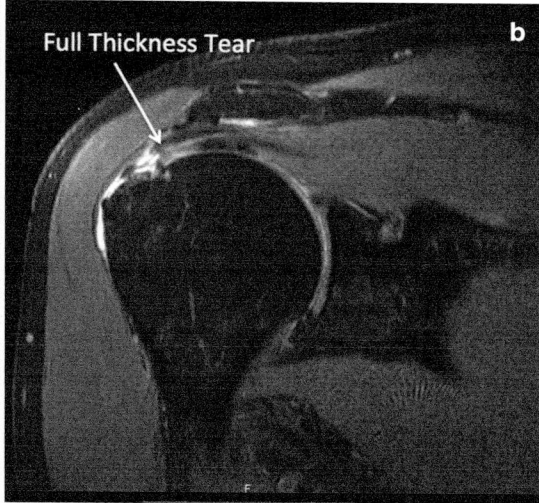

Fig. 13.1 Coronal magnetic resonance images from a shoulder with a partial-thickness, articular-sided supraspinatus tendon tear (**a**) and another patient with a full-thickness supraspinatus tendon tear (**b**)

can aid identifying subtle chondral wear and arthritis that may not be apparent on plain X-rays.

13.3.3.3 Ultrasonography

In recent years, ultrasound (US) has gained popularity as a method for evaluating rotator cuff disease. A number of studies have demonstrated comparable diagnostic capacity of US when compared to MRI when assessing dimensions and degree of retraction for full-thickness tears [36–38]. US has the benefits of allowing dynamic assessment and reduced cost compared to MRI; however, the accuracy and reliability is dependent upon user skill and experience, and it is not likely as reliable as MRI for assessing partial-thickness tears [39].

13.4 Treatment

13.4.1 Partial-Thickness Rotator Cuff Tears

13.4.1.1 Nonoperative Management

Nonoperative strategies are the mainstay of treatment for partial-thickness tears in overhead athletes. Although this approach includes activity modification, anti-inflammatory medications, and limited analgesics, the focus of nonoperative treatment is physical therapy. Therapy should begin with an initial assessment of the entire kinetic chain and targeted correction of any deficiencies. This includes, but is not limited to, lower extremity strengthening, balance, proprioception, and core strengthening. Significant attention must also be paid to peri-scapular strengthening and balance to eliminate scapular dyskinesia. It is critical that this is addressed in order to create a stable base upon which the shoulder can function [40].

Regarding the glenohumeral joint, the initial emphasis is on stretching and correction of motion deficits, particularly in the case of internal impingement and glenohumeral internal rotation deficiency. To overcome these deficiencies, sleeper stretches and horizontal adduction stretches are introduced and progressed as tolerated [40–42]. Once these rotational deficiencies are addressed and the kinetic chain is stabilized, closed-chain rotator cuff strengthening is instituted. As symptoms abate and strength and stability improve, sport-specific activities are gradually introduced. Generally speaking, athletes can begin with low reps of gentle groundstrokes and volleys. As these reps are slowly increased without symptoms, low-velocity overhead serving is introduced. As the patient tolerates, the number of serves per session and serving velocity are gradually increased.

13.4.1.2 Surgical Treatment

Because of the unique demands of the shoulder in these overhead athletes, surgical intervention for partial-thickness tears should be reserved only for those cases that have been recalcitrant to a comprehensive course of nonsurgical treatment. When determining the timing of operative intervention, a number of factors must be considered. These include the length and quality of nonoperative treatment attempted, timing of season, presence of significant mechanical symptoms, and overall patient goals. Once it is established that nonoperative treatment has failed and surgery is indicated, the primary treatment strategies include either debridement or repair.

For lesions with less than 50% of the tendon torn away from the tendon, debridement is generally the preferred surgical treatment (Fig. 13.2) [14, 17]. The extent of the tear is measured from medial to lateral for partial articular-sided tears. The normal width of the supraspinatus footprint is 12–14 mm, so lesions that involve less than 6 mm are generally considered candidates for debridement. Although the supraspinatus inserts just lateral to the articular margin of the humeral head, there is a bare spot on the humeral head that exists between the articular margin and the insertion site of the infraspinatus. The location and orientation of this region must be taken into consideration when assessing tear size. In cases were

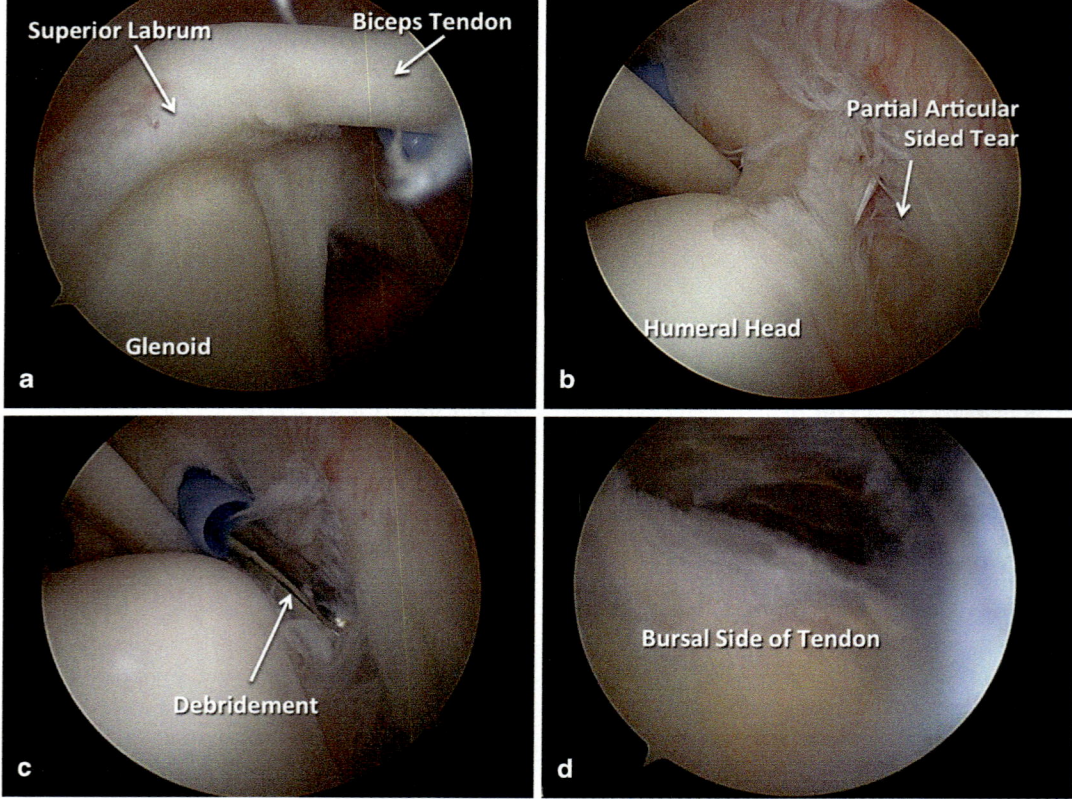

Fig. 13.2 Intra-articular images of right shoulder when viewing from a standard posterior viewing portal in an elite, 22-year-old tennis player. The biceps tendon and superior labrum were without significant pathology (**a**); however, a partial-thickness articular-sided tear of the supraspinatus was identified (**b**). This particular injury was treated with simple debridement without repair (**c**). When viewing from the subacromial space, there was no evidence of injury on the bursal side of the supraspinatus tendon (**d**)

internal impingement is suspected, the arm can be abducted and externally rotated into the "90/90" overhead position to assess for impingement of the cuff with the posterior superior labrum. When this phenomenon occurs, the posterior superior labrum may require concomitant debridement/repair.

Even in cases with less than 50% disruption of the footprint, a number of other factors must be taken into consideration before a final treatment strategy is determined. These include the presence of an intra-tendinous tear, quality of the remaining intact tissue, and presence of a bursal-sided tear in addition to the articular-sided injury. Lesions with articular-sided tears <50% of the footprint and an accompanying intra-tendinous tear can be treated with gentle debridement and intra-tendinous repair without the use of anchors into the bone (Fig. 13.3) [43–45]. If the remaining tissue is of poor quality, a substantial bursal-sided tear exists, or the articular portion involves more than 50% of the footprint, consideration is given to conversion of the tear to a full-thickness tear that is formally repaired using a double-row, transosseous equivalent technique. However, anytime a formal repair is performed in an

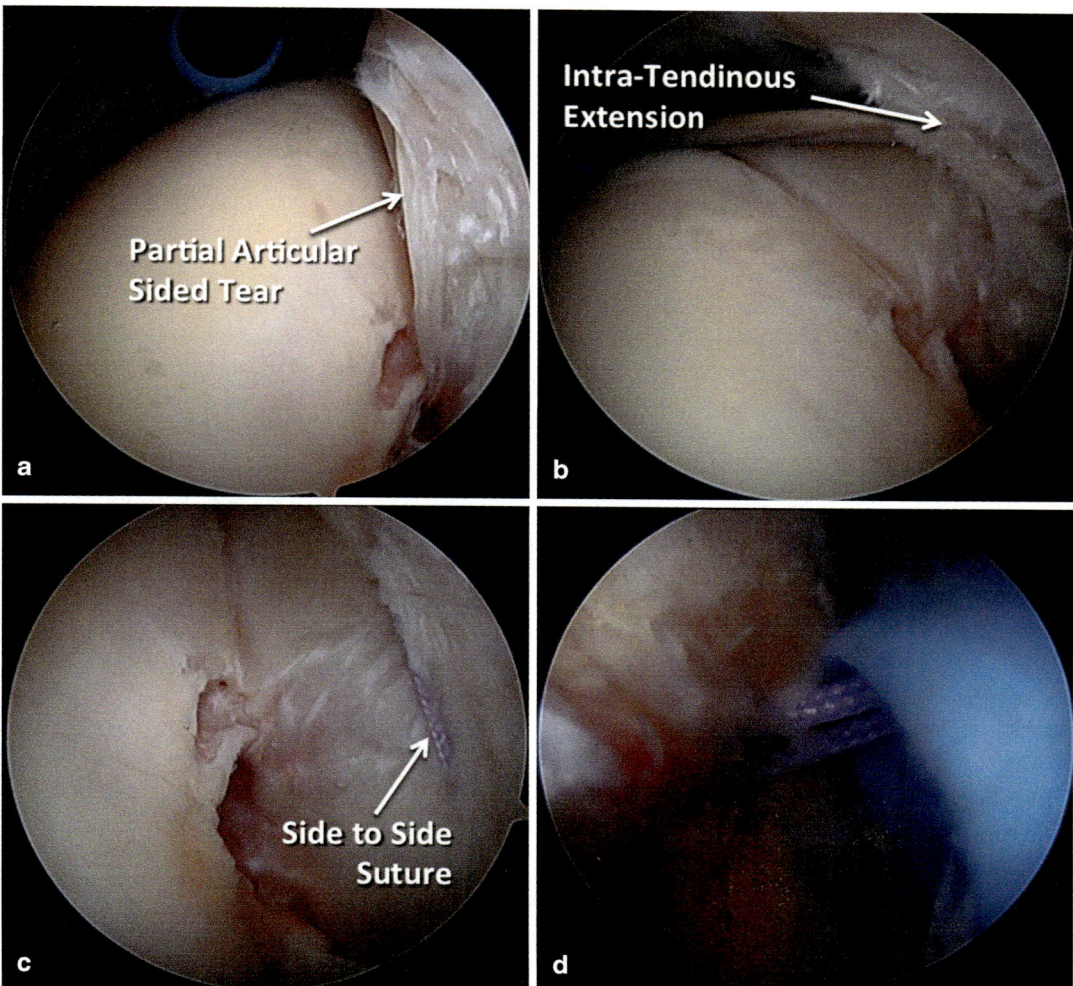

Fig. 13.3 In this athlete, a partial articular-sided tear (**a**) with medial intra-tendinous extension is identified (**b**). Because the lesion only involved a small portion of the footprint (<25%), it was treated with debridement and side-to-side intra-tendinous repair (**c**) that was tied in the subacromial space (**d**)

overhead athlete, it is critical to remember that if the repair site is too medial, the athlete is at a greater risk for dysfunction and failure secondary to internal impingement and restricted overhead motion. This phenomenon is unique to the overhead athlete and should always be taken into consideration during rotator cuff repairs in this population. To account for this, when a formal repair is actually indicated, it can be performed in a slightly lateralized position compared to standard techniques to limit the possibility of restricted overhead motion.

13.4.2 Full-Thickness Rotator Cuff Tears

13.4.2.1 Nonoperative Management

Similar to partial tear, nonoperative management is the initial treatment of choice for chronic, full-thickness tears in tennis players. Similarly, the focus of nonsurgical management is physical therapy focusing on the entire kinetic chain with gradual introduction of rotator cuff strengthening exercises and sport-specific exercises as able. Although the majority of chronic full-thickness tears are initially treated with a comprehensive course of nonoperative management, this is not always the case for acute injuries. Patients who sustain acute, full-thickness tears of a previously well-functioning rotator cuff are often considered for early surgical repair depending upon the patient demands and activity level.

13.4.2.2 Surgical Treatment

For patients with full-thickness tears that fail to respond to nonoperative treatment (or the high-demand athletes with acute tears), formal repair may be indicated. Our preferred technique is a double-row, transosseous equivalent repair. Although the steps of this technique have been published elsewhere [46–48], they include rotator cuff mobilization, footprint preparation, medial row fixation, suture passage ± knot tying, lateral row fixation, and subacromial decompression with acromioplasty as indicated (Fig. 13.4). Consideration must be given to the tear size, number of tendons involved, degree of retraction, and overall tendon quality. Large tears or those with an "L-shaped" tear pattern may require an element of marginal convergence in addition to repair to the footprint [49]. When multiple tendons are involved, it is critical that each tendon be addressed and repaired in an anatomic fashion. If cases of severe atrophy of the rotator cuff musculature, attempts at repair should be approached with caution as repair of this atrophic tissue is unlikely to lead to optimal outcomes.

As was stated previously, it is critical to remember that overhead athletes place very unique functional demands on their shoulders. Specifically, they require increased external rotation with the arm overhead and are prone to development of internal impingement. When formal cuff repairs are performed, one must be diligent to ensure that the repair is not performed too medial as this can reduce motion and lead to internal impingement.

13.4.3 Postoperative Rehabilitation

Following surgery, rehabilitation is primarily determined by the treatment rendered. In cases of debridement without formal repair, rehabilitation is accelerated. Patients are placed in a sling postoperatively, but range of motion exercises are initiated as soon as pain allows (typically 1–2 days following surgery). Full motion should be regained within 2–4 weeks, and a progressive strengthening program is introduced as tolerated. Patients are typically able to return to full, unrestricted activity within 3–4 months following surgery.

When formal repair is performed, postoperative rehabilitation is progressed at a slower pace. Generally speaking, there are four primary phases of the rehabilitation process including healing, motion, strengthening, and sport-specific activity. The rate in which patients progress through each of these phases is dependent upon the magnitude of the tear, quality of remaining tissue, integrity of the repair, and functional demands of the patient. For most patients with moderate-sized tears and robust repairs, a sling is worn for 4–6 weeks, and pendulum exercises are initiated

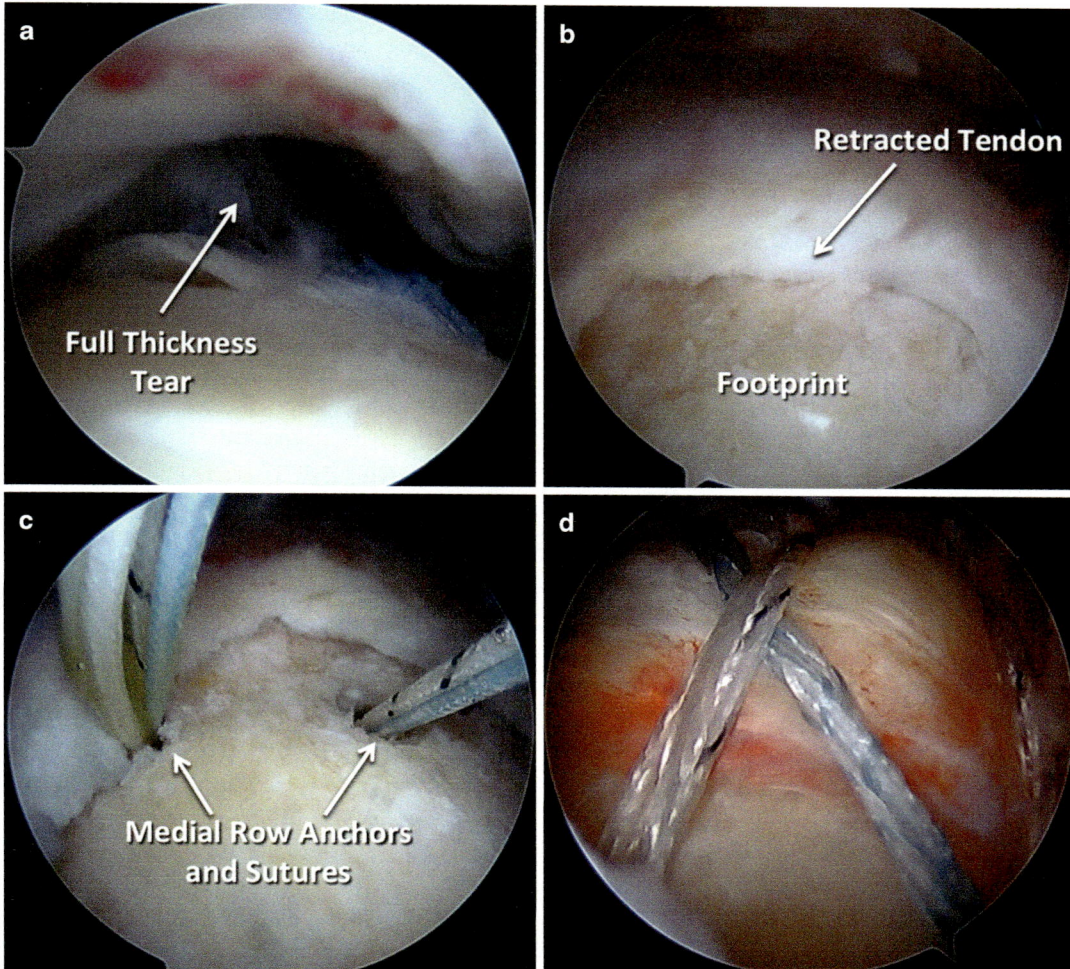

Fig. 13.4 In this patient with a full-thickness rotator cuff tear (**a**), the tendon was retracted approximately 2 cm medial (**b**). It was repaired using a double-row transosseous equivalent technique in which anchors are placed in the medial aspect of the footprint (**c**); sutures are passed through the tendon; and they are pulled into lateral row anchors to provide compression of the tendon against the entire surface area of the footprint (**d**)

right after surgery. Additional passive and active ROM exercises are instituted at 4–6 weeks. During this time, strengthening of the surrounding muscles (elbow flexors/extensors, wrist flexors/extensors, peri-scapular musculature) is typically instituted. Gentle strengthening of the rotator cuff begins around weeks 10–12 and is progressed as tolerated. This is followed by the introduction of sport-specific activities 4–6 months following surgery. A full return to tennis activity typically occurs around 6–8 months after surgery.

13.4.4 Outcomes

Although the literature reporting outcomes of rotator cuff injuries in elite tennis players is limited, a number of studies have reported results in mixed populations of athletes. For those with partial tears treated with simple debridement, the vast majority are able to return to sport. Although the overall satisfaction and general success rates range from 72% to 89% in the general athletic population, these results may not always hold up for overhead athletes [13–15, 50, 51]. When looking specifically at overhead athletes, Reynolds et al. [14] reported that 76% of professional pitchers were able to return to professional baseball, and this is further supported a previous study by Andrews et al. [15] in which 85% of throwers were able to return to competitive pitching. However, other studies have demonstrated inferior results with only 45–50% of overhead athletes returning to the same level of competition [50]. Ultimately, it appears that the vast majority of athletes are able to return to play following debridement of partial rotator cuff tears; however, results may not be as predictable in athletes participating in overhead sports.

For rotator cuff injuries requiring formal repair, a number of studies have been published on outcomes in overhead athletes. Conway et al. [18] reported on a series of overhead athletes (baseball players) who were able to return to the same level of competition at a rate of 89% following suture repair of intra-tendinous rotator cuff tears. For partial tears involving >50% of the footprint that are treated with tear completion and formal repair, the data is limited for the athletic population. While success rates in the general population have generally ranged from 85% to 100% [52–54], this may not be the case for competitive overhead athletes. In one study of trans-tendinous repair of partial-thickness cuff tears, Ide et al. found that of the six overhead throwers included, two returned to their previous level of competition, three returned to a lower level of play, and one did not return at all [55].

Full-thickness tears in overhead athletes have historically portended guarded results. In a recent study of professional pitchers, only 1 of 12 (8%) was able to return to his pre-injury level of play [56]. The results were slightly better for position players where three (one dominant side and two non-dominant) of four (75%) were able to return to professional baseball [56]. In another study, Tibone et al. [57] reported their results of treating partial- and full-thickness tears in overhead athletes. There were a total of three recreational tennis players included (two with partial tears and one with a complete tear). Following repair, all three (100%) experienced a good result and were able to return to recreational tennis. These results are limited, however, by the relatively small sample of tennis players included.

13.5 Summary

The high demands of the sport of tennis place a number of unique stresses on the shoulder joint. Effective play requires efficient transfer of energy along the entire kinetic chain of motion, and deficits in any link may place the shoulder at increased risk for injury. Accordingly, rotator cuff injuries are a common clinical concern for all overhead athletes, and tennis players are certainly no exception. The diagnosis is made by carefully considering the patient history, physical examination findings, and imaging results. The mainstay of treatment is a comprehensive course of nonsurgical management that focuses on activity modification, anti-inflammatory medications, and a robust physical therapy regimen to strengthen and stabilize the shoulder and entire kinetic chain. When these measures fail, surgery may be considered. Although the results of debridement for partial-thickness tears are encouraging in overhead athletes, the results of formal repair of full-thickness rotator cuff tears in this high-demand population are less optimistic.

References

1. Kovacs MS. Applied physiology of tennis performance. Br J Sports Med. 2006;40:381–5; discussion 386. https://doi.org/10.1136/bjsm.2005.023309.
2. Eygendaal D, Rahussen FTG, Diercks RL. Biomechanics of the elbow joint in tennis players and relation to pathology. Br J Sports Med. 2007;41:820–3. https://doi.org/10.1136/bjsm.2007.038307.
3. Kibler WB. Biomechanical analysis of the shoulder during tennis activities. Clin Sports Med. 1995;14:79–85.
4. Elliott B, Fleisig G, Nicholls R, Escamilia R. Technique effects on upper limb loading in the tennis serve. J Sci Med Sport. 2003;6:76–87.
5. van der Hoeven H, Kibler WB. Shoulder injuries in tennis players. Br J Sports Med. 2006;40:435–40. https://doi.org/10.1136/bjsm.2005.023218.
6. Dines JS, Bedi A, Williams PN, et al. Tennis injuries: epidemiology, pathophysiology, and treatment. J Am Acad Orthop Surg. 2015;23:181–9. https://doi.org/10.5435/jaaos-d-13-00148.

7. Pluim BM, Staal JB, Windler GE, Jayanthi N. Tennis injuries: occurrence, aetiology, and prevention. Br J Sports Med. 2006;40:415–23. https://doi.org/10.1136/bjsm.2005.023184.
8. Hutchinson MR, Laprade RF, Burnett QM, et al. Injury surveillance at the USTA Boys' Tennis Championships: a 6-yr study. Med Sci Sports Exerc. 1995;27:826–30.
9. Winge S, Jørgensen U, Lassen Nielsen A. Epidemiology of injuries in Danish championship tennis. Int J Sports Med. 1989;10:368–71. https://doi.org/10.1055/s-2007-1024930.
10. Lehman RC. Shoulder pain in the competitive tennis player. Clin Sports Med. 1988;7:309–27.
11. Perkins RH, Davis D. Musculoskeletal injuries in tennis. Phys Med Rehabil Clin N Am. 2006;17:609–31. https://doi.org/10.1016/j.pmr.2006.05.005.
12. Abrams GD, Renstrom PA, Safran MR. Epidemiology of musculoskeletal injury in the tennis player. Br J Sports Med. 2012;46:492–8. https://doi.org/10.1136/bjsports-2012-091164.
13. Economopoulos KJ, Brockmeier SF. Rotator cuff tears in overhead athletes. Clin Sports Med. 2012;31:675–92. https://doi.org/10.1016/j.csm.2012.07.005.
14. Reynolds SB, Dugas JR, Cain EL, et al. Débridement of small partial-thickness rotator cuff tears in elite overhead throwers. Clin Orthop Relat Res. 2008;466:614–21. https://doi.org/10.1007/s11999-007-0107-1.
15. Andrews JR, Broussard TS, Carson WG. Arthroscopy of the shoulder in the management of partial tears of the rotator cuff: a preliminary report. Arthroscopy. 1985;1:117–22.
16. Walch G, Boileau P, Noel E, Donell ST. Impingement of the deep surface of the supraspinatus tendon on the posterosuperior glenoid rim: an arthroscopic study. J Shoulder Elb Surg. 1992;1:238–45. https://doi.org/10.1016/S1058-2746(09)80065-7.
17. Neri BR, ElAttrache NS, Owsley KC, et al. Outcome of type II superior labral anterior posterior repairs in elite overhead athletes: effect of concomitant partial-thickness rotator cuff tears. Am J Sports Med. 2011;39:114–20. https://doi.org/10.1177/0363546510379971.
18. Conway JE. Arthroscopic repair of partial-thickness rotator cuff tears and SLAP lesions in professional baseball players. Orthop Clin North Am. 2001;32:443–56.
19. Reilly P, Amis AA, Wallace AL, Emery RJH. Supraspinatus tears: propagation and strain alteration. J Shoulder Elb Surg. 2003;12:134–8. https://doi.org/10.1067/mse.2003.7.
20. Reilly P, Amis AA, Wallace AL, Emery RJH. Mechanical factors in the initiation and propagation of tears of the rotator cuff. Quantification of strains of the supraspinatus tendon in vitro. J Bone Joint Surg Br. 2003;85:594–9.
21. Bey MJ, Song HK, Wehrli FW, Soslowsky LJ. Intratendinous strain fields of the intact supraspinatus tendon: the effect of glenohumeral joint position and tendon region. J Orthop Res. 2002;20:869–74. https://doi.org/10.1016/S0736-0266(01)00177-2.
22. Clark JM, Harryman DT. Tendons, ligaments, and capsule of the rotator cuff. Gross and microscopic anatomy. J Bone Joint Surg Am. 1992;74:713–25.
23. Nakajima T, Rokuuma N, Hamada K, et al. Histologic and biomechanical characteristics of the supraspinatus tendon: reference to rotator cuff tearing. J Shoulder Elb Surg. 1994;3:79–87. https://doi.org/10.1016/S1058-2746(09)80114-6.
24. Bey MJ, Ramsey ML, Soslowsky LJ. Intratendinous strain fields of the supraspinatus tendon: effect of a surgically created articular-surface rotator cuff tear. J Shoulder Elb Surg. 2002;11:562–9. https://doi.org/10.1067/mse.2002.126767.
25. Nho SJ, Yadav H, Shindle MK, Macgillivray JD. Rotator cuff degeneration: etiology and pathogenesis. Am J Sports Med. 2008;36:987–93. https://doi.org/10.1177/0363546508317344.
26. Hegedus EJ, Goode AP, Cook CE, et al. Which physical examination tests provide clinicians with the most value when examining the shoulder? Update of a systematic review with meta-analysis of individual tests. Br J Sports Med. 2012;46:964–78. https://doi.org/10.1136/bjsports-2012-091066.
27. Drakos MC, Rudzki JR, Allen AA, et al. Internal impingement of the shoulder in the overhead athlete. J Bone Joint Surg Am. 2009;91:2719–28. https://doi.org/10.2106/JBJS.I.00409.
28. Pearsall AW, Bonsell S, Heitman RJ, et al. Radiographic findings associated with symptomatic rotator cuff tears. J Shoulder Elb Surg. 2003;12:122–7. https://doi.org/10.1067/mse.2003.19.
29. Umans HR, Pavlov H, Berkowitz M, Warren RF. Correlation of radiographic and arthroscopic findings with rotator cuff tears and degenerative joint disease. J Shoulder Elb Surg. 2001;10:428–33. https://doi.org/10.1067/mse.2001.117123.
30. Tirman PF, Smith ED, Stoller DW, Fritz RC. Shoulder imaging in athletes. Semin Musculoskelet Radiol. 2004;8:29–40. https://doi.org/10.1055/s-2004-823013.
31. Parker BJ, Zlatkin MB, Newman JS, Rathur SK. Imaging of shoulder injuries in sports medicine: current protocols and concepts. Clin Sports Med. 2008;27:579–606. https://doi.org/10.1016/j.csm.2008.07.006.
32. Lee SY, Lee JK. Horizontal component of partial-thickness tears of rotator cuff: imaging characteristics and comparison of ABER view with oblique coronal view at MR arthrography initial results. Radiology. 2002;224:470–6. https://doi.org/10.1148/radiol.2241011261.
33. Meister K, Thesing J, Montgomery WJ, et al. MR arthrography of partial thickness tears of the undersurface of the rotator cuff: an arthroscopic correlation. Skelet Radiol. 2004;33:136–41. https://doi.org/10.1007/s00256-003-0688-z.
34. Tirman PF, Bost FW, Steinbach LS, et al. MR arthrographic depiction of tears of the rotator cuff: benefit of abduction and external rotation of the arm. Radiology. 1994;192:851–6. https://doi.org/10.1148/radiology.192.3.8058959.

35. van der Zwaal P, Thomassen BJW, Urlings TAJ, et al. Preoperative agreement on the geometric classification and 2-dimensional measurement of rotator cuff tears based on magnetic resonance arthrography. Arthroscopy. 2012;28:1329–36. https://doi.org/10.1016/j.arthro.2012.04.054.
36. Teefey SA, Rubin DA, Middleton WD, et al. Detection and quantification of rotator cuff tears. Comparison of ultrasonographic, magnetic resonance imaging, and arthroscopic findings in seventy-one consecutive cases. J Bone Joint Surg Am. 2004;86-A:708–16.
37. Teefey SA, Hasan SA, Middleton WD, et al. Ultrasonography of the rotator cuff. A comparison of ultrasonographic and arthroscopic findings in one hundred consecutive cases. J Bone Joint Surg Am. 2000;82:498–504.
38. Iannotti JP, Ciccone J, Buss DD, et al. Accuracy of office-based ultrasonography of the shoulder for the diagnosis of rotator cuff tears. J Bone Joint Surg Am. 2005;87:1305–11. https://doi.org/10.2106/JBJS.D.02100.
39. Lenza M, Buchbinder R, Takwoingi Y, et al (2013) Magnetic resonance imaging, magnetic resonance arthrography and ultrasonography for assessing rotator cuff tears in people with shoulder pain for whom surgery is being considered. Cochrane database Syst Rev CD009020. doi: https://doi.org/10.1002/14651858.CD009020.pub2.
40. Wilk KE, Meister K, Andrews JR. Current concepts in the rehabilitation of the overhead throwing athlete. Am J Sports Med. 2002;30:136–51.
41. Burkhart SS, Morgan CD, Kibler WB. The disabled throwing shoulder: spectrum of pathology Part III: The SICK scapula, scapular dyskinesis, the kinetic chain, and rehabilitation. Arthroscopy. 2003;19:641–61.
42. Kibler WB, McMullen J, Uhl T. Shoulder rehabilitation strategies, guidelines, and practice. Orthop Clin North Am. 2001;32:527–38.
43. Brockmeier SF, Dodson CC, Gamradt SC, et al. Arthroscopic intratendinous repair of the delaminated partial-thickness rotator cuff tear in overhead athletes. Arthroscopy. 2008;24:961–5. https://doi.org/10.1016/j.arthro.2007.08.016.
44. Greiwe RM, Ahmad CS. Management of the throwing shoulder: cuff, labrum and internal impingement. Orthop Clin North Am. 2010;41:309–23. https://doi.org/10.1016/j.ocl.2010.03.001.
45. Gonzalez-Lomas G, Kippe MA, Brown GD, et al. In situ transtendon repair outperforms tear completion and repair for partial articular-sided supraspinatus tendon tears. J shoulder Elb Surg. 2008;17:722–8. https://doi.org/10.1016/j.jse.2008.01.148.
46. Park MC, Tibone JE, ElAttrache NS, et al. Part II: Biomechanical assessment for a footprint-restoring transosseous-equivalent rotator cuff repair technique compared with a double-row repair technique. J Shoulder Elb Surg. 2007;16:469–76. https://doi.org/10.1016/j.jse.2006.09.011.
47. Park MC, Elattrache NS, Ahmad CS, Tibone JE. "Transosseous-equivalent" rotator cuff repair technique. Arthroscopy. 2006;22:1360.e1–5. https://doi.org/10.1016/j.arthro.2006.07.017.
48. Millett PJ, Mazzocca A, Guanche CA. Mattress double anchor footprint repair: a novel, arthroscopic rotator cuff repair technique. Arthroscopy. 2004;20:875–9. https://doi.org/10.1016/j.arthro.2004.07.015.
49. Davidson J, Burkhart SS. The geometric classification of rotator cuff tears: a system linking tear pattern to treatment and prognosis. Arthroscopy. 2010;26:417–24. https://doi.org/10.1016/j.arthro.2009.07.009.
50. Payne LZ, Altchek DW, Craig EV, Warren RF. Arthroscopic treatment of partial rotator cuff tears in young athletes. A preliminary report. Am J Sports Med. 1997;25:299–305.
51. Snyder SJ, Pachelli AF, Del Pizzo W, et al. Partial thickness rotator cuff tears: results of arthroscopic treatment. Arthroscopy. 1991;7:1–7.
52. Wright SA, Cofield RH. Management of partial-thickness rotator cuff tears. J Shoulder Elb Surg. 1996;5:458–66.
53. Deutsch A. Arthroscopic repair of partial-thickness tears of the rotator cuff. J Shoulder Elb Surg. 2007;16:193–201. https://doi.org/10.1016/j.jse.2006.07.001.
54. Shin S-J. A comparison of 2 repair techniques for partial-thickness articular-sided rotator cuff tears. Arthroscopy. 2012;28:25–33. https://doi.org/10.1016/j.arthro.2011.07.005.
55. Ide J, Maeda S, Takagi K. Arthroscopic transtendon repair of partial-thickness articular-side tears of the rotator cuff: anatomical and clinical study. Am J Sports Med. 2005;33:1672–9. https://doi.org/10.1177/0363546505277141.
56. Mazoué CG, Andrews JR. Repair of full-thickness rotator cuff tears in professional baseball players. Am J Sports Med. 2006;34:182–9. https://doi.org/10.1177/0363546505279916.
57. Tibone JE, Elrod B, Jobe FW, et al. Surgical treatment of tears of the rotator cuff in athletes. J Bone Joint Surg Am. 1986;68:887–91.

Labral Injury and Posterior Impingement in Elite Tennis Players

14

Giovanni Di Giacomo and Nicola de Gasperis

14.1 Introduction

The shoulder is the most mobile joint in the human body. Its anatomical design provides stability allowing a wide range of motion in all directions. This leads to a fragile equilibrium between stability and mobility, especially in the tennis player, who is trying to generate as much energy as possible for the serving motion. The repetition of the abduction-external rotation movement of the arm during the overhead action carries an increased risk of overloading various structures around the shoulder. The cause of shoulder pain in the overhead athlete is very difficult to identify and diagnose. Pathologic contact between the posterior margin of the glenoid and the articular surface of posterosuperior rotator cuff tendons is known as posterior internal impingement (PII) [1–3]. Young overhead athletes, continuously performing high velocity throwing actions over the years, usually go to specific osseous and soft tissue adaptations. Adaptive anatomic changes in throwers athletes that can lead to internal impingement include glenohumeral internal rotation deficit (GIRD), increased humeral and glenoid retroversion, acquired glenohumeral anterior-posterior instability, scapular weakness, and concomitant rotator cuff weakness. The chronic repeated compression or impingement leads to articular tears of the rotator cuff tendons as well as lesion of the superior labrum (SLAP lesions).

14.2 Biomechanical Aspects and Pathomechanics of Posterior Impingement and Labral Injuries in Tennis Players

To understand the function of the shoulder in the tennis serve, it is important to consider all aspects that contribute to this action. To create an optimal service motion with maximum power release, an intact kinetic chain function, a normal scapular function, and intact dynamic and static stabilizers of the shoulder are necessary. During the serve, the shoulder is part of a kinetic energy chain, in which the body is considered as a linked system of articulated segments, each part contributing to the final energy needed for hitting the ball. All segments (leg, hip, trunk, shoulder, elbow, and wrist) of the kinetic chain have to be in perfect shape to be able to transfer a sufficient level of energy to produce an effective serve. The kinetic chain allows generation, summation, and transfer of forces from the legs to the hand. Breakage of a link in the proximal part of the chain will lead to a higher demand on the more distally located segments. From this

G. Di Giacomo (✉)
Department of Orthopaedics and Trauma, Concordia Hospital, Rome, Italy

N. de Gasperis
Concordia Hospital for Special Surgery, Rome, Italy

mechanism, it is clear that the more distal parts of the kinetic chain (shoulder, elbow, and wrist) are more susceptible to overuse and injury than the proximal parts [4]. The scapula has a key role in the function of the shoulder. It acts as a stable base for the humeral head during the overhead motion. It also has to move around the thoracic wall while the arm moves from early cocking to late cocking and follow-through (retraction/protraction) and has to move in an upward direction (rotation) in order to clear the acromion from the moving humeral head. Finally, it forms a stable base for the intrinsic and extrinsic muscles that control arm motion and the position of the scapula against the thorax. Fine-tuning of scapular motion is provided by coupling of muscle action (serratus anterior, upper and lower trapezius, latissimus dorsi, and the rhomboideus muscles). Dysfunction of these muscles leads to scapular dyskinesis, caused by inflexibility, weakness, and imbalance of the muscles. This dysfunction can be either primary through direct injury of the muscles or secondary as a result of pain-induced muscular inhibition [5, 6]. The term "SICK scapula" was introduced to describe a pathological state of the scapula, characterized by scapular malposition, inferior medial border prominence, coracoid pain and malposition, and kinesis abnormalities of the scapula. This syndrome, characterized by a drooping shoulder, is often seen in overhead athletes and is thought to contribute to the development of shoulder injuries. In most tennis players, such an abnormal position of the scapula can be detected. Although it seems that the affected shoulder has a lower position compared with the healthy side, actually there is scapular malposition consisting of forward tilting and protraction. According to Kibler [7], this clinical picture is associated with anterior coracoid-based pain, posterosuperior localized pain, and pain at the superolateral side of the shoulder (subacromial space, acromioclavicular joint). The role of the capsulolabral complex in the development of a shoulder injury remains a topic of debate. The most important function of the ligaments is to limit the range of motion of the shoulder joint. At the beginning of abduction-external rotation, it is mainly the dynamic stabilizers that keep the shoulder in a central position in the glenoid socket. At the end of the range of motion, the ligamentous structures become more important. At maximal abduction and external rotation, the inferior glenohumeral ligament (IGHL) is taut and limits further movement [8]. In the IGHL, a distinctive reinforcement is present, called the anterior band, which moves in front of the humeral head, providing a restraint to anterior and inferior displacement. Behind this, the posterior part of the IGHL shifts in front of the posterior side of the humeral head in abduction and internal rotation, protecting the head against posterior displacement. This dynamic interplay of the ligaments means that, in the overhead athlete, the shoulder is often susceptible to injury. Several explanations have been developed to clarify the pathogenesis of shoulder injuries in overhead athletes. As mentioned above, one explanation is that the repetitive nature of the serve causes microtrauma of the anterior capsule. Elongation of the ligaments may be responsible for subtle instability. The anterior displacement of the humeral head shifts the center of rotation to a more anterior position. This probably brings, in abduction and external rotation (ABER) position, the greater tuberosity and rotator cuff tendons close to the posterior glenoid, causing posterior internal impingement (PII) [9]. Although PII occurs in healthy shoulders, it can become pathological in the tennis player. PII is characterized by pain in the posterior aspect of the glenohumeral joint of overhead-throwing athletes during the late cocking phase of the throw, where the arm is in a position of full external rotation and abduction of at least 90°. The pain is due to a compression of the supraspinatus and infraspinatus tendons by the posteriorly rotated greater tuberosity of the humeral head against the posterosuperior portion of the glenoid. This occurs when the humeral shaft moves posteriorly beyond the plane of the scapular body during the cocking phase of throwing [10]. In this phase, if the scapular body and the humeral shaft fail to remain on the same plane of movement, rotator cuff tendons could remain between the humeral head and the glenoid rim causing PII. Another common finding in tennis players is a change in the rotational arc of the shoulder. Usually, there is an

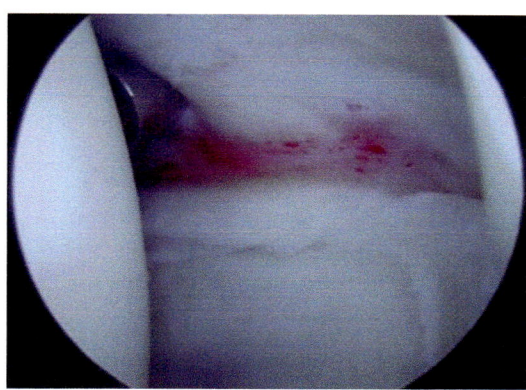

Fig. 14.1 Arthroscopic view of posterior capsule inflammation

increase in external rotation and a decrease in internal rotation caused by posteroinferior capsular contracture [11, 12]. It has been suggested that there is an association of glenohumeral internal rotation deficit (GIRD) with the development of shoulder injuries [13]. If the limitation of internal rotation exceeds the gain in external rotation, resulting in a decrease in rotational arc (>10% of the contralateral side), the shoulder is susceptible to injury [7]. The stiffness and shortening of the posterior structures have consequences for stabilization of the shoulder during abduction and external rotation (Fig. 14.1). According to O'Brien et al., the IGHL is the most important stabilizing capsular component in the shoulder (anterior band in abduction-external rotation; posterior band in internal rotation) [14]. In the position of abduction and external rotation of the shoulder, the posterior IGHL is positioned under the humeral head. In the case of a functionally shortened posterior IGHL, a posterosuperior directed force exists, shifting the center of rotation of the shoulder to a more posterosuperior location. This posterosuperior shift can lead to anatomical lesions of the labral complex (SLAP lesion).

14.3 Posterior Impingement

During the late cocking phase of throwing, the shoulder reaches a maximum external rotation of 170°–180°, while abduction is maintained at 90°–100°. In this ABER position, Walch et al. were the first to note that contact of the rotator cuff occurs between the greater tuberosity and the posterosuperior labrum [1]. This was called posterior internal impingement (PII). Following MRI studies showed that this contact is a physiological phenomenon and may occur in shoulders of normal individuals during the ABER position [15, 16]. However, as a result of the throwing biomechanics and the structural adaptations which occur in shoulders of these athletes, this contact is intensified and leads to pathological PII. This clinical syndrome is characterized by posterosuperior pain and glenohumeral joint dysfunction. Athletes participating overhead sports like tennis, baseball, water polo, and javelin are particularly at risk in developing PII. In these athletes, the pathological shift of the axis of glenohumeral joint contact/rotation occurs as the arm is brought in ABER position during the throwing or serving action, which leads to a no more physiological posterosuperior impingement [17]. There are two different theories which offer a biomechanical explanation for the change in the contact/rotational axis of the glenohumeral joint. In an earlier theory, Jobe postulated that anterior capsuloligamentous structures fail as a result of microtrauma caused by the repeated excessive strain occurring during the late cocking phase of throwing [3]. The injured anterior capsular structures are then less able to contain the humeral head leading to a posterior displacement of the contact point between the humeral head and glenoid which ultimately accentuates the contact of the rotator cuff between the posterosuperior labrum and the greater tuberosity in ABER position. In a more recent study, Burkhart proposed that the posteroinferior capsular contraction, caused by frequent microtrauma subsequent to repetitive distraction and rotational forces during the follow-through phase, was the initial mechanism of the glenohumeral contact point shift [11]. This theory is in line with the major clinical finding in patients with PII which is a glenohumeral internal rotational deficit (GIRD) [18]. Burkhart's theory also offers an explanation for the physiological adaptations in throwers as well as the pathologies commonly associated with PII. The new glenohumeral point of contact allows greater external rotation. This external rotation gain arises from the increased clearance of the greater tuberosity over the glenoid during rotation as well as a decrease in the cam effect of the anterior capsule. The thrower is then subject to rotator cuff tears due to a combination of impingement and increased torsional and shearing forces resulting from the fibers overtwisting. The increased external rotation in the late cocking phase of throwing also creates more torsional stress upon the biceps anchor leading to a greater risk of SLAP lesion [19]. Shear stress and impingement could result in posterosuperior labral tears. Young throwing athletes have an increased number and frequency of smaller labral tears [19]. It is important to note that abnormal MRI findings do not necessarily correlate with the existence of pain or the likelihood of developing PII in the throwing shoulder. Halbrect et al. noted abnormal MRI findings indicating potential pathological PII in asymptomatic shoulders of throwing athletes [16].Their study raises the suggestion that MRI findings may manifest prior to the clinical picture of pathological PII (Fig. 14.2a, b). The presentation of PII can be classified into three stages [3]. In stage 1 the athlete complains of poor throwing or serving performance and discomfort in warming up when the shoulder is placed in the ABER position. In stage 2 the thrower is able to localize pain to the posterior aspect of the shoulder during the late cocking phase. Stage 3 is described as the persistence of symptoms after the end of the rehabilitation program.

14.4 Clinical Evaluation and Treatment of Posterior Impingement

Internal impingement typically affects young to middle-aged adults; in most major case series of internal impingement, patients are under 40 years of age and participate in activities involving repetitive abducting and externally rotating arm motions or positions [20–23]. The majority of patients who have been identified with internal impingement are overhead athletes [24, 25]. Most patients present with a progressive decrease in throwing velocity or a loss of control and performance [10, 26, 27]. Chronic, diffuse posterior shoulder girdle pain is common in terms of the presenting complaint, but the pain may be localized to the joint line. Despite posterior shoulder pain being the most common complaint among patients with internal impingement, patients may also present with symptoms similar to those asso-

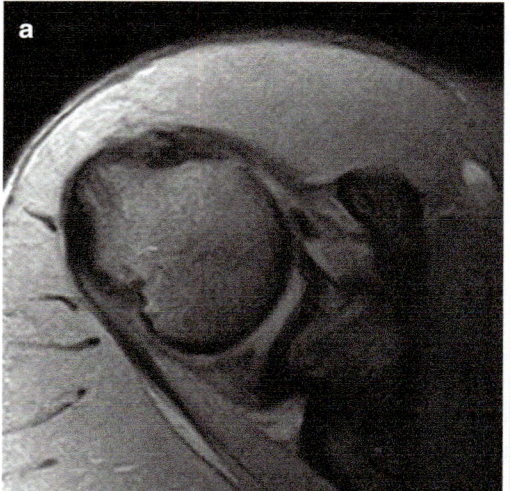
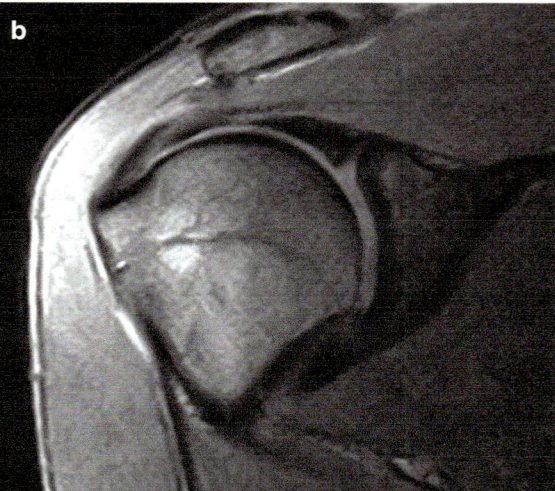

Fig. 14.2 (a) MRI axial view of a professional tennis player showing posterior impingement signs on the humeral head and on the posterior-superior aspect of the glenoid. (b) MRI frontal view of a professional tennis player showing SLAP lesion signs

ciated with classic rotator cuff disease [28, 29]. Alternatively, patients may also have instability symptoms, such as apprehension or the sensation of subluxation with the arm in an abduction and external rotation position. Burkhart et al. reported an 80% rate of anterior coracoid pain in their series of 96 athletes with a disabled throwing shoulder, rather than isolated posterior shoulder pain, described as the most common presenting symptom [5]. Posterior glenohumeral joint line tenderness, increased external rotation, and decreased internal rotation (GIRD) are the most common physical examination findings in throwing athletes. With regard to concomitant increased external rotation, Myers et al. recently emphasized that throwers with pathological internal impingement exhibiting significantly increased posterior shoulder tightness and glenohumeral internal rotation deficits do not necessarily gain significantly increased external rotation [18]. In addition, scapular dyskinesis is a commonly reported finding. Characteristic features include a prominent inferior medial border of the scapula and the appearance of an inferiorly dropped throwing shoulder compared to the non-throwing side [30]. Meister et al. investigated the ability of a single maneuver, referred to as the "posterior impingement sign," to detect the presence of articular-sided rotator cuff tears and posterior labrum lesions [31]. The subjects were tested for the presence of deep posterior shoulder pain when the arm was brought into a position similar to that noted during the late cocking phase of throwing. The sensitivity and specificity of the posterior impingement sign were 75.5% and 85%, respectively. MRI is considered the gold standard in the work-up of any young patient presenting with shoulder pain [9]. MR findings in internal impingement include articular-sided partial-thickness rotator cuff tears of the supraspinatus, infraspinatus, or both tendons and posterior or superior labral lesions [32]. The tears of the rotator cuff tendons are usually small and involve the articular surface. In addition, these athletes often present with associated posterosuperior labral abnormalities. Cysts and impaction deformity are also seen at the posterior greater tuberosity and can increase diagnostic confidence in the diagnosis of internal impingement. The vast majority of shoulder injuries in throwers should initially be treated with a conservative, nonoperative regime. Only significant structural injuries such as an acute rotator cuff tear, dislocation, or SLAP lesion deserve early surgical intervention. Every overhead athlete requires a training program that strengthens all elements of the kinetic chain of the throwing motion. Patients with mild symptoms and early phases of the disorder need active rest, including a complete break from throwing along with physical therapy. Anti-inflammatory measures to "cool down" the irritated shoulder can be beneficial in accelerating the rehabilitation process. This includes nonsteroidal anti-inflammatory drugs (NSAIDs) and occasionally a corticosteroid injection. Athletes with longer-lasting problems need a rehabilitation program emphasizing dynamic stability, rotator cuff strengthening, capsular stretching, and a scapular stabilization program [5, 33, 34]. Rehabilitation program Phase 1: the primary aims of the rehabilitation program are aimed at allowing the injured tissue to heal, modification of activity, decreasing pain and inflammation, on the re-establishment of a baseline dynamic stability, correction of the muscle balance, and restoration of proprioception. In addition, the athlete's activities (such as throwing and exercises) must be modified to a pain-free level. Active-assisted motion exercises may be used to normalize shoulder motion, particularly shoulder internal rotation and horizontal adduction. The thrower should also perform specific stretches and flexibility exercises for the benefit of the posterior capsule and rotator cuff muscles. Rehabilitation program Phase 2: the primary goals are to intensify the strengthening program, continue to improve flexibility, and facilitate neuromuscular control. During this phase, the rehabilitation program is progressed to more aggressive isotonic strengthening activities with emphasis on restoration of the muscle balance. Selective muscle activation is also used to restore muscle balance and symmetry. Contractures of the posterior structures, the pectoralis minor muscle, and the short head of the biceps muscle also contribute to a glenohumeral internal rotation deficit and increase the anterior tilting of the scapula. Borstad et al. found the "sleeper stretch" to be effective for a stretch on the posterior aspect of the shoulder [35]. Several authors have emphasized the importance of scapular muscle strength and neuromuscular control as a contribution to normal shoulder function [30]. Isotonic exercise techniques are used to strengthen the scapular muscles. Overhead-throwing athletes often exhibit external rotator muscle weakness. Also during this second rehabilitation phase, the overhead-throwing athlete is instructed to perform core-strengthening exercises for the abdominal and lower back musculature. In addition, the athlete should perform lower extremity strengthening and participate in a running program including jogging and sprints. Upper extremity stretching exercises are continued as needed to maintain soft tissue flexibility. Rehabilitation program Phase 3: the goals are to initiate aggressive strengthening drills, enhance power and endurance, perform functional drills, and gradually initiate throwing activities. Dynamic stabilization drills are also performed to enhance proprioception and neuromuscular control. An interval throwing program may be initiated in this phase of rehabilitation. Rehabilitation program Phase 4: this phase usually involves progression of the interval throwing program as well as neuromuscular maintenance. The goal is to return to the full throwing velocity over the course of 3 months. To prevent the effects of overtraining or throwing, it is essential to instruct the athlete what to do through specific exercises throughout the year. A lack of improvement after 3 months, or an inability to return to competition within 6 months, constitutes failure of the nonoperative conservative management and thus should result in an additional diagnostic testing, and, if necessary, operative intervention should be considered. The following arthroscopic examination is performed in terms of a systematic review of the entire shoulder. The surgeon should carefully evaluate the entire shoulder and look for evidence of instability in the biceps tendon, biceps anchor, labrum, capsule, rotator interval, and the rotator cuff insertion. Surgical intervention should be directed toward specific pathological lesions believed to correspond to the patient's symptoms or play a role in the complex pathophysiology of internal impingement. Despite this treatment, up to 90% of the patients can be expected to have persistent pain, although to a lesser degree, while playing tennis. Furthermore, only 50% of tennis players with posterosuperior glenoid impingement surgically treated can be expected to return to tennis at their preinjury level [25].

14.5 Labral Injury (SLAP Lesion)

The labrum is a fibrous structure strongly attached around the edge of the glenoid that increases the contact surface area between the glenoid and the humeral head [36]. The glenoid labrum enhances shoulder stability reducing humeral head translation, increasing the "concavity-compression" effect between the humeral head and the glenoid, increasing the overall depth of the glenoid fossa, and contributing to the stabilizing effect of the long head of the biceps anchor [36–41]. The superior labrum is rather loose and mobile and has a "meniscal-like" aspect, while the inferior labrum appears rounded and more tightly attached to the glenoid rim. The labrum is attached to the lateral portion of the biceps anchor superiorly. Additionally, approximately 50% of the fibers of the long head of the biceps originate from the superior labrum, and the remaining fibers originate from the superior glenoid tubercle. There are several injury mechanisms that are speculated to be responsible for creating SLAP lesions. These mechanisms range from single traumatic events to repetitive microtraumatic injuries. Repetitive overhead activity is maybe the most common mechanism of injury responsible for producing SLAP injuries. Andrews et al. originally described the detachment of the superior labrum in a subset of throwing athletes in 1985 [42]. Later Snyder et al. introduced the term SLAP lesion—indicating an injury located within the superior labrum extending anterior to posterior [43]. They originally classified these lesions into four distinct categories based on the type of lesion present, emphasizing that this lesion may disrupt the origin of the long head of the biceps. Over time, modifications have been made to the initial classification system such that ten different types of SLAP tears have now been identified [44–48]. Andrews et al. first hypothesized that SLAP pathology in overhead-throwing athletes was the result of the high eccentric activity of the biceps during the arm deceleration and follow-through phases of the overhead throw [42, 49]. Burkhart et al. and Morgan et al. have hypothesized a "peel back" mechanism that produces SLAP lesion in the overhead athlete. They suggest that when the shoulder is placed in a position of abduction and maximal external rotation, the rotation produces a twist at the base of the biceps, transmitting torsional force to the anchor [48, 50]. Furthermore, Jobe and Walch et al. have also demonstrated that when the arm is in a maximally externally rotated position, there is contact between the posterior-superior labral lesions and the rotator cuff [1, 3]. A recent study conducted at the authors' research center simulated each of these mechanisms using cadaveric models [40]. Nine pairs of cadaveric shoulders were loaded to biceps anchor complex failure in either a position of simulated in-line loading (similar to the deceleration phase of throwing) or simulated peel back mechanism (similar to the cocking phase of overhead throwing). Results showed that seven of eight of the in-line loading group failed in the midsubstance of the biceps tendon with one of eight fracturing at the supraglenoid tubercle. However, all eight of the simulated peel back group failures resulted in a type II SLAP lesion. The ultimate strength of the biceps anchor was significantly different when the two loading techniques were compared. The biceps anchor demonstrated significantly higher ultimate strength with the in-line loading (508 N) as opposed to the ultimate strength seen during the peel back loading mechanism (202 N). In theory, SLAP lesions most likely occur in overhead athletes from a combination of these two previously described forces. The eccentric biceps activity during deceleration may serve to weaken the biceps-labrum complex, while the torsional peel back force may result in the posterosuperior detachment of the labral anchor.

Several authors have also reported a strong correlation between SLAP lesions and glenohumeral instability. Normal biceps function and glenohumeral stability are dependent on a stable superior labrum and biceps anchor. Pagnani et al. found that a complete lesion of the superior portion of the labrum large enough to destabilize the insertion of the biceps was associated with significant increases in anterior-posterior and superior-inferior glenohumeral translation [37]. Reinold et al. reported that in a series of 130 overhead athletes with symptomatic hyperlaxity undergoing thermal-assisted capsular shrinkage (TACS) of the glenohumeral joint, 69% exhibited superior labral degeneration, while 35% had type II SLAP lesions [51]. Furthermore, Kim et al. reported that maximal biceps activity occurred when the shoulder was abducted to 90° and externally rotated to 120° in patients with anterior instability [52]. Because this position is remarkably similar to the cocking position of the overhand throwing motion, the finding of instability may cause or facilitate the progression of internal impingement (impingement of the infraspinatus on the posterosuperior glenoid rim) in the overhead athlete.

Although this tear pattern has been described and studied for quite some time, the ideal treatment of these injuries remains elusive. Indications for operative repair remain unclear with increasing reports of complications and suboptimal outcomes within the literature [53, 54]. With the knowledge that degenerative changes of the superior labrum occur commonly with age and improvements in magnetic resonance imaging quality, SLAP tears are becoming a more frequent diagnosis. Zhang et al. recently reviewed the demographic trends of SLAP repairs in the United States using a publicly available database and found that the number of SLAP repairs significantly increased over time from 2004 to 2009 [55]. This increase in the number of diagnosed SLAP tears that are treated with arthroscopic repair is interesting because the ideal treatment for SLAP tears has not been elucidated and several studies have shown increasing risk of complications and poor outcomes with inability to return to sport particularly in overhead-throwing athletes.

14.6 Clinical Evaluation and Treatment of SLAP Lesion

Clinical examination is essential to establishing the potential presence of glenoid labral pathology. Clinical examination to detect SLAP lesions is often difficult because of the common presence of concomitant pathology in patients presenting with this type of condition. Mileski and Snyder reported that 29% of their patients with SLAP lesions exhibited partial-thickness rotator cuff tears, 11% complete rotator cuff tears, and 22% Bankart lesions of the anterior glenoid [56]. Kim et al. prospectively analyzed the clinical features of different types of SLAP lesion as they vary with patient population in 139 cases [57]. They demonstrated that type I SLAP lesions are typically associated with rotator cuff pathology, while type III and IV lesions are associated with traumatic instability. They also note that injuries presenting concomitant with type II SLAP lesions vary by patient age, with older patients presenting more often with rotator cuff pathology and younger patients instability. Pain complaints are typically intermittent and are most frequently associated with overhead activity. Overhead athletes typically report a loss of velocity and accuracy along with general uneasiness of the shoulder. Probably the most predictive subjective complaint in the athlete is the inability to perform sporting activities at a high level. The physical examination should include a complete evaluation of bilateral passive and active range of glenohumeral motion with particular emphasis placed on determining the presence, persistence, and behavior of any painful arc of motion. A wide variety of potentially useful special test maneuvers have been described to help determine the presence of labral pathology in an overhead thrower, including the active compression test, the biceps load test, the biceps load test II, the pain provocation test, the resisted supination and external rotation test, the pronated load test, and the modified dynamic labral shear test [52, 58–62]. Several authors also recommend MR enhanced arthrography in order to detect SLAP lesions, but its reliability for the diagnosis is disputed [63–66]. Nevertheless definitive diagnosis of SLAP lesion requires arthroscopy. Conservative management of SLAP lesions is often the first line of treatment and has been shown to be successful. Edwards et al. showed that 10 of 15 overhead throwers with a known SLAP lesion who were treated with nonoperative management were able to return to play at the same level or better [67]. However, frequently, rehabilitation is unsuccessful; therefore, surgical intervention is often warranted to repair the labral lesion while addressing any concomitant pathology. Treatment in these patients remains somewhat controversial [68–71]. Not all SLAP tears require surgical intervention, and approximately 70–80% of patients who undergo surgical fixation can expect to return to their previous sports [44, 67, 72–74]. The marginal benefits of SLAP repair surgery have led some surgeons to consider biceps tenodesis as an alternative procedure [73, 75–79]. Several open and arthroscopic tenodesis techniques have been described, but none of them seem to be superior to another. To date the literature does not provide evidence to support one technique over the other, and there are advantages to each procedure. The lack of physical exam maneuvers and diagnostic tests to reliably diagnose SLAP tears has led to a significant increase in the number of SLAP repairs performed in the United States [55]. Most SLAP repairs are performed for type II SLAP tears (Figs. 14.3 and 14.4). The outcomes following debridement (without repair) of unstable type II and IV SLAP lesions have been poor, and thus these two types of lesions should be repaired in order to restore the normal anatomy [80]. In the presence of a type II SLAP lesion, the superior labrum should be reattached to the glenoid and the biceps anchor stabilized. The type II lesion is often stabilized utilizing suture anchors. Treatment of type IV SLAP lesions is generally based on the extent to which the biceps anchor is involved. When biceps involvement is less than approximately 30% of the entire anchor, the torn tissue is typically resected and the superior labrum reattached. If the biceps tear is more substantial, a side-to-side repair of the biceps tendon, in addition to reattachment of the superior

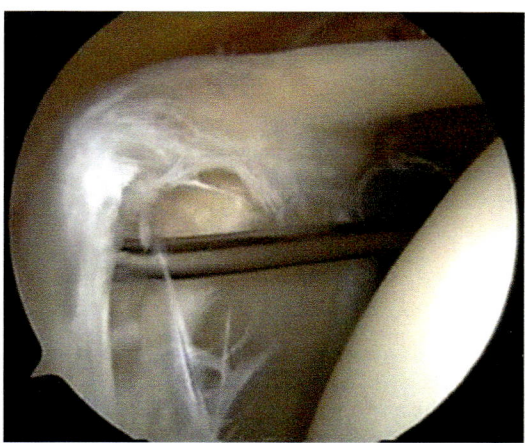

Fig. 14.3 Arthroscopic view of a type II SLAP lesion

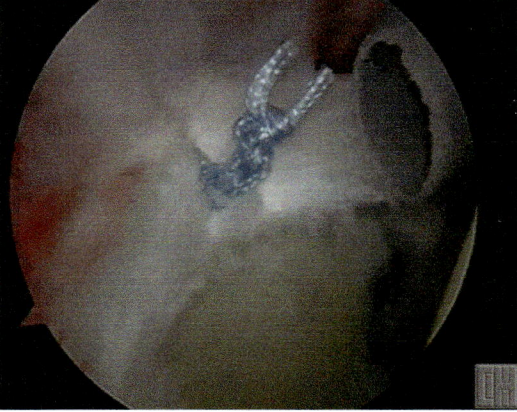

Fig. 14.4 Arthroscopic view of a type II SLAP lesion repair

labrum, is generally performed. However, if the biceps tear is extensive enough to substantially alter the biceps origin, a biceps tenodesis or tenotomy is more practical than a direct repair. Weber et al. recently reviewed data from the American Board of Orthopaedic Surgery Part II Database from 2003 to 2007 to determine the incidence rates, complications, and outcomes for SLAP repairs [53]. The most concerning conclusion was that only 26.3% of patients stated that they were pain-free, whereas only 13.1% rated their function as normal. Recently, multiple authors have reported outcomes of SLAP repairs as unpredictable [53, 54]. Provencher et al. reviewed 179 patients who underwent repair for a type II SLAP tear [81]. At a mean follow-up of 40.4 months, 37% were classified as a failure, and 28% underwent a revision. This study also found that the only risk factor that significantly increased a patient's risk of failure was age more than 36. Similarly, Boileau et al. found that 60% of patients who underwent repair for a type II SLAP tear were disappointed because of persistent pain and only 20% were able to return to sports at their preinjury level [73]. This was in comparison to a group of patients who underwent arthroscopic biceps tenodesis for a type II SLAP tear and showed a 93% satisfaction rate and an 87% return to the previous level of sport. Erickson et al. showed that the number of biceps tenodeses significantly increased over time, whereas that of SLAP repairs significantly decreased over time [82]. Although some argue that SLAP repairs restore arm function better than biceps tenodesis, Chalmers et al. proved this to be inaccurate [75]. The authors evaluated 18 pitchers (7 uninjured controls, 6 after a SLAP repair, and 5 after a subpectoral biceps tenodesis) and found that pitchers who underwent a SLAP repair had altered patterns of thoracic rotation compared with the controls and pitchers who had undergone a biceps tenodesis. Laughlin et al. similarly found altered mechanics in 13 collegiate and professional pitchers who underwent SLAP repairs compared with a group of control pitchers [83]. Therefore, in high-level athletes, biceps tenodesis is a reliable option compared with SLAP repair. Because overtreatment of SLAP tears may result in increased complications such as stiffness, persistent pain, and need for revision surgery, the future treatment of SLAP tears will likely see an increase in biceps tenodesis and a decrease in SLAP repairs based on the outcomes reported in the literature and the high risk of failure and complications seen with SLAP repairs.

Conclusion

The vast majority of shoulder injuries in overhead athletes should initially be approached with a conservative treatment. Only significant structural injuries deserve early surgical intervention. Every overhead athlete requires a training program that strengthens all elements of the kinetic chain of the throwing motion. Further investigation is needed to help determine which patients are likely to succeed with nonoperative treatment and those who will predictably do well with surgical repair. Most clinical studies on this topic are from single institutions and lack the power necessary to definitively draw conclusions about the superiority of specific management options.

References

1. Walch G, Boileau P, Noel E, Donell ST. Impingement of the deep surface of the supraspinatus tendon on the posterosuperior glenoid rim: an arthroscopic study. J Shoulder Elb Surg. 1992;1:238–45.
2. Walch G, Liotard JP, Boileau P, Noel E. Posterosuperior glenoid impingement. Another shoulder impingement. Rev Chir Orthop Reparatrice Appar Mot. 1991;77:571–4.
3. Jobe CM. Posterior superior glenoid impingement: expanded spectrum. Arthroscopy. 1995;11:530–6.
4. Van der Hoeven H, Kibler WB. Shoulder injuries in tennis players. Br J Sports Med. 2006;40:435–40. https://doi.org/10.1136/bjsm.2005.023218.
5. Burkhart SS, Morgan CD, Kibler WB. The disabled throwing shoulder: spectrum of pathology. Part III: The SICK scapula, scapular dyskinesis, the kinetic chain, and rehabilitation. Arthroscopy. 2003;19:641–61. S074980630300389X.
6. Burkhart SS, Morgan CD, Kibler WB. Shoulder injuries in overhead athletes. The "dead arm" revisited. Clin Sports Med. 2000;19:125–58.
7. Kibler WB. The role of the scapula in athletic shoulder function. Am J Sports Med. 1998;26:325–37.
8. Gagey OJ, Gagey N. The hyperabduction test: an assessment of the laxity of the inferior glenohumeral ligament. J Bone Joint Surg Br. 2001;83:69–74.
9. Heyworth BE, Williams RJ III. Internal impingement of the shoulder. Am J Sports Med. 2009;37:1024–37. https://doi.org/10.1177/0363546508324966.
10. Cools AM, Declercq G, Cagnie B, Cambier D, Witvrouw E. Internal impingement in the tennis player: rehabilitation guidelines. Br J Sports Med. 2008;42:165–71. https://doi.org/10.1136/bjsm.2007.036830.
11. Burkhart SS, Morgan CD, Kibler WB. The disabled throwing shoulder: spectrum of pathology. Part I: Pathoanatomy and biomechanics. Arthroscopy. 2003;19:404–20.
12. Jobe CM. Superior glenoid impingement. Current concepts. Clin Orthop Relat Res. 1996;330:98–107.
13. Myers JB, Laudner KG, Pasquale MR, et al. Posterior capsular tightness in throwers with internal impingement. Presented at the Annual Meeting of Orthopaedic Surgeons, February 23–27; 2005.
14. O'Brien SJ, Neves MC, Arnoczky SP, et al. The anatomy and histology of the inferior glenohumeral ligament complex of the shoulder. Am J Sports Med. 1990;18:449–56.
15. Gold GE, Pappas GP, Blemker SS, et al. Abduction and external rotation in shoulder impingement: an open MR study on healthy volunteers-initial experience. Radiology. 2007;244:815–22.
16. Halbrect JL, Tirman P, Atkin D. Internal impingement of the shoulder: comparison of findings between the throwing and non-throwing shoulders of college baseball players. Arthroscopy. 1999;15:253–8.
17. Fessa CK, Peduto A, Linklater J, Tirman P. Posterosuperior glenoid internal impingement of the shoulder in the overhead athlete: pathogenesis, clinical features and MR imaging findings. J Med Imaging Radiat Oncol. 2015;59:182–7. https://doi.org/10.1111/1754-9485.12276.
18. Myers JB, Laudner KG, Pasquale MR, Bradley JP, Lephart SM. Glenohumeral range of motion deficits and posterior shoulder tightness in throwers with pathologic internal impingement. Am J Sports Med. 2006;34:385–91. https://doi.org/10.1177/0363546505281804.
19. Jbara M, Chen Q, Marten P, Morcos M, Beltran J. Shoulder MR arthrography: how, why, when. Radiol Clin N Am. 2005;43:683–92.
20. Braun S, Kokmeyer D, Millett PJ. Shoulder injuries in the throwing athlete. J Bone Joint Surg Am. 2009;91:966–78. https://doi.org/10.2106/JBJS.H.01341.
21. Struhl S. Anterior internal impingement: an arthroscopic observation. Arthroscopy. 2002;18:2–7. S0749806302767625.
22. Tirman PF, Smith ED, Stoller DW, Fritz RC. Shoulder imaging in athletes. Semin Musculoskelet Radiol. 2004;8:29–40. https://doi.org/10.1055/s-2004-823013.
23. Kirchhoff C, Imhoff AB. Posterosuperior and anterosuperior impingement of the shoulder in overhead athletes - evolving concepts. Inter Orthop (SICOT). 2010;34:1049–58. https://doi.org/10.1007/s00264-010-1038-0.
24. Werner SL, Guido JA Jr, Stewart GW, McNeice RP, VanDyke T, Jones DG. Relationships between throwing mechanics and shoulder distraction in collegiate baseball pitchers. J Shoulder Elb Surg. 2007;16:37–42. https://doi.org/10.1016/j.jse.2006.05.007.
25. Sonnery-Cottet B, Edwards TB, Noel E, Walch G. Results of arthroscopic treatment of posterosuperior glenoid impingement in tennis players. Am J Sports Med. 2002;30:227–32.
26. Cools AM, Cambier D, Witvrouw EE. Screening the athlete's shoulder for impingement symptoms: a clinical reasoning algorithm for early detection of shoulder pathology. Br J Sports Med. 2008;42:628–35. https://doi.org/10.1136/bjsm.2008.048074.
27. Curtis AS, Deshmukh R. Throwing injuries: diagnosis and treatment. Arthroscopy. 2003;19(Suppl 1):80–5. https://doi.org/10.1016/j.arthro.2003.09.030.

28. Fleisig GS, Andrews JR, Dillman CJ, Escamilla RF. Kinetics of baseball pitching with implications about injury mechanisms. Am J Sports Med. 1995;23:233–9.
29. Gerber C, Sebesta A. Impingement of the deep surface of the subscapularis tendon and the reflection pulley on the anterosuperior glenoid rim: a preliminary report. J Shoulder Elb Surg. 2000;9:483–90. https://doi.org/10.1067/mse.2000.109322.
30. Kibler WB. Scapular involvement in impingement: signs and symptoms. Instr Course Lect. 2006;55:35–43.
31. Meister K. Internal impingement in the shoulder of the overhand athlete: pathophysiology, diagnosis, and treatment. Am J Orthop. 2000;29:433–8.
32. Wörtler K. Shoulder injuries in overhead sports. Radiologe. 2010;50(5):453–9.
33. Wilk KE, Meister K, Andrews JR. Current concepts in the rehabilitation of the overhead throwing athlete. Am J Sports Med. 2002;30:136–51.
34. Manske RC, Grant-Nierman M, Lucas B. Shoulder posterior internal impingement in the overhead athlete. Int J Sports Phys Ther. 2013;8(2):194–204.
35. Borstad JD, Ludewig PM. Comparison of scapular kinematics between elevation and lowering of the arm in the scapular plane. Clin Biomech. 2002;17:650–9. S0268003302001365.
36. Cooper DE, Arnoczky SP, O'Brien SJ, Warren RF, Di Carlo E, Allen AA. Anatomy, histology, and vascularity of the glenoid labrum. An anatomical study. J Bone Joint Surg Am. 1992;74(1):46–52.
37. Pagnani MJ, Deng XH, Warren RF, Torzilli PA, Altchek DW. Effect of lesions of the superior portion of the glenoid labrum on glenohumeral translation. J Bone Joint Surg Am. 1995;77(7):1003–10.
38. Wilk KE, Arrigo CA. Current concepts in the rehabilitation of the athletic shoulder. J Orthop Sports Phys Ther. 1993;18(1):365–78.
39. Wilk KE, Arrigo CA, Andrews JR. Current concepts: the stabilizing structures of the glenohumeral joint. J Orthop Sports Phys Ther. 1997;25(6):364–79.
40. Shepard MF, Dugas JR, Zeng N, Andrews JR. Differences in the ultimate strength of the biceps anchor and the generation of type II superior labral anterior posterior lesions in a cadaveric model. Am J Sports Med. 2004;32(5):1197–201.
41. Wilk KE, Andrews JR, Arrigo CA. The physical examination of the glenohumeral joint: emphasis on the stabilizing structures. J Orthop Sports Phys Ther. 1997;25(6):380–9.
42. Andrews JR, Carson WG Jr, McLeod WD. Glenoid labrum tears related to the long head of the biceps. Am J Sports Med. 1985;13(5):337–41.
43. Snyder SJ, Karzel RP, Del Pizzo W, Ferkel RD, Friedman MJ. SLAP lesions of the shoulder. Arthroscopy. 1990;6(4):274–9.
44. Knesek M, Skendzel JG, Dines JS, Altchek DW, Allen AA, Bedi A. Diagnosis and management of superior labral anterior posterior tears in throwing athletes. Am J Sports Med. 2013;41:444–60. https://doi.org/10.1177/0363546512466067.
45. Powell SE, Nord KD, Ryu RKN. The diagnosis, classification, and treatment of SLAP lesions. Oper Tech Sports Med. 2004;12:99–110.
46. Gartsman GM, Hammerman SM. Superior labrum, anterior and posterior lesions. When and how to treat them. Clin Sports Med. 2000;19(1):115–24.
47. Maffet MW, Gartsman GM, Moseley B. Superior labrum-biceps tendon complex lesions of the shoulder. Am J Sports Med. 1995;23(1):93–8.
48. Morgan CD, Burkhart SS, Palmeri M, Gillespie M. Type II SLAP lesions: three subtypes and their relationships to superior instability and rotator cuff tears. Arthroscopy. 1998;14(6):553–65.
49. Andrews JR, Broussard TS, Carson WG. Arthroscopy of the shoulder in the management of partial tears of the rotator cuff: a preliminary report. Arthroscopy. 1985;1(2):117–22.
50. Burkhart SS, Morgan CD. The peel-back mechanism: its role in producing and extending posterior type II SLAP lesions and its effect on SLAP repair rehabilitation. Arthroscopy. 1998;14(6):637–40.
51. Reinold MM, Wilk KE, Hooks TR, Dugas JR, Andrews JR. Thermal-assisted capsular shrinkage of the glenohumeral joint in overhead athletes: a 15- to 47-month follow-up. J Orthop Sports Phys Ther. 2003;33(8):455–67.
52. Kim SH, Ha KI, Ahn JH, Kim SH, Choi HJ. Biceps load test II: a clinical test for SLAP lesions of the shoulder. Arthroscopy. 2001;17(2):160–4.
53. Weber SC, Martin DF, Seiler JG III, Harrast JJ. Superior labrum anterior and posterior lesions of the shoulder: incidence rates, complications, and outcomes as reported by American Board of Orthopedic Surgery. Part II candidates. Am J Sports Med. 2012;40:1538–43.
54. Erickson J, Lavery K, Monica J, Gatt C, Dhawan A. Surgical treatment of symptomatic superior labrum anterior-posterior tears in patients older than 40 years: a systematic review. Am J Sports Med. 2015;43:1274–82.
55. Zhang AL, Kreulen C, Ngo SS, Hame SL, Wang JC, Gamradt SC. Demographic trends in arthroscopic SLAP repair in the United States. Am J Sports Med. 2012;40:1144–7.
56. Mileski RA, Snyder SJ. Superior labral lesions in the shoulder: pathoanatomy and surgical management. J Am Acad Orthop Surg. 1998;6(2):121–31.
57. Kim TK, Queale WS, Cosgarea AJ, McFarland EG. Clinical features of the different types of SLAP lesions: an analysis of one hundred and thirty-nine cases. J Bone Joint Surg Am. 2003;85-A(1):66–71.
58. O'Brien SJ, Pagnani MJ, Fealy S, McGlynn SR, Wilson JB. The active compression test: a new and effective test for diagnosing labral tears and acromioclavicular joint abnormality. Am J Sports Med. 1998;26(5):610–3.
59. Kim SH, Ha KI, Han KY. Biceps load test: a clinical test for superior labrum anterior and posterior lesions in shoulders with recurrent anterior dislocations. Am J Sports Med. 1999;27(3):300–3.

60. Mimori K, Muneta T, Nakagawa T, Shinomiya K. A new pain provocation test for superior labral tears of the shoulder. Am J Sports Med. 1999;27(2):137–42.
61. Myers TH, Zemanovic JR, Andrews JR. The resisted supination external rotation test: a new test for the diagnosis of superior labral anterior posterior lesions. Am J Sports Med. 2005;33(9):1315–20.
62. Kibler WB, Sciascia AD, Hester P, Dome D, Jacobs C. Clinical utility of traditional and new tests in the diagnosis of biceps tendon injuries and superior labrum anterior and posterior lesions in the shoulder. Am J Sports Med. 2009;37(9):1840–7. https://doi.org/10.1177/0363546509332505.
63. Bencardino JT, Beltran J, Rosenberg ZS, Rokito A, Schmahmann S, Mota J, et al. Superior labrum anterior-posterior lesions: diagnosis with MR arthrography of the shoulder. Radiology. 2000;214(1):267–71.
64. Nam EK, Snyder SJ. The diagnosis and treatment of superior labrum, anterior and posterior (SLAP) lesions. Am J Sports Med. 2003;31(5):798–810.
65. Green MR, Christensen KP. Magnetic resonance imaging of the glenoid labrum in anterior shoulder instability. Am J Sports Med. 1994;22(4):493–8.
66. Liu SH, Henry MH, Nuccion SL. A prospective evaluation of a new physical examination in predicting glenoid labral tears. Am J Sports Med. 1996;24(6):721–5.
67. Edwards SL, Lee JA, Bell JE, Packer JD, Ahmad CS, Levine WN, et al. Nonoperative treatment of superior labrum anterior posterior tears: improvements in pain, function, and quality of life. Am J Sports Med. 2010;38(7):1456–61. https://doi.org/10.1177/0363546510370937.
68. Bedi A, Allen AA. Superior labral lesions anterior to posterior - evaluation and arthroscopic management. Clin Sports Med. 2008;27:607–30. https://doi.org/10.1016/j.csm.2008.06.002.
69. Keener JD, Brophy RH. Superior labral tears of the shoulder: pathogenesis, evaluation, and treatment. J Am Acad Orthop Surg. 2009;17:627–37.
70. McCormick F, Bhatia S, Chalmers P, Gupta A, Verma N, Romeo AA. The management of type II superior labral anterior to posterior injuries. Orthop Clin North Am. 2014;45:121–8. https://doi.org/10.1016/j.ocl.2013.08.008.
71. Kibler WB, Sciascia A. Current practice for the surgical treatment of SLAP lesions: a systematic review. Arthroscopy. 2016;32(4):669–83. https://doi.org/10.1016/j.arthro.2015.08.041.
72. Steinhaus ME, Makhni EC, Lieber AC, Kahlenberg CA, Gulotta LV, Romeo AA, Verma NN. Variable reporting of functional outcomes and return to play in superior labrum anterior and posterior tear. J Shoulder Elb Surg. 2016;25(11):1896–905. https://doi.org/10.1016/j.jse.2016.04.020.
73. Boileau P, Parratte S, Chuinard C, Roussanne Y, Shia D, Bicknell R. Arthroscopic treatment of isolated type II SLAP lesions: biceps tenodesis as an alternative to reinsertion. Am J Sports Med. 2009;37:929–36. https://doi.org/10.1177/0363546508330127.
74. Voos JE, Pearle AD, Mattern CJ, Cordasco FA, Allen AA, Warren RF. Outcomes of combined arthroscopic rotator cuff and labral repair. Am J Sports Med. 2007;35:1174–9. https://doi.org/10.1177/0363546507300062.
75. Chalmers PN, Trombley R, Cip J, Monson B, Forsythe B, Nicholson GP, et al. Postoperative restoration of upper extremity motion and neuromuscular control during the overhand pitch: evaluation of tenodesis and repair for superior labral anterior-posterior tears. Am J Sports Med. 2014;42:2825–36. https://doi.org/10.1177/0363546514551924.
76. Denard PJ, Lädermann A, Parsley BK, Burkhart SS. Arthroscopic biceps tenodesis compared with repair of isolated type II SLAP lesions in patients older than 35 years. Orthopedics. 2014;37:e292–7. https://doi.org/10.3928/01477447-20140225-63.
77. Ek ET, Shi LL, Tompson JD, Freehill MT, Warner JJ. Surgical treatment of isolated type II superior labrum anterior-posterior (SLAP) lesions: repair versus biceps tenodesis. J Shoulder Elb Surg. 2014;23:1059–65. https://doi.org/10.1016/j.jse.2013.09.030.
78. Gottschalk MB, Karas SG, Ghattas TN, Burdette R. Subpectoral biceps tenodesis for the treatment of type II and IVsuperior labral anterior and posterior lesions. Am J Sports Med. 2014;42:2128–35. https://doi.org/10.1177/0363546514540273.
79. Tayrose GA, Karas SG, Bosco J. Biceps tenodesis for type II SLAP tears. Bull Hosp Jt Dis (2013). 2015;73:116–21.
80. Altchek DW, Warren RF, Wickiewicz TL, Ortiz G. Arthroscopic labral debridement. A three-year follow-up study. Am J Sports Med. 1992;20(6):702–6.
81. Provencher MT, McCormick F, Dewing C, McIntire S, Solomon D. A prospective analysis of 179 type 2 superior labrum anterior and posterior repairs: outcomes and factors associated with success and failure. Am J Sports Med. 2013;41:880–6.
82. Erickson BJ, Jain A, Abrams GD, Nicholson GP, Cole BJ, Romeo AA, Verma NN. SLAP lesions: trends in treatment. Arthroscopy. 2016;32(6):976–81. https://doi.org/10.1016/j.arthro.2015.11.044.
83. Laughlin WA, Fleisig GS, Scillia AJ, Aune KT, Cain EL Jr, Dugas JR. Deficiencies in pitching biomechanics in baseball players with a history of superior labrum anterior posterior repair. Am J Sports Med. 2014;42:2837–41.

Scapulothoracic Evaluation and Treatment in Tennis Players

Natalie L. Myers and W. Ben Kibler

15.1 Introduction

The scapula serves many roles in order for proper shoulder function to occur. It provides a stable base for muscle activation, a mobile platform for glenohumeral kinematics, a link between the core and the arm, and serves as a funnel to transmit forces to the distal upper extremity. Scapular movement is considered multi-planar and three-dimensional because as the arm elevates, the scapula undergoes a composite of motions [1, 2]. Rotary motions include upward/downward rotation around an axis perpendicular to the scapular body, anterior/posterior tilting around a horizontal axis along the scapular spine, and internal/external rotation around a vertical axis along with medial border. In conjunction with these rotary motions, the scapula also translates in the presence of intact clavicular anatomy, specifically at sternoclavicular (SC) and acromioclavicular (AC) joint. Scapula superior/inferior translation on the thorax wall is due to clavicular elevation/depression at the SC joint, while anterior/posterior translation corresponds to clavicular protraction/retraction at the SC joint.

Very little is known about scapular movement during overhead tasks such as a tennis serve or baseball throw despite the recognized importance of scapular movement during overhead activity. Three-dimensional (3D) scapular position during humeral elevation has been reported in healthy overhead athletes. As the arm moves into 120° of scapular plane elevation, the scapula has been found to upwardly rotate 28°, internally rotate 14°, retract 13°, and elevate 12° [3]. However, it must be noted that these scapular and clavicular movement patterns are specific to baseball players and do vary between studies [4]. At this time it is unknown if these findings can be translatable to a tennis population.

Abnormal scapular motion has been previously referred to as "scapular winging," [5] "snapping scapula," [6] scapula dyskinesia, and "scapular dyskinesis." Kuhn et al. [5] describes scapular winging as primary, secondary, or voluntary. Primary winging may be a result of neurological trauma, bony alterations, or thoracoscapulohumeral muscle weakness. Neurological trauma to the spinal accessory, long thoracic, or dorsal scapular can cause scapular winging. Damage to the spinal accessory and dorsal scapular nerves results in similar patterns as the scapula depresses and laterally translates with the inferior angle rotating laterally, while the exact opposite motions occur with long thoracic nerve damage [5]. Secondary scapular winging is a result of glenohumeral joint pathology, and patients will likely have normal

N. L. Myers (✉)
Department of Health & Human Performance,
Texas State University, San Marcos, TX, USA
e-mail: natalie.myers@txstate.edu

W. B. Kibler
Shoulder Center of Kentucky, Lexington Clinic Orthopedics, Lexington, KY, USA

EMG and nerve conduction examinations. Voluntary winging is the most rare and is associated with underlying psychological impairments. Therefore, the evaluation of a patient demonstrating scapular winging must be comprehensive in nature in order to determine the factors that may be causing the altered position or motion.

The "snapping scapula" is a term that represents audible and palpable crepitus along the superomedial border of the scapula during dynamic arm motion [6]. Possible causes of snapping scapula include bony pathology, soft tissue abnormality, or bursitis in the thoracoscapular space. Any of these alterations may create increased compressive pressure along the superomedial border and contribute to painful symptoms. Once again, a complete assessment incorporating flexibility and strength of the surrounding musculature is critical in identifying the causative factors.

Scapular dyskinesia implies a loss of voluntary motion [7]. However, scapular movement is both voluntary and involuntary, as rotational scapular movements are accessory in nature and cannot be controlled voluntarily like scapular translations (elevation/depression and retraction/protraction). Therefore, the term dyskinesia falsely represents abnormal scapular motion. Scapular dyskinesis ("dys" alteration of, "kinesis"—movement) is a more appropriate term that reflects the loss of control of normal scapular physiology, mechanics, and motion. Scapular dyskinesis has been identified as (1) abnormal static scapular position and/or dynamic scapular motion characterized by medial border prominence, (2) inferior angle prominence and/or early scapular elevation or shrugging on arm elevation, and/or (3) rapid downward rotation during arm lowering (Second Scapula Summit. Unpublished consensus statement. Lexington, KY July 20, 2006). Dyskinesis alone is not a diagnosis or injury, not a guarantee of injury, and not associated with one specific injury and may occur in both symptomatic and asymptomatic shoulders [8–10]. It is best categorized as an impairment of optimal shoulder function. Dyskinesis can alter shoulder function including subacromial space dimensions, muscle activation patterns, and optimal arm position and motion [11]. These alterations combined with overhead activities requiring repetitive joint motion, high joint loads, and large compression and distraction forces may diminish athletic performance or increase injury risk. Additionally, shoulder pathology (AC joint injury, superior labral tears, rotator cuff injury) along with proximal muscle and nerve trauma can promote scapular dyskinesis. Thus, dyskinesis should be assessed clinically to help clinicians determine if the movement dysfunction could be one factor responsible for symptom production.

15.2 Clinical Evaluation of the Scapula

The goal of a scapular evaluation is to identify the presence or absence of scapular dyskinesis at rest and during arm elevation to help determine relationships between altered motion and symptoms and identify potential proximal and distal causative factors of movement dysfunction [7]. Five main components should comprise the examination of the scapula: (1) location of pain, (2) observational assessment, (3) manual correction of dysfunction, (4) manual muscle testing, and (5) posture and flexibility [7, 12].

15.2.1 Location of Pain

Determining the location of pain through palpation can be helpful during the clinical examination. The medial scapular border is commonly sensitive to palpation as it serves as an attachment site for several major upper extremity muscles. In overhead athletes, the upper trapezius, levator scapula, and latissimus dorsi along the lateral scapular border, pectoralis minor, and short head of the biceps may also elicit pain to touch as these muscles tend to become shortened, tight, or spastic. Manual therapy and mobilization techniques can be initiated to improve flexibility.

15.2.2 Observational Assessment

Several techniques have been devised to quantify scapular dyskinesis objectively: measurement of scapular displacement (lateral scapular slide test) [13, 14], 3D electromagnetic assessment [3, 15], Moire topography [8], 3D wing computer tomography (CT) [16], and visual observation [10, 17, 18]. Much effort has been directed toward developing clinically useful methods as 3D assessment requires equipment that is not readily available to a clinician. The lateral scapular slide test is a static measure used to determine scapular position. The test requires minimal equipment; however, investigators have demonstrated that this test cannot be used reliably and is unable to discriminate between those with and without shoulder dysfunction (Odom CJ, Taylor AB et al. [14]). Thus, other clinically applicable methods of scapular assessment have been investigated in order to classify scapular movement [10, 17, 18].

The first visually based system for categorizing scapular dyskinesis was developed by Kibler et al. in 2002 [17]. The system incorporated three patterns that defined abnormal scapular motion at rest and during arm motion: type I, inferior medial border prominence patterns; type II, entire medial border prominence; and type III, superior medial border elevation and anterior translation. Patients were asked to perform three repetitions of bilateral arm elevations in scaption and abduction while being video recorded posteriorly. Four healthcare professionals (two physicians and two physical therapists) demonstrated varying degrees of fair to moderate reliability. With goals to improve the reliability, several authors simplified the categorization of scapular dyskinesis [10, 18].

Uhl et al. [10] collapsed all three dyskinesis categories (types I to III) into one single category of yes (an abnormal dyskinesis pattern) or no (normal scapular motion). They studied patients with and without shoulder pathology. The yes/no classification system demonstrated moderate interobserver reliability and demonstrated high sensitivity and positive predictive value when compared with 3D criterion. Additionally, symptomatic subjects (54%) had more multiple-plane asymmetries during forward flexion than asymptomatic subjects (14%). However, in scaption there was an equal distribution of multiple-plane scapular asymmetries of 45% in both groups.

The scapular dyskinesis test (SDT) put forth by McClure et al. [18] categorized scapular motion with a three-item rating scale. Division I overhead athletes performed weighted shoulder flexion and abduction and were categorized as either demonstrating (subtle or obvious abnormality) or not demonstrating scapular dyskinesis (normal motion). Dyskinesis was defined as the presence of dysrhythmia or winging. The SDT generated higher interobserver reliability than all other visually based test for scapular dyskinesis. This system also showed that overhead athletes visually categorized as having scapular dyskinesis demonstrated decreased scapular upward rotation, less clavicular elevation and retraction when measured using the gold standard of 3D motion tracking [19]. These results suggest that athletes with visual abnormalities in scapular motion do in fact demonstrate altered movement, especially in shoulder flexion.

15.2.3 Manual Correction of Dysfunction

The scapular assistance test (SAT) and scapular retraction (or reposition) test (SRT) are corrective maneuvers that can alter the injury-related symptoms and provide information on the role of scapular dyskinesis in the dysfunction that accompanies shoulder injury [9, 20, 21]. If the implementation of these maneuvers improves symptoms, this provides evidence that the dyskinesis is more than likely a driving factor to the shoulder symptoms. During the SAT the examiner assists the serratus anterior and lower trapezius muscles by manually assisting the scapula in upward rotation as the arm is elevated [9, 22]. Rabin et al. [23] later modified this test to incorporate scapular posterior tilting. Relief of painful symptoms indicates a positive test during the assisted maneuver. The test has been shown to have acceptable inter-rater reliability [23]. This test has been found to alter scapular motion by increasing scapular posterior tilt [24], so a positive test would point to the need for improvement in pectoralis flexibility and lower trapezius strength.

The scapular retraction test involves manually positioning and stabilizing the entire medial border of the scapula on the thorax [22]. In the SRT, the examiner grades the muscle strength in abduction following standard manual muscle testing procedures or by a handheld dynamometer or evaluates labral symptoms in patients with a positive modified dynamic labral shear (M-DLS) test [20]. The examiner then manually places and stabilizes the scapular in a retracted position (Fig. 15.1).

A positive test occurs when the demonstrated abduction strength is increased or the symptoms of internal impingement in the labral injury are relieved in the retracted position. The major kinematic result of this test is to increase scapular external rotation and posterior tilt, so a positive test would indicate that rotator cuff strengthening is not necessary, and focus should be on rhomboid strengthening and serratus function in retraction. The scapula reposition test is a modification of the scapular retraction test and emphasizes scapular posterior tilting and external rotation [25]. Tate et al. [25] conducted a study to determine if manual repositioning of the scapula would reduce pain and increase shoulder strength in a sample of 142 overhead athletes. Nearly 50% of the athletes with symptoms of shoulder impingement reported reduced pain with scapular repositioning, while 26% increased shoulder elevation strength. Although these tests are not capable of diagnosing a specific form of shoulder pathology, a positive SAT or SRT shows that scapular dyskinesis is directly involved in producing the symptoms and indicates the need for inclusion of early scapular rehabilitation exercises to improve scapular control.

15.2.4 Manual Muscle Testing

After determining the presence of scapular dyskinesis, it is imperative that the examiner assess the surrounding soft tissue to identify muscles that may be responsible for the alterations in scapular motion. Muscle imbalance can be an attributing factor to scapular dyskinesis, specifically excess upper trapezius activity combined with diminished lower/middle trapezius (LT UT) and serratus anterior (SA) activity [26, 27]. Thus, the LT, UT, and SA should be examined as part of the clinician's assessment as these are key muscles that contribute to scapular stabilization and movement. One test advocated to assess the integrity of the LT and SA is that of the low row [28]. To perform this maneuver, the patient is standing with the involved arm resting at the side with the palm facing posteriorly. The patient is instructed to extend his trunk and push his hand maximally against an examiners' resistance in the direction of shoulder extension and is instructed to retract and depress the scapula. This maneuver assesses both muscles' ability to actively stabilize the scapula while providing the examiner with a visual depiction of LT muscle contraction [28]. The LT can also be examined with the patient lying prone with the shoulder in 140° of elevation and resistance using a handheld dynamometer being applied to the spine of the scapula. The force on the scapula should be applied in the superior and lateral direction parallel to the long axis of the humerus [29]. This position has been shown to elicit high LT muscle activity. Other tests such as active scapular side-lying external rotation, side-lying forward flexion, prone horizontal abduction (LT/MT), and the push up plus (SA) have also been advocated as maneuvers to employ scapular muscle function [30].

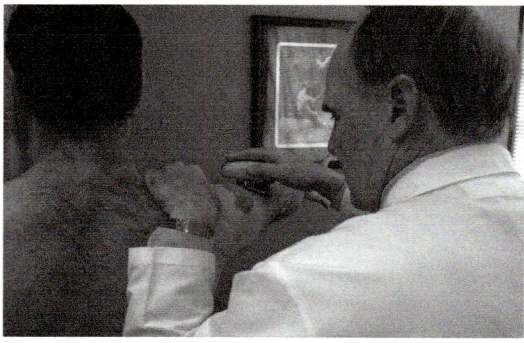

Fig. 15.1 The SRT performed with the medial border of the scapular stabilized

15.2.5 Posture and Flexibility

Forward head and rounded shoulder posture contributes to alterations in scapular kinematics and SA muscle activity which may lead to adaptive muscle shortening and/or muscle imbalance [31]. Shortening of the pectoralis minor has been implicated as a mechanics for forward head posture and for shoulder impingement [32]. Standing the patient against the wall and measuring the distance from the wall to the anterior acromial trip may obtain a rough measurement of pectoralis minor tightness. This can be done using a "double square" device with a patient standing with his or her back against the wall. There is evidence to suggest that anterior shoulder stretching and posterior shoulder strengthening in competitive swimmers reduce the distance from the anterior acromion to the wall [33]. Another assessment method involves using a tape measure or caliper to record the linear distance between the origin and insertion of the pectoralis minor [34]. Both methods have good intrarater reliability and validity.

Posterior shoulder tightness may contribute to abnormal scapular motion [35]. To obtain accurate glenohumeral internal rotation measurements, the patient should be positioned supine on a flat surface with the shoulder at 90° of abduction and approximately 10° of horizontal adduction (scapular plane). One examiner should stabilize the scapula by grasping the coracoid process and the spine of the scapula posteriorly. The same examiner will then passively move the extremity to end rage. A second examiner would take the measurement using a goniometer where the fulcrum is set at the olecranon process of the elbow, and the stationary arm perpendicular to the table [36].

15.3 Rehabilitation Considerations for Correction of Scapula Dyskinesis

Before treating scapular dyskinesis, it is important to individually assess patient-specific impairments, as the dyskinesis can either be a cause of symptoms or the result of shoulder pathology. Following evaluation, the rehabilitation of scapular dyskinesis should start proximally and end distally. The goal of initial therapy is to achieve the position of optimal scapular function—posterior tilt, external rotation, and upward rotation. Functional tasks involving the scapula and shoulder most frequently are dependent upon appropriate functioning of the kinetic chain as a unit. This requires optimization of the individual kinetic chain segments and appropriate coordination of the individual segments. A typical progression to follow in order to assure each segment is optimized is as follows: (1) acquire flexibility, (2) establish core strength and stability, (3) facilitate critical kinetic chain links via sequential activation, (4) utilize closed to open-chain sequence of exercise, (5) work in multiple planes, (6) apply eccentric upper limb exercise, and (7) develop activity-specific progressions.

15.3.1 Acquire Flexibility in Multiple Segments

Upper extremity dominant athletes may experience mobility deficits in the hamstrings, hip flexors, hip adductions, hip rotators, gastroc-soleus muscle groups, pectoralis minor, short head of the biceps, scalenes, levator scapulae, latissimus dorsi, and the posterior shoulder musculature [37–39]. Flexibility in multiple segments throughout the kinetic chain can be established through static, dynamic, or proprioceptive neuromuscular facilitation stretching. Improving flexibility has been shown to improve serve velocity among elite-level tennis players [40].

The dominant shoulder undergoes eccentric demands during the overhead motion that can diminish the amount of shoulder motion [41]. Acute changes in glenohumeral total range of motion and internal rotation on the dominant arm have been shown to decrease following an acute exposure to tennis play [42]. While these adaptations to motion are considered normal, the cause of the change in motion is of much discussion in the literature and should be monitored as total motion deficits between the dominant and nondominant arm have been linked to upper limb injury [43]. There are several different theories regarding motion alterations including bony adaptions [44, 45], posterior muscular tightness [46], and posterior capsule tightness [47]. A comprehensive assessment can help differentiate between bony, muscular, or capsular [48]. Once the culprit of the motion deficits is identified, the cross-body strength with scapular stabilization [49], muscle energy [50], joint mobilizations [51], and soft tissue mobilization may be implemented to improve shoulder mobility. Ellenbecker and Cools have developed a scapular rehabilitation algorithm in which they suggest flexibility deficits should be addressed with stretching and manual therapy techniques [52].

15.3.2 Establishing Core Strength, Stability, and Posture Control

The proximal segments of the kinetic chain are critical in the development of the force and energy distally. These segments create a stable base that is essential for distal mobility, power, energy transfer, and diminished upper limb loading. In order to create a stable base, the rehabilitation protocols must incorporate core stability. Optimal core stability requires a combination of motor control to the core musculature to maintain a neutral spine position and to resist motion through the lumbar spine [53]. The goal when working the core should be to increase strength and endurance in order to maintain a stable spine throughout activity. In order to maintain a stable spine, McGill developed a series of three exercises, entitled "The Big 3" (modified curl-up, side bridge, and the bird dog) [54]. These exercises can be introduced early on in the rehabilitation or training phase to promote neuromuscular control and spine neutral before more dynamic exercises are executed. Core stabilization training programs have been shown to improve dynamic postural control in tennis players [55]. Additionally, Myer et al. reported improvements in pelvic and trunk stability after a training program specific to the hip and trunk and suggested that the stability changes could translate into improved performance and injury reduction [56].

By emphasizing proximal stability, the hip and trunk musculature will be more effective during a specific task, such as overhead arm activity. In addition to generating force and transferring energy to distal segments, core training helps to develop a stable base for arm motion. This stage of rehabilitation is not only to restore core function itself but also is the first stage of extremity rehabilitation.

15.3.3 Facilitate Critical Kinetic Chain Links via Sequential Activation

Scapulohumeral muscles such as the serratus anterior and lower trapezius should be a point of focus in early training and rehabilitation. A fatigue of these muscles disrupts the normal kinematics leading to symptoms of impingement. The serratus and lower trapezius also form an important force couple that produces acromial elevation. If this force couple is dysfunctional, then scapulohumeral movement becomes abnormal [57]. Movement patterns that activate these two muscles should incorporate trunk and hip extension. Pelvic and trunk motion in conjunction with scapulothoracic movement promotes the kinetic chain proximal to distal sequence of muscle activation that is imperative for athletes engaged in repetitive overhead activity. Specific exercises known as the scapular stability series, low row, inferior glide, lawn mower, and robbery have been shown to activate the serratus and lower trapezius at safe levels of muscle activation and arm position and may be used in the early phases of rehabilitation [28].

Scapular stabilization protocols should focus on reeducating muscles to act as dynamic stabilizers. Maximal rotator cuff strength is achieved off a stabilized retracted scapula. It has been found that demonstrated rotator cuff strength increased as much as 24% when the scapula was stabilized and retracted [20, 25]. Consequently, rotator cuff exercises and more advanced exercises incorporating global muscles around the shoulder should occur after scapular control is achieved.

15.3.4 Closed to Open-Chain Progression

Kinetic chain-based training or rehabilitation has been segregated into either open or closed chain [58]. Characteristics of open chain incorporate free movement of the terminal segment. Characteristics of closed chain include fixed or minimal movement of the terminal segment. Examples of these are the scapular-clock exercise, quadruped, hand-supported weight shifts, and modified push-ups. These exercises can be useful in providing joint approximation forces, which promote co-contraction about the joint and enhance dynamic joint stability [59]. Force generation, force distribution, joint motion, muscle activation, and resultant tissue stress can be quite different in the two classes of exercises. Typically, when tissue is compromised, inflamed, or irritated, closed-chain exercises should be implemented early in the rehabilitation process due to the decreased amount of force and stress applied to the involved joints. Open-chain exercises should be incorporated later in the rehabilitation process as these exercises generate larger loads due to their increased demands on the body's joints and longer arm levers these exercises require [58].

The rationale behind the initial closed-chain emphasis is that the shoulder functions as a closed chain to transfer energy [60]. The hand is obviously moving in an open-chain fashion during throwing and serving. However, shoulder position, motion, and force transfer fit the physiological and biomechanical requirements of closed-chain activities. In throwing and serving, the scapula and shoulder display intersegmental coordination, with coupled movements that are predictable on the basis of arm position. As such, the shoulder acts as a funnel, transferring and regulating forces in the kinetic chain from the legs to the hand.

15.3.5 Work in Multiple Planes

Clinicians should incorporate multi-planar movements into the rehabilitation protocol. The overhead motion requires effort from multiple joints and muscle groups; thus, the use of single planar exercises that isolate muscles and joints should be minimized. Emphasis should be put on functional positions, motions, and muscle activation sequences, so normal physiological and biomechanical patterns can be restored. The goal is to establish coordinated muscle activation of the segments throughout the kinetic chain.

15.3.6 Apply Eccentric Upper Limb Exercise

When performed in isolation, eccentric muscle actions have shown to possess several distinct physiological properties as compared to concentric movement patterns. Compared with concentric actions, eccentric actions achieve higher contractile forces [61], reduced electromyography (EMG) amplitudes [62], and faster neural adaptions [63]. Furthermore, authors conducted a meta-analysis comparing the effects of eccentric versus concentric resistance training and found that eccentric training performed at high intensities has been shown to promote increased muscle mass and cross-sectional area compared to concentric training [64].

The shoulder is exposed to rapid decelerative eccentric contractions during overhead sport activity and should therefore not only be trained concentrically but eccentrically as well. Therefore, Kibler and collogues developed the "Kibler's eccentric six protocol." The protocol requires interaction between the clinician and player in order to be executed appropriately. All six exercises require eccentric muscle contractions to the upper limb and are illustrated in Figs. 15.2, 15.3, 15.4, 15.5, 15.6, and 15.7.

The exercises can be performed with a series of weighted balls or with a weighted wooden rod to lengthen the lever arm. Six repetitions of each exercise are performed. The first repetition is with a 1-lb weight; thereafter each repetition increases by a half a pound. Prone external rotation is the only exercise that is performed with 15 repetitions using a TheraBand. The eccentric phase of each exercise should incorporate an eight-second count.

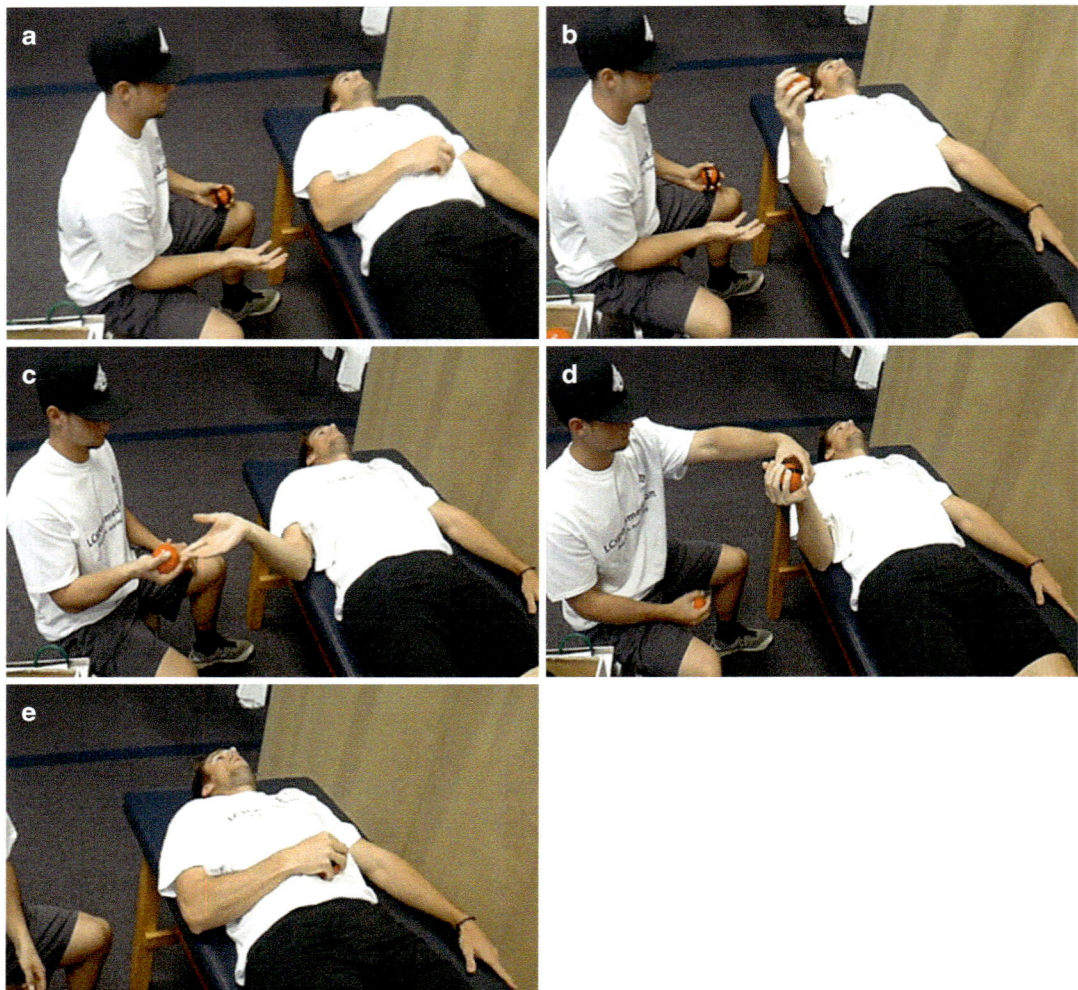

Fig. 15.2 Supine external rotation (ER). (**a**) Starting position in internal rotation with weighted ball. (**b**) The patient is instructed to externally rotate the shoulder (mid-range ER). (**c**) The patient then drops the weighted ball into the instructor's hand. (**d**) The instructor places a new weighted ball into the patient's hand. (**e**) Ending position

15.3.7 Develop Activity-Specific Progressions

Once the preceding components of the rehabilitation sequence have been satisfied, specific task and activity progression can be implemented. Functional movement tasks incorporating both the lower and upper extremity are imperative. The best activity-specific training is sport itself; however, specific skill exercises and drills can be executed to enhance sport performance. When implementing activity-specific progressions, clinicians must understand the demands of the sport. Clinicians training tennis players should

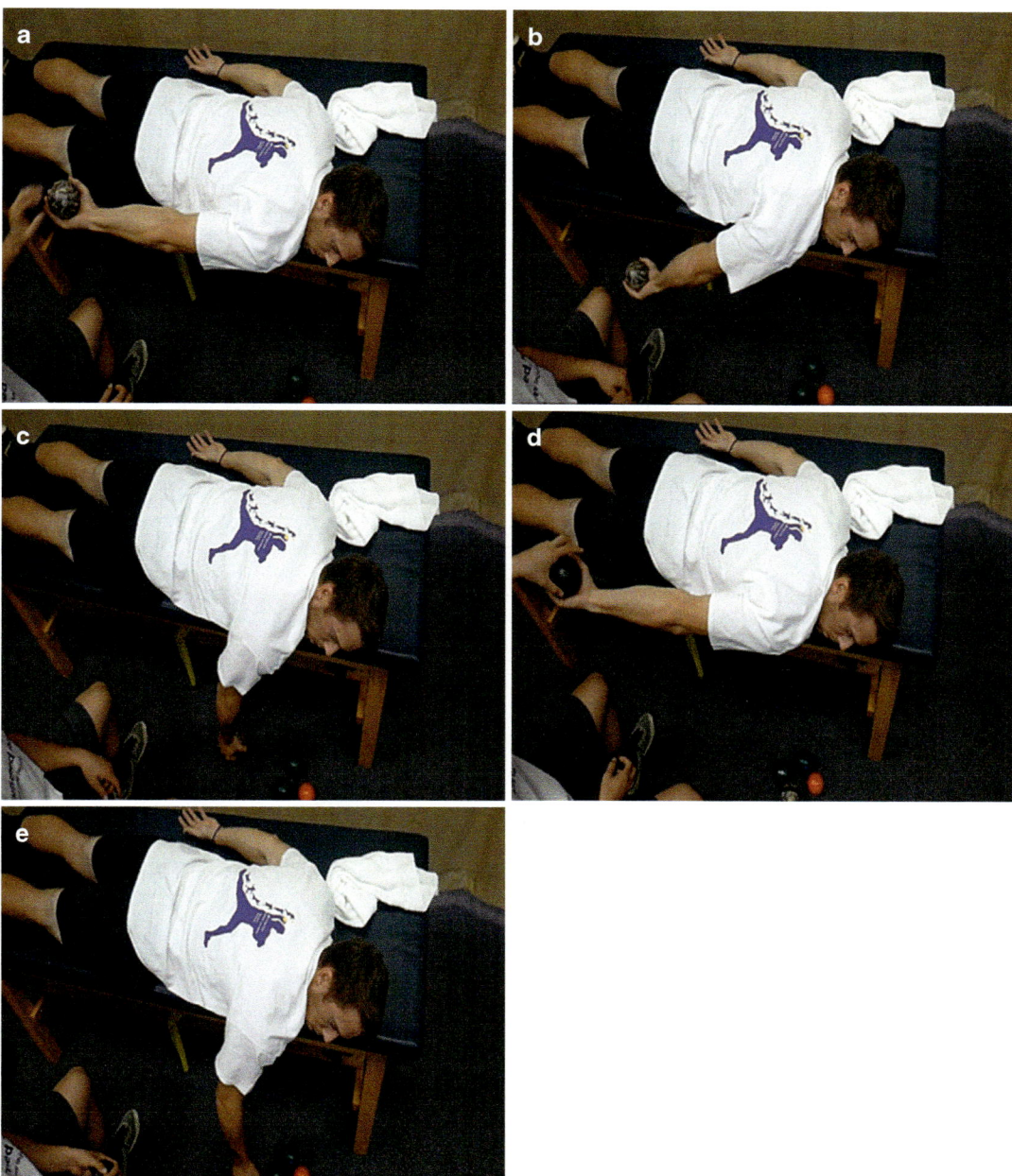

Fig. 15.3 Prone extension. (**a**) Starting position for extension with weighted ball. (**b**) The patient is instructed to lower the arm (mid-range extension). (**c**) When the arm is perpendicular with the table, the patient then drops the weighted ball. (**d**) The patient extends the arm so parallel with the table, and the instructor places a new weighted ball into the patient's hand. (**e**) Ending position

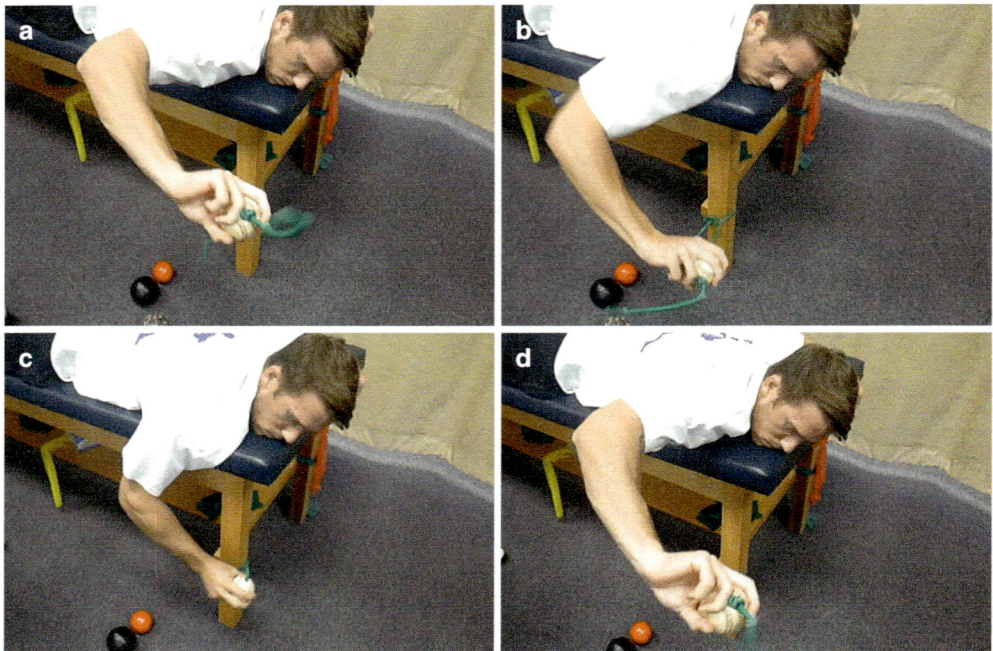

Fig. 15.4 Prone external rotation (ER). (**a**) Start patient in ER with TheraBand. (**b**) The patient is instructed to lower the arm while maintaining 90° of elbow flexion (mid-range ER). (**c**) When the upper arm is perpendicular with the table, the patient performs ER on a one second count. (**d**) Ending position

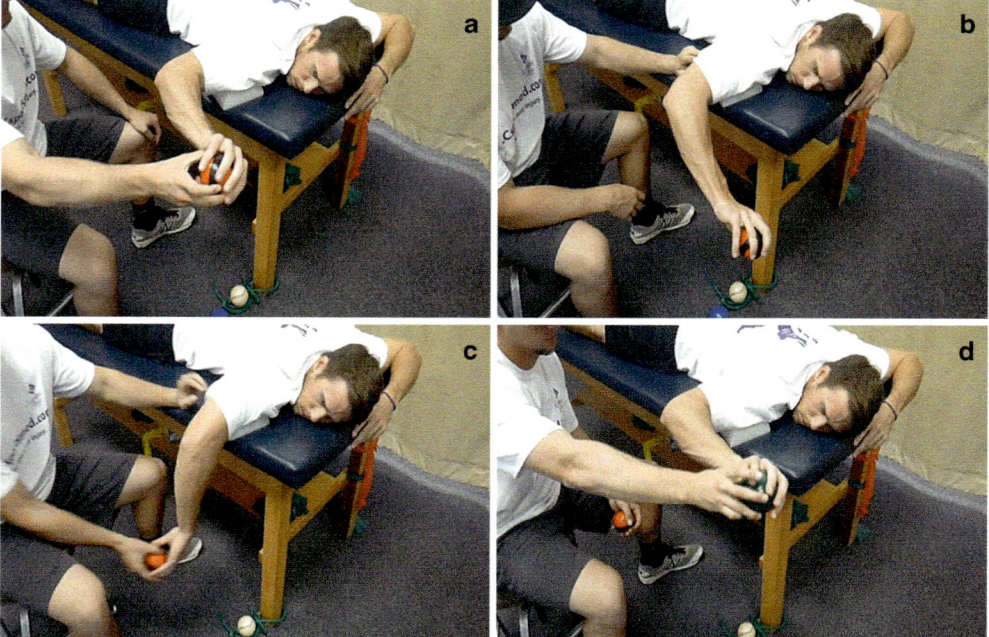

Fig. 15.5 90/90 external rotation (ER). (**a**) Start patient in ER with weighted ball. (**b**) The patient is instructed to lower the arm while maintaining 90° of elbow flexion (mid-range ER). (**c**) When the forearm is perpendicular with the table, the patient releases the ball. (**d**) The patient is then instructed to return to starting position, and the instructor places a new weighted ball into the patient's hand

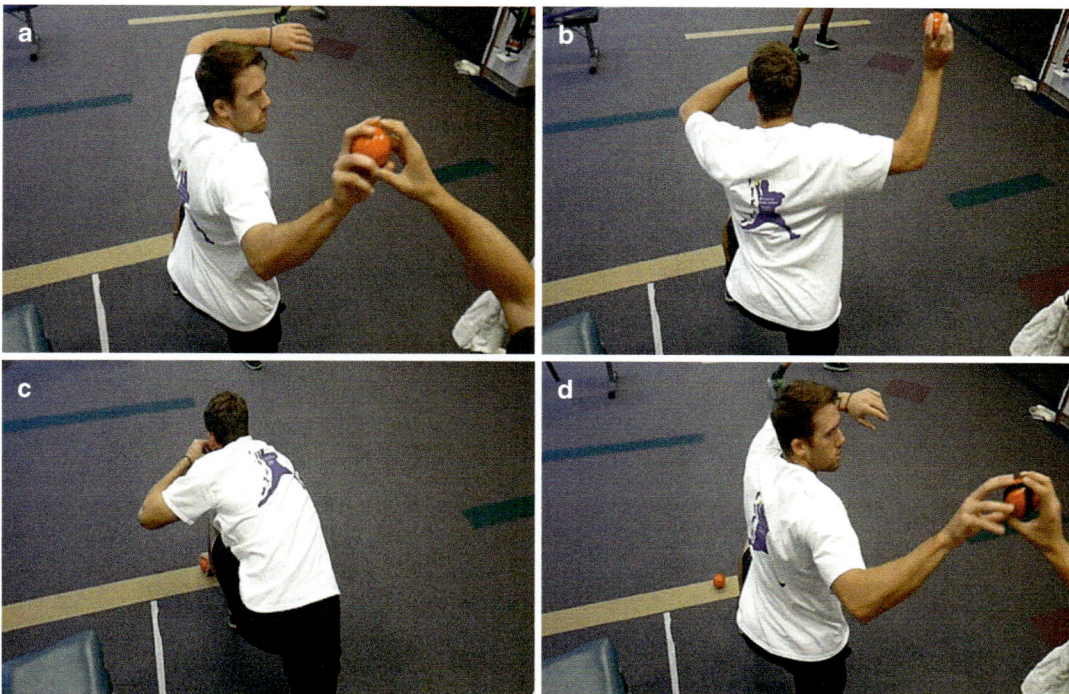

Fig. 15.6 Proprioceptive neuromuscular facilitation (PNF) pattern. (**a**) Starting position with weighted ball. (**b**) The patient is instructed to lower the arm toward the ground (similar to follow-through phase of tennis serve (mid-range movement). (**c**) When the hand reaches the ground, the patient is instructed to drop the ball. (**d**) The patient is then instructed to return to starting position, and the instructor places a new weighted ball into the patient's hand

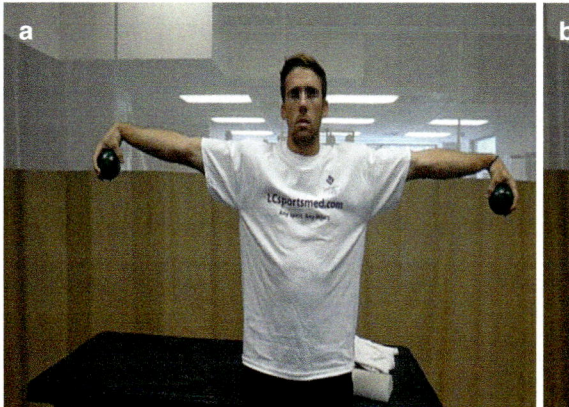
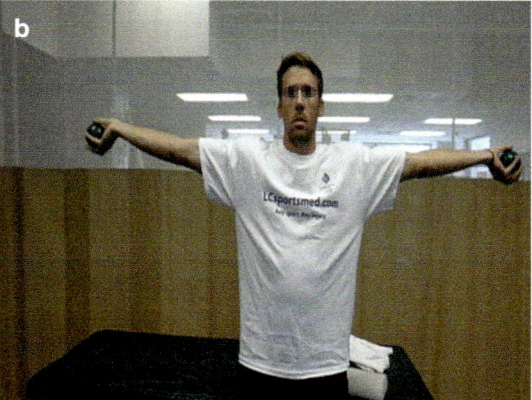

Fig. 15.7 Forearm and bicep exercise. (**a**) Start with arms at 0° of elbow extension and wrist flexed and pronated. (**b**) The patient is instructed to supinate and extend the wrist, while the elbow remained extended at 0°. (**c**) The patient is instructed to flex the elbow on a one count (mid-range elbow flexion). (**d**) The patient reaches full elbow flexion. (**e**) The patient is instructed to extend the elbows on an 8 count. (**f**) Ending position

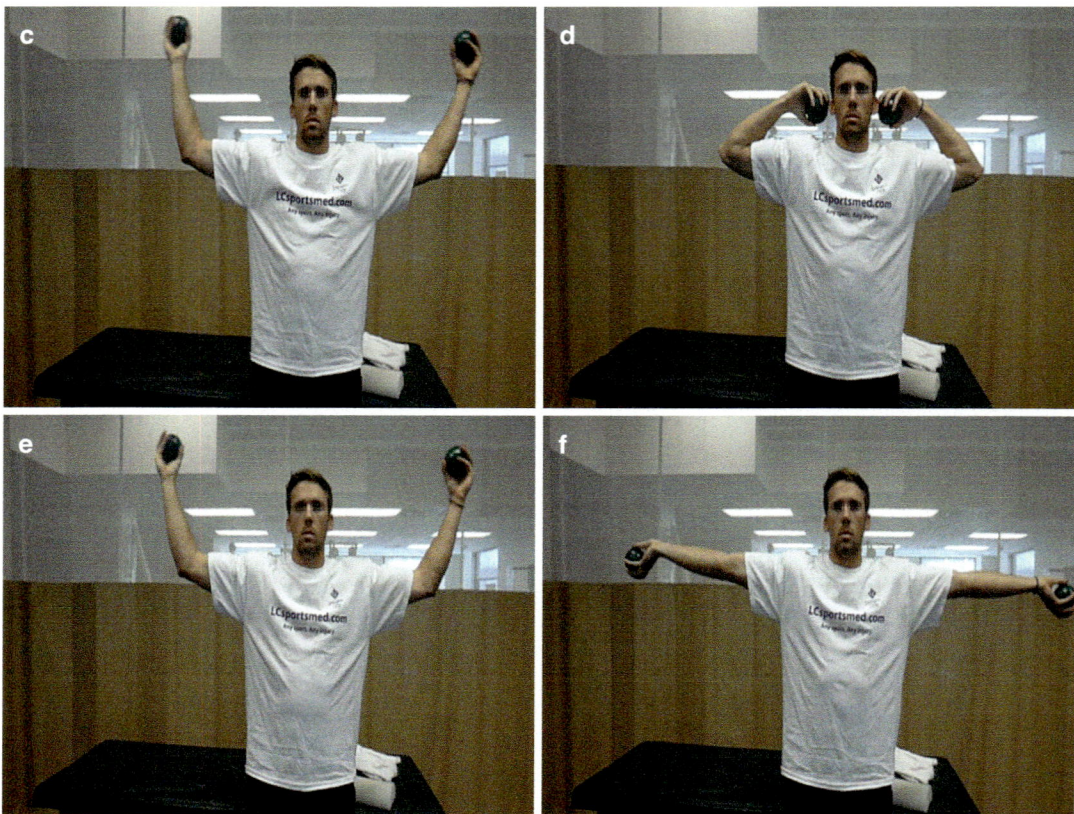

Fig. 15.7 (continued)

consider training programs that incorporate the sports main energy systems, muscular stresses (strength, power, speed, endurance, etc.), and volume demands. Data suggests that tennis singles competition has an aerobic as well as an anaerobic component [65]. Additionally, players must be able to exert muscular force at a high speed. Therefore, muscular strength and power should be challenged to accelerate the body around the court. As the lower extremity and core provide a stable base for distal mobility, these segments must not be neglected and should be trained to generate power. Agility and speed are critical to good court movement and correct positions on the court. Tennis depends on quick bursts of speed in multi-planar directions. Agility and speed drills should be executed on-court and incorporate high-intensity explosive movement. Parsons et al. [66] describe several speed and agility drills that can be used on-court and are shown in Figs. 15.8 and 15.9.

Furthermore, the volume of strokes should be integrated back into activity progression. Myers et al. [67] developed a three-phase volume-based interval training program specific to ground strokes and serves for elite-level tennis players (Table 15.1).

The 21-step progression can be incorporated into practice play where players mimic game-like scenarios. For example, during step 10, players are expected to hit 16 serves and 28 ground strokes. The players would compete in

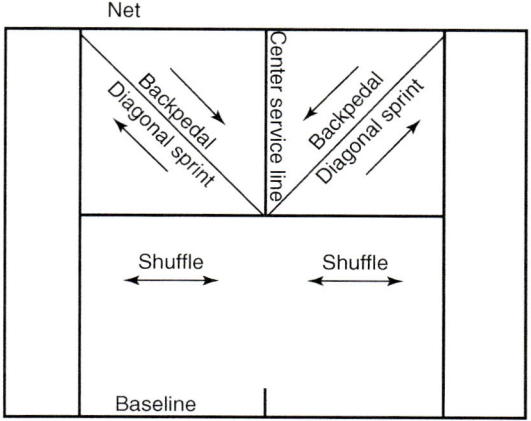

Fig. 15.8 Speed and agility drill (Adopted from Parsons et al.)

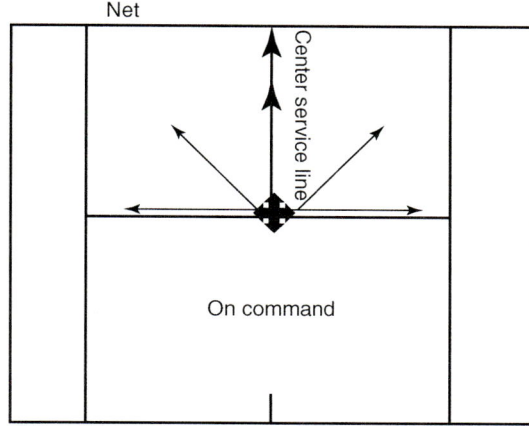

Fig. 15.9 Speed and agility drill (Adopted from Parsons et al.) *Represents player starting and ending position. Call out "sprint to left corner," then return as quickly as possible to starting position

Table 15.1 Elite-level tennis players' interval training program (Adopted from Myers et al.)

Phase	Step	Ground strokes	Serve	Stroke intensity (%)	Total stroke volume	Games played	First serves per game	Second serves per game	Ground strokes per game
1	1	10	–	–	10				
	2	10	2[a]	50	12				
	3	10	3[a]	50	13				
	4	12	4[a]	50	16				
	5	12	6[a]	50	18				
2	6	14	8	60	22	2	6	2	7
	7	18	10[b]	60	28				
	8	22	12[b]	60	34				
	9	26	14[b]	60	40				
	10	28	16	60	44	4[c]	6	2	7
3	11	28	16	80	44	4[c]	6	2	7
	12	42	24	80	66	6[c]	6	2	7
	13	56	32	80	88	8[c]	6	2	7
	14	42	24	90	66	6[c]	6	2	7
	15	56	32	90	88	8[c]	6	2	7
	16	84	48	90	132	10[c]	10[d]		8[e]
	17	112	64	90	176	12[c]	11[d]		9[e]
	18	56	32	100	88	8[c]	6	2	7
	19	168	96	100	264	14[c]	14[d]		12
	20	224	128	100	352	16[c]	12	4	14
	21	Simulated match							

[a]All second serves
[b]Combination of first and second serves
[c]Rest 90 s after two games
[d]Totals do no sum to serve column because of rounding, mathematically inappropriate to use a ratio of first to second serves
[e]Totals do not sum to ground stroke column because of rounding

four games, with two of those four representing service games. In each service game, the player would hit in total eight serves, and during each of the four games, the player would hit seven ground strokes. This approach allows for sport-specific training while diminishing the risk of boredom. The purpose of the protocol was to help players successfully return to tennis play after an injury or prepare for the demands of the strokes prior to or after competition. The program incorporates burst of intensity throughout a stepwise progression while following previously designed soreness and injury classification rules [68].

Conclusions

Scapular dyskinesis may directly cause, contribute to, or be the result of shoulder symptoms. It is a kinematic finding with no specific association to any single shoulder injury, and careful evaluation is required to identify it. Evaluation of the position and motion of the scapula and the results of corrective maneuvers should be a routine part of the overall assessment of all overhead athletes with shoulder pathology. Scapular rehabilitation should be comprehensive in nature and incorporate both the proximal and distal segments of the kinetic chain. The demonstration of the presence or absence of dyskinesis can indicate the need for a scapular rehabilitation program as part of the treatment plan and, in some cases, will actually indicate the direction for the treatment.

References

1. Ludewig PM, Cook TM, Nawoczenski DA. Three-dimensional scapular orientation and muscle activity at selected positions of humeral elevation. J Orthop Sports Phys Ther. 1996;24(2):57–65.
2. Ludewig PM, Behrens SA, Meyer SM, Spoden SM, Wilson LA. Three-dimensional clavicular motion during arm elevation: reliability and descriptive data. J Orthop Sports Phys Ther. 2004;34(3):140–9.
3. Myers JB, Laudner KG, Pasquale MR, Bradley JP, Lephart SM. Scapular position and orientation in throwing athletes. Am J Sports Med. 2005;33(2):263–71.
4. Laudner KG, Myers JB, Pasquale MR, Bradley JP, Lephart SM. Scapular dysfunction in throwers with pathologic internal impingement. J Orthop Sports Phys Ther. 2006;36(7):485–94.
5. Kuhn JE, Plancher KD, Hawkins RJ. Scapular winging. J Am Acad Orthop Surg. 1995;3(6):319–25.
6. Kuhne M, Boniquit N, Ghodadra N, Romeo AA, Provencher MT. The snapping scapula: diagnosis and treatment. Arthroscopy. 2009;25(11):1298–311.
7. Kibler WB, Sciascia A. Current concepts: scapular dyskinesis. Br J Sports Med. 2010;44(5):300–5.
8. Warner JJP, Micheli LJ, Arslanian LE, Kennedy J, Kennedy R. Scapulothoracic motion in normal shoulders and shoulders with glenohumeral instability and impingement syndrome. Clin Orthop Relat Res. 1992;285(191):199.
9. Kibler WB, Sciascia A, Wilkes T. Scapular dyskinesis and its relation to shoulder injury. J Am Acad Orthop Surg. 2012;20(6):364–72.
10. Uhl TL, Kibler WB, Gecewich B, Tripp BL. Evaluation of clinical assessment methods for scapular dyskinesis. Arthroscopy. 2009;25(11):1240–8.
11. Silva RT, Hartmann LG, de Souza Laurino CF, Biló JR. Clinical and ultrasonographic correlation between scapular dyskinesia and subacromial space measurement among junior elite tennis players. Br J Sports Med. 2010;44(6):407–10.
12. Kibler WB, Ludewig PM, McClure PW, Uhl TL, Sciascia A. Scapular summit. J Orthop Sports Phys Ther. 2009;39(11):A1–A13.
13. Kibler WB. Role of the scapula in the overhead throwing motion. Contemp Orthop. 1991;22((5)):525–32.
14. Odom CJ, Taylor AB, Hurd CE, Denegar CR. Measurement of scapular asymmetry and assessment of shoulder dysfunction using the lateral scapular slide test: a reliability and validity study. Phys Ther. 2001;81(2):799–809.
15. McClure PW, Michener LA, Sennett BJ, Karduna AR. Direct 3-dimensional measurement of scapular kinematics during dynamic movements in vivo. J Shoulder Elbow Surg. 2001;10(3):269–77.
16. Park J-Y, Hwang J-T, Kim K-M, Makkar D, Moon SG, Han K-J. How to assess scapular dyskinesis precisely: 3-dimensional wing computer tomography--a new diagnostic modality. J Shoulder Elbow Surg. 2013;22(8):1084–91.
17. Kibler WB, Uhl TL, Maddux JQ, McMullen J, Brooks PV, Zeller B. Qualitative clinical evaluation of scapular dysfunction. A reliability study. J Shoulder Elbow Surg. 2002;11(6):550–6.
18. McClure PW, Tate AR, Kareha S, Irwin D, Zlupko E. A clinical method for identifying scapular dyskinesis. Part 1: reliability. J Athl Train. 2009;44:160–4.
19. Tate AR, McClure PW, Kareha S, Irwin D, Barbe MF. A clinical method for identifying scapular dyskinesis. Part 2: validity. J Athl Train. 2009;44:165–73.
20. Kibler WB, Sciascia A, Dome D. Evaluation of apparent and absolute supraspinatus strength in patients with shoulder injury using the scapular retraction test. Am J Sports Med. 2006;34(10):1643–7.

21. Kibler WB. The role of the scapula in athletic shoulder function. Am J Sports Med. 1998;26(2):325–37.
22. Burkhart SS, Morgan CD, Kibler WB. Shoulder injuries in overhead athletes, the "dead arm" revisited. Clin Sports Med. 2000;19(1):125–58.
23. Rabin A, Irrgang JJ, Fitzgerald GK, Eubanks A. The intertester reliability of the Scapular Assistance Test. J Orthop Sports Phys Ther. 2006;36(9):653–60.
24. Seitz AL, McClure PW, Finucane S, et al. The scapular assistance test results in changes in scapular position and subacromial space but not rotator cuff strength in subacromial impingement. J Orthop Sports Phys Ther. 2012;42(5):400–12.
25. Tate AR, McClure PW, Kareha S, Irwin D. Effect of the Scapula Reposition Test on shoulder impingement symptoms and elevation strength in overhead athletes. J Orthop Sports Phys Ther. 2008;38(1):4–11.
26. Cools AM, Witvrouw EE, Declercq GA, Danneels LA, Cambier DC. Scapular muscle recruitment patterns: trapezius muscle latency with and without impingement symptoms. Am J Sports Med. 2003;31(4):542–9.
27. Cools AM, Dewitte V, Lanszweert F, et al. Rehabilitation of scapular muscle balance: which exercises to prescribe? Am J Sports Med. 2007;35(10):1744–51.
28. Kibler WB, Sciascia AD, Uhl TL, Tambay N, Cunningham T. Electromyographic analysis of specific exercises for scapular control in early phases of shoulder rehabilitation. Am J Sports Med. 2008;36(9):1789–98.
29. Michener LA, Boardman ND, Pidcoe PE, Frith AM. Scapular muscle tests in subjects with shoulder pain and functional loss: reliability and construct validity. Phys Ther. 2005;85(11):1128–38.
30. Moseley JB, Jobe FW, Pink M, Perry J, Tibone J. EMG analysis of the scapular muscles during a shoulder rehabilitation program. Am J Sports Med. 1992;20(2):128–34.
31. Thigpen CA, Padua DA, Michener LA, et al. Head and shoulder posture affect scapular mechanics and muscle activity in overhead tasks. J Electromyogr Kinesiol. 2010;20(4):701–9.
32. Ludewig PM, Cook TM. Alterations in shoulder kinematics and associated muscle activity in people with symptoms of shoulder impingement. Phys Ther. 2000;80(3):276–91.
33. Kluemper M, Uhl TL, Hazelrigg H. Effect of stretching and strengthening shoulder muscles on forward shoulder posture in competitive swimmers. J Sport Rehabil. 2006;15(1):58–70.
34. Borstad JD. Measurement of pectoralis minor muscle length: validation and clinical application. J Orthop Sports Phys Ther. 2008;38(4):169–74.
35. Burkhart SS, Morgan CD, Kibler WB. The disabled throwing shoulder: spectrum of pathology Part III: The SICK scapula, scapular dyskinesis, the kinetic chain, and rehabilitation. Arthroscopy. 2003;19(6):641–61.
36. Wilk KE, Reinold MM, Macrina LC, et al. Glenohumeral internal rotation measurements differ depending on stabilization techniques. Sports Health. 2009;1(2):131–6.
37. Cools AM, Johansson FR, Cambier DC, Velde AV, Palmans T, Witvrouw EE. Descriptive profile of scapulothoracic position, strength and flexibility variables in adolescent elite tennis players. Br J Sports Med. 2010;44(9):678–84.
38. Kibler WB, Chandler TJ. Range of motion in junior tennis players participating in an injury risk modification program. J Sci Med Sport. 2003;6:51–62.
39. Sauers E, August A, Snyder A. Fauls stretching routine produces acute gains in throwing shoulder mobility in collegiate baseball players. J Sport Rehabil. 2007;16(1):28–40.
40. Gelen E, Dede M, Bingul BM, Bulgan C, Aydin M. Acute effects of static stretching, dynamic exercises, and high volume upper extremity plyometric activity on tennis serve performance. J Sports Sci Med. 2012;11(4):600–5.
41. Reinold MM, Wilk KE, Macrina LC, et al. Changes in shoulder and elbow passive range of motion after pitching in professional baseball players. Am J Sports Med. 2008;36(3):523–7.
42. Moore-Reed SD, Kibler WB, Myers NL, Smith BJ. Acute changes in passive glenohumeral rotation following tennis play exposure in elite female players. Int J Sports Phys Ther. 2016;11(2):230–6.
43. Wilk KE, Macrina LC, Fleisig GS, et al. Correlation of glenohumeral internal rotation deficit and total rotational motion to shoulder injuries in professional baseball pitchers. Am J Sports Med. 2011;39(2):329–35.
44. Reagan KM, Meister K, Horodyski MB, Werner DW, Carruthers C, Wilk KE. Humeral retroversion and its relationship to glenohumeral motion in the shoulder of college baseball players. Am J Sports Med. 2002;30(3):354–60.
45. Crockett HC, Gross LB, Wilk KE, et al. Osseous adaptation and range of motion at the glenohumeral joint in professional baseball pitchers. Am J Sports Med. 2002;30(1):20–6.
46. Borsa PA, Wilk KE, Jacobson JA, et al. Correlation of range of motion and glenohumeral translation in professional baseball pitchers. Am J Sports Med. 2005;33(9):1392–9.
47. Thomas SJ, Swanik CB, Higginson JS, et al. A bilateral comparison of posterior capsule thickness and its correlation with glenohumeral range of motion and scapular upward rotation in collegiate baseball players. J Shoulder Elbow Surg. 2011;20(5):708–16.
48. Manske R, Wilk KE, Davies G, Ellenbecker T, Reinold M. Glenohumeral motion deficits: friend or foe? Int J Sports Phys Ther. 2013;8(5):537–53.
49. McClure P, Balaicuis J, Heiland D, Broersma ME, Thorndike CK, Wood A. A randomized controlled comparison of stretching procedures for posterior shoulder tightness. J Orthop Sports Phys Ther. 2007;37(3):108–14.
50. Moore SD, Laudner KG, McLoda TA, Shaffer MA. The immediate effects of muscle energy tech-

50. nique on posterior shoulder tightness: a randomized controlled trial. J Orthop Sports Phys Ther. 2011;41(6):400–7.
51. Manske RC, Meschke M, Porter A, Smith B, Reiman M. A randomized controlled single-blinded comparison of stretching versus stretching and joint mobilization for posterior shoulder tightness measured by internal rotation motion loss. Sports Health. 2010;2:94–100.
52. Ellenbecker TS, Cools A. Rehabilitation of shoulder impingement syndrome and rotator cuff injuries: an evidence-based review. Br J Sports Med. 2010;44(5):319–27.
53. McGill SM, Grenier S, Kavcic N, Cholewicki J. Coordination of muscle activity to assure stability of the lumbar spine. J Electromyogr Kinesiol. 2003;13(4):353–9.
54. McGill SM. Low back disorders: evidence based prevention and rehabilitation. 2nd ed. Champaign, IL: Human Kinetics; 2002.
55. Samson KM, Sandrey MA. A core stabilization training program for tennis athletes. Athletic Ther Today. 2007;12(3):41–6.
56. Myer GD, Chu DA, Brent JL, Hewett TE. Trunk and hip control neuromuscular training for the prevention of knee joint injury. Clin Sports Med. 2008;27(3):425–48. ix
57. Voight ML, Thompson BC. The role of the scapula in the rehabilitation of shoulder injuries. J Athl Train. 2000;35(3):364–72.
58. Kibler WB, Livingston B. Closed-chain rehabilitation for upper and lower extremities. J Am Acad Orthop Surg. 2001;9(6):412–21.
59. Wilk KE, Arrigo CA. Current concepts in the rehabilitation of the athletic shoulder. J Orthop Sports Phys Ther. 1993;18(1):365–77.
60. Veeger HE, van der Helm FC. Shoulder function: the perfect compromise between mobility and stability. J Biomech. 2007;40(10):2119–29.
61. Westing SH, Cresswell AG, Thorstensson A. Muscle activation during maximal voluntary eccentric and concentric knee extension. Eur J Appl Physiol Occup Physiol. 1991;62:104–8.
62. Tesch PA, Dudley GA, Duvoisin MR, Hather BM, Harris RT. Force and EMG signal patterns during repeated bouts of concentric or eccentric muscle actions. Acta Physiol Scand. 1990;138(3):263–71.
63. Fang Y, Siemionow V, Sahgal V, Xiong F, Yue GH. Greater movement-related cortical potential during human eccentric versus concentric muscle contractions. J Neurophysiol. 2001;86(4):1764–72.
64. Roig M, O'Brien K, Kirk G, et al. The effects of eccentric versus concentric resistance training on muscle strength and mass in healthy adults: a systematic review with meta-analysis. Br J Sports Med. 2009;43(8):556–68.
65. Morgans LF, Jordan DL, Baeyens DA, Franciosa JA. Heart rate responses during singles and doubles tennis competition. Phys Sportsmed. 1987;15(7):67–74.
66. Parsons LS, Jones MT. Development of speed, agility, and quickness for tennis athletes. Strength Condition J. 1998;20(3):14–9.
67. Myers NL, Sciascia AD, Kibler WB, Uhl TL. Volume-based interval training program for elite tennis players. Sports Health. 2016;8:536.
68. Axe MJ, Wickham R, Snyder-Mackler L. Data-based interval throwing programs for little league, high school, college, and professional baseball pitchers. Sports Med Arthrosc Rev. 2001;9:24–34.

Rehabilitation of the Shoulder in Tennis Players

16

Todd S. Ellenbecker and Ann Cools

16.1 Introduction: Incidence of Shoulder Injury in Elite Tennis Players

In epidemiologic studies of elite tennis players, the shoulder is frequently cited as one of the most often injured regions from high-level repetitive tennis play [1]. Ellenbecker et al. [2] reviewed many epidemiologic studies and reported high incidences (4–24%) of shoulder pain among elite players. Additionally, Kovacs et al. [3] surveyed 861 elite junior tennis players regarding their injury history. Shoulder pain was second only to lower back injury among the elite male and female players in their study. On the ATP World Tour, the evaluation and treatment of shoulder injury again are second only to spinal pathology in elite professional male players in injury frequency. Of the diagnoses commonly encountered in male professional players, rotator cuff impingement and tendonitis are most frequently reported. These studies identify the shoulder as a common site of injury and highlight the need for both rehabilitation and treatment programs as well as prevention programs for the shoulder.

16.2 Key Anatomical Adaptations Characteristic of Elite Tennis Players (TE)

Several anatomical adaptations have been reported in the musculoskeletal literature in elite tennis players. These adaptations have been identified in elite junior players as well as professional players. These adaptations include depression (lower) of the dominant shoulder when compared to the non-dominant shoulder [4, 5]. In male professional players on the ATP World Tour, Ellenbecker et al. [5] reported the dominant shoulder lower than the non-dominant shoulder through visual observation 82% of the time. Additionally the finding of visually observed infraspinatus atrophy on the dominant scapula has been reported in 73% of male professional players [5] and in 52% of professional female players [6]. Scapular dyskinesis diagnosed using the Kibler system of scapular classification [7] was present in 52% of male professional players on the dominant extremity and 38% in the non-dominant extremity [5]. In elite juniors, visual observation of scapular pathology was identified in 65% and 75% of male and female players,

T. S. Ellenbecker (✉)
ATP World Tour and Rehab Plus Sports Therapy, Scottsdale, AZ, USA
e-mail: tellenbecker@atpworldtour.com

A. Cools
Department of Rehabilitation Sciences & Physiotherapy, Faculty of Medicine and Health Sciences, Ghent University, Ghent, Belgium

Department of Occupational and Physical Therapy and Institute of Sports Medicine, Bispebjerg Hospital, University of Copenhagen, Copenhagen, Denmark

respectively, on their dominant extremities [8]. For the non-dominant extremity, significantly lower incidences of scapular dysfunction were identified (48–56% in males and females, respectively) [8].

In a recent study, performed on elite asymptomatic young tennis players in the age categories 12–20 years old, functional as well as structural sport specific adaptations were identified and reported. From a functional perspective, significant scapular position and scapular muscle strength differences or asymmetries between the dominant and non-dominant extremity were established, with age-dependent changes during adolescence, suggesting a relative decline of external rotator strength, total range of motion, scapular upward rotation, and strength in the scapular stabilizers, whereas increases were found in IR strength and strength in the scapular prime movers [9, 10].

Structural changes were apparent in the rotator cuff and proximal humerus in elite adolescent players, showing early signs of tendinosis in mainly the infraspinatus in more than 30% of the players [11], and growth plate alterations were established on the dominant proximal humerus compared to the non-dominant side [12]. Tendinosis of the rotator cuff seems to be correlated to lesser performance on the physical testing, possibly emphasizing the role of general fitness in adolescent tennis players to protect them from local musculoskeletal overload [13].

Finally, adaptations in shoulder ROM and strength have also been reported. The reader is referred to Chap. 10 for a more complete discussion of glenohumeral rotation and x-arm adduction ROM adaptations in elite professional and junior players. As a summary, dominant-arm internal-rotation ROM is less (mean 10–11°), and total rotation ROM loss (6–7°) has been reported in elite players [5, 8]. Additionally, in professional players, 7–8° less crossarm adduction ROM was reported in the uninjured dominant shoulder as compared to the non-dominant extremity [5, 8]. Isokinetic strength testing has identified significantly greater internal rotation strength, with no significant difference in external rotation strength when measured in 90° of glenohumeral joint abduction in several studies consistently [14–17]. This apparent preferential strength development of the internal rotators, without concomitant development of the external rotators on the dominant arm in elite players, creates an ER/IR muscle imbalance. This lower ER/IR unilateral strength ratio has been identified as a risk factor for shoulder injury in overhead athletes [18]. The desired ratio of ER to IR in the shoulder in normal shoulders and in the shoulder of the overhead athlete has been recommended to range between 66% and 75% [19, 20].

It is important for the clinician to understand these characteristic adaptations in the shoulder and scapula in elite-level tennis players to better interpret clinical examination findings and guide both preventative conditioning and injury rehabilitation programs [5, 20, 21].

16.3 Exercise Progression for Rotator Cuff and Scapular Exercise

A key part of any rehabilitation program for elite-level tennis players is to address strength and stabilization deficiencies in the rotator cuff and scapula [21]. From the perspective of prevention as well as rehabilitation of shoulder injuries, exercises for the tennis player should focus on restoration of rotator cuff (RC) strength as well as scapular muscle balance. The specific approach will depend upon the results of the clinical exam and additional measurements; however the following general guidelines may assist the clinician in the choice of exercises:

16.3.1 Rotator Cuff Training

In general, in view of their stabilizing role, and their ability to protect the joint against overload during throwing or serving, strengthening exercises for the rotator cuff muscles are mandatory. However, several research data point out the importance of strengthening in particular the posterior cuff muscles, performing external rotation (ER) exercises. Relative muscle weakness of the ER compared to the internal rotators (IR) has been established in healthy tennis players in different age categories [17, 22]. Loss of ER strength and decreased ER/IR ratio have been recognized as an intrinsic risk factor for throwing-related shoulder pain in baseball [18, 23, 24], volleyball [25], and handball [26]. In addition, early signs of infraspinatus (IS) tendinosis have been established in elite asymptomatic adolescent tennis players [27], and recently, decreased muscle activation of the IS was found in reaction to experimentally induced pain in the supraspinatus (SS) muscle [28]. In summary, the ER, in particular the IS, seems to be vulnerable to structural and functional changes in tennis players and in response to shoulder pain. Therefore the clinician should focus on ER training during rehabilitation and prevention of shoulder injuries.

In addition to the knowledge from risk factor analysis and the role of the IS in shoulder pain, several studies highlighted the importance of ER training based on biomechanical or electromyographic studies. ER exercises have a positive influence on the subacromial space, leading to decreased subacromial pressure [29] and decreased superior humeral head translations [30]. Townsend [31] showed that ER exercises are able to activate the posterior cuff muscles, whereas IR exercises activate the large glenohumeral muscles like the pectoralis major (PM) and latissimus dorsi (LD) rather than the subscapularis (SC). In other words IR exercises should only be performed if in general IR strength is the target of the exercise, and not to increase RC strength, and ER exercises should be favored. Additionally, ER exercises have been shown not only to activate the IS and teres minor (Tm) but also the SS, emphasizing the important role of the SS not only in maintaining inferior/superior glenohumeral stability but also controlling anterior/posterior translations [32]. Finally, external rotation components during exercises seem to activate the lower and middle trapezius [33, 34], which is in favor of scapular muscle exercises in case of muscular imbalance with relative weakness of these muscles.

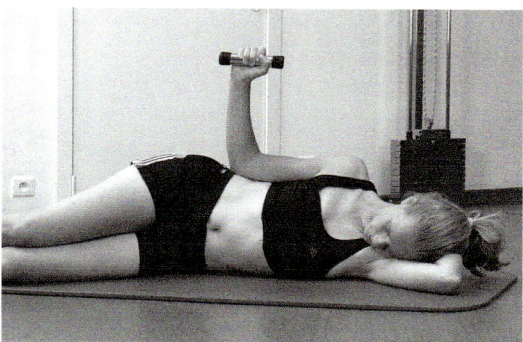

Fig. 16.1 Side-lying external rotation

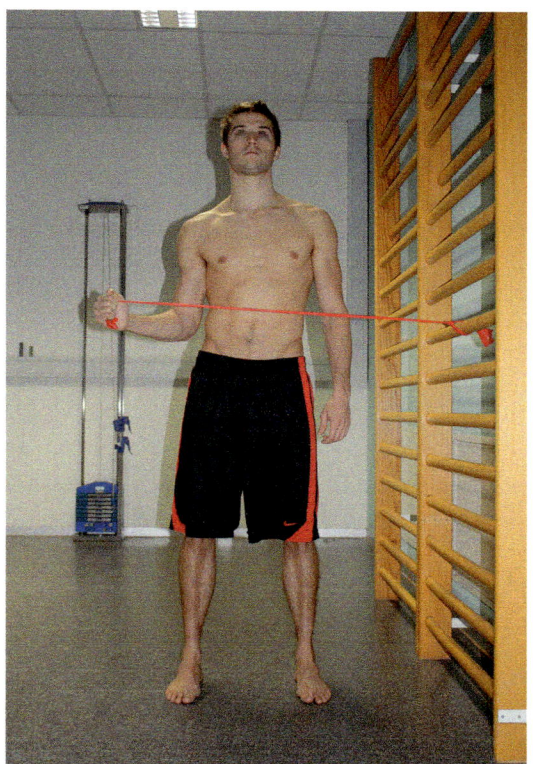

Fig. 16.2 Standing external rotation

The posterior cuff muscles may be activated by performing isolated ER exercises (Figs. 16.1 and 16.2 [35, 36]) or by performing combined movements such as horizontal abduction with ER (Fig. 16.3, [35, 36]). However, besides isolated ER movements, ER components may be implemented in functional elevation exercises (Fig. 16.4, [34]) or combined with activation of

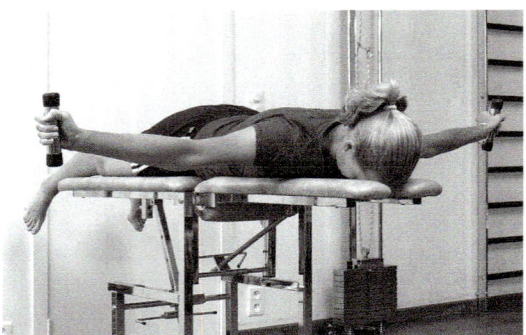

Fig. 16.3 Horizontal abduction with external rotation

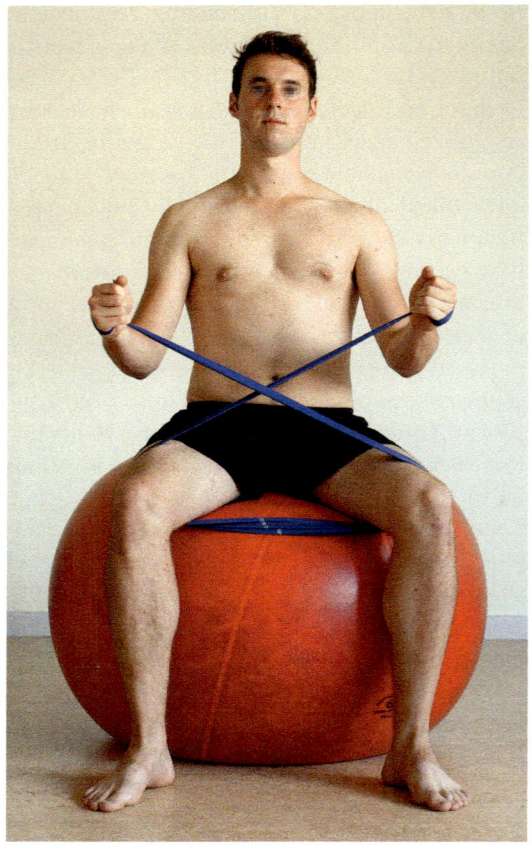

Fig. 16.5 External rotation with combined hip abduction

the hip abductors in order to optimize kinetic chain involvement (Fig. 16.5).

In view of the eccentric role of the posterior cuff muscles, training the eccentric capacity of these muscles is of extreme importance in tennis players [27]. These exercises may be performed in a slow (focusing on the load during the eccentric phase) or a more plyometric way (focusing on the decelerating characteristics of the posterior cuff).

For the eccentric loading, exercises may focus on higher loads during the eccentric compared to the concentric phase (Figs. 16.6 and 16.7) or on the deceleration role during quick movements. For the latter purpose, scapular muscle activity has been described [37, 38] during a variety of plyometric exercises. Based on the specific therapeutic goal (in view of scapular muscle balance),

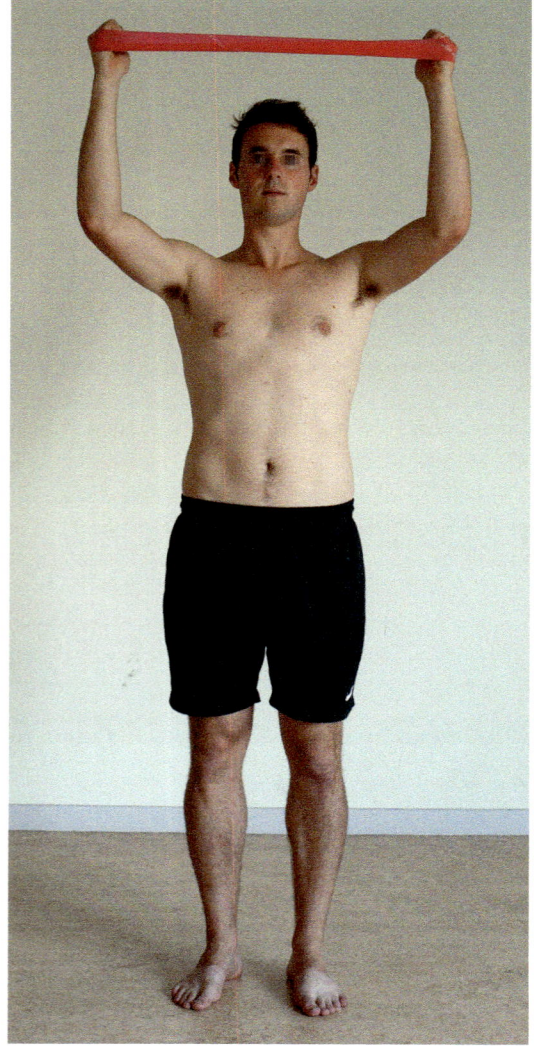

Fig. 16.4 Elevation with external rotation component

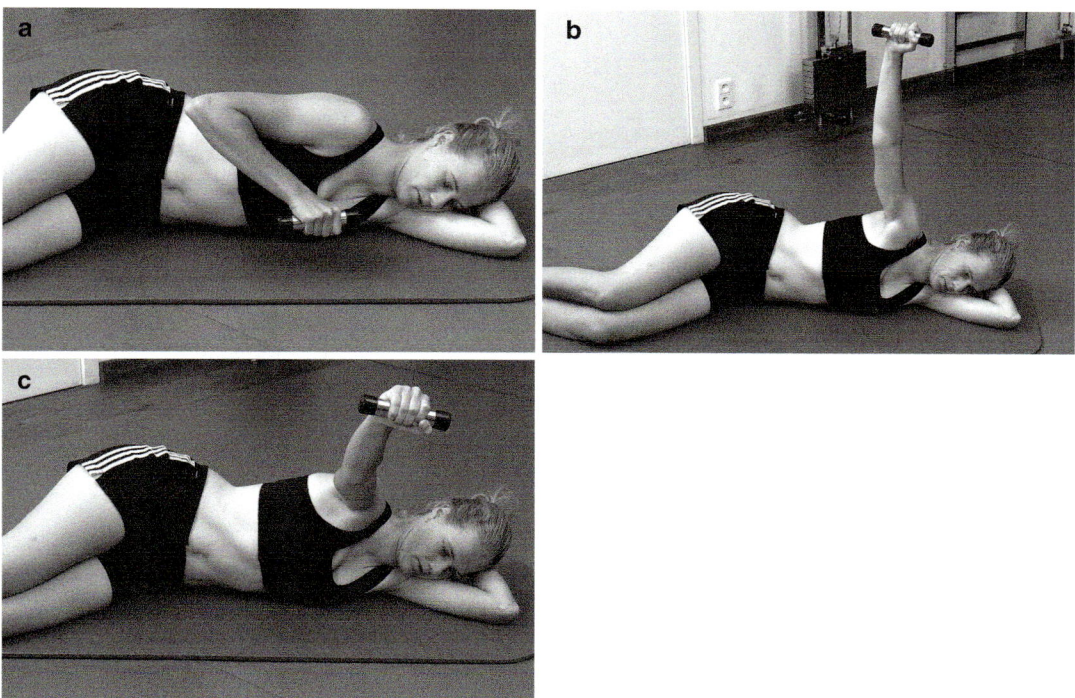

Fig. 16.6 (**a–c**) Eccentric exercise for the infraspinatus

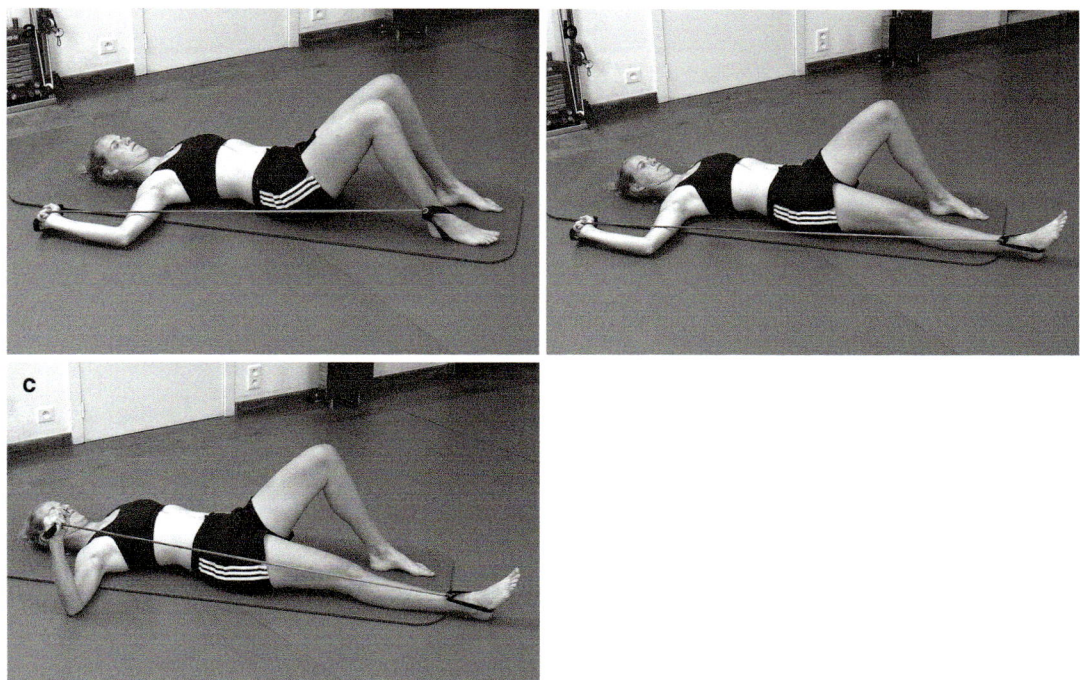

Fig. 16.7 (**a–c**) Eccentric exercise focusing in the abduction-ER position

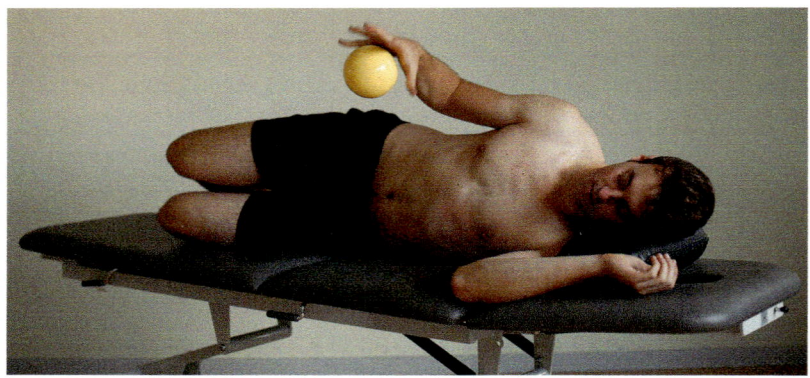

Fig. 16.8 Catching exercise in side lying with shoulder in neutral position

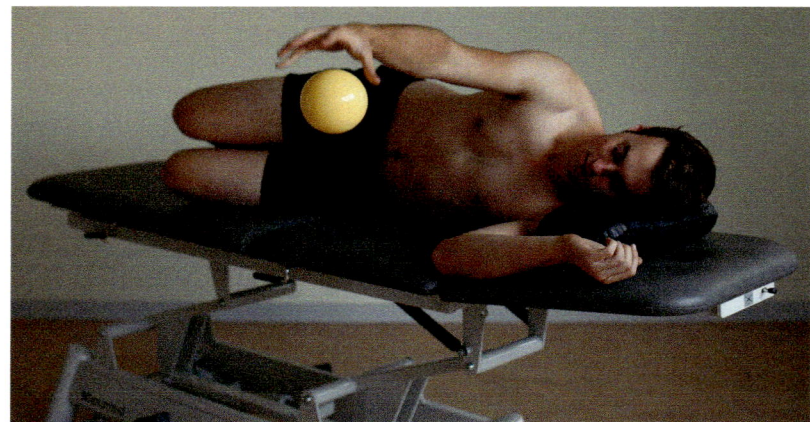

Fig. 16.9 Catching exercise in side lying with shoulder in forward flexion

exercises may be selected and a progression is proposed (Table 16.1).

16.3.2 Scapular Rehabilitation

For the rehabilitation of scapular dyskinesis in the tennis player, one should acknowledge that the muscles acting on the scapula may play various roles, as prime movers (mainly the upper trapezius (UT) and serratus anterior (SA)), dynamic stabilizers (for instance, MT and LT), or in a more postural role (pectoralis minor (Pm), levator scapulae (LS), rhomboids (RH)) [22, 39]. In view of this ascertainment, and in the knowledge that scapular dyskinesis related to shoulder pain is often characterized by a muscle imbalance rather than a lack of general muscle strength [22], rehabilitation of the tennis player with shoulder pain and scapular dysfunction should focus on

Table 16.1 Scapular muscle activity during progression in plyometric exercises for the posterior cuff

Hyperactive muscle	Hypoactive muscle	Proposed exercise
UT	LT or MT	Side-lying catching exercise with Plyoball with shoulder in neutral (Fig. 16.8)
		Side-lying catching exercise with Plyoball with shoulder in forward flexion (Fig. 16.9)
	SA	Plyometric push-up (Fig. 16.10)
None	Trapezius	Prone catching 90-90 (Fig. 16.11)
		Prone catching full elevation (Fig. 16.12)
None	SA + trapezius	Xco exercise (Fig. 16.13)
		Reversed catching (Fig. 16.14)

these clinically relevant muscle balances, activating the relative hypoactive muscles with simultaneous inhibition of the hyperactive muscle. Based on the available evidence [39, 40] and clinical experience, the clinically relevant balance ratios and most appropriate exercises are presented (Table 16.2).

The kinetic chain, in which the athlete functions, is highly sport-specific and needs to be reconsidered for every athlete. In ground-based sports, like tennis, all of the activities of the shoulder work within a kinetic chain linkage from the ground to the trunk, mostly in a diagonal pattern.

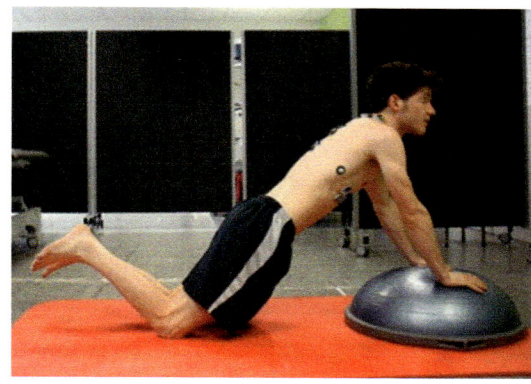

Fig. 16.10 Plyometric push-up

Table 16.2 Clinically relevant scapular muscle exercise ratios [22, 34, 36–39]

Hyperactive muscles	Hypoactive muscles	Clinically relevant balance ratios	Proposed exercises
Pm	SA	Pm/SA	Serratus punch standing (Fig. 16.15a)
	MT	Pm/MT	Elevation with ER
	LT	Pm/LT	Elevation with ER
	Rh	Pm/Rh	Elevation with ER
UT	SA	UT/SA	Elbow push-up (Fig. 16.16)
			Serratus punch supine (Fig. 16.15b)
			Elevation with ER
			Wall slide (Fig. 16.17)
	MT or LT	UT/MT or UT/LT	Elevation with ER
			Side-lying forward flexion (Fig. 16.18)
			Side-lying external rotation (Fig. 16.1)
			Prone hor abd with ER (Fig. 16.3)
			Prone extension (Fig. 16.19)
			Prone ER in 90° abd (Fig. 16.20)
	RH	UT/RH	Elevation with ER
LS	SA	LS/SA	Wall slide
	UT	LS/UT	Overhead shrug
	MT or LT or RH	LS/MT or LS/LT or LS/RH	Overhead retraction
RH	SA	RH/SA	Wall slide

These athletes benefit from diagonal patterns in closed as well as in open chain exercises. Research has shown that performing shoulder exercises standing on the contralateral leg enhances scapular muscle activity [41] and performing extension of the contralateral leg in a closed chain exercise (push-up) increases activity in the middle and lower trap of the involved shoulder [42].

Utilization of these exercises in a low-resistance/high-repetition format is applied to enhance relative activation of the rotator cuff [43, 44] and scapular stabilizer musculature [44].

16.3.3 Range of Motion and Mobilization Concepts for Rehabilitation of the Elite Tennis Player's Shoulder

The use and application of range of motion, stretching, and/or mobilization of the glenohumeral joint are predicated on a clear understanding of each player's range of motion profile gleaned during musculoskeletal evaluation. In cases where players have documented internal rotation ROM loss <5–8° (compared with the non-dominant uninjured extremity) without total rotation range of motion or total dominant arm total rotation <5–8°, stretching and range of motion are not typically a significant focus in the rehabilitation or maintenance program. Players who present with >6–8° of IR ROM loss coupled with total rotation ROM loss of 6–8° or more should receive stretches to enhance IR ROM gain. This cut point for range of motion is based on multiple descriptive studies from elite tennis players taking into account typical ROM adaptations that occur in healthy, uninjured elite players. This method requires careful isolated assessment of isolated bilateral glenohumeral joint internal rotation, external rotation, and total rotation ROM using scapular stabilization [20, 45] (Fig. 16.21).

Techniques used and recommended by these authors to increase internal rotation and crossarm adduction range of motion include the sleeper stretch and crossarm stretch [20, 46]. These stretches have been studied and shown to increase glenohumeral joint range of motion both acutely

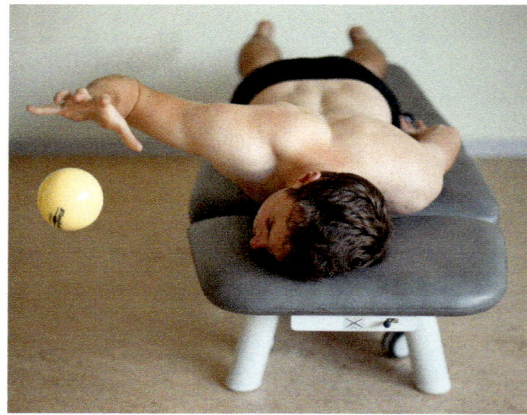

Fig. 16.11 Catching exercise in prone with shoulder in 90-90 position

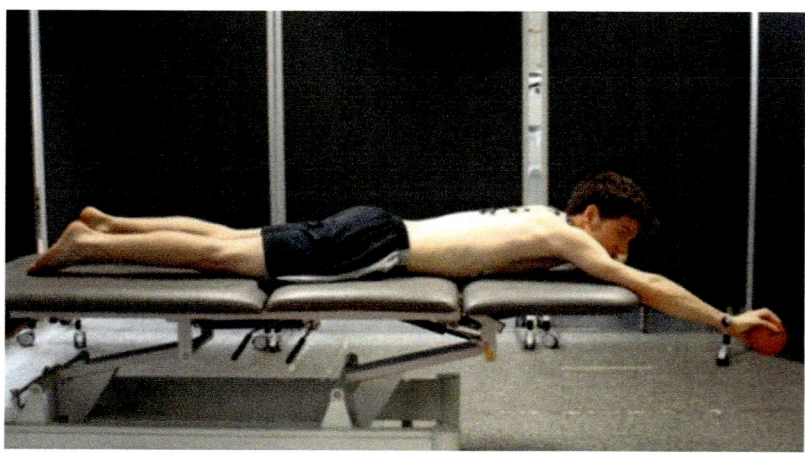

Fig. 16.12 Catching exercise prone with shoulder in full elevation

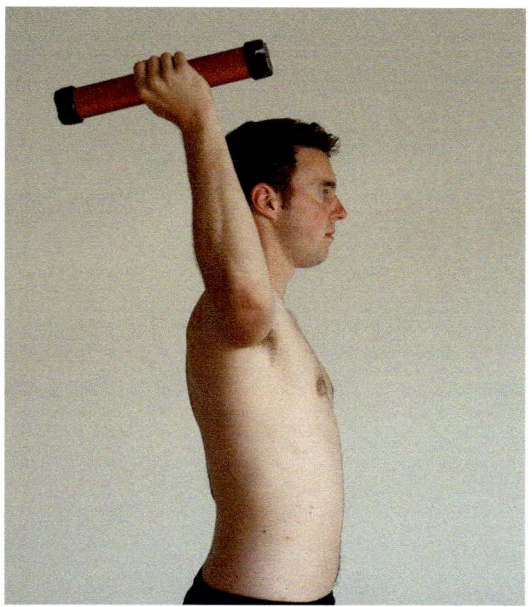

Fig. 16.13 Xco exercise

mobilization to increase internal rotation ROM in the overhead athlete would only be reserved for those individuals who had a significant reduction in manually assessed posterior translation using a posterior lateral assessment technique to ensure proper translation along the line of the glenohumeral joint. Excessive stretching or mobilization techniques applied to the overhead athlete's shoulder that is not range of motion restricted are not indicated.

16.3.4 Return to Play Considerations

One of the most critical final steps in the rehabilitation process of an elite tennis player is the determination of the return to tennis play. This is a step that is often overlooked and not completely integrated into the full rehabilitation program of the overhead athlete with a shoulder injury. Table 16.3 lists some of the criteria that can be used to provide an objective basis to aid the decision-making process for the clinician. These include clinical examination maneuvers, range of motion, and strength and functional tests/assessments that can be applied and reapplied to determine patient readiness. The additional objectivity afforded by the use of either a handheld dynamometer or an isokinetic dynamometer to obtain strength, endurance, and unilateral strength ratios can provide vital assistance to the clinician for this type of high-level clinical decision-making [19, 53].

[47, 48] as well as in training intervention studies [49, 50]. Several caveats for clinical application to enhance the patient response include use of the 30-degree rollback positon (Fig. 16.22) for the sleeper stretch in patients who have discomfort in the side-lying position [20, 51] as well as the use of scapular stabilization during the crossarm stretch (Fig. 16.23) [52]. These details may allow more optimal application of these specific shoulder stretches shown to enhance IR ROM in the human shoulder.

Finally, the concept of glenohumeral joint mobilization deserves discussion regarding its application in the rehabilitation of the overhead athlete. Manske et al. [50] studied the effect of adding a posterior glide mobilization by a physical therapist to crossarm adduction stretches over a 4-week experimental paradigm. Results after 4 weeks of posterior shoulder stretching or posterior shoulder stretching with posterior glide mobilization showed no significant difference between groups. This finding indicates that the posterior glide mobilization did not significantly increase internal rotation range of motion over posterior shoulder stretching (crossarm adduction stretching) alone. The use of posterior glide

The introduction of the interval tennis program follows several guidelines. While it is beyond the scope of this chapter to fully describe the interval tennis program, the program has been published elsewhere [20, 54], and several key components and concepts will be discussed here. First, the sequence of strokes applied for the patient following a shoulder injury is very important. Ground strokes (forehands and backhands) are the first tennis-specific movement patterns integrated into the interval tennis program. These strokes utilize lower levels of muscular activation and positions below 90° of shoulder elevation [55, 56] and are typically better tolerated in the initial introduction of the tennis program.

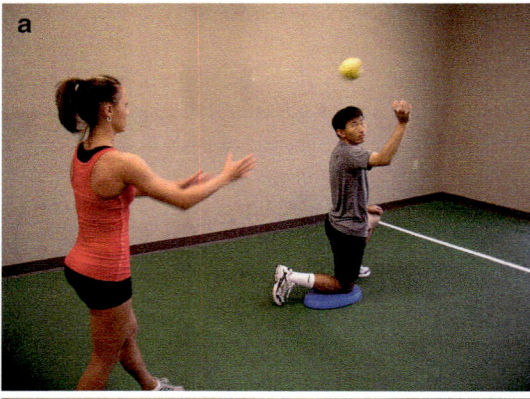
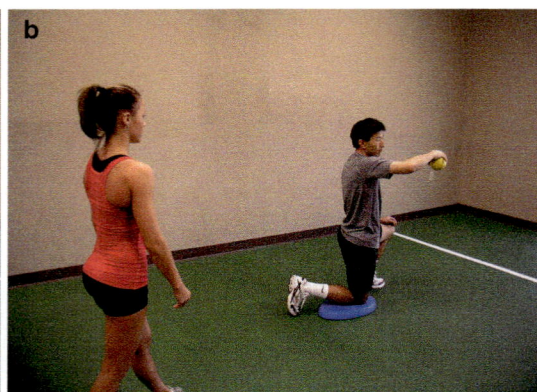
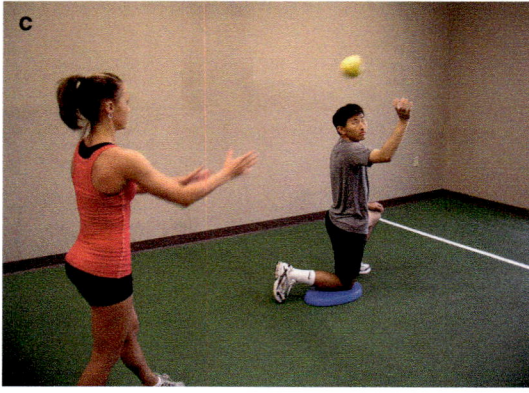

Fig. 16.14 (**a–c**) Reverse catch

Table 16.3 Objective criteria to progress to an interval tennis program

Satisfactory clinical examination and full non-painful ROM (appropriate and necessary ROM)
Acceptable muscular strength (especially of rotator cuff, scapular, and core muscles)
Special tests with acceptable results (subluxation-relocation test, SLAP tests)
Physician approval of initiation of interval tennis program
Satisfactory isokinetic test or handheld dynamometer manual muscle test
(a) External/internal rotation ratio
  - 66–75%
(b) Bilateral comparison
  - External rotation comparison: 95% or greater
  - Internal rotation comparison: 110–115% or greater
(c) Endurance ratios
  - 10–15% decrease in Peak Torque for ER and IR from first three reps to last three reps
Satisfactory functional tests
  - Single-leg squat, ten reps without loss of balance (squat to 45–50°)
  - Side-lying and prone ball flips for 30 s (satisfactory number and no pain)

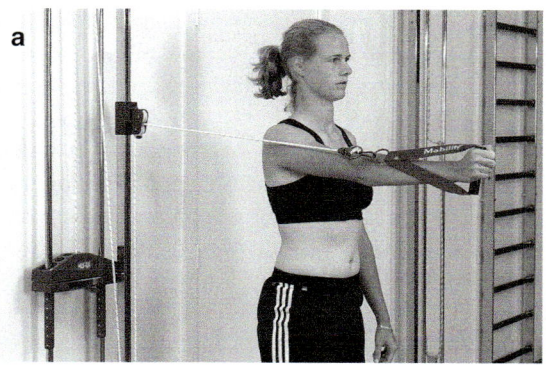 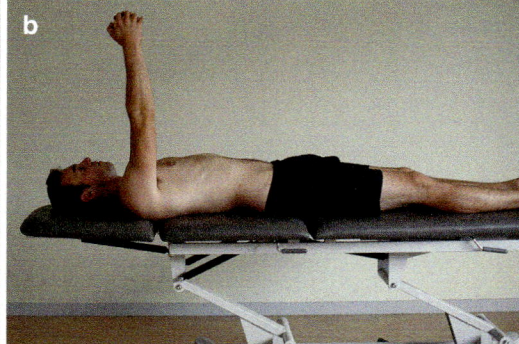

Fig. 16.15 Serratus punch standing (**a**) and supine (**b**)

Favoring of the backhand ground stroke (utilization of a 2:1 feeding/hitting ratio) is also recommended for players with a two-handed ground stroke to allow for greater kinetic chain contribution to both shock attenuation and force development in the early stages of the program. Gradual increase in the volume and intensity is followed using a stepwise-type progression.

In addition to careful selection of the initial tennis stroke pattern utilized, a specific pattern of tennis ball utilization is also followed. For the initial trials of tennis ground strokes, most often performed in the clinic under the direction of the physical therapist, foam balls are used. These balls are much lighter and provide a lower impact shock to the extremity. These foam balls can be obtained through many manufacturers and can also ensure that early phases of the program can be performed in the clinic in a limited space without jeopardizing safety. Progression from the foam ball to what are termed "low-compression" tennis balls is followed to gradually increase ball weight and stress to the extremity while also providing a closer, more realistic ball impact. These balls, used for teaching tennis to young children, again can be easily

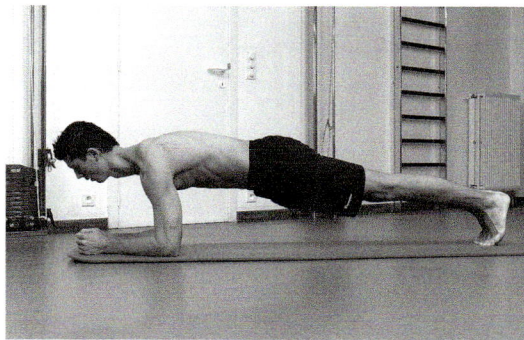

Fig. 16.16 Elbow push-up/prone bridging

purchased through tennis ball suppliers for clinical use and follow a progression from red-level balls (least amount of air) to orange-level balls and finally green-level balls (Fig. 16.24). These balls are all used in the progression of the patient through ground strokes initially with integration of volleys coming in the next phase of the program. Ground strokes are initially preferred as the ball bounces off the court surface and is decelerated providing a decreased preimpact ball velocity. When volleys are added, the ball is contacted prior to ball bounce with minimal

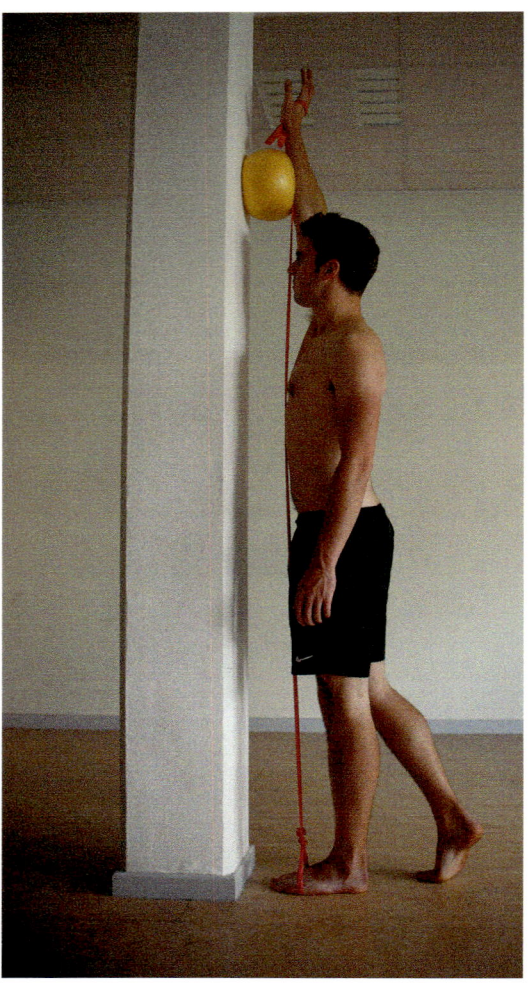

deceleration prior to impact. Therefore volleys are integrated only after successful progression through the ground strokes in the interval tennis program.

Serves, followed by overheads, are the last tennis-specific movement patterns integrated into the interval tennis program. The serve is performed and integrated first, prior to the overhead, even though many of the movement characteristics and muscle activity patterns are similar (see Chap. 1). The main difference between the serve and overhead smash is on the serve, careful positioning of the contact point through the patient's self-directed toss to hit the serve is preferable to the overhead which requires movement and positioning of the player's body in response to a lob and often less than optimal contact point utilization and frequent use of modified patterning of shoulder motion. The use of ball progression on the serve is again applied with foam used on the initial trials, followed by red, orange, green, and finally real tennis ball contacts. First serves are initiated and progressed prior to the introduction of second serves or "kick/spin" serves.

Successful progression through the interval tennis program is an essential final step to the player's return to the game following rehabilitation from shoulder injury or surgery.

Fig. 16.17 Wall slide

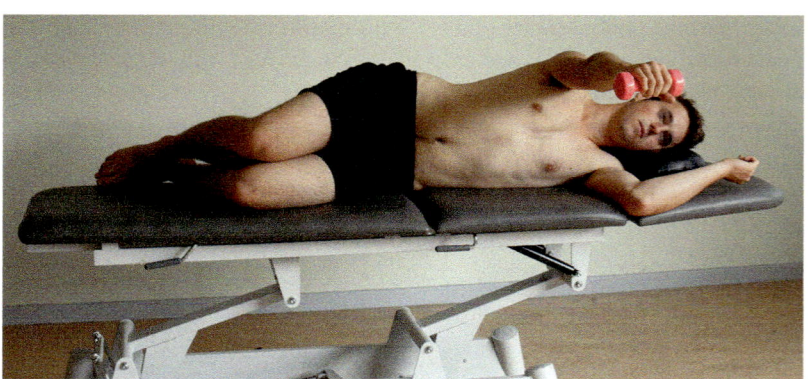

Fig. 16.18 Side-lying forward flexion

Fig. 16.19 Prone extension

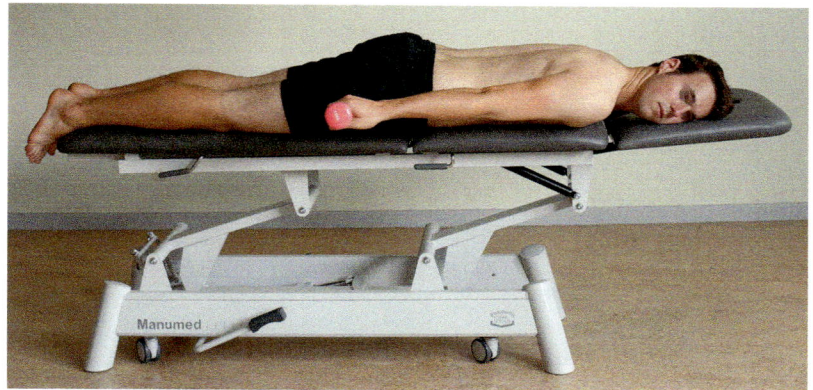

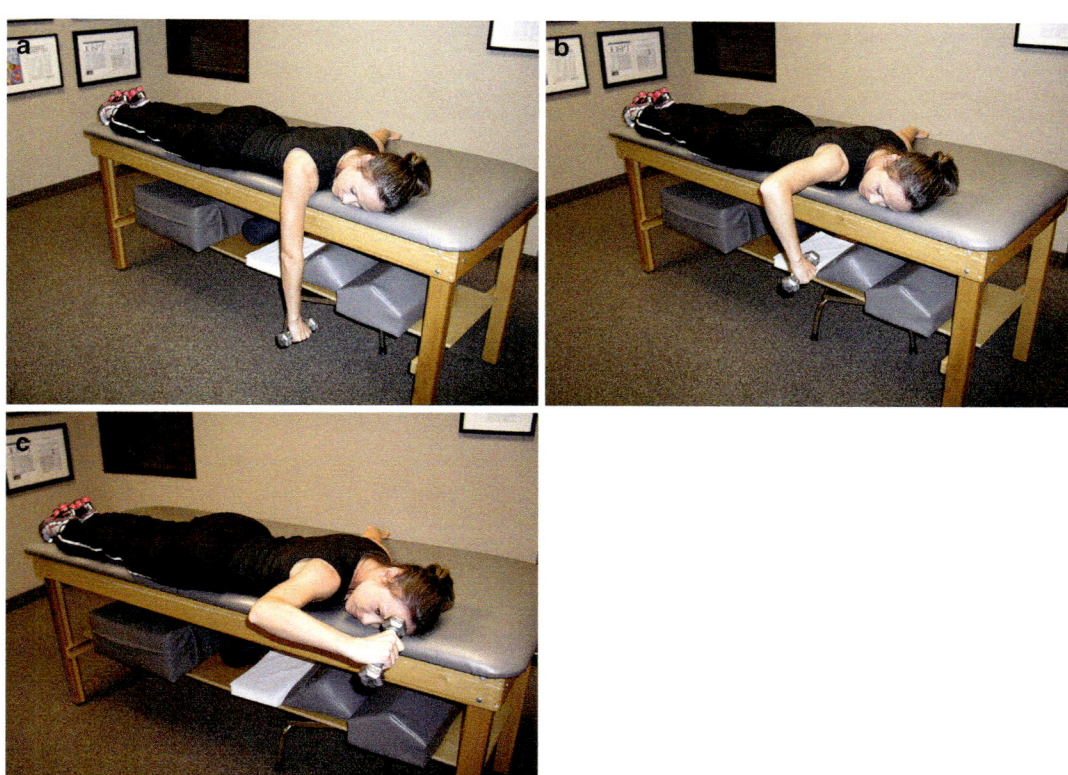

Fig. 16.20 Prone external rotation: (**a**) start position, (**b**) middle position, and (**c**) end position

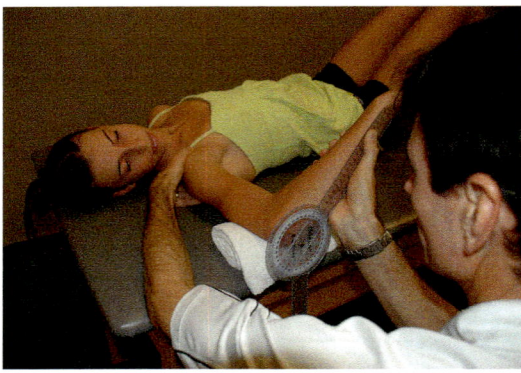

Fig. 16.21 Measurement of shoulder internal rotation with 90° of glenohumeral joint abduction

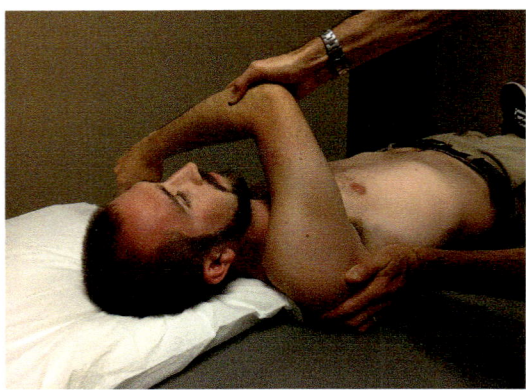

Fig. 16.23 Crossarm stretch with scapular stabilization

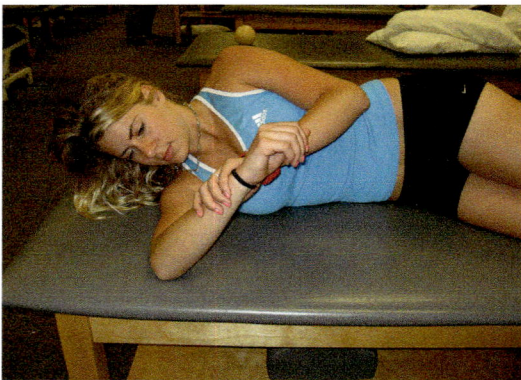

Fig. 16.22 Sleeper stretch with 30-degree rollback

Fig. 16.24 Tennis ball progression used with interval tennis program

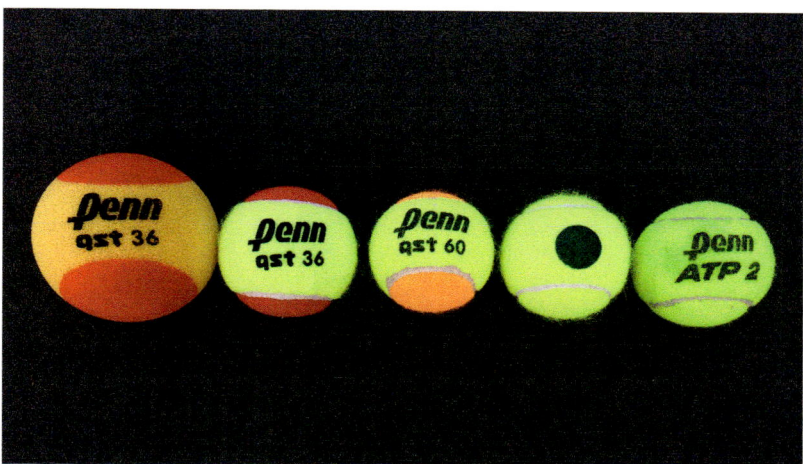

16.4 Summary

The concepts contained in this chapter serve to provide greater understanding of the characteristic musculoskeletal adaptations in the elite tennis player's shoulder as well as key rehabilitation concepts to improve muscular strength, balance, and stabilization. Careful evaluation of shoulder range of motion should lead to optimal application of interventions to increase shoulder motion using evidence-based guidelines based on descriptive musculoskeletal research on elite tennis players. Finally, the use of an interval tennis program after successful completion of a rehabilitation program and objective criterion can determine player readiness for a return to full activity following shoulder injury.

References

1. Pluim BM, Staal JB, Windler GE, et al. Tennis injuries: occurrence, aetiology, and prevention. Br J Sports Med. 2006;40:415–23.
2. Ellenbecker TS, Pluim B, Vivier S, Sniteman C. Common injuries in tennis players: exercises to address muscular imbalances and reduce injury risk. J Strength Condition. 2009;31(4):50–8.
3. Kovacs M, Ellenbecker TS, Kibler WB, Roetert EP, Lubbers P. Injury trends in American competitive junior tennis players. J Sci Med Tennis. 2014;19:19.
4. Priest JD, Nagel DA. Tennis shoulder. Am J Sports Med. 1976;4(1):28–42.
5. Ellenbecker TS, Windler G, Dines D, Renstrom P. Musculoskeletal profile of tennis players on the ATP World Tour: results of a 9-year screening program. J Med Sci Tennis. 2015;20(3):94–106.
6. Young SW, Dakic J, Stroia K, Nguyen ML, Harris AH, Safran MR. High incidence of infraspinatus muscle atrophy in elite professional female tennis players. Am J Sports Med. 2015;43(8):1989–93.
7. Kibler WB, Uhl TL, Maddux JW, Brooks PV, Zeller B, McMullen J. Qualitative clinical evaluation of scapular dysfunction: a reliability study. J Shoulder Elbow Surg. 2002;11:550–6.
8. Ellenbecker TS. Musculoskeletal examination of elite junior tennis players. Aspetar Sports Med J. 2014;3:548–56.
9. Cools AM, Johansson FR, Velde AV, Palmans T, Cambier DC, Witvrouw EE. Descriptive profile of scapulothoracic position-, strength- and flexibility variables in adolescent elite tennis players. Br J Sports Med. 2010;44(9):678–84.
10. Cools AM, Palmans T, Johansson FR. Age-related sport-specific adaptations of the shoulder girdle in elite adolescent tennis players. J Athl Train. 2014;49(5):647–53.
11. Johansson FR, Skillgate E, Adolfsson A, Jenner G, Debri E, Swärdh L, Cools AM. Asymptomatic elite adolescent tennis players show tendinosis signs on their dominant shoulder compared to their nondominant. J Athl Train. 2015;50(7):719–25.
12. Johansson FR, Skillgate E, Adolfsson A, Jenner G, Debri E, Swârdh L, Cools AM. Asymptomatic elite young tennis players show lateral and ventral growth plate alterations of proximal humerus on MRI. Knee Surg Sports Traumatol Arthrosc. 2016;25:3251.
13. Johansson F. The shoulder in the elite adolescent tennis player: Exploration of structural and functional

sport specific adaptations, Doctoral Thesis Ghent University, Supervisor Ann MJ Cools. 2017
14. Chandler TJ, Kibler WB, Stracener EC, Ziegler AK, Pace B. Shoulder strength, power and endurance in college tennis players. Am J Sports Med. 1992;20(4):455–8.
15. Ellenbecker TS. A total arm strength isokinetic profile of highly skilled tennis players. Isok Exer Sci. 1991;1:9–21.
16. Ellenbecker TS. Shoulder internal and external rotation strength and range of motion in highly skilled tennis players. Isokinet Exerc Sci. 1992;2:1–8.
17. Ellenbecker TS, Roetert EP. Age specific isokinetic glenohumeral internal and external rotation strength in elite junior tennis players. J Sci Med Sport. 2003;6(1):63–70.
18. Byrum IR, Bushnell BD, Dugger K, Charron K, Harrell FE, Noonan TJ. Preseason shoulder strength measurements in professional baseball pitchers: identifying players at risk for injury. Am J Sports Med. 2010;38(7):1375–82.
19. Ellenbecker TS, Davies GJ. The application of isokinetics in testing and rehabilitation of the shoulder complex. J Athl Train. 2000;35(3):338–50.
20. Ellenbecker TS, Wilk KE. Sport therapy for the shoulder: evaluation, rehabilitation and return to sport. Champaign, IL: Human Kinetics; 2017.
21. Ellenbecker TS, Cools A. Rehabilitation of shoulder impingement syndrome and rotator cuff injuries: an evidence based review. Br J Sports Med. 2010;44(5):319–27.
22. Cools AM, Struyf F, De Mey K, Maenhout A, Castelein B, Cagnie B. Rehabilitation of scapular dyskinesis: from the office worker to the elite overhead athlete. Br J Sports Med. 2014;48(8):692–7. (IF 4.17, ranking 6/81).
23. Wilk KE, Macrina LC, Fleisig GS, Porterfield R, Simpson CD II, Harker P, Paparesta N, Andrews JR. Correlation of glenohumeral internal rotation deficit and total rotational motion to shoulder injuries in professional baseball pitchers. Am J Sports Med. 2011;39:329–35.
24. Shanley E, Rauh MJ, Michener LA, Ellenbecker TS, Garrison JC, Thigpen CA. Shoulder range of motion measures as risk factors for shoulder and elbow injuries in high school softball and baseball players. Am J Sports Med. 2011;39:1997–2006.
25. Forthomme B, Wieczorek V, Frisch A, Crielaard JM, Croisier JL. Shoulder pain among high-level volleyball players and preseason features. Med Sci Sports Exerc. 2013;45(10):1852–60. https://doi.org/10.1249/MSS.0b013e318296128d.
26. Clarsen B, Bahr R, Andersson SH, Munk R, Myklebust G. Reduced glenohumeral rotation, external rotation weakness and scapular dyskinesis are risk factors for shoulder injuries among elite male handball players: a prospective cohort study. Br J Sports Med. 2014;48(17):1327–33. https://doi.org/10.1136/bjsports-2014-093702.
27. Johansson FR, Skillgate E, Lapauw ML, Clijmans D, Deneulin VP, Palmans T, Cools AM. Measuring eccentric strength of the shoulder external rotators using a hand-held dynamometer: reliability and validity. J Athl Train. 2015;50(7):719–25.
28. Castelein B, Parlevliet T, Cools CB. A The influence of induced shoulder muscle pain on rotator cuff and scapulothoracic muscle activity during elevation of the arm. J Shoulder Elbow Surg. 2017;26:497. https://doi.org/10.1016/j.jse.2016.09.005. pii: S1058-2746(16)30406-2.
29. Werner CM, Blumenthal S, Curt A, Gerber C. Subacromial pressures in vivo and effects of selective experimental suprascapular nerve block. J Shoulder Elbow Surg. 2006;15(3):319–23.
30. Mura N, O'Driscoll SW, Zobitz ME, Heers G, Jenkyn TR, Chou SM, Halder AM, An KN. The effect of infraspinatus disruption on glenohumeral torque and superior migration of the humeral head: a biomechanical study. J Shoulder Elbow Surg. 2003;12(2):179–84.
31. Townsend H, Jobe FW, Pink M, Perry J. Electromyographic analysis of the glenohumeral muscles during a baseball rehabilitation program. Am J Sports Med. 1991;19:264–72.
32. Boettcher CE, Ginn KA, Cathers I. The 'empty can' and 'full can' tests do not selectively activate supraspinatus. J Sci Med Sport. 2009;12(4):435–9.
33. Cools AM, Borms D, Cottens S, Himpe M, Meersdom S, Cagnie B. Rehabilitation exercises for athletes with biceps disorders and SLAP lesions: a continuum of exercises with increasing loads on the biceps. Am J Sports Med. 2014;42(6):1315–22.
34. Castelein B, Cagnie B, Parlevliet T, Cools AM. Superficial and deep scapulothoracic muscle EMG activity during different types of elevation exercises in the scapular plane. J Orthop Sports Phys Ther. 2016;11:1–26.
35. Reinold MM, Escamilla RF, Wilk KE. Current concepts in the scientific and clinical rationale behind exercises for glenohumeral and scapulothoracic musculature. J Orthop Sports Phys Ther. 2009;39(2):105–17. https://doi.org/10.2519/jospt.2009.2835.
36. Cools A, Dewitte V, Lanszweert F, Notebaert D, Roets A, Soetens B, Cagnie B, Witvrouw E. Rehabilitation of trapezius intramuscular balance: which exercises to prescribe? Am J Sports Med. 2007;35:1744–51.
37. Ellenbecker TS, Sueyoshi T, Bailie DS. Muscular activation during plyometric exercises in 90 degrees of glenohumeral joint abduction. Sports Health. 2015;7(1):71–9.
38. Maenhout A, Benzoor M, Werin M, Cools A. Scapular muscle activity in a variety of plyometric exercises. J Electromyogr Kinesiol. 2016;27:39–45.
39. Castelein B. The role of the deep scapular muscles in scapular dyskinesis in patients with shoulder or neck pain. Doctoral thesis, 2016.
40. Struyf F, Cagnie B, Cools A, Baert I, Van Brempt J, Struyf P, Meeus M. Scapulothoracic muscle activity and recruitment timing in patients with shoulder

impingement symptoms and glenohumeral instability, accepted for publication. J Electromyogr Kinesiol. 2014;24(2):277–84. https://doi.org/10.1016/j.jelekin.2013.12.002. Review. (IF 1.72, ranking 32/81).
41. De Mey K, Danneels L, Cagnie B, Vandenbosch L, Flier J, Cools AM. Kinetic chain influences on upper and lower trapezius muscle activation during eight variations of a scapular retraction exercise in overhead athletes. J Sci Med Sport. 2013;16(1):65–70. (IF 3.08, ranking 9/81).
42. Maenhout A, Van Praet K, Pizzi L, Van Herzeele M, Cools A. Electromyographic analysis of knee push up plus variations: what's the influence of the kinetic chain on scapular muscle activity? Br J Sports Med. 2010;44(14):1010–5. (Impactfactor 4.71; Ranking 6/81).
43. Bitter NL, Clisby EF, Jones MA, Magarey ME, Jaberzadeh S, Sandow MJ. Relative contributions of infraspinatus and deltoid during external rotation in healthy shoulders. J Shoulder Elbow Surg. 2007;16(5):563–8.
44. Andersen CH, Zebis MK, Saervoll C, et al. Scapular muscle activity from selected strengthening exercises performed at low and high intensities. J Strength Cond Res. 2012;26(9):2408–16. https://doi.org/10.1519/JSC.0b013e31823f8d24.
45. Wilk KE, Reinold MM, Macrina LC, Porterfield R, Devine KM, Suarez K, Andrews JR. Glenohumeral internal rotation measurements differ depending on stabilization techniques. Sports Health. 2009;1(2):131–6.
46. Manske R, Wilk KE, Davies G, Ellenbecker T, Reinold M. Glenohumeral motion deficits: friend or foe? Int J Sports Phys Ther. 2013;8(5):537–53.
47. Ellenbecker TS, Manske RM, Sueyoshi T, Bailie DS. The acute effect of a contract/relax horizontal cross-body adduction stretch on shoulder internal rotation. J Orthop Sports Phys Ther. 2016;46(1):A37.
48. Laudner KG Sipes RC, Wilson JT. The acute effects of sleeper stretch on shoulder range of motion. J NATA. 2008;43(4):359–63.
49. McClure P, Balaicuis J, Heiland D, Broersma ME, Thorndike CK, Wood A. A randomized controlled comparison of stretching procedures in recreational athletes with posterior shoulder tightness [abstract]. J Orthop Sports Phys Ther. 2005;35(1):A5.
50. Manske RC, Meschke M, Porter A, Smith B, Reiman M. A randomized controlled single-blinded comparison of stretching versus stretching and joint mobilization for posterior shoulder tightness measured by internal rotation motion loss. Sports Health. 2010;2(2):94–100.
51. Wilk KE, Hooks TR, Macrina LC. The modified sleeper stretch and modified cross-body stretch to increase shoulder internal rotation range of motion in the overhead throwing athlete. J Orthop Sports Phys Ther. 2013;43(12):891.
52. Salamh PA, Kolber MJ, Hanney WJ. Effect of scapular stabilization during horizontal adduction stretching on passive internal rotation and posterior shoulder in young women volleyball athletes: a randomized controlled trial. Arch Phys Med Rehabil. 2015;96(2):349–56. https://doi.org/10.1016/j.apmr.2014.09.038.
53. Riemann BL, Davies GJ, Ludwig L, Gardenhour H. Hand-held dynamometer testing of the internal and external rotator musculature based on selected positions to establish normative data and unilateral ratios. J Shoulder Elbow Surg. 2010;19(8):1175–83.
54. Ellenbecker TS, Reinold M, Nelson CO. Clinical concepts for treatment of the elbow in the adolescent overhead athlete. Clin Sports Med. 2010;29(4):705–24.
55. Ryu KN, McCormick FW, Jobe FW, Moynes DR, Antonell DJ. An electromyographic analysis of shoulder function in tennis players. Am J Sports Med. 1988;16:481–5.
56. Kovacs M, Ellenbecker TS. An 8-stage model for evaluating the tennis serve: implications for performance enhancement and injury prevention. Sports Health. 2011;3(6):504–13.

Osteoarthritis and the Senior Tennis Player

17

Keith T. Corpus, Evan W. James, Javier Maquirriain, and David M. Dines

17.1 Introduction

The benefits of tennis for promotion of health in older individuals have been well documented [1]. As players age, however, the cumulative effect of repetitive trauma to the joints and soft tissues may lead to chronic degenerative changes and overuse injuries. One such injury is osteoarthritis of the shoulder, which can cause progressive pain and decreased range of motion. Ultimately, these symptoms can lead to impaired participation and performance on the tennis court. As older individuals increasingly strive to remain active later in life, new diagnostic and treatment approaches have emerged to help tennis players stay active longer. This chapter will discuss current concepts regarding the progression of osteoarthritis in the shoulder of the senior tennis player, biomechanical considerations, diagnostic techniques, and current methods to treat this condition. Return to tennis statistics will be included along with outcomes of both surgical and nonsurgical methods of treatment.

17.2 Epidemiology

Injuries to the upper and lower extremities are common among senior tennis players, and the incidence may vary as a function of player's age, sex, volume of play, technique, and skill level [2]. A systematic review performed by Pluim et al. found that the incidence of all tennis injuries ranged from 0.05 to 2.9 injuries per player per year of play [3]. The incidence of primary shoulder osteoarthritis generally increases with age, particularly among those over 60 years of age [4]. Nakagawa and colleagues found the incidence of primary shoulder osteoarthritis was 0.4% and 4.6% among those presenting with a shoulder complaint. The authors also reported a higher incidence of shoulder arthritis among women compared to men [4]. Former elite-level tennis players may also have a higher incidence of shoulder osteoarthritis. A study by Maquirriain et al. compared 18 asymptomatic former elite tennis players to 18 sedentary control patients [5]. Results showed that 33% of former elite tennis players had evidence of mild to moderate osteoarthritis in their dominant shoulder, compared to 11% in the control group. This data suggests that volume and intensity of play early in life may predispose players to shoulder arthritis later in life.

K. T. Corpus (✉)
Department of Sports Medicine and Shoulder Surgery, Hospital for Special Surgery, New York, NY, USA

Attn: Academic Training Department, Hospital for Special Surgery, New York, NY, USA

E. W. James · D. M. Dines
Department of Sports Medicine and Shoulder Surgery, Hospital for Special Surgery, New York, NY, USA

J. Maquirriain
Centro Nacional de Alto Rendimiento Deportivo, Pilar, Buenos Aires, Argentina

17.3 Biomechanical Considerations

There are several biomechanical considerations unique to the tennis stroke which may predispose some individuals to osteoarthritis. Three basic strokes are employed in tennis: the overhead serve, forehand, and backhand [6]. The overhead serve can be further subdivided into five distinct phases: windup, early cocking, late cocking, acceleration, and follow-through [7, 8]. The serve can produce tremendous forces on the glenohumeral joint that when added over many matches over many years can increase risk of chronic degenerative changes in the shoulder.

Strokes can also be divided based on those that require power versus those that require precision [7]. For strokes that require power, the athlete combines leg drive, trunk rotation, and shoulder forward flexion to form a kinetic chain that, when functioning in tandem, produces power [9]. Proper form is essential to prevent overuse injuries. A study by Martin et al. recorded the serves of elite-level tennis players using an optoelectronic motion capture system to evaluate the amount of energy generated, absorbed, and transferred during a normal stroke [10]. Players were then given a questionnaire to identify injured (symptomatic) versus uninjured (asymptomatic) individuals. Motion capture system results demonstrated that players identified as injured had worse energy flow through the upper extremity kinetic chain, low ball velocity, and increased forces on the shoulder and elbow compared to their non-injured counterparts. Thus, players who continue to participate in tennis-related activities while injured are at increased risk of developing further injury to the shoulder. Over time, increased contact forces in the shoulder can lead to the development of osteoarthritis.

17.4 Diagnosis

The diagnosis of shoulder osteoarthritis in tennis players is best performed using a combination of history, physical exam, and imaging. While there is no classic presentation, symptoms suggestive of glenohumeral osteoarthritis include pain, loss of range of motion, instability, and mechanical symptoms such as clicking, catching, or popping. It is imperative to complete a full history when evaluating a patient with shoulder pain including onset of symptoms, activities that make symptoms better or worse, treatments, assessment of the quality and severity of discomfort, and timing of symptoms. Eliciting a history of prior shoulder trauma including history of dislocations is essential. A review of other medical problems, prior surgeries, history of trauma, activity level, and list of current medications should also be included.

17.4.1 Physical Exam

A thorough physical exam of the bilateral shoulders and cervical spine should be completed in all patients with suspected shoulder osteoarthritis. A comprehensive shoulder exam typically includes inspection, palpation, sensation, range of motion, and strength testing. Key structures to investigate on examination include the rotator cuff, glenohumeral cartilage, long head of the biceps brachii tendon, glenoid labrum, acromioclavicular joint, sternoclavicular joint, and scapula. Patients should disrobe from the mid-chest up such that the glenohumeral joint, scapula, and cervical spine are easily visualized. The examination begins by inspecting the shoulders and adjacent areas looking for gross asymmetry, differences in muscle bulk, and surgical scars. The relative position of the scapula should be noted. Evaluation of active scapular rotation during ROM of the glenohumeral joint is important in order to recognize primary or secondary scapular dyskinesia described in previous chapters. A careful assessment of the cervical spine and ipsilateral elbow and neurovascular examination are important in establishing referred pain patterns and help delineate differential diagnoses.

Next, range of motion testing is performed. Range of motion of the cervical spine should be performed including flexion, extension, lateral bending, and twisting. Active and passive range of motion of the shoulders should be assessed next. Movements include forward flexion, extension, abduction, adduction, internal rotation with the shoulder at 0 and 90° abduction, and external rotation with the elbow at 0 and 90° abduction. Forward flexion is performed. Internal rotation may be measured using vertebral level. Normal range of motion is to approximately the T4 to T8 vertebrae. Tennis players may have increased internal rotation and decreased external rotation in the dominant arm [11, 12]. Scapular motion is assessed either from a posterior or lateral position to examine for scapular internal and external rotation, upward and downward rotation, and anterior and posterior tilting, which together produce scapular protraction and retraction.

Finally, strength testing should be performed to assess individual muscle contributions to overall shoulder function. Specialized strength testing should be performed to test integrity of the supraspinatus, infraspinatus, teres minor, and subscapularis, which together comprise the shoulder rotator cuff. The supraspinatus is best assessed using Jobe's test. Jobe's test is performed with the shoulder forward flexed to 90°, the arms abducted 30° to coincide with the scapular plane, and the palm internally rotated with the thumb pointed downward. The examiner then applies a downward directed force while the patient resists. The infraspinatus can be tested using the external rotation lag sign. With this test, the arm is externally rotated with the elbow flexed to 90° and positioned at the patient's side. The arm is brought to maximal external rotation, and the patient is instructed to hold the position. If the arm begins to creep into internal rotation, the test is positive for weakness in the infraspinatus. The teres minor is assessed in a similar fashion with the elbow flexed at 90° and shoulder abducted to 90°. Again, the shoulder is placed in maximal eternal rotation, and any drift into internal rotation may be indicative of weakness in the teres minor. When positive, this test is called a positive Hornblower's sign. Finally, the subscapularis is tested by asking the patient to hold their arm in 90° of flexion at the elbow with the elbow at the side and internally rotate against resistance. The examiner should also evaluate the biceps brachii by flexing at the elbow against resistance, the triceps by extending at the elbow against resistance, and the deltoid by holding the shoulder at 90° of abduction against resistance.

17.4.2 Imaging

After completing a comprehensive history and physical exam, imaging is used to further assist with establishing a diagnosis. Common imaging modalities include plain radiographs, computed tomography (CT) scans, and magnetic resonance imaging (MRI). Plain radiographic views may include the Grashey, axillary, and scapular Y views. Nakagawa et al. proposed a radiographic classification scheme for glenohumeral osteoarthritis that progresses from grade 0 (no glenohumeral joint changes) to III (severe changes) [4]. Radiographic findings characteristic of glenohumeral osteoarthritis include joint space narrowing, subchondral sclerosis, cystic changes in the humeral head or glenoid, osteophytes, and posterior glenoid erosion [5]. Patients with osteoarthritis may also have a posteriorly subluxated humeral head relative to the glenoid, particularly as posterior glenoid erosion progresses. Superior migration of the humeral head can be present in patients with insufficiency of the rotator cuff.

In some instances, CT scans may also be employed to better quantify glenoid bone stock and assess version. Walch and colleagues proposed a classification scheme to characterize glenoid morphology that divides glenoid morphology into one of three types [13] (Table 17.1). Recently, they have amended this classification to broaden the existing definitions and introduce additional classes [14]. Classification is performed by examining images in the axial plane. Friedman et al. described a technique for measuring glenoid version, whereby a line is drawn down the long axis of the scapula on axial CT, a second line is drawn perpendicular to the long axis line, and a third line is drawn parallel to the glenoid rim [15]. The angle between the line perpendicular to the scapular axis and the line parallel to the glenoid represents the glenoid version. Increased glenoid retroversion may be seen in advanced glenoid bone loss with severe

Table 17.1 Walch classification of glenoid morphology [14]

Type A	A.1	Humeral head centered, minor central glenoid erosion (line drawn from anterior to posterior glenoid rim does not transect humeral head)
	A.2	Humeral head centered, major central glenoid erosion (line drawn from anterior to posterior glenoid rim transects humeral head)
Type B	B.1	Posterior humeral head subluxation, posterior joint space narrow, subchondral sclerosis, osteophytes present; no bony erosion
	B.2	Posterior humeral head subluxation, posterior erosion with biconcavity of the glenoid
	B.3	Monoconcave and posteriorly worn glenoid with at least 15° of retroversion or at least 70% posterior humeral head subluxation or both
Type C	C	Glenoid retroversion >25° (dysplastic, not caused by bony erosion)
Type D	D	Glenoid anteversion or anterior humeral head subluxation of <40%

osteoarthritis and posterior shoulder instability. Finally, magnetic resonance imaging (MRI) may help further define the integrity of the glenohumeral articular cartilage. It also provides excellent visualization of static and dynamic shoulder stabilizers adjacent to the glenohumeral articular cartilage. In practice, plain radiographs, CT, and MRI are often employed together during a diagnostic workup for shoulder osteoarthritis and provide essential information to track disease progression and assist in preoperative planning.

17.5 Treatment

Treatment options for osteoarthritis in the senior tennis player are largely similar to those available for osteoarthritis of the shoulder in the non-athlete population. Treatment is dictated by patient age, severity of symptoms, radiographic findings, and medical comorbidities. However, in addition to alleviating pain, treatment of the senior tennis player should also focus on restoration of function in order to allow the patient to return to sport.

17.5.1 Nonsurgical Treatment

The initial treatment for symptomatic glenohumeral OA is nonsurgical management. Nonsurgical management of shoulder OA in the senior tennis is not drastically different than that of the general population, consisting of activity modification, physical therapy (focusing on rotator cuff strengthening, periscapular strengthening, and range of motion), oral anti-inflammatory medications with the addition of multimodal pain regimens as needed, glenohumeral corticosteroid injections, glenohumeral viscosupplementation injections, or some combination thereof. The American Academy of Orthopaedic Surgeons released a clinical practice guideline (CPG) for the treatment of glenohumeral arthritis in 2010 [16]. This CPG is the result of meta-analysis data and provides several recommendations regarding the nonsurgical treatment of OA of the shoulder based on the current literature.

According to the CPG and based on the available literature, there is insufficient evidence to recommend for or against physical therapy in the initial treatment of patients with OA of the glenohumeral joint. However, given the relatively minimal risk associated with physical therapy, many physicians still employ the use of therapy in hopes of maintaining range of motion and strength about the shoulder. Similarly, the AAOS was unable to recommend for or against the use of oral nonsteroidal anti-inflammatory drugs, acetaminophen, opioids, and over-the-counter supplements. They are also unable to recommend for or against the use of intra-articular corticosteroid injections. Again, despite these recommendations, these modalities are the mainstay of nonsurgical treatment in mild to moderate OA for the majority of shoulder surgeons, given the relatively low risk associated with these interventions [16].

One nonsurgical treatment option which the AAOS endorses is the use of viscosupplementation. This recommendation is the result of one Level IV study by Silverstein et al. in which patients received three hyaluronic acid injections weekly for 3 weeks [17]. These injections resulted in a statistically significant benefit in pain reduction, range of motion, and quality of life across multiple subjective modalities. Of note, this recommendation received a "C" grade due to the poor quality of the evidence. Personal experience of the senior author (DMD) demonstrates that patients may get short-term relief of up to 6 months but rarely ask to undergo a second round of such injections.

17.5.2 Surgical Treatment

Surgical management of shoulder osteoarthritis in the senior tennis player can be lumped into two broad categories: joint preserving and joint replacing. Joint-preserving techniques involve arthroscopic debridement, glenoid and humeral chondroplasty, loose body removal, and capsular release (Fig. 17.1), while joint-replacing techniques most commonly involve the anatomic and reverse total shoulder replacement (Fig. 17.2).

The main goal of joint preservice procedures in the treatment of shoulder OA in the senior tennis player is pain relief and restoration of function. In addition, concomitant pathology such as rotator cuff tears, impingement, and acromioclavicular joint arthritis may also be addressed. These modal-

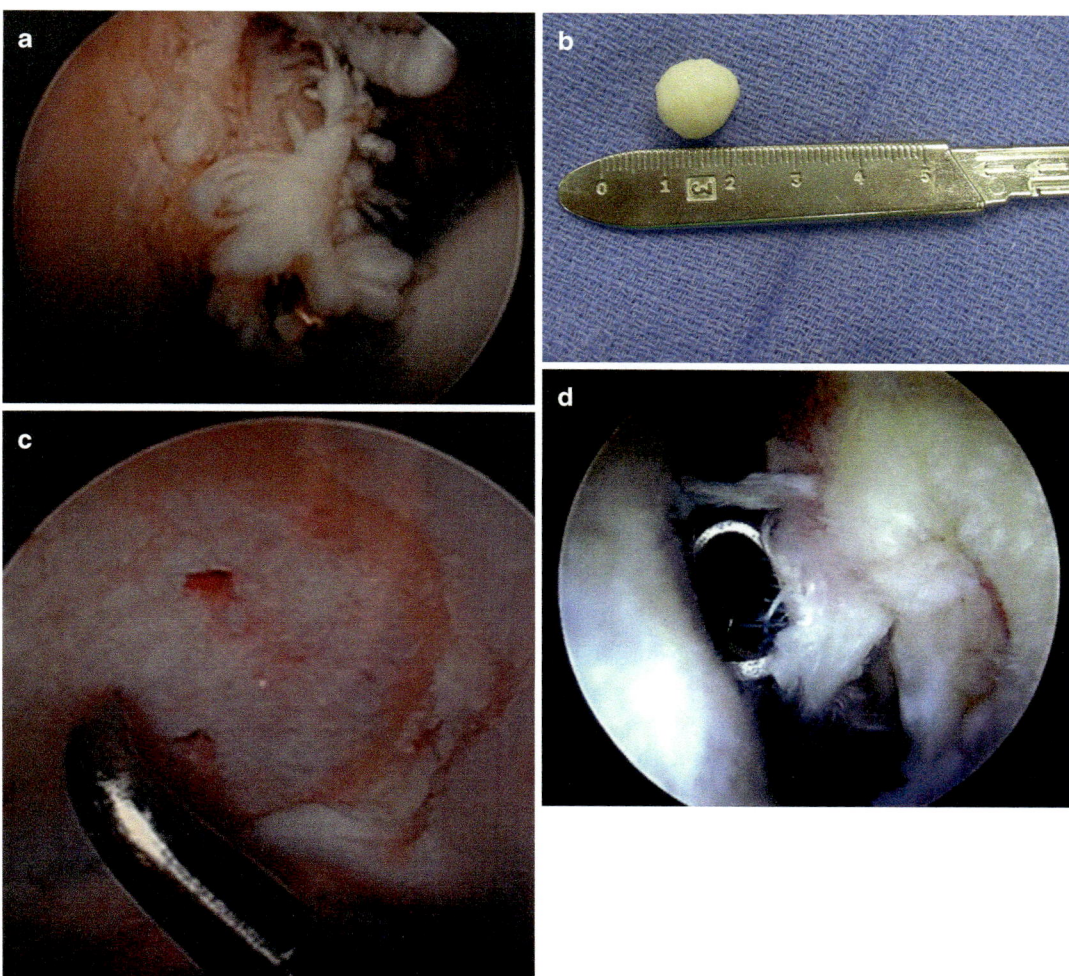

Fig. 17.1 (**a–d**) Arthroscopic techniques in glenohumeral DJD include synovectomy and capsular releases (**a**), excision of loose bodies (**b**), microfracture (**c**), and labral debridement (**d**) as well as dealing with rotator cuff tears, impingement lesions, and long head of biceps disease

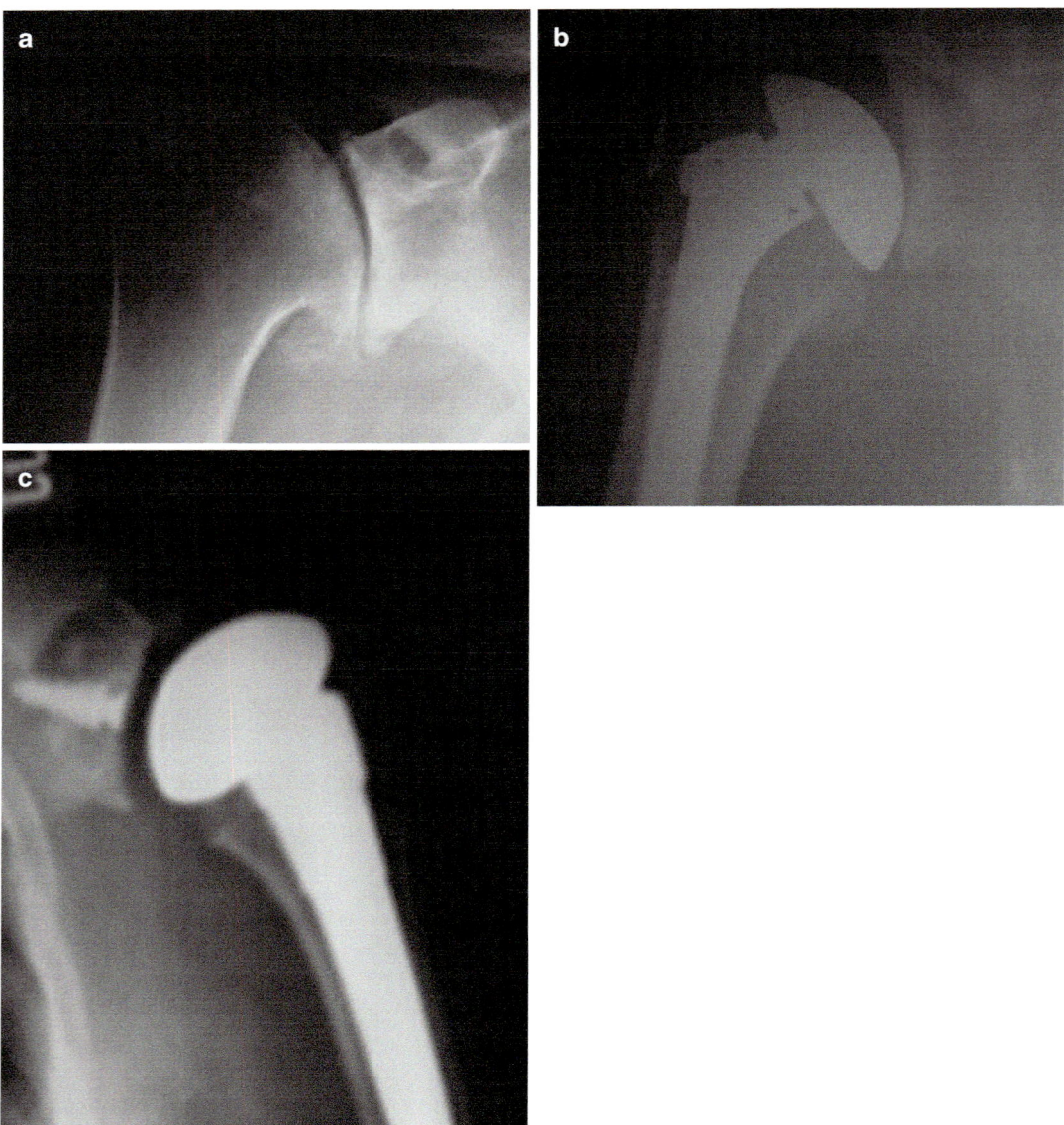

Fig. 17.2 (a–c) Severe glenohumeral arthritis with joint space narrowing and bone spurs (a) treated with hemiarthroplasty (b) or anatomic total shoulder arthroplasty (c)

ities are most commonly used in the younger patient population as a method of delaying the time to shoulder arthroplasty; therefore, the role of these joint-preserving techniques remains somewhat limited in the senior population.

Arthroscopic management of early shoulder arthritis has been shown to be an effective option in most studies, but these studies are geared toward short-term results. Weinstein et al. evaluated 25 patients with early shoulder OA (no severe changes on radiographs) that were treated with arthroscopic debridement, removal of loose bodies, and subacromial bursectomy [18]. At an average of 34 months, good to excellent results were found in 80% of the population. However, the authors did not recommend this procedure in patients with glenohumeral joint space narrowing.

Safran et al. also reported on 17 patients with severe degenerative shoulder OA (severe joint space narrowing and large osteophytes) that were treated with arthroscopic debridement, removal of loose bodies, and subacromial bursectomy (no osteophyte excisions or capsulectomies were performed) [19]. The population was followed for 2 years. Postoperatively, 82% had good to excellent results, and these results were maintained at 2–4 years in 78% of patients. Range of motion and functional gains were not significantly impacted.

Similarly, Weber et al. reported on 36 patients with severe shoulder OA that underwent debridement and subacromial bursectomy with a mean follow-up of 5 years [20]. Good to excellent results were shown in 86% of patients at 3 months, but only 33% had durable improvement in the long term. The time to progression to joint replacement was highest between 2 and 5 years post-op. It is this lack of durability in the long-term which has caused these non-arthroplasty techniques to be used only for younger patients as a method to delay time to joint replacement.

The mainstay for the surgical treatment of osteoarthritis of the shoulder in the senior tennis play is shoulder arthroplasty, including hemiarthroplasty, anatomic total shoulder arthroplasty, and reverse shoulder arthroplasty. While reverse shoulder arthroplasty has clear indications, no clear consensus exists regarding the use of hemiarthroplasty versus anatomic total shoulder arthroplasty. Similar to the joint-preserving techniques, the main goal of these procedures is pain relief and improvement in function. However, the goal of arthroplasty is to provide the patient with a stable and durable implant to improve outcomes in the long-term.

Hemiarthroplasty involves treatment with prosthetic replacement of the humeral head only, while the glenoid is left with its native articular surface. Anatomically, patients must either have a concentric glenoid or a nonconcentric glenoid that can be reamed intraoperatively to a concentric surface. Additionally, the humeral head must be well-centered in the glenoid preoperatively or after soft tissue releases have been completed. In contrast, anatomic total shoulder arthroplasty involves replacement of both the humeral head and the glenoid articular surface. Unlike hemiarthroplasty, anatomic total shoulder does have the ability to address nonconcentric glenoid surfaces and soft tissue imbalance resulting in subluxation of the humeral head. Due to the risk of glenoid component complications, total shoulder arthroplasty is typically used in the older patient population, whereas hemiarthroplasty with or without concomitant glenoid reaming or biologic resurfacing tends to be the treatment of choice for younger patients given the need for prolonged glenoid component survival. Most importantly, the surgeon must be proficient in techniques required to gain exposure to the glenoid in anatomic total shoulder arthroplasty.

The success of hemiarthroplasty in producing improvements in pain and function is well documented [21–24]. Anatomic total shoulder replacement has also shown excellent results in the treatment of primary OA, leading to dramatic pain relief, improved function, and high patient satisfaction [25–31]. As technology of implants and surgical techniques continue to improve, so do the outcomes of these excellent procedures.

Several studies have also compared hemiarthroplasty with total shoulder arthroplasty in the treatment of OA and found no difference in pain, function, range of motion, or patient satisfaction [21–23]. Gartsman et al. also completed a randomized controlled trial of total shoulder versus hemiarthroplasty and found that the total shoulder arthroplasty group achieved a post-op ASES score of 77.3, compared to 65.2 in the hemiarthroplasty group at 35 months (not statistically significant) [32].

Norris et al. completed a prospective study of 173 patients with primary OA of the shoulder treated with either hemiarthroplasty or total shoulder arthroplasty [24]. They found that total shoulder arthroplasty provided slightly better pain relief and motion, but ultimately the authors concluded that both procedures were successful.

A systematic review completed by Radnay et al. evaluated three randomized trials and 20 case series [33]. They found that total shoulder arthroplasty showed superior results for patient satisfaction, pain scores, and range of motion. They also showed a 1.7% revision rate for anatomic total shoulders, compared to a 10.2% revision rate for hemiarthroplasty (excluding metal-backed glenoid components which are a known risk factor for increased failure).

Lastly, for senior athletes with symptomatic glenohumeral OA associated with a massive rotator cuff tear who fail nonoperative treatment, the surgical treatment of choice is reverse total shoulder arthroplasty. Recently, expanding indications and improving technology are leading to a surge in reverse total shoulder replacements. More recently, reverse shoulder arthroplasty has gained popularity in fracture management and revision arthroplasty situations. Given this increase in usage, younger and more active patients are now being treated with reverse shoulder arthroplasty, including some older tennis players with severe concomitant rotator cuff insufficiency. In the general population, reverse total shoulder arthroplasty has been effective in decreasing pain and improving shoulder motion and function in these patients. The outcomes are highly dependent on the surgical indication. Additionally, complication rates among reverse total shoulder are higher than anatomic shoulder replacement, given the altered biomechanics, necessitating a need for careful surgical technique.

With specific attention to osteoarthritis in the senior tennis player, reverse shoulder arthroplasty, when indicated for rotator cuff arthropathy, shows as high as 96% of patients good to excellent results with improvement in pain, mobility, and strength [34]. These findings were echoed by Samuelsen et al. who showed patients had significant improvement in pain, range of motion, and strength at both 2 and 5 years after reverse shoulder arthroplasty with 99% and 91% revision-free survival at 2 years and 5 years, respectively [35]. Guery et al. also showed similar improvements [36].

17.6 Return to Sport

Improving techniques and implant survivorship have led to a large increase in shoulder arthroplasty for the management of glenohumeral OA. The excellent results published in the literature have given rise to greater patient expectations with regard to postoperative function, especially with respect to return to sport. As such, several publications have sought to determine the sporting ability of patients after glenohumeral arthroplasty.

With regard to surgeon expectations and preferences, several studies have sought to investigate the opinion of experienced shoulder surgeons with respect to return to sport after TSA. Golant et al. conducted a survey of the American Shoulder and Elbow Surgeons (ASES) to determine which types of activities they allow their patients to participate in after shoulder arthroplasty [37]. They grouped the sports into five categories based on impact and contact level. In this study, tennis was deemed a non-contact, high-impact sport. In this category, 19.6% of surgeons allowed patients to return to sport without limitation after anatomic TSA, and 39.7% of surgeons allowed patients to return with some limitations. Patients with hemiarthroplasty were allowed to return without limitation by 46.7% and with limitation by 31.9%. Reverse TSA had much lower return to sport allowance, as only 3.6% of surgeons allowed return to sport without limitation and only 19.4% allowed return with limitation. These numbers were lower for contact sports and higher for lower impact sports, showing that most surgeons do allow some return to sport after shoulder arthroplasty, but the amount modulates based on type of arthroplasty and contact/impact level of sport.

These limitations have more recently been called into question. A study by Liu et al. consisted of a retrospective review of 102 reverse TSA and 71 hemiarthroplasty patients [38]. All patients were participating in some sport preoperatively and had at least 1 year follow-up. They found that reverse TSA patients returned to sport at a significantly higher rate than hemiarthroplasty (85.9% versus 66.7%). They were also more satisfied with their ability to play sports. In addition, no sports-related complications were found.

A separate survey of members of the ASES, as well as the European Society for Surgery of the

Shoulder and Elbow (SECEC), was conducted by Magnussen et al. [39]. This survey contained 37 activities and asked surgeons to classify their postoperative activity recommendations based on the activity experience of the patient. Tennis was broken down into both singles and doubles. In summary, both singles and doubles tennis were "allowed with experience" for both the hemiarthroplasty group and the anatomic shoulder group. For patients undergoing reverse TSA, the majority of surgeons would not allow singles tennis regardless of experience level, but no consensus could be reached with regard to doubles tennis.

Return to sport after hemiarthroplasty was evaluated by Garcia et al. [40]. They conducted a retrospective review of 79 patients at an average of 63 months follow-up. Within the cohort, 58 patients played sports preoperatively, and 67.2% restarted at least one of those sports postoperatively. The average time to return to sport was 6.5 months. Fifty-seven percent of patients were able to return to doubles tennis. Younger age was associated with higher levels of sports achievement.

Another study by Schumann et al. evaluated 100 consecutive patients who had undergone anatomic total shoulder arthroplasty for postoperative sports activity [41]. Of the 55 patients in the cohort that played sports preoperatively, 49 (89%) were still able to participate at approximately 3 years follow-up. In addition, 11 patients that had given up sports preoperatively due to pain were able to resume sports after surgery. No patients were forced to cease sporting activity due to surgery. 36.7% of patients did still complain of sports restrictions secondary to shoulder problems. Specifically with regard to tennis, three patients in the cohort played tennis both before and after surgery. After surgery, all patients were able to return to their baseline frequency and duration of play, taking an average of 10 months to return to tennis. Pain was rated as mild in one patient, while the other two patients had no pain.

Similarly, McCarty et al. investigated a series of 75 patients with 86 shoulder arthroplasties (anatomic TSA or hemiarthroplasty) for return to sports activities at an average follow-up of 3.7 years [42]. The average frequency of participation in sporting activities prior to the onset of OA was 2.6 days/week, which decreased to 0.7 days/week after OA was diagnosed. In addition, 68% of patients were unable to participate in sports immediately before surgery due to pain and/or decreased function. One year postoperatively, the average frequency of sports participation increased to 1.7 days/week, with patients achieving a partial return to sport at 3.6 months and a full return to sport at an average of 5.8 months. Fifty percent of patients were able to increase their participation postoperatively, and 71% showed an improvement in their ability to play sport. *Tennis had a return to sport rate of 75%.* There were no differences with regard to return to sport between hemiarthroplasty and anatomic TSA.

A separate study by Garcia et al. evaluated return to sport after hemiarthroplasty versus anatomic TSA [43]. They evaluated 40 matched patients from each cohort at an average of approximately 62 months postoperative. They found that while 65.5% of hemiarthroplasty patients returned to at least one sport, 97.3% of anatomic TSA patients were able to return, at an average of approximately 5.5 months. They also found that a significantly higher number of TSA patients returned to higher upper extremity use sports than those with hemiarthroplasty. With respect to tennis in hemiarthroplasty patients, three of three patients were able to return to doubles tennis, and three of three were able to return to singles tennis. In the anatomic TSA cohort, four of four patients were able to return to doubles tennis, and four of five were able to return to singles tennis.

Labriola et al. provided some insight into the return to sport functionality after reverse TSA [44]. They report data on four senior athletes who underwent reverse TSA with more than 2 years follow-up. Postoperatively, three of the four were able to return to sports, including tennis. However, all reported that the level of play decreased and difficulty increased leading to frequent limitations in play. These patients displayed no evidence of hardware failure. The authors also endorse that patients undergoing reverse TSA for rotator cuff arthropathy do demonstrate better function and return to play than those undergoing reverse TSA for revision or fracture.

Lastly, Garcia et al. also evaluated return to sport after reverse TSA [45]. They evaluated 76 patients who underwent reverse TSA and played sports preoperatively with at least 1 year follow-up. They found that after reverse TSA, 85.5% of patients returned to at least one sport at an average of 5.3 months. Despite this high rate of return to sport, return to tennis numbers were not as impressive, with only 25% of patients returning to either singles or doubles tennis.

Conclusion

Osteoarthritis of the shoulder is a common phenomenon in the senior tennis player and easily diagnosed and classified based on physical examination and radiographic analysis. Treatment options include nonoperative and operative management. With effective treatment, senior athletes are able to return to tennis at high rates.

References

1. Pluim BM, Staal JB, Marks BL, Miller S, Miley D. Health benefits of tennis. Br J Sports Med. 2007;41(11):760–8.
2. Abrams GD, Renstrom PA, Safran MR. Epidemiology of musculoskeletal injury in the tennis player. Br J Sports Med. 2012;46(7):492–8.
3. Pluim BM, Staal JB, Windler GE, Jayanthi N. Tennis injuries: occurrence, aetiology, and prevention. Br J Sports Med. 2006;40(5):415–23.
4. Nakagawa Y, Hyakuna K, Otani S, Hashitani M, Nakamura T. Epidemiologic study of glenohumeral osteoarthritis with plain radiography. J Shoulder Elbow Surg. 1999;8(6):580–4.
5. Maquirriain J, Ghisi JP, Amato S. Is tennis a predisposing factor for degenerative shoulder disease? A controlled study in former elite players. Br J Sports Med. 2006;40(5):447–50.
6. Marx RG, Sperling JW, Cordasco FA. Overuse injuries of the upper extremity in tennis players. Clin Sports Med. 2001;20(3):439–51.
7. Elliott B, Fleisig G, Nicholls R, Escamilia R. Technique effects on upper limb loading in the tennis serve. J Sci Med Sport. 2003;6(1):76–87.
8. Dines JS, Bedi A, Williams PN, Dodson CC, Ellenbecker TS, Altchek DW, Windler G, Dines DM. Tennis injuries: epidemiology, pathophysiology, and treatment. J Am Acad Orthop Surg. 2015;23(3):181–9.
9. Kibler WB. Biomechanical analysis of the shoulder during tennis activities. Clin Sports Med. 1995;14(1):79–85.
10. Martin C, Bideau B, Bideau N, Nicolas G, Delamarche P, Kulpa R. Energy flow analysis during the tennis serve: comparison between injured and noninjured tennis players. Am J Sports Med. 2014;42(11):2751–60.
11. Ellenbecker T, Roetert EP. Age specific isokinetic glenohumeral internal and external rotation strength in elite junior tennis players. J Sci Med Sport. 2003;6(1):63–70.
12. Elliott B. Biomechanics and tennis. Br J Sports Med. 2006;40:392–6.
13. Walch G, Badet R, Boulahia A, Khoury A. Morphologic study of the glenoid in primary glenohumeral osteoarthritis. J Arthroplasty. 1999;14(6):756–60.
14. Bercik MJ, Kruse K, Yalizis M, Gauci MO, Chaoui J, Walch G. A modification to the Walch classification of the glenoid in primary glenohumeral osteoarthritis using three-dimensional imaging. J Shoulder Elbow Surg. 2016;25(10):1601–6.
15. Friedman RJ, Hawthorne KB, Genez BM. The use of computerized tomography in the measurement of glenoid version. J Bone Joint Surg. 1992;74(7):1032–7.
16. Izquierdo R, Voloshin I, Edwards S, Freehill MQ, Stanwood W, Wiater JM, Watters WC III, Goldberg MJ, Keith M, Turkelson CM, Wies JL, Anderson S, Boyer K, Raymond L, Sluka P, American Academy of Orthopedic Surgeons. Treatment of glenohumeral osteoarthritis. J Am Acad Orthop Surg. 2010;18(6):375–82.
17. Silverstein E, Leger R, Shea KP. The use of intra-articular hylan G-F 20 in the treatment of symptomatic osteoarthritis of the shoulder: a preliminary study. Am J Sports Med. 2007;35(6):979–85.
18. Weinstein DM, Bucchieri JS, Pollock RG, Flatow EL, Bigliani LU. Arthroscopic debridement of the shoulder for osteoarthritis. Arthroscopy. 2000;16(5):471–6.
19. Safran MR, Wolde-Tsadik G. Prospective outcome study of arthroscopic debridement for the treatment of grade IV glenohumeral arthritis. Presented at the American Academy of Orthopaedic Surgeons 68h Annual Meeting, 2002.
20. Weber SC, Kaufmann JI. Arthroscopic debridement in the management of glenohumeral arthritis. Presents at the American Academy of Orthopaedic Surgeons 70th Annual Meeting, 2004.
21. Bell SN, Gschwend N. Clinical experience with total arthroplasty and hemiarthroplasty of the shoulder using the Neer prosthesis. Int Orthop. 1986;10(4):217–22.
22. Boyd AD, Thomas WH, Scott RD, Sledge CB, Thornhill TS. Total shoulder arthroplasty versus hemiarthroplasty. Indications for glenoid resurfacing. J Arthroplasty. 1990;5(4):329–36.

23. Clayton ML, Ferlic DC, Jeffers PD. Prosthetic arthroplasties of the shoulder. Clin Orthop Relat Res. 1982;(164):184–91.
24. Norris TR, Iannotti JP. Functional outcome after shoulder arthroplasty for primary osteoarthritis: a multicenter study. J Shoulder Elbow Surg. 2002;11(2):130–5.
25. Rodosky MW, Bigliani LU. Indications for glenoid resurfacing in shoulder arthroplasty. J Shoulder Elbow Surg. 1996;5(3):231–48.
26. Neer CS, Watson KC, Stanton FL. Recent experience in total shoulder replacement. J Bone Joint Surg. 1982;64(3):319–37.
27. Iannotti JP, Norris TR. Influence of preoperative factors on outcome of shoulder arthroplasty for glenohumeral osteoarthritis. J Bone Joint Surg. 2003;85(2):251–8.
28. Godeneche A, Boileau P, Favard L, Le Huec JC, Levigne C, Nove-Josserand L, Walch G, Edwards TB. Prosthetic replacement in the treatment of osteoarthritis of the shoulder: early results of 268 cases. J Shoulder Elbow Surg. 2002;11(1):11–8.
29. Cofield RH. Total shoulder arthroplasty with the Neer prosthesis. J Bone Joint Surg. 1984;66(6):899–906.
30. Matsen FA. Early effectiveness of shoulder arthroplasty for patients who have primary glenohumeral degenerative joint disease. J Bone Joint Surg. 1996;78(2):260–4.
31. Torchia ME, Cofield RH, Settergren CR. Total shoulder arthroplasty with the Neer prosthesis: long-term results. J Shoulder Elbow Surg. 1997;6(6):495–505.
32. Gartsman GM, Roddey TS, Hammerman SM. Shoulder arthroplasty with or without resurfacing of the glenoid in patients who have osteoarthritis. J Bone Joint Surg. 2000;82(1):26–34.
33. Radnay CS, Setter KJ, Chambers L, Levine WN, Bigliani LU, Ahmad CS. Total shoulder replacement compared with humeral head replacement for the treatment of primary glenohumeral osteoarthritis: a systematic review. J Shoulder Elbow Surg. 2007;14(4):396–402.
34. Wall B, Nove-Josserand L, O'Connor DP, Edwards TB, Walch G. Reverse total shoulder arthroplasty: a review of results according to etiology. J Bone Joint Surg. 2007;89(7):1476–85.
35. Samuelsen BT, Wagner ER, Houdek MT, Elhassan BT, Sanchez-Sotelo J, Cofield R, Sperling JW. Primary reverse shoulder arthroplasty in patients aged 65 years or younger. J Shoulder Elbow Surg. 2016;16:e13.
36. Guery J, Favard L, Sirveaux F, Oudet D, Mole D, Walch G. Reverse total shoulder arthroplasty. Survivorship analysis of eighty replacements followed for five to ten years. J Bone Joint Surg. 2006;88(8):1742–7.
37. Golant A, Christoforou D, Zuckerman JD, Kwon YW. Return to sports after shoulder arthroplasty: a survey of surgeons' preferences. J Shoulder Elbow Surg. 2012;21(4):554–60.
38. Liu JN, Garcia GH, Mahony G, Wu HH, Dines DM, Warren RF, Gulotta LV. Sports after shoulder arthroplasty: a comparative analysis of hemiarthroplasty and reverse total shoulder replacement. J Shoulder Elbow Surg. 2016;25(6):920–6.
39. Magnussen RA, Mallon WJ, Willems WJ, Moorman CT. Long-term activity restrictions after shoulder arthroplasty: an international survey of experienced shoulder surgeons. J Shoulder Elbow Surg. 2011;20(2):281–9.
40. Garcia GH, Mahony GT, Fabricant PD, Wu HH, Dines DM, Warren RF, Craig EV, Gulotta LV. Sports- and work-related outcomes after shoulder hemiarthroplasty. Am J Sports Med. 2016;44(2):490–6.
41. Schumann K, Flury MP, Schwyzer HK, Simmen BR, Drerup S, Goldhahn J. Sports activity after anatomical total shoulder arthroplasty. Am J Sports Med. 2010;38(10):2097–105.
42. McCarty EC, Marx RG, Maerz D, Altchek D, Warren RF. Sports participation after shoulder replacement surgery. Am J Sports Med. 2008;36(8):1577–81.
43. Garcia GH, Liu JN, Mahony GT, Sinatro A, Wu HH, Craig EV, Warren RF, Dines DM, Gulotta LV. Hemiarthroplasty versus total shoulder arthroplasty for shoulder osteoarthritis: a matched comparison of return to sports. Am J Sports Med. 2016. https://doi.org/10.1177/0363546516632527. MID: 26960913.
44. Labriola JE, Edwards TB. Reverse total shoulder arthroplasty in the senior athlete. Oper Tech Sports Med. 2008;16(1):43–9.
45. Garcia GH, Taylor SA, DePalma BJ, Mahony GT, Grawe BM, Nguyen J, Dines JS, Dines DM, Warren RF, Craig EV, Gulotta LV. Patient activity levels after reverse total shoulder arthroplasty: what are patients doing? Am J Sports Med. 2015;43(11):2816–21.

Part IV

Elbow Wrist and Hand Injuries

Pathophysiology of Tendinopathy: Implications for Tennis Elbow

18

Per Renstrom and Paul W. Ackermann

18.1 Introduction

Tendinopathy accounts for a substantial part of all sports injuries and is increasing in prevalence. Despite the magnitude of the disorder, high-quality scientific data on etiology and available treatments have been limited. Repetitive exposure in combination with recently discovered intrinsic factors, such as genetic variants of matrix proteins, and metabolic disorders are risk factors for the development of tendinopathy [1].

Tendinopathy is a clinical syndrome, often implying overuse tendon injuries, characterized by a combination of pain, diffuse or localized swelling, and impaired performance. [2] Tendinopathy can also occur without signs of overuse and is then mostly associated with medical conditions [3]. Midportion and insertional tendinopathy (enthesopathy) should be distinguished as two different clinical diagnoses. The tendons most affected by overuse are the Achilles and patellar tendons and, in the upper extremities, the rotator cuff and extensor carpi radialis brevis (tennis elbow) tendons [4, 5].

The common pathological conditions associated with tendinopathy are tendinosis and peritendinitis. Tendinosis is the histopathological finding of collagen disorganization and fiber separation, increase in mucoid ground substance, hypercellularity, and nerve and vessel ingrowth but mostly without signs of intratendinous inflammation (tendinitis) [6]. However, lately, the noninflammatory etiology of tendinopathy has been questioned, as inflammation may play a role in the initial phase of the disease [7]. Tendinosis per se is not painful. Thus, histopathological alterations associated with degeneration, such as tendinosis, not correlated to pain must be separated from pain-generating pathophysiology.

Tendinitis, however, which is seen to a much lesser extent (<3%) is associated with classic inflammation usually observed during the early reparative phase [8]. Peritendinitis is an acute or chronic inflammation of the thin membrane, paratenon, surrounding the tendon, often induced by repetitive exercise and characterized by local swelling and infiltration of inflammatory cells [8]. The tendon insertion and bursae surrounding the tendon are common sites of classical inflammation in, e.g., chronic inflammatory conditions such as rheumatoid arthritis or as a response to repetitive stress, because of their greater density of blood vessels and nerves. The tendon proper

---

P. Renstrom
Department of Molecular Medicine and Surgery, Karolinska Institutet, Stockholm, Sweden

Stockholm Sports Trauma Research Center, Karolinska Institutet, Stockholm, Sweden
e-mail: per.renstrom@telia.com

P. W. Ackermann (✉)
Department of Molecular Medicine and Surgery, Karolinska Institutet, Stockholm, Sweden

Department of Orthopedic Surgery, Karolinska University Hospital, Stockholm, Sweden
e-mail: Paul.Ackermann@ki.se

meanwhile is mostly aneuronal and avascular and does not under normal conditions exhibit classical inflammatory responses [9, 10].

18.2 Etiology: Pathophysiology

Mechanical loading of tendon tissue is anabolic by upregulating collagen gene expression and increasing synthesis of collagen proteins. This peaks around 24 h after exercise and remains elevated for up to 70–80 h [6, 11, 12]. However, exercise also results in degradation of collagen proteins, although the timing of this catabolic peak occurs earlier than the anabolic peak. The result is catabolic, i.e., a net loss of collagen, around the first 24–36 h after training, followed by a net gain in collagen, i.e., anabolic [6]. Thus, a certain restitution time interval in between exercise bouts is critical for the tissue to adapt and to avoid a net catabolic situation (Fig. 18.1).

The tendon is able to adapt to load linked with the specific function of anatomic structures in and around the tendon—that is, the tendon cells, tenocytes, extracellular matrix, and nerve-ending receptors. Repetitive strain causes tenocytes to produce inflammatory molecules and microruptures of collagen fibrils. Increased levels of inflammatory mediators (e.g., prostaglandin E2 [PGE2]) are found in tendons after repetitive mechanical loading [14]. Intratendinous injections of PGE2 cause intense degenerative changes, and peritendinous injections of PGE1 result in a histological pattern of tendinopathy [15, 16].

Today, several studies confirm a partly inflammatory background to tendinopathy with granulation alterations of capillary vessels and a significant inflammatory infiltrate consisting of macrophages, mast cells, and B and T lymphocytes [1, 17, 18]. These findings suggest a role for intrinsic immune pathways in the events that mediate early tendinopathy. Presumably, the inflammatory cells activate a cascade of proinflammatory cytokines (e.g., IL-18, IL-15, and IL-6) found in tendinopathy [19]. Tendon cells and fibroblasts, subjected to repetitive mechanical stress in combination with proinflammatory cytokines and transforming growth factor β (TGF-β) stimulation, can transform into myofibroblasts. Myofibroblasts are important cells for tendon healing, possibly also for tissue adaptations. After the healing process is completed and the mechanical stress is released on the myofibroblasts, these cells undergo pro-

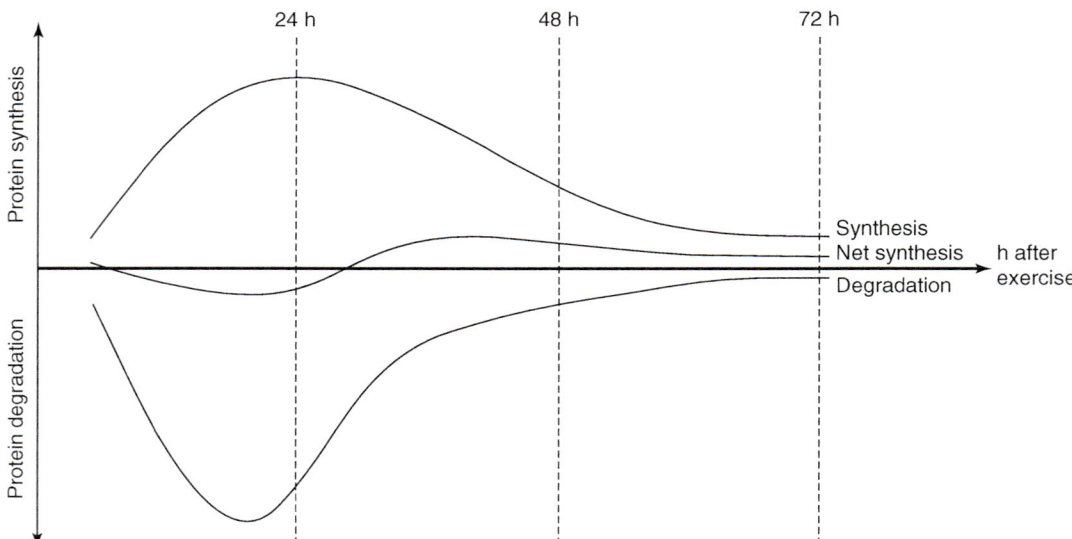

Fig. 18.1 Diagram depicting collagen synthesis and degradation after acute exercise in humans. The first 24–36 h after exercise results in a net loss of collagen. However, 36–72 h after exercise, a net synthesis of collagen follows. Hence, repetitive training without enough resting time in between may result in a net catabolic situation with degradation of the matrix and lead to tendinopathy. Reproduced with permission from Magnusson et al. 2010 [6]

grammed cell death (apoptosis) [20]. If this mechanism fails, the myofibroblasts will propagate a hyperproliferative process, fibrosis, seen as a prominent histological feature of tendinopathy.

Another factor that may cause fibroblast hyperproliferation is hypoxia, which can upregulate matrix metalloproteinases, leading to altered material properties of the tendon [21, 22]. Hypoxia upregulates vascular endothelial growth factor, which may initiate microvessel ingrowth (neoangiogenesis) into the tendon—a major finding in tendinopathy. Neoangiogenesis has been speculated to be a causative factor for pain since sclerotherapy relieves pain in tendinopathy [13]. However, blood vessels per se are not painful, but ingrowth of sensory nerve fibers alongside of blood vessels may elicit pain responses on mechanical or chemical stimulation (Fig. 18.2)

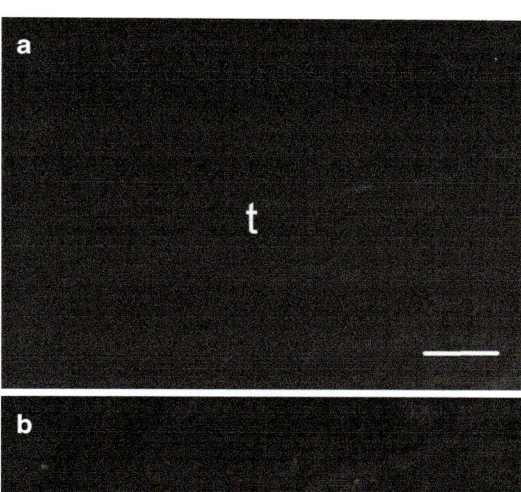

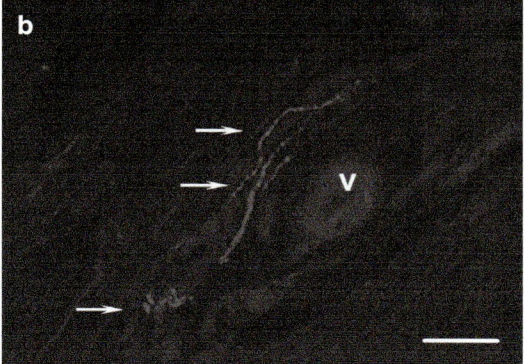

Fig. 18.2 Achilles tendon of healthy control (**a**) and painful tendinopathy (**b**) after immunostaining for substance P (SP) and picture taken with immunofluorescence microscopy. Arrows denote free nerve endings. The micrograph illustrates sensory SP-positive free nerve fibers in close vicinity to a proliferated vessel (**b**). v = blood vessel. Bar = 50 μm. Reproduced with permission from Ackermann et al. 2014 [10]

[18, 23, 24]. Healthy nonpainful tendons are almost aneuronal within the tendon proper, i.e., the intrafascicular matrix [23, 24]. Chronic painful tendons, however, show ingrowth of sensory nerves from the surrounding structures, i.e., the interfascicular matrix, e.g., paratenon, with release of nociceptive substances. Restricting pathological nerve ingrowth by denervation (e.g., mini-invasive surgery or release of the paratenon) can cause pain relief [25]. Interestingly, sensory nerve ingrowth in the tendon can be a reaction to repetitive loading and also a response to injury [26]. In normal tendon repair, sensory nerve ingrowth is correlated with increased nociception, followed by autonomic nerve ingrowth, coinciding with decreased nociception and subsequent nerve retraction [23]. In tendinopathy, though, the ingrown sensory nerves do not retract, as in normal healing. Thus, neuronal dysregulation in tendinopathy, characterized by aberrant sensory nerve sprouting, may reflect a failed healing response (Fig. 18.2), leading to increased pain signaling and possibly to the hyperproliferative changes associated with tendinopathy [24]. In addition to pain transmission, peripheral nerve fibers react to mechanical stimuli and release several chemical substances, which are normally involved in healing and homeostasis but can cause fibrosis during prolonged release [10]. The presence of essential neuromediators in tendon was established more than 10 years ago, and recent studies have verified a diverse group of nerve mediators and receptors in tendon [10]. Tendinopathic tendons exhibit increased levels of the sensory neuropeptide, substance P (SP), which may, in addition to its role in nociception, reflect proinflammatory and trophic actions [27]. SP regulates vasodilation, plasma extravasation, and release of cytokines by binding to its receptor, neurokinin 1, found in tendon and upregulated by loading [27–32]. SP stimulates proliferation of fibroblasts and endothelial cells and possibly also transforms fibroblasts into myofibroblasts by increasing the production of TGF-β in fibroblasts [30]. Hence, abnormal upregulation of SP may contribute to tendinosis (fibrosis), tenocyte transformation, hypercellularity, and hypervascularization observed in tendinopathic patients [33].

Other neuronal factors, highly upregulated in tendinopathy, are the neurotransmitter glutamate and its receptor, NMDAR1, which are implicated in various painful diseases [9, 34, 35]. Furthermore, the localization of the increased glutamate signaling has just lately been established in tendinopathic patients, suggesting a pathological role [35]. Thus, upregulated glutamate/NMDAR1 is observed in morphologically transformed tenocytes, in the endothelial and adventitial layers of neovessel walls, and in ingrown sprouting nerve fibers [35]. Activated NMDA, phospho-NMDA, is seen in the tendon proper of tendinopathic biopsies but not in controls, suggesting a role in pathologic tenocyte transformation, neovessel formation, and pain signaling [35–37]. These may be hypothetically mitigated by blocking of NMDAR1. Systematic investigation of the pathophysiological processes in tendinopathy may lead to novel therapies, which are targeted to the underlying pathomechanisms [38].

18.3 Implications for "Tennis Elbow": Humeral Epicondylar Lateral Tendinopathy

Tendon injuries to the elbow are common, especially in the overhead athlete due to the repetitive loads and forceful muscular activations inherent in tennis serving, badminton smashes, but also in baseball pitching, handball throwing, etc. [39, 40]. The most common injury in the athletic elbow is "tennis elbow"—humeral epicondylar lateral tendinopathy. Other elbow injuries involve valgus extension overload and ulnar collateral ligament injury [34, 41].

18.3.1 Etiology of Tennis Elbow

As early as 1873, Runge described humeral epicondylitis, or "tennis elbow," as it is more popularly known [42]. Cyriax and Cyriax in 1936 listed 26 causes of tennis elbow, while an extensive study by Goldie in 1964 reported hypervascularization of the extensor aponeurosis and increased free nerve endings in the subtendinous space [43]. Leadbetter later described humeral epicondylitis as a degenerative time-dependent process including vascular, chemical, and cellular events that lead to a failure of the cell matrix healing response in human tendon [44]. This description of tendon injury differs from earlier theories where an inflammatory response was considered a primary factor; hence, the term tendonitis was used, as opposed to the term recommended by Leadbetter [44] and Nirschl and Sobel [8]. Since 1998 the term tendinopathy is mostly used. It is a clinical syndrome, often implying overuse tendon injury, characterized by a combination of pain, diffuse or localized swelling, and impaired performance [2]. Hence the term humeral epicondylar lateral tendinopathy may be used for tennis elbow.

18.3.2 Functional Anatomy and Pathoanatomy of the Elbow

The stability of the elbow is provided by the collateral ligaments and the fibrous capsules, as well as by the bones, articulations, muscles, and tendons. The passive stability of the elbow is guaranteed by the adjacent bones, i.e., humerus, radius, and ulna, and the surrounding collateral ligaments and joint capsules. On the lateral aspect of the elbow are the muscles and tendons that extend the wrist, i.e., extensor carpi radialis longus and brevis, digitorum communis, digiti minimi, and carpi radialis brevis, and originate from the lateral epicondyle (Fig. 18.3). These muscles and tendons contribute to the active stability [45].

The normal range of motion (ROM) of the elbow is flexion and extension 0–145° with a functional arc of 0–130°. Pronation and supination can be carried out with 70–90° of pronation to 90° of supination. The axial rotation is around the center of the radial head. At full extension, there is an extra twist (valgus carrying angle) of the elbow in valgus of 10–15° [45].

The pathoanatomy of lateral elbow tendinopathy related to tennis involves primarily the extensor carpi radialis brevis (ECRB) and secondarily the extensor digitorum communis muscle tendons. The lateral epicondyle of the humerus forms a common origin for at least parts of all the extensors of the wrist and fingers.

18.3.3 Incidence of Tennis Elbow

The incidence of lateral humeral epicondylar tendinopathy is far greater than that of medial epicondylar tendinopathy in recreational tennis players and in the leading arm (left arm in a right-handed golfer), while medial humeral epicondylar tendinopathy is far more common in elite tennis players and throwing athletes due to the powerful loading of the flexor and pronator muscle tendon units during the valgus extension overload inherent in the acceleration phase of those overhead movement patterns [8, 46]. The trailing arm of the golfer (right arm in a right-handed golfer) is more likely to have medial symptoms than lateral.

The exact incidence and prevalence of injuries caused by tennis have been difficult to determine as there is a variety of methodologies used and different populations involved. Pluim et al., in a comprehensive meta-analysis across all player levels, reported tennis-injury incidence as ranging from 0.04 to 3.0 injuries per 1000 h played [47]. In top-level players under 18 years of age, injury rates have been estimated to be anywhere from 2 to 20 injuries per 1000 h of tennis played. In a very recent study, the incidence of acute injuries was 1.2/1000 h of tennis play (95% CI, 0.7–1.7) [48]. The high occurrence of overuse injuries among elite junior tennis players suggests that an early focus on preventative measures is warranted, with a particular focus on the monitoring and management of workload.

Tennis elbow is most common in recreational players in tennis, who are often 30–50 years of age and have a high activity level, i.e., playing tennis more than three times a week for hour-long sessions. The overall incidence of lateral epicondylitis has been reported to be anywhere from 35% to 51% [49]. "Tennis elbow" has an incidence of 4.7 events per 1000 patients in primary care [4].

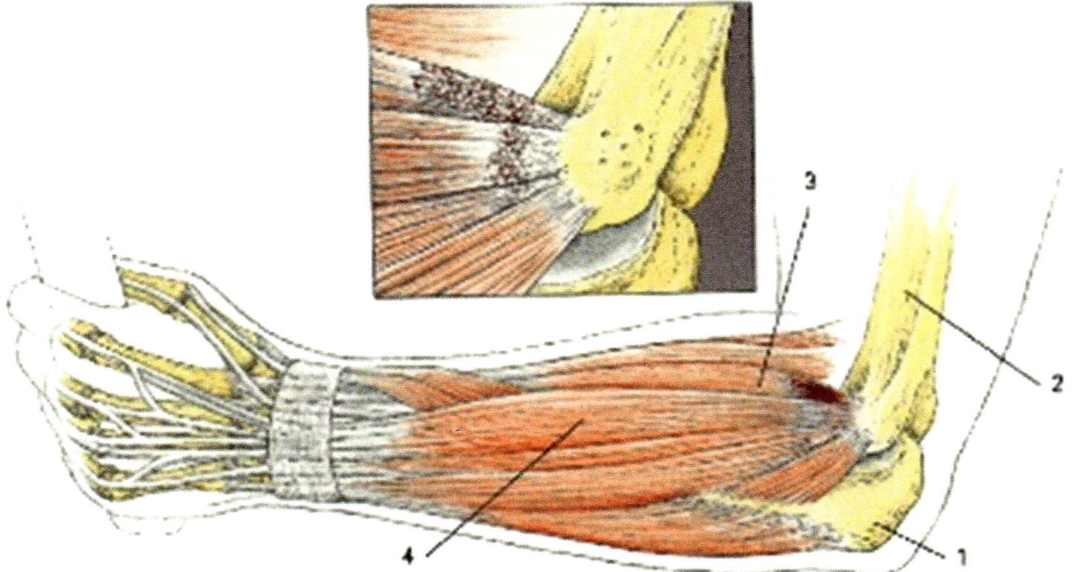

Fig. 18.3 Tennis elbow with degenerative changes in the extensor carpi radialis muscle tendon where it attaches to the lateral epicondyle of the humerus. 1—Ulna; 2—humerus; 3—extensor radialis brevis muscle and its tendon; 4—extensor digitorum communis muscle (with permission by Peterson L., Renström P., Sports injuries, CRC Press, Taylor & Francis, London 2017) [45]

18.3.4 Injury Mechanism

The serving motion in tennis can be divided into different phases. In the *preparation phase*, the elbow is flexed to 45°. In the *cocking phase*, the arm is pulled backward, as well as the trunk. The shoulder externally rotates to 150–180°, causing the anterior capsule of the shoulder to stretch and increase in flexibility. In the *acceleration phase*, the forward movement is started for the arm. During this explosive phase, the rotator cuff stabilizes the shoulder joint, which results in valgus stress on the elbow. This phase is stressful for athletes with elbow pain. The *deceleration phase* is a short phase with the shoulder internally rotated to 0 degrees. This is the most harmful phase of the tennis serve. This typical throwing movement can cause injuries in, e.g., tennis and baseball such as tennis elbow, stretch laxity on the medial collateral ligaments, and overuse injury on the lateral side, with possible cartilage damage on the capitellum [45].

In tennis the symptoms of recreational players are located around the lateral epicondyle, but for top players it is more often on the medial epicondyle. Other problems around the elbow are the "Golfer's elbow" tendinopathy, i.e., problems usually localized to the medial epicondyle. In baseball players, the problems occur at the posterior part where the olecranon hits the humerus, s.c., "posterior tennis elbow." In the tennis serve, this may occur in the follow-through phase when the arm is extended and internally rotated. The forearm goes into pronation. The elbow is maximally extended so that the posterior upper part of the ulna, i.e., the olecranon, is pressed against the back of the upper arm and can cause impingement.

18.3.5 Risk Factors

Although not proven in clinical investigations, some authors believe that the rate of lateral epicondylar tendinopathy is lower in those with two-handed backhands as the nondominant arm is able to absorb some of the forces associated with the stroke and using the second arm lessens the likelihood of faulty mechanics of the trailing and flexed wrist. One investigation examining the electromyographic (EMG) profile of the ECRB between single- and two-handed backhands, however, did not show any significant differences in activity.

The degree of symptoms is directly related to how much they play tennis, with a direct connection between game sessions and pain. Even experienced players, who play longer and more frequent sessions, can suffer pain in the elbow. The tennis player who most easily is subjected to tennis elbow is working with a demanding technique that is not matched by fitness level. Improper technique is one of the most common causes, and particularly common are incorrect backhand strokes [45].

The serve can also cause elbow pain. Of the 75% of the recreational players with tennis elbow, 40% received this affliction by a faulty backhand stroke combined with muscle weakness. Fifty percent of female and 30% of the male professional players have had this problem caused by an overuse on the forehand and/or backhand [45]. It is the combination of extending the elbow and rotating the wrist in the ulnar (pronation) direction that causes the extensor carpi radialis brevis tendon to erode the lateral epicondyle.

Other risk factors associated with lateral epicondylitis have been demonstrated in rotator cuff pathology (OR 4.95), De Quervain's disease (OR 2.48), carpal tunnel syndrome (OR 1.50), oral corticosteroid therapy (OR 1.68), and previous smoking history (OR 1.20). [50]

18.3.6 Tennis Elbow: Humeral Lateral Epicondylar Tendinopathy

Humeral epicondylar tendinopathy is an extra-articular tendinous injury characterized by excessive vascular granulation and an impaired healing response in the tendon, "angiofibroblastic hyperplasia" [46, 51, 52]. In a thorough histopathological analysis, specimens of injured tendon from areas of chronic overuse did not contain large numbers of lymphocytes, macrophages, and neutrophils [53]. Instead, tendons were characterized by large populations of fibroblasts, disorganized collagen, and vascular hyperplasia, and therefore a description of a degenerative process was given, i.e., tendinosis. The primary tendon in lateral humeral epicondylitis is the extensor carpi radialis brevis [46, 51, 52]. Approximately one-third of cases involve the tendon of the extensor communis [48]. The extensor carpi radialis longus and extensor carpi ulnaris can be involved as well. The primary sites of medial humeral epicondylar tendinopathy are the flexor carpi radialis, pronator teres, and flexor carpi ulnaris tendons [46, 52].

18.3.7 Structural Adaptations

Adaptation occurs in the overhead athlete's elbow in range of motion, laxity, and muscular compensation. Comparison to the contralateral nondominant extremity is often complicated by these asymmetric anatomic developments.

Elite-level tennis players had significantly less internal rotation and no significant difference in external rotation on the dominant arm, as well as an overall decrease in total rotation range of motion on the dominant arm of approximately 10° [53].

In baseball 50% of pitchers have a flexion contracture of the dominant elbow, with 30% demonstrating a cubitus valgus deformity [54]. Elbow flexion contractures averaging 5° were common in 40 healthy professional baseball pitchers [55]. In 33 throwing athletes prior to the competitive season, the average loss of elbow extension was 7°, and the average loss of flexion was 5.5° [56]. Directly related to elbow function was wrist flexibility, which was 3° less on the dominant arm for extension and 3° greater on the dominant side for flexion compared with the nondominant extremity [55].

Careful monitoring of glenohumeral range of motion is recommended for the athlete with an elbow injury.

18.3.8 Tennis Elbow: Symptoms and Diagnosis

A history of repetitive activity or overuse, such as playing tennis intensively at a training camp or resuming playing after a period of little activity, is often observed. Problems can often occur after activities such as painting a house and the like. Pain mainly affects the lateral aspect of the elbow but can also radiate upward along the upper arm and downward along the outside of the forearm. Weakness in the wrist can cause difficulty in carrying out such simple movements as lifting a plate or a coffee cup, opening a car door, wringing out a wet dishcloth, and shaking hands. A distinct tender point is elicited by pressure or percussion over the lateral epicondyle [45].

In the "coffee cup" test, i.e., when the injured person lifts a cup of coffee, pain arises over the lateral epicondyle. Pain occurs over the lateral epicondyle when the hand is dorsiflexed at the wrist against resistance. This sign alone is sufficient to justify a diagnosis of "tennis elbow." In a positive middle finger test, there is pain over the lateral elbow when the middle finger is extended against resistance. Involvement of the extensor carpi radialis brevis is typical in tennis players. In lateral elbow tendinosis due to other causes, e.g., industrial work, it seems that the extensor digitorum communis is typically involved. This also leads to a positive middle finger test. In other words, there may be two different etiologies of lateral elbow tendinopathy with different locations of the problem. An accurate diagnosis of tendinopathy includes an evaluation of the magnitude of pathological change, which is helpful as a prognostic predictor, as well as formulating the treatment protocol. The patient's description of time and intensity of pain is the best guide to evaluation [45].

The elbow can be X-rayed to exclude a loose body in the joint or a fracture. Other possible diagnoses are rheumatic disorders, trapping of a nerve (the deep branch of the radial nerve), and radiating pain caused by degenerative changes in the spine in the region of the fifth and sixth cervical vertebrae.

A thorough evaluation of the athlete's elbow is necessary to rule out other concomitant injured structures and, most important, to identify the underlying cause of the tendon injury. Evaluation of the entire upper extremity kinetic chain with a particular focus on shoulder and scapular strength, motion, and stabilization, coupled with diagnostic imaging and clinical tests for the distal upper extremity, is needed [45].

18.4 Prevention

Correct playing and working techniques are the most important preventive measures. Asymmetrical training techniques should be avoided. In tennis, the following points should be emphasized: good footwork so that the player approaches the ball correctly.

Equipment: The ball should be hit correctly with the racquet and at the right moment. The shoulder and the whole of the body should take part in every stroke so that deceleration does not occur when the ball is hit. The stroke should be followed through, and the wrist should be firm.

The court surface should be slow in order to decrease the velocity of the ball. Fast surfaces such as grass or concrete cause the ball to hit the racquet with increased force, resulting in increased load on the player's arm. The balls should be light. Wet or dead balls become heavy.

Correct equipment should be used. The racquet should be individually selected with regard to playing technique. It should be well-balanced and easy to handle, e.g., when making angled drop shots. The arm is likely most safe with a relatively heavy racquet, which is not balanced overly headlight, as more weight in the racquet head provides more resistance to torsion, which also enhances control. A tightly strung racquet increases the impact and tension forces. The stringing of the racquet should be individually adjusted and should not be too taut. Anyone troubled by tennis elbow should have the racquet strung more loosely as it spreads the force of the ball's impact over a longer period of time. The main disadvantage of looser strings is less control. Gut strings give more resilience and less vibration than nylon ones. The size of the racquet grip should be carefully chosen to fit the hand comfortably. A grip that is too large or too small may force the player to grab the handle too tightly and thereby increase the strain on the forearm. A too small grip is likely to be worse, as it more likely will try to twist the hand. A grip that is too small can easily be corrected by adding an overwrap. The impact between racquet and ball produces shock transmission from the racquet to the player. This may be increased unless the ball is hit exactly on the racquet's so-called sweet spot (center of percussion). This is the area of the racquet face where minimal torsion occurs on impact. Hits outside this spot will increase torsion and unwanted forces and vibrations. These may not directly cause tennis elbow but is considered to worsen this condition when established.

18.5 Treatment Concepts

Treatment should follow the healing response; this includes three phases: (1) an acute inflammatory phase, (2) a collagen and ground substance production phase, and (3) a maturation and remodeling phase. [57]

Based on the healing response of the human tendon, several specific phases can be followed during nonoperative treatment of elbow tendinosis: protected function, total arm strength, and return to activity. Each plays a critical part in the comprehensive treatment of elbow tendinopathy.

Protected Function: During this first phase, care is taken to protect the injured muscle tendon unit from stress but not from function. Often, all sport activity must cease temporarily to allow the muscle tendon unit time to heal and to allow formal rehabilitation to progress. Immobilization can atrophy the musculature and negatively affect the upper extremity kinetic chain [46, 52]. Cessation of serving for medial-based humeral symptoms is indicated. Allowing hitting double-handed backhands in tennis continues activity while minimizing stress to the injured area. Continued work or sports may slow the progression of resistive exercise and physical therapy.

The athlete should reduce pain and inflammation when the injury is in its acute stage by the use of cooling for about 2 days (elevation and compression are not needed, as swelling is not a problem). Rest actively, i.e., rest the injured area and avoid movements that trigger pain, but continue with conditioning activity such as running or cycling. Continue with tennis, but avoid the strokes that cause pain. Apply local heat and use a heat retainer when the injury is no longer in its acute stage. Treat with ice massage, perhaps alternating with heat treatment. Try taping the wrist to support the elbow joint under load. Reduce the load on the extensors with the help of a brace, which should be applied when the arm is relaxed and kept in position until the rehabilitation period is over.

Counterforce bracing constrains key muscles groups. An air-filled bladder has been developed as a counterpressure element. This constrictive band caused a significant reduction in integrated electromyography (EMG) activity of the extensor carpi radialis brevis and the extensor digitorum communis when compared with controlled values and a standard band. More research is needed to confirm the effect of braces for the treatment of tennis elbow. Clinical experience indicates, however, that the use of such braces is a valuable complementary tool in the treatment of tennis elbow. The elbow bands can be combined with heat-retaining neoprene sleeves which add the positive effects of heat in stimulating healing.

Resistive exercise for humeral epicondylitis focuses on the principle that "proximal stability is needed to promote distal mobility" [58]. It should be said that the initial nonoperative treatment should involve eccentric exercise, which should be the cornerstone (basis) of treatment of tendinopathy [59]. Strength, stamina, and mobility should be improved by exercises once the pain and inflammation are under control, i.e., the athlete can tolerate the pain of a handshake. The training program should follow the guidelines set out below.

Eccentric training by flexing the wrist with a load of 1–2 kg 20 times per day is the central component of the training [60]. This can be combined with the corresponding stretch at training of the wrist. Eccentric training combined with extracorporeal shockwave treatment has in some reports shown higher success rates compared to any therapy alone. One study showed that 71% reported full recovery in the eccentric exercise group, with 39% in the contract-relax stretching group. Eccentric exercise produced a significant reduction in pain and eliminated strength deficits in the wrist extensors and forearm supinators [60, 61].

Electrophysical modalities may be helpful during the rehabilitation period. In a multicenter prospective randomized control study, extracorporeal shockwave therapy was, however, ineffective in 272 patients with humeral epicondylar tendinopathy [62]. Similarly, low-intensity Nd:YAG laser irradiation at 7 points along the forearm, 3 times a week for 4 weeks, did not demonstrate any significant benefits [63].

Agreement on a superior modality does not exist [64–66]. A meta-analysis of 185 studies on treatment of humeral epicondylar tendinopathy showed major deficits in the scientific quality of the investigations, with no superior treatment approach [65]. In a comprehensive review of the treatment for humeral epicondylar tendinopathy, no significant difference was found with low-energy lasers, acupuncture, extracorporeal shockwave therapy, or steroid injection [64]. A recent systematic review demonstrated potential effectiveness of ultrasound and laser for the management of tennis elbow; however, more high-quality studies are needed. [67]

Local steroid injections have been used for long time in the treatment of tennis elbow. Today, however, research evidence demonstrate that corticosteroid injections are ineffective and may even delay the recovery of tennis elbows. [68, 69] Moreover, high-quality research not only demonstrate local detrimental effects [70] but also the potential systemic harmful effects of corticosteroid therapy [71].

The use of autologous blood injections as treatment for tendinopathy is a therapy with ancient history, which over the last decade has gained increasing interest modified as platelet-rich plasma (PRP) injections [72]. Although there have been some promising studies, currently there is no evidence to support the use of autologous blood injections for tennis elbow [73]. Moreover, while PRP injections have demonstrated positive results from animal studies and experience an increasing interest from the general public, there is no evidence to support its use for tennis elbow [74].

Failed healing is considered to have occurred if there are chronic symptoms of tendinopathy/

pain for more than 6–12 months. If there is poor response to a rehabilitation program, if there is a history of persistent pain, or if the patient has not been able to return to an acceptable quality of life, surgery may be indicated. Different types of surgery in patients with humeral epicondylar lateral tendinopathy have been proposed including open, arthroscopic, as well as percutaneous release of the extensor origin. Functional outcomes of open and arthroscopic releases may be superior to those of percutaneous release; however, the differences may not be clinically noticeable [75]. All surgical techniques report around 90% patient satisfaction rate. [75]

In patients undergoing surgery, it has been found that in 100% the tissue involved was from the extensor carpi radialis brevis. Tissue from the extensor digitorum communis, especially the anterior edge, was involved in 35%, and there was osteophyte formation of the lateral epicondyle in 20%.

Surgical Concepts: The principles of surgical intervention are total excision of the unhealthy pain producing angiofibroblastic tendinosis tissue, enhancement of vascular access to the surgical site, and preservation of normal tissue [55]. Techniques that fail to identify and excise tendinosis tissue and release normal tendons are not recommended. Failed surgery is almost always related to inadequate excision of tendinosis tissue with or without excessive release of normal tissue (e.g., lateral epicondyle, extensor digitorum communis, and lateral ligaments) [55, 61]. The mini-open techniques have reported success rates of 95% and 97% for medial and lateral tissue, respectively [62]. The key pathological tissues are in the extensor carpi radialis brevis and extensor digitorum communis lateral, pronator teres and flexor carpi radialis medial, triceps posterior, and distal biceps anterior [55, 62]. There should then be quality postoperative rehabilitation. The elbow is protected at 90° for 1 week in a counterforce elbow immobilizer. Strength and endurance resistance exercises usually start 3 weeks after surgery.

Ulnar nerve neurapraxia is often associated (50%) with medial elbow tendinosis and may require decompression of the cubital tunnel [55, 62].

Today surgery is less indicated because of successful conservative therapies. New minioperative procedures that, via the endoscope, remove pathological tissue or abnormal neoinnervation demonstrate promising results but need confirmation by Level 1 studies.

Treatment Summary: The recommended treatment strategies for tendinopathy vary. Exercise enhances tendon repair and nerve withdrawal from the tendon proper. Eccentric loading may result in the tendon resistance to injury. Heavy, slow strength training, specifically eccentric, is effective for Achilles and patellar tendinopathy, with encouraging results for epicondylalgia. Physical therapy supervision increases compliance and quality since management of tendinopathy is difficult and time-consuming and may lead to frustration and reinjury. Exercise should be the cornerstone of tendinopathy treatment. Adjuvant biophysical procedures, such as extracorporeal shockwave therapy, may initiate healing of the failed tendon repair by selective denervation of sensory nerves. Injection therapies with blood products, sclerosing agents, and cortisone may have good short-term effects, but all have limited long-term results. There are no Level 1 or high-quality studies to support any of the injection therapies. Thus, there is a limited role for injection treatments in the management of tendinopathy. Surgery may occasionally be indicated in recalcitrant cases and may allow 60–85% of patients to return to preinjury activity levels. Rehabilitation after surgery, however, may take quite some time [76]. Mini-invasive surgery addressing the pathological nerve and vessel ingrowth in tendinopathy shows good initial results.

New techniques addressing tendon repair, such as tissue engineering and regeneration, seem promising. These methods include molecular approaches by which genetically modified cells, including stem cells, synthesize growth factors or other mediators needed for healing. However, molecular procedures are not yet ready for routine clinical use. Novel mini-invasive procedures that target underlying pathology, such as abnormal neoinnervation, are being developed and are initially promising but necessitate high-quality randomized controlled trials before these can be recommended.

18.5.1 Healing

A genuine tennis elbow is self-limited and mostly heals spontaneously, and the prognosis is generally good. The symptoms can, however, persist for anything from 2 weeks to 2 years, especially if the athlete continues to load the arm. Strenuous activity can be resumed when the arm is fully mobile, has regained normal strength, and is pain-free. After surgery, 8–10 weeks should elapse before tennis is resumed.

> **Conclusion**
>
> Humeral epicondylitis is an extra-articular tendon injury that is common in athletes subjected to repetitive upper extremity loading. There is no association between age, sex, and skill level on injury rate in tennis players. Volume of play, however, is clearly associated with an increased risk of injury. Factors for which the literature is mixed include the association between tennis participation and long-term arthritis in joints other than the knee as well as the effect of court surface, racquet grip, and racquet properties on the rate of injury.
>
> Research is limited on the identification of treatment modalities that can reduce pain and restore function to the elbow. Eccentric exercise has been studied in several investigations and, when coupled with a complete upper extremity strengthening program, can produce positive results in patients with elbow tendon injury. Further research is needed in high-level study to delineate optimal treatment methods.

References

1. Ackermann PW, Hart D. Metabolic influences on risk for tendon disorders. Cham: Springer; 2016. 298 p.
2. Khan KM, Maffulli N. Tendinopathy: an Achilles' heel for athletes and clinicians. Clin J Sport Med. 1998;8(3):151–4.
3. Ackermann PW, Hart DA. General overview and summary of concepts regarding tendon disease topics addressed related to metabolic disorders. Adv Exp Med Biol. 2016;920:293–8.
4. Sanders TL, Maradit Kremers H, Bryan AJ, Ransom JE, Smith J, Morrey BF. The epidemiology and health care burden of tennis elbow: a population-based study. Am J Sports Med. 2015;43(5):1066–71.
5. Woo SL-Y, Renström PAFH. Tendinopathy: a major medical problem in sport. In: Woo SL-Y, Renström PAFH, Arnoczky SP, editors. Tendinopathy in athletes. Oxford: Blackwell Publishing Ltd; 2008.
6. Magnusson SP, Langberg H, Kjaer M. The pathogenesis of tendinopathy: balancing the response to loading. Nat Rev Rheumatol. 2010;6(5):262–8.
7. Battery L, Maffulli N. Inflammation in overuse tendon injuries. Sports Med Arthrosc. 2011;19(3):213–7.
8. Nirschl RP, Sobel J. Conservative treatment of tennis elbow. Phys Sportsmed. 1981;9(6):43–54.
9. Alfredson H, Forsgren S, Thorsen K, Fahlström M, Johansson H, Lorentzon R. Glutamate NMDAR1 receptors localised to nerves in human Achilles tendons. Implications for treatment? Knee Surg Sports Traumatol Arthrosc. 2001;9(2):123–6.
10. Ackermann PW, Franklin SL, Dean BJ, Carr AJ, Salo PT, Hart DA. Neuronal pathways in tendon healing and tendinopathy--update. Front Biosci. 2014;19:1251–78.
11. Heinemeier KM, Olesen JL, Haddad F, et al. Expression of collagen and related growth factors in rat tendon and skeletal muscle in response to specific contraction types. J Physiol. 2007;582(Pt 3):1303–16.
12. Miller BF, Olesen JL, Hansen M, et al. Coordinated collagen and muscle protein synthesis in human patella tendon and quadriceps muscle after exercise. J Physiol. 2005;567(Pt 3):1021–33.
13. Ohberg L, Alfredson H. Ultrasound guided sclerosis of neovessels in painful chronic Achilles tendinosis: pilot study of a new treatment. Br J Sports Med. 2002;36(3):173–5. discussion 176–177.
14. Wang JH, Jia F, Yang G, et al. Cyclic mechanical stretching of human tendon fibroblasts increases the production of prostaglandin E2 and levels of cyclo-oxygenase expression: a novel in vitro model study. Connect Tissue Res. 2003;44(3-4):128–33.
15. Khan MH, Li Z, Wang JH. Repeated exposure of tendon to prostaglandin-E2 leads to localized tendon degeneration. Clin J Sport Med. 2005;15(1):27–33.
16. Sullo A, Maffulli N, Capasso G, Testa V. The effects of prolonged peritendinous administration of PGE1 to the rat Achilles tendon: a possible animal model of chronic Achilles tendinopathy. J Orthop Sci. 2001;6(4):349–57.
17. Millar NL, Hueber AJ, Reilly JH, et al. Inflammation is present in early human tendinopathy. Am J Sports Med. 2010;38(10):2085–91.
18. Schubert TE, Weidler C, Lerch K, Hofstädter F, Straub RH. Achilles tendinosis is associated with sprouting of substance P positive nerve fibres. Ann Rheum Dis. 2005;64(7):1083–6.
19. Millar NL, Wei AQ, Molloy TJ, Bonar F, Murrell GA. Cytokines and apoptosis in supraspinatus tendinopathy. J Bone Joint Surg Br. 2009;91(3):417–24.
20. Tomasek JJ, Gabbiani G, Hinz B, Chaponnier C, Brown RA. Myofibroblasts and mechano-regulation

of connective tissue remodelling. Nat Rev Mol Cell Biol. 2002;3(5):349–63.
21. Freeman TA, Parvizi J, Dela Valle CJ, Steinbeck MJ. Mast cells and hypoxia drive tissue metaplasia and heterotopic ossification in idiopathic arthrofibrosis after total knee arthroplasty. Fibrogenesis Tissue Repair. 2010;3:17.
22. Pufe T, Petersen WJ, Mentlein R, Tillmann BN. The role of vasculature and angiogenesis for the pathogenesis of degenerative tendons disease. Scand J Med Sci Sports. 2005;15(4):211–22.
23. Ackermann PW, Li J, Lundeberg T, Kreicbergs A. Neuronal plasticity in relation to nociception and healing of rat achilles tendon. J Orthop Res. 2003;21(3):432–41.
24. Lian Ø, Dahl J, Ackermann PW, Frihagen F, Engebretsen L, Bahr R. Pronociceptive and antinociceptive neuromediators in patellar tendinopathy. Am J Sports Med. 2006;34(11):1801–8.
25. van Sterkenburg MN, van Dijk CN. Mid-portion Achilles tendinopathy: why painful? An evidence-based philosophy. Knee Surg Sports Traumatol Arthrosc. 2011;19(8):1367–75.
26. Messner K, Wei Y, Andersson B, Gillquist J, Räsänen T. Rat model of Achilles tendon disorder. A pilot study. Cells Tissues Organs. 1999;165(1):30–9.
27. Scott A, Bahr R. Neuropeptides in tendinopathy. Front Biosci. 2009;14:2203–11.
28. Andersson G, Danielson P, Alfredson H, Forsgren S. Presence of substance P and the neurokinin-1 receptor in tenocytes of the human Achilles tendon. Regul Pept. 2008;150(1-3):81–7.
29. Bring DK, Reno C, Renstrom P, Salo P, Hart DA, Ackermann PW. Joint immobilization reduces the expression of sensory neuropeptide receptors and impairs healing after tendon rupture in a rat model. J Orthop Res. 2009;27(2):274–80.
30. Hoffmann P, Hoeck K, Deters S, Werner-Martini I, Schmidt WE. Substance P and calcitonin gene related peptide induce TGF-alpha expression in epithelial cells via mast cells and fibroblasts. Regul Pept. 2010;161(1-3):33–7.
31. Ljung BO, Alfredson H, Forsgren S. Neurokinin 1-receptors and sensory neuropeptides in tendon insertions at the medial and lateral epicondyles of the humerus. Studies on tennis elbow and medial epicondylalgia. J Orthop Res. 2004;22(2):321–7.
32. Schizas N, Li J, Andersson T, et al. Compression therapy promotes proliferative repair during rat Achilles tendon immobilization. J Orthop Res. 2010;28(7):852–8.
33. Fong G, Backman LJ, Hart DA, Danielson P, McCormack B, Scott A. Substance P enhances collagen remodeling and MMP-3 expression by human tenocytes. J Orthop Res. 2013;31(1):91–8.
34. Molloy TJ, Kemp MW, Wang Y, Murrell GA. Microarray analysis of the tendinopathic rat supraspinatus tendon: glutamate signaling and its potential role in tendon degeneration. J Appl Physiol (1985). 2006;101(6):1702–9.
35. Schizas N, Lian Ø, Frihagen F, Engebretsen L, Bahr R, Ackermann PW. Coexistence of up-regulated NMDA receptor 1 and glutamate on nerves, vessels and transformed tenocytes in tendinopathy. Scand J Med Sci Sports. 2010;20(2):208–15.
36. Dean BJ, Snelling SJ, Dakin SG, Javaid MK, Carr AJ. In vitro effects of glutamate and N-methyl-D-aspartate receptor (NMDAR) antagonism on human tendon derived cells. J Orthop Res. 2015;33(10):1515–22.
37. Spang C, Backman LJ, Le Roux S, Chen J, Danielson P. Glutamate signaling through the NMDA receptor reduces the expression of scleraxis in plantaris tendon derived cells. BMC Musculoskelet Disord. 2017;18(1):218.
38. Ackermann PW, Salo P, Hart DA. Tendon Innervation. Adv Exp Med Biol. 2016;920:35–51.
39. Fleisig GS, Andrews JR, Dillman CJ, Escamilla RF. Kinetics of baseball pitching with implications about injury mechanisms. Am J Sports Med. 1995;23(2):233–9.
40. Ryu RK, McCormick J, Jobe FW, Moynes DR, Antonelli DJ. An electromyographic analysis of shoulder function in tennis players. Am J Sports Med. 1988;16(5):481–5.
41. Ellenbecker T, AJ M. The elbow in sport. Champaign, IL: Human Kinetics; 1997.
42. Runge F. Zur genese und behandlung des schreibekrampfes. Berlin Klin Wochensch. 1873;21:245.
43. Cyriax J, Cyriax P. Illustrated manual of orthopaedic medicine. London: Butterworth; 1983.
44. Leadbetter WB. Cell-matrix response in tendon injury. Clin Sports Med. 1992;11(3):533–78.
45. Peterson L, Renström P. Sport injuries. London: CRC Press, Taylor & Francis Ltd; 2017.
46. Ollivierre CO, Nirschl RP. Tennis elbow. Current concepts of treatment and rehabilitation. Sports Med. 1996;22(2):133–9.
47. Pluim BM, Staal JB, Windler GE, Jayanthi N. Tennis injuries: occurrence, aetiology, and prevention. Br J Sports Med. 2006;40(5):415–23.
48. Pluim BM, Clarsen B, Verhagen E. Injury rates in recreational tennis players do not differ between different playing surfaces. Br J Sports Med. 2018;52(9):611–5.
49. Carroll R. Tennis elbow: incidence in local league players. Br J Sports Med. 1981;15(4):250–6.
50. Titchener AG, Fakis A, Tambe AA, Smith C, Hubbard RB, Clark DI. Risk factors in lateral epicondylitis (tennis elbow): a case-control study. J Hand Surg Eur Vol. 2013;38(2):159–64.
51. Nirschl RP, Rodin DM, Ochiai DH, Maartmann-Moe C. Group D-A--S. Iontophoretic administration of dexamethasone sodium phosphate for acute epicondylitis. A randomized, double-blinded, placebo-controlled study. Am J Sports Med. 2003;31(2):189–95.
52. Nirschl RP, Ashman ES. Tennis elbow tendinosis (epicondylitis). Instr Course Lect. 2004;53:587–98.
53. Ellenbecker TS, Roetert EP, Bailie DS, Davies GJ, Brown SW. Glenohumeral joint total rotation range

of motion in elite tennis players and baseball pitchers. Med Sci Sports Exerc. 2002;34(12):2052–6.
54. King JW, Brelsford HJ, Tullos HS. Analysis of the pitching arm of the professional baseball pitcher. Clin Orthop Relat Res. 1969;67:116–23.
55. Ellenbecker TS, Mattalino AJ, Elam EA, Caplinger RA. Medial elbow joint laxity in professional baseball pitchers. A bilateral comparison using stress radiography. Am J Sports Med. 1998;26(3):420–4.
56. Wright RW, Steger-May K, Wasserlauf BL, O'Neal ME, Weinberg BW, Paletta GA. Elbow range of motion in professional baseball pitchers. Am J Sports Med. 2006;34(2):190–3.
57. Ackermann PW. Healing and repair mechanism. In: Karlsson J, Calder J, van Diek N, editors. Achilles tendon disorders. Current concepts. 2nd ed. Guildford: DJO Publications; 2014. p. 17–26.
58. Ellenbecker TS, Nirschl R, Renstrom P. Current concepts in examination and treatment of elbow tendon injury. Sports Health. 2013;5(2):186–94.
59. Cullinane FL, Boocock MG, Trevelyan FC. Is eccentric exercise an effective treatment for lateral epicondylitis? A systematic review. Clin Rehabil. 2014;28(1):3–19.
60. Peterson M, Butler S, Eriksson M, Svardsudd K. A randomized controlled trial of eccentric vs. concentric graded exercise in chronic tennis elbow (lateral elbow tendinopathy). Clin Rehabil. 2014;28(9):862–72.
61. Croisier JL, Foidart-Dessalle M, Tinant F, Crielaard JM, Forthomme B. An isokinetic eccentric programme for the management of chronic lateral epicondylar tendinopathy. Br J Sports Med. 2007;41(4):269–75.
62. Haake M, König IR, Decker T, et al. Extracorporeal shock wave therapy in the treatment of lateral epicondylitis : a randomized multicenter trial. J Bone Joint Surg Am. 2002;84A(11):1982–91.
63. Basford JR, Sheffield CG, Cieslak KR. Laser therapy: a randomized, controlled trial of the effects of low intensity Nd:YAG laser irradiation on lateral epicondylitis. Arch Phys Med Rehabil. 2000;81(11):1504–10.
64. Boyer MI, Hastings H. Lateral tennis elbow: "Is there any science out there?". J Shoulder Elbow Surg. 1999;8(5):481–91.
65. Labelle H, Guibert R, Joncas J, Newman N, Fallaha M, Rivard CH. Lack of scientific evidence for the treatment of lateral epicondylitis of the elbow. An attempted meta-analysis. J Bone Joint Surg Br. 1992;74(5):646–51.
66. Trudel D, Duley J, Zastrow I, Kerr EW, Davidson R, MacDermid JC. Rehabilitation for patients with lateral epicondylitis: a systematic review. J Hand Ther. 2004;17(2):243–66.
67. Dingemanse R, Randsdorp M, Koes BW, Huisstede BM. Evidence for the effectiveness of electrophysical modalities for treatment of medial and lateral epicondylitis: a systematic review. Br J Sports Med. 2014;48(12):957–65.
68. Coombes BK, Connelly L, Bisset L, Vicenzino B. Economic evaluation favours physiotherapy but not corticosteroid injection as a first-line intervention for chronic lateral epicondylalgia: evidence from a randomised clinical trial. Br J Sports Med. 2016;50(22):1400–5.
69. Claessen FM, Heesters BA, Chan JJ, Kachooei AR, Ring D. A meta-analysis of the effect of corticosteroid injection for enthesopathy of the extensor carpi radialis brevis origin. J Hand Surg Am. 2016;41(10):988–998.e982.
70. Dean BJ, Carr AJ. The effects of glucocorticoid on tendon and tendon derived cells. Adv Exp Med Biol. 2016;920:239–46.
71. Waljee AK, Rogers MA, Lin P, et al. Short term use of oral corticosteroids and related harms among adults in the United States: population based cohort study. BMJ. 2017;357:j1415.
72. de Vos RJ. Does platelet-rich plasma increase tendon metabolism? Adv Exp Med Biol. 2016;920:263–73.
73. de Vos RJ, Windt J, Weir A. Strong evidence against platelet-rich plasma injections for chronic lateral epicondylar tendinopathy: a systematic review. Br J Sports Med. 2014;48(12):952–6.
74. de Vos RJ, Weir A, van Schie HT, et al. Platelet-rich plasma injection for chronic Achilles tendinopathy: a randomized controlled trial. JAMA. 2010;303(2):144–9.
75. Pierce TP, Issa K, Gilbert BT, et al. A systematic review of tennis elbow surgery: open versus arthroscopic versus percutaneous release of the common extensor origin. Arthroscopy. 2017;33(6):1260–1268.e1262.
76. Pascarella A, Alam M, Pascarella F, Latte C, Di Salvatore MG, Maffulli N. Arthroscopic management of chronic patellar tendinopathy. Am J Sports Med. 2011;39(9):1975–83.

Humeral Epicondylitis in Elite Tennis Players and Indications for Elbow Arthroscopy

19

David M. Dare, Christopher L. Camp, Ioonna Felix, and Joshua S. Dines

19.1 Introduction

Tennis players are frequently exposed to repetitive, sudden, and explosive stressors during competition, resulting in demands on their musculoskeletal system that are unique to the sport. During a tennis stroke, the elbow is subject to extraordinarily high loads and forces. Not surprisingly, then, it is believed that elbow symptoms and injuries occur in at least 40–50% of tennis players at some point in their career [1, 2]. First described by Runge in 1873, lateral epicondylitis, or "tennis elbow," is the most common upper extremity diagnosis in recreational tennis players, with injury rates ranging from 75% to 85% of elbow injuries [3–6].

Lateral epicondylitis more commonly affects novice tennis players compared to professional-

D. M. Dare
Raleigh Orthopaedic Clinic, Raleigh, NC, USA

C. L. Camp
Department of Orthopedic Surgery and Sports Medicine, Mayo Clinic, Rochester, MN, USA

I. Felix
Sports Medicine and Shoulder Service, Hospital for Special Surgery, New York, NY, USA

J. S. Dines (✉)
Sports Medicine and Shoulder Service, Hospital for Special Surgery, New York, NY, USA

Orthopedic Surgery, Weill Cornell Medical College, New York, NY, USA

Aspetar Sports Medicine Hospital, Doha, Qatar

or elite-level players. Recreational players are more likely to hit their backhand strokes with their wrists in a more flexed position, while elite-level players increase wrist extension just prior to ball contact [7, 8]. Recreational players have also been shown to eccentrically contract their extensor muscles, causing repetitive microtrauma to the tendon [7, 9].

Rather than an inflammatory condition, humeral epicondylitis is an extra-articular tendon injury characterized by proliferative vascular granulation and an impaired healing response in the tendon, a process termed "angiofibroblastic hyperplasia" [6, 10]. Histologic studies of the injured tendon have shown a degenerative tendon featuring fibroblasts, disorganized collagen, and vascular hyperplasia [11]. The application of stress on a tendon typically leads to increased cross-linkage and collagen deposition [12]. Microtears result, though, when the rate of stretching exceeds the tendon's tolerance. There are four well-defined histological stages that result from such repetitive microtrauma and microtearing [11].

- Stage 1: acute inflammatory phase. Patients may seek treatment during this phase. If given time and rest, this phase may resolve completely.
- Stage 2: if microtrauma continues, there is increased concentration of fibroblasts, vascular hyperplasia, and disorganized collagen. Together these factors are called angiofibroblastic hyperplasia and result in

tendinosis. This is the most common phase at which patients present for treatment.
- Stage 3: continued microtrauma causes persistent development and accumulation of pathologic changes ultimately leading to tendon failure, manifested as a partial or complete tear.
- Stage 4: it contains aspects of stage 2 and stage 3 with other more advanced changes like fibrosis and soft-tissue calcification.

The tendon's altered structure alone, however, is not sufficient to explain the variability in patients' symptoms. It is believed that part of the pain in lateral epicondylitis is attributable to an increased concentration of neurotransmitters, which magnify the pain response, and lactate or other chemicals that cause direct irritation [13]. Both of these mechanisms can initiate a cascade of alterations in neurons in the peripheral nervous system that promote sensitization of the central nervous system [14]. This may explain why athletes with tennis elbow have pain in neurologic regions distant from the elbow. It has been noted that of patients with lateral epicondylitis, 56% also have associated discomfort in the neck [15]. Of course, though, associated neck, shoulder, or wrist pain may simply represent a breakdown in the kinetic chain.

19.2 Biomechanics of the Elbow in Tennis

Elbow stability is maintained by articular congruity, capsuloligamentous competency, and dynamic muscle control. Bony constraints provide primary stability at flexion angles <20° or more than 120°. While the ulnar collateral ligament serves as the primary static stabilizer to valgus stress, the forearm flexor tendons—namely, the flexor carpi ulnaris and flexor digitorum superficialis—provide important dynamic stability to the elbow.

Tennis play includes three basic strokes:

- The overhead serve
- The forehand
- The backhand [16]

The overhead serve and the ground stroke (forehand and backhand) can be further subdivided into several critical phases unique to each stroke. The overhead serve is comprised of the windup, cocking, and deceleration/follow-through (Fig. 19.1) [17]. The ground stroke includes racquet preparation, acceleration, and follow-through [18]. Each phase demands that

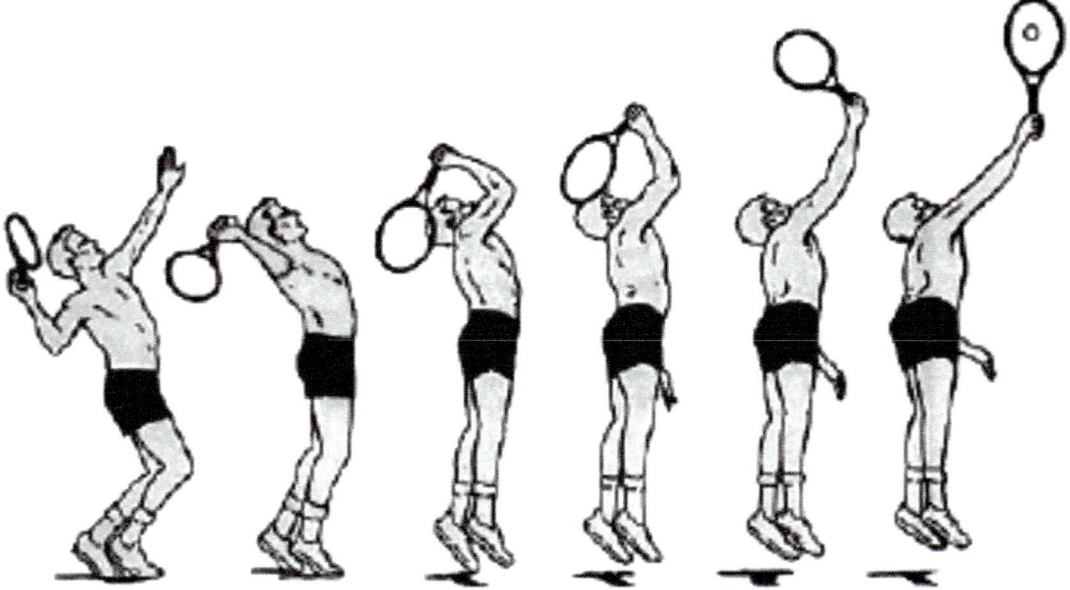

Fig. 19.1 Different phases of the tennis service motion. Van der Hoeven H, Kibler WB. Shoulder injuries in tennis players. *Br J Sports Med 2006*; 40: 435–440

energy is generated by and transmitted through the elbow. This complex interplay of energy transfer is understood in the framework of the kinetic chain.

The elbow functions as a link in the kinetic chain of both the ground stroke and the serve (Fig. 19.2) [19]. Kinetic energy is generated and transferred sequentially through the chain. The elbow is the penultimate link in this chain, accepting and then adding energy and force before transferring them on to the wrist and racquet. Inefficiencies in any of the more proximal links will cause inefficient biomechanics and may lead to increased injury risk.

Motion at the elbow link is comprised of flexion/extension and varus/valgus at the elbow and supination/pronation at the forearm. During the service motion, the elbow moves from 116° of flexion to 20° of flexion, with ball impact at 35°. This flexion arc occurs in just 0.21 s. The flexion/extension arc is much smaller with ground strokes, averaging 11° (46–35°) on the forehand and 18° (48–30°) on the backhand. The angular velocity of the extended elbow during overhead service was determined to be 982°/s [19]. Kibler's data highlights the extraordinary forces that pass through the elbow during tennis play.

The muscles and tendons around the elbow actively produce the energy and force necessary for efficient biomechanics. Muscle activity in the forehand stroke reflects the need for active supination/pronation, along with elbow and wrist stabilization through the acceleration phase. As such, there is increased activity in the biceps, pronator teres, and wrist flexors and extensors. Wrist extensors are active in the acceleration and follow-through phases of both the one-hand and two-handed backhand. Wrist flexors and the pronator teres, however, are also activated in the two-handed backhand [19].

Clearly, tennis confers extreme stress on both the elbow flexors and extensors. The purpose of this chapter is to describe the etiologies associated with both lateral and medial epicondylitis, in addition to keys of diagnosis and treatment options.

19.3 Lateral Epicondylitis

While tennis elbow is not exclusive to tennis players, it is reported that up to 50% of recreational tennis players will develop lateral elbow tendinopathy at some point in their careers [10].

19.4 Etiology

Biomechanical analysis has shown that eccentric contractions of the extensor carpi radialis brevis (ECRB) muscle during the backhand swing, particularly in recreational players, cause repetitive microtrauma and tearing to the tendon's origin, ultimately resulting in lateral epicondylitis (Fig. 19.3). During the backhand, the ball transmits a force to the racket that imparts a force on the player's hand and in turn the wrist extensor muscles, namely, the ECRB and extensor digitorum communis (EDC).

The force is then passed from the extensor muscles to the common tendinous origin at the lateral epicondyle [20]. There are several factors associated with the development of this problem in tennis players [21]:

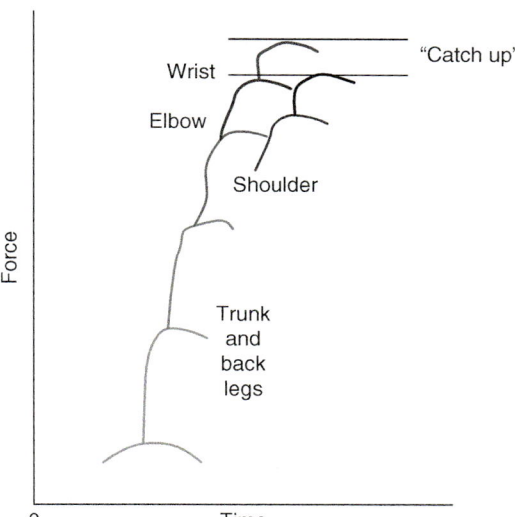

Fig. 19.2 A schematic illustration of the kinetic chain theory. Van der Hoeven H, Kibler WB. Shoulder injuries in tennis players. *Br J Sports Med 2006*; 40: 435–440

- Improper technique: snapping of the wrist in backhand play, incorrect feet positioning, and

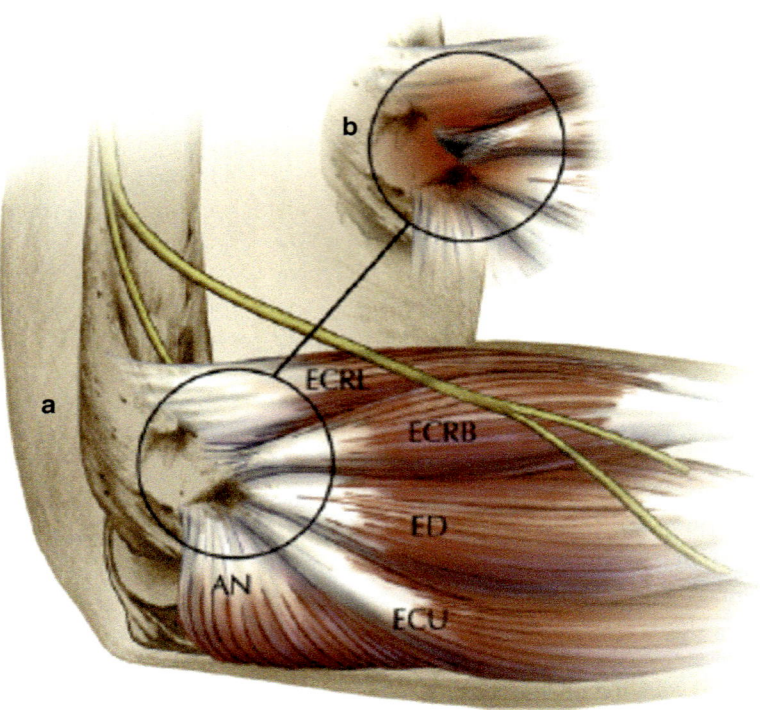

Fig. 19.3 (**a**) Normal anatomy and (**b**) location of pathologic tendinosis at ECRB origin. *ECRL* extensor carpi radialis longus, *ECRB* extensor carpi radialis brevis, *ED* extensor digitorum, *ECU* extensor carpi ulnaris, *AN* anconeus. Van Hofwegen C, Baker CL, Baker CL (2010) Epicondylitis in the Athlete's Elbow. Clin Sports Med 29:577–597

hitting the ball late or with a bent elbow. These improper techniques result in force generation from the forearm extensors rather than the core muscles or rotator cuff.
- Extended duration and frequency of play, leading to overuse.
- Racquet weight.

While tennis elbow more frequently affects novice players, professional athletes are not immune. Professional tennis players are particularly affected by increased vibrational loads at ball strike coupled with an inappropriate racquet weight [22]. Despite previous reports, though, recent data suggests that racquet grip size does not influence the development of lateral epicondylitis [20].

19.5 Presentation

Athletes most often complain of pain at or around the lateral epicondyle that often radiates down the forearm in line with the common extensor muscles. The pain is typically triggered or made worse by contraction of the common extensor mass. The intensity and frequency of the pain varies and may affect activities of daily living and sleep. Tennis players may also complain of grip strength weakness.

Inspection alone is unlikely to uncover obvious abnormalities. The exception is the patient who has had numerous corticosteroid injections, resulting in muscle wasting and thinning of the overlying skin. This presentation is very unusual in an elite athlete. There is frequently tenderness to palpation at the ECRB insertion just anterior to the anterior border of the lateral epicondyle. The tenderness, however, may be more diffuse, with particular point tenderness over the lateral epicondyle itself.

Full range of motion is usually maintained. However, in more severe cases, patients may experience elbow pain in maximal extension in a fully pronated forearm. Passive maximal wrist flexion, which tensions the ECRB, may cause pain. There are several provocative tests that may reproduce the player's symptoms. Resisted wrist extension with the elbow fully extended and pronated stresses the common extensor origin and can reproduce pain in even mild cases [23]. The classic "chair test" asks that the patient lift a chair with the forearm pronated. A positive test is one that reproduces the patients' complaints [24]. And as mentioned previously, tennis players may also complain of diminished grip strength.

Other diagnoses with clinical features similar to lateral epicondylitis must be ruled out. In the athlete, these conditions include:

- Cervical radiculopathy causing pain in the elbow and forearm.
- Breakdown of a more proximally located link in the kinetic chain leading to elbow overuse.
- Posterior interosseous nerve (PIN) entrapment in the lateral forearm can produce pain in the lateral elbow and forearm. PIN entrapment, or radial tunnel syndrome, does not generate pain with resisted wrist extension. Pain may be provoked by resisted supination and relieved by a local injection. Electromyography may also be used to help exclude PIN entrapment.
- Lateral pain in the elite tennis player may be related to degenerative or chondral changes in the radiocapitellar joint.

19.6 Imaging

Imaging studies are usually more helpful in excluding other causes of lateral elbow pain than in making the diagnosis of lateral epicondylitis. Plain radiographs can help to exclude loose bodies, osteochondritis dissecans, or osteoarthritis. An accumulation of calcium may be visualized at the origin of the common extensor.

Ultrasound is useful in assessing structural changes in the tendon, including thickening or thinning, degeneration, full-thickness tearing, or calcific deposits. Doppler ultrasound, more specifically, can evaluate neovascularization. It has been reported that the absence of neovascularization and gray-scale changes rules out the diagnosis of lateral epicondylitis [25].

While ultrasound has proven to be a useful tool in the evaluation of tennis elbow, MRI is more reproducible and can also investigate for concomitant intra-articular pathology [26]. MRI reliably confirms the presence of degenerative tissue or tears within the tendon, and these imaging findings correlate well surgical and histological findings [27] (Fig. 19.4). Coel et al. [28] reported increased MRI signal in the anconeus muscle in cases of recalcitrant lateral epicondylitis but were unable to determine if this edema was related to the chronicity of symptoms or to abnormal elbow motion secondary to the patient's symptoms. MRI findings, in contrast, correlate poorly with patient's symptoms—the size of the tear does not clearly relate to the severity of symptoms [29].

While imaging has proven to be a useful adjunct in the diagnosis of lateral epicondylitis, it should not supplant clinical judgment. Imaging findings must be correlated with the clinical presentation and examination in order to provide an accurate diagnosis.

19.7 Treatment

As always, treatment should begin with prevention. The tennis player must focus on racquet striking techniques; in particular, the wrist must be in extension during ball impact. Emphasis should be placed on balanced concentric and eccentric training of the forearm musculature, as muscle imbalances can create injury [30]. Perhaps most importantly, attention must be paid to the efficiency of the entire kinetic chain, as deficits in a single link may have downstream effects.

The principles of treatment are not unlike other orthopedic problems: (1) pain control, (2) preserve motion, (3) improve grip strength and endurance, (4) return to activity, and (5) prevent further clinical and histological deterioration.

19.8 Nonoperative Treatment

Most patients with lateral epicondylitis respond well to nonoperative treatment. Rest, avoidance of aggravating activities, and behavior modification typically result in resolution of symptoms [31]. Compared to rest alone, physical therapy

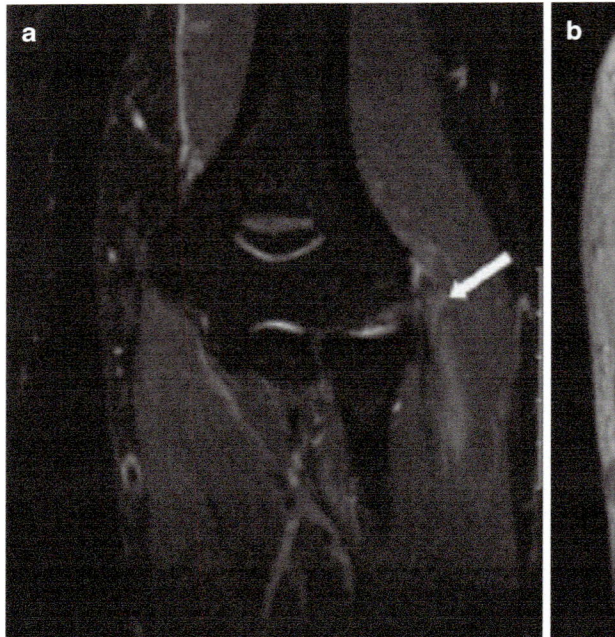 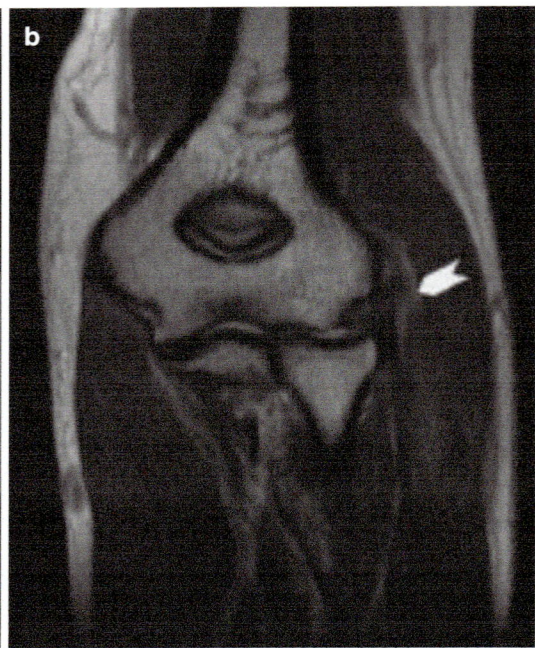

Fig. 19.4 (**a**) MRI of the left elbow shows extracapsular soft tissue edema (*arrow*) on a coronal inversion recovery sequence. (**b**) A high-grade proximal tear is noted in the ECRB tendon (arrowhead) on the coronal proton density sequence. Images courtesy of Hollis G. Potter, MD. Attending Radiologist, Hospital for Special Surgery, 535 E 70th Street, NY, NY 10021

has proven to be more effective at 6 weeks [32]. Physical therapy should include a comprehensive subjective history and assessment of musculoskeletal health, which includes shoulder, forearm, core, and lower body strength, flexibility, and endurance [33, 34]. In addition to the musculoskeletal assessment, the clinician must consider the extrinsic factors that contribute to lateral epicondylitis. These factors include overtraining, grip strength, string tension, playing style, and stroke mechanics. Deficits in shoulder kinematics may contribute to elbow pathology. Therefore, physical therapy should include strengthening and stabilizing the scapula [35, 36]. Fatigue of the scapular stabilizers can cause a change in elbow kinematics, such as increase in elbow motion in the serve's cocking phase. In short, physical therapy for humeral epicondylitis should emphasize scapular muscle strength, endurance, neuromuscular control, and efficient movement patterning, as tennis is a sport that optimizes the kinetic chain. A successful rehabilitation plan must include the entire upper extremity, the core, and the legs. Once the player has met the criteria to return to play, an interval program should be implemented. Utilizing an interval tennis program can gradually return the player to hitting as long as the player remains asymptomatic.

Epicondylar counterforce braces work to reduce the tension in the forearm extensors. Compared to placebo orthoses or wrist splints, counterforce braces (elbow straps, clasps, sleeves, etc.) have proven superior in relieving pain and improving grip strength [37]. Wrist extension splints were found to significantly improve the pain component of the ASES score compared to counterforce braces [38]. While a wrist splint may expedite the acute improvement of pain, it is impractical for an elite tennis player to play or practice in a wrist splint.

Nonsteroidal anti-inflammatory drugs (NSAIDs) are also used frequently and may improve short-term function. Local injection of corticosteroid should be used with caution in elite tennis players but may allow for an expedited, albeit transient, resolution of symptoms. In fact, corticosteroids were demonstrated to be superior to NSAIDs at 4 weeks but possess no advantages in the long-term [39]. Injections may be administered using a single-injection technique or peppered injections into multiple parts of the tendon. A randomized, controlled trial revealed only slightly better improvements in the disabilities of the arm, shoulder, and hand (DASH) score and visual analogue score (VAS) for pain and grip strength, in the peppered group.

There are numerous alternative methods of treatment. These include extracorporeal shock wave (ECSW) therapy, laser therapy, acupuncture, botox, topical nitrates, autologous blood injection, and platelet-rich plasma (PRP) injection.

ECSW therapy delivers shock wave through the tissue. Its mechanism is not fully understood, but it is believed to activate a cycle of inflammation that is required for healing. A 2006 Cochrane review investigated nine studies. While five studies showed ECSW to be superior to sham therapy, the authors did not find an overall statistically significant benefit [33]. Low-level laser therapy may be clinically beneficial if an optimal dose and wavelength are used [40].

While the long-term benefits are uncertain, acupuncture has been shown to reduce pain at 2–8 weeks after the treatment [41]. Botulinum toxin may reduce pain in the short-term but is associated with side effects, such as finger extension weakness [42]. A separate study showed no difference between botox injection and saline injection [43]. Nitric oxide is an important factor in tendon healing. Not surprisingly, then, topical nitrates, which stimulate blood flow and perhaps stimulate collagen production, have proven effective in the reduction of pain in tennis elbow [44].

Autologous blood and PRP injection have both been studied. Autologous blood has been shown to reduce pain in patients with tennis elbow [45, 46]. Additionally, in a randomized, controlled trial, autologous blood injections were found to be superior to corticosteroid at 4 and 8 weeks [47]. Nonetheless, these studies are all fairly small in scale, and it is therefore difficult to draw conclusions on its efficacy. PRP is a concentrate of platelets that contains a high concentration of growth factors that may enhance tendon healing. Several studies have demonstrated that PRP is superior to autologous blood and local anesthetic [48, 49]. There is, though, enormous variation in the methods by which PRP is prepared and activated, thus confounding reports on its clinical effect. Future work must aim to minimize this variability, as PRP has shown promise in the treatment of recalcitrant lateral epicondylitis [50–52].

19.9 Operative Treatment

Surgery should be reserved for patients who have failed nonoperative treatments. Operative treatment may be achieved with open, percutaneous, or arthroscopic techniques. There is no consensus regarding the optimal surgical technique. Nirschl and Pettrone excised the tendinotic tissue within the ECRB, decorticated or drilled the lateral epicondyle, and repaired the extensor carpi radialis longus (ECRL) and EDC. In 88 patients, they reported that 97.7% improved [53]. Other authors have advocated for a simple release of the common extensor tendon, as described by Spencer and Herndon [54], and found good results in 80% [55] and 89% [56] of patients. ECRB lengthening at the wrist and percutaneous release have also been described separately and resulted in good to excellent results in 78% and 91% of patients, respectively [57, 58].

The most frequently used open technique, and the one endorsed by the authors, includes excision of any abnormal or degenerative tissue at the extensor tendon origin, followed by decortication to prepare a bleeding bony bed, and reapproximation of the overlying aponeurosis. Prior to repairing that aponeurosis, the authors prefer to reduce the ECRB to its origin using a suture anchor [59].

Open surgery has provided a high rate of successful outcomes and a high rate of return to sport [56]. In a large series of 92 elbows, 93% of athletes were able to return to sporting activities. The advantages of an open procedure are that it permits inspection of the ECRB undersurface, which may reveal tears, and allows separation of the ECRL from the extensor aponeurosis, allowing anatomical repair.

Many have suggested that the primary advantage of arthroscopic treatment is the ability to address concomitant intra-articular pathology. Additionally, the arthroscopic approach offers a quicker rehabilitation and lower morbidity [60–63]. Moreover, the undersurface of the ECRB can be debrided without violating the common extensor aponeurosis [64].

Not unlike that for open surgery, the arthroscopic technique is also associated with good results. Baker and Baker [65] reported a satisfaction rate of 87% at an average of 130 months in 42 elbows after arthroscopic debridement. Solheim et al. [66] recently compared the outcome of patients treated with open versus arthroscopic ECRB tendon release. Both methods proved to be effective treatment options, but the arthroscopic technique provided a small, but not insignificant, improvement in outcomes, as measured by the QuickDASH score.

A recent study confirmed no difference between percutaneous, open, and arthroscopic techniques with regard to recurrence, complications, failures, or postoperative functional scores [62]. Regardless of the technique employed, successful operative treatment is contingent on proper patient selection, identification of the pathology, and comprehensive resection of the diseased tendon.

19.10 Rehabilitation

The authors immobilize the elbow in a split for 7–10 days after open surgery. This is followed by progressive range of motion exercises. A progressive strengthening program is then initiated when full and painless motion is achieved, typically at around 3 weeks. Light hitting and ground strokes can be resumed with caution at approximately 6 weeks. Rehabilitation and strengthening should continue for at least 2–3 months prior to returning to competitive play.

19.11 Medial Epicondylitis

Medial epicondylitis, or medial tennis elbow, or golfer's elbow, is an injury at the myotendinous junction at the medial elbow. While lateral epicondylitis is more common in novice tennis players, medial elbow tendinopathy is more common in elite-level players. There are three layers of tissue at the medial epicondyle. The pronator teres (PT), flexor carpi radialis (FCR), palmaris longus, and flexor carpi ulnaris (FCU) originate from the supracondylar ride and comprise the superficial layer. The flexor tendons' deeper fibers and anterior portion of the ulnar collateral ligament (UCL), which attach to the base of the medial epicondyle, comprise the middle layers. The deep layer includes the UCL and the elbow capsule, which attaches to the anterior inferior epicondyle. The interface of the pronator teres and flexor carpi radialis (FCR) is the site most commonly involved but may also include the origins of the FCU and flexor digitorum sublimis [67, 68] (Fig. 19.5).

19.12 Etiology

Medial epicondylitis may be caused by excessive wrist snap on serve and forehand strokes, in addition to open-stance hitting and short-arming strokes [69]. All of these factors result in repetitive valgus overload at the elbow. The tennis serve occurs in four stages: windup, cocking, acceleration, and follow-through. The medial elbow withstands significant stress during the cocking and acceleration phases of the serve, largely due to valgus stress, forearm pronation, and wrist flexion [68].

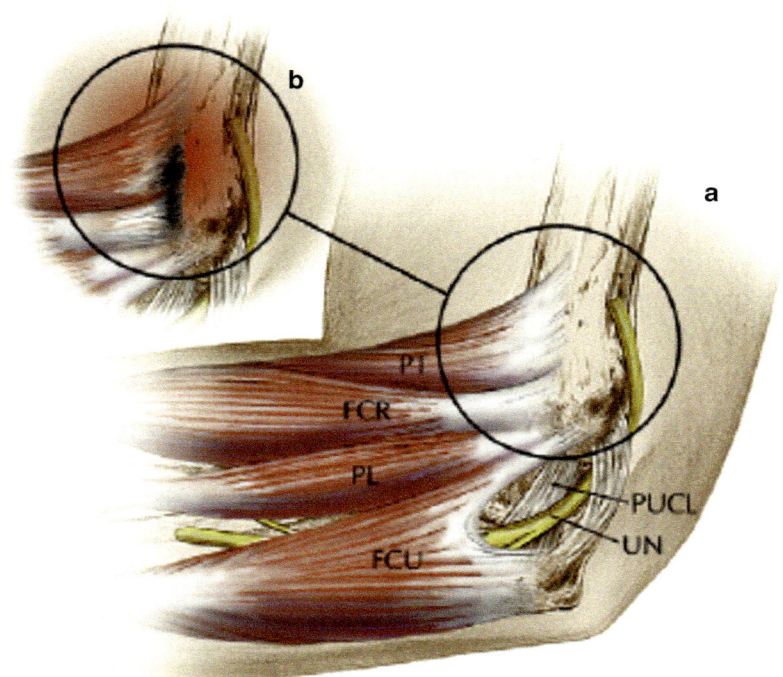

Fig. 19.5 (**a**) Normal anatomy and (**b**) the typical location of pathology at the FCR-PT origin. *PT* pronator teres, *FCR* flexor carpi radialis, *PL* palmaris longus, *FCU* flexor carpi ulnaris, *PUCL* posterior bundle of the ulnar collateral ligament, *UN* ulnar nerve. Van Hofwegen C, Baker CL, Baker CL (2010) Epicondylitis in the Athlete's Elbow. Clin Sports Med 29:577–597

Ground strokes, on the other hand, are comprised of racquet preparation, acceleration, and follow-through. The medial elbow is exposed to substantial valgus load during the acceleration phase of the forehand and is most commonly seen in players that use abundant topspin, which requires aggressive forearm pronation [68]. Unrelenting tension through the microtears in FCR and pronator teres origins results in a pathologic healing response called angiofibroblastic tendinosis, analogous to the above description of lateral elbow tendinopathy. Similar to lateral epicondylitis, medial epicondylitis consists of degenerative, fibroblastic tendinosis [10].

19.13 Presentation

Evaluation of medial-sided elbow pain in the athlete must include pathologies such as ulnar nerve entrapment, intra-articular disease, or ulnar collateral ligament injury. The diagnosis is challenging, as one pathologic entity does not preclude, but more often includes, another diagnosis. In fact, ulnar neuritis is reported to accompany medial epicondylitis in 60% of cases [70].

Pain is usually insidious in onset and without a particular inciting event. Tenderness is typically present at or just distal to the flexor-pronator common tendon attachment. Resisted wrist flexion may elicit pain. Resisted forearm pronation, though, is the most sensitive provocative test for medial tendon injury [71].

Range of motion should be scrutinized, as players with medial tennis elbow have a mild flexion contracture in 20% of cases. A loss in flexion may also be accompanied by a loss in supination [72]. Valgus laxity must be ruled out with valgus testing. Also, a thorough neurological examination should be performed to rule out ulnar nerve irritation, as it is not infrequently associated with medial elbow tendinopathy [10, 71, 72].

19.14 Imaging

Radiographs are obtained to detect associated loose bodies or calcification within the medial tendon [67, 71]. MRI typically shows a thickened common flexor tendon origin with increased signal intensity on T1- and T2-weighted images. Some patients, on the other hand, demonstrate areas of thinning in the tendon origin with intensely increased fluid signal on T2-weighted images.

19.15 Treatment

Treatment for medial epicondylitis largely mirrors that of lateral epicondylitis with a few exceptions. Nonoperative and operative treatment options are outlined below.

19.16 Nonoperative

Nonsurgical management is the mainstay of treatment and should include relative rest, ice, physiotherapy, and nonsteroidal medications or acetaminophen for pain relief. Review of stroke mechanics to minimize overload may also be helpful. Counterforce bracing is effective in some patients but should be used judiciously, as it can worsen ulnar nerve compressive neuropathy.

Local corticosteroid injection provides good results in the short-term, but there is no long-term benefit compared to conservative treatment alone. Stahl et al. [73] demonstrated that steroid injections significantly improved pain scores and symptoms at 6 weeks compared to control patients. These improvements, however, were not sustained at 3 and 12 months. Additionally, medial epicondylar injections are associated with complications, including skin atrophy, chemical neuritis [73], pigment changes, and attenuation of the UCL from direct inoculation.

Alternative methods of treatment parallel those used for lateral epicondylitis. These include ECSW therapy, laser therapy, acupuncture, botox, topical nitrates, autologous blood injection, and PRP injection [74]. Well-designed studies on these alternative treatments are lacking. All local treatments of medial epicondylitis must consider with caution the proximity of the ulnar nerve. Injuries to the ulnar and medial antebrachial cutaneous nerves have been reported [73, 75].

19.17 Operative

Surgery is reserved for those with persistent pain and disability despite at least 6 months of nonoperative management [67, 72]. Similar to the operative treatment of lateral epicondylitis, the goal of surgery is to remove the degenerative, diseased tendon and to subsequently repair the remaining tendon. The tendinosis is often found deep to and in the interval between the pronator teres and flexor carpi radialis.

There are few published reports describing the operative management of medial epicondylitis. These include percutaneous epicondylar muscle release [58], open detachment of the flexor muscle origin without debridement [72], open detachment of the flexor origin with debridement and repair [67, 76], open medial epicondylectomy, and open resection of the pathologic tissue [77]. We would caution, specifically, against the use of medial epicondylectomy in tennis players.

The author's preferred technique is similar to that described by Ollivierre et al. [77]. It is crucial to reevaluate for ulnar nerve symptoms prior to surgical intervention. Depending on the severity of the neurological symptoms, an ulnar nerve decompression alone or decompression and transposition may be performed. A 6-cm longitudinal incision is made centered over the medial epicondyle. The incision is extended if ulnar nerve decompression is required. Special care must be taken to protect the posterior branch of the medial antebrachial cutaneous nerve, which lies just anterior to the medial epicondyle. The common flexor tendon is exposed. Either a longitudinal split is made in the tendon or the pronator teres/FCR interval is used. The diseased tendinotic tissue is often readily exposed as the dissection is deepened. An elliptical resection of the dull, gray pathologic tissue is performed. Ollivierre et al. [77] describe the scratch test to help identify abnormal tissue. Once all diseased tissue has been excised, the underlying bone is gently debrided and prepared to stimulate healing at the bony bed of the tendon footprint for later repair. Then, one or two double-loaded SuperQuick G2 anchors (DePuy Mitek; Raynham, Massachusetts) are used at the site of the medial epicondyle. The number of anchors needed is determined by the size of the medial epicondyle. Sutures are then passed through the remaining tendon in a horizontal mattress configuration to advance healthy tendon back down to its footprint. Closure is then completed in a layered fashion. Lastly, the patient is placed in a compressive dressing and posterior splint at 90° of flexion.

Patients with symptoms refractory to nonoperative management that ultimately require surgery will likely experience improvement in pain but may not return to their pre-injury sporting activities. Ollivierre et al. [77] reported on 50 patients treated with surgery. All patients described partial or complete pain relief, but notably, 26% were unable to return to their previous level of sporting activity. Four of six professional athletes were able to return to their pre-injury level following surgery. Grawe et al. [78] reported that 24 of 28 patients returned to their premorbid sporting activities at a median of 4.5 months.

Vangsness et al. [67] describe a more extensive medial flexor tendon detachment, debridement, and reattachment with suture through bone tunnels. These authors reported 97% good to excellent results with 98% relief of pain. Thirteen of the athletically-inclined patients were college or professional level. Nineteen of these 20 athletes returned to their pre-injury level.

Cases in which ulnar neuritis accompanies medial epicondylitis have a less favorable outcome compared to those with isolated medial epicondylitis. Kurvers et al. [72] reported on concomitant ulnar nerve symptoms in 24 of 38 elbows. Subjective outcome scores were significantly lower in the group with preoperative ulnar neuritis. In this cohort, three of 24 patients with ulnar neuritis were symptom free at final follow-up, compared with 11 of 16 with isolated medial epicondylitis. This observation has been reported in other studies [71, 79, 80].

While it was proven safe in a cadaver study [81], elbow arthroscopy is rarely used in the treatment of medial epicondylitis.

19.18 Rehabilitation

The splint is removed within 7–10 days. A supervised rehabilitation program is started at the first postoperative visit, and the patient is transitioned to a low-profile hinged elbow brace to protect the healing tendon for 6–8 weeks. Early rehabilitation focuses on elbow and wrist range of motion, while passive wrist extension and active wrist flexion are limited. At 4–6 weeks, a tennis elbow rehabilitation program should begin with a focus on return to full strength and activity by approximately 3 months. Return to full-level function usually requires 6 months.

19.19 Indications for Elbow Arthroscopy

As mentioned above, elbow arthroscopy offers several purported advantages in the treatment of lateral epicondylitis. These cited advantages include the ability to debride the ECRB undersurface without violating the common extensor tendon, the ability to evaluate for intra-articular pathology, and a potentially shortened rehabilitation [64, 65]. Previous studies suggest that 18–58% of patients undergoing elbow arthroscopy for lateral epicondylitis had concomitant intra-articular pathology, usually synovitis [62, 65, 82, 83]. It is unclear, however, what criteria are used to make this diagnosis and how treatment of it influences outcomes.

Patient complaints of mechanical symptoms may warrant elbow arthroscopy. Loose bodies have been noted to be present in 3–5% of elbow arthroscopies performed for lateral epicondylitis [62, 83]. In the authors' experience, though, the incidental discovery of symptomatic concomitant intra-articular pathology is rare. Moreover, despite generally positive outcomes, the learning curve, along with the risks of neurovascular injury or inadvertent release of the lateral ulnar collateral ligament, is not insignificant [64, 84].

Hyperextension overload, which is not uncommon in elite tennis players, generates excessive forces in the posterior aspect of the elbow joint [85], resulting in chondromalacia and spurring on the posterior trochlea and olecranon. As the disease progresses, players have limited extension and describe pain during the follow-through phase of serving. Additional symptoms include crepitus and locking. Posterior impingement is readily treated arthroscopically, and, as such, a tennis player with concomitant lateral epicondylitis and posterior impingement may be best treated with elbow arthroscopy.

In the authors' experience, isolated lateral or medial epicondylitis is best treated with an open technique, as it has proven to be reliable, operator-independent, and safe.

19.20 Summary

Humeral epicondylitis in the athlete is caused a pathologic healing response to repetitive eccentric contraction of the extensor and flexor muscles at their origins on the elbow. Rather than an inflammatory condition, humeral epicondylitis is an extra-articular tendon injury characterized by proliferative vascular granulation, called angiofibroblastic hyperplasia. Lateral epicondylitis is more common in novice tennis players, while medial epicondylitis is more common in elite-level players.

Lateral epicondylitis involves the base of the ECRB and usually exists in isolation. Medial epicondylitis is encountered at the base of FCR and pronator teres origins. Medial tennis elbow must be distinguished from other causes of medial elbow pain, such as ulnar collateral ligament instability or ulnar neuritis.

Nonoperative management, which includes rest, ice, oral anti-inflammatories, bracing, physical therapy, and injections is the mainstay of treatment. In recalcitrant cases, surgery is recommended. Lateral epicondylitis is treated with both open and arthroscopic techniques. Medial epicondylitis is more frequently treated with open surgery, given the proximity of the ulnar nerve and ulnar collateral ligament. Irrespective of the technique, pain relief is fairly predictable, whereas return to sport with complete resolution of symptoms is less reliable.

The authors prefer an open technique for humeral epicondylitis, but note that elbow arthroscopy is indicated when concomitant intra-articular pathology is suspected.

References

1. Adelsberg S. The tennis stroke: an EMG analysis of selected muscles with rackets of increasing grip size. Am J Sports Med. 1986;14:139–42.
2. Groppel JL, Nirschl RP. A mechanical and electromyographical analysis of the effects of various joint counterforce braces on the tennis player. Am J Sports Med. 1986;14:195–200.
3. Cabrera JM, McCue FC. Nonosseous athletic injuries of the elbow, forearm, and hand. Clin Sports Med. 1986;5:681–700.
4. Giangarra CE, Conroy B, Jobe FW, et al. Electromyographic and cinematographic analysis of elbow function in tennis players using single- and double-handed backhand strokes. Am J Sports Med. 1993;21:394–9.
5. Gruchow HW, Pelletier D. An epidemiologic study of tennis elbow. Incidence, recurrence, and effectiveness of prevention strategies. Am J Sports Med. 1979;7:234–8.
6. Nirschl RP, Ashman ES. Elbow tendinopathy: tennis elbow. Clin Sports Med. 2003;22:813–36.
7. Blackwell JR, Cole KJ. Wrist kinematics differ in expert and novice tennis players performing the backhand stroke: implications for tennis elbow. J Biomech. 1994;27:509–16.
8. Dines JS, Bedi A, Williams PN, et al. Tennis injuries: epidemiology, pathophysiology, and treatment. J Am Acad Orthop Surg. 2015;23:181–9. https://doi.org/10.5435/jaaos-d-13-00148.
9. Riek S, Chapman AE, Milner T. A simulation of muscle force and internal kinematics of extensor carpi radialis brevis during backhand tennis stroke: implications for injury. Clin Biomech. 1999;14:477–83. https://doi.org/10.1016/S0268-0033(98)90097-3.
10. Nirschl RP. Elbow tendinosis/tennis elbow. Clin Sports Med. 1992;11:851–70.
11. Kraushaar BS, Nirschl RP. Tendinosis of the elbow (tennis elbow). Clinical features and findings of histological, immunohistochemical, and electron microscopy studies. J Bone Joint Surg Am. 1999;81:259–78.

12. Sharma P, Maffulli N. Tendon injury and tendinopathy: healing and repair. J Bone Joint Surg. 2005;87:187–202. https://doi.org/10.2106/JBJS.D.01850.
13. Waugh EJ. Lateral epicondylalgia or epicondylitis: what's in a name? J Orthop Sports Phys Ther. 2005;35:200–2. https://doi.org/10.2519/jospt.2005.0104.
14. Ahmad Z, Siddiqui N, Malik SS, et al. Lateral epicondylitis: a review of pathology and management. Bone Joint J. 2013;95(B):1158–64. https://doi.org/10.1302/0301-620X.95B9.
15. Coombes BK, Bisset L, Vicenzino B. A new integrative model of lateral epicondylalgia. Br J Sports Med. 2009;43:252–8. https://doi.org/10.1136/bjsm.2008.052738.
16. Perry J. Anatomy and biomechanics of the shoulder in throwing, swimming, gymnastics, and tennis. Clin Sports Med. 1983;2:247–70.
17. Morris M, Jobe FW, Perry J, et al. Electromyographic analysis of elbow function in tennis players. Am J Sports Med. 1989;17:241–7. https://doi.org/10.1177/036354658901700215.
18. Ryu RK, McCormick J, Jobe FW, et al. An electromyographic analysis of shoulder function in tennis players. Am J Sports Med. 1988;16:481–5. https://doi.org/10.1177/036354658801600509.
19. Kibler WB. Clinical biomechanics of the elbow in tennis: implications for evaluation and diagnosis. Med Sci Sports Exerc. 1994;26:1203–6.
20. Hatch GF, Pink MM, Mohr KJ, et al. The effect of tennis racket grip size on forearm muscle firing patterns. Am J Sports Med. 2006;34:1977–83. https://doi.org/10.1177/0363546506290185.
21. Smidt N, van der Windt DA. Tennis elbow in primary care. BMJ. 2006;333:927–8. https://doi.org/10.1136/bmj.39017.396389.BE.
22. Marx RG, Sperling JW, Cordasco FA. Overuse injuries of the upper extremity in tennis players. Clin Sports Med. 2001;20:439–51.
23. Van Hofwegen C, Baker CL, Baker CL. Epicondylitis in the Athlete's Elbow. Clin Sports Med. 2010;29:577–97. https://doi.org/10.1016/j.csm.2010.06.009.
24. Gardner RC. Tennis elbow: diagnosis, pathology and treatment. Nine severe cases treated by a new reconstructive operation. Clin Orthop Relat Res. 1970;72:248–53.
25. du Toit C, Stieler M, Saunders R, et al. Diagnostic accuracy of power Doppler ultrasound in patients with chronic tennis elbow. Br J Sports Med. 2008;42:572–6. https://doi.org/10.1136/bjsm.2007.043901.
26. Miller TT, Shapiro MA, Schultz E, Kalish PE. Comparison of sonography and MRI for diagnosing epicondylitis. J Clin Ultrasound. 2002;30:193–202. https://doi.org/10.1002/jcu.10063.
27. Tuite MJ, Kijowski R. Sports-related injuries of the elbow: an approach to MRI interpretation. Clin Sports Med. 2006;25:387–408. https://doi.org/10.1016/j.csm.2006.02.002.
28. Coel M, Yamada CY, Ko J. MR imaging of patients with lateral epicondylitis of the elbow (tennis elbow): importance of increased signal of the anconeus muscle. Am J Roentgenol. 1993;161:1019–21. https://doi.org/10.2214/ajr.161.5.8273602.
29. Savnik A, Jensen B, Nørregaard J, et al. Magnetic resonance imaging in the evaluation of treatment response of lateral epicondylitis of the elbow. Eur Radiol. 2004;14:964–9. https://doi.org/10.1007/s00330-003-2165-4.
30. Eygendaal D, Rahussen FTG, Diercks RL. Biomechanics of the elbow joint in tennis players and relation to pathology. Br J Sports Med. 2007;41:820–3. https://doi.org/10.1136/bjsm.2007.038307.
31. Bisset L, Beller E, Jull G, et al. Mobilisation with movement and exercise, corticosteroid injection, or wait and see for tennis elbow: randomised trial. BMJ. 2006;333:939–0. https://doi.org/10.1136/bmj.38961.584653.AE.
32. Bisset L, Paungmali A, Vicenzino B, Beller E. A systematic review and meta-analysis of clinical trials on physical interventions for lateral epicondylalgia. Br J Sports Med. 2005;39:411–22. https://doi.org/10.1136/bjsm.2004.016170.
33. Buchbinder R, Green SE, Youd JM, et al. Systematic review of the efficacy and safety of shock wave therapy for lateral elbow pain. J Rheumatol. 2006;33:1351–63.
34. Stasinopoulos D, Stasinopoulos I. Comparison of effects of exercise programme, pulsed ultrasound and transverse friction in the treatment of chronic patellar tendinopathy. Clin Rehabil. 2004;18:347–52.
35. Decker MJ, Hintermeister RA, Faber KJ, Hawkins RJ. Serratus anterior muscle activity during selected rehabilitation exercises. Am J Sports Med. 1999;27:784–91.
36. Kibler WB, Sciascia AD, Uhl TL, et al. Electromyographic analysis of specific exercises for scapular control in early phases of shoulder rehabilitation. Am J Sports Med. 2008;36:1789–98. https://doi.org/10.1177/0363546508316281.
37. Jafarian FS, Demneh ES, Tyson SF. The immediate effect of orthotic management on grip strength of patients with lateral epicondylosis. J Orthop Sport Phys Ther. 2009;39:484–9. https://doi.org/10.2519/jospt.2009.2988.
38. Garg R, Adamson GJ, Dawson PA, et al. A prospective randomized study comparing a forearm strap brace versus a wrist splint for the treatment of lateral epicondylitis. J Shoulder Elbow Surg. 2010;19:508–12. https://doi.org/10.1016/j.jse.2009.12.015.
39. Wolf JM, Ozer K, Scott F, et al. Comparison of autologous blood, corticosteroid, and saline injection in the treatment of lateral epicondylitis: a prospective, randomized, controlled multicenter study. J Hand Surg Am. 2011;36:1269–72. https://doi.org/10.1016/j.jhsa.2011.05.014.
40. Bjordal JM, Lopes-Martins RA, Joensen J, et al. A systematic review with procedural assessments and meta-analysis of Low Level Laser Therapy in lateral elbow tendinopathy (tennis elbow). BMC

41. Trinh KV. Acupuncture for the alleviation of lateral epicondyle pain: a systematic review. Rheumatology. 2004;43:1085–90. https://doi.org/10.1093/rheumatology/keh247.
42. Wong SM, Hui ACF, Tong P-Y, et al. Treatment of lateral epicondylitis with botulinum toxin: a randomized, double-blind, placebo-controlled trial. Ann Intern Med. 2005;143:793–7.
43. Hayton MJ, Santini AJA, Hughes PJ, et al. Botulinum toxin injection in the treatment of tennis elbowa double-blind, randomized, controlled, pilot study. J Bone Joint Surg. 2005;87:503. https://doi.org/10.2106/JBJS.D.01896.
44. Paoloni JA, Appleyard RC, Nelson J, GAC M. Topical nitric oxide application in the treatment of chronic extensor tendinosis at the elbow: a randomized, double-blinded, placebo-controlled clinical trial. Am J Sports Med. 2003;31:915–20.
45. Edwards SG, Calandruccio JH. Autologous blood injections for refractory lateral epicondylitis. J Hand Surg [Am]. 2003;28:272–8. https://doi.org/10.1053/jhsu.2003.50041.
46. Creaney L, Wallace A, Curtis M, Connell D. Growth factor-based therapies provide additional benefit beyond physical therapy in resistant elbow tendinopathy: a prospective, single-blind, randomised trial of autologous blood injections versus platelet-rich plasma injections. Br J Sports Med. 2011;45:966–71. https://doi.org/10.1136/bjsm.2010.082503.
47. Kazemi M, Azma K, Tavana B, et al. Autologous blood versus corticosteroid local injection in the short-term treatment of lateral elbow tendinopathy. Am J Phys Med Rehabil. 2010;89:660–7. https://doi.org/10.1097/PHM.0b013e3181ddcb31.
48. Mishra A, Collado H, Fredericson M. Platelet-rich plasma compared with corticosteroid injection for chronic lateral elbow tendinosis. PM R. 2009;1:366–70. https://doi.org/10.1016/j.pmrj.2009.02.010.
49. Mishra A, Pavelko T. Treatment of chronic elbow tendinosis with buffered platelet-rich plasma. Am J Sports Med. 2006;34:1774–8. https://doi.org/10.1177/0363546506288850.
50. Rodik T, McDermott B. Platelet-rich plasma compared with other common injection therapies in the treatment of chronic lateral epicondylitis. J Sport Rehabil. 2016;25:77–82. https://doi.org/10.1123/jsr.2014-0198.
51. Nichols AW. Two-year follow-up of injection with platelet-rich plasma versus corticosteroid for lateral epicondylitis. Clin J Sport Med. 2012;22:451–2. https://doi.org/10.1097/JSM.0b013e31826a091f.
52. Palacio EP, Schiavetti RR, Kanematsu M, et al. Effects of platelet-rich plasma on lateral epicondylitis of the elbow: prospective randomized controlled trial. Rev Bras Ortop. 2016;51:90–5. https://doi.org/10.1016/j.rboe.2015.03.014.
53. Nirschl RP, Pettrone FA. Tennis elbow. The surgical treatment of lateral epicondylitis. J Bone Joint Surg Am. 1979;61:832–9.
54. Spencer GE, Herndon CH. Surgical treatment of epicondylitis. J Bone Joint Surg Am. 1953;35A:421–4.
55. Calvert PT, Allum RL, Macpherson IS, Bentley G. Simple lateral release in treatment of tennis elbow. J R Soc Med. 1985;78:912–5.
56. Verhaar J, Walenkamp G, Kester A, et al. Lateral extensor release for tennis elbow. A prospective long-term follow-up study. J Bone Joint Surg Am. 1993;75:1034–43.
57. Kumar VS, Shetty AA, Ravikumar KJ, Fordyce MJ. Tennis elbow--outcome following the Garden procedure: a retrospective study. J Orthop Surg (Hong Kong). 2004;12:226–9.
58. Baumgard SH, Schwartz DR. Percutaneous release of the epicondylar muscles for humeral epicondylitis. Am J Sports Med. 1982;10:233–6.
59. Thornton SJ. Treatment of recalcitrant lateral epicondylitis with suture anchor repair. Am J Sports Med. 2005;33:1558–64. https://doi.org/10.1177/0363546505276758.
60. Owens BD, Murphy KP, Kuklo TR. Arthroscopic release for lateral epicondylitis. Arthroscopy. 2001;17:582–7. https://doi.org/10.1053/jars.2001.20098.
61. Peart RE, Strickler SS, Schweitzer KM. Lateral epicondylitis: a comparative study of open and arthroscopic lateral release. Am J Orthop (Belle Mead NJ). 2004;33:565–7.
62. Szabo SJ, Savoie FH, Field LD, et al. Tendinosis of the extensor carpi radialis brevis: an evaluation of three methods of operative treatment. J Shoulder Elbow Surg. 2006;15:721–7. https://doi.org/10.1016/j.jse.2006.01.017.
63. Yeoh KM, King GJW, Faber KJ, et al. Evidence-based indications for elbow arthroscopy. Arthrosc J Arthrosc Relat Surg. 2012;28:272–82. https://doi.org/10.1016/j.arthro.2011.10.007.
64. Kuklo TR, Taylor KF, Murphy KP, et al. Arthroscopic release for lateral epicondylitis: a cadaveric model. Arthroscopy. 1999;15:259–64.
65. Baker CL, Baker CL. Long-term follow-up of arthroscopic treatment of lateral epicondylitis. Am J Sports Med. 2008;36:254–60. https://doi.org/10.1177/0363546507311599.
66. Solheim E, Hegna J, Øyen J. Arthroscopic versus open tennis elbow release: 3- to 6-year results of a case-control series of 305 elbows. Arthrosc J Arthrosc Relat Surg. 2013;29:854–9. https://doi.org/10.1016/j.arthro.2012.12.012.
67. Vangsness CT, Jobe FW. Surgical treatment of medial epicondylitis. Results in 35 elbows. J Bone Joint Surg Br. 1991;73:409–11.
68. Field LD, Altchek DW. Elbow injuries. Clin Sports Med. 1995;14:59–78.
69. Elliott B, Fleisig G, Nicholls R, Escamilia R. Technique effects on upper limb loading in the ten-

nis serve. J Sci Med Sport. 2003;6:76–87. https://doi.org/10.1016/S1440-2440(03)80011-7.
70. Field LD, Savoie FH. Common elbow injuries in sport. Sports Med. 1998;26:193–205.
71. Gabel GT, Morrey BF. Operative treatment of medical epicondylitis. Influence of concomitant ulnar neuropathy at the elbow. J Bone Joint Surg Am. 1995;77:1065–9.
72. Kurvers H, Verhaar J. The results of operative treatment of medial epicondylitis. J Bone Joint Surg Am. 1995;77(9):1374.
73. Stahl S, Kaufman T. The efficacy of an injection of steroids for medial epicondylitis. A prospective study of sixty elbows. J Bone Joint Surg Am. 1997;79:1648–52.
74. Hechtman KS, Uribe JW, Botto-vanDemden A, Kiebzak GM. Platelet-rich plasma injection reduces pain in patients with recalcitrant epicondylitis. Orthopedics. 2011;34:92. https://doi.org/10.3928/01477447-20101221-05.
75. Richards RR, Regan WD. Medial epicondylitis caused by injury to the medial antebrachial cutaneous nerve: a case report. Can J Surg. 1989;32:366–7. 369.
76. Jobe C. Lateral and medial epicondylitis of the elbow. J Am Acad Orthop Surg. 1994;2:1–8.
77. Ollivierre CO, Nirschl RP, Pettrone FA. Resection and repair for medial tennis elbow. A prospective analysis. Am J Sports Med. 1995;23:214–21.
78. Grawe BM, FaBricant PD, Christopher C, et al. Clinical outcomes after suture anchor repair of recalcitrant medial epicondylitis. Orthopedics. 2016;39:e104. https://doi.org/10.3928/01477447-20151222-09.
79. Chen FS, Rokito AS, Jobe FW. Medial elbow problems in the overhead-throwing athlete. J Am Acad Orthop Surg. 2001;9:99–113.
80. Grana W. Medial epicondylitis and cubital tunnel syndrome in the throwing athlete. Clin Sports Med. 2001;20:541–8.
81. Zonno A, Manuel J, Merrell G, et al. Arthroscopic technique for medial epicondylitis: technique and safety analysis. Arthroscopy. 2010;26:610–6. https://doi.org/10.1016/j.arthro.2009.09.017.
82. Grewal R, MacDermid JC, Shah P, King GJW. Functional outcome of arthroscopic extensor carpi radialis brevis tendon release in chronic lateral epicondylitis. J Hand Surg [Am]. 2009;34:849–57. https://doi.org/10.1016/j.jhsa.2009.02.006.
83. Lattermann C, Romeo AA, Anbari A, et al. Arthroscopic debridement of the extensor carpi radialis brevis for recalcitrant lateral epicondylitis. J Shoulder Elbow Surg. 2010;19:651–6. https://doi.org/10.1016/j.jse.2010.02.008.
84. Smith AM, Castle JA, Ruch DS. Arthroscopic resection of the common extensor origin: anatomic considerations. J Shoulder Elbow Surg. 2003;12:375–9. https://doi.org/10.1016/mse.2003.S1058274602868239.
85. Moskal MJ, Savoie FH, Field LD. Arthroscopic treatment of posterior elbow impingement. Instr Course Lect. 1999;48:399–404.

Minimally Invasive Treatment of Wrist and Hand Lesions in Tennis Players

20

Alejandro Badia

20.1 Introduction

Hand and wrist injuries are exceedingly common in tennis players because the tennis racket serves as a conduit for force transmission to the entire upper limb and ultimately the entire body. The hand/wrist unit absorbs that blow initially and can suffer acute (suprathreshold) injury or overuse issues due to cumulative trauma over time during this intense sport. Currently, more of these injuries are being seen due to the increasingly powerful nature of the elite game, and also due to the aging population which continues to engage, fortunately, in intense sport during later decades. A clear diagnosis, often requiring a subspecialist, is necessary in order to keep the player active, even competing, often via minimally invasive treatments and procedures. This chapter will focus on minimally invasive treatments, often arthroscopic, for both acute and chronic injury to the hand and wrist.

20.2 Anatomic Basis

The hand and wrist are comprised of 27 carpal bones, metacarpals, and phalanges, all connected to the upper limb via the radius and ulna, now considered the "forearm joint" given the wrist interplay with the elbow during pronosupination, naturally a critical function in the game of tennis. While forearm and elbow issues are ubiquitous, it is the hand/wrist that often suffers the first manifestation of injury and overuse syndromes.

It is important to keep in mind that the hand/wrist unit is largely a skeletal/tendinous conduit of this force transmission during racket impact, since the major muscles reside in the forearm (flexor and extensor surfaces) and mostly originating at the elbow level. The intrinsic muscles within the hand contribute a great deal to grip; however, these are actually much more important for dexterity and fine manipulation, key factors in sports outside of tennis. The grip and swing of the racket are much more extrinsic muscle/tendon dependant. Consequently, soft tissue injury of the hand and wrist is common due to this force transfer including ligamentous or tendon failure.

Tennis is also a unique sport enjoyed and played by athletes of virtually all ages. There are few sports that can count on participants from ages 3 to 93. This implies that injuries to the hand/wrist can have various manifestations within these age groups. Children can suffer from occult growth plate issues, while older players will have to deal with degenerative conditions, often apart from the activity itself. These are very different injuries than those sustained by elite players in their teens, third and fourth decade players. It is these latter lesions that we will focus our attention on.

A. Badia
Badia Hand to Shoulder Center, OrthoNOW®
Orthopedic Urgent Care Centers, Miami, FL, USA
e-mail: alejandro@drbadia.com

20.3 Hand Lesions

Injuries to the hand most typically occur during a fall on the court. Otherwise, the dominant hand might suffer from excessive grip, usually due to poor forearm strength, and the non-dominant hand rarely suffers.

Overuse injuries can result from heavy grip activity but not typically in the younger, elite athlete. Older athletes may suffer exacerbations of such common entities as flexor tenosynovitis, carpal tunnel syndrome, and focal joint pains often related to osteoarthritis, such as of the basal joint of the thumb. However, these common entities among the general population are well beyond the scope of this chapter.

A brief discussion of digit injuries is warranted since they may occur in non-tennis related activities, having a profound effect on players racket grip, and they occasionally occur in falls on the court.

Digit trauma can be divided into fractures and the more ubiquitous soft tissue injuries such as sprains, avulsions, and strains.

20.4 Fractures of the Digits

Fractures of the phalanges and metacarpals occasionally occur on tennis-related falls but also commonly during other sports or daily activity. However, appropriate treatment is critical, since the tennis grip requires strong/painless prehension [1].

Distal phalanx fractures may occur during a direct impact to the fingertip or an axial-directed force to the finger in a fall or even being struck by the ball. Most are minimally or non-displaced, and my preferred treatment is a directly applied finger cast since this is custom made and much better tolerated than the custom or off-the-shelf splints that are made of thermoplast (Fig. 20.1). A well-applied cast can often allow the player to even continue training while the fracture heals. Postfracture rehab is minimal and the patient recovers DIP (distal interphalangeal) flexion fairly quickly.

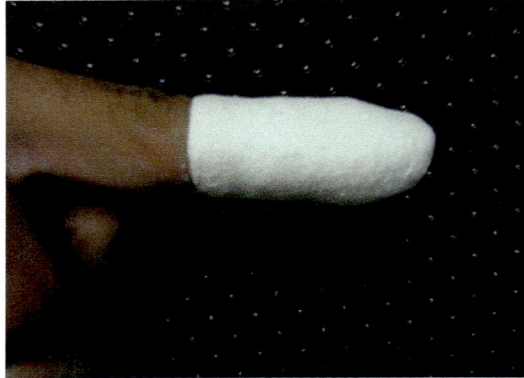

Fig. 20.1 Plaster of Paris can be directly applied to a digit fracture at either the DIP or PIP interval and can be custom molded and well tolerated by the skin

Fractures of the middle or proximal phalanges are much more troubling since these can affect the critical PIP (proximal interphalangeal) joint, critical to grip and racket control. Non-displaced fractures near the PIP joint may be amenable to PIP casting, much like the DIP, but it must be in full extension to avoid contracture. The displaced fractures are much more challenging since they can lead to malunion or nonunion, and this will greatly affect tennis play.

Fractures of the proximal phalanx condyles require open reduction/internal fixation (ORIF) if at all displaced. Even a minimal step-off can lead to chondral erosion and post-traumatic arthrosis that can end a tennis player's career, particularly if in the dominant hand. The key is to avoid this via anatomic reduction via either pins or rigid screw fixation. The latter is preferred since it allows early motion to be instituted but requires exacting technique best done via nearly percutaneous approaches. Less common articular fractures combined with neck/diaphysis fractures usually need plate fixation. The current armamentarium of rigid but low-profile titanium plates can lead to excellent result in combination of precise technique and early, aggressive hand therapy.

Comminuted (fragmented) fractures at the PIP joint, usually of the base of the middle phalanx, are often not amenable to open reduction since the fragments are too small to allow fixation, and the technique itself of fully exposing the joint can be detrimental to joint function in and of itself. The principle of ligamentotaxis, where traction on the joint helps align the fragments, is critical here and has been used in other joints. However, early motion is particularly important in the sensitive PIP joint, and dynamic external fixation with a precisely constructed frame has proven to be very effective even in the most severe of fracture-dislocations [2]. This assumes timely intervention, usually no later than 2 weeks after injury so that the articular surface can be reconstituted.

Delayed presentation, as often when patients present to "general urgent care centers" or even the hospital ER, can be disastrous. The process of the patient finding the "right surgeon" is particularly critical here since many of these patients and their families are simply told the athlete has a "jammed finger." The consequent delay in definitive care then leads to early malunion and treatment options are limited. In the athlete there is little choice at this point and a joint reconstruction must be performed, and this is currently best done using the hemi-hamate arthroplasty (HHA) technique [3]. The still novel method requires the use of taking the dorsal/distal articular surface of the hamate (at CMC joint) and transposing this to the substantial defect at the middle phalanx base after the malunion is resected. It is a very exact and somewhat unpredictable surgery which is why early recognition and appropriate treatment of PIP articular fractures are needed. The coach/trainer must seek out care of the hand surgeon with any so-called "jammed finger" injuries.

Shaft fractures, of both middle and proximal phalanx, are often non- or minimally displaced and require 3–4 weeks of immobilization, usually in an MCP (knuckle) block cast. This "functional position" of the hand is where the MCP joints are flexed to near 90°, and the interphalangeal joints are held in extension or allowed early mobilization [4]. This position is called the intrinsic plus position and is critical to allow early restoration of hand function and subsequent tennis grip. Complications arising from not following this protocol are actually quite common, and a typical scenario is the hand being immobilized with all digits completely straight, ala "karate chop" positioning, and this can be disastrous for hand function often requiring surgical care via joint capsulectomies. It is easy to avoid with simple awareness and some attention to detail.

Shaft fractures that are displaced, often angulated or rotational, do require ORIF and can often be done with percutaneous pins or minimally invasive screw fixation. Plates can usually be avoided as they often lead to stiffness and may require removal, extensor tenolysis, and other subsequent procedures. Early rehabilitation is key to have the player minimize time away from the court.

Metacarpal fractures are more common and a significant degree of displacement can often be accepted in the non-athlete. However, angulated fractures can be easily corrected with a more recently described technique of intramedullary flexible rod fixation (Fig. 20.2). This allows for anatomic restoration and rapid healing also within an MCP block cast to protect this nonrigid but minimally invasive method [5]. Weekend "boxing fractures" often occur when the player strikes a wall or gets in an altercation although these fractures can occur when the hand strikes the court, particularly if holding the racket.

20.5 Soft Tissue Injuries of the Hand

While fractures in the hand are relatively common and often fairly benign, it is the ubiquitous soft tissue injuries that can keep a player out of play for an extended period of time, particularly if in the dominant hand. A major issue remains the inexact diagnosis and consequently ill-defined treatment plan that results from many of these injuries. A perfect example is the term "jammed finger" often assigned to digit injuries that may actually represent a wide range of clinical diagnoses, some of them potentially devastating. While a typical playground term, it should be stricken from clinical lexicon as it provides no specificity as to the actual lesion sustained.

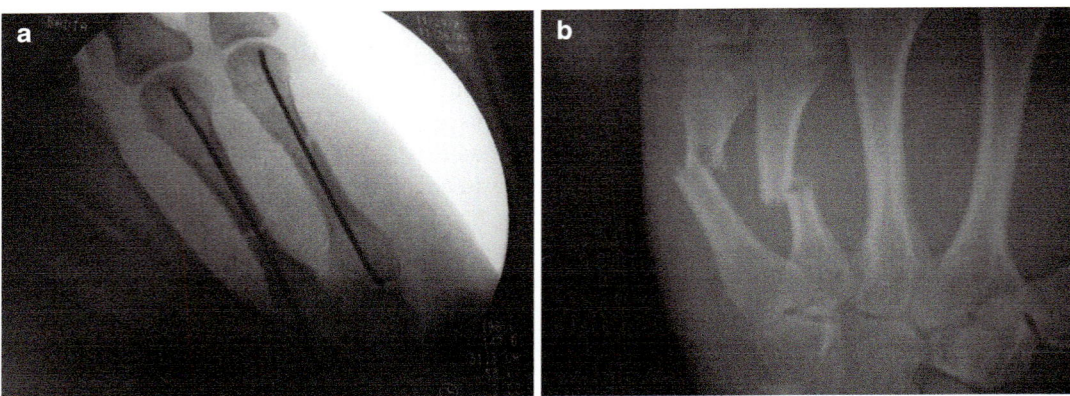

Fig. 20.2 Intramedullary rod fixation for metacarpal shaft and neck fractures allows near anatomic reduction while minimizing compromise to blood supply or excessive scarring due to minimally invasive nature

The so-called "jammed finger" injury must be fully analyzed to elicit an accurate diagnosis and give it the attention it deserves. The most common injury is a sprain of the PIP collateral ligaments and likely represents the classic "jammed finger" presentation. The joint is swollen, stiff, and usually tender over one collateral ligament more than the opposite, either radial or ulnar. Severe injuries require X-ray and only days of immobilization and ice. A stable joint, best deemed fluoroscopically, warrants early mobilization, either by the patient actively flexing/extending or a buddy splint to adjacent non-injured digit that can hasten recovery. Much like ankle sprains, most PIP sprains need early movement but light usage.

Severe proximal interphalangeal (PIP) joint injuries can include a central slip avulsion which can then become a boutonniere, which is where the joint loses extension and can lead to subsequent hyperextension of the more distal joint. The biomechanics of this are beyond the scope of this chapter, but important to institute immediate immobilization of the PIP joint alone, in full extension, and have assessment by the hand surgeon. When deemed to be a partial tear, or without retraction, a PIP plaster finger cast can be applied for 3–4 weeks, encouraging early DIP motion so that the lateral bands remain mobile. In severe cases, early reattachment of the central slip extensor mechanism is a simple procedure that can avoid serious long-term sequelae to the hand if not addressed in a timely and appropriate fashion.

DIP soft tissue injuries can also include collateral ligament sprains but are less common. At this location, mallet finger injuries often occur with an axial impact to the finger, usually being struck by the ball or the fingertip hitting the ground. This is where the terminal extensor tendon is ruptured off its insertion on the distal phalanx base. Soft tissue mallet injuries require 6–8 weeks of continuous immobilization in full extension with no interruption. Most surgeons/therapists will use a stack splint, a thermoplast off-the-shelf, or custom-made, device that holds the finger in extension. However, the plastic is poorly tolerated by the skin for that period of time, and I greatly prefer a custom-made finger cast, as described, where the skin tolerates this very well and is fashioned to the circumferential anatomy of the digit. Early PIP range of motion should be allowed and encouraged.

Bony mallet finger injuries often require repair, and a multitude of techniques are available although a minimally invasive option is best in order to not disrupt the blood supply to the small fragment. I have described a simple technique with two small pins that allow for anatomic reduction with well-documented good results (Fig. 20.3) [6].

Tendon avulsions of the flexor can also occur at the distal level and should not be missed. The "jersey finger" is aptly named because they com-

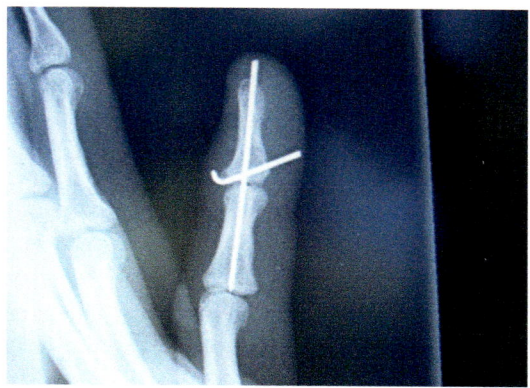

Fig. 20.3 Radiograph demonstrating placement of longitudinal extension k-wire and joystick avulsed fragment pin to allow percutaneous anatomic reduction of troublesome bony mallet finger injury

monly occur in sports where tackling is performed, like rugby or American football. The inability to actively flex the DIP joint, often in the ring finger, requires immediate referral to the hand surgeon for reattachment.

Soft tissue injuries at the metacarpophalangeal joint are relatively uncommon, but a hyperextension injury can cause rupture to the volar plate on the palmar side. More common are injuries to the extensor hood or even the collateral ligaments. Acute rupture of the sagittal band on either side of the extensor can lead to a painful swollen knuckle and causes painful and/or weak extension of the finger. A forceful backhand can cause this injury leading to the extensor tendon deviating from the midline. A true rupture, best diagnosed by ultrasound exam at time of consultation, will need repair much like a classic "boxer's knuckle" lesion [7]. Immobilization for 4 weeks with the MCP joints in extension is necessary but encouraging early active motion of the IP joints. Similarly, a collateral ligament injury at this location can also lead to a swollen, painful knuckle, but open repair is not warranted and can actually be detrimental due to scarring in the athlete's hand. Arthroscopic debridement, perhaps coupled with radiofrequency shrinkage, has led to painless recovery in more chronic cases and certain severe, acute lesions, as long as the hand is then immobilized in MCP block flexion, contrary to a boxer's knuckle lesion.

Arthroscopy of these small joints is still a vastly underutilized technique but has wide-ranging applications in all metacarpophalangeal joints as both a diagnostic and therapeutic procedure. This includes the thumb where the most common MCP soft tissue injury occurs: the skier's (gamekeepers) thumb. This is a tear to the ulnar collateral ligament and most commonly seen among skiers who hold onto their pole when falling, leading to a hyperabduction moment when the pole/thumb strikes the snow. However, this can also occur when the tennis athlete falls on their dominant hand and the racket forcibly deviates the thumb upon impact. The diagnosis is often clinical, although live fluoroscopic exam of both thumbs will demonstrate the joint line widening seen on the ulnar side, and MRI can confirm the clinical suspicion also noted on physical exam by an experienced hand specialist. A Stener lesion, the avulsed ligament sitting outside the adductor aponeurosis, is diagnostic and can be palpated and then confirmed by ultrasound. It is a clear indication for surgical reattachment, usually via small lazy S incision, using a bone anchor to reattach the ligament to its insertion on the proximal phalanx. Lesser lesions, and often chronic ones, can be addressed by arthroscopic debridement and placing the ligament at insertion site to create healing [8]. Thermal shrinkage can also be beneficial, particularly in chronic lesions where the ligament/capsular complex is lax, redundant, and inflamed. Regardless of technique, a thumb spica short-arm cast is required between 4 and 6 weeks depending on clinical severity and other factors.

Thumb injuries can also occur at the basal joint (trapeziometacarpal), often the site of painful synovitis or arthritis in older, active players. Elite players can have deep pain in the area, however, and this can be due to occult injuries to the capsule or 1 of the 11 named ligaments at the critical trapeziometacarpal joint [9]. This most commonly occurs in a fall but can be considered an "overuse" injury where heavy repetitive stress to the area leads to subtle injury to the surrounding soft tissues. The diagnosis is often clinical, and negative studies (MRI, bone scan, X-ray) should not be considered definitive. Despite scant awareness even in the orthopedic community, thumb arthroscopy of the basal joint has been very effective in both diagnosing and treating occult lesions to this critical joint [10]. A 1.9 or 2.7 mm arthroscope is used to assess the joint surfaces, capsule, and ligaments within the painful joint. Debridement of frayed issue, often including radiofrequency shrinkage, is very effective in stimulating the healing process so necessary to relieve the pain, much like the MCP joints previously mentioned (Figs. 20.4 and 20.5). A thumb spica cast is generally applied for a 4–6-week period to allow for healing and is a protocol not uncommonly utilized in the active player.

The thumb and digits can present a wide array of bony and soft tissue lesions, as seen, that can obviously hamper a players performance due to the resultant loss in strength or dexterity so critical for the tennis athlete. However, it is the wrist that is often the bane of the elite tennis player/coach's existence and requires an in-depth discussion.

20.6 Wrist Bony Lesions/Fractures

The wrist is comprised of eight carpal bones interconnected by a complex array of both intrinsic (intercarpal) and extrinsic ligaments. While chronic wrist lesions are usually ligamentous, carpal bone fractures are frequently seen in falls and can represent a challenging diagnosis for the non-hand surgeon.

The hand is connected to the wrist (carpus) via the critical carpometacarpal joints. This is a frequently injured area in the fighting sports, but pain and even acute injury can occur in the dominant hand of tennis athletes. These joints are virtually immobile, except ring and small, but are stabilized by thick ligaments that can be injured. On occasion, severe sprains or articular fractures can occur at this interval and generally respond well to a 1-month period of immobilization. Grip strength can suffer considerably; hence, a strengthening program will be vital for return to effective play. The index and middle finger CMC joints can also suffer from an obscure but common malady termed a carpal boss [11]. The bossing represents a breaking of the base of the metacarpal that spans the joint and is essentially a painful mass that is often confused with a wrist ganglion cyst. It is more distal than the latter, and can often be treated with a corticosteroid injection, particularly if there is an associated painful cyst. Resistant cases may need excision of the mass and often arthrodesis (fusion) of that joint to eliminate pain and avoid recurrence. This does not affect hand function adversely and should be considered in the tennis athlete whose grip strength is being affected.

Falls on the outstretched hand occasionally injure the hand, as previously discussed, but the wrist carpal bones usually bear the brunt of the energy transmitted. A contusion, usually to the thenar or hypothenar region, typically heals within days to weeks and can be accelerated by immediate ice to the affected area, and subsequent anti-inflammatory modalities as instituted by the trainer or therapist (physical or occupational). Recovery of grip strength is then progressed as imperative for the dominant (racket hand), while dexterity for the ball toss is needed during the serve.

Persistent pain will require a more thorough work-up. It is important that the hand undergoes a comprehensive, stepwise physical exam by an experienced clinician. Unfortunately, many athletes present to the subspecialist with a myriad of diagnostic studies, including MRI, CT, and

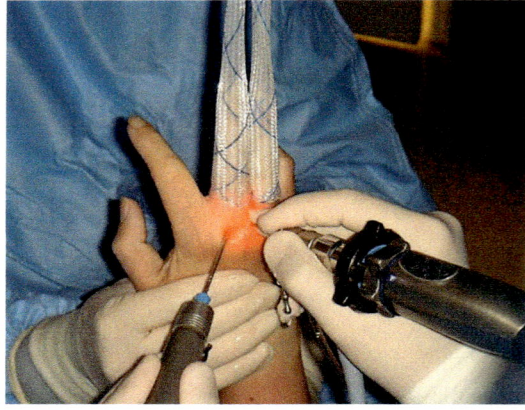

Fig. 20.4 View of middle finger metacarpophalangeal arthroscopic debridement utilizing 1.9 mm arthroscope and small joint shaver

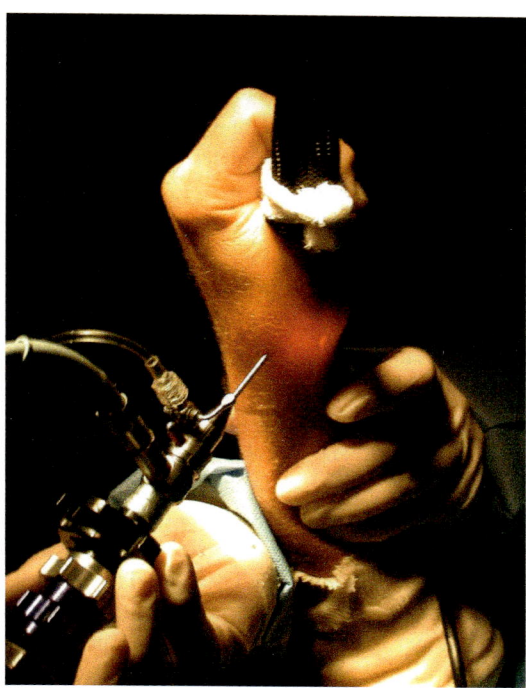

Fig. 20.5 Arthroscopy of the thumb carpometacarpal joint utilizing small joint scope and shaver allows true assessment of possible articular causes for thumb basal joint pain in the tennis athlete

ultrasound that are less helpful when performed, and viewed, out of context. The hand specialist can often determine the likely lesion simply by physical exam, and subsequent studies are then done to rule in, determine extent, identify concomitant injuries, etc.

The dreaded scaphoid (carpal navicular) is by far the most commonly fractured bone of the carpus. This occurs mainly because it is the largest bone, longitudinally oriented, and spans the proximal and distal carpal rows [12]. Hyperextension wrist injuries typically cause a fracture in the mid-waist of this bone, although distal and proximal pole injuries also occur. The former represents a usually benign injury since the blood supply enters the scaphoid radiodistally, and healing typically occurs within a 4–8-week period in a thumb spica cast. Conversely, proximal pole fractures have a high propensity to nonunion due to precarious blood supply, and many require surgery to stabilize and compress the fracture site. Many of these fractures will be indicated for some type of bone healing system. This can be electrical or ultrasound depending upon clinicians' preference.

Scaphoid fractures are not only problematic due to challenges in healing but also because they are often missed. Patients typically go to an emergency room where only two views of the wrist are performed, and the patient is sent away being told it is a "wrist sprain" by the busy ER physician who is likely managing a myocardial infarction or hip fracture patient. This was the genesis of the OrthoNOW concept; the term "wrist sprain" is perhaps the most overused description in orthopedic medicine. Wrist sprains are simply capsular or minor ligamentous injuries that heal within days to weeks. Any persistent wrist pain needs much more thorough evaluation by a wrist specialist since subtle injuries can be career threatening to many laborers and, of course, athletes, particularly tennis players. Pain on the radial side of the wrist requires multiple X-ray views, including the scaphoid view (slight extension with ulnar deviation). In office fluoroscopy is very helpful since it allows the wrist to be visualized in multiple views and with real-time dynamic motion. Significant pain with normal images, typically localized in the anatomic snuffbox (proximal to base of thumb), should undergo MRI imaging since subtle scaphoid fractures are often not seen in plain X-ray views in the acute stage. Controversy now exists as to treatment when non-displaced fractures are found, particularly in the typical mid-waist location. Most wrist surgeons now recommend that a percutaneous screw be inserted to not only increase chance of healing but to accelerate that process, so critical for the tennis athlete. This relatively simple outpatient procedure under local anesthesia entails placement of a compression headless screw that is placed via a stab wound incision and can also permit early motion. I typically accompany this with wrist arthroscopy that allows assessment in the wrist of any concomitant soft tissue injuries (later discussed) and ensures anatomic reduction by assessing the scaphoid articular surface. Any displacement on plain X-ray is by definition an "unstable fracture" and therefore naturally requires percutaneous or open reduction/internal fixation. Bony healing is assessed by serial radiographs although CT scan may be indicated when the athlete wants to return to hitting earlier since the X-ray picture typically lags behind actual bony union. Naturally, a player should not return to any hitting during this process until actual fracture union occurs. During this period, vigorous conditioning can be maintained, particularly when the fracture is stabilized. The days of bulky, long-arm thumb spica casts are long gone, and one should be wary when an athlete is placed into this restrictive device that can compromise a tennis career so greatly.

Scaphoid fractures require such aggressive, early treatment because the nonunion rate is so high. In cases, where a fracture was missed, or conservative treatment failed, a more invasive surgical procedure that includes bone grafting is often necessary. However, if done correctly, even these patients can potentially return to a tennis career. Early diagnosis and appropriate treatment are keys to avoid these later challenges.

While scaphoid fractures are the most common carpal bone fracture, there are lesions in other areas of the wrist that should be understood. Often mimicking the scaphoid injury, trapezial ridge fractures can often be seen in falls on the tennis court. The tenderness is on the palmar base of the thumb and only requires 1 month of thumb spica cast immobilization. Equivalent injury on the opposite, hypothenar, side of the palm can lead to a hook of hamate fracture [13]. This is also seen in baseball players and golfers where the butt of the bat/club can cause fracture at the base of this carpal bone projection. Diagnosis is often made by carpal tunnel view X-ray or CT scan/MRI axial views. The treatment is almost always wide excision of the hook of hamate since it has little role in hand function, and this will expedite return to sport. Also on the ulnar side, but dorsum of the wrist, is the relatively common triquetral avulsion fracture. This can be a misnomer since the small fracture may also occur with hyperextension of the wrist where the dorsum of the triquetrum is knocked off, along with a portion of capsule. This painful injury can be thought of as a severe wrist capsular sprain, and the healing is usually quite rapid since bone heals well to bone [14]. Casting for 4 weeks usually suffices, and any persistent pain should be an indication for wrist arthroscopy where redundant scar and painful synovitis can be ablated.

Other carpal bone fractures (capitate, lunate, etc.) are exceedingly rare and don't merit discussion; however, the most common adult fracture requiring surgery must be mentioned. The distal radius fracture is a ubiquitous bony injury that has been fraught with complications up until fairly recently. It has a bimodal incidence distribution, in this case being common in both children and older adults. However, the age group of elite tennis players can also be subjected to this fracture in the case of high-energy falls. Motor vehicle accidents, falls from a height, or extreme sports can lead to typical dorsally displaced distal radius fractures that will greatly impact the tennis game if not aggressively treated. During my early career, most fractures were treated conservatively and often went on to subtle malunion, affecting hand and wrist function. More displaced fractures were often treated by external fixation, a method of indirect reduction and prolonged treatment that ruined many an athlete's career. It was in the late 1990s that I and my colleagues at our now defunct Miami Hand Center developed the concept that volar plate fixation, via a fixed-angle locking plate, was preferable to all other techniques [15]. This concept soon spurred an international treatment revolution that I proudly watched, and now this is the standard of care treatment for most fractures of this bone. While not common in the younger tennis athletes, one should be well aware that the vast majority of distal radius fractures should undergo locked plate internal fixation via a palmar approach in the majority of cases. Older tennis athletes, occasionally in bilateral injuries sustained in falls on a court, have universally returned to play within months in my hands using this now established technique. Elite tennis players often sustain other injuries about the distal radius, as discussed, due to the excellent bone quality of the distal radius in this age group. However, a displaced distal radius fracture (previously termed Colles) can certainly occur in any demographic, and the same aggressive approach should be utilized. Stable,

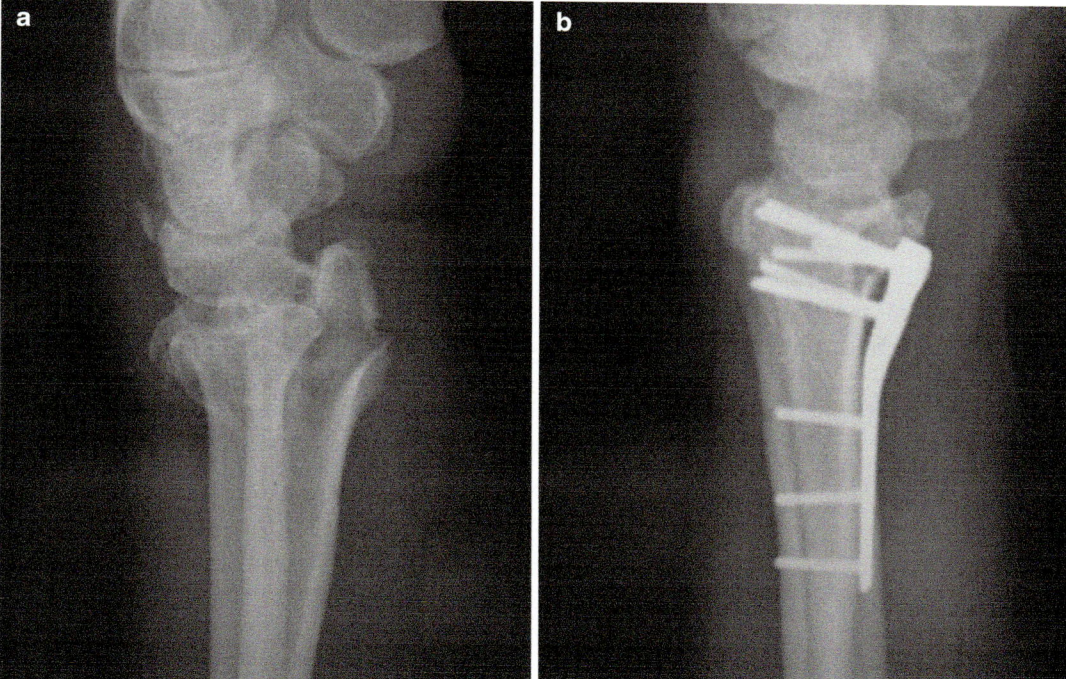

Fig. 20.6 Pre- and post-op radiographs of a reduced distal radius fracture secured with a volar locking titanium plate/screw fixation device

anatomic reduction with internal fixation should lead to return of gradual tennis play within an 8–12-week period (Fig. 20.6).

20.7 Soft Tissue Injuries About the Wrist

While bony injuries may occur in the wrist, it is the more subtle soft tissue injuries that perhaps afflict most players at some point in their careers and remain among the most difficult to accurately diagnose as well as the most challenging to treat. The reason is simple: the tennis racket is a long lever arm extending from the athlete's hand/wrist unit, often required to sustain blows of up to 140 mph in returning a serve. Forces from this activity are transmitted via strings to handle to hand, with the wrist often being the weak link in the receipt of that force. The hand is strongly gripping the racket, and the elite players' forearm musculature is generally well developed enough to sustain that force impact. However, soft tissue structures such as tendons, ligaments, and fibrocartilage cannot be directly trained and consequently remain the weak link in this racket/upper limb functioning unit. The goal should be early recognition, and accurate diagnosis so that further injury is not sustained, and to embark upon recovery as soon as possible. Many an elite player's career has been hampered or even terminated by these injuries, occasionally due to misdiagnosis or inaccurate treatment. The hand and wrist specialist should have open dialogue with tennis coaches, trainers, and team doctors thus facilitating early, appropriate diagnosis/treatment. The frequent challenges seen in the tennis athlete's wrist was one principal driving force in the creation of ISSPORTH (International Society for Sport Traumatology of the Hand).

Tendonitis of the wrist is perhaps an overdiagnosed entity among athletes but, nonetheless, is extremely common and particularly frequent in female elite players. Ulnar-sided wrist pain is considered "the low back" of the upper limb, exhibiting frequent occult pain that is as challenging to diagnose as it may be to treat. In many instances, the cause is tendonitis of the extensor carpi ulnaris (ECU) [16]. The most common tendonitis of the wrist in tennis players is in fact ECU tendonitis, although in the general population, tendonitis of the first extensor compartment (abductor pollicis longus/extensor pollicis brevis) is by far the most commonly encountered. Occasionally, the so-called crossover tendonitis is seen, where the thumb long extensor begins to chafe and becomes inflamed as it obliquely crosses the wrist extensors [17]. Careful physical exam, often coupled with in-office ultrasound assessment, can establish the diagnosis and even provide treatment via a directed corticosteroid injection. I recall a particular case in a former top ten female who had a "crossover" tendonitis from the thumb first compartment as it rubbed over the long wrist extensor. After symptom recurrence, despite two steroid injections, open debridement and partial tendon excision led to complete resolution and rapid return to play. While these forms of radial-sided wrist tendonitis are often seen in tennis players, it is the ECU tendon that generally hampers play.

The cause of ECU tendinosis is complex, multifactorial, and still not fully understood. This is thought to be an attritional issue where microtears due to heavy suprathreshold demands are placed on this large tendon, so critical for wrist extension and ulnar deviation: key motions for the leading wrist in the backhand shot. Precarious blood supply is often thought to be related to tendinosis where this poor perfusion not permit microhealing. This explains why rest, ice/heat, and other modalities are so critical to treating early stage tendinosis. More recalcitrant lesions may require surgical debridement. Naturally, there are intermediate stages where simple anti-inflammatory modalities may not suffice. It is in these cases where infiltration of corticosteroids is often considered. The trade-off, naturally, is that the steroid medication can lead to further tendon degeneration since it promotes a catabolic state within the tissues. While the anti-inflammatory properties lead to short-term pain relief, the long-term detrimental effects must be considered. In acute cases, one can consider 1–2 steroid injections in the course of a year, but there remains equivocal literature on how many injections can be safely given. The key is to promote tendon strengthening and modalities directed at augmenting tendon perfusion, therefore minimizing the chance of relapse. There are cases where an important tournament or match may justify a low-dose injection in order to permit effective play. This is a personal decision the player and trainer must make, ensuring that the ramifications are clearly understood. I typically use ultrasound guidance in order to precisely place the medication within the tendon sheath and into the tenosynovium where the inflammatory process is active. This not only maximized effectiveness but also minimizes the amount of steroid being use and therefore the deleterious effect. If the player sustains skin atrophy or hypopigmentation in the area, too much steroid is being administered. A less common form of ECU tendinosis is an insertional enthesopathy, where the tendon can degenerate at its insertion on the fifth metacarpal base. Conservative measures to augment tendon perfusion are usually effective in reversing this problem, assuming early diagnosis (Figs. 20.7 and 20.8).

ECU problems can also manifest from injury to the actual tunnel the tendon runs within, the sixth extensor compartment, but more specifically the subsheath. This thick, fibrous structure

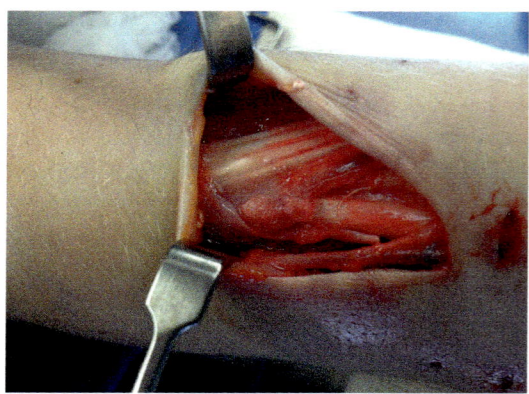

Fig. 20.7 Intraoperative evidence of extensor tendon crossover chafing in this patient with recurrent symptoms of radial-sided wrist/forearm pain despite injection at point where strap muscles cross over the wrist extensor tendons. Simple debridement and partial excision of a tendon strip resolved the problem promptly

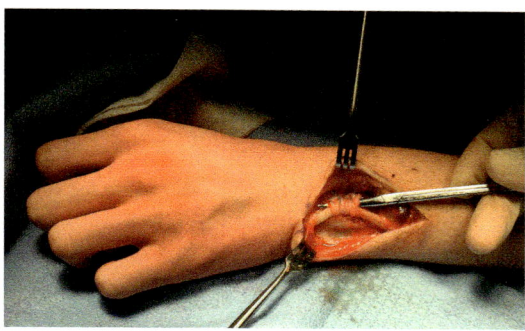

Fig. 20.8 ECU tendinosis coupled with subsheath attritional rupture is a common cause of ulnar-sided wrist pain in the tennis athlete

maintains the tendon within the shallow groove of the dorsal ulna, critical to maximizing tendon efficiency. Attritional, or even acute, rupture can occur and leads to a snapping ECU tendon [18]. The tendon not only becomes unstable and secondarily inflamed but can lose its biomechanical efficiency for extension and ulnar vector pull, thereby affecting critical strength needed in the tennis stroke. At this point, debride of the tendon and tendon subsheath reconstruction is usually needed. Direct repair of the ECU subsheath is usually not possible since the injury occurs over the course of time and the tissue themselves have limited tensile strength. A reconstruction is usually done, whether by advancing local tissue, often in a z-plasty manner, or utilizing the extensor retinaculum to augment the repair. Regardless, the wrist will need to be immobilized for a minimum of 6 weeks, usually in supination. Therefore, a just above elbow cast, termed a Muenster cast, can be used that allows for some elbow flexion/extension in order to minimize elbow stiffness and disuse atrophy.

While ECU issues are ubiquitous in tennis athletes, it is generally not the cause of potentially career-ending injuries. The triangular fibrocartilage complex (TFCC) is a now better understood anatomic structure that can lead to disabling wrist pain and loss of strength in tennis players and other athletes [19]. Recent attention to this structure has certainly increased awareness of its role in wrist pain, but it should be placed in context as there are many other causes of ulnar-sided pain as we are now discussing. Furthermore, disruption of this structure must be viewed as a spectrum of injury since there are many components.

The TFCC is a confluence of two ligaments, the palmar and dorsal radioulnar ligaments, that run from the ulnar side of the radius to then insert on the foveal depression of the ulnar head, which is at the base of the ulnar styloid. Between them sits the articular disc, a fibrocartilaginous structure that histologically resembles the meniscal cartilage of the knee. These structures, together, comprise the major stabilizing component of the distal radioulnar joint. This allows for stable pronosupination of the wrist/forearm complex, allowing the critical motion necessary for the mechanically sound tennis stroke. It is perhaps the increasing emphasis on topspin shots that has led to the increasing prevalence of ulnar wrist pain among tennis athletes, although the increasing power of strokes may contribute to this. Furthermore, there is now increased awareness of this structure, and perhaps overdiagnosis is occurring.

TFCC injury typically occurs with sudden pronation motion, although hypersupination and ulnar deviation can also cause the structure to fail. Dr. Andrew Palmer first described the types of lesions, assigning a number to whether acute (I) or chronic (II) and a letter depending on where the lesion occurs in relation to the articular disc [20, 35]. Tennis athletes typically suffer a Palmer type IB, which represents an acute detachment of the peripheral attachment of the disc, whether from the capsular insertion or at the actual foveal attachment in bone. The former can often heal with a period of immobilization and avoidance of activity, typically maintaining the wrist in supination to take stress off the structure, or may be so minor as to simply be considered a "wrist sprain," and the injury is short lived. Most lesions can be identified by an experienced wrist clinician, and imaging studies are more for confirmation and more precise identification of the type and grade of the tear. MRI has the greatest sensitivity but the specificity remains modest; therefore, the study should be ordered and interpreted by the clinician examining the patient [21]. Once a tear is suspected, the treatment will depend on many factors and may vary considerably depending upon clinician experience and training.

The history and clinical exam is paramount in assessing a patient for TFCC injury and, in fact, ulnar-sided wrist complaints in general. Most diagnostic studies are frequently normal, or the radiologist's interpretation may have little relevance to the patient's complaints.

Palpation of the principal point of tenderness is key. A peripheral tear (Palmer 1B lesion) will usually be specifically tender just palmar to the ECU and distal to the ulnar styloid. The pain is aggravated usually by two maneuvers: ulnar deviation and hypersupination. Any player with this constellation of symptoms for greater than 4 months warrants a wrist arthroscopic exam assuming that conservative measures and a period of wrist have not resolved the symptoms. While imaging studies, such as MRI, may or may not show the lesion, it is the arthroscopic evaluation that not only makes the definitive diagnosis but also allows the treating surgeon to definitively address the pathology found. A prime benefit is that this is minimally invasive; therefore, even minimal pathology can be discounted, and the player can return to play potentially within weeks. When dealing with elite players whose livelihood depends on their wrist, it is perhaps better to have an occasional false positive than miss potentially fixable injuries that should have been scoped earlier in their evolution.

Wrist arthroscopy has revolutionized how carpal soft tissue injuries are diagnosed and treated. While akin to the paradigm shift in treatment at the knee level, it is different in that many clinicians who examine tennis wrist injuries are not trained in this methodology. Conversely, most orthopedic surgeons are well versed in multiple arthroscopic procedures of the knee. Many clinicians, from athletic trainer to therapist to team orthopedic surgeon or sports medicine physician, may examine a player's wrist. However, a hand surgeon with wrist arthroscopy may be vital to that players' potential recovery. Early assessment can allow the clinical team to take the decision to understand "why" is the player's wrist still hurting.

Like many other techniques in surgery, wrist arthroscopy is typically done in a stepwise fashion, assessing virtually all parts of the wrist, finally focusing on the pathology found during the latter half of the procedure, which can be done outpatient and with wrist block anesthesia and minimal IV sedation [22]. Photographs of the pathologic findings, and how it is managed, can then be shown to the player and his training/treatment team so everyone is on the same page.

I generally perform wrist arthroscopy with 10 lb of vertical traction via two Chinese finger traps that allow distraction of both radiocarpal and midcarpal joints. I begin with the 2.7 mm 30° arthroscope inserted into the 3–4 portal, so named since it lies between the third and fourth extensor tendon compartments. Initial assessment of the wrist is started on the radial side, assessing the scaphoid and distal radius articular surfaces, volar ligaments, and then the critical scapholunate ligament. This latter structure can occasionally be injured, and the clinical exam may be muted, thinking that the pathology is toward ulnar compartment. Therefore, wrist arthroscopy may be the first moment when an occult tear of the SL ligament is detected allowing immediate treatment. Another frequent pathology is the dorsal ganglion cyst. A small subcapsular cyst often emanates from the dorsal aspect of the SL ligament and is a common cause of occult wrist pain, albeit, normally midline dorsum [23]. Simple resection arthroscopically can give rapid relief of chronic, disabling wrist pain where the diagnosis remained elusive until the arthroscopy is performed. It is important to address concomitant soft tissue pathologies, no matter how minor, as the player may experience ongoing lesser pain in the wrist if only the primary pathology is addressed. Once radial and midline wrist anatomic structures are evaluated, we now look ulnarward and get our first glimpse of the ulnar compartment of the wrist. In players with ongoing ulnar wrist pain, we typically see profuse synovitis that actually obscures the dorsal capsule and even TFCC complex. At this point, we introduce a 2.9 mm full-radius shaver, which is a mechanical ablation device connected to suction, that allows rapid removal of the inflamed, abnormal tissue. Once synovectomy is done, we can assess the anatomic structures. We begin with the dorsal capsule as this may be the only point of injury, allowing the player to continue hitting, but greatly limits the effectiveness and can be the cause of ongoing discomfort. While lesser capsular injuries (sprains) respond to conservative measures including rest, the significant capsular tear becomes a vicious cycle of pain since the tissue becomes redundant and limited perfusion limits healing [24]. The key is to generate a healing response, brought on by scar that will stabilize the capsuloligamentous complex via aggressive debridement, followed by limited thermal shrinkage capsulorrhaphy. The latter technique is where high-energy radio frequency is used to alter the collagen cross-linking, effectively "tightening" the soft tissues and creating a stable, nonredundant capsule. This requires a period of immobilization, usually 4 weeks in a waterproof, fiberglass cast where the player can continue conditioning. I recall a specific top 50 ranked player who managed to win the first round of Wimbledon within 9 weeks after a thermal shrinkage capsulorrhaphy. Prior to the shrinkage procedure, however, or any other intervention, one must rule out midcarpal pathology. This is done by moving the arthroscope into the radial midcarpal portal. This entry site is just distal to the 3-4 portal and is crucial to assess for intercarpal ligament tears (Fig. 20.9).

It is now important to further discuss tears of the scapholunate ligament and, more importantly for the elite tennis player, the lunotriquetral ligament. The latter is often the culprit for undiagnosed and chronic ulnar-sided wrist pain of the athlete and is best identified via midcarpal joint arthroscopy of the wrist.

The scapholunate ligament is far and away the most commonly injured deep ligament of the wrist, whether athletic or otherwise [25]. It is generally caused by a fall on the outstretched hand and leads to tensile overload of the small transverse fibers of the ligament that spans the 2–4 mm interval between proximal pole of the scaphoid and the lunate. The capitate drives proximally, leading to a distraction moment at this intercarpal ligament, where the lunate typically

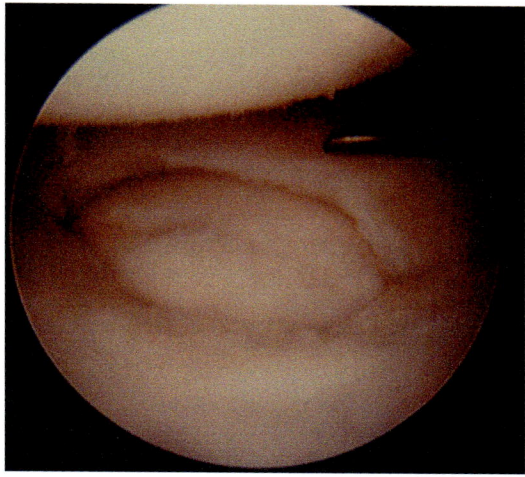

Fig. 20.9 TFCC central tear noted in this radiocarpal arthroscopic view from the 3–4 portal and addressed by combination of mechanical shaver and radiofrequency shrinkage of the articular disc defect edges

hyperextends, and the scaphoid flexes or remains neutral, avoiding will fracture to the scaphoid itself. In older patients, or with higher-energy injuries than typically sustained on the tennis court, the distal radius will fracture as previously discussed. These are generally not attritional ruptures, and the athlete will immediately note severe, usually midline, dorsal wrist pain. In fact, the player will likely not be able to continue play or even perform simple gripping activities of daily life. These injuries are generally recognized quickly due to the fact that this can be so disabling. Plain X-rays may show a diastasis (widening) of the interval, and lateral X-rays will often demonstrate a DISI (dorsal intercalated segmental instability) pattern where the scaphoid is flexed relative to the lunate which is tilted dorsally. Consequently, the scapholunate angle is usually increased, and a well-done MRI will generally show the avulsed ligament. There are four grades of a SL tear, the most severe (grade 4) should likely undergo an open ligament reconstruction; actual ligament repair is not feasible. This is generally not done arthroscopically, and surgeons tend to have their favored open approach. I typically will reduce the SL interval, correct the anatomic deformity, and then pin the bones in the reduced position. I utilize the dorsal capsule to then "reconstruct" the ligament utilizing bone anchors to position the new reconstructed ligament. Details are beyond the scope of this chapter, but understand that the player must remain in a thumb spica short-arm cast for 8 weeks, followed by pin removal and subsequent physiotherapy. While a player will typically take 6 months to return to play after this devastating injury, it should be understood that this can be an elite career-ending injury regardless of the integrity of ligament reconstruction.

It is much more common to see partial, dynamic SL ligament tears. These are difficult to diagnose, often hard to pinpoint when the exact injury occurred, and typically are delayed in treatment since the player is often told they have a "wrist sprain." While MRI may identify the lesion, it is often at time of arthroscopy, as previously mentioned, that the tear is identified. This explains why midcarpal arthroscopy is so crucial, even when clinicians are convinced this is an ulnar compartment, perhaps TFCC problem. The ligament disruption is manifested by seeing either a step-off or frank widening, at the space between the scaphoid and lunate in the midcarpal view. A hook probe can be placed into the ulnar midcarpal portal and the tip easily inserted within the SL interval. If that tip can be rotated 90 degrees, this constitutes a grade 3 tear, as first described by Geissler and Haley [26]. Many times a step-off can also be seen at the interval. Regardless, any significant dynamic instability will lead to chronic pain, at either racket impact or dorsiflexion of the wrist, and needs to be addressed. Once the diagnosis is made, the frayed ligament is aggressively debrided, even creating a bleeding surface of the carpal bones on either side of the dorsal ligament portion, the most critical of the SL ligament. This will lead to bleeding and scar formation at that location of the ligament, since the interval will be immobilized via two k-wires (0.045″ is my preference) that cross the interval from scaphoid to lunate [27]. These pins are driven by a k-wire driver, once the scope is removed and sterile mini-fluoroscopy is brought into the field. Therefore, this represents the conclusion of the surgical intervention, and the arthroscope is typically placed back into the radiocarpal joint to address ulnar compartment pathology if indicated, prior to pinning. Combined lesions are not uncommon; therefore, any pinning of intercarpal injuries is performed at the end, prior to application of the splint-dressing. In the case of scapholunate pathology, a thumb spica splint is utilized since the scaphoid needs to be immobilized via the thumb axis.

Much like the open SL ligament reconstruction, dynamic tears treated by arthroscopic debridement and pinning require 8 weeks of cast immobilization. This is simply due to the basic science premise that collagen cross-linking and, consequently, scar formation will take 8 weeks. The player will naturally have a stiff wrist, and the first weeks of rehabilitation are dedicated to recovering supple wrist range of motion. Forearm muscle atrophy naturally occurs, and I now try to minimize that by instituting ENMT (electroneuromuscular therapy) Neurotherapy in the immediate post-op period. This will increase perfusion via neurovascular mechanisms but also stimulate the forearm flexor/extensors directly in order to minimize muscle mass loss. This concept has been well accepted in the elite sports community, although only now being introduced to the layperson and weekend warriors via OrthoNOW orthopedic urgent care centers. Suffice to say that further developments are occurring in the rehabilitation, and sports conditioning phase of recovery and details are outside the goals of this chapter. Assuming no additional interventions or adjunctive treatments, a seasoned tennis player should return to play within a 4–6-month period after a scapholunate ligament injury.

Despite the prevalence of scapholunate ligament tears among the sporting population, it is likely that the lunotriquetral (LT) ligament is the most commonly injured among tennis players [28]. It is also a likely cause of ongoing ulnar-sided wrist pain, despite the contention that the player suffers from a TFCC injury. Furthermore, patients with persistent ulnar-sided pain, even after surgical intervention, may actually be suffering from an undiagnosed LT ligament tear, hence the necessity for midcarpal arthroscopic evaluation. I recall a top ranked junior player who had severe ulnar-sided wrist pain where I debrided a minimal TFCC border injury, but neglected to stabilize a lesser LT ligament injury. The presumption was made that the minor instability would heal with simple immobilization after midcarpal debridement. Needless to say, the player's pain recurred within a year and repeat arthroscopy was needed. At this point, the ligament injury was more pronounced, and definitive pinning was now performed. This patient went on to a brilliant college career and is currently entering the pros rank. Defined pathology seen at the time of wrist arthroscopy must be fully addressed (Fig. 20.10).

The lunotriquetral ligament is often injured in more insidious fashion, where the player often cannot recall the exact moment of injury. It usually occurs when the wrist is forcibly pronated, often with ulnar deviation and a dorsiflexion moment. This load can surpass the tensile strength of the LT ligament, and a disruption of the critical volar component of the ligament then leads to significant motion between the two carpal bones, rarely with any diastasis. Classically, a complete LT ligament tear should demonstrate a VISI (opposite of SL tear's DISI) pattern on lateral X-ray; however, I have found this to be rarely the case. The diagnosis is clinical and often first detected at the time of midcarpal arthroscopic evaluation.

On physical exam, the player will usually have point tenderness just distal to the TFCC disc and accentuated by palpating the wrist in flexion. Ulnar deviation with dorsiflexion is usually quite painful, and grip strength, as in SL tears, can be greatly diminished. The player may describe a subtle click or clunk with wrist motion or with racket-ball impact. The joint can be directly stressed by manipulating the lunate against the triquetrum which is secured between the thumb

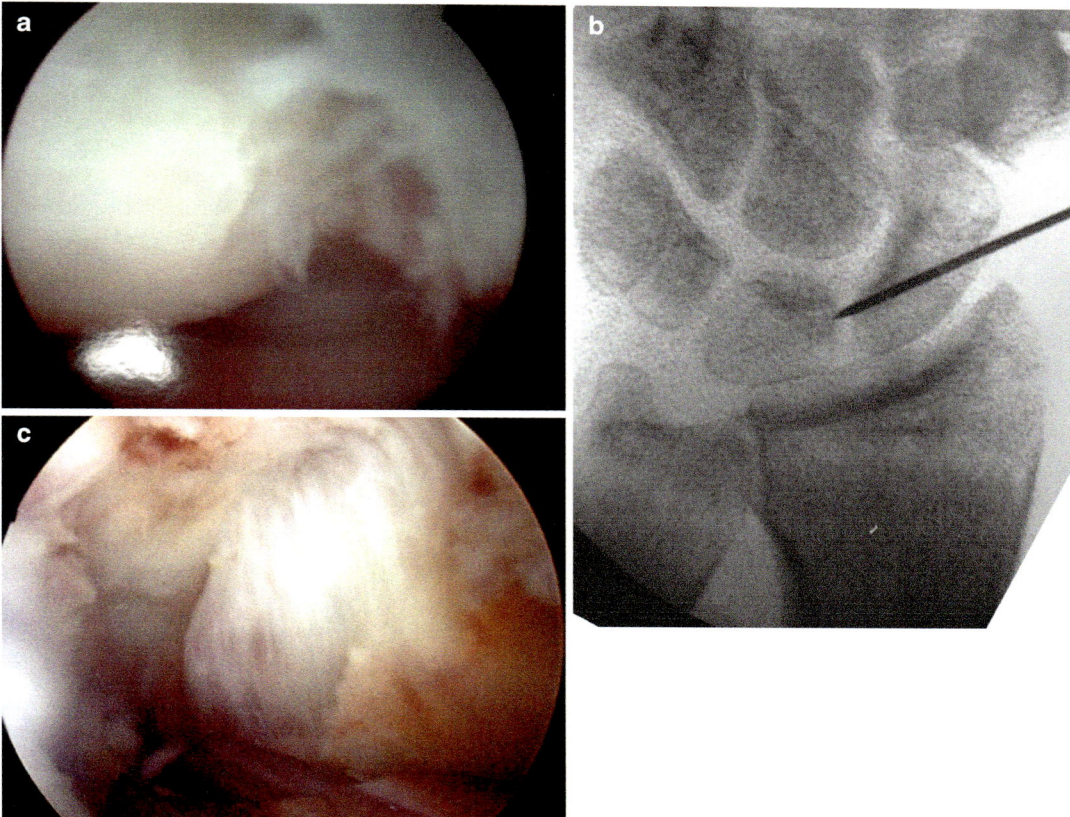

Fig. 20.10 Scapholunate occult ligament tear in a Venezuelan player who was initially felt to have an isolated TFCC lesion and the arthroscopic appearance of the reconstituted SL ligament at time of pin removal as shown here

while the index finger is on the pisiform. The pisotriquetral complex is now rocked, or shucked, against the lunate which should elicit pain in the event of a tear. This lunotriquetral shuck test is nearly as sensitive as a coronal MRI image but likely much more specific. This physical finding will be corroborated at the time of arthroscopy and is often accompanied by the appearance of a bare triquetrum dorsally, where the ulnocarpal capsule has been avulsed. After arthroscopic debridement, with particular attachment to the volar LT, the interval is pinned, much like the SL interval. Pins remain similarly in place for an 8-week period while the player is protected in a simple short-arm cast. If the patient has a concomitant peripheral TFCC tear that is repaired, the long arm Muenster cast will be shortened at 5 weeks, and that cast/pin is removed 2–3 weeks later. One cannot emphasize how common these injuries are, and I can recall an episode where a young Russian couple both had the same injury, neither being able to play for the prior 6 months to a year from when I first evaluated them. They each had combined TFCC/LT repairs but 2 weeks apart. Apparently the male player first wanted to see how the girlfriend fared after surgery (Fig. 20.11).

Given the relative high prevalence of these ligament injuries, it is important to recognize that some players may actually sustain simultaneous injury of the SL and LT ligaments. I first published this concept, calling it the "floating lunate lesion" [29]. It has since been substantiated in the literature, termed a grade 0 PLIND lesion by Herzberg [30]. The treatment is similar as to isolated lesions, with debridement now of both SL and LT intervals, followed by four pins, all meeting and crossing within the lunate. The aftercare is similar although recovery may take longer given the fact that this is a more global lesion to the wrist soft tissue structures.

Understanding that LT lesions are often occult and missed and can occur alongside TFCC cartilage tears, we must still recognize that the isolated small peripheral tear of the TFCC articular disc likely represents the most common acute

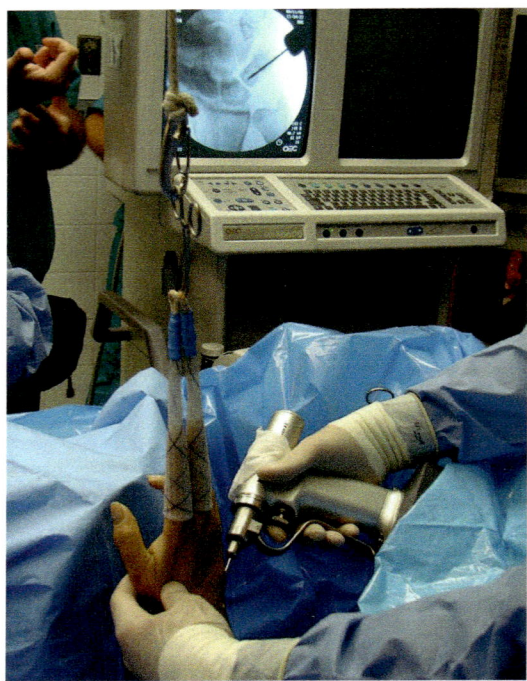

Fig. 20.11 Lunotriquetral pins being placed in the operating room under fluoroscopic control after LT ligament debridement was performed arthroscopically

soft tissue injury of the tennis athlete's dominant wrist. It is important to know how to recognize this pathology, and understand the myriad of treatment options, often depending on stage and complexity of tear, chronicity, and impact on play.

The athlete with a TFCC tear will complain of ulnar side wrist discomfort and loss of grip strength. There is often a discrete recollection of when the injury occurred, but it can be insidious in nature and gradually worsen to the point that play is not possible. Pain is exacerbated when initiating the forehand in the dominant wrist or the backhand if non-dominant wrist is involved. Difficulty supinating the wrist is a classic finding, as is extreme ulnar deviation. Physical findings also include vague puffiness over the ulnar compartment, just distal to ulnar styloid, and diminished grip strength compared to contralateral wrist. As previously mentioned, the diagnostic studies may not be very helpful as plain X-rays are normal, and ultrasound assessment will show increased fluid but with little anatomic significance. A well-done MRI will usually show the lesion but can be deceiving.

Recent onset of pain usually calls for a period of rest, perhaps immobilization with a cockup splint and anti-inflammatory modalities. The unknown variable is for how long to cease play and when a lesion can be deemed a failure of conservative treatment. In the elite tennis player, early MRI is recommended only because one must rule out a massive peripheral tear, or other finding, and therefore the evaluating hand surgeon can proceed directly to arthroscopic assessment and repair. The player's career can be severely impacted by waiting a prolonged time to definitive treatment in the scenario of a major lesion. Early intervention is what accelerates return to play.

The smaller tears tend to be the clinical dilemma. The Palmer classification separates tears as to location and chronicity, type I being acute (post-traumatic) and type II degenerative.

Type IA tears are central tears, often due to anatomic findings such as ulnar-positive variance (ulna long relative to radius) and very poor perfusion of the central articular disc. These lesions tend to be of moderate pain but long-standing in nature. Conservative measures can usually minimize symptoms, and it is only the resistant cases that require surgery. The tear is immediately recognized during radiocarpal arthroscopy and is managed by debridement, typically followed by RF shrinkage of the periphery of the lesion as to stabilize it [31]. Redundant, frayed edges need to be annealed, and the pain usually resolves quickly. Actual repair is not possible since the central disc has poor perfusion and any attempt at suturing is doomed to failure, much like many meniscal tears of the knee.

Type IB tears are the classic tennis athlete's tear, where the peripheral edge of the disc is torn away from the capsular insertion and more severe injuries actually tear the insertion on the fovea of the ulnar head. The latter disruption can actually cause an instability of the distal radioulnar joint (DRUJ) and may need reinsertion with a bone anchor or bone tunnels. However, the typical injury is capsular detachment where the TFCC articular disc loses its "trampoline effect" and suture repair is now indicated [32]. Naturally, small tears can be treated only by debridement, usually accompanied with shrinkage, and brief immobilization. However, large tears are not uncommon and require anatomic repair, implying restoration of the trampoline effect, thereby stabilizing the DRUJ. Much like the peripheral meniscal tears, suture repair is now possible due to evolution of techniques and the fact that healing will occur due to vigorous perfusion of the peripheral areas of the cartilage. For many years, I used a simple "out to in" type of suture repair where the edge of the disc tear was pierced with a large bore needle, allowing a nonabsorbable suture to be passed through that needle canal and then retrieved with a small joint grasper device. This allowed placement of a "simple stitch" which was then retrieved and tied down onto the capsule to restore tension on the articular disc. Most tears required passage of a second stitch, followed by tying both of these down tightly as the wrist is held in supination, minimizing tension on the repair. This immediately restored trampoline effect, and the supinated position was held for about 6 weeks, allowing for healing to the capsule. Since the ulnar capsule is immediately subcutaneous, many times the sutures were irritating and even caused irritation to the dorsal sensory branch of the ulnar nerve. This was a common complaint among wrist arthroscopists and alternative methodologies were sought. In the early 2000s, I published a technique whereby the suture, nylon in this case, was "welded" so that the painful knot was effectively eliminated, avoiding the complication [33]. Despite a significant series being compiled, the ultrasonic welding technology was acquired by a larger company and the instrumentation vanished from the market. I am hopeful this may represent the future of knot management in many branches of surgery. Consequently, other methods to avoid external

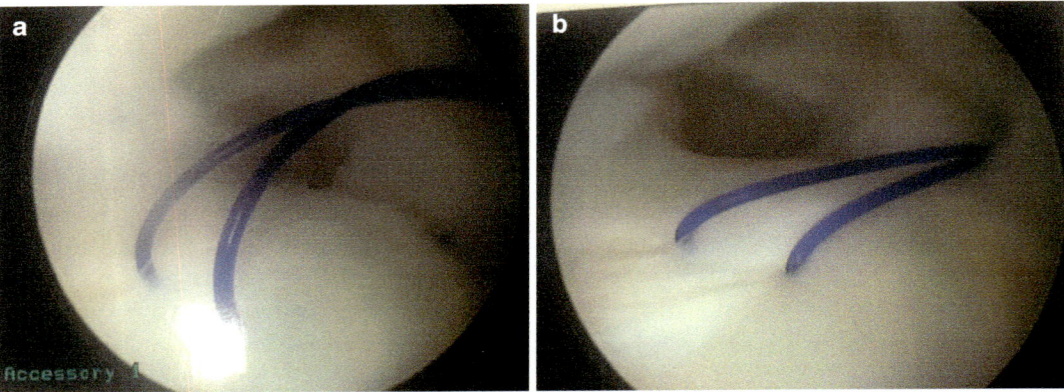

Fig. 20.12 TFCC peripheral tear being repaired with classic out-in technique utilizing Nylon suture

capsule knots have been devised. Myself, and many wrist arthroscopists, now uses an all-inside repair that allows placement of a bioabsorbable tack which is placed external to the capsule, while a second one is placed on the peripheral aspect of the articular disc [34]. Sutures are preloaded into the device that deploys these tacks, including a slip knot that the surgeon pulls, approximating the detached disc to the capsular insertion site. Post-op immobilization is similar as capsular healing needs to occur, but a much more anatomic repair is achieved, in a minimally invasive manner. Recovery of pronosupination tends to be rapid, and athletes can usually go back to mini-tennis and then light hitting by 6 weeks after cast removal. I can recall a number of athletes on the tour who returned to successful play by 5 months after arthroscopic TFCC repair (Fig. 20.12).

Palmer type 1C and 1D represent tears of the volar ligament/disc complex and radial side of articular disc, respectively. The former is fairly uncommon, and the latter is now treated similarly to a central type tear with simple debridement and frequently coupled with radiofrequency shrinkage. The radial side of the TFCC is also poorly vascularized; therefore, attempted repairs with bone tunnels, suture passage, is likely a fruitless exercise when tissue healing will likely not occur (Fig. 20.13).

Conclusion

The demanding sport of tennis has led to recognition of a wide range of athletic injuries to the hand and wrist that can sideline the player. Early diagnosis coupled with appropriate, often minimally invasive, treatment has now seen many players return to their premorbid level of play. Communication and consultation with the hand specialist provide the best chance for the injured player to achieve successful clinical outcome and subsequent athletic performance.

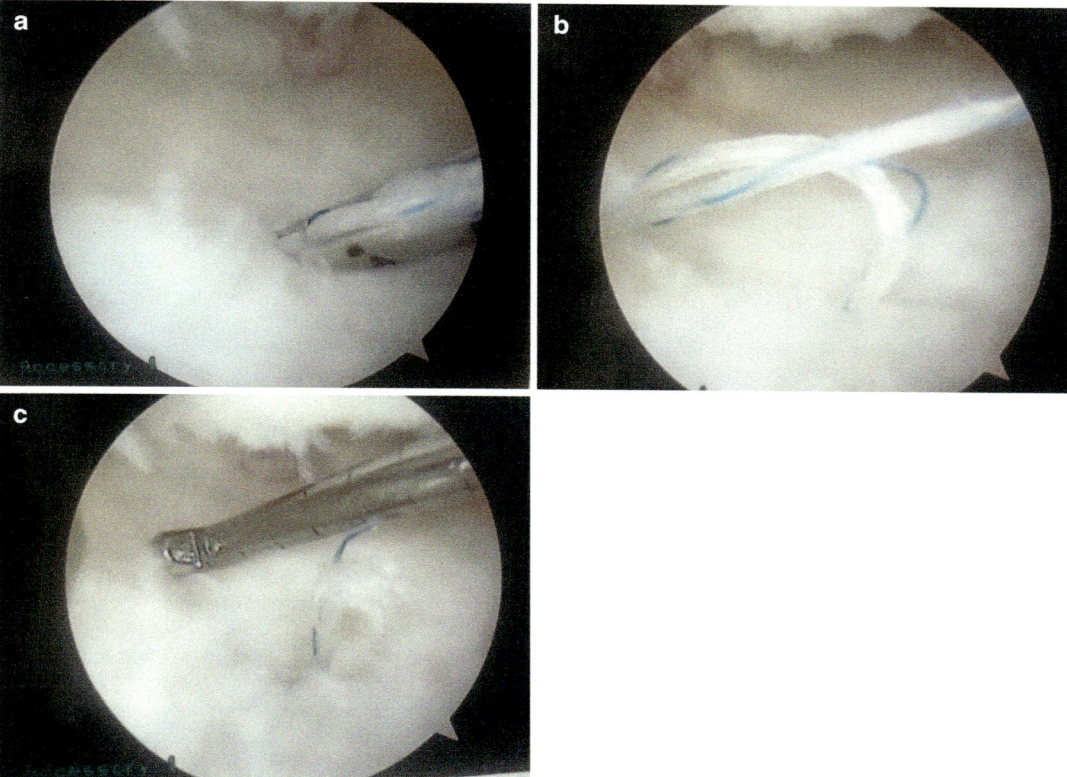

Fig. 20.13 Intra-articular view of TFCC peripheral detachment tear secured with Fast-Fix device

References

1. Cotterell IH, Richard MJ. Metacarpal and phalangeal fractures in athletes. Clin Sports Med. 2015;34(1):69–98.
2. Badia A, Riano F, Ravikoff J. Dynamic intra-digital external fixation for proximal interphalangeal joint fracture dislocations. J Hand Surg Am. 2005;30(1):154–60.
3. Calfee RP, Kiefhaber TR, Sommerkamp TG, Stern PJ. Hemi-hamate arthroplasty provides functional reconstruction of acute and chronic proximal interphalangeal fracture-dislocations. J Hand Surg. 2009;34:1232–41.
4. Burkhalter WE, Reyes FA. Closed treatment of fractures of the hand. Bull Hosp Jt Dis Orthop Inst. 1984;44(2):145–62.
5. Foucher G. "Bouquet" osteosynthesis in metacarpal neck fractures: a series of 66 patients. J Hand Surg Am. 1995;20(3 Pt 2):S86–90.
6. Badia A, Riano F. A simple fixation method for unstable bony mallet finger. J Hand Surg Am. 2004;29(6):1051–5.
7. Hame SL, Melone CP Jr. Boxer's knuckle in the professional athlete. Am J Sports Med. 2000;28(6):879–82.
8. Badia A. Arthroscopy of the trapeziometacarpal and metacarpophalangeal joints. J Hand Surg Am. 2007;32:707–24.
9. Bettinger PC, Linscheid RL, Berger RA, Cooney WP 3rd, An KN. An anatomic study of the stabilizing ligaments of the trapezium and trapeziometacarpal joint. J Hand Surg Am. 1999;24(4):786–98.
10. Badia A. Trapeziometacarpal arthroscopy: a classification and treatment algorithm. Hand Clin. 2006;22(2):153–63.
11. Park MJ, et al. The carpal boss: review of diagnosis and treatment. J Hand Surg. 2008;33A:446–9.
12. Riester JN, Baker BE, Mosher JF, et al. A review of scaphoid fracture healing in competitive athletes. Am J Sports Med. 1985;13:159–61.
13. Stark HH, Jobe FW, Boyes JH, et al. Fracture of the hook of the hamate in athletes. J Bone Joint Surg Am. 1977;59:575–82.
14. Levy M, Fischel RE, Stern GM, et al. Chip fractures of the os triquetrum: the mechanism of injury. J Bone Joint Surg Br. 1979;61:355–7.

15. Badia A, Khanchandani P. Volar plate fixation. In: Slutsky DJ, Osterman AL, editors. Distal radial fractures and carpal injuries: the cutting edge. 1st ed. Philadelphia: Saunders, Elsevier; 2008. p. 149–56.
16. Chun S, Palmer AK. Chronic ulnar wrist pain secondary to partial rupture of the extensor carpi ulnaris tendon. J Hand Surg Am. 1987;12:1032–5.
17. Hanlon DP, Luellen JR. Intersection syndrome: a case report and review of literature. J Emerg Med. 1999;17(6):969–71. https://doi.org/10.1016/S0736-4679(99)00125-0.
18. MacLennan AJ, Nemechek NM, Waitayawinyu T, et al. Diagnosis and anatomic reconstruction of extensor carpi ulnaris subluxation. J Hand Surg Am. 2008;33:59–64. https://doi.org/10.1016/j.jhsa.2007.10.002.
19. Nagle DJ. Triangular fibrocartilage complex tears in the athlete. Clin Sports Med. 2001;20(1):155–66. https://doi.org/10.1016/S0278-5919(05)70253-2.
20. Palmer AK. Triangular fibrocartilage complex lesions: a classification. J Hand Surg Am. 1989;4:594–606. https://doi.org/10.1016/0363-5023(89)90174-3.
21. Haims AH, Schweitzer ME, Morrison WB, Deely D, Lange R, Osterman AL, et al. Limitations of MR imaging in the diagnosis of peripheral tears of the triangular fibrocartilage of the wrist. AJR Am J Roentgenol. 2002;178:419–22.
22. Whipple TL, Marotta JJ, Powell JH III. Techniques of wrist arthroscopy. Arthroscopy. 1986;2(4):244–52.
23. Luchetti R, Badia A, Alfarano M, Orbay J, Indriago I, Mustapha B. Arthroscopic resection of dorsal wrist ganglia and treatment of recurrences. J Hand Surg Br. 2000;25(1):38–40.
24. Slutsky DJ. Arthroscopic dorsal radiocarpal ligament repair. Arthroscopy. 2005;21(12):1486.
25. Manuel J, Moran SL. The diagnosis and treatment of scapholunate instability. Hand Clin. 2010;26:129–44. https://doi.org/10.1016/j.hcl.2009.08.006.
26. Geissler WB, Haley T. Arthroscopic management of scapholunate instability. Atlas Hand Clin. 2001;6:253–74.
27. Darlis NA, Kaufmann RA, Giannoulis F, Sotereanos DG, et al. Arthroscopic debridement and closed pinning for chronic dynamic scapholunate instability. J Hand Surg Am. 2006;31:418–24.
28. Weiss LE, Taras JS, Sweet S, Osterman AL. Lunotriquetral injuries in the athlete. Hand Clin. 2000;16:433–8.
29. Badia A, Khanchandani P. The floating lunate: arthroscopic treatment of simultaneous complete tears of the scapholunate and lunotriquetral ligaments. Hand (N Y). 2009;4:250–5.
30. Herzberg G. Perilunate injuries, not dislocated (PLIND). J Wrist Surg. 2013;2(4):337–45.
31. Wallace AL, Hollinshead RM, Frank CB. The scientific basis of thermal capsular shrinkage. J Shoulder Elb Surg. 2000;9:354–60.
32. Estrella EP, Hung LK, Ho PC, Tse WL. Arthroscopic repair of triangular fibrocartilage complex tears. Arthroscopy. 2007;23:729–37. 737.e1
33. Badia A, Jiménez A. Arthroscopic repair of peripheral triangular fibrocartilage complex tears with suture welding: a technical report. J Hand Surg Am. 2006;31(8):1303–7.
34. Yao J. All-arthroscopic triangular fibrocartilage complex repair: safety and biomechanical comparison with a traditional outside-in technique in cadavers. J Hand Surg Am. 2009;34(4):671–6.
35. Palmer AK. Triangular fibrocartilage complex lesions: a classification. J Hand Surg Am. 1989;4:594–606. https://doi.org/10.1016/0363-5023(89)90174-3.

Pathophysiology of Wrist and Hand Injuries in Tennis Players: Tendons, Ligaments and TFCC Lesions

Andrea De Vita, R. A. Purnachandra Tejaswi, and Paolo Scarso

21.1 Introduction

The final, crucial link in the kinetic chain between the body and racket is the wrist and hand, a complex structure that executes several roles essential to the production of all tennis strokes. There is no question that modern tennis players themselves in their striving through trial and error for more power, more control and more variety in stroke production are the primary factors in determining changes to stroke mechanics. Within this scenario, the wrist plays an important role in achieving the best strokes. General theory provides a basis upon which modifications can be made; an understanding of individual stroke mechanics leads to improved performance [1]. An increase in the incidence of wrist problems among tennis players in the last 20 years can be attributed to changes in equipment, grip, velocity and performance. Musculoskeletal injuries related to tennis may be tied to either a single event in which a macrotrauma is responsible for acute injury or to chronic overuse [2].

Unlike lower limb injuries, most wrist and other upper limb injuries in tennis are associated with overuse and a chronic time course [3], with repeated loading during the tennis stroke often described as a contributing factor [4–6].

21.2 Biomechanics

It is important to consider the wrist and the hand, the final parts of kinetic chain. The role of both structures is to achieve the correct power transfer from inferior part of the body to the racquet. To obtain maximal performance and minimal risk of injury, it requires optimum activation of all the links in the kinetic chain [7]. Injury is often associated with alterations in the flow of energy across segments, such that if one segment is removed from the chain, then there is an increased reliance on the others to accommodate this loss, which may lead to tissue overload [1]. The loading of the body in tennis, to achieve a strong hit of the ball, is obtained by applying external and internal forces that means to have a good ground reaction forces and good forces and torques of the muscles. According to Elliott [1] in a stretch-shorten cycle, elastic energy stored during the eccentric phase of the action (the stretch) is partially recovered, such that the concentric phase (shorten) is enhanced. This is also supported by the fact that the concentric action begins with the appropriate muscles under higher tension than would be created if they were to contract purely

A. De Vita (✉)
Concordia Hospital for Special Surgery, Roma, Italy

R. A. P. Tejaswi
Kasturba Medical College, Manipal University, Manipal, India

P. Scarso
Concordia Hospital for Special Surgery, Rome, Italy

concentrically from a resting state [1]. Papers have shown that muscle pretension is most important in tennis to have strong service and groundstrokes [8]. In service the eccentric stretch and pretensing of the anterior shoulder muscles (particularly the internal rotators) is maximised by a vigorous leg drive which positions the racquet "down behind and away from the lower back" in preparation for the drive to the ball. In the forehand strokes, the rotation of the shoulders, greater than the hips (creating a separation angle) and the positioning of the upper limb relative to the trunk during the backswing phase of these strokes, places appropriate muscles on stretch. This is why in the backhand a separation angle (one-handed 30°; two-handed 20°) is created in the backswing in preparation for the swing to the ball [9].

The key to the recovery of the elastic energy is the timing between the stretch and shorten phases of the motion. Therefore, in tennis it will be essential to have a short pause between the backswing and forward swing phases of stroke to produce the best transmission of power from the eccentric phase to concentric phase. This means, increasing the velocity from eccentric to concentric phases of the strokes permits to hit the ball with stronger power. The perfect coordination (movement and timing) between all the links in the kinetic chain can achieve an ideal strokes (service, forehand, backhand and volley), but we have to consider variability in stroke production for different players. Sometimes this variability (depending on body elasticity, strength of the muscles, etc.) must be considered by the coaches to achieve good strategies for successful playing.

Consider to this, it is simple to understand that biomechanics of the tennis play is a perfect combination between muscles in work in eccentric and concentric phases and that involve all the joints in different way during different times of the stroke. For example, classic service starts with backswing. During this phase there are specific foot positions, knee in flexion, trunk and hip in rotation, shoulder in external rotation and wrist in extension. In this phase, all the external rotator muscles work in concentric fashion and internal rotators muscles in eccentric fashion; the forward swing continues with knee in extension, trunk and hip in de-rotation, shoulder in internal rotation, elbow in extension, wrist in flexion and hand in pronation. In this phase the internal rotator muscles work in concentric fashion and the external rotator muscles in eccentric fashion.

Regarding wrist biomechanics it is important to consider different phases during the different strokes. The role of the wrist and hand in tennis is to transfer energy from the body to the racquet and to deliver good spin and direction to the ball.

During the serve, the wrist starts in extension and supination of the hand in the cooking phase and then continues with flection and ulnar deviation during the acceleration phase with pronation of the hand. This movement gives more stable link between the wrist and racquet at the time of the strike with the ball and permits to give direction and spin to the ball at the same time. The muscles, FRC and FUC involved in flexion and ulnar deviation of the wrist, work in eccentric fashion during the cooking phase and concentric fashion during the acceleration phase. However, during the follow-through, the extensor muscles work in eccentric fashion to rapidly decelerate the wrist.

During the forehand and backhand strokes, the wrist moves in different fashion if the player is skill or novice. The position of the wrist in the last 10 years has completely changed during the forehand stroke according to grip changes. Most of the tennis players, in particular young players, use a Western or semi-Western grip. This extreme grip gives the possibility to give to the ball a topspin effect. During the hit, the wrist is positioned in extension and ulnar deviation and rapidly moved to flection and pronation. The flexor muscles (flexor carpi ulnaris and flexor carpi radialis) work in concentric fashion after eccentric loading. Extensor muscles (extensor carpi ulnaris) play an important role during the backswing for positioning the wrist in extension and ulnar deviation. Most of the modern tennis athletes practice the two-handed backhand stroke. Skilled players impact the ball with a hyperextended wrist and extend the hand through impact. That is, the extensor muscles about the wrist joint act concentrically to develop racquet speed through impact. However, novice players often strike the ball with the wrist flexed (13°), while moving the hand at the wrist joint into further flexion. That is, the extensor muscles about the wrist joint contract eccentrically, before the contraction concentrically following impact [1]. At the same time, during the two-handed backhand stroke, the distal hand moves (close to the racquet head) in same way of the hand of forehand stroke and becomes the leading hand. The non-dominant hand is moved from supination to pronation and from extension to flexion very quickly with the wrist in ulnar deviation. This movement is responsible for most of the wrist injuries in the non-dominant wrist during two-handed backhands.

21.3 Equipment

Modern racquets have enabled the ball to be hit with a higher speed than was possible with previous designs. Lighter racquets with larger "areas of percussion" and new string designs have all affected modern technique and are the primary reason for a number of changes to stroke production discussed below. Until the 1970s, the racquets were made of wood. The modern racquets are composed mainly of graphite and increase in head size, which was possible because of the greater strength of the new materials (from 27 × 9 in. [68.6 × 22.9 cm] to 29 × 12.5 in. [73.7 × 31.8 cm]). A second change was a decrease in mass, as wood is considerably denser than modern composite materials. Racquet mass has decreased from about 400–250 g today, despite being larger. This decrease in mass has the important spin off that players are able to swing the racquet faster, which generates higher impact speeds, resulting in faster ball speeds. By being wider, modern racquets have a greater polar moment of inertia (the resistance of the racquet to rotation about its longitudinal axis), which makes them more accommodating to off-centre hits. This not only renders play easier for the novice but also allows them to more rapidly improve technique [10]. Despite being lighter, modern racquets are also stiffer than wooden ones. As a result, they deform less and transmit vibration with high frequency to the hand and wrist. The ball-racket contact time is about 5–6 ms, which means that a racket needs to vibrate at a frequency of 166–200 Hz. Old wooden racquets vibrate at about 90 Hz.

Today's professional tennis is based on power. The increase in the size of racket heads makes it easier to apply topspin: a fact which has arguably contributed to today's playing style being based on power hitting. Power is not constant at all points on the racquet face. The physical characteristics described above contribute to the presence of what has become known as the "sweet spot". To fully understand the meaning of this term, the following are important:

Node—that point on the head of the racket where the vibration transmitted to the hand produced when the ball impacts the racket is minimum.

Centre of percussion—impacts at this location produce no acceleration of the handle in the hand, and thus no "shock" is transmitted to the player.

Maximum coefficient of restitution—the location on the strings where maximum ball speed is produced.

Because the locations described above are not coincident, the sweet spot is more of a "sweet area", with power peaking towards the centre of the head and dropping away towards the tip and throat. It does not follow, however, that the maximum ball speed will always result from hitting at the point where power is at its peak. Both synthetic and natural strings are used. Natural gut strings are made of cow gut and have superb elasticity, tension stability, and "liveliness". Synthetic strings are high-tech products that are now similar to natural gut strings but keep the advantage of synthetic materials' higher durability. Hybrid strings are a combination of two different strings for mains and crosses; we recorded strings as "hybrid" when the main strings were of natural gut and the cross ones synthetic or vice versa [2]. It is generally accepted that lower string tension generates more power, whereas higher tension gives more control. The choice of material is solely a matter of personal preference. Although modern racquet technology has produced many positive effects, it is arguable that injury rates have increased as a result. Anecdotal evidence suggests that the vast majority of upper limb injuries are chronic, having been developed over time through repetition [10].

21.4 Grips

It is important to describe the grip types because it is generally accepted that modification in technical equipment and grip is the reason of the high percentage of wrist injuries in modern tennis players. According to Tagliafico et al. [2], there are four basic single-handed grips used to hit the forehand: Continental, Eastern, semi-Western and full Western. For each grip, the player places the base knuckle of the index finger and the heel pad of the palm on the grip bevel of the racquet. Grips are defined according to the location of the base knuckle of the index finger on the eight faces of the racquet grip.

Continental (Fig. 21.1). The base knuckle is placed on face number 2, and the heel pad is between 1 and 2. Once the universal grip used to hit almost all strokes: forehands, backhands, special shots, volleys and the serve. It originated on the soft, low-bouncing clay courts of Europe. Today, it is usually employed only for serves and volleys.

Eastern (Fig. 21.2). In the Eastern grip, the base knuckle is on face 3, and the heel pad is between 2 and 3. This grip arose on the medium-bouncing courts in the eastern United States and represents the classic forehand grip as it is appropriate for different styles of play, comfortable for beginners and adaptable for all surfaces. The advantages of the Eastern grip are that it is easy for beginners to learn, generates power easily, is ideal for waist-high balls and can be used to hit a variety of topspin, underspin and flat drives. The disadvantage is that it is difficult to powerfully hit very high.

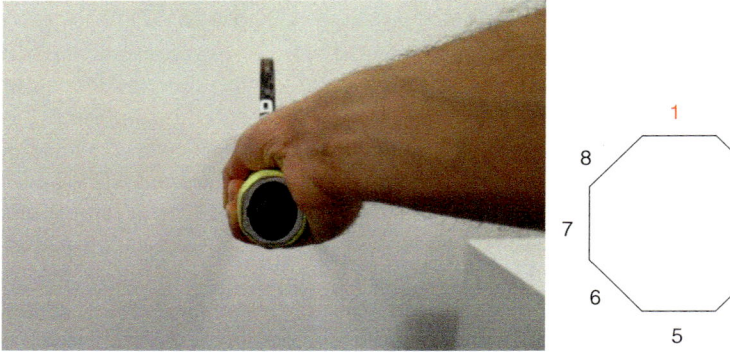

Fig. 21.1 Continental grip. At the side the position of base knuckle and heel pad on the racquet handle

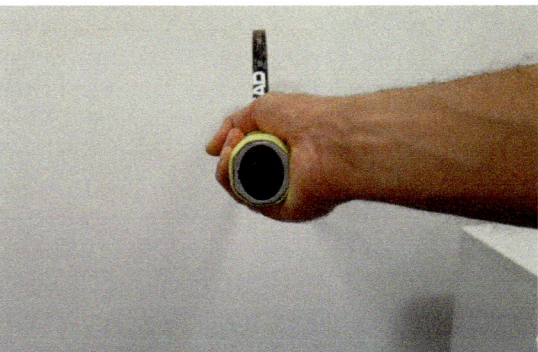
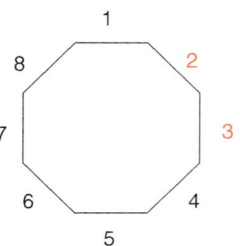

Fig. 21.2 Eastern grip. At side the position of the base knuckle and the heel pad on the racquet handle

Fig. 21.3 Semi-Western grip. At side the position of the base knuckle and the heel pad on the racquet handle

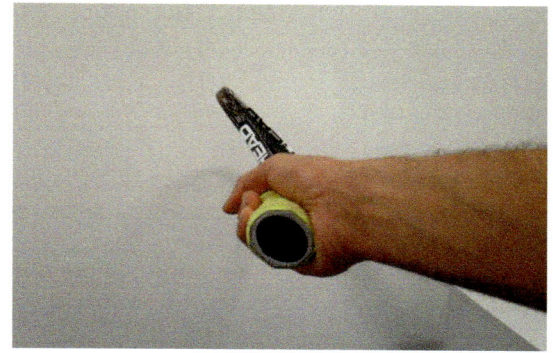
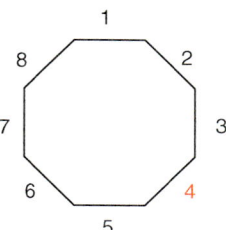

Fig. 21.4 Western grip. At side the position of the base knuckle and heel pad on the racquet handle

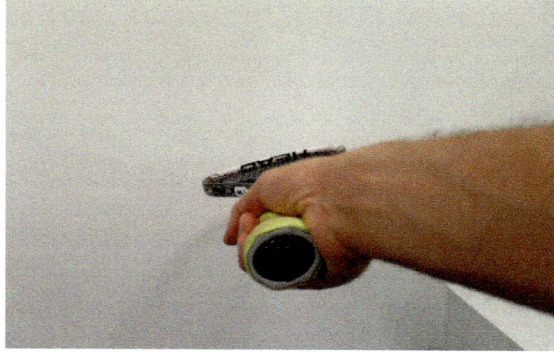
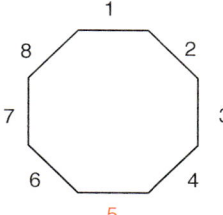

Semi-Western (Fig. 21.3). Both the base knuckle and the heel pad are on face 4. This grip guarantees both strength and control in the forehand, particularly facilitating powerful topspin forehands. Beginners feel comfortable because the palm of the hand supports the racquet, providing additional stability at contact. Powerful topspin forehands are the strokes facilitated by this grip. An advantage to this grip is that high balls are easy to hit; however, low balls and backspins are difficult, and grip changes are necessary to hit volleys and overheads.

Western (Fig. 21.4). Both the base knuckle and heel pad are located on face 5. Originating on the high-bouncing cement courts of the western United States, the drawback of this grip is that it closes the racket face too soon before contact. Excellent for high balls and topspin, it is however awkward for low balls and underspin. It is widely accepted that this grip is the most dangerous for the wrist and that a strong wrist and perfect timing are essential to avoid wrist injuries [2].

Most often the backhand stroke is executed using the two-handed backhand; it is generally accepted that this grip is correlated to injuries in the non-dominant hand.

21.5 Wrist Injuries

In the last 20 years, the tennis has become one of the most popular sport. Scores of non-professional athletes have improved and developed a more effective and aggressive game, thanks to changes in equipment and technique. Yet, they have done so without adequate physical training. The imbalance between the power of the strokes and the level of physical conditioning, which includes coordination, power, strength, speed, endurance and flexibility, is responsible for negative adaptive changes that may determine the injury pattern.

Wrist injuries, according to Tagliafico et al. [2], are correlated to the change in the grip. No statistical correlation was observed, in the same paper, between the group of injured players and the non-injured ones regarding body mass index, years of practice, weekly hours of training, racket weight and kind of strings [2]. Some evidence suggests that wrist pain/injury accounts for a higher percentage of total injuries reported in more recent studies (2014–2015; 7.6–11.8%) [11, 12] than in early studies (1986–1995; 2.3–3.8%) [13, 14]. Second, in 1986, Reece et al. [14] found that the relative frequency of wrist pain/injury (2.3%) was considerably less than that observed in well-recognized problem areas for tennis players, such as the shoulder complex (9.1%), elbow (7.4%) and lumbar spine (5.1%). However, a change in some of the more recent studies is noticeable, particularly among females [11, 15].

The most important groundstroke for professional and novice tennis players is the forehand. It is played with an open stance position: here the wrist plays a key role in developing angular momentum to increase the speed of the racquet head. Today's forehand is usually executed using extreme grips such as semi-Western or Western having considerable rotational motion (Fig. 21.5).

The ball is hit very hard with a significant topspin [16]. In this phase, it is possible to create sufficient stress on the wrist ulnar side to result in acute or repetitive trauma. It is also clear the association between ulnar-sided wrist pain in the non-dominant wrist and the use of a two-handed backhand [4] (Fig. 21.6).

The most important structure involved is extensor carpi ulnaris (ECU) tendon and its sheath and TFCC. The most common problem recorded by different authors is inflammation of the tendons and, rarely, lesions. As regards an Eastern grip, the increased wrist flexion described by Elliott et al. [17] could explain the flexor carpi radialis (FCR) tenosynovitis and the de Quervain syndrome, which typically occur in repeated flexion and extension movements. The dissimilar injury pattern associated with the different grips reflects the diverse biomechanical loads on the wrist joint developed by the traditional and modern strokes. Moreover, in Tagliafico article [2],

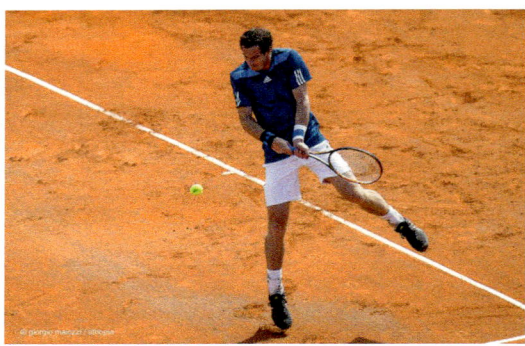

Fig. 21.6 The two-handed backhand

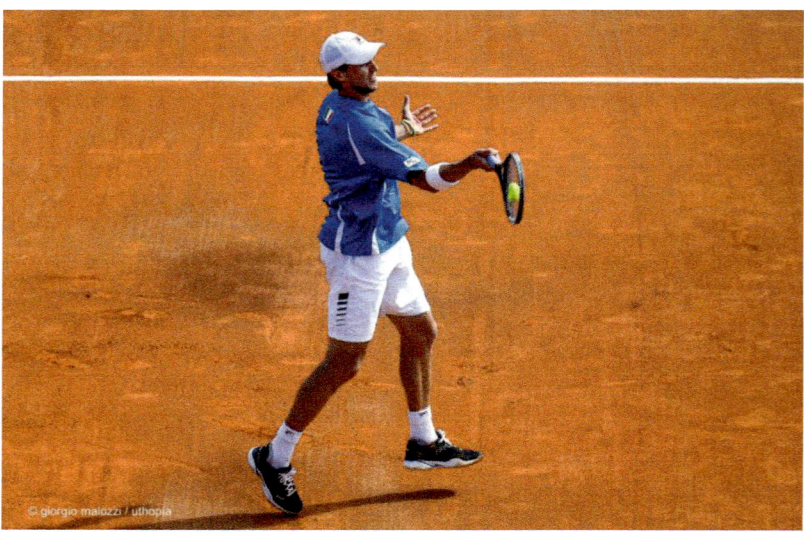

Fig. 21.5 The forehand stroke with Western grip

the Eastern grip players were significantly older (42 years) if compared to semi-Western and Western grip players (22) when they developed wrist injuries. This means that Eastern players had a significantly longer duration of activity that of semi-Western and Western grip players (20 years of activity vs. 8 years; $P < 0.01$).

21.5.1 ECU Injuries

The muscle fibres of the ECU tendon are described as ending in a tendon a little above the wrist. The tendon passes behind the lower end of the ulna in an osteofibrous sheath which runs through an osseous groove between the head of the ulna and its articular process. The tendon inserts on to the internal process of the fifth metacarpal [18]. The ECU tendon is stabilized in the osseous groove. It lies in the sixth compartment formed by duplication of the deep antebrachial fascia inserted on to the osseous groove, forming a tunnel (ECU subsheath) [19]. The dorsal retinaculum, which runs over the five dorsal compartments, passes above it, like a bridge. The retinaculum is not attached to the inferior ulna and inserts on to the triquetrum and pisiform, allowing both pronation and supination [19]. This tendon moves less freely than the other extensor tendons resulting in stress on the ECU tendon during pronation and supination. During pronation, the ECU tendon is situated on the inner surface of the ulnar head, far from the extensor digiti minimi. A gap is therefore created between the two tendons, with the ECU tendon having a direct course. During supination, the ECU tendon moves closer to the extensor digiti minimi, obliterating the space between the two. The ECU tendon is subjected to maximal traction and has to adopt an approximately 30° angle to reach the base of the fifth metacarpal. Changes in modern tennis play can explain severe stress on this tendon because of pronation-supination of the wrist in forehand and two hand backhand strokes. An interesting paper of Mantalvan [18] studied 28 cases of wrist pain in professional tennis players reporting 11.2% of wrist injuries in men and 15.7% in women in 5 years. Of this injuries, ECU pain accounts for 76% in men and 45% in women. Three distinct clinical entities which differed in their onset, clinical presentation and imaging and finally their outcome are described:

1. Traumatic instability of the ECU tendon. In this case, pain occurred suddenly, corresponding to a traumatic instability of the ECU tendon within the osteofibrous groove at the inferior section of the ulna.
2. Tendinopathy of the ECU. Here no initial trauma was reported. Pain occurred gradually and the clinical picture suggested ECU tendinopathy.
3. Rupture of the ECU tendon. Rare cases of complete ECU tendon rupture were described following a classic pattern.

21.5.2 Traumatic Instability of ECU

This injury occurs suddenly during a forehand or a backhand stroke. It is more common in non-dominant hand for two hand backhand stroke. In this case pain at the ulnar side of the wrist was severe, and the player was unable to resume play for a few minutes. Players most often describe the pain as violent but rarely reported rebound pain in the ulnar styloid. Recurrence of the pain can be seen as soon as the player tried to put topspin on the ball again. During the clinical examination, the patient has:

1. Intense pain on passive supination
2. Pain on palpation of the ECU tendon where it passes into the ulnar groove
3. Slight local swelling, which disappears after a few days

At times, upon evaluation, the wrist appears normal, and no pain is elicited during palpation of the ulnar groove. In this case, it is necessary to reproduce the instability through isometric stress in both resisted supination and pronation. Anatomically, two problems may present: (a) the ECU retinaculum has completely ruptured and the tendon left its sheath; (b) the tendon leaves the sheath during supination and recovers its

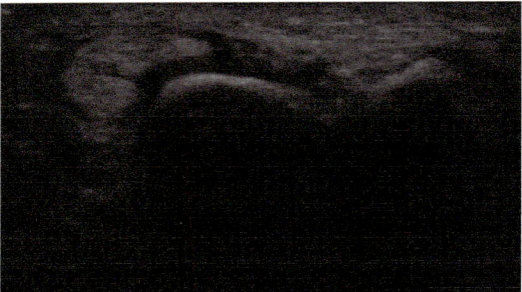

Fig. 21.7 Ultrasound view. ECU instability. Ulnar lesion of the sheath

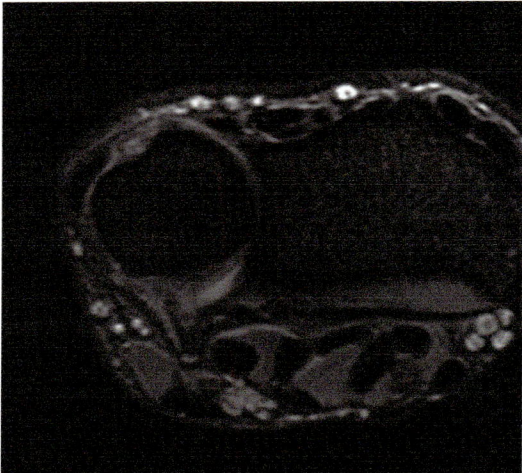

Fig. 21.8 MRI view. ECU instability. Ulnar lesion of the sheath

position during pronation. This is full ECU luxation [20, 21]. Three possible kinds of damage to the actual retinaculum are described in the literature [22]: ulnar rupture of the fibro-osseous sheath, whereby the torn sheath lies superficial to the tendon (type A) (Figs. 21.7 and 21.8); radial disruption of the fibro-osseous sheath, whereby the sheath lies in the ulnar groove beneath the tendon (type B); detachment of the periosteum from the ulnar side of the ulna, whereby the fibro-osseous sheath forms a false pouch (type C). Both training and experience are essential to an accurate and precise diagnosis of sheath lesions. Two imaging techniques are particularly useful: the first choice being an ultrasound scan at rest and during supination, using the method developed by JLB. In this case, two physicians are involved: one scans while the second attempts to exert stress during wrist supination. It is not always possible to reproduce ECU instability. MRI with millimetric slices of the ulnar sheath in T1, T1 STIR, T2, T2 and FATSAT GADO modes and comparative films obtained during pronation and supination of the wrist can also be useful.

21.5.3 Tendinopathy of the ECU

ECU tendinopathy develops gradually. The medical history is negative for an initial violent trauma or fall. It is the commonly occurring ECU injury; repeated microtrauma, the cause of the pain. In general, it is possible to continue to play tennis despite the pain, because, although the first strokes are painful, the pain lessens after warm up. Clinical examination shows ulnar-sided wrist pain. Pain with forced isometric supination is found in most of the cases. Slight swelling of the ulnar sheath associated with pain on palpation was sometimes observed. Ultrasound scan and MRI, using the same method described above, show normal stability of the ECU tendon without ulnar or radial-sided retinacular detachment. Fluid around the tendon, sometimes associated with tendon thickening or even intratendon fissures, was occasionally found in ultrasound and in MRI.

21.5.4 Rupture of the ECU Tendon

Rupture of ECU is a rare condition. It is possible after repetitive microtraumas and after corticosteroid injections. An initial accident was usually noted followed by recurrent pain and alternating periods of enforced rest and play. Players reported that the impact on daily life was minimal, but they were unable to use a double-handed backhand because of a lack of power in the wrist. During wrist examination, the tendon could not be palpated in its sheath. Ultrasound and MRI confirm that the ECU tendon sheath was empty. Relative literature [23–26] describes this problem in elite athletes [24–26], an initial violent trauma, several episodes of ulnar-sided wrist pain, several local corticosteroid injections and eventually ending in tendon rupture.

21.5.5 Treatment of ECU Injuries

Many cases described can be managed by conservative measures and rehabilitation. The necessarily long rest period involved in a conservative treatment approach might suggest, at times, surgical management for professional tennis players. A distinction must be made between stable and unstable conditions of the tendon. Tendon subluxation is a difficult condition to evaluate and may occur in asymptomatic patients. Management remains controversial.

21.6 Triangular Fibrocatilage Complex (TFCC) Injuries

The triangular fibrocartilage complex is the ligamentous and cartilaginous structures that separates the radio-carpal from the distal radio-ulnar joint. The TFCC consists of an articular disc, meniscus homologue, ulnocarpal ligament, dorsal and volar radio-ulnar ligament and extensor carpi ulnaris sheath. It originates from firm attachments on medial border of distal radius and inserts into the base of the ulnar styloid. The vascular supply is only in the peripheral 15–20% of the TFCC. Ulnar attachment of the TFCC is anchored by two bands inserting to the styloid process and fovea (base of the styloid). Volar ulnocarpal ligaments run from the base of the ulnar styloid process across the volar surface of the TFCC and then insert on the lunate and triquetrum; ulnocarpal ligaments include volar ulno-lunate and ulnotriquetral ligaments. These ligaments prevent dorsal migration of the distal ulna and are more stretched during supination of the wrist. The TFCC is responsible for stabilizing the distal radio-ulnar joint, as well as contributing to ulnocarpal stability; it is important in loading and stabilizing of distal radio-ulnar joint. TFCC normally, not only stabilizes the ulnar head in sigmoid notch of radius, but also acts as a buttress to support proximal carpal row. Volar TFCC prevents dorsal displacement of ulna and is tight in pronation. Dorsal TFCC prevents volar displacement of ulna and is tight in supination. During axial loading, the radius carries the majority of load (82%) and the ulna a smaller load (18%). Increasing the ulnar variance to a positive 2.5 mm increases the load transmission across the TFCC to 42%. If the TFCC is excised, the radial load increases to 94%. The occurrence of sports-related injuries of the TFCC can be due to both acute trauma and overuse and is a common cause of ulnar-sided wrist pain in the athlete. Acute traumatic injuries result from significant axial load through the wrist but are rare in tennis players. Repetitive microtrauma of the wrist, like that occurring in tennis players, with wrist in extension, ulnar deviation and supination, can create TFCC lesions, specially if there is a positive ulnar variance. The relationship between TFCC injury and the use of Western or semi-Western forehand grips has been attributed to increased loading of the ulnar wrist structures [2]. Clinical examination of the wrist with ulnar pain starts with TFCC palpation directly at the ulnar side of the wrist. Testing the wrist with ulnar deviation combined with axial load, supination and pronation may also reproduce the symptoms. At time, TFCC tears that are symptomatic often note a painful click during wrist motions. As the TFCC is a major stabilizer to the distal radio-ulnar joint (DRUJ), its stability should be checked on examination by assessing motion of the ulna relative to the radius. DRUJ motion should be compared with that of the contralateral wrist in a similar position of forearm rotation to differentiate normal from pathologic laxity.

It is important to demonstrate a pathognomonic abnormality of the bone on radiographic evaluation. Secondary findings, such as positive ulnar variance or ulnar styloid fracture, also may be demonstrated, which may aid in diagnosis. Fractures of the ulnar styloid base may destabilize the TFCC and DRUJ. MRI evaluation, with or without arthrography, is sensitive for detection of TFCC pathology. Various articles disagree regarding the accuracy of MRI for TFCC lesion evaluation. Recent studies suggest that MRI can detect abnormalities in many asymptomatic wrists [27, 28]. It is quite likely that peripheral TFCC injuries (Fig. 21.9) may be more difficult

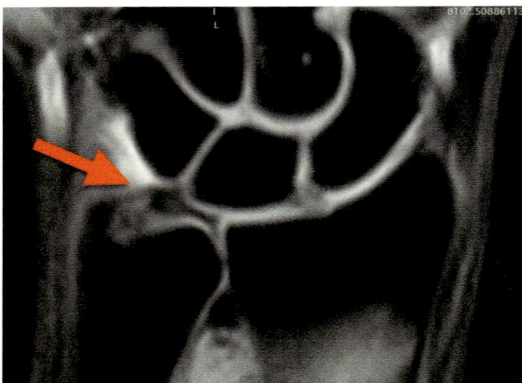

Fig. 21.9 Ulnar side lesion of TFCC (L. Pegoli M.D. courtesy)

Table 21.1 Palmer Classification of the TFCC lesions

Palmer classification for triangular fibrocartilage complex (TFCC) lesions is based on the cause, location and degree of injury

Class 1—traumatic injury
(a) Central perforation
(b) Ulnar avulsion with or without distal ulnar fracture may involve the proximal or distal lamina (foveal and styloid attachment, respectively) or both
(c) Distal avulsion
(d) Radial avulsion with or without sigmoid notch fracture

Class 2—degenerative injury (ulnocarpal abutment syndrome)
(a) TFCC wear
(b) TFCC wear with lunate and/or ulnar chondromalacia
(c) TFCC perforation with lunate and/or ulnar chondromalacia
(d) TFCC perforation with lunate and/or ulnar chondromalacia and lunotriquetral ligament perforation
(e) TFCC perforation with lunate and/or ulnar chondromalacia, lunotriquetral ligament perforation and ulnocarpal arthritis

to detect than central or radial tears due to the more complex anatomy and focal synovitis at the ulnar TFCC attachment. This was also reported in a study by Oneson et al. [29], in which the sensitivity for detection of ulnar-sided tears was only 25–50% compared with 86–100% for central and radial tears. The physician should always be aware of false positives case and make a careful clinical examination to confirm diagnosis. Arthroscopy remains the gold standard for diagnosis of TFCC pathology [30]. In Palmer classification system (Table 21.1), tears of the TFCC are classified as either traumatic or degenerative [31]. Blood supply to the TFCC is more robust peripherally and relatively avascular centrally [31, 32]. This anatomy guides surgical treatment.

21.6.1 Treatment of TFCC Injuries

Nonoperative treatments are usually the initial form of management for the TFCC lesions and consist of rest, immobilization, physical therapy and cortisone injection. Arthroscopic debridement or repair for tears of the TFCC has proven successful for patients who fail to respond to the usual nonoperative treatments.

A study by McAdams [33] shows that arthroscopic debridement or repair of the TFCC is successful in competitive athletes who require a high level of wrist function for performance.

Depending on the type of TFCC lesions, if there are ulnar or radial lesions, it is useful to suture using specific technique. All inside techniques, like the meniscus repair, showed the best results. Sutures give good results due of the good vascular supply of the peripheral portions of the TFCC. When the lesion affects central portion of the TFCC, only debridement is performed because of the absence of vascularity supply. Wrist immobilization time depends on the procedure performed. After TFCC suture 6 weeks of immobilization in a short arm splint is recommended. Subsequently 6 weeks of progressive range-of-motion and strengthening exercises with full return to sport allowed at 3 months postoperatively. Postoperatively, patients with debrided central lesions of the TFCC are splinted for 1 week and range of motion is begun. Bednar and Osterman [34] reported 90% good-to-excellent results with debridement of the centrum. In degenerative triangular fibrocartilage complex lesions or acute or chronic injuries, the ulnar variance must be carefully assessed. In neutral and positive variance, the option of ulnar shortening, either by a Feldon wafer resection [35] or formal ulnar shortening with plate fixation, should be discussed with the athlete. The Feldon wafer technique is indicated in cases of an ulnar variance of <3 mm and may be performed open or arthroscopically [36]. In cases with more than 3 mm positive variance, a formal open ulnar shortening with 3.5 compression plate fixation is indicated, accompanied by wrist arthroscopy. Several articles have demonstrated a high rate of the recurrent ulnar synovitis if the patient was allowed to return too quickly to play tennis, even after TFCC debridement alone. For example, the patients with ECU tendonitis were not allowed to return to play until 7 months postoperatively [33].

21.7 Hook of the Hamate Fractures

Fractures of the hook of the hamate are more common in athletes. The incidence of hook of the hamate fractures is 2–4% of all carpal fractures [37–41]. The mechanism of injury is thought to be caused by abutment of the hook on an object or by a shearing force applied by the flexor tendon of the small and ring fingers [41, 42].

The injury usually occurs in athletes who participate in baseball, golf and racquet sports because of the position of the instrument of play in the hand. Repetitive microtrauma can lead to a stress fracture (Fig. 21.10). Fracture anatomy has been studied: of note is a watershed area that may explain the high incidence of nonunion postfractures [43, 44].

Hook of the hamate fracture should be suspected in athletes participating in racquet sports, golf or baseball who are seen with ulnar wrist pain. Physical examination reveals pain over the hook of the hamate during palpation. The hook of the hamate is found a line between the pisiform and second metacarpal head. X-ray for carpal tunnel (30° of wrist extension) (Fig. 21.11) and lateral views of the wrist can help in correct diagnosis. A high density CT scan (Fig. 21.12) with the wrists in the "praying position" using 2 mm cuts in the axial and sagittal plane allows

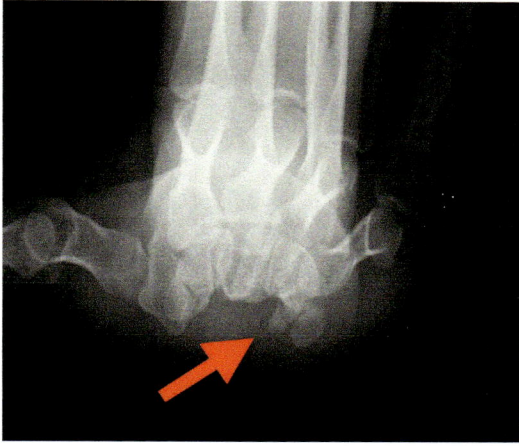

Fig. 21.11 X-ray of the wrist. The carpal tunnel view shows the fracture of the hook of hamate

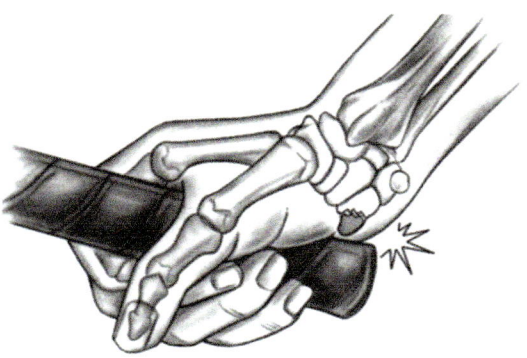

Fig. 21.10 The repetitive trauma during the tennis play on the heel pad of the hand can create a stress fracture of the hook of the hamate

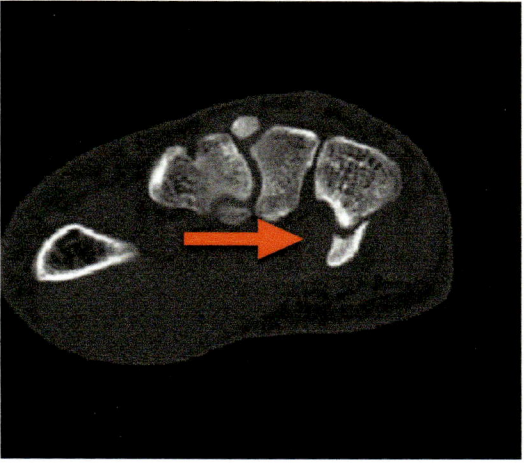

Fig. 21.12 CT scan of the wrist. The red arrow indicates the hook of the hamate fracture

comparison between the two wrists, have a sensitivity of 100%, specificity of 98.4% and accuracy of 97.2% [45], and is the radiographic technique of choice in the diagnosis of hook of the hamate fractures.

21.7.1 Treatment of Hook of the Hamate Fracture

Treatment of hook of the hamate fractures in athletes varies from casting to open reduction and internal fixation to excision. The fixation with screw is possible with volar or dorsal approach. Excision is the most popular procedure and gives good results. Fractures can be treated also conservatively with immobilization involving the fourth and fifth fingers for 5/6 weeks with specific cast.

> **Conclusion**
>
> The increase in the incidence of wrist complications in tennis players over recent years requires that closer attention be paid to these pathologies. Changes in grip, equipment and the pressing request for ever higher performance in modern play is clearly an important factor in the increase in wrist injuries. Both players and coaches need more information so as to improve technical gestures and prevent serious problematics from arising.

References

1. Elliott B. Biomechanics and tennis. Br J Sports Med. 2006;40:392–6.
2. Tagliafico A, Ameri P, Michaud J, Derchi LE, Sormani MP, Martinoli C. Wrist injuries in nonprofessional tennis players: relationships with different grips. Am J Sports Med. 2009;37(4):760–7.
3. Pluim BM, Staal JB, Windler GE, et al. Tennis injuries: occurrence, aetiology, and prevention. Br J Sports Med. 2006;40(5):415–23.
4. Kibler WB, Safran MR. Tennis injuries. Med Sport Sci. 2005;48:120–37.
5. Loosli AR, Leslie M. Stress fractures of the distal radius. Am J Sports Med. 1991;19(5):523–4.
6. Rettig AC. Stress fracture of the ulna in an adolescent tournament tennis player. Am J Sports Med. 1983;11(2):103–6.
7. Kibler B. Kinetic Chain contributions to elbow function and dysfunction in sports. Clin Sports Med. 2004;23:545–52.
8. Walshe A, Wison G, Ettema G. Stretch-shorten cycle compared with isometric preload: contributions to enhanced muscular performance. J Appl Physiol. 1998;89:97–106.
9. Reid M, Elliott B. The one- and two-handed backhands in tennis. Sports Biomech. 2002;1:47–68.
10. Miller S. Modern tennis rackets, balls, and surfaces. Br J Sports Med. 2006;40:401–5. https://doi.org/10.1136/bjsm.2005.023283.
11. Stuelcken M, Mellifont D, Gorman A, Sayers M. Wrist injuries in tennis players: a narrative review. Sports Med. 2016;47(5):857.
12. Lynall RC, Kerr ZY, Djoko A, et al. Epidemiology of national collegiate athletic association men's and women's tennis injuries, 2009/2010–2014/2015. Br J Sports Med. 2016;50(19):1211–6.
13. Hutchinson MR, Laprade RF, Burnett QM, et al. Injury surveillance at the usta boys' tennis championships: a 6-yr study. Med Sci Sports Exerc. 1995;27(6):826–31.
14. Reece LA, Fricker PA, Maguire KF. Injuries to elite young tennis players at the Australian Institute of Sport. Aust J Sci Med Sport. 1986;18:11.
15. Sell K, Hainline B, Yorio M, et al. Injury trend analysis from the us open tennis championships between 1994 and 2009. Br J Sports Med. 2014;48(7):546–51.
16. Bahamonde R, Knudson D. Kinematics analysis of the open and square stance in tennis forehand. J Sci Med Sport. 2003;6(1):88–101.
17. Elliott B, Marsh T. A biomechanical comparison of the top-spin and back-spin forehand approach shots in tennis. J Sports Sci. 1989;7:215–27.
18. Montalvan B, Parier J, Brasseur JL, Le Viet D, Drape JL. Extensor carpi ulnaris injuries in tennis players: a study of 28 cases. J Sports Med. 2006;40:424–9. https://doi.org/10.1136/bjsm.2005.0232759.
19. Spinner M, Kaplan EB. Extensor carpi ulnaris. Its relationship to the stability of the distal radio-ulnar joint. Clin Orthop Relat Res. 1970;68:124–9.
20. Rayan GM. Recurrent dislocation of the extensor carpi ulnaris in athletes. Am J Sports Med. 1983;11:183–4.
21. Vulpius J. Habitual dislocation of the extensor carpi ulnaris tendon. Acta Orthop Scand. 1964;34:105–8.
22. Inoue G, Tamura Y. Recurrent dislocation of the extensor carpi ulnaris tendon. Br J Sports Med. 1998;32:172–4.
23. Allende C, Le Viet D. Extensor carpi problems at the wrist: classification, surgical treatment and results. J Hand Surg Br. 2005;30:265–72.
24. Palmer AK, Shaken JR, Werner FW, et al. The extensor retinaculum of the wrist; an anatomical and biomechanical study. J Hand Surg Br. 1985;10:11–6.

25. Solomon L. Tenovaginitis of the extensor carpi ulnaris. South Afr Med J. 1964;38:42–4.
26. Angerman P. Post traumatic partial rupture of the extensor carpi ulnaris tendon. Scand J Hand Surg. 1993;27:321–2.
27. Blazar PE, Chan PS, Kneeland JB, Leatherwood D, Bozentka DJ, Kowalchick R. The effect of observer experience on magnetic resonance imaging interpretation and localization of triangular fibrocartilage complex lesions. J Hand Surg Am. 2001;26:742–8.
28. Iordache SD, Rowan R, Garvin GJ, Osman S, Grewal R, Faber KJ. Prevalence of triangular fibrocartilage complex abnormalities on MRI scans of asymptomatic wrists. J Hand Surg Am. 2012;37:98–103.
29. Oneson SR, Timins ME, Scales LM, Erickson SJ, Chamoy L. MR imaging diagnosis of triangular fibrocartilage pathology with arthroscopic correlation. AJR Am J Roentgenol. 1997;168:1513–8.
30. Rosner JL, Zlatkin MB, Clifford P, Ouellette EA, Awh MH. Imaging of athletic wrist and hand injuries. Semin Musculoskelet Radiol. 2004;8:57–79.
31. Palmer AK. Triangular fibrocartilage complex lesions: a classification. J Hand Surg Am. 1989;14:594–606.
32. Nagle DJ. Triangular fibrocartilage complex tears in the athlete. Clin Sports Med. 2001;20:155–66.
33. McAdams TR, Swan J, Yao J. Arthroscopic treatment of triangular fibrocartilage wrist injuries in the athlete. Am J Sports Med. 2009;37(2):291–7. https://doi.org/10.1177/0363546508325921.
34. Bednar JM, Osterman AL. The role of arthroscopy in the treatment of traumatic triangular fibrocartilage injuries. Hand Clin. 1994;10:605–14.
35. Rettig AC. Athletic injuries of the wrist and hand. Part I: traumatic injuries of the wrist. Am J Sports Med. 2003;31:1038–48.
36. Feldon P, Terrono AL, Belsky MR. Wafer distal ulna resection for triangular fibrocartilage tears and/or ulna impaction syndrome. J Hand Surg. 1992;17A:731–7.
37. Bishop AT, Beckenbaugh RD. Fracture of the hamate hook. J Hand Surg. 1988;13A:135–9.
38. Bowen TL. Injuries of the hamate bone. Hand. 1973;5:235–8.
39. Bryan RS, Dobyns JH. Fractures of the carpal bones other than lunate and navicular. Clin Orthop. 1980;(149):107–11.
40. Murray PM, Cooney WP. Golf-induced injuries of the wrist. Clin Sports Med. 1996;15:85–109.
41. Weber ER, Chao EY. An experimental approach to the mechanism of scaphoid waist fractures. J Hand Surg. 1978;3A:142–8.
42. Stark HH, Jobe FW, Boyes JH, et al. Fracture of the hook of the hamate in athletes. J Bone Joint Surg. 1977;59A:575–82.
43. Failla JM. Hook of hamate vascularity: vulnerability to osteonecrosis and nonunion. J Hand Surg. 1993;18A:1075–9.
44. Panagis JS, Gelberman RH, Taleisnik J, et al. The arterial anatomy of the human carpus. Part II: The intraosseous vascularity. J Hand Surg. 1983;8A:375–82.
45. Egawa M, Asai T. Fractures of the hook of the hamate: report of six cases and the suitability of computerised tomography. J Hand Surg. 1983;8:393.

Wrist and Hand Rehabilitation

Belinda Herde and Kathleen A. Stroia

22.1 Wrist Pathology and Diagnosis

Wrist injuries can be traumatic or overuse [1], while most wrist injuries are reported to be overuse in tennis. Injuries to the wrist may include ganglion cyst from repetitive overuse, tendinopathy, stress fractures, ligament sprains, and cartilage injuries. Wrist injuries can generally be classified as radial or ulnar sided. Common ulnar-sided complaints include the extensor carpi ulnaris (ECU) tendon and/or the triangular fibrocartilage complex (TFCC). Repetitive trauma may also cause injury to the hook of hamate bone. Radial-sided injuries may include dorsal carpal ganglion cyst, de Quervain's tenosynovitis, scapholunate injury, and scaphoid fracture. A thorough history, clinical examination, and sound diagnosis are required to comprehensively rehabilitate a wrist and hand injury. Clinical examination and history may guide diagnosis; however, medical imaging may be required for further investigation. Once a diagnosis is made, a thorough treatment plan needs to be established with the athlete, coach, and medical team. See Chap. 21 for further pathophysiology of wrist and hand injuries.

22.2 Management

A treatment plan needs to be established including required rest (if any from sport/activity), workload management, treatment interventions, and any potential operative treatment. Predisposing factors to wrist injury need to be identified, and then the early goals of management include reducing pain and restoring normal range of motion and strength. Assessment and review of proper technique is a primary goal for rehabilitation and to prevent injury recurrence. Treatment options to include in a wrist management plan include manual therapy, taping, splinting, anti-inflammatory medications, exercise therapy, biomechanics, and equipment assessment [2]. Prior to returning to competition, adequate rehabilitation including a progressive strengthening program, core stabilization inclusive of the kinetic chain, and sports-specific training is required. Prevention of recurrence of injury may also require addressing stroke biomechanics, equipment (string type and tension, weight balance of racquet, grip size, and overgrip), and grip placement (Continental, Eastern, semi-Western, or Western grip) [3].

B. Herde
Primary Health Care Provider, WTA Women's Tennis Association, St. Petersburg, FL, USA

Director and Sports Physiotherapist,
Grand Slam Physiotherapy, Geelong, Australia
e-mail: BSmith@wtatennis.com

K. A. Stroia (✉)
Sport Sciences and Medicine and Transitions,
WTA Women's Tennis Association,
St. Petersburg, FL, USA
e-mail: KStroia@wtatennis.com

22.3 Manual Therapy

Manual therapy aims to restore normal pain-free range of motion by applying techniques to the musculoskeletal system. Manual therapy to the wrist may include therapies such as nerve gliding, stretching, joint mobilization, soft tissue and massage techniques, and Mulligan therapy. Manual therapy techniques may have positive treatment effects such as increased range of motion of the wrist, release of tissue adhesions, and improvements in blood flow through increased joint motion [4]. Thorough assessment is essential to assess for restrictions in movement, and treatment efficacy can be evaluated through reassessment following treatment. Combinations of treatment techniques and individualization are more likely to be successful than single techniques, combined with thorough clinical reasoning.

Following a sustained period of immobilization, athletes are generally stiff with a loss of mobility and considerable muscle wasting. Using the management guidelines of the attending physician, mobilization of the wrist and strengthening should occur as soon as able following immobilization. After either operative or non-operative immobilization, early range of motion particularly to fingers and swelling should be emphasized. Once adequate tissue healing or fracture healing, wrist and forearm range of motion should be a focus with progressive strengthening when adequate range of motion is established.

22.3.1 Joint Mobilization

The mechanism of treatment effects within the wrist is unknown; however, joint mobilization based on the Maitland technique is thought to have biomechanical, neurological modulation and activate central nervous system mechanisms that control pain and modulation of autonomic function [5]. Joint mobilization to the wrist may include general distractions and glides to the radiocarpal joint and both the proximal and distal row of carpals as a group (Fig. 22.1). For a restriction in flexion, a dorsal glide may be applied to the radiocarpal joint, whereas a volar glide may target increasing extension range of

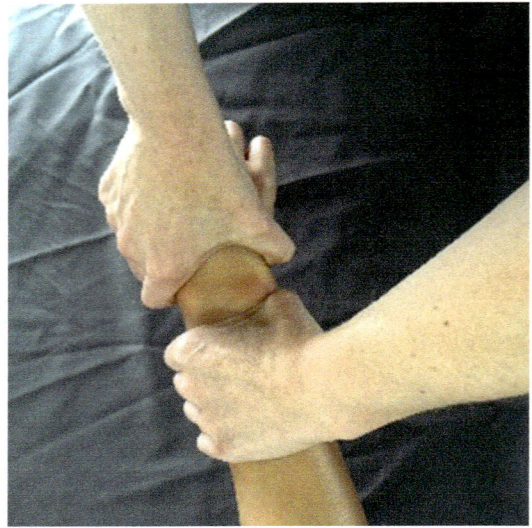

Fig. 22.1 Radio-carpal joint mobilization: the radius and ulnar are stabilized, while a posterior-anterior glide is applied to the carpals

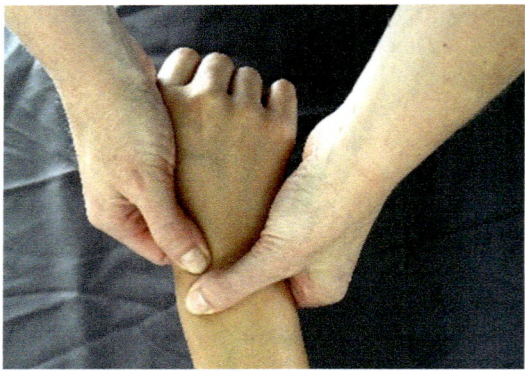

Fig. 22.2 Carpal glide: individual carpal bones may be mobilized, whereby adjacent carpal bone is stabilized while a glide is applied to restricted carpal bone

motion. A radial glide may increase ulnar deviation, and ulnar glide increases radial deviation to the radiocarpal joint. If there is a segmental restriction within the intercarpal joints, individual carpal joint mobilizations may be required (Fig. 22.2). Assessment may find a specific carpal restriction, and then treatment may be applied in volar or dorsal direction by stabilizing proximal carpal bone and gliding distal bone. To increase mobility of the hand, carpometacarpal, intermetacarpal, metacarpophalangeal, and interphalangeal joint mobilization of the digits may be applied with glides and distraction. Joint mobilization when combined with therapeutic ultrasound is reported to be effective at restoring full active range of movement in the wrist following wrist injury or surgery [6]. Manual therapy, carpal bone joint mobilization, and nerve gliding exercises have also been reported to be effective in the treatment of carpal tunnel syndrome [7, 8].

22.3.2 Proximal-Directed Treatment

Tennis shot play requires interplay of multiple proximal and distal joint segments to produce a stroke. A breakdown or restriction in a proximal segment may place excess stress on the distal segments such as the wrist. Therefore, thorough assessment of the kinetic chain including neck, shoulder, and trunk mobility is required including motor control and strength of these areas. Treatment can then be applied to any deficits. Treating proximal structures may have some efficacy in treatment of the wrist, with some evidence supporting neck manipulation in the treatment of lateral epicondylagia [9]. Proximal treatment techniques may include joint mobilization and/or manipulation, neural glides, and soft tissue therapy.

22.3.3 Soft Tissue Therapy

There are a number of soft tissue techniques that may be applied in and around the upper extremity with the goal of improving wrist function including Active Release Technique, digital ischemic pressure, massage, trigger point therapy, friction, connective tissue techniques (e.g., skin rolling), and myofascial release. Soft tissue techniques were found to have clinical efficacy in improving nerve conduction latencies, wrist strength, and motion in carpal tunnel syndrome with both Graston instrument-assisted soft tissue mobilization and soft tissue mobilization being effective [4]. Active trigger points, hypertonicity, and muscle shortening may be found in the forearm and hand in athletes with wrist pathology. Forearm posterior compartment muscles to direct treatment toward may include brachioradialis, extensor carpi radialis longus and brevis, extensor digitorum, extensor carpi ulnaris, extensor digiti minimi, and anconeus. Forearm anterior compartment muscles to assess for treatment include pronator teres and quadratus, flexor carpi radialis and ulnaris, palmaris longus, flexor digitorum superficialis, and profundus. Some of the hand muscles to assess include abductor digiti minimi, interosseous muscles, abductor/adductor/extensor, and flexor pollicis muscles, to name a few. Symptoms should be reassessed after treatment.

22.3.4 Stretching

Stretching may include static or proprioceptive neuromuscular facilitation (PNF) with the aim of improving muscle flexibility, reducing stiffness, and improving stretch tolerance. Following injury or to prevent injury, flexibility may need to be restored to normal range of movement. Stretching may play a role in injury prevention in dynamic sports involving the stretch-shortening cycle [10]. Static stretching is reported to be most effective with at least a 30–60 s duration and is required to be performed at least once a day for benefits. PNF uses muscle inhibition by relaxing the muscle prior to stretching, and may commonly use an agonist contraction. Figure 22.3 shows a stretch of the wrist extensors and flexors; a static stretch should be held for 30–60 s with 2–3 sets daily, while a PNF technique may involve an isometric contraction of the wrist extensors followed by a stretch of wrist extensors to point of resistance.

22.3.5 Muscle Energy Technique

There is no known research into muscle energy technique at the wrist; however, this may be another adjunctive treatment option to restore normal movement in local and proximal segments. Muscle energy technique aims to identify and treat asymmetry or dysfunction within the musculoskeletal system by applying low-intensity isometric contractions of the agonist or antagonist muscle in an attempt to relax the muscle and restore symmetry.

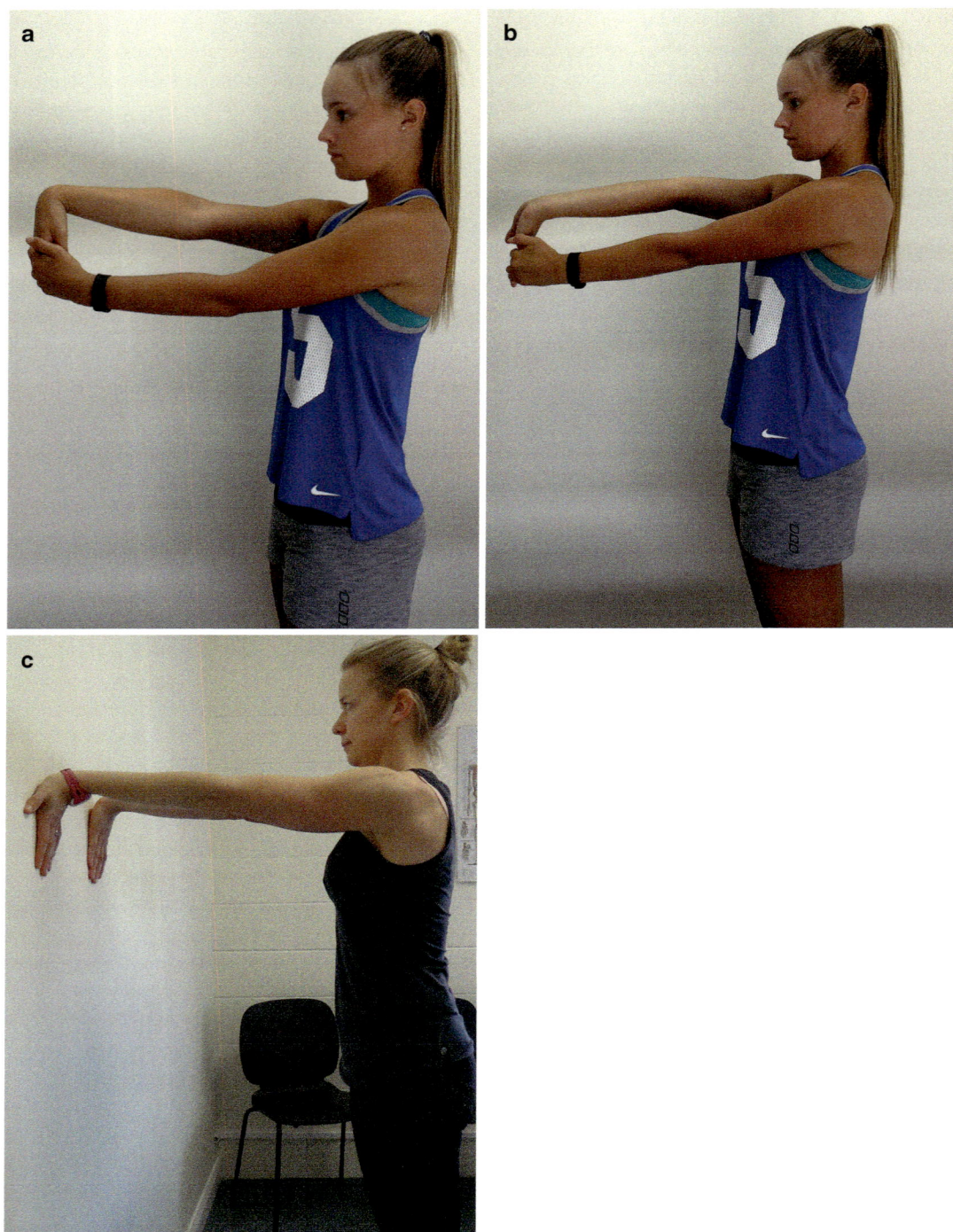

Fig. 22.3 Wrist extensor (**a**) and wrist flexor/pronator (**b**, **c**) stretches. The wall stretch is also effective in restoring supination range of motion

22.3.6 Mulligan Mobilization with Movement

Brian Mulligan developed a joint mobilization combined with movement technique, which is reported to improve function while reducing pain [11]. Various techniques can be applied to the hand, wrist, forearm, and elbow in an attempt to normalize range of motion. Figure 22.4 demonstrates a volar glide to the radiocarpal joint combined with extension to target increasing extension range of motion.

22.3.7 Neural Tissue Mobilization

Abnormality to neural tension should be assessed through the upper limb tension tests. If adverse neural tension is contributing to symptoms, neural mobilization and treatment to adjacent tissues such as the fascia, muscle, skin, and joints may be an effective treatment to restore neural tension and mechanics of the nervous system [12]. Neural symptoms may be irritable; therefore, treatment techniques should monitor symptoms closely and may include passive neural mobilization techniques and home mobilizing exercises such as gliders and sliders (Fig. 22.5). Treatment of neurodynamics was found to be effective in carpal tunnel syndrome [7].

22.3.8 Dry Needling

Dry needling is where a fine filament needle is placed intramuscular or into a myofascial trigger point causing a local twitch response, with a goal of reducing pain and muscle tension. There is emerging literature supporting dry needle insertion in neuromusculoskeletal conditions throughout the body at non-trigger point sites with the goal of stimulating neural, muscular, and connective tissues while reducing pain and improving function. Varying research exists into the effectiveness of dry needling; however, it is reported to have a positive effect on pain [13, 14] and alter myofascial trigger points [14]. In their systematic review of dry needling, Dunning et al. suggest more high-quality trials are required to determine long-term efficacy of dry needling and to determine optimal frequency, duration, and intensity. Techniques may include sustained dry needling where needles are left in situ for 5–40 min and in-and-out techniques that target trigger points such as pistoning or sparrow pecking. A paucity of literature exists into treating wrist pain with dry needling, although it has been advocated in wrist extensors in lateral epicondylagia [15]. Dry needling has been supported in treating Achilles tendinopathy [16]; however, more research is required in the wrist to determine efficacy. Treatment with dry needling may be to local hypertonic or taut muscles, with the goal of reducing muscle tension and inhibiting activity of myofascial trigger points (Fig. 22.6). Treating myofascial trigger points proximal to wrist may also have some benefit, whereby dry needling of myofascial trigger points in patients with shoulder pain was found to inhibit activity of myofascial trigger points in the shoulder, elbow, and forearm [17].

22.3.9 Electrotherapy

Electrotherapy modalities may be used in the treatment of sporting injuries including ultrasound, transcutaneous electrical stimulation, interferential stimulation, laser, and extracorporeal shock wave therapy. Electrotherapy is

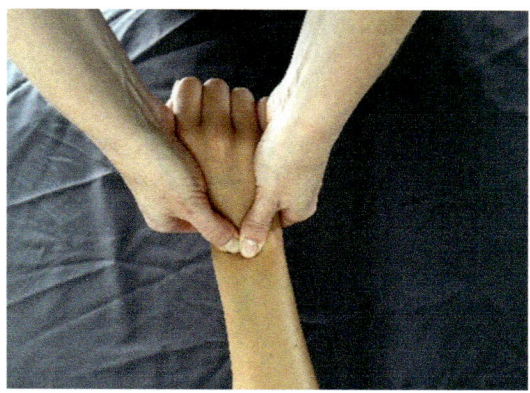

Fig. 22.4 Mulligan technique: a glide is applied to carpal bones, while active or passive extension of the wrist is simultaneously applied

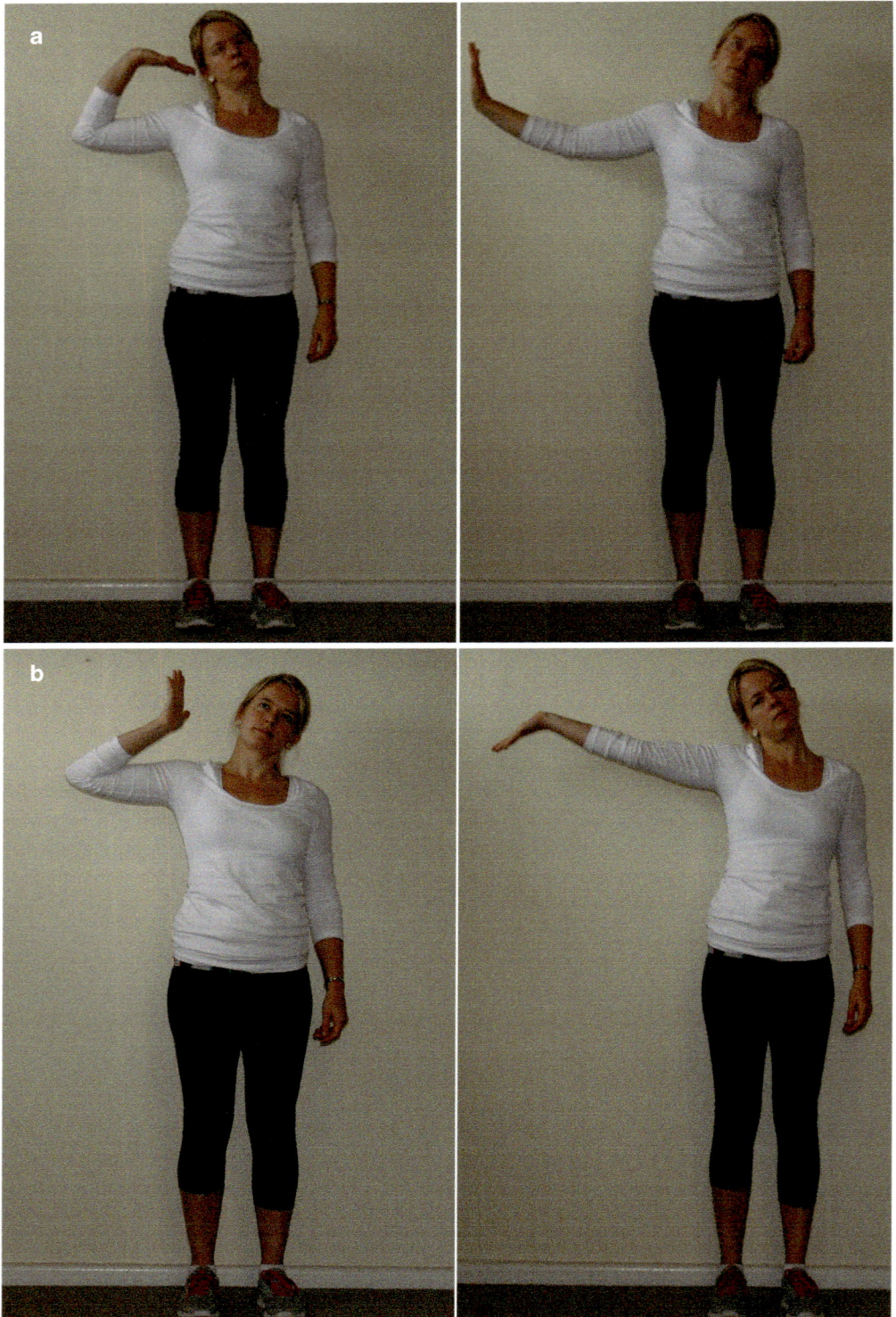

Fig. 22.5 Neurodynamics: (**a**) an ulnar nerve glide and (**b**) median nerve glide home exercise technique; 1–2 sets of 10–15 repetitions may be performed in an attempt to improve neural mobility

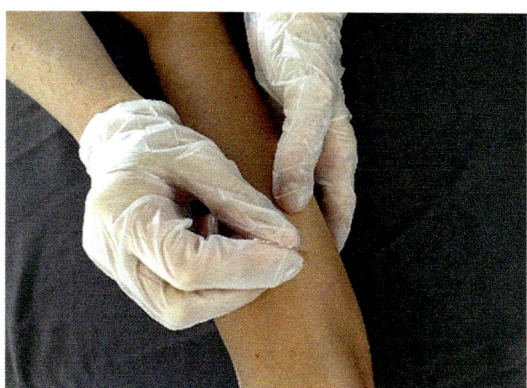

Fig. 22.6 Dry needling technique to the extensor carpi radialis brevis muscle

reported to promote healing and reduce inflammation. The use of these modalities is varied among health professionals, with varying and limited scientific evidence to support use of electrotherapy. Therefore, clinical experience should drive the use of electrotherapy, and it would be advised to use as an adjunctive treatment option.

22.3.10 Cryotherapy

Icing is effective following acute injury with a goal of reducing tissue metabolism, pain, and inflammation [18]. It may also be used as a therapeutic modality to provide pain relief, in the later stages of injury. High-quality evidence is lacking for duration of ice application; however, it is suggested at least 10 min [19] of ice therapy is required every 1–2 h after acute injury and may be applied following activity when used subacutely in injury with either sustained application for 10 min or 5–10 min of ice massage.

22.4 Exercise Therapy

Exercise therapy may initially include active assisted, active, or mobility exercises to restore range of movement then progressing through a strengthening program to restore full strength. Exercise protocols will be highly individualized depending on pathology, severity, and treating surgeon/physician preferences. Progressions should be guided by pain, mobility, and healing status.

22.4.1 Early Stage Exercises

Early-stage exercises following injury may be directed to restoring full range of motion, including:

- Active or active-assisted exercises of the wrist and forearm (flexion, extension, radial deviation, ulnar deviation, pronation, and supination).
- These may be completed twice daily, two sets of 15–20 repetitions, or may include a sustained hold.

22.4.2 Strength and Resistance Training

Resistance exercises can be commenced once full mobility is restored; prior to regaining mobility, isometrics may be appropriate to commence strengthening in midrange positions. Both concentric and eccentric modes should be trained as these are both required in stroke play [20]. Muscle imbalances should be addressed through thorough musculoskeletal assessment and screening. Performing the below exercises will challenge all muscles supporting the wrist joint while also improving elbow strength with their origins near or over the elbow joint. Exercises may include:

- Wrist extension (Fig. 22.7)
- Wrist flexion (Fig. 22.8)
- Supination/pronation of forearm (Fig. 22.9)
- Wrist ulnar deviation (Fig. 22.10)
- Radial deviation (Fig. 22.11)
- Grip strength (Fig. 22.12)
- Wrist endurance and oscillations (Fig. 22.13)

If commencing these exercises on a low level of strength, endurance dosage may be appropriate to develop adequate neuromuscular control, commencing with 2–3 sets of 12–15 repetitions

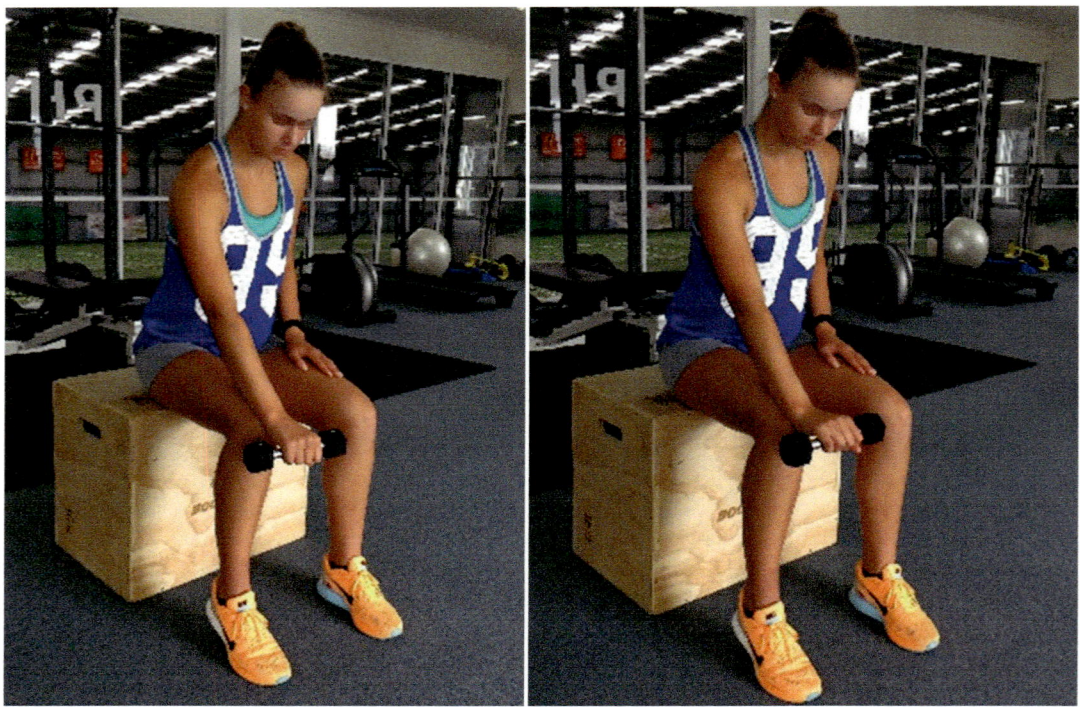

Fig. 22.7 Wrist extension with dumbbell: an upright posture should be maintained and scapula/shoulder set in good posture. Wrist extension may also be performed with elbow extension and in supination to strengthen in alternate position

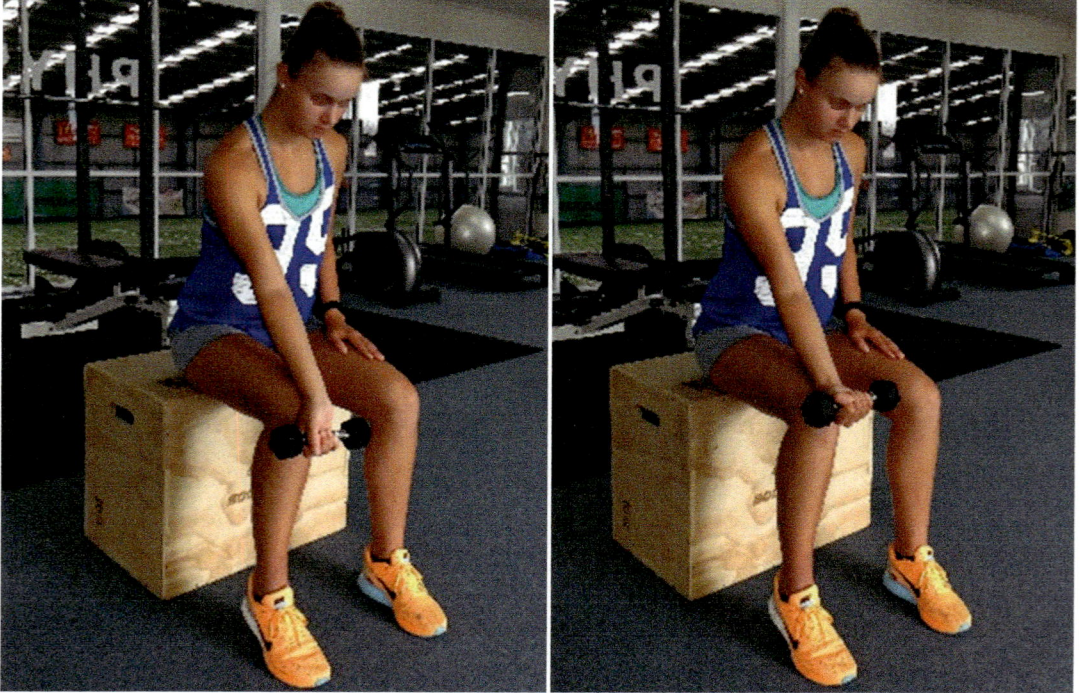

Fig. 22.8 Wrist flexion with dumbbell

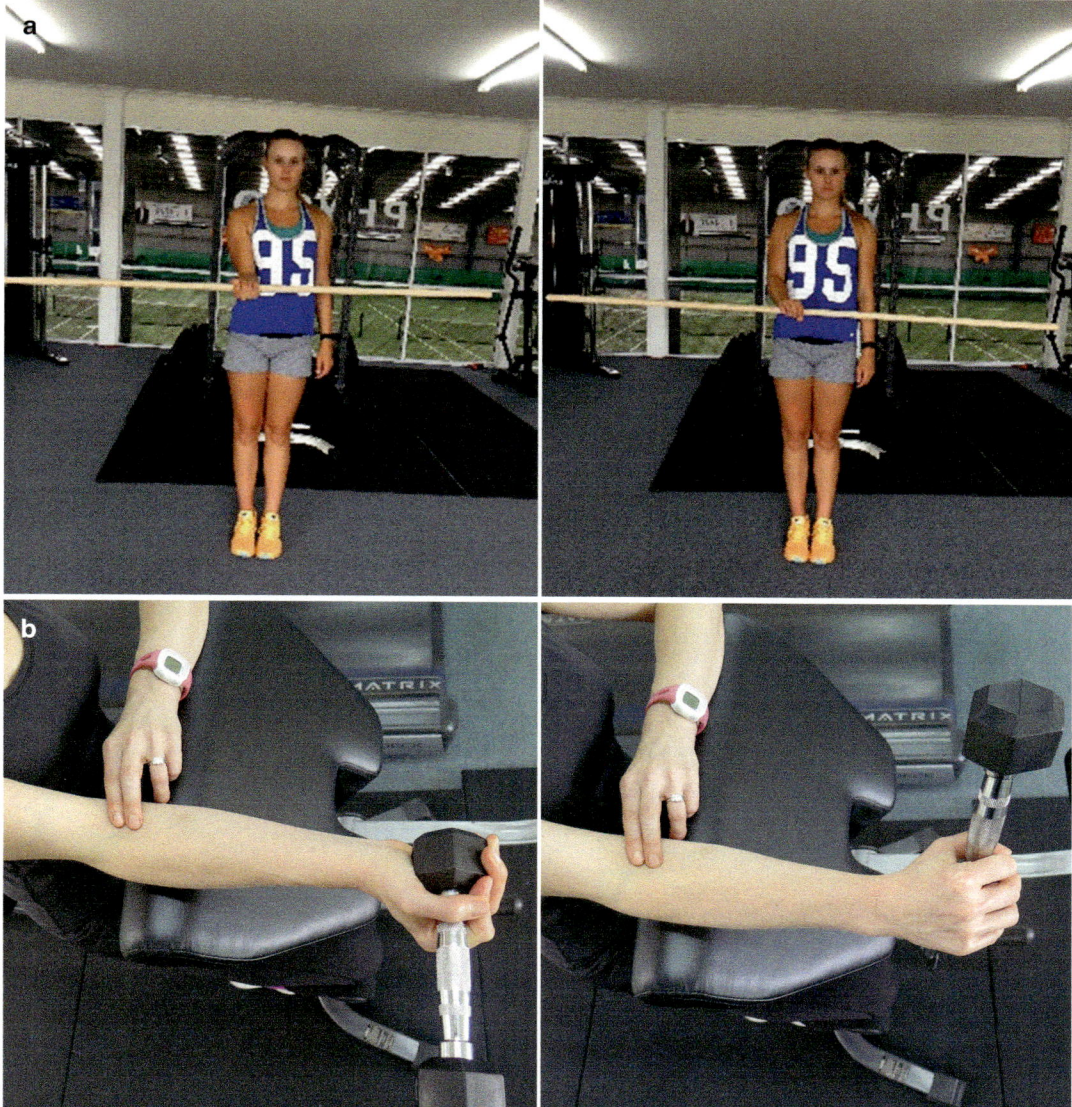

Fig. 22.9 (**a**) Use a broomstick, increasing the length of the lever arm to make the load heavier. Alternatively use a dumbbell. (**b**) Use a dumbbell or a broomstick. Increase lever arm of weight/ broomstick to increase load

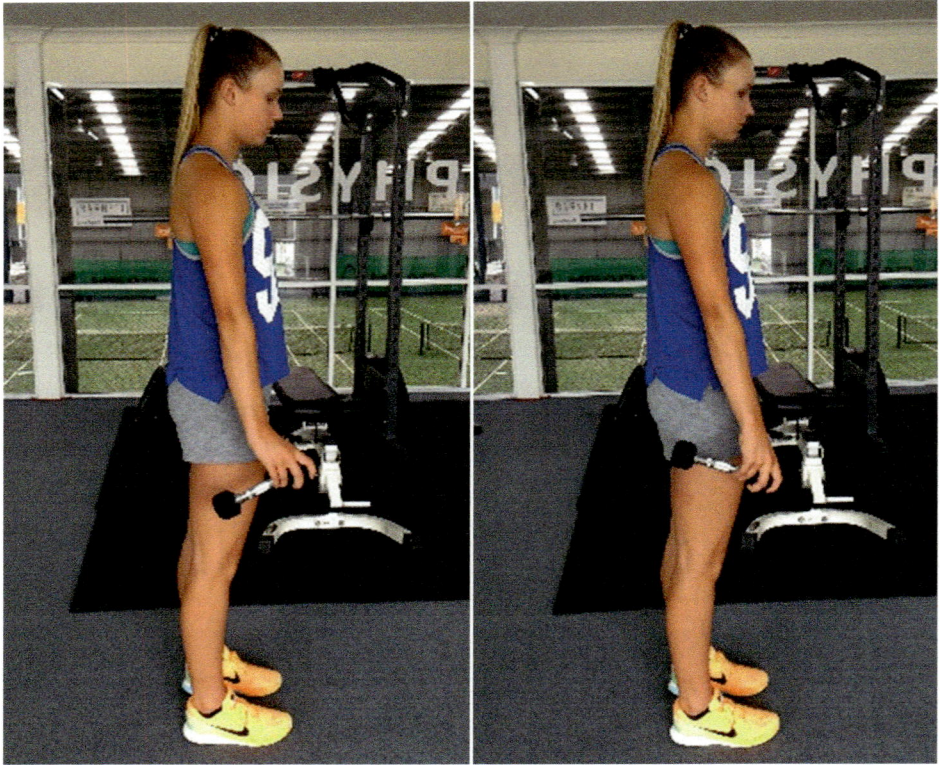

Fig. 22.10 Wrist ulnar deviation with a dumbbell. Resistance tubing or a cable pulley may be substituted

at approximately 70% 1RM. Strength training may reduce injury risk by protecting joints, ligaments, and muscles while also improving performance. Grip strength is required in tennis to keep the racquet head in projected path for optimal stroke execution [21]. Wrist strength has been found to be greater in dominant arm wrist extension, flexion, and forearm pronation compared to non-dominant side in elite female junior tennis players [22]. Grip strength was also found to be higher in dominant wrist in WTA athletes, dominant 36.9 kg and non-dominant 33.2 kg (unpublished data). This is a good reference point when performing screening of athletes, whereby greater strength muscular adaptations may be expected in the dominant wrist in tennis players in addition to greater dominant side wrist strength being restored following injury.

Once symptoms are resolved, preventative exercises should be continued and included in the tennis training program to minimize loading stresses [23] and maintain strength. During the off-season three to four times weekly and one to two times weekly in-season, preventative strengthening exercises of the wrist are advantageous.

22.4.3 Sport-Specific Exercises

When adequate foundation of strength has been developed, exercises incorporating rotational components and tennis-specific movements can be implemented to develop the kinetic chain, eccentric control, and the stretch-shorten cycle. Training tennis-specific movements with the aim

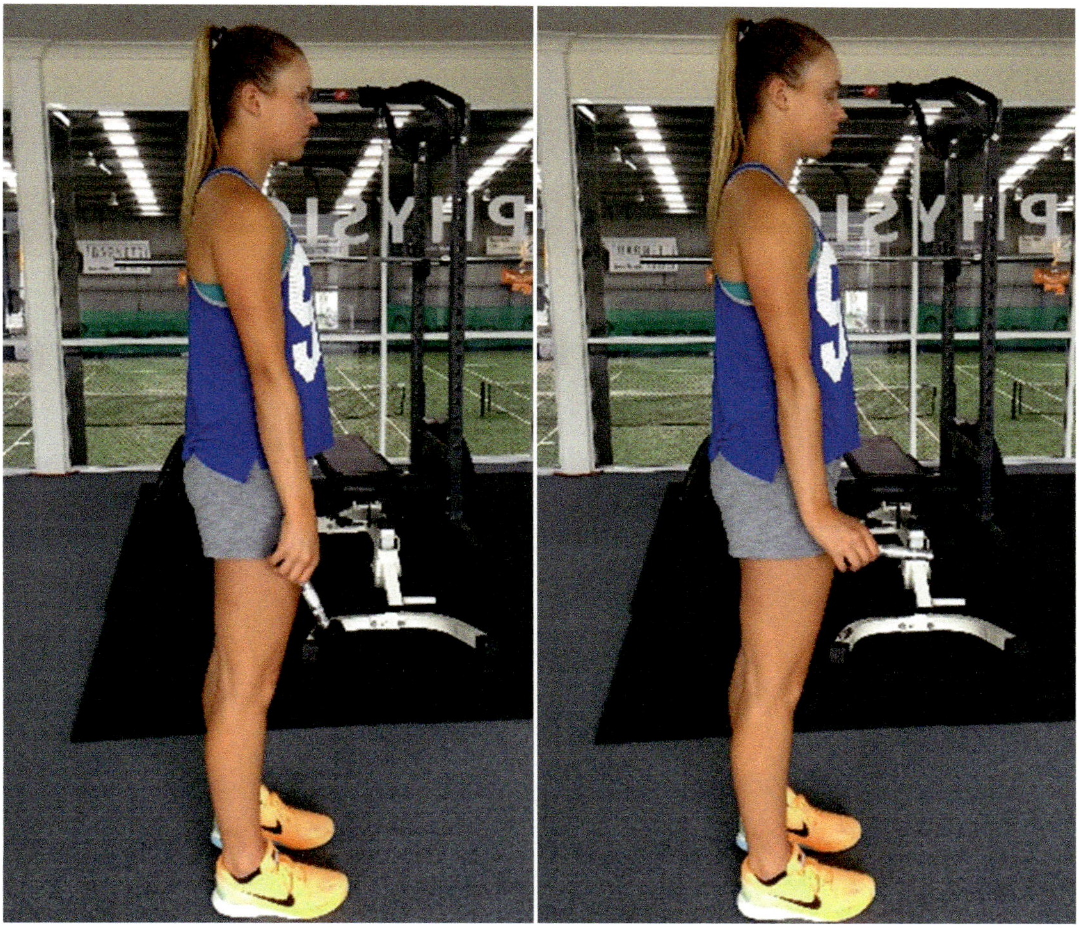

Fig. 22.11 Wrist radial deviation

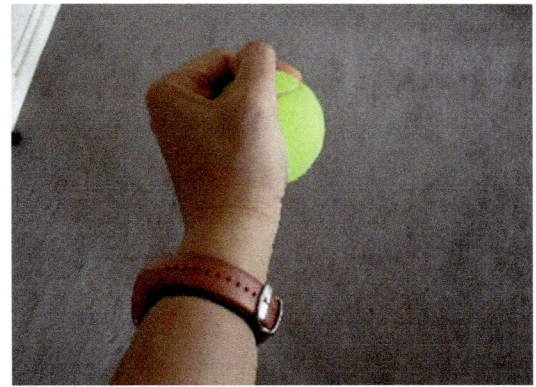

Fig. 22.12 Grip strength may be used to develop general isometric strength around wrist and hand. Start in mid-pronated position or pain-free position

to develop strength and power will improve performance by coordinating movements used in tennis and also prevent injury. Medicine ball exercises are effective at allowing tennis-specific movements to be trained. The forehand and backhand shots in open stance or closed stance positions are able to be trained and should be individualized to the technique of the athlete. Wide stance positions mimicking the forehand may also be trained to weight transfer from the lower extremities and develop rotational trunk strength and control [24] (Fig. 22.14). More high-level fundamental exercises for the wrist may include:

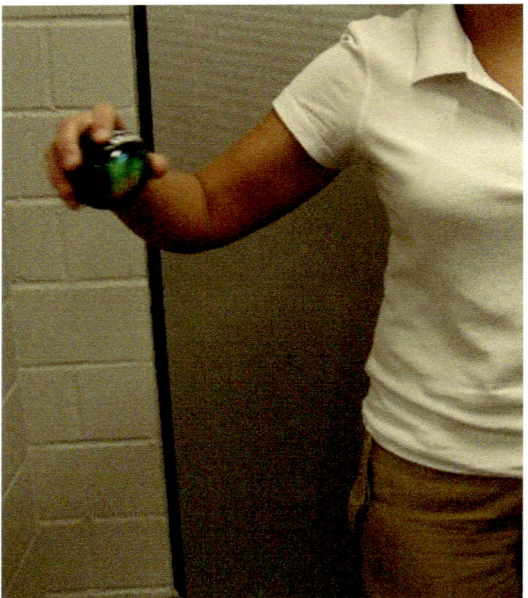

Fig. 22.13 Wrist ball oscillation, to train endurance and control in the wrist and scapula. Progress to functional positions. Using a circular motion, oscillate for 15–30 s and complete two to four sets

- Dynamic ball bounce (Fig. 22.15)
- Pronation and supination drop and catch (Fig. 22.16)
- Tennis wrist roller drill (Fig. 22.17)
- Wrist kickbacks (at speed) (Fig. 22.18)

22.4.4 Rotational Core Control

The ground strokes and serve have a large rotary component that is required to be trained for efficient use of the kinetic chain to reduce reliance on distal segments. These exercises aim to encourage the use of kinetic chain through transference of power from legs through trunk to upper extremity.

- Cable rotations focus on both acceleration and deceleration phases (Fig. 22.19).
- Wood chop: high to low, low to high (Fig. 22.20).
- Cocking diagonals and follow through diagonals: aim to mimic weight transference and the use of kinetic chain (Fig. 22.21).

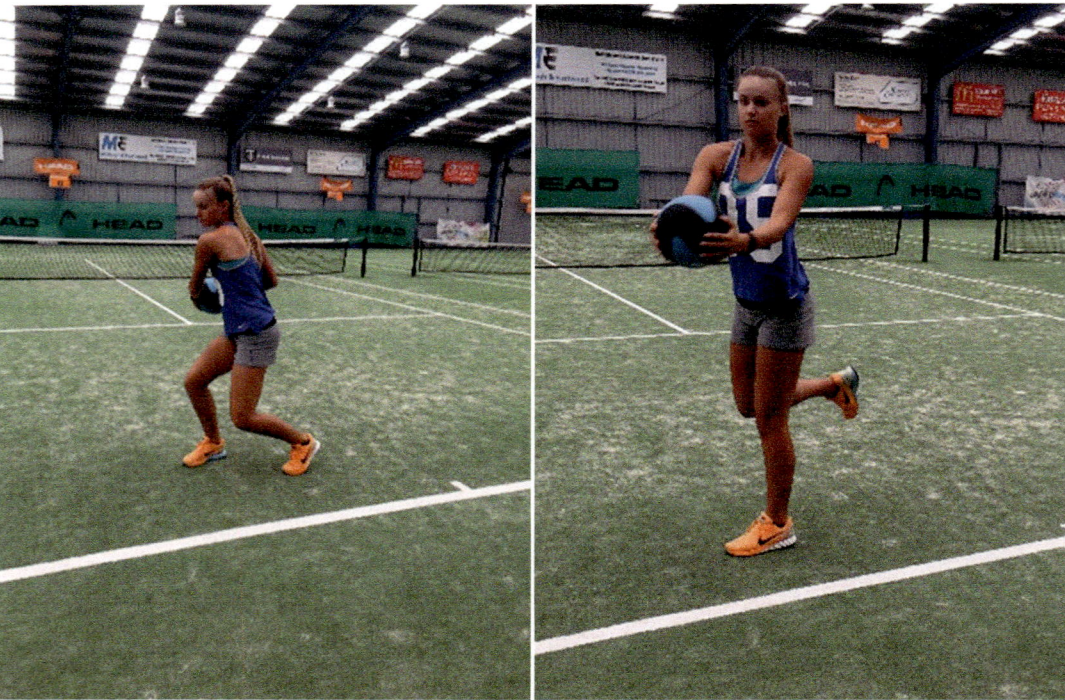

Fig. 22.14 Medicine ball rotations. Perform in forehand and backhand positions. Rotation throws can also be performed against wall. Rotate through hips and trunk to load legs and encourage use of kinetic chain

Fig. 22.15 Dynamic ball bounce: various sized and weighted medicine balls can be dynamically bounced against ground in neutral (**a**) and progressed into range against wall (**b**)

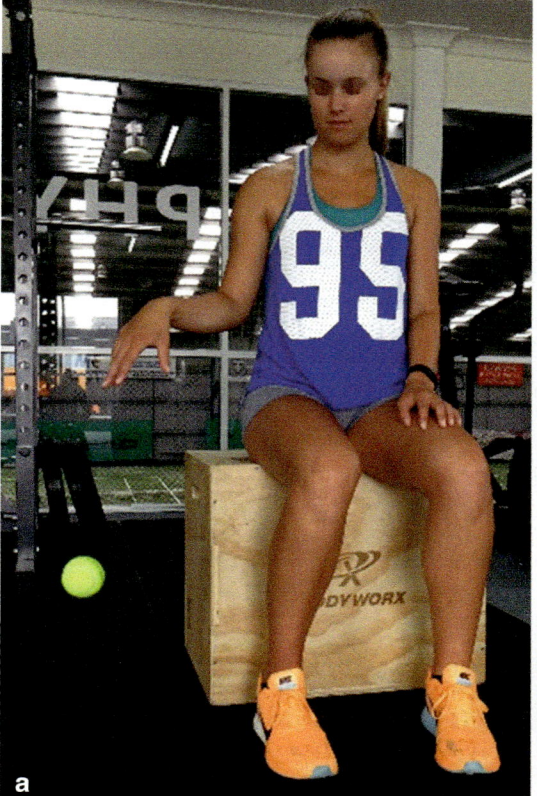
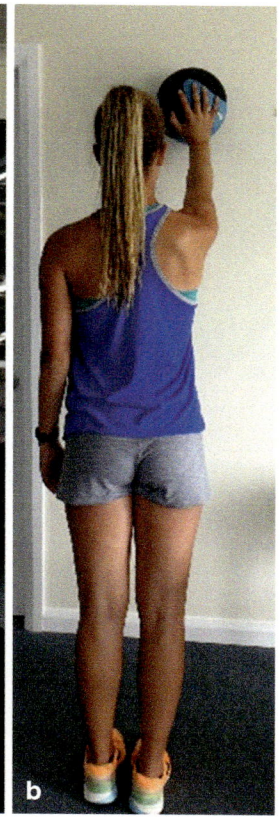

Fig. 22.16 Supination/pronation drop and catch. To build dynamic strength, from a pronated or mid-pronated position, dynamically drop into supination; progress into functional ranges at shoulder height

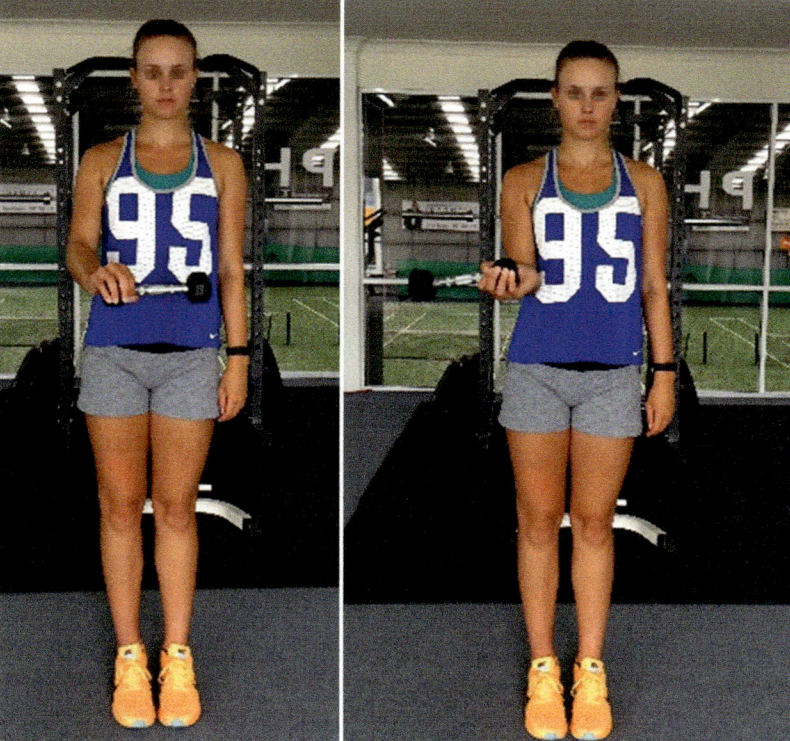

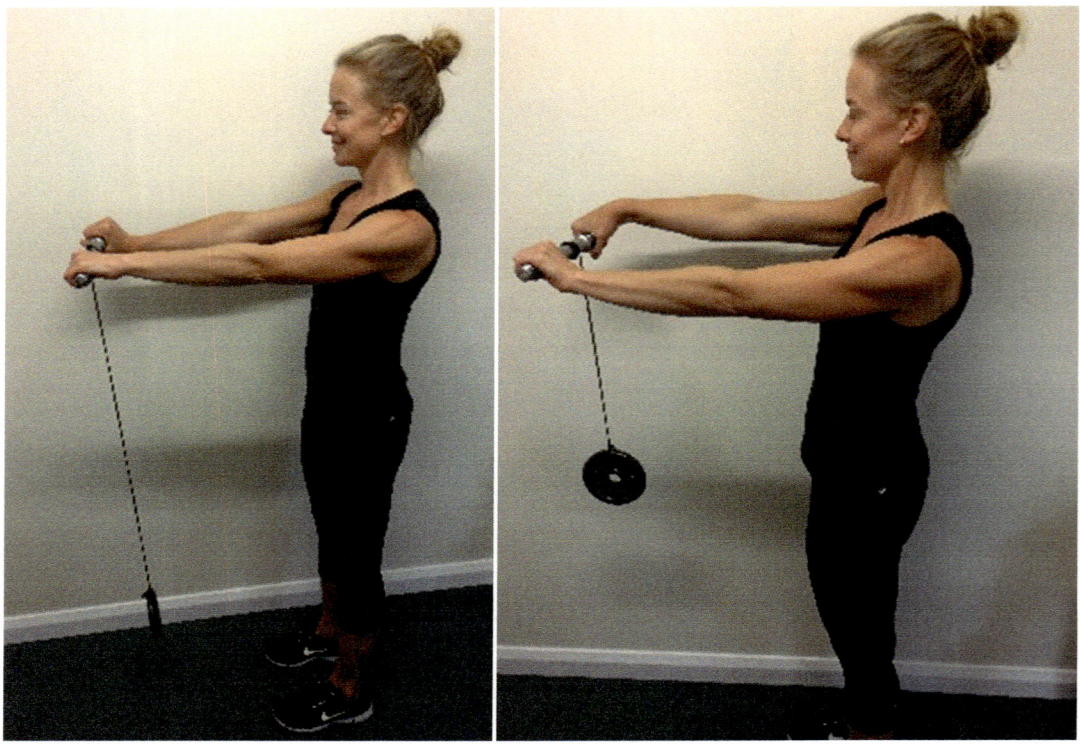

Fig. 22.17 Tennis wrist roller drill: dynamically extend/flex wrist to lower and raise weight

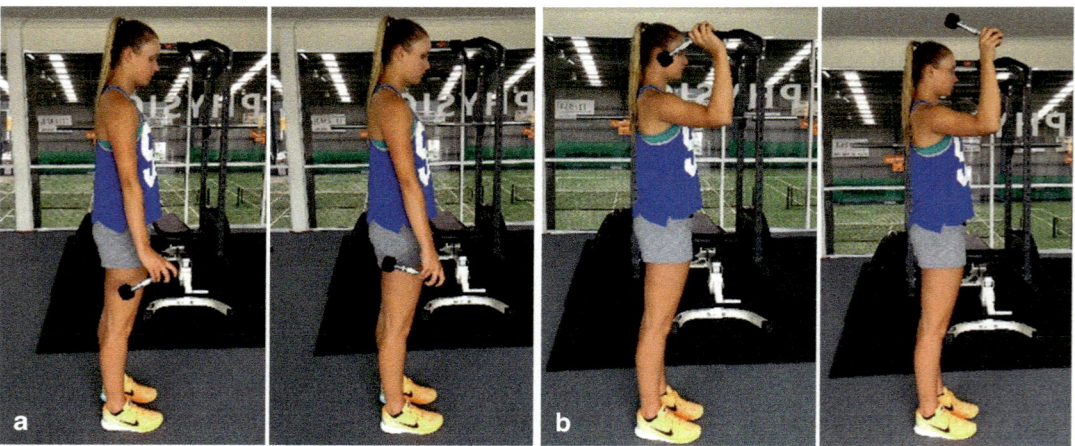

Fig. 22.18 Wrist kickbacks: holding weight by side, palm facing inward, ulnar deviate wrist rapidly with soft hand to build plyometric strength. Start by side (**a**); progress to overhead (**b**)

22.4.5 Kinetic Chain

Optimization of the kinetic chain is advantageous in tennis strokes for efficiency and to power strong stroke play from the legs while reducing injury risk. The kinetic chain refers to the combined complex movement integration of body segments to achieve function [25]. In tennis an

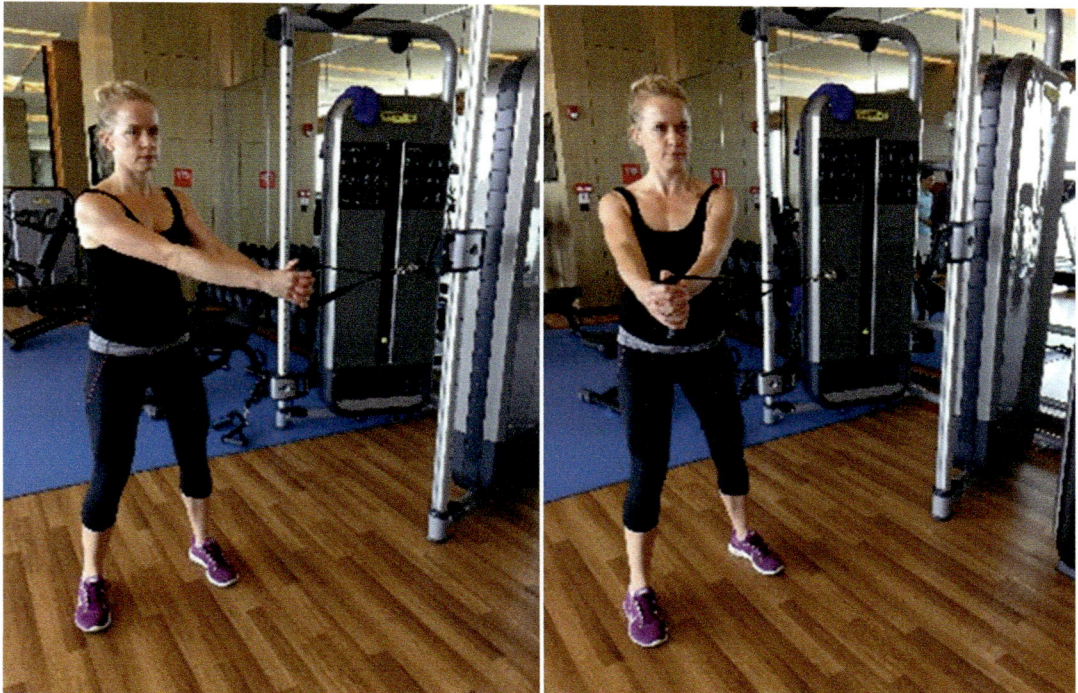

Fig. 22.19 Cable rotations

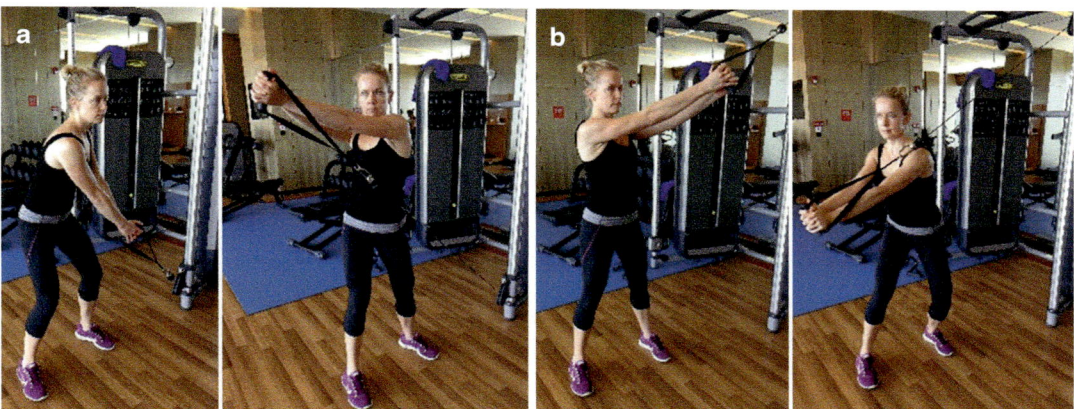

Fig. 22.20 Wood chop: low to high (**a**), high to low (**b**)

optimal kinetic chain will use the legs and trunk to generate power, while distal segments will be used for precision. Over 50% of kinetic energy and force should be generated from the trunk and leg during the serve while <15% from the wrist (see Table 22.1) [26]. Trunk mobility restrictions may reduce the ability to sequence and use the kinetic chain during strokes, potentiating in overload of the upper extremities [27, 28]. Furthermore, reduced knee flexion and leg drive during the service motion have been shown to increase torques on the upper extremity [29]. Maximizing techniques using the kinetic chain and strengthening should be a focal point in rehabilitation of the wrist and hand to reduce overload of the wrist.

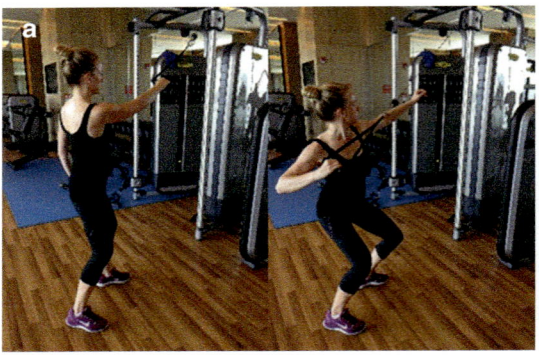
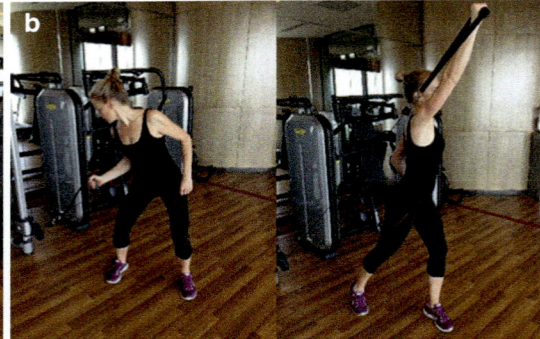

Fig. 22.21 Cocking diagonal (**a**) and follow through diagonal (**b**)

Table 22.1 Kinetic energy and force of kinetic chain during tennis serve

	Kinetic energy (%)	Force (%)
Trunk and Leg	51	54
Shoulder	13	21
Elbow	21	15
Wrist	15	10

Adapted from Kibler [26]

22.4.5.1 Trunk and Hip

Trunk and hip mobility need to be assessed as deficits may contribute to increases in upper extremity loads [30]. Deficits in trunk and hip mobility should be addressed with rehabilitative mobility exercises, local mobilization, and soft tissue and manual techniques. Hip and lumbo-pelvic weakness has been suggested to play a role in poor kinetic chain function [31, 32]; therefore, any deficits should be included in a training program to address lumbo-pelvic and hip core control and strength.

22.4.5.2 Shoulder and Scapula

For optimal function of strokes in tennis, the upper extremity requires a stable base, whereby it can move distally to provide precision in shot play [33]. Implementing scapula control and shoulder exercises to provide a stable proximal base for the upper extremity should be considered in wrist rehabilitation. Shoulder mobility including glenohumeral internal rotation deficit (GIRD) and total range of motion deficit have been associated with shoulder injury and may create poor pathomechanics [34]. GIRD may alter optimal biomechanics of the upper extremity, potentially altering joint loads on the wrist.

Mobility exercises and local manual therapy may address deficits in the management program.

22.4.6 Foot Work Drills

Tennis athletes require explosive first step speed, fast reaction times, and excellent multidirectional movement. Foot work drills are a necessity to be trained to enable athletes to move efficiently on the court but also get into position early, as hitting late or not being in the correct position may place increased stress on the wrist.

22.5 Technique/Biomechanics

To comprehensively manage a wrist injury and to reduce recurrence risk, biomechanical adjustments may be implemented including stroke analysis and equipment assessment. Technical factors including grip type, size, string tension, racquet type, and weight balance are fundamental when rehabilitating the injured wrist and hand. A qualified tennis coach or professional may be able to assist with biomechanical assessment and technique modification.

22.5.1 Serve Biomechanics

Technique is fundamental to having a successful tennis game; hence, an athlete's biomechanics needs to be assessed and optimized for performance and injury treatment and or prevention.

High wrist forces and torques have been reported in upper limb joint kinetic analysis during the tennis serve suggesting the serve may potentially impact wrist injuries. Analysis of the serve [32], particularly looking at the use of the kinetic chain and legs to push from the ground to generate force, is fundamental in reducing excess loads on the upper extremity and should be a part of wrist management. Inadequate hip counter rotation and tilt has been reported to reduce loading of the back leg, which is a key component in using the kinetic chain to generate force in the serve [32]. The Observational Tennis Serve Analysis Tool [32, 35] is one method to analyze the serve to detect inefficiencies in particular nodes that may reduce effectiveness of kinetic chain and place increased stress on the upper extremity. Stroke correction exercises may be implemented by coaches, clinicians, and fitness trainers in an attempt to optimize the use of the kinetic chain, while a thorough assessment may identify any muscle weaknesses or joint restrictions limiting optimal mechanics. See Chap. 1 for further information on serve biomechanics.

22.5.2 Forehand

Modern tennis play has seen an increase in speed and power; this increase in speed has also seen an increased use of the open stance forehand technique compared to the more traditional square stance [36]. Peak torques in upper extremity kinetics are reported to be to be similar between open and square stance forehands [37]. Similar to the serve, optimal performance of ground strokes will use the kinetic chain while reducing injury risk [20, 38]. However, this transfer of forces from the lower extremity and trunk to the smaller distal segments of the upper extremity may place these tissues under stress [24]. Trunk rotation, horizontal shoulder adduction, and internal rotation are the main kinetic chain motions that create racquet head speed in the forehand [39]. The Western grip (Fig. 22.22) enables athletes to hit with more top spin; however, the wrist is placed in more extreme motions, whereas the Eastern grip (Fig. 22.22) affords a more flat shot. Grip technique may require modification prior

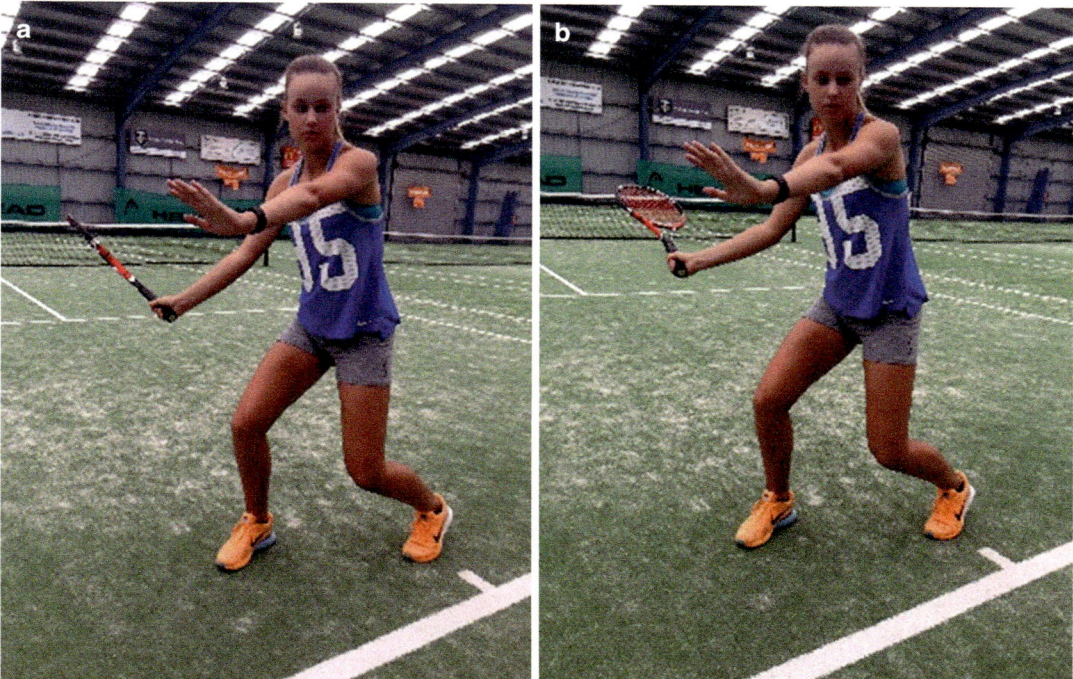

Fig. 22.22 Eastern (**a**) and Western (**b**) grip on forehand: note the more extreme extension and ulnar deviation in the Western grip

to return to play in recurrent injuries. Both grip types in forehand technique involve the use of the stretch-shorten cycle by using sequential coordinated movements [24]. A great deal of eccentric control and strength is also required in the follow through to decelerate the racquet on the follow through [24]. Exercises to strengthen the kinetic chain mimicking the action of the stretch-shorten cycle muscle action of the forehand should be trained in addition to eccentric control. Acute injury may occur to the ECU tendon or subsheath with rapid extension and ulnar deviation load that is typical of a low forehand [1], which may occur due to low bounce on grass. Quick footwork, speed and explosive power, and eccentric control of the lower extremity to stay low are physiological components that need to be trained for grass court play [40] and should be emphasized in athletes returning from wrist injury.

22.5.3 Backhand

The modern two-handed backhand also has a more open stance posture than the traditional square stance backhand. Similar racquet head speeds are able to be created in one- and two-handed backhands [41]. The one-handed backhand has higher torques on the wrist extensors and therefore requires high strength and control in the wrist and upper extremity. The one-handed backhand uses more front leg extensor torque [41], less trunk rotation, and more coordination of upper extremity rotational sequences to create the backhand compared to two-handed backhands [24]. The two-hand backhand has more trunk rotation and back leg drive with larger axial torques for trunk and hip rotation than the one-handed backhand [41]. Poor timing and poor technique are thought to contribute to ulnar-sided wrist injury in the non-dominant wrist [42]. Furthermore, inadequate trunk and thoracic rotation may limit the motion during a two-handed backhand leading to excessive loading of the ulnar side of the wrist due to compensatory supination, ulnar deviation, and extension [2]. In the non-professional tennis athlete, a common one-hand backhand error includes leading with the elbow, causing the wrist to be in a non-optimal length tension position (Fig. 22.23).

22.6 Equipment

Racquet type, weight, and size, string tension, and grip size may be related to upper extremity injury with changes or inappropriate equipment potentially leading to injury. Modern racquets are stiffer and lighter, this may have facilitated a change in playing style with more power and spin being prevalent in the modern game [8]. While increased stiffness of racquets may increase playing power, they may also be associated with upper extremity injury [8].

22.6.1 String Tension

String tension may also impact the upper extremity. Typically it is strung to 50–70 lb or 23–32 kg. Ulnar wrist pain may be exacerbated by higher string tension [42]. The ball deforms less when it impacts on looser strings and therefore will rebound at higher speed due to reduced energy loss; therefore, racquets are typically strung at low tension (loose) for increased power and high tension (tight) for increased control. Lower tensions result in a softer string bed and therefore reduced shock and vibration to upper extremity [43]. Therefore, athletes may consider stringing the racquet looser if injured to reduce vibration to upper extremity and wrist. When treating upper extremity injuries, discuss these factors with athletes and encourage gradual increase in workload with new equipment/changes.

22.6.2 Grip Technique

Modern advancements in technique with extreme Western grips becoming more prevalent and the dominance of the double backhand may be associated with the recent increases in wrist injuries in epidemiology studies [44]. This increase is also more common in females, suggesting increases in wrist injuries with the modern game. Ulnar-sided wrist injuries have been reported to be associated with Western or semi-Western grips, while radial-sided wrist injuries are more common in athletes who use Eastern grips [45]. Extreme grip positions may place the wrist into excessive wrist extension and/or ulnar deviation. This extreme wrist position may occur in the dominant hand

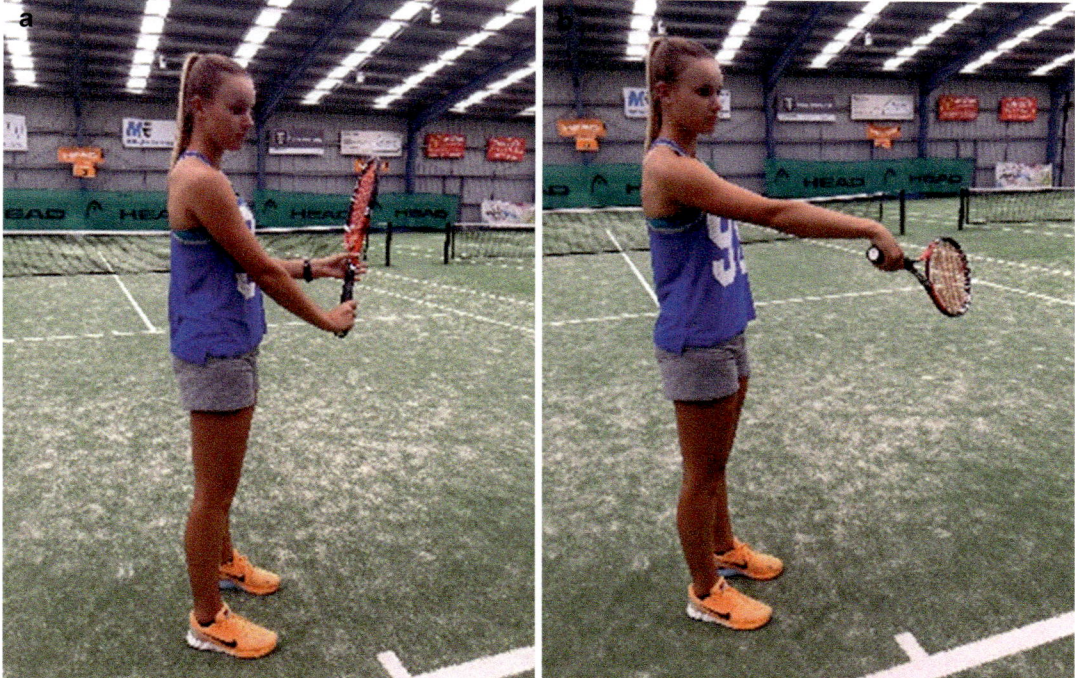

Fig. 22.23 One-handed back hand technique: (**a**) leading with wrist, (**b**) leading with elbow may overload elbow and/or wrist

forehand and in the non-dominant hand during double-hand backhand causing overload or stress to the extensor carpi ulnaris tendon [42]. These extreme wrist positions are typically associated with increased top spin; therefore, changing grip technique to afford a flatter shot with reduced top spin may reduce load on ulnar side of wrist.

To enable adequate grip on the racquet, there are eight sides called bevels on a racquet handle (Fig. 22.24).

- Continental Grip
  - The continental grip is commonly used for volleys and the serve and is obtained by having the base of the index finger on the second bevel. This grip is commonly taught to beginners; however, it is less popular in seasoned players with less ability to hit top spin on ground strokes.
- Eastern Grip
  - The Eastern forehand grip is obtained by placing the base of index finger on bevel 3.
- Semi-Western Grip

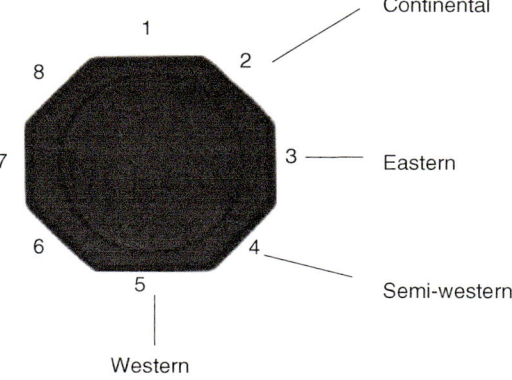

Fig. 22.24 Forehand (right handed) bevel grip and knuckle position of base of index finger

  - The base knuckle of index finger is on bevel 4 in the semi-Western forehand and is popular in baseliners with top spin and power.
- Western Grip
  - The base knuckle of index finger is on bevel 5 in the Western forehand grip and enables extreme top spin (Fig. 22.25).

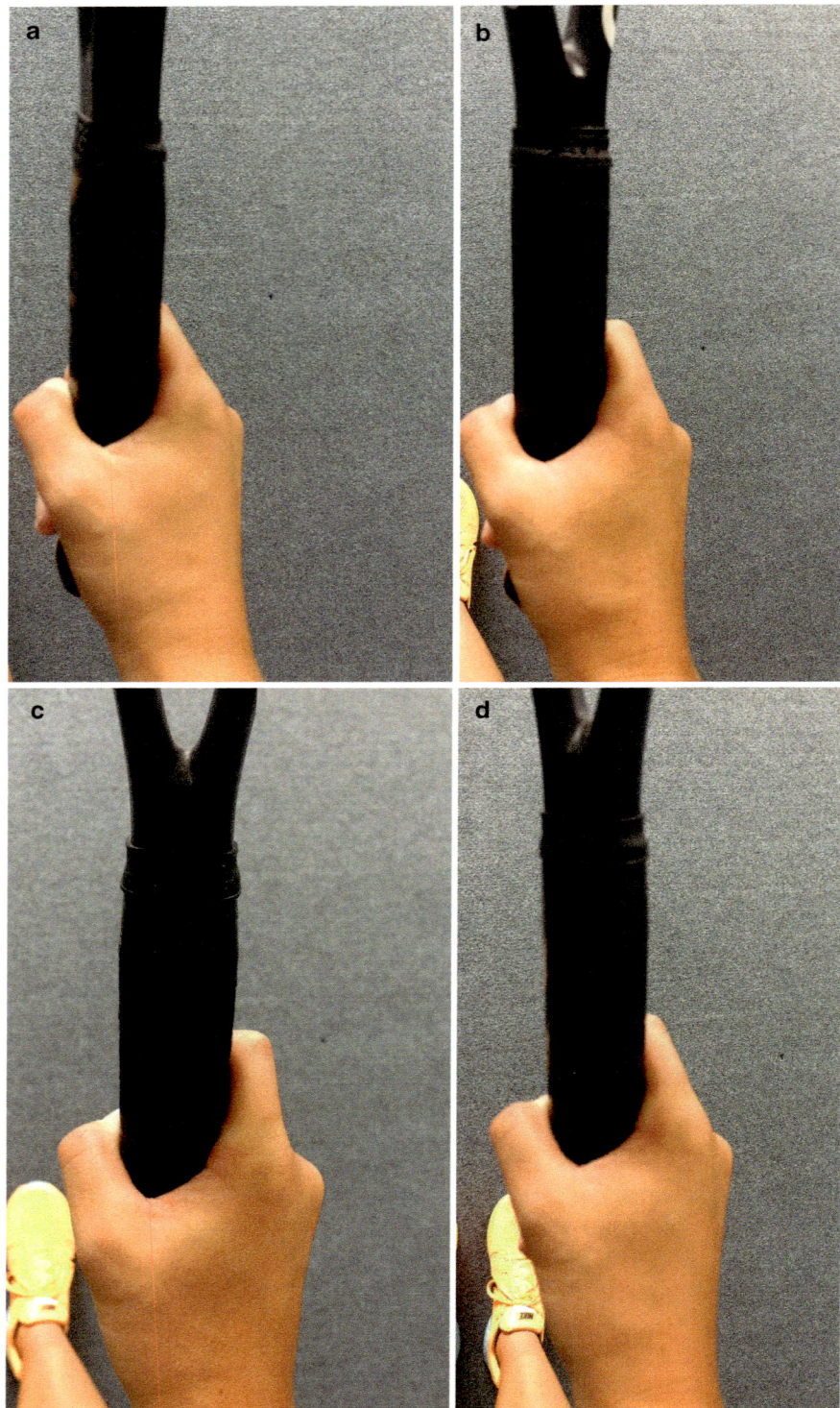

Fig. 22.25 Forehand grip positions: (**a**) Continental, (**b**) Eastern, (**c**) semi-Western, (**d**) Western

22.7 Taping and Splinting

22.7.1 Splinting and Bracing

Wrist splinting may be beneficial to immobilize the wrist to reduce pain and allow pathology to heal by reducing movement through the wrist. A brace may be worn during nonplaying times to reduce movement through the joint and excessive loads, when sleeping to prevent sustained positions of extreme flexion and/or extension, or to settle pathology allowing healing and reductions in pain [46]. A Physician will guide requirements for splinting/bracing to the injured wrist.

22.7.2 Taping

Athletic tape is a method often utilized by physiotherapists and athletic trainers to support and to also prevent injuries [47–49]. Tape may reduce pain and promote tissue healing [50 while providing stability, facilitating normal structural alignment, and providing increased proprioception [47]. In tennis the wrist is involved in all stroke play, transferring high forces from the kinetic chain to the racquet, which may place high stresses on the wrist [24]. In the injured wrist, taping may be used to protect and support the joint and may be used continually to prevent injury recurrence once pathology has resolved [2].

There are a number of methods to tape wrists, with a conventional compression technique to the distal radioulnar joint applied using white athlete tape that aims to restrict motion in all directions (Fig. 22.29). Inflamed tissue may not tolerate this compression tape. The WTA developed a number of tennis-specific taping techniques primarily using McConnell principles [2] with a goal of unloading irritated tissues, protecting injured structures while restricting desired motions. These techniques include an unload, block to motion, and redirection tape. Taping should be individualized to the individual and pathology, with combinations of these methods used and a functional test should be reassessed following the application of tape to test effectiveness such as a manual muscle test or a particular provocative stroke. The combination of the unload, block, and redirection tapes to apply to TFCC and/or ECU tendon injuries [2] has been found to be more effective than conventional techniques at reducing wrist pain [51]. This method involves TFCC unload, with unload tape applied along the ulnar border of wrist either side of ECU tendon. Optional extras will then include an extension and/or ulnar deviation block and supination redirection tape (Figs. 22.26, 22.27, and 22.28). Tape adhesive will prevent application of tape loosening from sweat or repetitive use prior to play.

Other taping methods other than conventional athletic tape include Dynamic and Kinesio taping methods. Dynamic tape is a more recent taping method, with a four-way stretch designed to assist movement mechanically by absorbing load and then aiming to facilitate movement through elastic energy stored being released [52]. More research is required to assess the efficacy of Dynamic tape; however, it appears to be a taping option when restriction of motion is not required. Kinesio tape is another taping method that is anecdotally reported to have facilitation or inhibitory effects to muscle [53]. Kinesio tape lacks rigidity therefore will not support a joint or restrict motion; however, it may have some efficacy in joint movement promotion [54], increasing muscle activity [55], and enhancing performance [56].

22.7.3 Taping Methods

1. Unload (Fig. 22.26):
   - Aim: unload underlying tissue by lifting and/or shortening underlying tissue.
   - One centimeter wide strips of brown athlete tape are applied in an alternating diagonal pattern, tensioning from the anchor to application, while applying lift to soft tissue beneath to shorten underlying tissue.
   - For irritable areas, foam padding or gutters may be applied to disperse force and avoid direct pressure from tape.

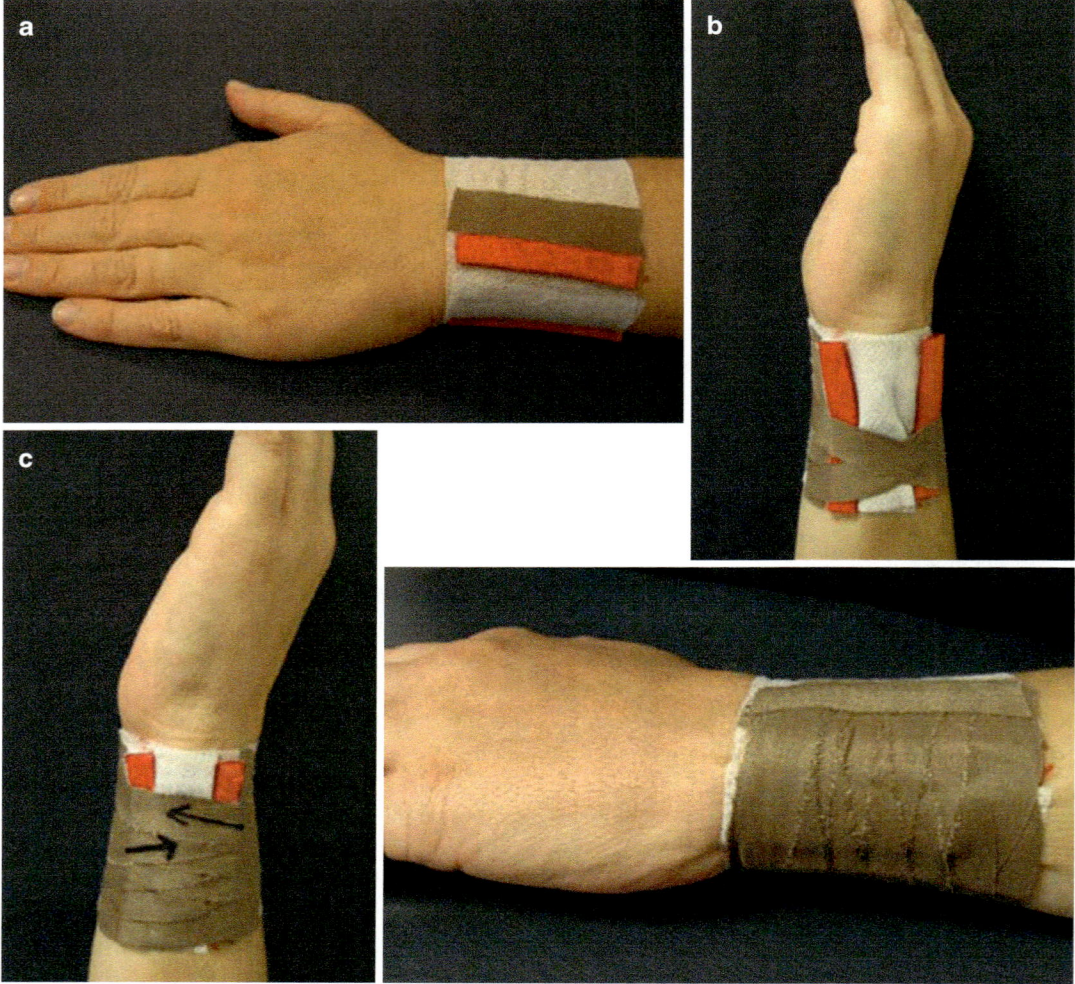

Fig. 22.26 Unload tape (**a**) gutters applied, (**b**) unload strips are applied in herring bone pattern in direction of arrow, (**c**) unload tape. Additional tape may be applied over top such as blocks, redirection, or compression wrap

2. Blocks (Fig. 22.27):
   - Aim: limit wrist from moving into painful range of motion and or limit extreme range of motion.
   - Blocks can be applied to flexion, extension (Fig. 22.27b), ulnar deviation (Fig. 22.27a), radial deviation, or a combination of these.
   - Tape (brown tape approximately 2 cm wide) is applied by instructing the athlete to hold their wrist in neutral position, while tape is applied with equal pressure from both ends
3. Redirection tape (Fig. 22.28):
   - Aim is to redirect the wrist from painful range of motion while restricting end range of motions.
   - A redirection technique may include a supination redirection or pronation assist, which restricts end range supination.
4. Compression wrap (Fig. 22.29):

22 Wrist and Hand Rehabilitation

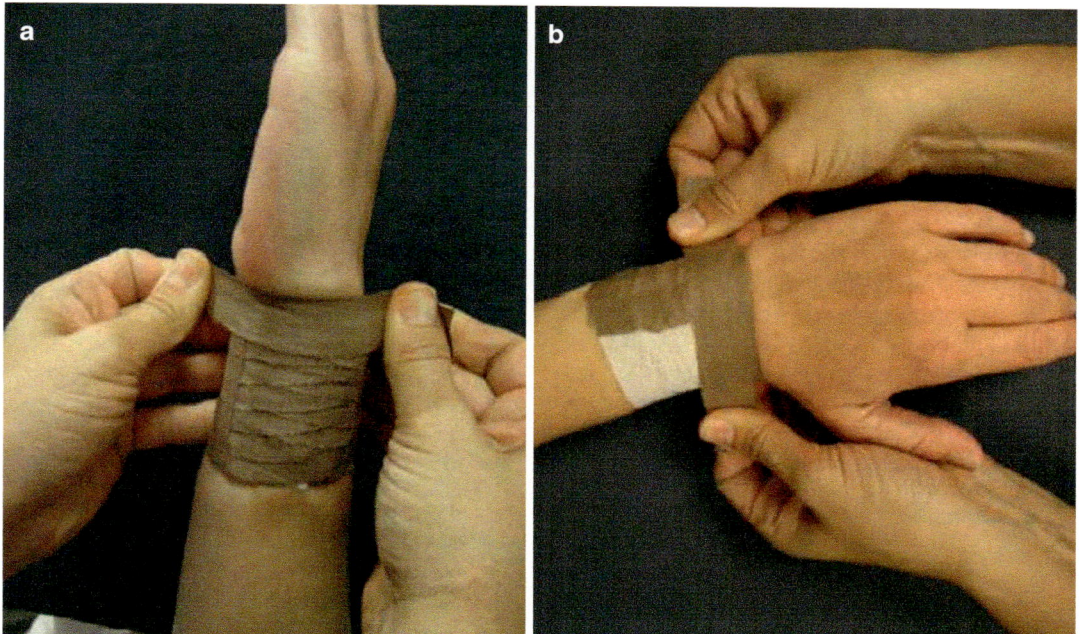

Fig. 22.27 Wrist block tape, (**a**) ulnar deviation block, (**b**) extension block. May be applied over unload or without unload tape

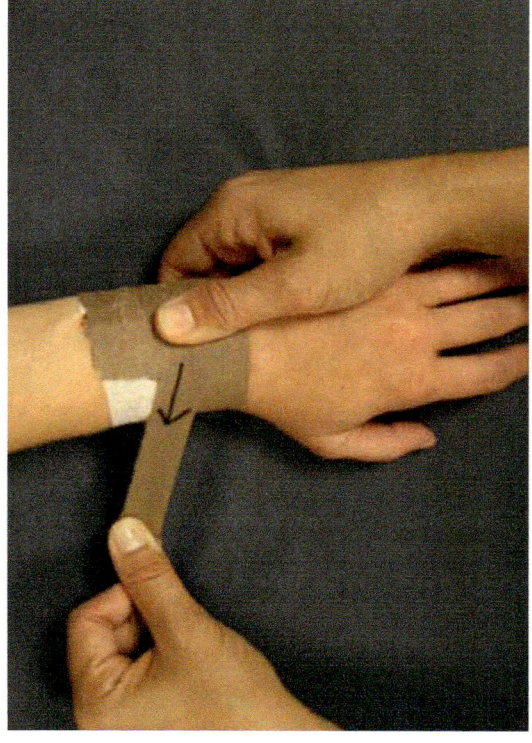

Fig. 22.28 Redirection tape, pronation assist

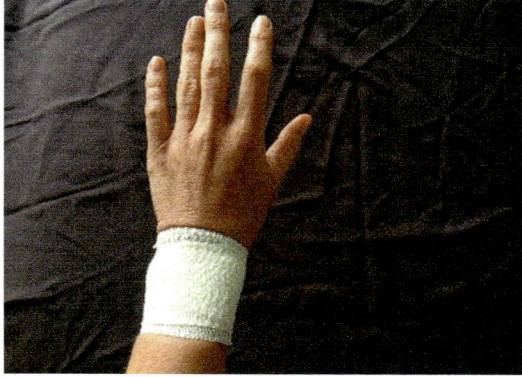

Fig. 22.29 Compression wrap

- Aim: to provide light compression and slight restriction to all movements.
- Lightplast tape is applied over other tape to reinforce or may be used over under-wrap or Cover-Roll base as a light supportive wrist tape.
- To increase compression, white athletic tape may be applied.

5. Carpal approximation tape (Fig. 22.30):
   - Aim: with TFCC instability to approximate carpal bones to distal ulna to stabilize distal radioulnar joint (with or without presence of a carpal lag).
   - Cover-Roll base applied over wrist approximately 6 cm wide.
   - Two centimeter brown tape is applied diagonally from palmar surface of wrist, while manually approximating carpal to ulnar tape is applied over carpals to dorsal surface of wrist.

6. Dynamic tape application:
   - Aim: to facilitate movement.
   - Dynamic tape is an elastic tape with recoil that aims to assist motion.
   - May be applied to any joint; in the wrist is effective if not wanting to restrict motion. It can be applied to the wrist extensors to assist motion, with long anchors which may be applied with up to 40% stretch with the muscle in a shortened position.
   - A dynamic tape course is recommended prior to applying tape clinically.

7. Thumb spica (Fig. 22.31):
   - Aim: to stabilize the first metacarpal-phalangeal joint.
   - A base of Cover-Roll is applied around the proximal first phalanx and the wrist. Two centimeter wide brown stability strips are applied with the thumb in a neutral position, and a closing strip over top of stability strips is applied.

8. Blister tape (Fig. 22.32):
   - Aim: to protect/pad blister preventing pain and reducing further friction/injury.
   - Cover-Roll, with brown tape edges, is applied over blister to protect during play and may require further padding directly on the blister prior to applying Cover-Roll, such as second skin and/or gauze. Brown edges can be applied to reinforce tape to stop it rolling during play.

9. Finger taping techniques (Fig. 22.33):
   - Buddy taping
     - For interphalangeal joint sprains, buddy taping allows immobilization of the joint by taping to adjacent finger.
   - Interphalangeal joint stabilization
     - To stabilize collateral ligament sprains to the interphalangeal joint, 1/3 of centimeter tape can be applied in X with apex over the joint line.

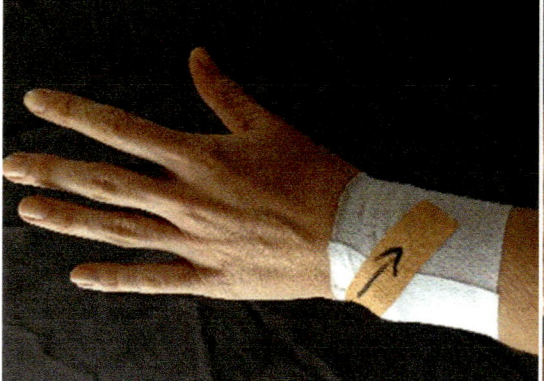 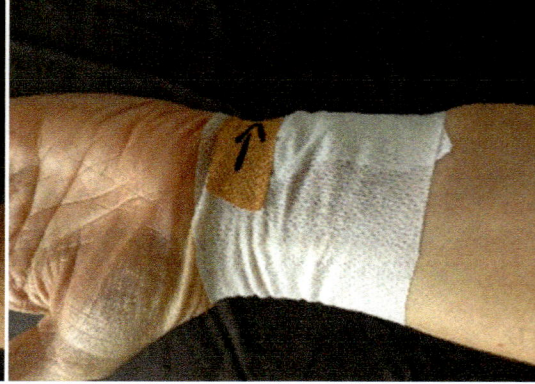

Fig. 22.30 Carpal approximation tape. Therapist manually approximates carpals to ulnar and applies tape from volar to dorsal surface of wrist

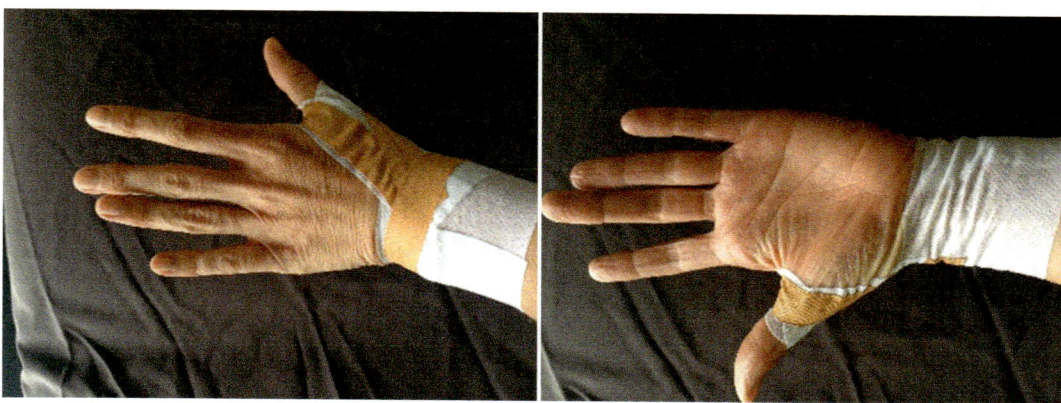

Fig. 22.31 Thumb spica

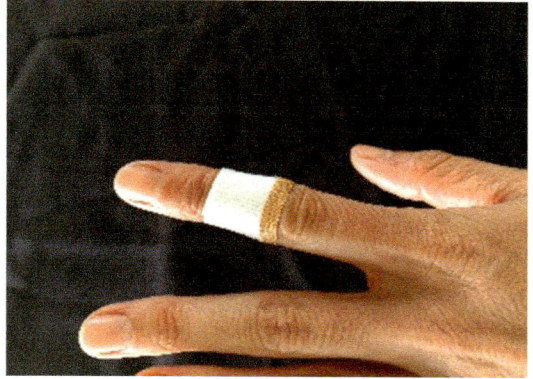

Fig. 22.32 Finger blister tape

22.8 Return to play

There are specific guidelines for return to play for different wrist pathologies; however, these will be largely varied with individuals and treating health professionals. The optimal time for return to play will vary individually; however, medically satisfactory bone and soft tissue healing are required in conjunction with adequate rehabilitation [57] and restoration of full strength and movement. Athletes may choose to defer surgery until the end of season, which if choosing to return to play early, the athlete with their medical team will need to factor protecting the wrist from further injury, social factors, and the relative stability of injury [58]. The overall long-term health of the athlete must be considered by the athlete and physician when deciding on deferral of surgical management and debating risks of early return to play [57]. Dominant wrist injuries are often difficult to manage in-season with the requirement of holding a racquet for all shot play, and often protective splinting is not amenable to being able to hold the racquet adequately for play. Individual pathologies and return to play are discussed below.

22.8.1 Return to Play Guideline

A guideline following immobilization and rest from play from wrist injury may include (note this is a guideline and time frames will be dependent upon individual pathology, severity, and treating health practitioner/physician/surgeon protocols):

Stage 1: 0–6 weeks
Goal: Maintain cardiovascular fitness

- While immobilized in splint, athletes should continue strengthening rest of the body, whereby not having to hold weights in the affected wrist. Fitness work such as stationary bike (not holding onto handle with affected limb) may be continued.

Stage 2: 6–12 weeks
Goal: Range of motion

- When out of wrist splint, begin gentle range of motion exercises; if no increase in symptoms

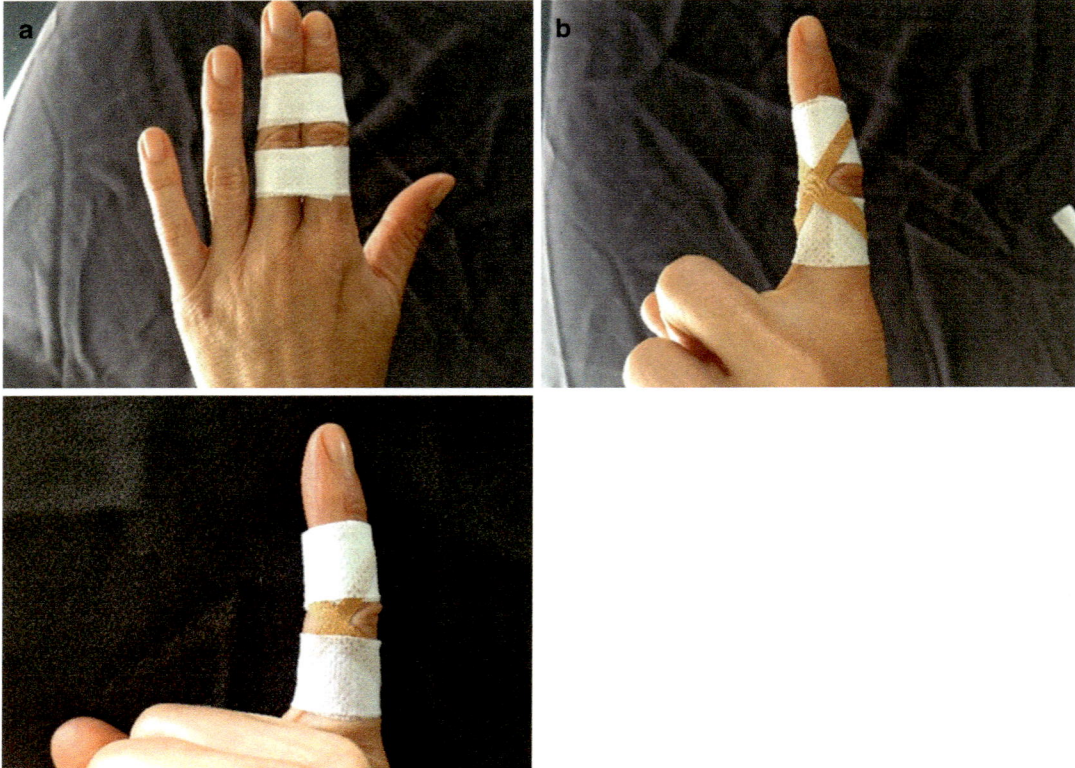

Fig. 22.33 Finger buddy taping (**a**), interphalangeal joint stabilization tape (**b**)

after 1–2 weeks, you may commence strengthening exercises. Initially strengthen with isometric contractions, building to through range isotonic strengthening in inner ranges as tolerated.
- Tennis activity may include visualization, strategic planning, and video analysis with coach.
- Later stage may commence some on court fitness training without hitting, focusing on movement and agility, however taking care to not aggravate or risk falling on wrist.

Stage 3: 3–4 months
Goal: Strengthening

– Commence with basic concentric-eccentric exercises building to advanced exercises with increased weights and resistance.
– Tennis-specific exercises should be introduced when strength is improving toward normal with exercises that mimic tennis strokes and finally exercises with your racket in hand.
– Fitness and conditioning should continue building up to more interval-based exercises.
– Start hitting with foam balls once full strength and mobility are achieved and treating physician gives clearance.

Stage 4: 4–5 months
Goal: Return on court tennis practice

– Prior to returning to tennis practice, consultation should be made with treating physician. The time frame will be dependent on progress and advice of surgeon. Wrist is required to be pain-free with full range of motion and strength prior to hitting, and tape should be

worn to support wrist, which may be weaned off in 4–8 weeks.
- Start practice with a good warm up.
- Begin with 1/2 court activities and progress to full court activities.
- Begin with gentle forehands and backhands for 5–10 min and gradually increase length of practice.
- If no pain with playing, gradually increase to 45 min practice once a day depending on symptoms.
- Advance to hitting two times per day, building up to 1 h per session.
- Ice after every practice.
- Continue with rehab and advance strength training of the wrist, elbow, and shoulder inclusive of core and kinetic chain.
- Progress to play practice sets and practice matches as symptoms and workload tolerance allow.
- Once an athlete is able to play a practice match (three sets) without wrist pain with no latent pain, the athlete may return to competition with clearance from physician.

Stage 5: Return to competition

- Once returning to competition, a maintenance wrist strengthening program should be implemented to keep the wrist strong and prevent recurrence.
- A biomechanical and technique review of strokes may be beneficial to improve stroke mechanics and any potential contributors to pain.

22.8.2 Specific Pathology

22.8.2.1 Scaphoid Fractures
Displaced scaphoid fractures require surgical intervention with anatomical reduction and internal fixation, while non-displaced fractures may have percutaneous fixation or be treated with cast immobilization [46]. Return to play will vary for the severity of the fracture and rate of healing, and caution should be taken with the risk of nonunion and malunion [59] with the poor blood supply in scaphoid fractures. Due to impact forces in tennis, early return to play with a brace may be less of an option compared to other sports.

22.8.2.2 Hook of Hamate Fractures
Large fractures or displacement of hook of hamate may require internal fixation or excision, while small fractures may be immobilized for management [46]. Return to sport is generally 6–8 weeks postoperatively [57]. The injury is generally brought about by repetitive forces from the racquet to the palm causing the fracture [57]; therefore, some modification may be required to the grip technique or grip itself to reduce transmission of forces to the palm prior to return to play.

22.8.2.3 Dorsal Wrist Ganglions
There is variation in dorsal wrist ganglion management depending on presenting symptoms. Immobilization in a splint and 2–3 weeks rest may be adequate for reducing symptoms, or a corticosteroid injection plus or minus aspiration may reduce symptoms [46, 60]. These nonsurgical options may have high recurrence rates [60]; therefore, arthroscopic surgical excision of the ganglion cyst is reported to have lower recurrence rate [61]. Following aspiration or surgical intervention, immobilization in a splint may occur for 1–2 weeks, and it may then take anywhere from 2 to 8 weeks for swelling and full mobility to be restored [60], and return to sport can take place when full mobility and strength is available.

22.8.2.4 TFCC
In the absence of distal radioulnar joint or ECU instability, isolated TFCC tears may have definitive management deferred until the off-season [57], and non-operative management may include taping, splinting, nonsteroidal anti-inflammatory drugs, and intra-articular corticosteroid injections. If conservative management fails, arthroscopic surgery may be indicated either requiring debridement or repair depending on the extent of the TFCC tear [62]. Several weeks of recovery is required following a TFCC repair to allow adequate healing, whereas debridement surgery may have a faster return to

play [57]. Wrist splinting and or taping may be applied upon return to play from conservative or surgical management, to preventatively support the distal radioulnar joint and the TFCC.

22.8.2.5 ECU Subluxation

ECU tendon subluxation has a suggested period of immobilization which may be 6–12 weeks depending on recovery [42]. If initial conservative management fails, surgery may be indicated [63], with immobilization for several weeks required, and return to play will depend on the state of healing of the tendon sheath [57].

22.8.2.6 ECU Tendinopathy

ECU tendinopathy has been described to take between 2 weeks and 9 months to resolve [42, 64]. Depending on injury severity and pain tolerance, athletes may be able to continue match play with a tendinopathy injury. Training load may need to be modified avoiding aggravating tensile loads; this is highly individualized but may involve reduced serve training or shot play minimization during training. Reducing aggravating high workloads will aim to reduce tendon cell response and prevent further disruption to the tendon matrix. Introducing pain relieving loads may assist in controlling pain and stimulate tendon healing while also maintaining strength of the musculotendinous unit [65, 66]. Intense plyometric loads and excessive tensile load should be avoided until adequate tolerance to high workloads is reached within the tendon. Normal tendons adapt to high loads within 8 weeks; however, adaptations can take more than 12 weeks [67]; therefore, rehabilitation can be lengthy. Isometric exercises may be an appropriate introductory exercise as they have been found to be pain-relieving in-season [68, 69] while maintaining tendon load capacity. Isometric supination with a broomstick/weight or racquet may be an ideal exercise to strengthen the wrist extensors inclusive of ECU (Fig. 22.9). Progressing to strength training once tendon load is controlled will improve tendon load-bearing capacity of the musculotendinous unit while stimulating tendon adaptations [67]. Strength exercises should be heavy and performed slowly on non-playing days [70], inclusive of supination/ pronation and wrist extensors while also addressing any muscle imbalances. High tendon workloads such as plyometric exercises involve store and release of energy and may take 3 days for adequate tendon recovery and adaptation [71]. Therefore, these exercises are best introduced out of competition or in the pre-season when high workloads can be controlled. Focus should initially be on speed with all exercises in inner range with a later progression to plyometrics. The ECU tendon requires both mobility and stability as it's position changes during supination and pronation [72]. It lies in a more dorsal position during supination therefore has a greater contribution to extension. Whereas it is positioned in a more palmar position in pronation and has reduced contribution to extension. The ECU tendon is angulated during supination as it exits the subsheath during supination and flexion. This position of supination and flexion may be required to be avoided in early stages of rehabilitation due to stress on the ECU subsheath and tendon. Early stage rehabilitation may include isometric supination in more pronated position and wrist extension avoiding supinated positions. Taping to protect and unload the ECU tendon may be advantageous during all play [2], while wearing a wrist splint when not playing or at night may further reduce stress to tendon.

22.9 Summary

The wrist plays an enormous role in tennis, as the final segment in the body to interact with the racquet in stroke play. High forces are imparted from the kinetic chain on the wrist in addition to impact forces from the racquet, necessitating requirement for a strong wrist. Rehabilitation should involve sound clinical reasoning addressing any contributing factors such as musculoskeletal deficits in strength or mobility both locally or proximally in the kinetic chain, addressing any biomechanical or technique deficits that may contribute to recurrence of injury, and modifying any equipment variables that could reduce risk of injury recurrence including racquet type and weight, string tension and type, and grip type and size.

References

1. Rettig AC. Athletic injuries of the wrist and hand: Part II: Overuse injuries of the wrist and traumatic injuries to the hand. Am J Sports Med. 2004;32:262–73.
2. Stroia K, Baudo M, et al. Taping techniques for TFCC and ECU injuries on the Sony Ericsson WTA Tour. Med Sci Tennis. 2009;14(1):15–9.
3. Maquirriain J, Ghisi JP. Stress injury of the lunate in tennis players: a case series and related biomechanical considerations. Br J Sports Med. 2007;41:812–5.
4. Burke J, Buchberger DJ, Carey-Loghmani T, et al. Manual therapy interventions for Carpal Tunnel Syndrome. J Manipulative Physiol Ther. 2011;30(1):50–61.
5. Schmid A, Brunner F, Wright A, Bachmann LM. Paradigm shift in manual therapy? Evidence for a central nervous system component in the response to passive cervical joint mobilization. Man Ther. 2008;13:387–96.
6. Draper DO. Ultrasound and joint mobilizations for achieving normal wrist range of motion after injury or surgery: a case series. J Athl Train. 2010;45(5):486–91.
7. Tal-Akabi A, Rushton A. An investigation to compare the effectiveness of carpal bone mobilisation and neurodynamic mobilisation as methods of treatment for carpal tunnel syndrome. Man Ther. 2000;5:214–22.
8. Muller M, Tsui D, Schnurr R, Biddulph-Deisroth L, Hard J, MacDermid JC. Effectiveness of hand therapy interventions in primary management of carpal tunnel syndrome: a systematic review. J Hand Ther. 2004;17:210–28.
9. Fernandez-Carnero J, Cleland JA, Arbizu RL. Examination of motor and hypoalgesic effects of cervical vs thoracic spine manipulation in patients with lateral epicondylalgia: a clinical trial. J Manipulative Physiol Ther. 2011;34(7):432–40.
10. Witrouw E, Mahieu N, Danneels L, McNair P. Stretching and injury prevention: an obscure relationship. Sports Med. 2004;34(7):443–9.
11. Vicenzino B, Paungmali A, Teys P. Mulligan's mobilization-with-movement, positional faults and pain relief: current concepts from a critical review of literature. Man Ther. 2007;12(2):98–108.
12. Butler DS. Mobilisaiton of the nervous system. Melbourne, VIC: Churchill Livingstone; 1994.
13. Cagnie B, Castelein B, Pollie F, Steelant L, Verhoeyen H, Cools A. Evidence for the use of ischemi compression and dry needling in the management of trigger points of the upper trapezius in patients with neck pain: a systematic review. Am J Phys Med Rehabil. 2015;94(7):573–83.
14. Gerber LH, Shah J, et al. Dry needling alters trigger points in the upper trapezius muscle and reduces pain in subjects with chronic myofascial pain. PM R. 2015;7(7):711–8.
15. Gonzalez-Iglesias J, Cleland JA, del Rosario Gutierrez-Vega M, Fernandez-de-las-Penas C. Multimodal management of lateral epicondylalgia in rock climbers: a prospective case series. J Manipulative Physiol Ther. 2011;34(9):635–42.
16. Kubo K, Yajima H, Takayama M, Ikebukuro T, Mizoguchi H, Takakura N. Effects of acupuncture and heating on blood volume and oxygen saturation of human Achilles tendon in vivo. Eur J Appl Physiol. 2010;109(3):545–50.
17. Hsieh YL, Kao MJ, Kuan TS, Chen SM, Chen JT, Hong CZ. Dry needling to a key myofascial trigger point may reduce the irritability of satellite MTrPs. Am J Phys Med Rehabil. 2007;86(5):397–403.
18. Bleakley C, McDonough S, MacAuley D. The use of ice in the treatment of acute so-tissue injury: a systematic review of randomized controlled trials. Am J Sports Med. 2004;32(1):251–61.
19. MacAuley DC. Ice therapy: how good is the evidence? Int J Sports Med. 2001;22(5):379–84.
20. Elliott B. Biomechanics and tennis. Br J Sports Med. 2006;40:392–6.
21. Behm DG. A kinesiological analysis of the tennis service. NSCA J. 1988;10:4–14.
22. Ellenbecker TS, Roetert EP, Riewald S. Isokinetic profile of wrist and forearm strength in elite female junior tennis players. Br J Sports Med. 2006;40(5):411–4.
23. Kibler B. Rehabilitation of rotator cuff tendinopathy. Clin Sports Med. 2003;22:837–47.
24. Roetert EP, Kovacs M, Knudson D, Groppel JL. Biomechanics of the tennis groundstrokes: implications for strength training. Strength Condition J. 2009;31(4):41–9.
25. Kibler WB, Press J, Sciascia AD. The role of core stability in athletic function. Sports Med. 2006;36(3):189–98.
26. Kibler WB. Biomechanical analysis of the shoulder during tennis activities. Clin Sports Med. 1995;14:79–85.
27. Campbell A, Straker L, O'Sullivan P, et al. Lumbar loading in the elite adolescent tennis serve: link to low back pain. Med Sci Sports Exerc. 2013;45(8):1562–8.
28. Campbell A, Straker L, Whiteside D, et al. Lumbar mechanics in tennis groundstrokes: differences in elite adolescent players with and without low back pain. J Appl Biomech. 2016;32(1):32–9.
29. Elliott B, Fleisig G, Nicholls R, et al. Technique effects on upper limb loading in the tennis serve. J Sci Med Sport. 2003;6(1):76–87.
30. Robb AJ, Fleisig GS, Wilk KE, et al. Passive ranges of motion of the hips and their relationship with pitching biomechanics and ball velocity in professional baseball pitchers. Am J Sports Med. 2010;38(12):2487–9.
31. Nadler SF, Malanga GA, Feinberg JH, et al. Relationship between hip muscle imbalance and occurrence of low back pain in collegiate athletes: a prospective study. Am J Phys Med Rehabil. 2001;80(8):572–7.
32. Kibler WB, Wilkes T, Sciasca A. Mechanics and pathomechanics in the overhead athlete. Clin Sports Med. 2013;32:637–51.
33. Van der Hoeven H, Kibler WB. Shoulder injuries in tennis players. Br J Sports Med. 2006;40:435–40.

34. Wilk KE, Macrina LC, Fleisig GS, et al. Loss of internal rotation and the correlation to shoulder injuries in professional baseball pitchers. Am J Sports Med. 2011;39(2):329–35.
35. Myers N, Kibler WB, et al. Validity and reliability of a biomechanically based analysis method for the tennis serve. Int J Sports Phys Ther. 2017;12(3):437–49.
36. Milano S. Should our students be teaching us? TennisPro. 1993;1.
37. Bahamonde R, Knudson D. Kinetics of the upper extremity in the open and square stance tennis forehand. J Sci Med Sport. 2003;6:88–101.
38. Kibler WB. Kinetic chain contributions to elbow function and dysfunction in sports. Clin Sports Med. 2004;23:545–52.
39. Elliott B, Takahashi K, Noffal G. The influence of grip position on the upper limb contributions to racket head speed in the tennis forehand. J Appl Biomech. 1997;13:182–96.
40. Kuganesan K. Analysis of the effect of the different types of tennis court training on physical fitness. Res J Phys Educ Sci. 2015;3(10):1–5.
41. Reid M, Elliott B. The one- and two- handed backhand in tennis. Sports Biomech. 2002;1:47–68.
42. Montalvan B, Parier J, Brasseur JL, et al. Extensor carpi ulnaris injuries in tennis players: a study of 28 cases. Br J Sports Med. 2006;40:424–9.
43. Bower R, Cross R. Player sensitivity to changes in string tension in a tennis racket. J Sci Med Sport. 2003;6(1):120–31.
44. Stuelcken M, Mellifont D, Gorman A, Sayers M. Wrist injuries in tennis players: a narrative review. Sports Med. 2017;47:857. https://doi.org/10.1007/s40279-016-0630-x.
45. Tagliafico AS, Ameri P, Michaud J, et al. Wrist injuries in tennis players: relationships with different grips. Am J Sports Med. 2009;37:760–7.
46. Umansky S. Wrist injuries in tennis: evaluation and treatment. Aspetar Sports Med J. 2014;3:540–4.
47. Alexander CM, MacMullan M, Harrison PJ. What is the effect of taping along or across a muscle on motoneurone excitability? A study using triceps surae. Man Ther. 2008;13:57. https://doi.org/10.1016/j.math.2006.08.003.
48. Cools AM, Witvrouw EE, Daneels LA, Cambie DC. Does taping influence electromyographic muscle activity in the scapular rotators in healthy shoulders? Man Ther. 2002;7(3):154–62.
49. Cook JL, Purdam CR. The Challenge of managing tendinopathy in competing athletes. Br J Sports Med. 2014;48:506–9.
50. Constantinou M, Brown M. Therapeutic taping for musculoskeletal conditions. Melbourne, VIC: Churchill Livingstone; 2010.
51. Dar SM, Arunmozhi R, Sharma B. Effect of McConnell taping on pain, ROM and grip strength in patients with triangular fibrocartilage complex injury. Sci Res J India. 2013;2(1):1–9.
52. McNeil W, Pedersen C. Dynamic tape. Is it all about controlling load? Bodywork Move Ther. 2016;20(1):179–88.
53. Cai C, Au IPH, An W, Cheung RTH. Facilitatory and inhibitory effects of Kinesio tape: factor or fad? J Sci Med Sport. 2016;19:109–12.
54. González-Iglesias J, Fernández-de-Las-Peñas C, Cleland Joshua A, et al. Short-term effects of cervical kinesio taping on pain and cervical range of motion in patients with acute whiplash injury: a randomized clinical trial. J Orthop Sports Phys Ther. 2009;39(7):515–21.
55. Hsu Y-H, Chen W-Y, Lin H-C, et al. The effects of taping on scapular kinematics and muscle performance in baseball players with shoulder impingement syndrome. J Electromyogr Kinesiol. 2009;19(6):1092–9.
56. Jaraczewska E, Long C. Kinesio taping in stroke: improving functional use of the upper extremity in hemiplegia. Top Stroke Rehabil. 2006;13(3):31–42.
57. Chen NC, Jupiter JB, Lebson PJL. Sports-related wrist injuries in adults. Sports Health. 2009;1(6):469–77.
58. Morgan WJ, Slowman LS. Acute hand and wrist injuries in athletes: evaluation and management. J Am Acad Orthop Surg. 2001;9(6):389–400.
59. Amadio PC, Berquist TH, Smith DK, Ilstrup DM, Cooney WP III, Linscheid RL. Scaphoid malunion. J Hand Surg Am. 1989;14(4):679–87.
60. Meena S, Gupta A. Dorsal wrist ganglion: current review of literature. J Clin Orthop Trauma. 2014;5(2):59–64.
61. Kang L, Weiss AP, Akelman E. Arthroscopic vs open dorsal ganglion cyst excision. Op Tech Orthop. 2012;22:131–5.
62. Estrella EP, Hung LK, Ho PC, Tse WL. Arthroscopic repair of triangular fibrocartilage complex tears. Arthroscopy. 2009;23(7):729–37.
63. Inoue G, Tamura Y. Surgical treatment for recurrent dislocation of the extensor carpi ulnaris tendon. J Hand Surg. 2001;26:556–9.
64. Futami T, Moritoshi I. Extensor carpi ulnaris syndrome. Acta Orthop Scand. 1999;66:538–9.
65. Kjaer M. Role of extracellular matrix in adaptation of tendon and skeletal muscle to mechanical loading. Physiol Rev. 2004;84:649–98.
66. Knudson D. Forces on the hand in the one-handed backhand. Int J Sports Biomech. 1991;7:282–92.
67. Bohm S, Mersmann F, Arampatzis A. Human tendon adaptation in response to mechanical loading: a systematic review and meta-analysis of exercise intervention studies on healthy adults. Sports Med Open. 2015;1:7.
68. Rio E, Cook J. Clinical implementation of isometric exercise for patellar tendinopathy: is it successful on the road? J Sci Med Sport. 2013;18S:e141.
69. Rio E, Kidgell D, Purdam C, Gaida J, Moseley GL, Pearce AJ, Cook J. Isometric exercise induces analgesia and reduces inhibition in patellar tendinopathy. Br J Sports Med. 2015;49:1277–83.

70. Bohm S, Mersmann F, Tettke M, Kraft M, Arampatzis A. Human Achilles tendon plasticity in response to cyclic strain: effect of rate and duration. J Exp Biol. 2014;217:4010. https://doi.org/10.1242/jeb.112268.
71. Langberg H, Skovgaard D, Asp S, Kjaer M. Time pattern of exercise-induced changes in type I collagen turnover after prolonged endurance exercise in humans. Calcif Tissue Int. 2000;67:41–4.
72. Campbell D, Campbell R, O'Connor P, Hawkes R. Sports-related extensor carpi ulnaris pathology: a review of functional anatomy, sports injury and management. Br J Sports Med. 2013;47:1105–11.

Part V

Lower Extremity Injuries

Principles of Hip Arthroscopy in Elite Tennis Players

23

J. W. Thomas Byrd

23.1 Introduction

The first challenge is to recognize the existence of a hip joint problem. In 2001, the first scientific article on hip arthroscopy in athletes noted that 60% of intra-articular disorders were treated for an average of 7 months before it was recognized that the joint might be the source of symptoms [1]. The continued allusive nature of hip problems is reflected by the statistic that patients suffering from hip problems see an average of four clinicians before a diagnosis is reached [2]. A contributing explanation may be that hip problems infrequently occur in isolation. For example, femoroacetabular impingement (FAI) is a common causative factor for joint problems among athletes [3, 4]. Athletes are likely compensating for the effects of FAI long before the joint becomes symptomatic. Accompanying compensatory problems may be more evident and thus obscure the presence of an underlying joint problem.

Compensatory problems may be especially relevant in the tennis game. An association between FAI and athletic pubalgia is well recognized in athletes [5, 6]. The association is easy to explain as limited hip motion is compensated by increased pelvic movement, overworking the pelvic stabilizers, and resulting in the breakdown of these structures characterized by athletic pubalgia. An association between lumbar spine and hip disorders has been recognized, especially in sports where rotational velocity is a premium, most commonly implicated in golf and baseball [7]. As one area breaks down, the athlete loses the ability to compensate for the other, resulting in a constellation of problems within the lumbopelvic complex. Tennis would be similarly implicated, since slightly greater than half of the kinetic energy is calculated to be derived from the leg-hip-trunk link [8]. There is no limit to how far up or down the kinetic chain the negative implications of hip dysfunction can be experienced. Among major league baseball pitchers, 75% of those treated with arthroscopic correction of FAI also had ulnar collateral ligament surgery of their throwing elbow.

Although not well documented, it is likely that equipment including shoe wear and racket design could have both negative and positive influences on hip disorders. These should be kept in consideration when treating a specific injury as well as when attempting to understand the epidemiology of tennis-related hip problems. Additionally, the style of the game play by an athlete may have ramifications. An open stance has been implicated in increased anterior translational forces and anterior labral pathology [9].

The role of physical therapy should not be underestimated. Even among athletes with symptomatic FAI, there is much more to the pathological process than simply the static bony

J. W. Thomas Byrd
Nashville Sports Medicine Foundation, Nashville, TN, USA
e-mail: byrd@nashvillehip.org

architecture. There are likely significant dynamic influences. Pelvic stabilization can alter the orientation of the pelvis, potentially opening the anterior aspect of the acetabulum and reducing FAI-related forces [10]. In fact, just the concept of FAI is too simple. It easily explains why some athletes get into trouble with joint damage but how are some Masters athletes able to function in a well-compensated manner for decades [11]. It is likely that pathological FAI is a perfect storm with enough factors coming together just wrong, resulting in intra-articular damage. As a clinician, it is likely that not all factors can be identified. But if enough can be targeted and addressed, both with surgical and nonsurgical means, to reach critical mass for successful treatment in terms of reduced symptoms and improved function that may be a reasonable goal.

For a clinician, it can be a time-consuming process to decipher the various compensatory problems that may compound primary joint damage. A skilled physical therapist can often systematically identify and isolate various contributing components. Correcting the compensatory patterns alone can often reduce symptoms and regain an athlete's ability to compensate.

When surgery is contemplated, thorough understanding of associated compensatory patterns is imperative. It is best if these can be corrected prior to surgery. Like most surgical procedures, the success of operations on the joint is dependent on the rehab process afterward. Thus, front end correction of compensatory issues offers a greater chance of successful postoperative recovery. There can reach a point where compensatory problems are simply not correctable until the joint has been addressed. However, it is best to be aware of this so that it is understood by the athlete/patient, that the postoperative recovery may be more prolonged and complex, necessitating correction of compensatory patterns even after the joint itself has healed.

With this brief introduction, there are seven steps to successful hip arthroscopy or virtually any surgical procedure around the hip region. Each step must be successfully completed before proceeding to the next. Inadequate completion of one step will result in more challenges for the next and reduce the chance for a successful outcome.

23.2 Step One: Pick the Right Patient

Successful hip arthroscopy is most clearly dependent on proper patient selection. The best operation will fail when performed for the wrong reason. History and physical examination are the most powerful clinical assessment tools for determining the presence of a joint problem [12]. Imaging generally helps to substantiate the diagnosis but is fraught with many pitfalls in both false-positive and false-negative findings. Ultrasonography is the single greatest adjunct to the history and exam (Fig. 23.1) [13–15]. The

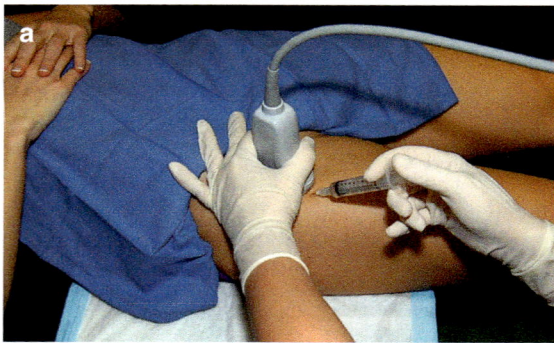
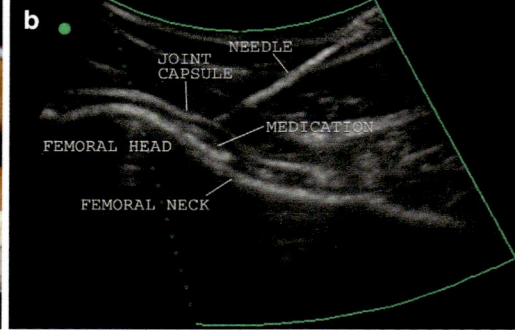

Fig. 23.1 (**a**, **b**) Ultrasound-guided injections such as this one in the joint can be performed in the office with diagnostic value differentiating various sites of pain generation and can have therapeutic benefit

response to ultrasound-guided diagnostic injections in and around the hip helps to establish the clinical relevance of various findings and potentially has therapeutic value in efforts to exhaust conservative treatment. Attempting to assess complex hip disorders without ultrasonography is akin to practicing cardiology without a stethoscope.

There are a few objective contraindications to hip arthroscopy: Tönnis III radiographic changes, less than 2 mm of joint space, and dysplasia significant enough to warrant a periacetabular osteotomy (PAO) as a potentially lifelong solution [16, 17]. However, there are many more subjective contraindications. Paramount among these is reasonable expectations on the part of the athlete. Unreasonable expectations will assure a disappointing outcome. Among athletes who are unable or unwilling to modulate their goals, arthroscopy may be contraindicated. Physical therapists are a further asset in this regard as they can help to assess and modulate patient goals and get a sense for the patient's level of commitment to their own recovery.

23.3 Step Two: Plan the Procedure

Try to understand as completely as possible the various factors that have led to an athlete being a candidate for surgical intervention (Fig. 23.2). Know how each will be addressed and especially the specifics of the components that will be corrected with surgical intervention.

23.4 Step Three: Patient Positioning

If the patient is positioned properly, then there is a reasonable chance the case will go well, while poor positioning will assure a difficult and challenging procedure. Hip arthroscopy has been well described with both supine and lateral decubitus positioning of the patient (Fig. 23.3) [18, 19]. Distraction of the joint is necessary for access to the central/intra-articular compartment of the joint. Although arthroscopy has been described without a peroneal post, most methods include a distraction device or a fracture table [20]. The principal components are a well-padded perineal post to protect the perineum, a boot for applying longitudinal traction, and some method for altering the intraoperative position of the leg. Various methods are available, and it is important to adopt a reliable technique that works in each surgeon's hands.

23.5 Step Four: Portal Placement

Proper portal placement is essential, both for safety and efficacy of the procedure. The dense soft tissue envelope and constrained architecture of the hip lends itself to greater risk of iatrogenic injury compared to other joints (Fig. 23.4). Similarly, there is less maneuverability for the instrumentation, and thus having the portals in the correct position is also more important for accessing the pathology.

Numerous portals have been described for both the central and peripheral compartments (Figs. 23.5 and 23.6) [18, 21, 22]. It is important for each surgeon to select those that work best for him or her and to become facile in their placement. Consistency in portal placement is also important for being properly oriented to the three-dimensional anatomy of the hip, which is often being corrected in conjunction with FAI.

23.6 Step Five: Proper Visualization

Next to poor patient selection, poor visualization is the root of all evil in hip arthroscopy. If the surgeon cannot see well, it is unlikely that a well-performed procedure will result. This is partly dependent on portal placement for optimal viewing and then meticulous soft tissue preparation. Tissue preparation for visualization is often the most tedious, time-consuming portion of the procedure. It is wise to fully discern the pathology to be addressed, visualizing exactly where any corrective procedure will begin and end.

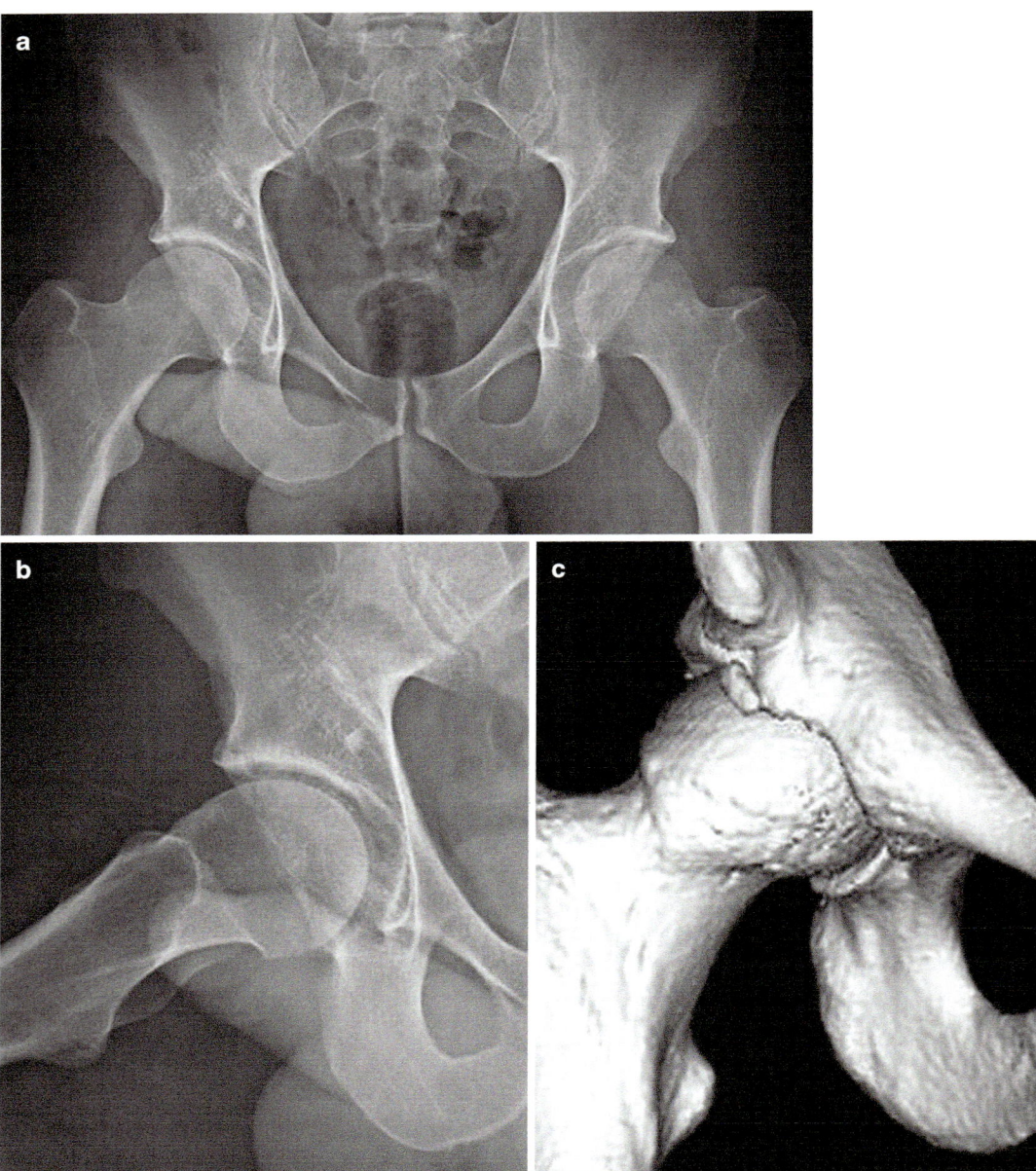

Fig. 23.2 AP (**a**) and lateral (**b**) radiographs illustrate presence of FAI, especially cam type. 3D CT scan (**c**) more clearly delineates presence of pincer lesion with accompanying on acetabulum

Visualization is also dependent on controlling hemostasis. A high flow volume fluid management system is important for helping to keep a clear field without having to use high pressures. Modestly hypotensive anesthesia (systolic BP <100 mmHg) is advantageous when not contraindicated. A dilute solute of epinephrine is added to the arthroscopy fluid. Meticulous coagulation of small vessels aids as well (Table 23.1).

23 Principles of Hip Arthroscopy in Elite Tennis Players

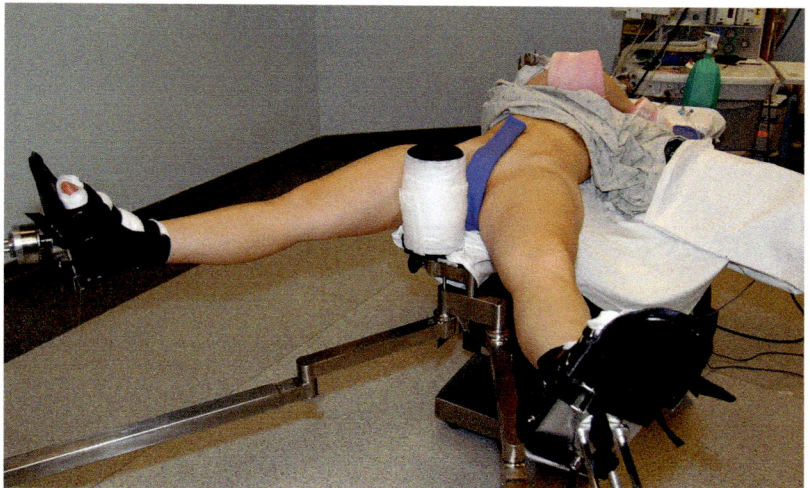

Fig. 23.3 An example of supine positioning. A well-padded perineal post is lateralized against the medial thigh of the operative hip. This helps to achieve the optimal traction vector and moves the post away from the pudendal nerve

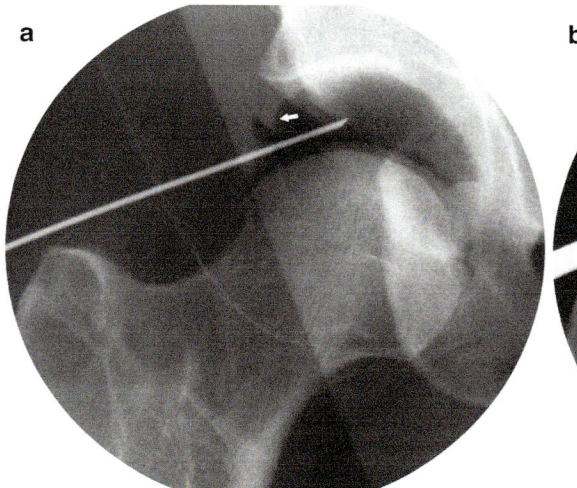
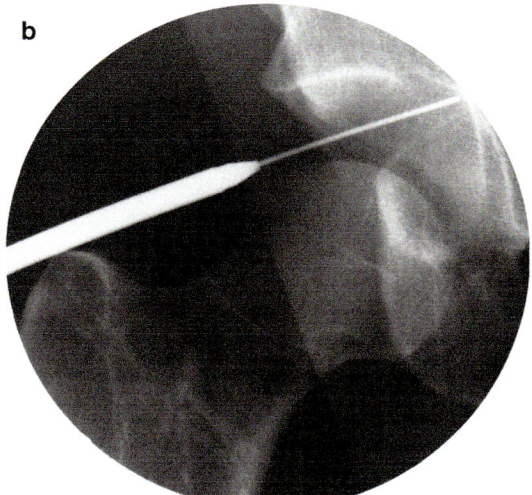

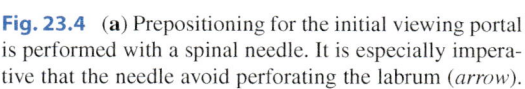

Fig. 23.4 (**a**) Prepositioning for the initial viewing portal is performed with a spinal needle. It is especially imperative that the needle avoid perforating the labrum (*arrow*). (**b**) Wherever the needle is placed is where the cannula will then go over the guidewire

23.7 Step Six: Perform the Procedure

A tentative plan is established preoperatively. The definitive treatment may be influenced by findings at arthroscopy. The extent and pattern of damage may be only partly revealed by preoperative studies.

An interportal capsulotomy is commonly used to effectively maneuver between the central and peripheral compartments for addressing most forms of pathology (Fig. 23.7a and b). Thus, an integral part of the procedure is proper capsular management. Capsular preservation with repair at the completion of the procedure is important when there may be concerns of iatrogenic instability:

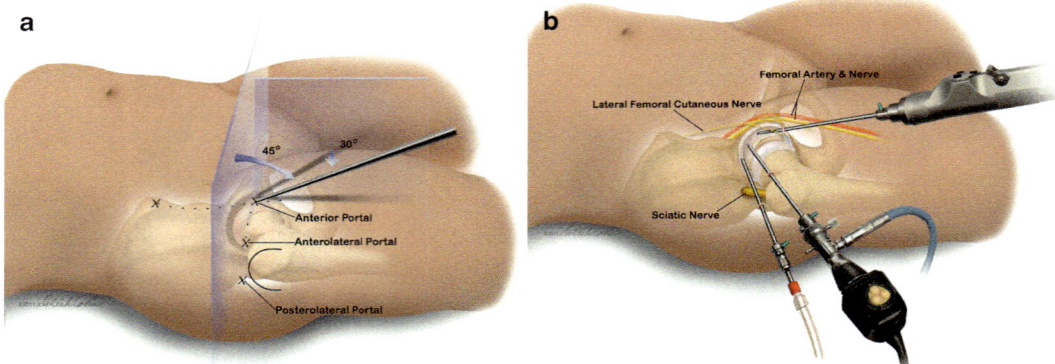

Fig. 23.5 (a) The anterior portal roughly coincides with the intersection of a sagittal line drawn distally from the anterior superior iliac spine and a transverse line across the superior margin of the greater trochanter. Generally, it is directed approximately 45° cephalad and 30° toward the midline. Depending on the patient's anatomy, it may be chosen to place this slightly more lateral and distal in order to properly intersect the joint. The anterolateral and posterolateral portals are positioned at the anterior and posterior borders of the trochanteric tip, converging slightly as they enter the joint. (b) The relationship of the major neurovascular structures to the three standard portals is demonstrated. The femoral artery and nerve lie well medial to the anterior portal. The sciatic nerve lies posterior to the posterolateral portal. Small branches of the lateral femoral cutaneous nerve lie close to the anterior portal. Injury to these is avoided by utilizing proper technique in portal placement. The anterolateral portal is established first since it lies most centrally in the safe zone for arthroscopy

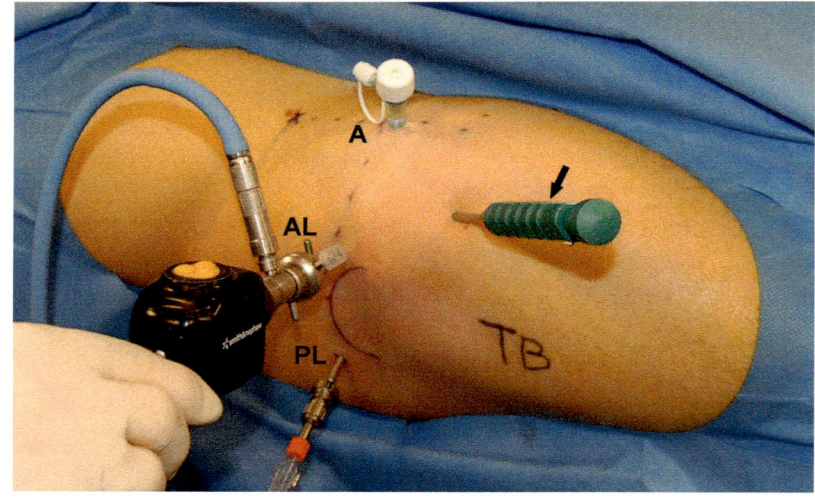

Fig. 23.6 Portals are placed for greatest utility within the joint. Suture anchors for labral repair can be placed percutaneously independent of conventional portals. Here, the anchor delivery system (*arrow*) is placed distally, equidistant between the anterior and anterolateral portals

Table 23.1 Seven steps to successful hip arthroscopy

1.	Pick the right patient
2.	Plan the procedure thoughtfully
3.	Position the patient properly
4.	Proper portal placement
5.	Clear visualization
6.	Execute the procedure
7.	Titrate the rehabilitation

low acetabular coverage of the femoral head, underlying physiologic laxity, or returning to activities that require extremes of motion. A variety of strategies on capsular restoration have been described (Fig. 23.7c) [23, 24]. For excessively stiff hips, especially those with degenerative changes, more of a therapeutic capsulectomy may be performed as part of the treatment.

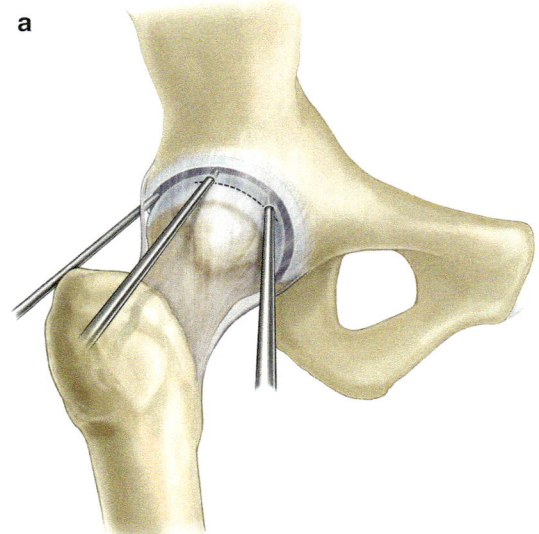
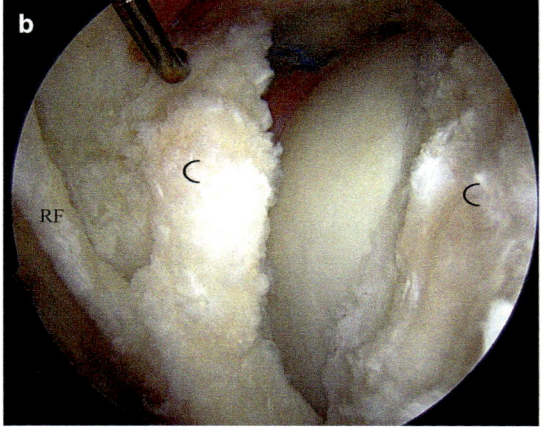
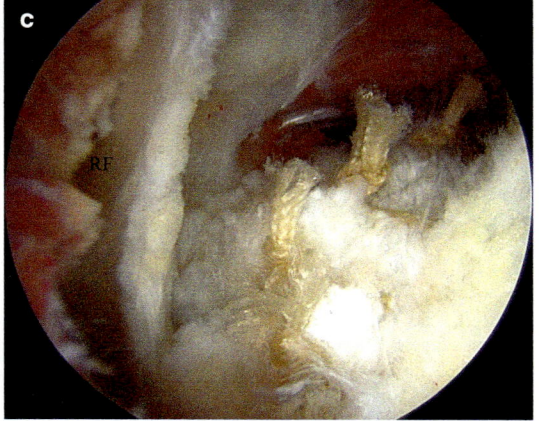

Fig. 23.7 (**a**) A capsulotomy is performed by connecting the anterior and anterolateral portals (dotted line). (**b**) Arthroscopic view of the capsulotomy through the capsule (**c**) and the relationship to the reflected head of the rectus femoris tendon (RF). The capsulotomy has been closed with absorbable #2 sutures

23.8 Step Seven: Titrate the Rehabilitation

Most postoperative problems are associated with misguided rehabilitation. This may be too much or too little or just improperly timed stepwise progression. When patients are having difficulties, close scrutiny of the rehab process may often provide answers and solutions for getting the patients back on track [25–27].

References

1. Byrd JWT, Jones KS. Hip arthroscopy in athletes. Clin Sports Med. 2001;20(4):749–62.
2. Clohisy JC, Knaus ER, Hunt DM, Lesher JM, Harris-Hayes M, Prather H. Clinical presentation of patients with symptomatic anterior hip impingement. Clin Orthop Relat Res. 2009;467(3):638–44.
3. Lynch TS, Bedi A, Larson CM. Athletic hip injuries. J Am Acad Orthop Surg. 2017;25(4):269–79.

4. Byrd JWT. Femoroacetabular impingement in athletes: current concepts. Am J Sports Med. 2014;42(3):737–51.
5. Hammoud S, Bedi A, Magennis E, Meyers WC, Kelly BT. High incidence of athletic pubalgia symptoms in professional athletes with symptomatic Femoroacetabular impingement. Arthroscopy. 2012;28(10):1388–95.
6. Larson CM, Pierce BR, Giveans MR. Treatment of athletes with symptomatic intra-articular hip pathology and athletic pubalgia/sports hernia: a case series. Arthroscopy. 2011;27(6):768–75.
7. Byrd JWT. Hip arthroscopy in the athlete. Oper Tech Sports Med. 2012;20(4):310–9.
8. Kibler WB. Biomechanical analysis of the shoulder during tennis activities. Clin Sports Med. 1995;14(1):79–85.
9. Byrd JWT. Hip arthroscopy in the athlete. Oper Tech Sports Med. 2005;13(1):24–36.
10. Ross JR, Tannenbaum EP, Nepple JJ, Kelly BT, Larson CM, Bedi A. Functional acetabular orientation varies between supine and standing radiographs: implications for treatment of femoroacetabular impingement. Clin Orthop Relat Res. 2015;473(4):1267–73.
11. Anderson LA, Anderson MB, Kapron A, Aoki SK, Erickson JA, Chrastil J, Grijalva R, Peters C. The 2015 frank Stinchfield Award: radiographic abnormalities common in senior athletes with well-functioning hips but not associated with osteoarthritis. Clin Orthop Relat Res. 2016;474(2):342–52.
12. Byrd JWT, Jones KS. Diagnostic accuracy of clinical assessment, magnetic resonance imaging, magnetic resonance arthrography, and intra-articular injection in hip arthroscopy patients. Am J Sports Med. 2004;32(7):1668–74.
13. McCarthy E, Hegazi TM, Zoga AC, Morrison WB, Meyers WC, Poor AE, Nevalainen MT, Roedl JB. Ultrasound-guided interventions for core and hip injuries in athletes. Radiol Clin N Am. 2016;54(5):875–92.
14. Byrd JWT, Potts EA, Allison RK, Jones KS. Ultrasound-guided hip injections: a comparative study with fluoroscopy-guided injections. Arthroscopy. 2014;30(1):42–6. https://doi.org/10.1016/j.arthro.2013.09.083.
15. Jones KS, Potts EA, Byrd JWT. Perioperative care. In: Byrd JWT, editor. Operative hip arthroscopy. 3rd ed. New York: Springer; 2013. p. 441–54.
16. Philippon MJ, Briggs KK, Carlisle JC, Patterson DC. Joint space predicts THA after hip arthroscopy in patients 50 years and older. Clin Orthop Relat Res. 2013;471(8):2492–6.
17. Horisberger M, Brunner A, Herzog RF. Arthroscopic treatment of femoral acetabular impingement in patients with preoperative generalized degenerative changes. Arthroscopy. 2010;26(5):623–9.
18. Byrd JWT. Routine arthroscopy and access: central and peripheral compartments, iliopsoas bursa, peritrochanteric, and subgluteal spaces. In: Byrd JWT, editor. Operative hip arthroscopy. 3rd ed. New York: Springer; 2012. p. 131–60.
19. Glick JM. Hip arthroscopy by the lateral approach. Instr Course Lect. 2006;55:317–23.
20. Mei-Dan O, McConkey MO, Young DA. Hip arthroscopy distraction without the use of a perineal post: prospective study. Orthopedics. 2013;36(1):e1–5.
21. Bond JL, Knutson ZA, Ebert A, Guanche CA. The 23-point arthroscopic examination of the hip: basic setup, portal placement, and surgical technique. Arthroscopy. 2009;25(4):416–29.
22. Robertson WJ, Kelly BT. The safe zone for hip arthroscopy: a cadaveric assessment of central, peripheral, and lateral compartment portal placement. Arthroscopy. 2008;24(9):1019–26.
23. Domb BG, Philippon MJ, Giordano BD. Arthroscopic capsulotomy, capsular repair, and capsular plication of the hip: relation to atraumatic instability. Arthroscopy. 2013;29(1):162–73.
24. Frank RM, Lee S, Bush-Joseph CA, Kelly BT, Salata MJ, Nho SJ. Improved outcomes after hip arthroscopic surgery in patients undergoing T-capsulotomy with complete repair versus partial repair for femoroacetabular impingement: a comparative matched-pair analysis. Am J Sports Med. 2014;42(11):2634–42.
25. Coplen EM, Voight M. Rehabilitation of the hip. In: Byrd JWT, editor. Operative hip arthroscopy. 3rd ed. New York, NY: Springer; 2013. p. 441–0.
26. Cheatham SW, Enseki KR, Kolber MJ. Postoperative rehabilitation after hip arthroscopy: a search for the evidence. J Sport Rehabil. 2015;24(4):413–8.
27. Domb BG, Sqroi TA, VanDevender JC. Physical therapy protocol after hip arthroscopy: clinical guidelines supported by 2-year outcomes. Sports Health. 2016;8(4):347–54.

Treatment of Femoroacetabular Impingement and Labral Injuries in Tennis Players

24

Marc R. Safran and Alberto Costantini

24.1 Introduction

Tennis participation continues to grow and has quickly become one of the most popular sports in the world with over 75 million players globally [1]. The unique functional demands of the sport require multidirectional movements, repetitive loading, and rapid torsional forces across the lower extremity for on-court performance. Importantly, the ability to generate energy from the lower extremity and trunk muscle groups can translate to greater force applied to the eventual racquet strike via the kinetic chain. However, these same gameplay characteristics can also lead to an increased risk for lower extremity injury in tennis players [2]. Anecdotally, we have seen an increase in the diagnosis and treatment of hip-related pain in these athletes. While traditionally hip injuries have been thought of being muscular in origin (hip flexor and adductor), intra-articular sources of hip pain have become more commonplace. Furthermore, professional tennis players are undergoing hip arthroscopy more frequently for related injuries. While early experiences with hip arthroscopy showed more modest results, recent reports demonstrate the growing success with this modality of treatment. Nonetheless, hip injuries in this population can be particularly difficult to manage, often due to the high-demand activity and the innate desire for earlier return to play.

Femoroacetabular impingement (FAI) has emerged as a well-recognized cause of hip dysfunction in the athletic population [3–7]. FAI has been described as repetitive abutment of a morphologically abnormal proximal femur and/or acetabulum during terminal range of motion of the hip [8]. These terminal ranges of motion include internal rotation, hip flexion, and adduction, depending on the location of offset loss from the femoral head-neck junction and/or acetabular overcoverage. In addition, recent findings demonstrate increased axial and anterior forces on the hip with open-stance forehand strokes [9]. During an external rotation moment, subsequent anterior femoral head translation can cause stretching of the anterior labrum. The presence of FAI or increased INTERNAL rotation forces at the hip can lead to labral and chondral injuries, hindering recovery and placing the patient at risk for further degenerative changes [10]. Still, treatment of FAI and the associated soft-tissue injuries can help to decrease abnormal contact stresses and provide improved stability [11, 12]. While our current understanding of the process continues to grow, treatment directives to alter the natural history could lead to joint preservation for this group. In this chapter we focus on

M. R. Safran (✉)
Department of Orthopaedic Surgery, Stanford University, Redwood City, CA, USA
e-mail: msafran@stanford.edu

A. Costantini
Department of Orthopaedic Surgery, Concordia Hospital for Special Surgery, Rome, Italy

hip injuries in tennis players, highlighting the impact of FAI and labral injuries in the athletic population. In addition, we highlight our current understanding of the etiology of these injuries and highlight the current treatment strategies available.

24.2 Etiology of FAI and Labral Injuries in Tennis Players

While tennis players are susceptible to injuries throughout the musculoskeletal system, hip injuries have been reported to occur in 1–27% of tennis players [2]. At the junior tennis level, hip pain has been reported in 1.3 per 100 players, though often these injuries are muscular in origin [13]. Similarly, Lynall et al. reported that the incidence of hip pain in college tennis players was 8.8% in males and 6.6% for females [14]. The pathomechanism for injuries in tennis players is related to the high forces placed across lower extremity joints during competitive play. Groin pain is common in tennis players and could signify impingement or labral injury, often related to torsional maneuvers [15]. Still, multiple factors specific to sporting demands and training regimens will invariably affect those tennis athletes at risk for injury of the hip.

FAI has emerged as a common cause of hip pain in the young adult population [16], with pain linked to FAI affecting both athletic participation and overall quality of life [17]. However, our current understanding of FAI has evolved rapidly over the last two decades. Previously described as an abnormal contact between the proximal femur and acetabulum due to excessive or supraphysiologic motion, Ganz et al. were one of the first to propose a possible link of FAI leading to chondral damage [10]. The repetitive motion of the hip, commonly seen in tennis, can lead to morphologic changes consistent with FAI. The subtypes of FAI are represented as pincer lesions, cam deformities, or a mixed combination of both. The pincer lesion is identified by overcoverage of the acetabulum (Figs. 24.1 and 24.4a), while cam deformities will lose

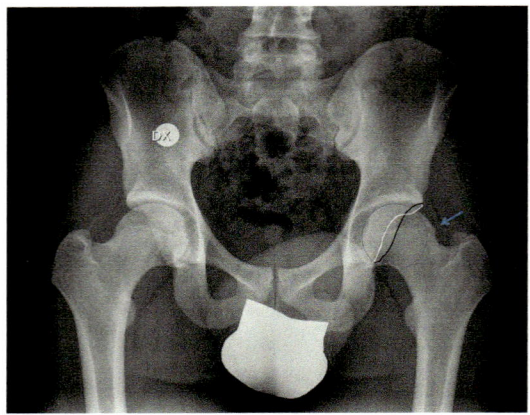

Fig. 24.1 AP radiograph of a male professional tennis player. This player has combined FAI. The acetabulum demonstrates retroversion, with decreased posterior coverage, a crossing sign, and increased center-edge angle. The proximal femur also demonstrates loss of femoral head-neck offset (*arrow*), diagnostic of cam morphology

the normal spherical shape of the femoral head at the head-neck junction, giving rise to what is often described as a bump or pistol grip deformity (Figs. 24.1 and 24.3a). Pincer lesions tend to predominate in active middle-aged women, while cam deformities are often found in young athletic males. Still the majority of FAI patients will have components of both cam and pincer morphologies present.

While debate exists over the etiology of FAI, it likely results from a combination of both genetic and acquired causes [18]. Pollard et al. showed that familial relationships are present in those with FAI, with an increased relative risk for cam and pincer deformities in siblings [19]. In addition, osteoarthritis was more proliferative in this group as compared to the controls. Ethnic differences in hip morphology may also contribute to the development of FAI. Van Houcke et al. showed that 56% of asymptomatic white patients had radiographic alpha angles >55°, diagnostic of cam impingement, as compared to only 34% of Chinese patients [20]. Furthermore, Safran et al. delved into specific genetic components potentially linked to FAI, focusing on single nucleotide polymorphisms also connected to osteoarthritis [21]. While no clear link could be established for FAI, it is likely that further efforts in this area will help uncover potential genetic relationships.

There has also been growing support to suggest that athletic activities, particularly at vulnerable stages of development, may lead to morphologic changes of FAI. Frank et al. demonstrated that the athletic population were more likely to show cam deformities (55%) than those considered nonathletes (23%) [22]. Siebenrock et al. reviewed findings of the hip in 37 athletes and compared this to 38 age-matched volunteers who did not participate in high-level sport [23]. They found that the high-intensity athletics led to a substantial increase in symptomatic FAI by both exam and radiographic findings. Athletes in this group also had a tenfold increased likelihood of having radiographs meeting diagnostic criteria of cam impingement. Increased activity coupled with physeal closure of the hip may also lead to morphologic changes of the hip. In support of this notion, Agricola et al. showed that adolescent soccer players were more likely to develop cam deformities than their nonathletic peers [24]. Kapron et al. also evaluated 67 male college football players for radiographic FAI, finding signs of impingement in 95% of this cohort [25]. The authors suggested that morphologic changes were potentially attributed to the athletic competition in football with increased demand on the hip and increased body mass index.

Adaptations around the hip joint can also place the tennis player at risk. Sanchis-Moysi et al. demonstrated asymmetric hypertrophy of the iliopsoas in professional tennis players [26], which could lead to groin pain. Many in the tennis community have long known that the rectus abdominis muscle is hypertrophied on the non-dominant side of high-level tennis players. Further, professional women tennis players were shown to develop flexion contractures of the hip with iliopsoas tightness also and subsequently be prone to abdominal strain injury [27]. While no detriments in hip range of motion was found, adaptive changes around the hip may present an environment that places the tennis athlete at risk for further injury. Similarly, Ellenbecker et al. assessed hip range of motion in 147 elite tennis athletes and 101 professional baseball players. They found that no significant differences were found between measured internal and external rotation of the hip in these groups. Moreno-Perez et al. also looked at range of motion in 109 elite level tennis players from Spanish tennis academies [28]. In contrast, they found small bilateral differences in motion to exist between dominant and non-dominant hip flexion and abduction, as well as internal rotation for males.

24.3 Clinical Evaluation and Imaging

Hip pain in the athlete can include a broad differential diagnosis. However, understanding the intra-articular and extra-articular components of hip pain can help narrow down the potential causes. Utilizing a systematic approach to evaluate hip pain in these athletes, by combining a thorough history, physical examination, and directed imaging, will help to uncover the underlying issues. In this section, we do not provide a comprehensive approach to the evaluation of hip pain, which is discussed earlier in Chap. 7, but aim to highlight specific clinical findings associated with FAI and labral injury in the athletic population.

The first step is obtaining a detailed history of the injury. FAI and resultant labral injuries are examples of intra-articular pathology and will typically present with groin pain or mechanical symptoms. Specific details about activity regimens should be inquired. This will include onset of symptoms, severity of the pain, whether intensity or duration of training has changed, playing surfaces used, or provocative motions during play that can elicit pain. The playing mechanics utilized should also be part of the discussion, for example, whether a one-handed or two-handed backhand stroke is used. A significant difference in hip joint moments has been found between these two backhand strokes, with one-handed hits exerting large forces on the lead leg compared to greater forces on the back leg with a two-handed shot [29]. In contrast, a forehand stroke will demand greater external rotation of the back hip, potentially leading to posterior impingement and stress along the anterior capsule [30]. Open-stance forehands produce increased anterior translational forces, with both down the line and crosscourt shots, in the dominant hip (Fig. 24.2) [9]. These anterior forces and the anterior translation of the femoral head will cause increased stress on the anterior labrum, producing anterior labral tears. Also, this increased external rotation can subsequently lead to laxity of the anterior capsule [31]. Playing surfaces have also contributed to injury risk, as grass and hard courts led to more athletes seeking medical treatment than those who played on clay [32]. Nonetheless, a thorough history should encompass details specific to the active tennis athlete.

Physical examination can be focused based on information garnered from the history. Intra-articular pathology, such as FAI and labral injuries, will often be reproduced with passive maneuvers of the hip joint. In contrast, extra-articular pain sources can usually be reproduced with palpation or by resisting muscular contraction. The most sensitive test for detecting FAI is the flexion, adduction, and internal rotation (FADIR), demonstrated as having value as a screening test for FAI; however, it is not specific for FAI [33]. Decreased internal rotation of the hip (as measured in flexion or extension), particularly in the setting of normal motion in all the other planes, is associated with FAI [34]. Restricted range of motion may also show predilection for injury, as decreased internal rotation of the hip can lead to anterior cruciate ligament (ACL) injury [35]. However, despite a focused physical examination, there seems to be just modest agreement among experienced hip surgeons in using history and examination for the diagnosis of hip disorders [36]. This suggests that examination maneuvers still need improvement and could benefit from a standardized approach.

Imaging evaluation for athletes with intra-articular injuries, such as FAI and labral pathology, will often include various modalities to delineate the structural and soft-tissue disruptions. Plain radiographs are usually involved in this initial work-up. Our preference is an anteroposterior (AP) of the pelvis, along with cross-table lateral view of the affected hip. This allows one to ascertain osseous changes in the acetabulum and proximal femur, along with other contributing extra-articular factors that could contribute. Cam deformity of the proximal femur and acetabular overcoverage seen with pincer impingement can then be measured. In addition, there should be close attention given to joint congruence, arthritic changes present, and findings suggestive of version abnormalities.

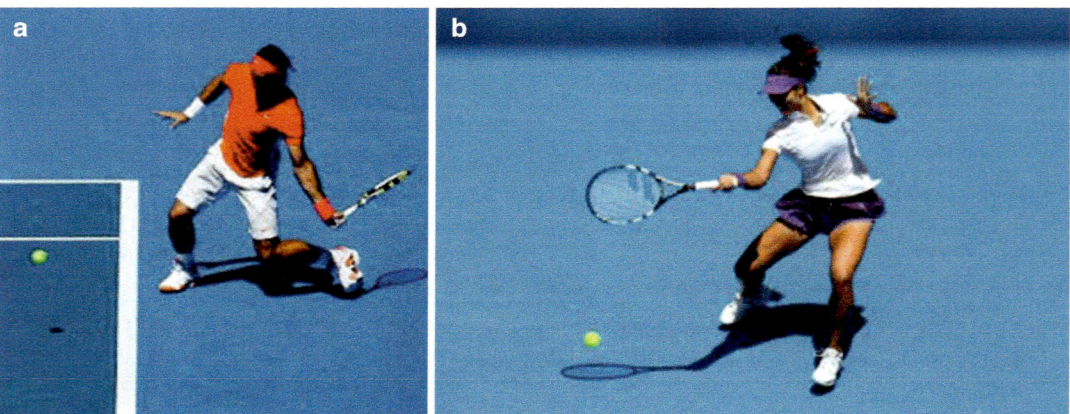

Fig. 24.2 (**a**) Closed-stance forehand—the feet (and hips) are aligned nearly perpendicular to the net. (**b**) Open-stance forehand—the feet and pelvis/hip, oblique or parallel to the net

The benefits of MR imaging include providing details on both osseous and soft-tissue changes. For patients with FAI, evaluation of the proximal femur with axial views can help elicit head-neck offset changes by measurement of the alpha angle [37]. Described by Nötzli et al. as alpha-angle measurements greater than 55° signifying cam impingement [37], controversy still surrounds what threshold value should be used. Nonetheless, combining this measurement and associated morphologic changes can help aid in the diagnosis. Likewise, osseous acetabular changes can be delineated using MR imaging, particularly by version and depth analysis [38].

Direct magnetic resonance arthrography (MRA) of the hip has been shown to be more sensitive than standard MR imaging for the detection of labral and cartilage lesions [39]. In addition, intra-articular injection of anesthetic can be performed at the same time, providing additional diagnostic and therapeutic benefits. If extra-articular pathology exists as well, the anesthetic will not mask these symptoms [40]. Changes in the labrum can also be detected with MR imaging; however, tear pattern differentiation can be difficult with MRI or MRA [41].

While beyond the scope of this chapter, ultrasound may also have a limited role in visualizing the periarticular structures and allow for guided injections. Computed tomography (CT) can also be beneficial, especially in more clear visualization of bony morphology, surgical planning, or assessment of AIIS subspine impingement. While we do not routinely use CT, this modality can be useful in select cases or revision scenarios.

24.4 Other Causes of Intra-Articular Hip Pain in the Athlete

While our current understanding of FAI in athletes has continued to expand, symptomatic hip microinstability has begun to gain traction as a potential source of dysfunction in athletes. Shu and Safran have defined this as extra-physiologic hip motion that causes pain with or without joint unsteadiness [42]. The presence of symptomatic microinstability, admittedly, has remained difficult to evaluate due to symptoms that are less overt and not clearly defined by examination. However, tennis athletes have been identified as a particular group of athletes at risk for developing microinstability of the hip [43, 44]. This proposed mechanism is related to subtle anatomic abnormalities coupled with repetitive hip rotation and axial loading [44]. Diagnosis can be quite difficult to ascertain, although examination, imaging findings, and strong history for microinstability are necessary for confirming the cause. In these patients who fail conservative management, capsular plication has been shown to provide reliable results for symptomatic relief [45]. While FAI is widespread in the athletic population, future research may grow to show that high-demand athletes may also be prone to intra-articular changes due to microinstability that occurs at the hip capsule.

24.5 Nonoperative Management

Conservative management for FAI is frequently directed at activity modification and supplementation with nonsteroidal anti-inflammatory (NSAID) medication. If the inciting mechanism for pain can be found, then avoidance can be used to prevent recurrent symptoms. Nonetheless, the goal is aimed at alleviating pain for the patient. Often focused physical therapy regimens can help to strengthen the surrounding musculature and improve proprioception. In this scenario, the decision in returning to sport should be individualized as symptom management and adequate strength need to be obtained first.

Wall et al. performed a systematic review of nonoperative treatments for FAI. They included just five studies that discussed nonoperative management, yet no single study focused exclusively on nonoperative management. They note that numerous studies promote the use of nonoperative care, yet little evidence exists in its support. Another option is intra-articular injections for the treatment of FAI. This can be used for diagnostic purposes but has shown utility in therapeutic pain relief [46]. Krych et al. investigated intra-articular steroid injections in 54 patients. In this group, average pain relief was 9.8 days, yet only 6% had relief at 6 weeks after injection. Abate et al. used hyaluronic acid alone in 23 patients for FAI. Interestingly, clinical improvements were found to be maintained at 1 year after injection by visual analog scale (VAS) and Harris hip scores (HHS). In addition, ten of these patients decreased their use of NSAIDs by more than 50%. Another direction was taken by Ayeni et al., who showed that intra-articular injections had predictive value in equating pain relief to subsequent success with arthroscopic surgery [47].

Despite a lack of strong support in the literature, we still advocate for initial nonoperative care when appropriate. This period of conservative management should also entail a frank discussion about goals for returning to sport. Currently, the protocol for the Femoroacetabular Impingement Trial (FAIT) is trying to scientifically prove whether operative or nonoperative intervention is more effective at improving symptoms and preventing the development and eventual progression of osteoarthritis [48]. It is possible that results from this multicenter randomized controlled trial will better elucidate potential benefits with conservative care.

24.6 Operative Management

The aims of surgical treatment for FAI and labral injuries in athletes are to restore function, alleviate symptoms, and allow for successful return to sport. For those that undergo surgery, nonoperative options have often been exhausted, and yet they remain sidelined by persistent symptoms. The principles of operative treatment for FAI include correction of the underlying bony abnormalities and associated chondrolabral injuries. In cam deformities, the structural abnormalities of the proximal femur occur at the head-neck junction which leads to labral and chondral injury at the anterosuperior region of the acetabulum [49]. In contrast, the pathomechanism of pincer impingement often relates to overcoverage phenomena of the acetabulum. This can be caused by acetabular retroversion, focal anterior overcoverage, coxa profunda, or protrusio [50]. While a circumferential pattern of disease is commonly found in pincer pathology, posteroinferior lesions are also common in this group [49]. These posterior lesions can occur with subluxation of the femoral head once flexion blocks impingement at the anterosuperior rim.

Surgical correction of cam pathology involves resection of the deformity present at the head-neck junction (Figure 24.3), which has been shown to restore motion of the hip [51]. For symptoms related to overcoverage, as seen in pincer impingement, acetabuloplasty or rim trimming can alter the morphology of the acetabular rim (Figure 24.4). While planning for rim resection, it is important to quantify the intraoperative rim reduction to reach a planned center-edge angle of acetabulum [52]. In cases of more severe torsional deformities of the acetabulum or retroversion, open periacetabular osteotomy can be used to address these more complex deformities. Femoral derotational osteotomy may be required for management of impingement due to severe femoral rotational or version abnormalities.

In addition to FAI, subsequent changes in the labrum occur with repeated microtrauma [53]. Labral injuries represent an intra-articular injury that can cause significant limitations for athletes. The loss of femoral head-neck offset in cam impingement can lead to shearing stresses at the acetabular rim that result in chondrolabral separation and chondral delamination, while pincer impingement often follows compression patterns of the labrum and nearby cartilage. Depending on tear characteristics, options can include labral debridement, labral refixation (repair), or labral reconstruction. As described, ideal indications for labral repair include minimal degeneration, little ossification, or absence of complex tearing (Figure 24.5) [54]. For stable focal tears, debridement can be safely performed if less than 3 mm [54, 55], although studies suggest that preservation of labral tissue is optimal in comparison [54, 56]. Larson et al. investigated 36 females undergoing hip arthroscopy for pincer or combined FAI morphology with associated labral injury. Comparison between labral repair and labral debridement in this population revealed that repair resulted in superior clinical outcomes at

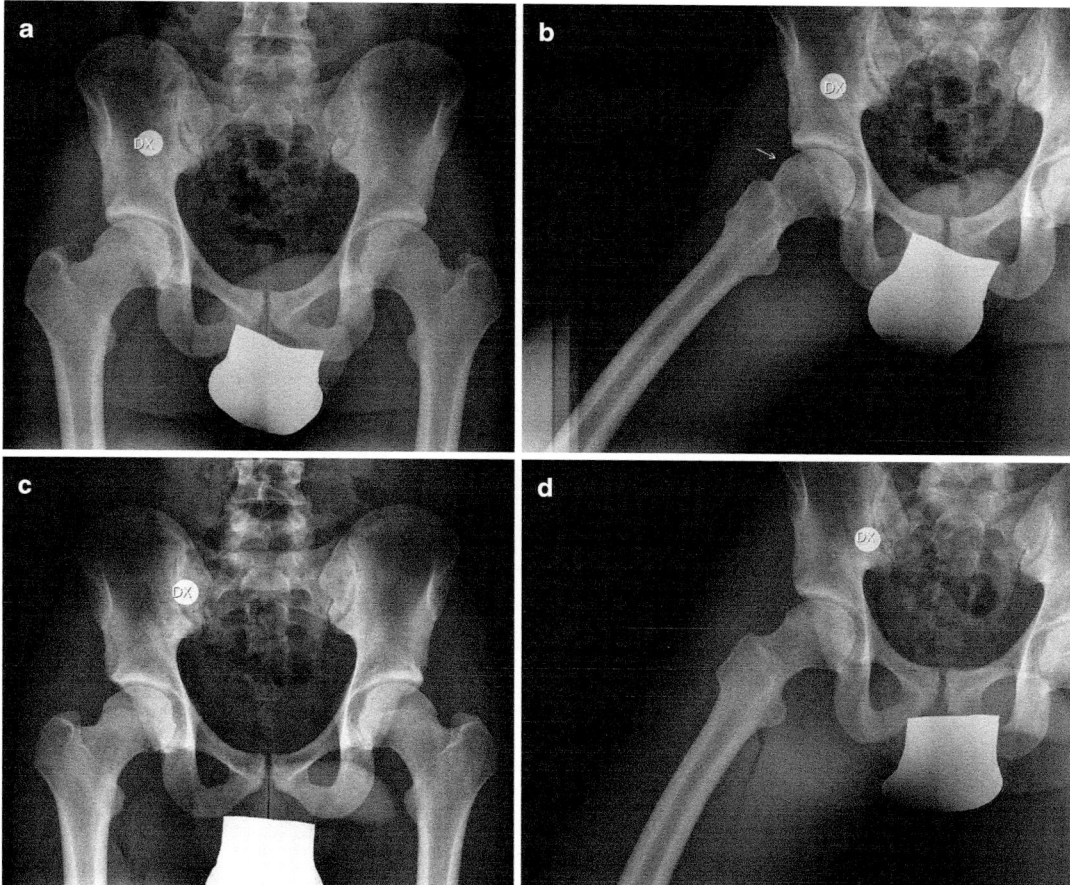

Fig. 24.3 (**a**) 21-year-old athlete with bilateral cam and pincer FAI. Figure **a** is the preoperative radiographs showing the combined FAI. Figure **b** is a cross-table lateral radiograph of the right hip preoperatively. The arrows point to the cam lesion where the femoral head-neck junction has loss of offset. Figure **c** and **d** is the postop images, demonstrating restoration of femoral head-neck offset on AP (**c**) and cross-table lateral (**d**) radiograph

3.5 years postoperatively. Philippon et al. specifically looked at repair and FAI treatment in professional hockey players [57]. Similarly, significant improvements in functional outcomes were seen in this select group of athletes.

In revision settings after failure of labral repair, there is growing support for labral reconstruction [58]. Boykin et al. performed a retrospective review of elite athletes who underwent arthroscopic iliotibial band labral reconstruction for irreparable labral tears. In this group, 86% returned to sport, with 81% returning to the same level of play with improved satisfaction after surgery [59].

Approaches for surgical management of FAI originally included open surgical dislocation of the hip, which has been proven successful [51, 60–62]. However, current data exists for both open surgery and hip arthroscopy in being able to return the athlete to sport after surgery [63]. Still, there has been a strong trend toward hip arthroscopy as it continues to grow in popularity [64–66]. Bozic et al. evaluated the incidence of hip arthroscopy procedures between 2006 and 2010 in board-eligible surgeons who were taking the American Board of Orthopaedic Surgery (ABOS) Part II exam [64]. They found that there was an over 600% increase in arthroscopic treatment of FAI. Invariably, exposure to arthroscopic management of hip disorders in residency and fellowship has contributed to this growth. While there is support for both approaches

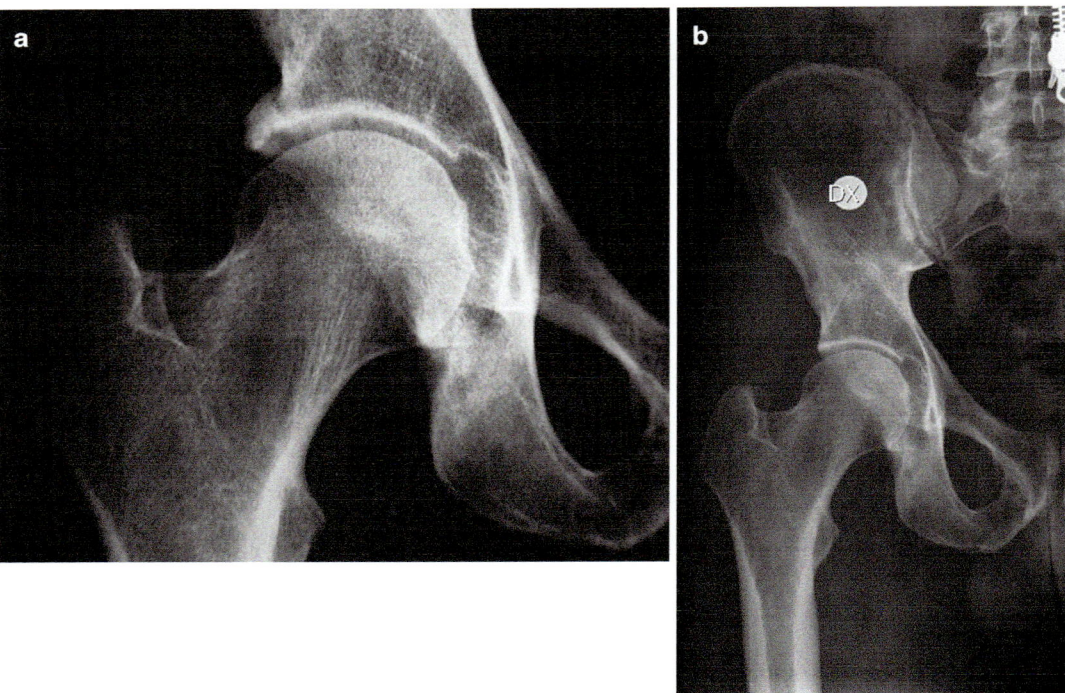

Fig. 24.4 A 24-year-old athlete with right hip pain. Figure **a** demonstrated the lateral extent of the acetabular socket. Figure **b** is 2 years after acetabuloplasty to reduce acetabular depth

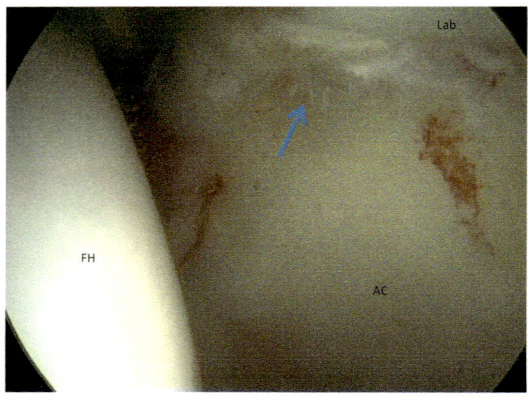

Fig. 24.5 Arthroscopic photograph of the hip joint in a collegiate athlete. Labeling shows the femoral head (FH) is to the left and acetabulum (AC) on the right. The labrum (Lab) is on the top . A labral-chondral separation and frying are present (*arrow*). This type of injury is amenable to labral repair

with equivalent outcomes for return to sport, it is likely that further studies will continue to focus on arthroscopic management as the field continues to expand.

Nwachukwu et al. recently performed a systematic review to determine differences in clinical outcomes or progression to total hip arthroplasty between hip arthroscopy and open dislocation for FAI [67]. It was found that both techniques provided excellent long-term clinical outcomes along with equivalent hip survival rates at medium-term follow-up. However, hip arthroscopy demonstrated significantly higher general health-related quality of life (HRQoL) compared to open surgical dislocation. The progressive development of arthroscopic techniques, improved training, and along with careful patient selection may lead to the comparable results now being seen. Additionally, advantages of hip arthroscopy can include less soft-tissue disruption, earlier recovery for the patient, and better short-term outcome [68].

Recent data suggests that athletes may be affected by symptomatic FAI and labral injuries greater than the general population [24, 25, 69], with high-level male athletes being most likely to undergo hip arthroscopy [70].

Casartelli et al. performed a systematic review on athletes who underwent hip surgery for the treatment of FAI. This aggregate review of 18 studies, including open surgery and hip arthroscopy, showed that 87% athletes returned to sport and 82% achieved the same level of sport [63]. The elite-level athlete may even find greater success with FAI surgery, as return rates at 1 year have been reported to be much higher when compared to recreational athletes [71]. We recently reviewed the outcomes of hip arthroscopy, for FAI and hip instability for elite athletes [72]. In this study cohort, 80 college, professional, and Olympic athletes from various sports, including tennis, were followed for return to sport after hip arthroscopy. In this group, 84% were able to return to sports at the same level at an average of just over 8 months. Also, Philippon et al. reported on professional athletes undergoing hip arthroscopy, with 93% returning to professional sport and 76% remaining in professional competition at 1.6 years postoperatively [7]. Still, these findings may not be limited to adult high-level athletes, as Byrd et al. also revealed favorable outcomes in arthroscopic treatment of FAI in adolescent athletes. This group of 104 adolescents at average age of 16 revealed that 94% obtained good to excellent results [73]. While there are many factors that can influence eventual return to sport, these findings suggest successful outcomes can be achieved with operative management in this select group.

Additional benefits of corrective FAI surgery can include improved biomechanics of the hip [74]. Rylander et al. demonstrated that FAI patients exhibited abnormalities of their gait when compared to controls [75]. However, following FAI surgery, kinematics were largely restored, including sagittal plane motion and maximum internal rotation of the hip. Similarly, Lamontagne et al. evaluated postoperative changes in FAI patients with respect to lower extremity joint and pelvic displacement during squatting [76]. It was found that postoperative gains were made in maximal squatting depth, affecting the hip, knee, and ankle joints in the group. While there is no direct correlation to athletic performance, presumption may be made that increased mobility due to biomechanical improvements could lead to potential advantages for performance on the court.

Conclusion

The tennis athlete can be susceptible to injuries of the hip due to the high demands of their sport. As our current understanding grows, we have learned that FAI and labral injury can be quite common in this athletic population. Recognizing symptoms of impingement and risk factors for injury can help guide diagnosis and subsequent management. While the etiology appears to be influenced by genetic and acquired mechanisms, symptomatic athletes with FAI may be placing their joint at risk if symptoms are ignored. Conservative management can include activity modification, NSAIDs, and intra-articular injections that can be both diagnostic and therapeutic. However, in scenarios where nonoperative care has failed, there is growing support for surgical management that has provided excellent results. In addition, we suspect that hip arthroscopy will continue to gain traction over open surgery as the more commonly utilized approach. Future directives should also be focused on standardizing our diagnostic approaches and helping to elucidate whether intervention can provide long-term preservation of the hip joint in the active athlete.

References

1. Pluim BM, Miller S, Dines D, et al. Sport science and medicine in tennis. Br J Sports Med. 2007;41(11):703–4.
2. Abrams GD, Renstrom P, Safran MR. Epidemiology of musculoskeletal injury in the tennis player. Br J Sports Med. 2012;46(7):492–8.
3. Byrd JWT. Femoroacetabular impingement in athletes: current concepts. Am J Sports Med. 2014;42(3):737–51.
4. Byrd JW, Jones KS. Arthroscopic management of femoroacetabular impingement: minimum 2-year follow-up. Arthroscopy. 2011;27(10):1379–88.
5. Vaughn ZD, Safran MR. Arthroscopic femoral osteoplasty/chielectomy for cam-type femoroacetabular

impingement in the athlete. Sports Med Arthrosc. 2010;18(2):90–9.
6. Nho SJ, Magennis EM, Singh CK, Kelly BT. Outcomes after the arthroscopic treatment of femoroacetabular impingement in a mixed group of high-level athletes. Am J Sports Med. 2011;39(Suppl(1_suppl)):14S–9S.
7. Philippon M, Schenker M, Briggs K, Kuppersmith D. Femoroacetabular impingement in 45 professional athletes: associated pathologies and return to sport following arthroscopic decompression. Knee Surg Sports Traumatol Arthrosc. 2007;15(7):908–14.
8. Anderson CN, Riley GM, Gold GE, Safran MR. Hip-femoral acetabular impingement. Clin Sports Med. 2013;32(3):409–25.
9. Bondi E. Using the open stance forehand may subject tennis players to increased hip joint force. In: Presented at Society for Tennis Medicine & Science, Amelia Island, FL; December 5, 2016.
10. Ganz R, Parvizi J, Beck M, Leunig M, Notzli H, Siebenrock KA. Femoroacetabular impingement: a cause for osteoarthritis of the hip. Clin Orthop Relat Res. 2003;(417):112–20.
11. Crawford MJ, Dy CJ, Alexander JW, et al. The 2007 Frank Stinchfield Award. The biomechanics of the hip labrum and the stability of the hip. Clin Orthop Relat Res. 2007;465:16–22.
12. Freehill MT, Safran MR. The labrum of the hip: diagnosis and rationale for surgical correction. Clin Sports Med. 2011;30(2):293–315.
13. Hutchinson MR, Laprade RF, Burnett QM, Moss R, Terpstra J. Injury surveillance at the USTA boys' tennis championships: a 6-yr study. Med Sci Sports Exerc. 1995;27(6):826–30.
14. Lynall RC, Kerr ZY, Djoko A, Pluim BM, Hainline B, Dompier TP. Epidemiology of National Collegiate Athletic Association men's and women's tennis injuries, 2009/2010–2014/2015. Br J Sports Med. 2015;50(7):1–6.
15. Dines JS, Bedi A, Williams PN, et al. Tennis injuries: epidemiology, pathophysiology, and treatment. J Am Acad Orthop Surg. 2015;23(3):181–9.
16. Samora JB, Ng VY, Ellis TJ. Femoroacetabular impingement: a common cause of hip pain in young adults. Clin J Sport Med. 2011;21(1):51–6.
17. Diamond LE, Dobson FL, Bennell KL, Wrigley TV, Hodges PW, Hinman RS. Physical impairments and activity limitations in people with femoroacetabular impingement: a systematic review. Br J Sports Med. 2015;49(4):230–42.
18. Packer JD, Safran MR. The etiology of primary femoroacetabular impingement: genetics or acquired deformity? J Hip Preserv Surg. 2015;2(3):249–57.
19. Pollard TCB, Villar RN, Norton MR, et al. Genetic influences in the aetiology of femoroacetabular impingement: a sibling study. J Bone Joint Surg Br. 2010;92(2):209–16.
20. Van Houcke J, Yau WP, Yan CH, et al. Prevalence of radiographic parameters predisposing to femoroacetabular impingement in young asymptomatic Chinese and white subjects. J Bone Joint Surg Am. 2015;97(4):310–7.
21. Safran M, Hariri S, Smith L. Paper 31: Is there a genetic link to FAI: a DNA pilot study of GDF5 and frizzle single nucleotide polymorphisms. YJARS. 2010;27:e18.
22. Frank JM, Harris JD, Erickson BJ, et al. Prevalence of femoroacetabular impingement imaging findings in asymptomatic volunteers: a systematic review. Arthroscopy. 2015;31(6):1199–204.
23. Siebenrock KA, Ferner F, Noble PC, Santore RF, Werlen S, Mamisch TC. The cam-type deformity of the proximal femur arises in childhood in response to vigorous sporting activity. Clin Orthop Relat Res. 2011;469(11):3229–40.
24. Agricola R, Bessems JHJM, Ginai Z, et al. The development of cam-type deformity in adolescent and young male soccer players. Am J Sports Med. 2012;40(5):1099–106.
25. Kapron AL, Anderson AE, Aoki SK, et al. Radiographic prevalence of femoroacetabular impingement in collegiate football players: AAOS Exhibit Selection. J Bone Joint Surg Am. 2011;93-A(19):e111(1–10).
26. Sanchis-Moysi J, Idoate F, Izquierdo M, Calbet JAL, Dorado C. Iliopsoas and gluteal muscles are asymmetric in tennis players but not in soccer players. PLoS One. 2011;6(7). https://doi.org/10.1371/journal.pone.0022858.
27. Young SW, Dakic J, Stroia K, Nguyen ML, Harris AHS, Safran MR. Hip range of motion and association with injury in female professional tennis players. Am J Sports Med. 2014;42(11):2654–8.
28. Moreno-Pérez V, Ayala F, Fernandez-Fernandez J, Vera-Garcia FJ. Descriptive profile of hip range of motion in elite tennis players. Phys Ther Sport. 2016;19:43–8.
29. Akutagawa S, Kojima T. Trunk rotation torques through the hip joints during the one- and two-handed backhand tennis strokes. J Sports Sci. 2005;23(8):781–93.
30. Klingenstein GG, Martin R, Kivlan B, Kelly BT. Hip injuries in the overhead athlete. Clin Orthop Relat Res. 2012;470:1579–85.
31. Martin RL, Sekiya JK. The interrater reliability of 4 clinical tests used to assess individuals with musculoskeletal hip pain. J Orthop Sports Phys Ther. 2008;38(2):71–7.
32. Kulund DN, McCue FC 3rd, Rockwell DA, Gieck JH. Tennis injuries: prevention and treatment. A review. Am J Sports Med. 1979;7(4):249–53.
33. Reiman MP, Goode AP, Cook CE, Holmich P, Thorborg K. Diagnostic accuracy of clinical tests for the diagnosis of hip femoroacetabular impingement/labral tear: a systematic review with meta-analysis. Br J Sports Med. 2015;49(12):811.
34. Kapron AL, Aoki SK, Peters CL. In-vivo Hip arthrokinematics during supine clinical exams: application to the study of femoroacetabular impingement. J Biomech. 2016;116(8):1477–90.

35. Vandenberg C, Crawford EA, Enselman ES, Robbins CB, Wojtys EM, Bedi A. Restricted hip rotation is correlated with an increased risk for anterior cruciate ligament injury. Arthroscopy. 2016;33:317–25.
36. Martin RL, Kelly BT, Leunig M, et al. Reliability of clinical diagnosis in intraarticular hip diseases. Knee Surg Sport Traumatol Arthrosc. 2010;18(5):685–90.
37. Nötzli HP, Wyss TF, Stoecklin CH, et al. Ovid: the contour of the femoral head-neck junction as a predictor for the risk of anterior impingement. J Bone Joint Surg Br. 2002;84(4):556–60.
38. Riley GM, McWalter EJ, Stevens KJ, Safran MR, Lattanzi R, Gold GE. MRI of the hip for the evaluation of femoroacetabular impingement; past, present, and future. J Magn Reson Imaging. 2015;41(3):558–72.
39. Sutter R, Zubler V, Hoffmann A, et al. Hip MRI: how useful is intraarticular contrast material for evaluating surgically proven lesions of the labrum and articular cartilage? Am J Roentgenol. 2014;202(1):160–9.
40. Kivlan BR, Martin RL, Sekiya JK. Response to diagnostic injection in patients with femoroacetabular impingement, labral tears, chondral lesions, and extra-articular pathology. Arthroscopy. 2011;27(5):619–27.
41. Blankenbaker DG, Tuite MJ. Acetabular labrum. Magn Reson Imaging Clin N Am. 2013;21(1):21–33.
42. Jiajue R, Jiang Y, Wang O, et al. Suppressed bone turnover was associated with increased osteoporotic fracture risks in non-obese postmenopausal Chinese women with type 2 diabetes mellitus. Osteoporos Int. 2014;25(8):1999–2005.
43. Shu B, Safran MR. Hip instability: anatomic and clinical considerations of traumatic and atraumatic instability. Clin Sports Med. 2011;30(2):349–67.
44. Kalisvaart MM, Safran MR. Microinstability of the hip—it does exist: etiology, diagnosis and treatment. J Hip Preserv Surg. 2015;2(2):123–35.
45. Kalisvaart MM, Safran MR. Hip instability treated with arthroscopic capsular plication. Knee Surg Sport Traumatol Arthrosc. 2016. https://doi.org/10.1007/s00167-016-4377-6.
46. Byrd JWT, Jones KS. Diagnostic accuracy of clinical assessment, magnetic resonance imaging, magnetic resonance arthrography, and intra-articular injection in hip arthroscopy patients. Am J Sports Med. 2004;32(7):1668–74.
47. Ayeni OR, Farrokhyar F, Crouch S, Chan K, Sprague S, Bhandari M. Pre-operative intra-articular hip injection as a predictor of short-term outcome following arthroscopic management of femoroacetabular impingement. Knee Surg Sport Traumatol Arthrosc. 2014;22(4):801–5.
48. Palmer a JR, Ayyar-Gupta V, Dutton SJ, et al. Protocol for the femoroacetabular impingement trial (FAIT): a multi-centre randomised controlled trial comparing surgical and non-surgical management of femoroacetabular impingement. Bone Joint Res. 2014;3(11):321–7.
49. Beck M, Kalhor M, Leunig M, Ganz R, Surgeon O. Hip morphology influences the pattern of damage to the acetabular cartilage femoroacetabular impingement as a cause of early osteoarthritis of the hip. J Bone Joint Surg Br. 2005;87:1012–8.
50. Tönnis D, Heinecke A. Acetabular and femoral anteversion: relationship with osteoarthritis of the hip. J Bone Joint Surg Am. 1999;81(12):1747–70.
51. Beck M, Leunig M, Parvizi J, Boutier V, Wyss D, Ganz R. Anterior femoroacetabular impingement: Part II. Midterm results of surgical treatment. Clin Orthop Relat Res. 2004;418:67–73.
52. Philippon MJ, Wolff AB, Briggs KK, Zehms CT, Kuppersmith DA. Acetabular rim reduction for the treatment of femoroacetabular impingement correlates with preoperative and postoperative center-edge angle. Arthroscopy. 2010;26(6):757–61.
53. Seldes RM, Tan V, Hunt J, Katz M, Winiarsky R, Fitzgerald RH. Anatomy, histologic features, and vascularity of the adult acetabular labrum. Clin Orthop Relat Res. 2001;382:232–40.
54. Larson CM, Giveans MR. Arthroscopic debridement versus refixation of the acetabular labrum associated with femoroacetabular impingement. Arthroscopy. 2009;25(4):369–76.
55. Kelly BT, Weiland DE, Schenker ML, Philippon MJ. Arthroscopic labral repair in the hip: surgical technique and review of the literature. Arthroscopy. 2005;21(12):1496–504.
56. Krych AJ, Thompson M, Knutson Z, Scoon J, Coleman SH. Arthroscopic labral repair versus selective labral debridement in female patients with femoroacetabular impingement: a prospective randomized study. Arthroscopy. 2013;29(1):46–53.
57. Philippon MJ, Weiss DR, Kuppersmith DA, Briggs KK, Hay CJ. Arthroscopic labral repair and treatment of femoroacetabular impingement in professional hockey players. Am J Sports Med. 2010;38(1):99–104.
58. White BJ, Patterson J, Herzog MM. Revision arthroscopic acetabular labral treatment: repair or reconstruct? Arthroscopy. 2016;32(12):2513–20.
59. Boykin RE, Patterson D, Briggs KK, Dee A, Philippon MJ. Results of arthroscopic labral reconstruction of the hip in elite athletes. Am J Sports Med. 2013;41(10):2296–301.
60. Ganz R, Gill TJ, Gautier E, Ganz K, Krügel N, Berlemann U. Surgical dislocation of the adult hip. J Bone Joint Surg. 2001;83(8):1119–24.
61. Lavigne M, Parvizi J, Beck M, Siebenrock KA, Ganz R, Leunig M. Anterior femoroacetabular impingement: Part I. Techniques of joint preserving surgery. Clin Orthop Relat Res. 2004;418(February):61–6.
62. Cohen SB, Huang R, Ciccotti MG, Dodson Christopher C, Parvizi J. Treatment of femoroacetabular impingement in athletes using a mini-direct anterior approach. Am J Sports Med. 2012;40(7):1620–8.
63. Casartelli NC, Leunig M, Maffiuletti NA, Bizzini M. Return to sport after hip surgery for femoroacetabular impingement: a systematic review. Br J Sports Med. 2015;49(12):819–24.
64. Bozic KJ, Chan V, Valone FH, Feeley BT, Vail TP. Trends in hip arthroscopy utilization in the United States. J Arthroplast. 2013;28(8 Suppl):140–3.

65. Colvin AC, Harrast J, Harner C. Trends in hip arthroscopy. J Bone Joint Surg. 2012;94(4):e23.
66. Montgomery SR, Ngo SS, Hobson T, et al. Trends and demographics in hip arthroscopy in the United States. Arthroscopy. 2013;29(4):661–5.
67. Nwachukwu BU, Rebolledo BJ, McCormick F, Rosas S, Harris JD, Kelly BT. Arthroscopic versus open treatment of femoroacetabular impingement: a systematic review of medium- to long-term outcomes. Am J Sports Med. 2016;44(4):1062–8.
68. Zingg PO, Ulbrich EJ, Buehler TC, Kalberer F, Poutawera VR, Dora C. Surgical hip dislocation versus hip arthroscopy for femoroacetabular impingement: clinical and morphological short-term results. Arch Orthop Trauma Surg. 2013;133(1):69–79.
69. Gerhardt MB, Romero AA, Silvers HJ, Harris DJ, Watanabe D, Mandelbaum BR. The prevalence of radiographic hip abnormalities in elite soccer players. Am J Sports Med. 2012;40(3):584–8.
70. Nawabi DH, Bedi A, Tibor LM, Magennis E, Kelly BT. The demographic characteristics of high-level and recreational athletes undergoing hip arthroscopy for femoroacetabular impingement: a sports-specific analysis. Arthroscopy. 2014;30(3):398–405.
71. Malviya A, Paliobeis CP, Villar RN. Do professional athletes perform better than recreational athletes after arthroscopy for femoroacetabular impingement? Clin Orthop Relat Res. 2013;471:2477–83.
72. Shibata KR, Safran MR. Arthroscopic hip surgery in the elite athlete: comparison of female and male elite athletes. Am J Sports Med. 2017;45(8):1730–9.
73. Byrd JWT, Jones KS, Gwathmey FW. Arthroscopic management of femoroacetabular impingement in adolescents. Arthroscopy. 2016;32(9):1800–6.
74. Sampson JD, Safran MR. Biomechanical implications of corrective surgery for FAI: an evidence-based review. Sports Med Arthrosc. 2015;23(4):169–73.
75. Rylander J, Shu B, Favre J, Safran M, Andriacchi T. Functional testing provides unique insights into the pathomechanics of femoroacetabular impingement and an objective basis for evaluating treatment outcome. J Orthop Res. 2013;31(9):1461–8.
76. Lamontagne M, Brisson N, Kennedy MJ, Beaulé PE. Preoperative and postoperative lower-extremity joint and pelvic kinematics during maximal squatting of patients with cam femoroacetabular impingement. J Bone Joint Surg. 2011;93(2):40–5.

Tennis Injuries of the Hip and Thigh

25

Ioonna Félix, Pete Draovitch, Todd S. Ellenbecker, and Joshua Dines

25.1 Etiology and Epidemiology of Hip and Thigh Injuries in Elite Tennis Players

Injuries to the hip and thigh in the elite tennis player are common and deserve great attention from both an injury prevention and rehabilitation standpoint. The modern game of tennis imparts repetitive stresses to the hip complex through multidirectional repetitive movement patterns required for successful elite-level performance.

I. Félix
Sports Medicine and Shoulder Service, Hospital for Special Surgery, New York, NY, USA
e-mail: felixi@hss.edu

P. Draovitch
Hospital for Special Surgery, New York, NY, USA
e-mail: pdraovitch@comcast.net

T. S. Ellenbecker
Rehab Plus Sports Therapy Scottsdale, Scottsdale, AZ, USA

Medical Services ATP World Tour, Scottsdale, AZ, USA
e-mail: tellenbecker@atpworldtour.com

J. Dines (✉)
Sports Medicine and Shoulder Service, Hospital for Special Surgery, New York, NY, USA

Orthopedic Surgery, Weill Cornell Medical College, New York, NY, USA

Aspetar Sports Medicine Hospital, Doha, Qatar
e-mail: dinesj@hss.edu

An average point in tennis requires 4.2 directional changes and requires maximal level exertion and sprinting speeds over short- to mid-range distances [1]. Pluim et al. [2] published a review of epidemiological studies in tennis players. Their review found 10 of 13 epidemiological studies reporting a greater number of lower extremity injuries than in the upper extremity. Four of six of the studies comparing acute versus chronic injuries reported greater incidence of acute injuries in the lower extremity in tennis players. Additionally injuries to the trunk and core accounted for a range of 5–25% of all tennis injuries. This chapter will show the interplay and kinetic chain dependence of evaluation and treatment of hip injuries indicating the need for core stability evaluation and treatment technique utilization in the management of hip and thigh injuries.

In a 5-year study of musculoskeletal injuries on the ATP World Tour, Ellenbecker et al. [3] report that injuries to the hip account for on average 6% of injuries evaluated and treated in men's professional tennis. With respect to the most common diagnosis, femoroacetabular impingement (FAI) was the most common hip injury diagnosis (32%). Muscular injuries in the thigh accounted for 11% of all injuries on the ATP World Tour. The breakdown of these thigh injuries by location for the years 2014–2016 is shown in Fig. 25.1.

As can be seen in the graphic in Fig. 25.1, adductor, hamstring, and quadriceps muscle injuries are the most common injuries reported in male professional tennis players [4]. Consistent

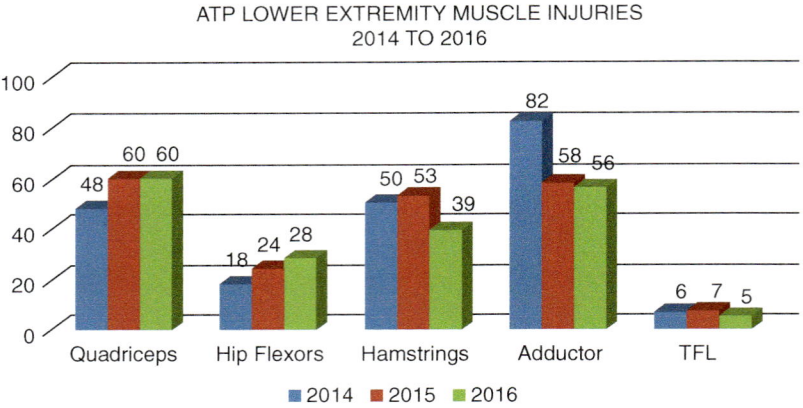

Fig. 25.1 Number of thigh muscle injuries in 2014 to 2016 ATP World Tour

numbers for these three muscle groups have been reported and are greater than hip flexor and TFL injuries in this population. Information on the most common injuries in the hip and thigh coupled with knowledge of expected anatomical adaptations of muscular strength and range of motion [5] presented in other chapters of this book will assist the clinician in the design and implementation of optimal rehabilitation programs for the hip and thigh. This chapter will present key rehabilitation and kinetic chain concepts used in the treatment of hip and thigh injuries in elite tennis players. The keen understanding of the interplay of the key mechanics between the spine, core musculature, hip, and lower extremity is essential to preventing and treating these injuries in elite tennis players.

25.2 The Layer System and Regional Interdependence

The layer concept of the hip was developed to identify pain generators, determine pathology, and design treatment protocols based on structure and function [6]. The layers include osteochondral, capsulolabral, muscular, and neuromechanical and are categorized from Layer I to IV, respectively [6]. Although pathology may exist in isolation or in combination at any layer, regional interdependence may also exist. Simply put, injuries or interventions at one part of the body may affect forces, movements, or compensations at other parts of the body [7].

The osteochondral layer consists of the structures of the femur, acetabulum, and innominate with the purpose of joint congruity and articular mechanics. The capsulolabral layer consists of the structures of the capsule, labrum, ligamentous complex, and ligamentum teres with the purpose of static joint stability. The muscular layer consists of periarticular, lumbosacral, and pelvic floor musculature with the purpose of dynamic stability. We will later discuss the roles these first three layers play when we compare FAI and dysplasia. The neuromechanical layer consists of the vasculature, spinal nerves, mechanoreceptors, and thoracolumbar and lower extremity mechanics.

Pathology of Layer I can be classified into static and dynamic causes. Static causes include developmental dysplasia, femoral/acetabular version, femoral inclination, and acetabular profunda and protrusio. Dynamic causes include cam/rim impingement, trochanteric impingement, subspine impingement, and delamination. Pathology of Layer II consists of labral tears, capsular instability, ligamentum teres tears, and adhesive capsulitis. Pathology of Layer III can be categorized based on anatomic location. Pubalgia, hip flexor strain, and psoas/rectus femoris impingement can be identified anteriorly. Adductor tendinopathy and rectus abdominis enthesiopathy can be identified medially. Hamstring strains and deep gluteal syndrome can be found posteriorly, while gluteus medius tears and peri-trochanteric space pathologies can be found laterally. Pathology of Layer IV can be classified into neural and mechanical causes. Neural issues range from nerve entrapments and referred spinal pathology to neuromuscular dysfunction and regional pain syndromes. Mechanical issues range from spine, pelvic, and lower extremity structural issues to the same areas being affected by mechanical dysfunction.

The last concept that must be addressed in this section is regional interdependence. Erhard and Bowling [8] alluded to this concept in 1977 when they stated: "Dysfunction in any unit of the system will cause delivery of abnormal stresses to other segments of the system with the development of a subsequent dysfunction here as well." This can be seen many times throughout the literature as it relates to the hip. Robb et al. [9] showed the relationship that existed in the overhead athlete and loss of hip range of motion. Ellera-Gomes et al. [10] showed the relationship between noncontact ACL injuries in soccer players who presented with decreased hip ROM radiologically. Vad et al. [11] demonstrated decreased hip ROM of the lead hip in golfers and its relationship to low back pain. Bedi et al. [12, 13] showed possible knee, back, and foot injury relationships that may exist among collegiate football players who had less than 10° of measured hip internal rotation. Lastly, Larson et al. [14, 15] presented a case series demonstrating outcomes of players presenting with both hip and core muscle symptoms. The concept of regional interdependence could not be demonstrated or applied more appropriately than it is for the hip joint. Knowing in tennis that forces are created from the ground up and that these forces are unable to be generated or transferred in the overhead athlete when weak hips and core exist, it would be safe to conclude that regional interdependence is an important concept to consider in design of rehab and performance training programs for tennis players.

25.3   FAI vs Dysplasia

Repetitive athletic motions and forces of structurally noncongruent joint surfaces can lead to joint structure pathology [16]. This can be seen in the hip when femoral-acetabular impingement (FAI) or dysplasia exists [12, 13]. FAI can be found on the femoral or the acetabular side. Femoral-sided involvement is commonly referred to as a CAM lesion, while acetabular side involvement is clinically referred to as a RIM lesion. The deformities may occur in isolation or, more commonly, in combination. The CAM lesion presents radiographically as a loss of head neck offset, while local or global acetabular "overcoverage" would be more indicative of the potential for a RIM lesion [17]. Dysplasia, on the other hand, is a local or global acetabular "undercoverage." FAI can be considered a dynamic impingement issue, while dysplasia is considered as static overload issue and is differentiated by structure, location of problem, or mechanism of anatomical damage [12, 13, 18].

Since it is still unclear as to whether the CAM structural changes that occur are developmental, morphological, or repetitively based, designing rehab and training programs for specializing young tennis players must be given careful consideration. Avoiding unnecessary stress to these areas at risk would demonstrate prudence.

25.4   Kinetic Chain Concepts for Hip Rehabilitation and Injury Prevention

Under ideal conditions the lumbopelvic-hip complex creates a stable base where the extremities can simultaneously move and transfer load. This stable base allows the trunk and lower extremities to move in multiple directions with minimal energy, a necessity for the game of tennis. A comprehensive preoperative musculoskeletal and movement assessment serves as a guide to the clinician to point out where the impairments in the chain exist. The goal is to determine where the system's failed load transfer occurred and the relevant source of this dysfunction [19]. In addition, we must assess the elements of force closure, the active muscle system, and form closure, the passive structure system. Frequently hip dysfunctions can be tied to a lack of stability or an excessive degree of mobility. These types of impairments will frequently lead to the creation of inhibitory patterns as a form of compensation. Similarly, we have seen the facilitation of different muscle groups that are in line with the lower cross syndrome of Janda [20]. This population tends to exhibit over-recruitment of the iliopsoas, rectus femoris, and thoracolumbar extensors while simultaneously inhibiting the abdominals and gluteal muscles. In response, we see changes in muscle tone that result in muscle imbalances and movement dysfunctions.

It is also possible for compensatory strategies to exist as a result of asymmetrical motion in one region of the body. Earlier cited, this concept has been described by Wainner et al. [21] as "regional interdependence." As an example, we know that both the thoracic spine and the hip joint are made to allow for rotation in the transverse plane [22]. Subsequently, any limitation in one of these joints will affect the motion as a whole. Our clinical evaluation must include an assessment of the ROM of the thoracic spine and hip as well as the foot and ankle in order to gather a complete understanding of the motion and any restrictions that may be present.

Preoperative screening will establish a baseline for these athletes' adaptations and compensations in the presence of pain and injury. Screening becomes even more important when considering that research has shown a correlation between physical and functional impairments in the pre- and postoperative states. In this respect, clinicians must act as detectives looking to find the cause and not just the source of hip pain. You must find the *driver*.

Open-stance groundstrokes have become a standard in the modern game of tennis as they allow players to generate tremendous force while simultaneously recovering faster. Optimizing the kinetic chain is essential for this power development as efficiency in the lower extremities is responsible for the development of 54% of total force in groundstrokes [23]. Additionally, there must exist a good balance in strength between the upper and lower body in order to minimize injury. Weakness and imbalances in the upper body or trunk will increase the demand on the lower body thus increasing the risk of injuries [24].

Sports that involve repetitive hip rotation and loading commonly create hip weakness and instability symptoms not related to trauma. In order to hit open-stance groundstrokes successfully, players must drive into the ball while simultaneously rotating their body. This creates the loaded hip rotation that may lead frequently to injury. In particular, the weighted dominant leg is most at risk and is frequently the symptomatic side (R hip on an R hand dominant player). One negative side effect of this action is that it forces the hip into an abducted and externally rotated position. In order to perform this movement successfully and repetitively, the individual must have the available ROM as well as the control, strength, power, and endurance to produce a greater arc of motion with increasing amounts of force [25]. This is all driven from the core, pelvis, and hips.

Evaluation of the player must include a movement and biomechanical analysis to be fully comprehensive [26]. The service mechanics are as important as the groundstrokes in the health and vitality of the hip. An efficient serve is able to optimize the entire body, utilizing the lower extremities and synchronizing the kinetic chain. An efficient serve is often compared to a bow and arrow. If the bowstring is too inflexible to pull back, then it cannot generate flight for the arrow. When the bowstring is both strong and flexible, it has the range and control to generate the speed and force necessary to adequately propel the arrow. This is the same requirement for the spine, hips, and legs in the tennis serve. The back hip (R hip on R handed player) must flex, internally rotate, and adduct in order to maximize ground reaction forces and generate leg drive in the acceleration phase of the serve. This position, even when optimal, exposes players to soft tissue and structural hip impingements.

Coaches can play a role in changing a player's biomechanics. For example, a player with a structural femoroacetabular impingement (FAI) will commonly present with pain and restrictions in hitting open-stance groundstrokes. It is known that players with hip joint limitations in ROM will subconsciously seek mobility from somewhere else in the kinetic chain in order to continue competing [27]. The lumbar spine is commonly a site of compensatory movement. Research has shown that a decrease of hip internal rotation ROM is a predictive factor in low back pain [11]. These players who lack hip IR can benefit in changing their stance to a semi-open or even a square (more closed) position thereby decreasing the demand on hip ROM. These biomechanical changes can minimize the effects above and below the kinetic chain.

25.5 Postoperative Hip Arthroscopy Rehabilitation Strategies

Once an injury occurs, an individual's neuroplasticity is altered yielding nonoptimal movement strategies. Over time these nonoptimal strategies increase the load and stress on the lumbopelvic-hip complex, and this, in turn, creates soft tissue changes. Hip pain and dysfunction present for more than 6 months is known to result in lower extremity deconditioning and a reduction in function and performance [28]. In addition research has shown that a unilateral pain stimuli in the body creates a chain of events in the central nervous system including activation of the cerebellum bilaterally as well as neural firing of the contralateral motor area and ipsilateral premotor area [29, 30]. These changes in the central nervous system will in turn affect the musculoskeletal system and movement patterns [31].

Motor patterning is the foundation for movement. In the authors' clinical experience, successful outcomes stem from relearning movement patterns starting week one following surgery. The longer an injury has been present, the more established a faulty movement pattern would be and subsequently the longer the required timeframe to naturalize a new movement.

Postoperative rehabilitation can be broken down into several different formats ranging from phases or stages to named categories such as stage I "protected phase" to the end stage of "return to play and maintenance." Phases I and II are clearly to restore normal arthro-kinematics, normal resting muscle length, build strength, and develop proper timing of normal movement patterns. Since there is overlap between the phases, time-based protocols could limit the appropriate advancement from one phase to another. As long as the biology of soft tissue is respected, phase time periods can and will vary between individuals. Phases III and IV are more about developing muscular endurance and power in preparation for returning to both an artificial controlled and competitive uncontrolled environment, respectively. Phases II and III are about establishing a strength and conditioning base that will carry the individual through the competitive season. Many people fail to comply with an in season maintenance program which could also invite soreness and symptoms to the affected side. The most important factors in designing the post-op program is management, modification when appropriate, workload monitoring, and maintenance (see below).

The following hip arthroscopy guidelines were developed by the Sports Rehabilitation and Performance Center staff at Hospital for Special Surgery, and were modified for this chapter. **Progression is both criteria-based and patient-specific. Phases and time frames are designed to give the clinician a general sense of progression.** The rehabilitation program following hip arthroscopy must be tailored to the exact surgical procedure performed, taking into account tissue and bone healing properties. The program is developed to balance healing, while gently restoring hip range of motion and developing muscular balance and stability in the core, pelvic floor, and hip. Special attention is given to not irritating the psoas muscle during patient education of ADLs and in physical therapy exercises. Underlying etiology to this hip pathology is closely examined during the rehabilitation process to ensure that mechanics throughout the kinematic chain are not contributing factors in this pathological process.

25.6 Follow Physician's Modifications as Prescribed

25.6.1 Postoperative Phase I (Day 1–Week 6)

Goals
- Patient education.
- Compliance with self-care, home management, activity modification.
- Normalize gait with appropriate assistive device.
- 0/10 pain at rest and ambulation.
- 75% full ROM, all planes.

> Emphasize
> - PROTECTING SURGICAL SITE.
> - Minimizing pain and inflammation.
> - Patient compliance with activity modification.

Precautions
- Capsular irritation.
- Ambulation to fatigue.
- Pivoting or rotating hip during ambulation.
- Symptom provocation during ambulation, ADLs, therapeutic exercise.
- Active hip flexion with long lever arm, such as SLR as well as protected hip ER with A/PROM.
- NO open chain or isolated hip muscle activation, unless isometric.
- Protective progressive WB (20% to start) × 2–3 weeks, as per MD.

Treatment Recommendations
- Treatment focus on core and hip stability activation exercises utilizing isometrics and co-contractions of muscle groups.
- Short crank or regular bike with minimal resistance for 10–20 min without pain. Patients who have had a psoas release or pelvic floor pain: it is not contraindicated, however proceed with caution. Stop if they have pain.
- Range of motion progress as tolerated. Quadruped rocking into hip flexion and AAROM IR/ER may begin at 5–10 days.
- Home exercise program to include: abdominal setting supine, prone abdominal setting with gluteal setting with pillow under hips, quadriceps setting, long arc quads. Patient education: activity modification, bed mobility, positioning, transitional movements. Gait training with appropriate assistive device on level surfaces and stairs; instruct in a step-to gait pattern progressing to a normalized gait pattern. Initiate short crank bike, light resistance as tolerated.

Criteria for Advancement
- Control of pain.
- Normalized gait with or without assistive device, depending on the extent of surgical findings.
- Program may be advanced prior to 6 weeks as per MD.

25.6.2 Postoperative Phase 2 (Weeks 6–12)

Goals
- Normalize gait.
- 0/10 pain during ADLs.
- Avoid kinetic collapse with SL squat and steps.
- Core control during low-demand exercises.
- Adequate pelvic stability to meet demands of ADLs.

> Emphasize
> - Minimizing pain and inflammation.
> - Patient compliance with activity modification.
> - Continued protection of hip flexor and faulty movement patterns.

Precautions
- Symptom provocation during ADLs or therapeutic exercise.
- Faulty movement patterns, posture.
- Active hip flexion if symptomatic.
- Premature use of gym equipment for hip strengthening.

Treatment Recommendations
- Core control progression either from upper extremity movement patterns or functional, closed chain movements. Hip strengthening in closed chain function and stability movements; open chain for hip extension to neutral and abduction. Functional strength to include: leg press, squats, step-ups/step-downs, contralateral stability with elastic bands, windmills. Hip range of motion with a stable pelvis: bent knee fall out, heel slides. Proprioception and balance exercises: progress from double-limb to single-limb support. Incorporate developmental progressions from supine through standing, being sure to include high and half kneeling. Remember to use exercise variables of repetitions, sustained holds, timed work sessions, and speed when appropriate. If appropriate, think about initiating modified skill training progressions.

Criteria for Advancement:
- Range of motion within functional limits.
- SL squat and steps without kinetic collapse.
- Good pelvic control during single-limb stance.
- Normalized gait with improved functional endurance.

Modifications to Phase II: Per exam, symptoms, and MD findings

25.6.3 Postoperative Phase 3 (Weeks 12–16)

Goals
- Independent home exercise and gym program, as instructed.
- Optimize range of motion.
- Core control: Level II–III/V based on *Sahrmann scale or Bunkey scale or McGill scale.
- 5/5 lower extremity strength.
- Good dynamic balance.
- Pain-free ADLs.

*Core strength scales are used as a measuring tool of progress, not as an exercise progression.

Precautions
- Symptom provocation.
- Ignoring functional progression.
- Sacrificing quality of movement for quantity.

Treatment Recommendations
- Instruction of range of motion at end range. Demonstration of moderate-level core exercises in functional patterns in quadruped, standing diagonals. Cross training: elliptical trainer and bicycle, observing for good core and pelvic control. Initiate plyometrics with an adequate strength base. May begin running if appropriate.

Criteria for Advancement
- Good dynamic balance.
- 5/5 lower extremity strength for single and multiple reps.
- Level II–III/V core control (Sahrmann progression) or Bunkey Scale or McGill Scale.
- Range of motion to meet demands of activities.
- Pelvic control with single-limb activities.

Uncompensated movement patterns.

Modifications to Phase III: Per exam, symptoms, and MD findings

25.6.4 Postoperative Phase 4 (Weeks 16–24)

Goals
- Independent home exercise and gym program, as instructed.
- Minimize post-exercise soreness.

Precautions
- Symptom provocation.
- Ignoring functional progression.
- Maintaining adequate strength base.

Treatment Recommendations
- Home exercise and gym program, as instructed: strength training and flexibility exercises. Advance plyometric training and running program: interval training. Dynamic balance activities, cutting/agility skills. Advance training of core for strength and endurance. Continue to address muscle imbalances. Also, remember to incorporate high-level skill training.

Criteria for Advancement
- Core and hip strength and stability to maintain pelvic control.
- 0/10 pain with advanced activities.
- Optimal range of motion days following intense exercise sessions.
- Ability to maintain optimal movement patterns.

Modifications to Phase IV: Per exam, symptoms, and MD findings

Post-Op Program Design Factors
- Management
- Modification
- Monitoring
- Maintenance

Clinically, we have observed that to successfully return an athlete to play, the rehabilitation must correct all the components that created the hip injury including faulty movement patterns. It is important to keep in mind the philosophy "one size does not fit all." This mantra applies to the demands of different sports. A linesman or hockey goalie should not have the same return to play criteria as a tennis player. Tennis is unique as it encompasses all characteristics of sports: speed, endurance, control, power, agility, movement, mental toughness, conditioning, and flexibility. In this sport a point can last anywhere from 5–20 s and can require more than 100 bursts of explosive energy during extended rallies. Matches, however, can regularly last over 2 h. Preparing an athlete to return to play requires sport-specific rehabilitation that mimics the demands of that sport. This stage of rehab should only be initiated when the athlete is asymptomatic and has demonstrated full strength, endurance, balance, control, stability, and mastery of fundamental motions and movement patterns like squatting, cutting, and sprinting without any compensation.

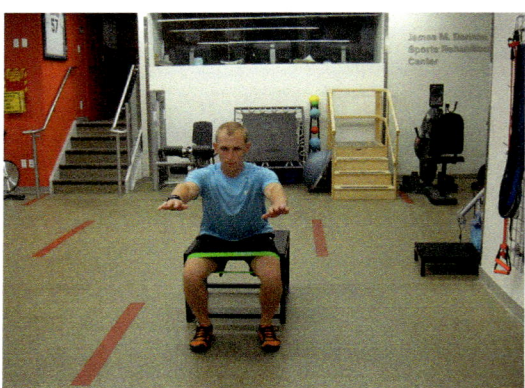

When returning to tennis after a hip injury, a primary component must be the retraining of movement. This means establishing new motor patterns that the individual can rely on under duress. Motor patterning exercises demand the individual to improve static and dynamic stability in order to be efficient [32]. As tennis demands control of many complex and high-speed movements, our retraining must simulate these movements in order to be effective. The movements of most importance will depend on an individual's playing style but must include multidirectional, lateral, and linear movements of short distance, usually less than 20 yards, that replicate the demands of the game. Loaded positions such as the half-kneel, squat, lunge, and athletic position require lumbopelvic stability and should be performed in a slow, controlled fashion that will increase muscle strength without stressing the soft tissue. It is necessary to create a new mind-body connection that performs the movement habitually and under pressure. Once a player is able to train under load, the athletic position is an ideal start. This position allows one to maintain their center of mass between the feet and establishes a base of support from the pelvis and hips. As an individual progresses, more advanced movement drills should be incorporated. These can include drills such as the lateral shuffle, lateral shuffle with crossover focusing on balance, fast response, and quick recovery.

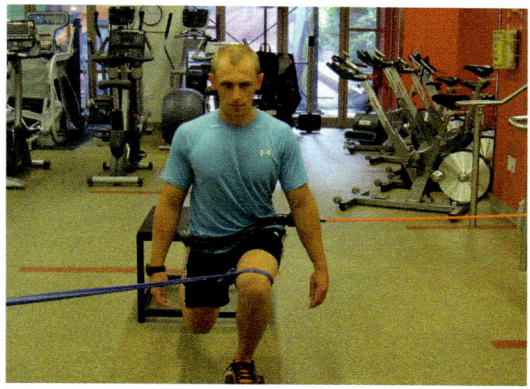

Flexibility and range of motion are crucial components in maximizing function. The player must have the appropriate joint range of motion and muscular flexibility in order to be able to rotate into the ball when hitting groundstrokes. Tennis players aim to achieve an optimal separation angle (defined as the difference in rotation between the shoulders and the hips), which allows for better performance in both the forehand and backhand groundstroke in addition to the serve [33]. In addition to the inert and dynamic layers, the myofascial system plays a role in tissue length. This system consists of lines of connective tissue that form meridians in the body [31]. These lines can provide postural and movement function stability. An example is the front functional line described by Myers as the fascial connection originating from the pectoralis muscle and extending to the external oblique, rectus abdominis, and pubis before finally culminating with the adductor longus [31]. This line is fully active during the serve. If the front line has the length to stay vertical, one can produce a stronger drive into the serve. Incorporating soft tissue techniques such as foam rolling, cupping, ball release, or gentle pressure can help to lengthen these tissues. The hip adductors and gluteal muscles are especially responsive to this. It is critical that any gain in soft tissue length is adapted into a new movement pattern and end range strength development, in order to maintain the new functional length. Range of motion may be achieved with things such as conventional techniques such as static stretching, dynamic warm-up, and PNF, as well as unconventional techniques such as animal flow, active release, or resistive stretching.

As previously mentioned the modern game is characterized by power, speed, and strength. It goes without saying that resistance training is crucial to compete at this level, both to enhance performance and to protect from injury. Competitive training should emphasize core and proximal hip strengthening with a particular emphasis on the gluteus maximus, obliques, and spinal extensors. Dr. Kibler defines core stability as, "the ability to control the trunk over the planted leg to allow optimum production, transfer, and control of force and motion to the terminal limbs" [23]. It is this core stability that allows a player to effectively generate and transfer force from his lower body. Training hip strength and power will allow the player to split step and change directions explosively without compensations [34]. The hip muscles must be trained both concentrically and eccentrically to best mimic their activity during groundstrokes.

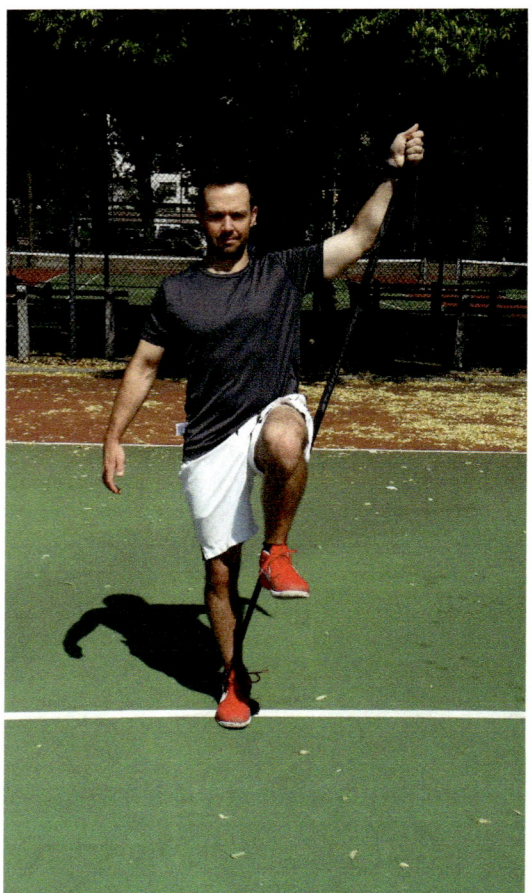

ball throws (both rotational and overhead), chest passes, and whole body functional movements. At this stage of the rehabilitation process, more sport-specific drills should be incorporated such as running, reaction drills, bounding, and even hitting live balls on the court. Additionally a comprehensive dynamic warm-up should include aerobic training as well as dynamic flexibility exercises. Examples of some excellent activities to include are running for 10 min, sprint drills for 20 m, alternating lunges, accelerations for 20 m, and progressive power jumps.

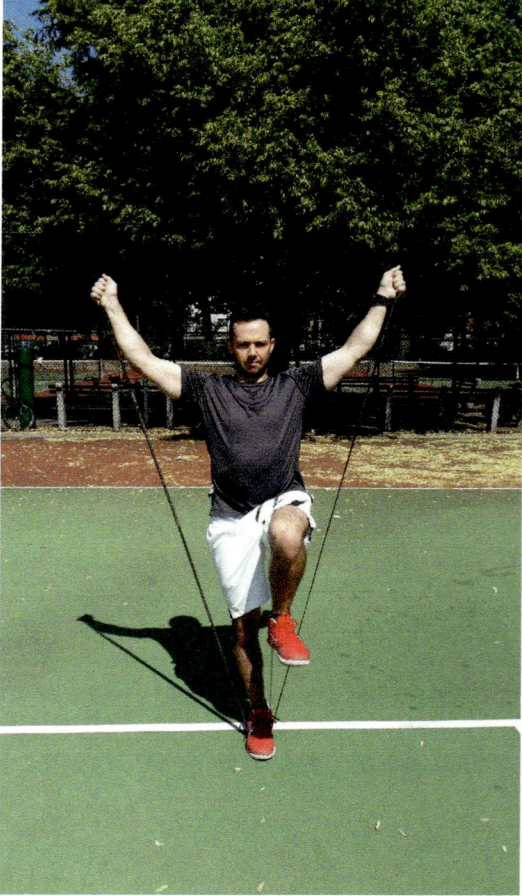

There are some common patterns of imbalance and asymmetry that emerge in tennis players. The ready position is the competitive posture in tennis. This position naturally shortens the hip flexors while lengthening the hip extensors. Additionally, we frequently observe difference in strength and flexibility between the dominant and nondominant sides. True symmetry in this realm might not be realistic, and so clinically we advise a balanced muscular training approach.

Plyometric training is another vital component in postoperative rehab. Plyometric training will improve the hip's ability to absorb shock and generate forces which are necessary because of the many directional changes involved in the sport. Plyometrics specific to tennis include box jumps, squat jumps, lunge jumps, push presses, medicine

In addition to strength and movement training, endurance is another crucial component of the sport. Fatigue is a factor that increases an individual's susceptibility to injuries both during longer matches and as the season progresses. Players will maximize their endurance by training both their aerobic and anaerobic capacity since both systems play a role in the sport [35]. Aerobic conditioning should be tailored to the individual and the court surface of the next competition. Longer rallies and physically demanding service games are characteristic of slow surfaces, while shorter and quicker points are seen on faster surfaces. This indicates that play on slower surfaces requires a greater aerobic capacity compared to play on faster courts.

The last stage of rehabilitation is returning the tennis player to competition. After the hip injury, the tennis player must be conscious of foot, body, and racquet work to ensure proper kinetic linkage. However due to the lack of data on return-to-play criteria, this phase is a daunting task for many multidisciplinary teams. The current return-to-play guidelines only necessitate asymptomatic full range of motion (ROM) and strength as the minimal criteria. Clearly this is not sufficient to play tennis at the most competitive levels. This institution's return-to-play criteria should include endurance, firing sequence, ROM/flexibility throughout the kinetic chain, proprioception, coordination, power, agility, and considerations of fatigue protocol, as well as concentric and eccentric strength that adequately meets the demands of a given sport. Additionally, the player should be able to meet metabolic and biomechanical demands of the sport in a progressive fashion. Furthermore, an interval program can safely guide the transition back to the courts. The player begins this transition with mini-tennis for approximately 10 min focusing on foot work. Over the course of several weeks, the distance is gradually extended toward the baseline. At this point groundstrokes begin in the middle of the court steadily progressing toward hitting on the run and stretching out wide. Incorporating open-stance slalom drills and neutral-stance pivot recovery drills will reteach the hip how to stabilize when stretched out wide for a shot and build its ability to abruptly stop and change direction as the player recovers for the next shot. Eventually serves are incorporated and games can be played.

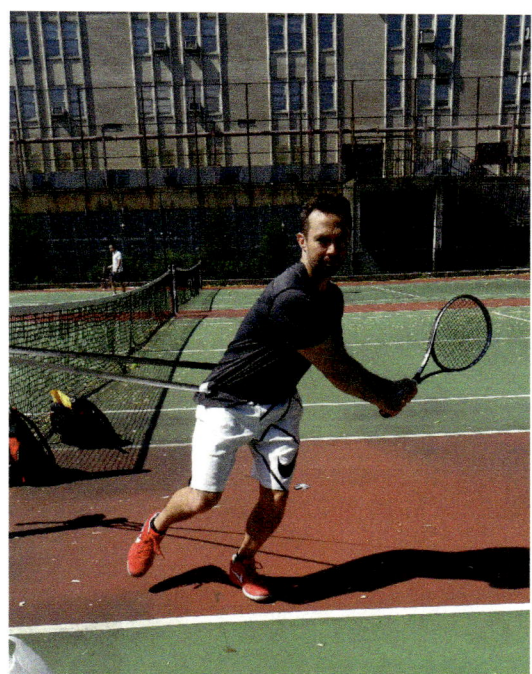

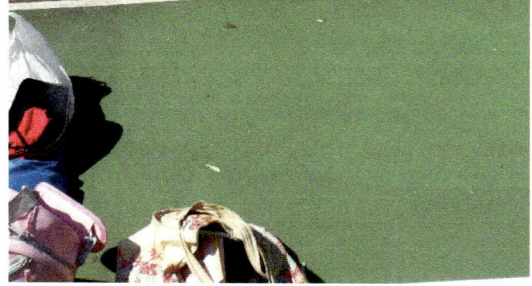

25.7 Soft Tissue Injuries About the Hip: Anterior

The open-stance forehand has increased the demands on the hip. This shot is hit with the weight loaded on the dominant leg while simultaneously rotating the upper body and pelvis over this stable base. These mechanics increase the stress on all of the hip's anterior structures. The individual must have the strength, flexibility, control, and endurance to provide dynamic stability of the hip joint while to perform this repetitive uncoiling mechanism. Research has shown us that repetitive loading of the hip frequently results in nontraumatic motion loss.

Muscular strains of the anterior hip compartment are one of the most common lower body injuries in tennis. Two joint muscles such as the rectus femoris are the most susceptible to these injuries especially at the myotendinous junction. The mechanism for this injury is generally due to a contraction of excessive force or an extreme stretch while muscle activation occurs [36]. The rectus femoris is the only quadriceps muscle that flexes the hip while also extending the knee, and so it can become strained when it attempts to counter its anatomical function, as it commonly does when sprinting on the tennis court.

Management of a hip flexor or quad strain must begin with a comprehensive assessment of the individual's history and a musculoskeletal examination that includes range of motion (ROM), flexibility, strength, functional testing, movement strategies, and groundstroke mechanics analysis. Clinical presentation may include palpable tenderness in the anterior thigh/groin, swelling seen below the anterior superior iliac spine (ASIS), and pain with resistive muscle testing of hip flexion and knee extension. Assessing hip ROM is of utmost importance because this can help to differentiate the hip injury from a structural impingement. Conservative treatment in the acute phase includes rest, ice, compressive wraps, and elevation. NSAIDs might be prescribed to reduce swelling and pain. Assistive devices, like crutches, are provided if the individual exhibits an antalgic gait or painful loading. Once the acute pain has resolved, the clinician can initiate gentle ROM exercises. Typically symptoms begin to subside over the first 2 weeks, and the individual regains full ROM. Strengthening is then initiated through the entire range using a combination of isometric, isokinetic, and isotonic exercises as well as light functional activities. Clinically we will progress the individual though functional movements such as rolling → quadruped → half kneel → tall knee → lunge → standing loaded stance [32]. Following functional and sport-specific progressions, the player is gradually ramped into greater volumes and a higher intensity of play while being monitored for any signs of injury recurrence [37]. Average recovery spans 4–6 weeks before the individual is able to return to tennis at his previous level of play.

Anterior hip injuries also include iliopsoas or AIIS impingement. The iliopsoas consists of the iliacus and the psoas major and minor muscles. Anatomically this muscle is in a position to create dysfunction above and below the chain. It originates from the transverse processes of T12-L5, passes under the inguinal ligament, and finally inserts onto the respective lesser trochanter. When the IT band snaps across the femoral head and acetabulum this is the reason, iliopsoas impingement is referred to as "internal snapping hip." When inflamed, the tendon can also compress the labrum of the hip resulting in labral tears. Clinically those with iliopsoas impingement will complain of hip pain and soreness and will present with possible swelling. In addition they usually present with anterior hip tightness or pain with movements that require hip extension. A "snapping" feeling may be felt in the front part of the hip.

Conservative treatment of iliopsoas impingement includes rest, NSAIDs, and a comprehensive flexibility program. Slow and gradual strengthening of the muscle will help protect the hip from reinjury. In some cases, the use of a steroid injection into the hip may help decrease the inflammation of the tendon, reduce pain, and allow for ease in returning to normal activity. When a psoas tendon is symptomatic, injections can be performed under ultrasound. As mentioned, a painful psoas tendon often results in compression and tearing of the labrum. A comprehensive assessment of the kinetic chain should be performed along with the correction of any mechanical impairments that are discovered. Similar to the treatment of other diagnoses, rehabilitation should further emphasize core and proximal hip strengthening as well as neuromuscular reeducation and movement patterning.

25.7.1 Medial Soft Tissues

Since tennis is a sport that is characterized by lateral movements, sudden stops, and explosive changes of direction, the medial hip compartment is at high risk of injury. In an efficient system, the lower back, pelvis, and hip engage in a symbiotic, codependent relationship. As mentioned the pelvis is the gateway of the body where we transfer load between the lower and upper extremities. In this analogy, the pubic symphysis serves as the gatekeeper to the anterior pelvis. Among its many roles, it acts as a fulcrum and insertional point for important stabilizing muscles such as the rectus abdominis superiorly and the adductor longus inferiorly. It is for this reason that injuries involving the medial hip compartment and the pubic symphysis can potentially lead to an imbalance of force with subsequent dysfunction and instability producing core muscle injuries [38–40].

Patho-anatomical hip injuries can occur anywhere from the superficial to the deep layers of the system. In tennis the most common medial soft tissue injury is an adductor strain or "groin strain." The hip adductors make up 22.5% of the total mass of the lower extremity [41] and include the pectineus, adductor brevis, adductor longus, adductor magnus, and the gracilis muscles. In general the majority of muscle strains occur at the musculotendinous junction. However, adductor strains tend to occur at the tendinous origin at the pubis. The adductor longus is the most frequently affected of these muscles because its lack of mechanical advantage makes it the most vulnerable. In open chain movements, the adductors' primary function is to adduct the thigh, but they become stabilizers of the lower extremity in closed kinetic chain movements, especially in the frontal plane if the gluteus medius is not activated or is being amnesic. Research has demonstrated that the adductor longus is the primary pelvic stabilizer during cutting movements [42]. Subsequently the constant side-to-side movements in tennis demand a strong contraction from the adductors. Injury of this muscle group occurs most frequently when a player loses his or her step while reaching for a ball, ending in a "split" stance. This leads to an overextension of the adductors.

Clinical presentation of adductor strains will include sharp pain in the groin area or thigh. Palpation at the insertion of the pubic bone, passive abduction, and resistive testing of the adductors will elicit tenderness and/or pain. Frequently there will be some palpable tone in the belly of the adductor group as well. Research has shown that any preseason deficit in adductor strength increases the risk of strains [43]. Edema and ecchymosis might also be present but can appear days after the injury dependent upon the severity. Clinically, grade one and two strains are the most prevalent.

Acute adductor muscle strains are managed similar to iliopsoas muscle strains. An initial period of rest, ice, and compression is beneficial to the injured muscle group. Typically, after several days, the symptoms will subside. Athletes, from a young age, are taught to push through pain. In rehabilitation, however, the athlete must be informed that any pain they experience is a warning sign and must be relayed to the clinician immediately. Exceeding one's pain threshold will only delay the healing process and create an inhibitory cascade of events throughout the body. After symptoms subside, the next goal is to normalize function while focusing on pain-free strengthening of the short adductors and proximal hip muscles. Core training, stretching, proprioceptive balance training, and soft tissue techniques should be added and progressed as the individual advances through the stages of rehab.

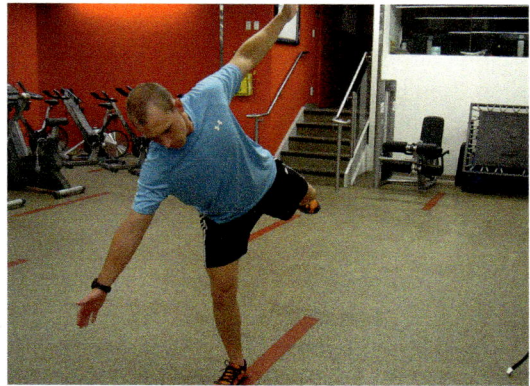

Once the athlete demonstrates confidence and is asymptomatic with all loaded movements, we can transition the player to the tennis court. Progressive strengthening at this point should continue by increasing the lever arm of the long adductors. This will prepare the muscles for the demands of competition. Once on the court, the player must be taught to take short, alternating yet explosive steps. Long strides should be avoided initially as this is too much strain to place on the injured muscle when first returning to play. Sport-specific exercises should include lunges, side lunges, and lunges with rotation eventually progressing toward light jogging and sideway hops. Pivots, quick turns, leaps, side jumping, and short sprints must all be included over time as the individual advances.

The individual's playing style and primary court surface is a factor in injury rehabilitation and return to play. Clay generally creates a higher bouncing ball and often calls for players to slide into a shot. The ability to slide successfully demands appropriate strength of the anterior and posterior hip muscle groups as well as the medial compartment. Both the hip abductors and adductors must be trained to effectively stabilize the hips and pelvis in the sliding position while allowing the transfer of force from the lower body to the upper body. This requires adequate flexibility, strength, and power output [34].

Remember that with any injury we are ultimately responsible for returning the athlete to their pre-injury level of performance. Transitioning to tennis the player should begin by hitting against a wall or playing mini-tennis with a partner. Over time the player extends him/herself toward the baseline and gradually begins hitting more difficult shots from more advanced positions. If practicing continues to be asymptomatic, the player should be able to compete in approximately 2 weeks. Usually after 6 weeks, the player is able to return to competition. At this time the player can consider taping the thigh as a preventative measure.

25.7.1.1 Core Muscle Injury

The abdominal wall consists of both muscles and fascia. The muscles include the obliques (both external and internal) and the transversus abdominis, while the fascia consists of the oblique fascia and the transversalis fascia. The conjoined tendon, comprised of the internal oblique and the aponeurosis of the transversus abdominis, inserts onto the pubic tubercle and is located anterior to the rectus abdominis. Core muscle injury is a broad term that is used for an injury to any of the abovementioned structures. The terms athletic pubalgia and sports hernia, although both outdated, are still seen in the literature. These phrases describe a specific injury to the rectus abdominis and the insertion of the conjoined tendon onto the pubic symphysis. In this disorder there is no palpable hernia, but there is often an accompanying injury to the adductor longus. The inadequacy of the posterior inguinal wall combined with muscle imbalances creates a subtle instability throughout the pelvis. Research has alluded to the possibility that an imbalance between the adductor muscles and the abdominal muscles may be the underlying cause of athletic pubalgia, but there is no concrete evidence to support this.

The prevailing thought is that these core muscle groups are constantly in a tug-of-war among themselves. During a hyperextension moment of the rectus abdominis, as we see in a tennis serve, we can see these contradictory forces at work. Hyperextension creates micro-tears throughout the muscle and increases stress on the pubic symphysis. In response, the adductors attempt to stabilize the pelvis with a strong contraction of their own. This creates a shear force across the pelvis and hip that results in attenuation of the tendon at its insertion [44]. The presence of a femoroacetabular impingement or a decrease in hip internal rotation ROM will also create a compensatory overload to the pubic symphysis. This can cause strain on the symphysis as well as the lower back and adductors. Research among Aussie rules footballers has shown a correlation between reduced hip internal rotation and osteitis pubis [45]. We also know from research that there exists a population of athletes with concomitant hip pathologies including FAI and athletic pubalgia [14, 15].

Repetitive rotational movements of the trunk, quick changes of direction, and turning on a loaded extremity increase the risk for core muscle injuries. Clinical presentation of these injuries includes complaints of pain localized to the lower abdominal/inguinal area with referral pain possible in the adductors, rectus abdominis, or the testicles. The pain is usually present during play but subsides as soon as the activity is stopped. Movements such as sit-ups, coughing, the

Valsalva maneuver, or the squeeze test can also elicit the pain [38, 39].

The mechanics of the groundstrokes and the violent nature of the serve place tennis players at risk for core muscle injuries. A well-crafted service motion requires adequate ankle dorsiflexion in addition to sufficient hip and low back extension in order to explode upward while simultaneously rotating the pelvis and laterally tilting the trunk. Stabilization is required throughout the abdominals and trunk while torque is generated.

An optimal tennis serve places the abdominals in a stretched position which is quickly followed by a forceful concentric contraction. Studies have shown that elite servers are able to achieve pelvic rotation at speeds of 440°/s and lateral trunk tilt at speeds of 280°/s [46]. As a result, the rectus abdominis and the external oblique of the nondominant arm side are shown to have the highest muscle activation during the serve regardless of the type of serve being hit [47].

Apart from the serve, oblique abdominal strains are also common when hitting open-stance strokes. The nature of the open stance demands that the obliques are in a position of maximal contraction. "Sports hernias" are most common in junior players. Physical deficits in these young players, such as a lack of hip internal rotation, trunk extension of less than 30°, or poor abdominal conditioning, increase the load on the abdominals.

Conservative management of core muscle injuries includes NSAIDs, activity modification, and cryotherapy. When physical therapy is initiated, there is an emphasis on core and hip strengthening, neuromuscular reeducation, and restructuring of movement patterns. If conservative treatment fails after 6–12 weeks, then the individual is considered a surgical candidate.

25.7.2 Posterior Soft Tissues

25.7.2.1 Hamstring

The acute injury of the hamstring complex can occur in sports requiring rapid acceleration and deceleration with the motions of simultaneous hip flexion and knee extension [48]. Acute muscle belly injuries will present with localized pain and eventual ecchymosis that can travel down into the calf and foot, depending on its severity. This patient will usually be seen "pulling up" and grabbing the back of their leg.

Proximal hamstring injuries can range from tendinous avulsions to apophyseal avulsions to degenerative micro-tears leading to tendinous [49]. These proximal injuries may also present with nerve-like symptoms similar to sciatica and will have poor control of the eccentric swing phase of gait [17]. It may be so painful that they can present to the clinic walking sideways to avoid the pain from the swing phase of gait.

A patient may also present with localized pain in the buttocks or near the ischial tuberosity and report pain and alteration with sitting. Although symptoms may mimic a proximal hamstring injury, differential diagnosis may suggest ruling out ischial bursitis.

Examination of these types of injuries would initially look for obvious deformity such as changes in muscle contour, changes in gait, ecchymosis, and weakness with knee flexion and hip extension. Imaging of the area include plain radiographs to rule out fractures and avulsions, while MRI will be used to assess the extent of soft tissue and tendon involvement. Ultrasound may also be used to do a dynamic assessment if indicated.

25.7.2.2 Nonoperative

Although there has been much literature published on the topic ranging on forces during running to suggested treatment protocols, the single paper that changed the direction of nonoperative hamstring rehabilitation was published by Sherry and Best [50]. In their study they compared treatment using an accepted isolated hamstring stretching and strengthening protocol or a progressive agility and trunk stabilization program. The results for reinjury were compared at 2 weeks and 1 year post-injury. The reinjury rates were found to be higher for the group receiving the isolated hamstring treatment. Reinjury rates for this group were found to be 54% at 2 weeks and 70% at 1 year versus the progressive agility group whose values were recorded at 0% reinjury rate at 2 weeks and 8% at 1 year [51]. These results suggested the importance of pelvic control exercise integration in the treatment of this group.

25.7.2.3 Operative

Generally speaking, when the decision is made for surgical repair or reconstruction of the hamstring, management and patient compliance are two very important variables that must be considered [52]. Postoperatively, there will be a period of bracing that limits hip flexion and knee extension for a period of 4–6 weeks. Weight bearing will be restricted 2–6 weeks depending on the surgical procedure and protocol. Hamstring strengthening usually begins between 6 and 10 weeks, while jogging and training may begin around the ()month mark, if indicated. One can expect a return to sport and vigorous activities somewhere between 6 and 9 months [53, 54].

25.7.3 Lateral Soft Tissues

Lateral soft tissue problems about the hip can affect both inert and contractile tissue (Pfirrmann, Williams). These pathologies can range from bursitis to muscle tears to pain and snapping syndromes. The greater trochanter facets are the sites for both gluteal muscle and trochanteric bursa attachment [55]. In addition, the iliotibial band can become irritated when it snaps back and forth over the trochanter [56].

The bursa is isolated and can be palpated on the posterior facet of the greater trochanter. People experiencing bursal pain will complain of pain when lifting the leg to don pants, using stairs, and laying directly on their side [57].

Gluteus medius tears and tendinous issues can be palpated on the posterior superior facet of the greater trochanter [18]. Gluteus medius tendon tears are more common in women than in men and are obviously going to have difficulty with frontal plane control during side-to-side activities. A positive Trendelenburg will often be noticeable, while hip abduction manual muscle testing should also be performed in a fatigued state.

Iliotibial band syndrome may present as either hip or knee pain and, in some instances, will be reported as a hip dislocation when the IT band snaps over the greater trochanter [17].

The load and force demands of tennis, combined with constant irregular changes in speed and direction, will expose the hips of tennis players to bony, inert, and contractile tissue issues during both competition and training.

25.8 Bony Injuries About the Hip

The rectus femoris originates from the anterior inferior iliac spine (AIIS or subspine) of the ilium. This bony process lies deep underneath several layers of soft tissue and has a sloping orientation toward the hip joint. Abnormal contact between the AIIS and the femoral neck during hip flexion can result in subspine impingement which is another form of extra-articular dynamic impingement [14, 15]. Differences in the AIIS morphology as well as previous avulsion fractures of the AIIS have been associated with an increased risk of subspine impingement [58].

Subspine impingements typically begin with an insidious onset of dull, aching anterior groin pain. The pain occurs during straight hip flexion beyond 90° and is provoked with activities like prolonged walking, running, and jumping. On examination there might be palpable tenderness in the groin. The player may also present with crepitus and a positive impingement test. It is not uncommon for this diagnosis to coexist with the presence of a FAI.

Similar to other hip disorders, conservative management of subspine impingement includes activity modification, rest, NSAIDs, and rehabilitation with an emphasis on core and hip strengthening and ROM.

Although not common in tennis players, stress fractures do occur as a result of the repetitive nature of the sport and high volume of training involved. "Bone stress injury" is a global term that encompasses the spectrum from bone stress reaction injuries to stress fractures. Repetitive strain over a prolonged period of time upon a normal bone structure is the most common cause of stress fractures. The bone simply fatigues. The hip and pelvis are afforded stability by their joint structure and the muscle forces acting upon them. These components allow us to endure the constant loading and the many forces placed on our hips and pelvis. Activities as simple as running and jumping create stress that is sent through the body. A stable pelvic base allows an individual to efficiently receive this shock while also creating the necessary stability for the shock to be counteracted. However an imbalance between bone structure and muscle force does make the pelvis susceptible to injuries [59]. Femoral neck stress fractures are an example of what can happen when this imbalance exists. Weak hip muscles decrease the ability to absorb impactful forces subsequently leading to an increase in stress at the femoral neck. Pelvis stress fractures, on the other hand, occur at a low rate and are seen almost exclusively in females. These typically occur at the attachment site of the proximal adductor magnus on the inferior pubic ramus.

The best management of stress injuries is prevention. Recognizing the risk factors and correcting them in time is the goal. Intrinsic factors include gender (females are at greater risk), metabolic issues, biomechanics, and musculoskeletal abnormalities. Extrinsic risk factors include training factors and errors, variable surface play, a sudden increase in distance or intensity, faulty equipment, and sudden changes in activity. An athlete with a stress fracture of the hip will complain of a deep ache while playing tennis and relief when resting. The complaints of pain are typically vague and nonlocalized, but pain with weight bearing is always a red flag. When suspecting this diagnosis, a comprehensive examination that includes identification of risk factors and training history is warranted. When components of female athlete triad are suspected, a comprehensive menstrual history, activity level, and nutrition must be included. Once the source of the pain and the risk factors of the injury have been determined, then an appropriate individualized treatment plan can be implemented.

Conclusion

A comprehensive and detailed evaluation is essential to the success of any rehabilitation program. The management of hip pathologies and dysfunctions in tennis players is no different. A key component, however, must be the assessment of the entire kinetic chain in order to properly determine both the source and the cause of impairment. You must find the driver or, in some cases, the drivers. In the presence of hip pain and injury, an individual will seek the path of least resistance despite the ensuing consequences this has on the rest of the body. Athletes, above all, will find ways to compensate for their injuries in order to compete. This is why it is crucial that we, as rehab professionals, break down their movement patterns and identify their restrictions and limitations. Successfully returning the tennis player to competition will be a process of developing an essential neuromuscular and physiologic base in order to prevent reinjury and improve skill and performance.

References

1. Kovacs M, Roetert EP, Ellenbecker TS. Complete conditioning for Tennis. Champaign, IL: Human Kinetics Publishing; 2017.
2. Pluim BM, Staal JB, Windler GE, Jayanthi N. Tennis injuries: occurrence aetiology, and prevention. BR J Sports Med. 2006;40:415–23.
3. Ellenbecker TS, Dines DD, Renstrom P, Windler GE. Injury and illness data from the ATP World Tour 2012 to 2016: a five year analysis. Unpublished Data, 2017
4. Maquirrian J, Baglione R. Epidemiology of tennis injuries: an eight year review of Davis Cup retirements. Eur J Sport Sci. 2016;16:266–70.
5. Ellenbecker TS, Ellenbecker GA, Roetert EP, Silva R, Keuter G, Sperling F. Descriptive profile of hip rotation range motion in elite tennis players and professional baseball pitchers. Am J Sports Med. 2007;35(8):1371–6.
6. Draovitch P, Edelstein J, Kelly BT. The layer concept; utilization in determining the pain generators, pathology and how structure determines treatment. Curr Rev Musculoskelet Med. 2012;5(1):1–8.
7. Sueki DG, Cleland AJ, Wainner RS. A regional interdependence model of musculoskeletal dysfunction: research, mechanisms and clinical implications. J Man Manip Ther. 2013;21(2):90–102.
8. Erhard R, Bowling R. The recognition and management of the pelvic component in low back and sciatic pain. Bulletin of Orthopedic Section-APTA, 1977
9. Robb AJ, Fleisig G, Wilk K. Passive ranges of motion of the hips and their relationship with pitching biomechanics and ball velocity in professional baseball players. Am J Sports Med. 2010;38:2487–93.

10. Ellera-Gomes JL, de Castro JV, Becker R. Decreased hip range of motion and non-contact injuries of the anterior cruciate ligament. Arthroscopy. 2008;24(9):1034–7.
11. Vad VB, Bhat AL, Basari D. Low back pain in professional golfers. Am J Sports Med. 2004;32(2):494–7.
12. Bedi A, Warren RF, Oh YK, Wojtys EM, Oltean HN, Kelly BT. Restriction of hip internal rotation is associated with an increased risk of ACL injuries in NFL combine athletes: a clinical and biomechanical study. Orthop J Sports Med. 2013;1(4 suppl) https://doi.org/10.1177/2325967113S00062.
13. Bedi A, Dolan M, Leunig M, Kelly BT. Static and dynamic mechanical causes of hip pain. Arthroscopy. 2011;27(2):235–51.
14. Larson CM, Pierce BR, Giveans MR. Treatment of athletes with symptomatic intra-articular hip pathology and athletic pubalgia/sports hernia: a case series. Arthroscopy. 2011a;27(6):768–75.
15. Larson CM, et al. Making a case for anterior inferior iliac spine/subspine hip impingement: three representative case reports and proposed concept. Arthroscopy. 2011b;27(12):1732–7.
16. Tibor LM, Sekiya J. Differential diagnosis of pain around the hip joint. Arthroscopy. 2008;24(12):1407–21.
17. Kelly BT, Larson CM. Femoroacetabular impingement: pathoanatomy, clinical evaluation and arthroscopic treatment strategies. In Sports hip injuries; diagnosis and management. SLACK. 2015. p. 27–8.
18. Narveson J, et al. Management of a patient with acute acetabular labral tear and femoral acetabular impingement with intra-articular steroid injection and a neuromotor training program. J Orthop Sports Phys Ther. 2016;46(11):965–76.
19. Lee D, et al. The pelvic girdle. Churchill Livingstone: Elsevier; 2011.
20. Page P, Frank C, Lardner R. Assessment and treatment of muscle imbalance: The Janda approach. Champaign, IL: Human Kinetics Publishing; 2010.
21. Wainner RS, Whitmann JM, Cleland JA, Flynn TW. Regional interdependence: a musculoskeletal examination model whose time has come. JOSPT. 2007;37(11):658–60.
22. Sizer P, Cook C. Coupling behavior of the thoracic spine: a systematic review of the literature. J Manipulative Physiol Ther. 2007;30(5):390–9.
23. Kibler WB. Biomechanical analysis of the shoulder during tennis activities. Clin Sports Med. 1995;14(1):79–85.
24. Hjelm N, et al. Injury risk factors in junior tennis players: a prospective 2-year study. Scand J Med Sci Sports. 2012;22:40–8.
25. Kibler WB. The 4000-watt tennis player: power development for tennis. Med Sci Tennis. 2009;14(1):5–8.
26. Kibler WB, Chandler TJ. Range of motion in junior tennis players participating in an injury risk modification program. J Sci Med Sport. 2003;6(1):51–62.
27. Azevedo D, et al. Pelvic rotation in femoroacetabular impingement is decreased compared to other symptomatic hip conditions. J Orthop Sports Phys Ther. 2016;46(11):957–64.
28. Kemp J, et al. Patients with chondrolabral pathology have bilateral functional impairments 12 to 24 months after unilateral hip arthroscopy: a cross-sectional study. J Orthop Sports Phys Ther. 2016;46(11):947–56.
29. Coghill RC, Sang CN, Maisog JM, Ladrola NJ. Pain intensity processing within the human brain: a bilateral, distributed mechanism. J Neurophysiol. 1999;82(4):1934–43.
30. Pelletier R, et al. Is neuroplasticity in the central nervous system the missing link to our understanding of chronic musculoskeletal disorders? BMC Musculoskelet Disord. 2015;16:25.
31. Myers T. Anatomy trains: myofascial meridians for manual and movement therapists. Churchill Livingstone: Elsevier; 2009.
32. Hoogenboom B, Voight M, Cook G, Gill L. Using rolling to develop neuromuscular control and coordination of the core and extremities of athletes. N Am J Sports Phys Ther. 2009;4(2):70–82.
33. Landlinger J, Stoggl T, Lindinger S, Wagner H, Muller E. Differences in ball speed and accuracy of tennis groundstrokes between elite and high performance players. Eur J Sport Sci. 2012;12(4):301–8.
34. Roetert E, et al. Tennis anatomy. Champaign, IL: Human Kinetics Publishing; 2011.
35. Kovacs M. Tennis training: enhancing on-court peformance. USRSA, 2007.
36. Garret WE. Muscle strain injuries. Am J Sports Med. 1996;24:S2–8.
37. Anderson. Hip and groin pain in athletes. Am J Sports Med. 2001;29(4):521–33.
38. Meyers WC, Foley DP, Garrett WE, Lohnes JH, Mandlebaum BR. Management of severe lower abdominal or inguinal pain in high-performance athletes. Am J Sports Med. 2000;28:2–8.
39. Meyers WC, McKechnie A, Philippon MJ, Horner MA, Zoga AC, Devon ON. Experience with "sports hernia" spanning two decades. Ann Surg. 2008;248:656–65.
40. Weir A, Brukner P, Delahunt E, Ekstrand J, Griffin D, Khan K, et al. Doha agreement meeting on terminology and definitions in groin pain in athletes. Br J Sports Med. 2015;49(12):768–74.
41. Levangie P, et al. Joint structure and function: a comprehensive analysis. VitalSource eBook. 5th ed. Philadelphia: F. A. Davis; 2011.
42. Neptune RR. Muscle coordination and function during cutting movements. Med Sci Sports Exerc. 1999;31(2):294–302.
43. Tyler T, et al. The effectiveness of a preseason exercise program to prevent adductor muscle strains in professional hockey players. Am J Sports Med. 2002;30(5):680–3.
44. Caudill P, Nyland J, Smith C, Yerasimides J, Lach J. Sports hernias: a systematic literature review. Br J Sports Med. 2008;42:954–64.

45. Verrall GM. Hip joint range of motion reduction in sports-related chronic groin injury diagnosed as pubic bone stress injury. J Sci Med Sport. 2000;8(1):77–84.
46. Fleisig G, Nicolls R, Elliot B, Escamilla R. Kinematics used by world class tennis players to produce high-velocity serves. Sports Biomech. 2003;2(1):51–64.
47. Chow JW. Lower trunk muscle activity during the tennis serve. J Sci Med Sport. 2003;6(4):512–8.
48. Neuschwander TB, Benke MT, Gerhardt MB. Anatomic description of the origin of the proximal hamstring. Arthroscopy. 2015;31(8):1518–21.
49. Lempainen L, Johansson K, Banke IJ, Ranne J, Mäkelä K, Sarimo J, et al. Expert opinion: diagnosis and treatment of proximal hamstring tendinopathy. Muscles Ligaments Tendons J. 2015;5(1):23–8.
50. Sherry MA, Best TM. A comparison of 2 rehabilitation programs in the treatment of acute hamstring strains. J Orthop Sports Phys Ther. 2004;34(3):116–25.
51. Mica L, Schwaller A, Stoupis C, Penka I, Vomela J, Vollenweider A. Avulsion of the hamstring muscle group: a follow up of 6 adult non-athletes with early operative treatment: a brief report. World J Surg. 2009;33(8):1605–10.
52. Klingele KE, Sallay PI. Surgical repair of complete proximal hamstring tendon rupture. Am J Sports Med. 2002;30(5):742–7.
53. Sallay PI, Ballard G, Hamersly S, Schrader M. Subjective and functional outcomes following surgical repair of complete ruptures of the proximal hamstring complex. Orthopedics. 2008;31(11):1092.
54. Cohen SR, Rangavajjula A, Vyas A, Bradley JP. Functional results and outcomes after repair of proximal hamstring avulsions. Am J Sports Med. 2012;40(9):2092–8.
55. Williams BS, Cohen SP. Greater trochanteric pain syndrome: a review of anatomy, diagnosis and treatment. Anesth Analg. 2009;108(5):1662–70.
56. Strauss EJ, Nho SJ, Kelly BT. Greater trochanteric pain syndrome. Sports Med Arthrosc. 2010;18(2):113–9.
57. Pfirrmann CW, Chung CB, Theumann NH, Trudell DJ, Resnick D. Greater trochanter of the hip: attachment of the abductor mechanism and a complex of three bursae—MR imaging and MR bursography in cadavers and MR imaging in asymptomatic volunteers. Radiology. 2001;221(2):469–77.
58. Hestroni I, Larson CM, Dela Torre K, Zbdea RM, Magennis E, Kelly BT. Anteriro inferior iliac spine deformity as an extra-articular source for hip impingement: a series of 10 patients treated with arthroscopic decompression. Arthroscopy. 2012;28(11):1644–53.
59. Vleeming A, Schuenke M, Masi A, Danneeis L, Willard F. The sacroiliac joint: an overview of its anatomy, function and potential clinical implications. J Anat. 2012;221(6):537–67.

Physiotherapy Management of Patellar Tendinopathy in Tennis Players

Hio Teng Leong, Jill Cook, Sean Docking, and Ebonie Rio

26.1 Introduction

Patellar tendinopathy (often called jumper's knee) is a common cause of knee pain in both recreational and elite tennis players, a sport that requires repetitive side-to-side movements, quick stops and starts, or changing directions [1–3]. It is commonly seen in younger athletes, both children and adolescents, and increases in prevalence with age up to 18 years [4]. Patellar tendinopathy is more common in male athletes [4], and they are almost two to four times more likely to develop patellar tendinopathy than females [5–7].

Characteristics of patellar tendinopathy include pain localized to the inferior pole of the patella and load-related pain that is aggravated by energy storage and release within the tendon such as jumping, landing, cutting, and pivoting [8]. Also, given that tennis is a sport that can be played on a variety of surfaces (grass, artificial grass, hard court surfaces, and clay), changes in surface or shoes may affect the amount of shock absorption as harder surfaces can increase the risk of patellar tendinopathy [9–11].

Patellar tendinopathy can affect playing ability or even prevent a player from being on court. Indeed, more than a third of patients presenting to a sports medicine clinic with patellar tendinopathy were unable to return to sport within 6 months [12], and more than 50% of athletes with patellar tendinopathy were forced to retire from sport but continue to have pain with stairs climbing when surveyed 15 years later [13]. Management of patellar tendinopathy relies on understanding the pathophysiology of patellar tendinopathy, a detailed history and assessment of an individual with patellar tendinopathy to differentiate it from other potential diagnoses of anterior knee pain, recognizing the possible risk factors, and then prescribing appropriate treatment and rehabilitation for patellar tendinopathy.

26.2 Pathophysiology

The continuum model of tendon pathology is the most clinically relevant and provides a framework to stage the presentation of patellar tendinopathy [14] (Fig. 26.1). Normal tendon is pain-free and capable of absorbing and releasing energy like a spring in functional tasks such as jumping, running, cutting, and pivoting. Tendons have a specific capacity to withstand load and, when loaded appropriately, will adapt in adults

H. T. Leong (✉)
Department of Orthopaedics and Traumatology, Prince of Wales Hospital, The Chinese University of Hong Kong, Shatin, Hong Kong
e-mail: annieleonght@cuhk.edu.hk

J. Cook · S. Docking · E. Rio
La Trobe Sport and Exercise Medicine Research Centre, La Trobe University, Melbourne, VIC, Australia
e-mail: j.cook@latrobe.edu.au;
S.Docking@latrobe.edu.au; e.rio@latrobe.edu.au

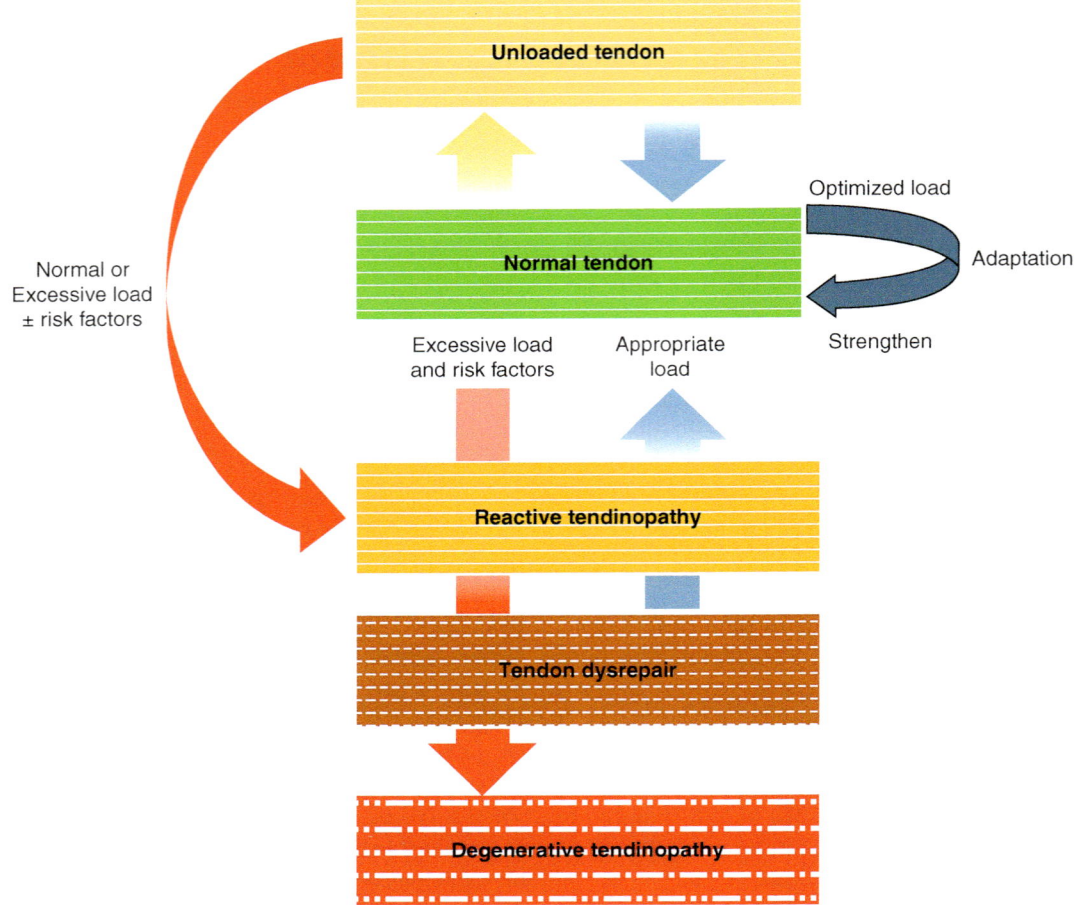

Fig. 26.1 The tendon pathology continuum model. Reproduced from 'Is tendon pathology a continuum? A pathology model to explain the clinical presentation of load-induced tendinopathy', Cook JL and Purdam CR, 43, 409–416, 2009 in British Journal of Sports Medicine

by increasing stiffness without thickening of the tendon. If excessive load is placed on a tendon, with insufficient rest, pathology may develop. The continuum of tendinopathy suggests that there are three stages of tendinopathy: *reactive tendinopathy*, *tendon disrepair*, and *degenerative tendinopathy* [14].

26.2.1 Reactive Tendinopathy

Reactive tendinopathy is the first stage of tendon pathology and is predominantly seen in an acutely overloaded tendon. This usually occurs with a sudden increase in training or returning to a normal training volume after an injury or holiday. This may also be seen in tennis players when changing suddenly from a soft (grass) to hard court surface (clay or En-Tout-Cas), which increases the amount of shock absorption in the tendon. Reactive tendinopathy is a noninflammatory proliferative response in the tendon cell and matrix, driven by tenocytes to increase protein production such as proteoglycans. These large hydrophilic proteoglycans can increase the tendon dimension by increasing the amount of bound water [15, 16]. This reactive cellular response is a short-term adaptation to overload—the thickened tendon reduces stress (force/unit area) and increases stiffness, while the collagen structure remains intact. If sufficient time is given for the tendon to adapt, or the load is reduced or modified appropriately, the tendon has the potential to revert back to normal tendon structure [17, 18].

26.2.2 Tendon Disrepair

If the tendon continues to be excessively loaded, the tendon will progress toward *tendon disrepair*. It is characterized by a failed healing response of the tendon with greater matrix breakdown. The tenocytes will continue to respond to excessive load, resulting in an overall increase in the number of chondrocytic cells and protein production (proteoglycan and collagen). This marked increase in ground substance (non-collagenous proteins and water) causes separation of the collagen fibers and disorganization of the matrix. At this stage, the areas of matrix changes are more focal rather than diffuse changes seen in reactive tendon pathology. There is also an increase in type III collagen that results in a tendon less resilient to tensile strain [19]. Some increased vascularity may be observed [20].

26.2.3 Degenerative Tendinopathy

If a tendon is continuously overloaded and unable to repair itself, the tendon will progress to the final stage of tendon pathology: *degenerative tendinopathy*. In this stage, focal areas of pathology will develop and are characterized by extensive matrix breakdown [21, 22]. These changes are irreversible [14]. Nevertheless, a degenerative tendon appears to be compensated by increase in cross-sectional dimension around the lesion to maintain a sufficient amount of load-bearing aligned fibrillar structure [23]. Thus, increasing the load capacity in the normal portion of the tendon by strengthening will allow the player to become pain-free and return to full activity [24].

26.2.4 Other Pathologies

Clinically, athletes with patellar tendinopathy often have a combination of pathology stages at

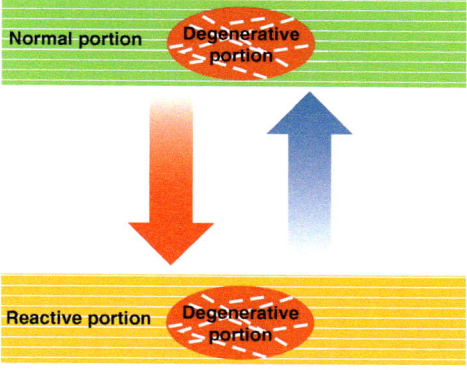

Fig. 26.2 Schematic representation of "reactive-on-degenerative" tendinopathy. Reproduced from *'Revisiting the continuum model of tendon pathology: what is its merit in clinical practice and research? Cook JL, Rio E, Purdam CR, et al, doi:10.1136/bjsports-2015-095422, 2016 in British Journal of Sports Medicine*

one time: *reactive-on-degenerative tendinopathy* (Fig. 26.2). The degenerative portion of the tendon does not bear load and is mechanically silent; hence, excessive load may lead to reactive changes in the structurally normal portion of the patellar tendon [24, 25]. As with reactive tendon pathology, this is reversible, and the tendon will revert to having areas of degeneration surrounded by normal tendon.

26.3 Diagnosis

Patellar tendinopathy is a clinical diagnosis of pain and dysfunction in the patellar tendon. A detailed history and assessment of an individual with patellar tendinopathy is essential to differentiate it from other potential diagnoses of anterior knee pain and to provide prognostic value and direction for the rehabilitation program.

26.3.1 History

The first clinical challenge is to identify whether the tendon is the source of pain. Players with patellar tendinopathy should point with one finger to the proximal attachment of the patellar tendon to the patella [25]. This feature of localized pain (with loading not palpation) is used clinically to differentiate it from other potential diagnoses of anterior knee pain.

Second, patellar tendinopathy is characterized by a history of an insidious onset of pain that is usually due to tendon overload. Clinically, tendon overload occurs with a sudden increase in training or sudden change of surface (from a soft (grass) to hard court surface (clay or sand)), which may increase the amount of shock absorption in the tendon. It may also occur in tennis players who return to a normal training volume after an injury or training break.

Pain behavior of patellar tendinopathy has a classic presentation. Pain or discomfort in the patellar tendon occurs at the beginning of activity, with variable response to warm-up [25], and will be worst the next day [25, 26]. Players with patellar tendinopathy will rarely complain of night pain and morning stiffness (unless symptoms are severe) [25]. Other signs and symptoms such as pain with prolonged sitting (especially in a car) and daily activities such as squatting and stairs can be provocative [25–27].

In addition, there are a number of extrinsic and intrinsic risk factors that are associated with patellar tendinopathy (Table 26.1). Extrinsic factors such as the training volume and frequency may trigger the onset of patellar tendinopathy [6]. Also, tennis is a sport that can be played on a variety of surfaces (grass, artificial grass, hard court surfaces, and clay), and change in surface or shoes may affect the amount of shock absorption as harder surfaces can increase the risk of patellar tendinopathy [9]. A number of intrinsic factors may predispose an individual to developing tendon pain and include systemic, medical, and genetic factors. Increased adiposity [40] and diabetes [39]elevate the risk of tendinopathy by altering tendon structure and immune responses. Other conditions such as rheumatological diseases and rare hereditary conditions such as Marfan syndrome and Ehlers-Danlos syndrome may also predispose an individual [41]. Finally medications such as fluoroquinolones (a class of antibiotic) are also a risk factor for development of tendinopathy [42]. Many of these are non-modifiable and will be uncommon in the young fit player but may be a contributing factor in the older and recreational player.

Other specific anthropometric characteristics are also linked with patellar tendinopathy such as taller body stature and higher BMI [7], increased waist circumference [32] or waist-to-hip ratio [29–31], lower foot arch height [33], reduced ankle dorsiflexion [34], greater leg length discrepancy [35], and less extensible hamstring and stiffer quadriceps muscles [36].

Table 26.1 Risk factors for patellar tendinopathy

Extrinsic risk factors	Intrinsic risk factors

• Training volume and frequency [6]
• Change in surface or shoes [9]
	• Adolescent jumping athletes [28]
	• Men are two to four times higher risk than females [6]
	• Taller body stature [7]
	• Higher body weight [7]
	• Increased wait circumference or waist-to-hip ratio [29–32]
	• Lower foot arch height [33]
	• Reduced ankle dorsiflexion [34]
	• Greater leg length discrepancy [35]
	• Less extensible hamstrings [36]
	• Stiffer quadriceps muscles [36]
	• Better jumping ability [37]
	• Greater fat pad size [38]
	• Medical conditions:
	  – Rheumatologic conditions
	  – Diabetes [39]
	  – Increased adiposity [40]
	  – Genetic-based conditions that affect the connective tissue such as Marfan syndrome and Ehlers-Danlos syndrome [41]

26.3.2 Physical Assessment

Patellar tendinopathy is a clinical diagnosis based on the presence of (1) pain localized to the inferior pole of the patella and (2) load-related pain that is aggravated by energy storage and release within the tendon [26, 27]. Patients with patellar tendinopathy should point with one finger to the proximal attachment of the tendon to the patella [25]. This feature of localized pain is used clinically to differentiate it from other potential diagnoses of anterior knee pain (Table 26.2) [50]. Tenderness on palpation is an unreliable diagnostic test as mild tenderness is frequently present in asymptomatic athletes [51].

The single-leg decline squat is the best clinical pain provocation test which preferentially loads the patellar tendon [52, 53]. While standing on the affected leg on decline board (25°), the patient is asked to maintain an upright trunk and squat up to 90° if possible [53]. The test is repeated on the unaffected leg for comparison. The maximal angle of knee flexion is recorded, and the pain level can be rated on an 11-point numeric rating scale, where 0 indicates no pain and 10 indicating the worst pain. Importantly, the pain should remain localized at the inferior pole of the patella and not spread, as this test may also be provocative for other anterior knee pain conditions.

It is also important to examine the lower extremity to identify any deficits at the hip, knee, and ankle/foot region. Atrophy or reduced strength of the gluteal, quadriceps, and calf muscles may be apparent [25]. A decrease in thigh and calf bulk can

Table 26.2 Differential diagnosis in relation to anterior knee pain

Differential diagnosis	History	Symptoms and signs	Examination
Patellofemoral pain [43]	• Common in adolescents and both younger and older adults • Gradual onset of pain	• Characteristics of pain is generally located diffusely around the patella • Pain during low tendon load such as walking, descending stairs, running, or cycling • Discomfort while sitting with bent knees • Patellofemoral crepitus and knee stiffness	• Diffuse pain around the patella during squatting maneuvers [44] • Pain reduction when using patellofemoral taping with provocative maneuvers [45]
Tibial apophysitis or Osgood-Schlatter lesion	• Common in growing adolescents • History of growth spurt	• Localized pain and tenderness at the tibial tuberosity • Swelling at the tibial tuberosity	• Pain is reproduced with resisted active extension or passive hyperflexion of the knee • Tender point at the tibial tuberosity
Infrapatellar fat pad [46]	• Common in adolescents • Repetitive end-range knee extension or forceful extension maneuver	• Diffuse pain located in the anterior inferior region of the knee • Pain during end-range extension	• Positive Hoffa test • Pain is exacerbated by both flexion and extension maneuvers
Plica syndrome or injuries [47, 48]	• Blunt or twisting trauma [47] • Acute onset after a marked increase of activities	• Intermittent, dull, and aching pain located in the anteromedial region of the knee • Snapping and clicking sensation • Locking and catching • Aggravation of symptoms by stair climbing, prolonged standing, squatting, or sitting	• Tenderness and mobile nodularity are present along the medial and inferior aspect of the patella [48]
Patellar subluxation [49]	• Young women • Increased quadriceps angle (Q-angle), usually greater than 15°	• Achy pain with painful popping or giving-way episodes • Mild effusion	• Positive subluxation test and apprehension test [49]

be observed when compared to the contralateral side [5, 26, 54]. Muscle strength can be assessed with clinical tests such as single-leg squat, resisted knee extension, and repeated calf raises [27]. Foot alignment, quadriceps and hamstring flexibility, and ankle dorsiflexion range of movement have been associated with patellar tendinopathy (Table 26.1) and should also be assessed.

Deficits in lower limb kinetic chain function, lumbo-pelvic control, and energy-storage activities such as jumping and landing can be seen in patients with patellar tendinopathy [26]. Patients with patellar tendinopathy tend to have a stiff knee during landing and are softer at the ankle and hip during these tasks to compensate for the lower force absorption at the knee. This can be assessed by various functional tests such as hopping and specific change of direction tasks that load the patellar tendons.

26.3.3 Patient-Reported Outcome Measures (PROMs)

The VISA-P (Victorian Institute of Sport Assessment for patellar tendinopathy) questionnaire is used to quantify pain, function, and ability to participate in sports [55]. The VISA-P is a 100-point scale, with higher score indicating better function and less pain [55]. The VISA-P has good test-retest reliability (ICC = 0.91–0.99) [56, 57], and the minimum clinically important difference is a change in score of greater than 13 points [58]. It can be used to assess severity of symptoms and to monitor treatment outcomes at regular intervals of 4 weeks or more [27, 59].

26.3.4 Imaging

The imaging of patellar tendon with conventional ultrasound and magnetic resonance imaging (MRI) allows for the visualization of the tendon structure and is used to identify structural disorganization within the tendon. Although both ultrasound and MRI have good to excellent accuracy in confirming clinically diagnosed patellar tendinopathy [60–62], there is the lack of a valid clinical gold standard and no direct relationship between tendon structural changes visualized on imaging and tendon pain [60]. The diagnosis of patellar tendinopathy should not rely solely on the imaging of the patellar tendon and requires the features of pain and the aggravating factors [63]. Furthermore, imaging may be helpful in differential diagnoses of anterior knee pain (such as plica) when the clinical picture is unclear [27, 50, 63].

26.4 Physiotherapy Management of Patellar Tendinopathy

The key management of patellar tendinopathy is to develop load tolerance of the tendon by reducing pain initially, followed by progressive loading rehabilitation to target musculotendinous strength and function in the kinetic chain during sport-specific activities [26]. The principle of managing patellar tendinopathy consists of a staged rehabilitation program that addresses *pain management, strength progression, energy-storage loading, progressive return to sport, and maintenance* (Table 26.2) [25, 27]. It is important that rehabilitation should vary according to the stages of pathology or presentation. For example, reactive tendinopathy requires load modification and pain reduction, which may be achieved by prescription of isometric exercises [64]. In contrast, reactive-on-degenerative tendinopathy requires early pain management and then progressive loading to target the muscle-tendon strength and functional deficits [26].

Endurance needs to be built into each level, to ensure that the person can manage longer exposures to load required in tennis matches. The program aims to completely relieve pain during training and playing, but there are occasions where there is residual pain even when function has been restored; these players can continue to play without increasing pain.

26.4.1 Pain Management

Load modification. Load modification to reduce pain and symptoms requires reducing the training frequency, decreasing training volume, and removing high-load energy-storage activities such as running or jumping. It is important to note that complete rest should be avoided as unloading a tendon may further reduce the load capacity of the tendon [25–27].

Isometric exercises. Heavy sustained isometric exercises have been shown to induce immediate analgesia in painful patellar tendinopathy [64]. Pain relief can be obtained for several hours after five repetitions of 45-s isometric midrange (around 30° to 60° of knee flexion) quadriceps exercise (preferably single leg) at 70% of maximal voluntary contraction on a leg extension machine [64]. When there is limited or no access to gym equipment, the Spanish squat [65] is an alternative way in which a double-leg squat (around 70–90° of knee flexion) can be performed with the assistance of a rigid strap fixating at the lower legs [27]. Both exercises can be done during in-season training or playing [25] and can be performed several times a day to reduce pain and maintain loading of the muscle-tendon unit [66].

26.4.2 Stage 2: Strength Progression

Eccentric training and heavy resistance training have been investigated in patellar tendinopathy rehabilitation. Heavy slow isotonic exercise program has been shown to have short-term and long-term effects on pain reduction and function [67–69], accompanied by improvement in pathology on imaging [67], increased collagen turnover [67], and normalization of fibril morphology [70]. van Ark et al. (2015) reported that 4 weeks of isotonic exercises can decrease pain in athletes with patellar tendinopathy in-season [68]. The strengthening program in this chapter incorporates both of these strengthening strategies.

Isotonic exercise. Heavy slow isotonic exercise restores muscle bulk and strength of the lower limb (including quadriceps, gluteal, and calf muscles) and should be started when it can be performed with minimal pain [27]. These exercises include single-leg seated knee extension (leg extension machine), leg press, hip extension and abduction (hip machine), and calf raise exercise (both soleus and gastrocnemius) for both the affected and unaffected leg. For each exercise, 4 sets of 6–8 repetitions at 80% of 8 repetition maximum (RM) are required, with a 3-s concentric phase immediately followed by a 4-s eccentric phase. It is important to progress the loading every week by increasing the initial weight as tolerated [68]. The heavy slow isotonic exercise program can be performed 3–5 times per week for at least 12 weeks and should be continued throughout the remaining stages of rehabilitation and return to sport [27].

26.4.3 Stage 3: Energy-Storage and Release Loading

When good strength has been restored, it is crucial to train energy-storage loading to ensure a successful return to sport. At this stage, energy-storage exercises are the most irritable and pain provocative, and progression of the volume and intensity (depth, speed, and repetition) depends on load tolerance of the individual patients (guided by pain experienced 24 h after exercise preferably using the decline squat) and the demands of the sport [27]. Initially, exercises such as split squats and up-and-down stairs can be performed. These may be followed by skipping; jumping; forward hops, with progression to side-to-side movements; change of direction tasks; and quick stops and starts as required in tennis. The energy-storage exercises can be performed every third day, while the isometric loading and isotonic exercises are maintained on alternate days to manage pain and maintain muscle strength.

26.4.4 Stage 4: Progressive Return to Sport

When the player can tolerate sport-specific energy-storage loading, the player can progressively return to sports training and eventually competition. Initially, the training volume and intensity should be similar to the final progression of energy-storage activities and gradually progress to training drills that require the demand of sports training [27].

26.4.5 Stage 5: Maintenance

Once the player has returned to sport, it is important they monitor their symptoms, manage their load, and adjust participation in training/competition to prevent flare-ups. Isometric exercises and Spanish squat exercises can be continued while training and playing [27] if flare ups occur and for cortical inhibition [64]. Isotonic exercises such as seated knee extension, leg press, split squats, and gluteal and calf strengthening exercises (preferably single leg) are performed at least twice a week to maintain lower limb strength [25, 27] (Table 26.3).

26.5 Adjunct Treatments

Many adjuncts carry risk or require downtime (e.g., a period of enforced rest after an injection). We would advocate noninvasive adjuncts

Table 26.3 Rehabilitation progression for patellar tendinopathy

Phase	Aim	Intervention	Example of exercises	Indication to initiate
Pain management	Reduce pain	• Load modification • Heavy sustained single-leg isometric midrange quadriceps exercise	• Reduce training frequency and volume • Remove high-load energy-storage activities such as jumping and running • Leg extension, 45 s, 70% maximal voluntary contraction, five repetitions, two times/day • Spanish squat	• Pain >3/10 on a numeric pain-rating scale
Strength progression	Improve strength	• Heavy slow isotonic exercise	• Seated knee extension, leg press, split squat, hip extension and abduction, calf raises, four sets of eight repetitions, 80% of eight repetition maximum (RM), three times/week, 12 weeks	• Pain <3/10 on a numeric pain-rating scale during exercise
Energy-storage loading	Develop stretch-shorten cycle	• Whole kinetic chain patterns • Plyometric exercises	• Walk lunge • Skipping • Jumping • Split squat jumps • Single-leg hops • Forward hops • Change of direction tasks • Side-to-side movements • Quick stops and starts	• Good strength (ability to perform four sets of eight repetitions of single-leg press with 150% body weight • Pain <3/10 on a numeric pain-rating scale during initial-level energy-storage exercise
Progressive return to sport	Return to training and competition	• Sport-specific training drills	• Progressively add training drills similar to the demand of sports training and competition	• Load tolerance to energy-storage exercise
Maintenance	Management of symptoms and prevention of flare-ups	• Continue strengthening exercise, manage load tolerance, education	• Isotonic exercises such as seated knee extension, leg press, hip extension and abduction, calf raises • Isometric exercises and Spanish squat exercise while training and playing	• Load tolerance to return to sports

that allow loading (such as tape may be used) over invasive interventions or those that simply remove pain and may place the athlete at risk. Furthermore, there is very little evidence directing clinicians for in-season management in terms of these adjuncts. There is evidence for isometric and isotonic exercise in-season [71, 72].

26.5.1 Extracorporeal Shock Wave Therapy

Two systematic reviews showed there is limited evidence on the effectiveness of ESWT in the short-term and long-term improvements in pain and function for patellar tendinopathy [73, 74]. Zwerver et al. [7] reported that there was no benefit of ESWT compared to placebo treatment for in-season athletes with patellar tendinopathy. Based on the literature, there is no specific treatment protocol of ESWT for patellar tendinopathy [74].

26.5.2 Injections

Corticosteroid injections, platelet-rich plasma (PRP), and other injections (sclerosis, high-volume, aprotinin, dry needling, and autologous blood injections) are often used for patellar tendinopathy to reduce pain and are proposed to improve tendon structure. A systematic review showed overall positive outcomes for injection treatments for patellar tendinopathy; however, only a small number of high-quality studies have been conducted [76].

Corticosteroid can act as an inhibitor of cell activity and proliferation. Unlike other injection treatments, corticosteroid injections appear to be effective in the short term for a reactive tendon to relieve pain and decrease swelling and vascularization [67, 75, 76, 77], but the long-term outcomes (4 weeks to 6 months) were poorer [67, 77].

PRP injection is a current treatment option for patellar tendinopathy. PRP is an autologous blood fraction rich in platelets, and their associated growth factors promote tendon healing [78].

A systematic review in 2015 showed that PRP injection is a safe and promising therapy in the treatment of patellar tendinopathy [79]. However, its superiority over other physiotherapy treatments is unknown. A combination of PRP injection followed by eccentric exercises program has been shown to have both short-term (12 weeks) and long-term (6–12 months) improvements in pain and function [78, 80], although results should be interpreted with caution as it is unclear whether the benefits are as a result of the injection or the exercise program. It is also worth noting that the efficacy of this treatment in-season for athletes is unknown.

Given this, caution should be taken with analgesic injection in athletes with painful patellar tendinopathy. Removing pain and allowing the athlete to continue to play may cause maximal loading on the pathologic tendon. This may progressively overload the tendon and cause tendon rupture [81].

26.5.3 Strapping or Bracing

Strapping or bracing can also be considered in managing the athletes with patellar tendinopathy. Strapping has been shown to decrease patellar tendon strain by altering the angle of the patellar tendon [82] although no better than placebo taping [83]. It can also be considered as one of the adjunct treatment in managing the athletes with in-season patellar tendinopathy [66]. Different strapping techniques and materials may be experimented with, to help players decrease pain and feel more confident on the affected limb.

26.5.4 Kinetic Chain Deficits

Patellar tendinopathy is often seen in the contralateral limb to the serving arm, as a result of the force absorption of the front leg during the service action. Anecdotally, tennis players often seek treatment for muscle tightness around the hip of the front leg (such as psoas or tensor fasciae latae), and soft tissue release through these muscles may help decrease the load on the patellar tendon, by balancing force absorption through the whole kinetic chain. Mobilization techniques to help maintain hip internal rotation may also be helpful.

Another aspect of the kinetic chain to consider is ankle dorsiflexion. Incidence of ankle sprains in tennis players is significant, and often, full dorsiflexion may not be regained after injury. Assessment for any deficit and appropriate treatment by mobilization of the talocrural and subtalar joints may be beneficial for restoring full range of motion and in turn decreasing patellar tendon loading.

Conclusion

Patellar tendinopathy is a clinical diagnosis of pain and dysfunction in the patellar tendon. Management of patellar tendinopathy relies on understanding the pathophysiology of patellar tendinopathy, and the continuum model of tendon pathology has the most clinical relevance and provides a framework to stage the continuity of patellar tendinopathy. A detailed history and assessment of an individual with patellar tendinopathy is essential to differentiate it from other potential diagnoses of anterior knee pain and to prescribing appropriate treatment approaches and direction for the rehabilitation program according to the stages of pathology or presentation. Exercise is the cornerstone of patellar tendinopathy rehabilitation. The key to management of patellar tendinopathy is to develop load tolerance of the tendon by addressing pain reduction initially, followed by a progressive loading rehabilitation to target strength followed by energy-storage loading to increase load tolerance, before a progression to return to sport.

References

1. Abrams GD, Renstrom PA, Safran MR. Epidemiology of musculoskeletal injury in the tennis player. Br J Sports Med. 2012;46:492–8.
2. Hjelm N, Werner S, Renstrom P. Injury profile in junior tennis players: a prospective two year study. Knee Surg Sports Traumatol Arthrosc. 2010;18:845–50.
3. Sell K, Hainline B, Yorio M, Kovacs M. Injury trend analysis from the US Open Tennis Championships between 1994 and 2009. Br J Sports Med. 2014;48:546–51.
4. Simpson M, Rio E, Cook J. At what age do children and adolescents develop lower limb tendon pathology or tendinopathy? A systematic review and meta-analysis. Sports Med. 2016;46(4):545–57.
5. Cook JL, Khan KM, Kiss ZS, Purdam CR, Griffiths L. Prospective imaging study of asymptomatic patellar tendinopathy in elite junior basketball players. J Ultrasound Med. 2000b;19:473–9.
6. Visnes H, Bahr R. Training volume and body composition as risk factors for developing jumper's knee among elite volleyball players. Scan J Med Sci Sports. 2013;23:607–13.
7. Zwerver J, Bredeweg SW, van der Akkler-Scheek I. Prevalence of jumper's knee among nonelite athletes from different sports: a cross-sectional survey. Am J Sports Med. 2011;39(9):1984–8.
8. Lian Ø, Refsnes P-E, Engebretsen L, Bahr R. Performance characteristics of volleyball players with patellar tendinopathy. Am J Sports Med. 2017;31(3):408–13.
9. Ferretti A. Epidemiology of jumper's knee. Sports Med. 1986;3:289–95.
10. Maquirrianin J, Baglione R. Epidemiology of tennis injuries: an eight-year review of Davis Cup retirements. Eur J Sport Sci. 2016;16(2):266–70.
11. Tiemessen IJ, Kuijer PP, Hulshof CT, Frings-Dresen MH. Risk factors for developing jumper's knee in sport and occupation: a review. BMC Res Notes. 2009;8(2):127.
12. Cook JL, Khan KM, Harcourt PR, Grant M, Young DA, Bonar SF. A cross sectional study of 100 athletes with jumper's knee managed conservatively and surgically. The Victorian Institute of Sport Tendon Study Group. Br J Sportd Med. 1997;31:332–6.
13. Kettunen JA, Kvist M, Alanen E, Jujala UM. Long-term prognosis for jumper's knee in male athletes. A prospective follow-up study. Am J Sports Med. 2002;30(5):689–92.
14. Cook JL, Purdam CR. Is tendon pathology a continuum? A pathology model to explain the clinical presentation of load-induced tendinopathy. Br J Sports Med. 2009;43:409–16.
15. Corps AN, Robinson AH, Movin T, Costa ML, Hazleman BL, Riley GP. Increased expression of aggrecan and biglycan mRNA in Achilles tendinopathy. Rheumatology. 2006;45(3):291–4.
16. Samiric T, Parkinson J, Ilic MZ, Cook J, Feller JA, Handley CJ. Changes in the composition of the extracellular matrix in patellar tendinopathy. Matrix Biol. 2009;28(4):230–6.
17. Docking SI, Daffy J, van Schie HT, Cook JL. Tendon structure changes after maximal exercise in the Thoroughbred horse: use of ultrasound tissue characterisation to detect in vivo tendon response. Vet J. 2012;194(3):338–42.
18. Rosengarten SD, Cook JL, Bryant AL, Cordy JT, Daffy J, Docking SI. Australian football players'

Achilles tendons respond to game loads within 2 days: an ultrasound tissue characterisation (UTC) study. Br J Sports Med. 2015;49(3):183–7.
19. Maffuli N, Ewen SW, Waterston SW, Reaper J, Barrass V. Tenocytes from ruptured and tendinopathic Achilles tendons produce greater quantities of type III collagen than tenocytes from normal Achilles tendons. An in vitro model of human tendon healing. Am J Sports Med. 2000;28(4):499–505.
20. Danielson P, Alfredson HK, Forsgren S. Distribution of general (PGP 9.5) and sensory (substance P/CGRP) innervations in the human patellar tendon. Knee Surg Sports Traumatol Arthrosc. 2006;14:125–32.
21. Kraushaar BS, Nirschl RP. Current concepts review - Tendinosis of the elbow (tennis elbow). Clinical features and findings of histological, Immunohistochemical, and Electron microscopy studies. J Bone Joint Surg Am. 1999;81(2):259–78.
22. Lian Ø, Scott A, Engebretsen L, Bahr R, Duronio V, Khan K. Excessive apoptosis in patellar tendinopathy in athletes. Am J Sports Med. 2017;35(4):605–11.
23. Docking SI, Cook J. Pathological tendons maintain sufficient aligned fibrillar structure on ultrasound tissue characterization (UTC). Scand J Med Sci Sports. 2016;26(6):675–83.
24. Cook JL, Rio E, Purdam CR, Docking SI. Revisiting the continuum model of tendon pathology: what is its merit in clinical practice and research? Br J Sports Med. 2016;0:1–7.
25. Rudavsky A, Cook J. Physiotherapy management of patellar tendinopathy (jumper's knee). J Physiother. 2014;60(3):122–9.
26. Kountouris A, Cook J. Rehabilitation of Achilles and patellar tendinopathies. Best Pract Res Clin Rheumatol. 2007;21(2):295–316.
27. Malliaras P, Cook J, Purdam C, Rio E. Patella tendinopathy: clinical diagnosis, load management, and advice for challenging case presentations. J Orthop Sports Phys Ther. 2015;45(11):887–98.
28. Cook JL, Khan KM, Kiss ZS, Griffiths L. Patellar tendinopathy in junior basketball players: a controlled clinical and ultrasonographic study of 268 patellar tendons in players aged 14-18 years. Scand J Med Sci Sports. 2000;10(4):216–20.
29. Cook JL, Kiss ZS, Khan KM, Purdam CR, Wbster KE. Anthropometry, physical performance, and ultrasound patellar tendon abnormality in elite junior basketball players: a cross-sectional study. Br J Sports Med. 2004;38:206–9.
30. Gaida JE, Alfredson H, Kiss ZS, Bass SL, Cook JL. Asymptomatic Achilles tendon pathology is associated with a central fat distribution in men and a peripheral fat distribution in women: a cross sectional study of 298 individuals. BMC Musculoskelet Disord. 2010;11:41.
31. Gaida JE, Cook JL, Bass SL, Austen S, Kiss ZS. Are unilateral and bilateral patella tendinopathy distinguished by differences in anthropometry, body composition, or muscle strength in elite female basketball players? Br J Sports Med. 2004;38:581–5.
32. Malliaras P, Cook JL, Kent PM. Anthropometric risk factors for patellar tendon injury among volleyball players. Br J Sports Med. 2007;41:259–63.
33. Crossley KM, Thancanamootoo K, Metcalf BR, Cook JL, Purdam CR, Warden SJ. Clinical features of patellar tendinopathy and their implications for rehabilitation. J Orthop Res. 2007;25:1164–75.
34. Malliaras P, Cook JL, Kent P. Reduced ankle dorsiflexion range may increase the risk of patellar tendon injury among volleyball players. J Sci Med Sport. 2006;9:304–9.
35. Kujala UM, Osterman K, Kvist M, Aalto T, Friberg O. Factors predisposing to patellar chondropathy and patellar apicitis in athletes. Int Orthop. 1986;10:195–200.
36. Witvrouw E, Bellemans J, Lysens R, Danneels L, Cambier D. Intrinsic risk factors for the development of patellar tendinitis in an athletic population. Am J Sports Med. 2017;29(2):190–5.
37. Lian O, Refsnes PE, Engebretsen L, Bahr R. Performance characteristics of volleyball players with patellar tendinopathy. Am J Sports Med. 2003;31:408–13.
38. Culvenor AG, Cook JL, Warden SJ, Crossley KM. Infrapatellar fat pad size but not patellar alignment, is associated with patellar tendinopathy. Scand J Med Sci Sports. 2011;21:e405–11.
39. Ranger TA, Wong AMY, Cook JL, Gaida JE. Is there an association between tendinopathy and diabetes mellitus? A systematic review with meta-analysis. Br J Sports Med. 2015;0:1–10.
40. Gaida JE, Ashe MC, Bass SL, Cook JL. Is adiposity an under-recognized risk factor for tendinopathy? A systematic review. Arthritis Rheum. 2009;61(6):840–9.
41. Callewaert B, Malfait F, Loeys B, de Paepe A. Ehlers-Danlos syndromes and Marfan syndrome. Best Pract Res Clin Rheumatol. 2008;22:165–89.
42. Lewis T, Cook J. Fluoroquinolones and tendinopathy: a guide for athletes and sports clinicians and a systematic review of the literature. J Athl Train. 2014;49(3):422–7. https://doi.org/10.4085/1062-6050-49.2.09.
43. Crossley KM, Callaghan MJ, van Linschoten R. Patellofemoral pain. BMJ. 2015;451:h3939.
44. Nunes GS, Stapait EL, Kirsten MH, et al. Clinical test for diagnosis of patellofemoral pain syndrome: systematic review with meta-analysis. Phys Ther Sport. 2013;14:54–9.
45. Ng GYF, Cheng JMF. The effects of patellar taping on pain and neuromuscular performance in subjects with patellofemoral pain syndrome. Clin Rehabil. 2016;16(8):821–7.
46. Eymard F, Chevalier X. Inflammation of the infrapatellar fat pad. Joint Bone Spine. 2016;83(4):389–93.
47. Hardaker W, Whipple TL, Bassett FH. Diagnosis and treatment of the plica syndrome of the knee. J Bone Joint Surg Am. 1980;62(2):221–5.
48. McConnell J. Running injuries: the infrapatellar fat pad and plica injuries. Phys Med Rehabil Clin N Am. 2016;27(1):79–89.

49. McCarthy MA, Bollier MJ. Medial patella subluxation: diagnosis and treatment. Iowa Orthop J. 2015;35:26–33.
50. Calmback WL, Hutchens M. Evaluation of patients presenting with knee pain: Part II. Differential diagnosis. Am Fam Physician. 2003;68(5):917–22.
51. Cook JL, Khan KM, Kiss ZS, Purdam CR, Griffiths L. Reproducibility and clinical utility of tendon palpation to detect patellar tendinopathy in young basketball players. Victorian Institute of Sport tendon study group. Br J Sports Med. 2001;35:65–9.
52. Kongsgaard M, Aagaard P, Roikjaer S, Olsen D, Jensen M, Langberg H, Magnusson SP. Decline eccentric squats increases patellar tendon loading compared to standard eccentric squats. Clin biochech 2006;21:748-54. Clin Biomech (Bristol, Avon). 2006;21:748–54.
53. Purdam C, Cook J, Hopper D, Khan K, VTS G. Discriminative ability of functional loading tests for adolescent jumper's knee. Phys Ther Sport. 2003;4:3–9.
54. Cook J, Khan K, Maffulli N, Purdam C. Overuse tendinosis, not tendinitis: applying the new approach to patellar tendinopathy. Phys Sportsmed. 2000a;28(6):31–46.
55. Visentini PJ, Khan KM, Cook JL, Kiss ZS, Harcourt PR, Wark JD. The VISA score: an index of the severity of jumper's knee (patellar tendinosis). J Sci Med Sport. 1998;1(1):22–8.
56. Frohm A, Saartok T, Edman G, Renstrom P. Psychometric properties of a Swedish translation of the VISA-P outcome score for patellar tendinopathy. BMC Musculoskelet Disord. 2004;18(5):49.
57. Wageck BB, de Noronha M, Lopes AD, da Cunha RA, Takahashi RH, Costa LO. Crosscultural adaptation and measurement properties of the Brazilian Portuguese version of the Victorian Institute of Sport Assessment-Patella (VISA-P) scale. J Orthop Sports Phys Ther. 2013;43:163–71.
58. Hernandez-Sanchez S, Hidalgo MD, Gomez A. Cross-cultural adaptation of VISA-P score for patellar tendinopathy in Spanish population. J Orthop Sports Phys Ther. 2011;41:581–91.
59. Macdermid JC, Silbernagel KG. Outcome evaluation in tendinopathy: foundations of assessment and a summary of selected measures. J Orthop Sports Phys Ther. 2015;45(11):950–64.
60. Cook JL, Khan KM, Harcourt PR, Kiss ZS, Fehrmann MW, Griffiths L, Wark JD. Patellar tendon ultrasonography in asymptomatic active athletes reveals hypoechoic regions: a study of 320 tendons. Victorian Institute of Sport Tendon Study Group. Clin J Sport Med. 1998;8:73–7.
61. Khan KM, Cook JL, Kiss ZS, et al. Patellar tendon ultrasonography and jumper's knee in female basketball players: a longitudinal study. Clin J Sport Med. 1997;7:199–206.
62. Warden SJ, Kiss ZS, Malara FA, Cook JL, Crossley KM. Comparative accuracy of magnetic resonance imaging and ultrasonography in confirming clinically diagnosed patellar tendinopathy. Am J Sports Med. 2007;35(3):427–36.
63. Docking SI, Ooi CC, Connell D. Tendinopathy: is imaging telling us the entire story? J Orthop Sports Phys Ther. 2015;45(11):842–52.
64. Rio E, Kidgell D, Purdam C, Gaida J, Moseley GL, Pearce AJ, Cook J. Isometric exercise induces analgesia and reduces inhibition in patellar tendinopathy. Br J Sports Med. 2015;49(19):1277–83. https://doi.org/10.1136/bjsports-2014-094386.
65. Basas Garcia A, Fernandez de las Penas C, Martin Urrialde JA. Tratamiento fisioterapico de la rodilla. Madrid, Spain: McGraw-Hill-Interamericana; 2003.
66. Cook JL, Purdam CR. The challenge of managing tendinopathy in competing athletes. Br J Sports Med. 2014;48:506–9.
67. Kongsgaard M, Kovanen V, Aagaard P, Doessing S, Hansen P, Laursen AH, Kaldau NC, Kjaer M, Magnusson SP. Corticosteroid injections, eccentric decline squat training and heavy slow resistance training in patellar tendinopathy. Scand J Med Sci Sports. 2009;19(6):790–802.
68. van Ark M, Cook JL, Docking SI, Zwerver J, Gaida JE, van den Akker-Scheek I, Rio E. Do isometric and isotonic exercise programs reduce pain in athletes with patellar tendinopathy in-season? A randomised clinical trial. J Sci Med Sport. 2016;19(9):702–6.
69. Cannell LJ. A randomised clinical trial of the efficacy of drop squats or leg extension/leg curl exercises to treat clinically diagnosed jumper's knee in athletes: pilot study. Br J Sports Med. 2001;35(1):60–4.
70. Kongsgaard M, Qvortrup K, Larsen J, Aagaard P, Doessing S, Hansen P, Kjaer M, Peter Magnusson S. Fibril morphology and tendon mechanical properties in patellar tendinopathy. Am J Sports Med. 2017;38(4):749–56.
71. Rio E, van Ark M, Docking S, Moseley GL, Kidgell D, Gaida JE, et al. Isometric contractions are more analgesic than isotonic contractions for patellar tendon pain: an in-season randomized clinical trial. Clin J Sport Med. 2016. https://doi.org/10.1097/jsm.0000000000000364.
72. van Ark M, Cook JL, Docking SI, Zwerver J, Gaida JE, van den Akker-Scheek I, Rio E. Do isometric and isotonic exercise programs reduce pain in athletes with patellar tendinopathy in-season? A randomised clinical trial. J Sci Med Sport. 2016;19(9):702–6. https://doi.org/10.1016/j.jsams.2015.11.006.
73. Mani-Babu S, Morrissey D, Waugh C, Screen H, Barton C. The effectiveness of extracorporeal shock wave therapy in lower limb tendinopathy. Am J Sports Med. 2015;43(3):752–61.
74. van Leeuwen MT, Zwerver J, van den Akker-Scheek I. Extracorporeal shockwave therapy for patellar tendinopathy: a review of the literature. Br J Sports Med. 2009;43(3):163–8.
75. Fredberg U. Local corticosteroid injection in sport: review of literature and guidelines for treatment. Scand J Med Sci Sports 1997;7:131–39.

76. van Ark M, Zwerver J, van den Akker-Scheek I. Injection treatments for patellar tendinopathy. Br J Sports Med. 2011;45(13):1068–76.
77. Fredberg U, Bolvig L, Pfeiffer-Jensen M, et al. Ultrasonography as a tool for diagnosis, guidance of local steroid injection and, together with pressure algometry, monitoring of the treatment of athletes with chronic jumper's knee and Achilles tendinitis: a randomized, double-blind, placebo-controlled study. Scand J Rheumatol. 2004;33(2):94–101.
78. Dragoo JL, Wasterlain AS, Braun HJ, Nead KT. Platelet-rich plasma as a treatment for patellar tendinopathy. A double-blind, randomized controlled trail. Am J Sports Med. 2014;42(3):610–8.
79. Liddle AD, Rodriguez-Merchan EC. Plasma-rich plasma in the treatment of patellar tendinopathy: a systematic review. Am J Sports Med. 2015;42(10):2583–90.
80. Kaux J-F, Bruyete O, Croisier J-L, Forthomme B, Le Goff C, Crielaard JM. One-year follow-up of platelet-rick plasma infiltration to treat chronic proximal patellar tendinopathies. Acta Orthop Belg. 2015;81(2):251–6.
81. Chen S-K, Lu C-C, Chou P-H, Guo L-Y, Wu W-L. Patellar tendon ruptures in weight lifters after local steroid injections. Arch Orthop Trauma Surg. 2009;129(3):369–72.
82. Lavagnino M, Arnoczky SP, Dodds J, Elvin N. Infrapatellar straps decrease patellar tendon strain at the site of the jumper's knee lesion: a computational analysis based on radiographic measurements. Sports Health. 2011;3(3):296–302.
83. de Vries A, Zwerver J, Diercks R, Tak I, van Berkel S, van Cingel R, et al. Effect of patellar strap and sports tape on pain in patellar tendinopathy: a randomized controlled trial. Scand J Med Sci Sports. 2016;26(10):1217–24. https://doi.org/10.1111/sms.12556.

Rehabilitation of Knee Injuries

27

Robert C. Manske and Mark V. Paterno

27.1 Introduction

Tennis is a sport when placed at high levels places players at risk for multiple musculoskeletal injuries. Tennis is a physically demanding sport that can be played on multiple surfaces. Due to the repetitive jarring compressive forces during match play which can last for hours, knee injuries are commonplace. Tennis players move in all directions oftentimes pivoting and rotating on surfaces that are non-yielding. Lateral movements followed by quick anterior or posterior transitions are common and place tremendous stress on the musculoskeletal system. Acute injuries to muscles, tendons, menisci, ligaments, and articular cartilage can occur with fast cutting-type movements inherent in match play. Through the years, reported incidence and prevalence of injury in tennis have varied widely due to differences in the definition of injury study populations, methods of data collection, and duration and or frequency of follow-up between investigations. Overuse tendon injuries also abound as competitive tennis players, like other competitive athletes, continue workouts and play for in some instances weeks at a time without a break. Chard and Lachmann [1] report that knee injuries are very common in all racquet sports. Collateral ligament, cruciate ligament, and meniscal injury occurred in about 24% of their population, while patellofemoral pain and patellar dislocation occurred in about 60% of tennis players. One large epidemiologic study documented 17,397 athletes of all skill levels and ages with 19,530 sports injuries over a 10-year period. There were nearly 300 knee injuries related to tennis, and of these, 11% incurred injury to the anterior cruciate ligament (ACL). This same study also reported injuries to the lateral collateral ligament, and medial meniscus pathology was frequent in tennis players [2]. Still others have reported findings that 10–13% of tennis players with knee injuries incur intra-articular anterior cruciate ligament injury [3, 4]. Hjelm and colleagues [5, 6] report that knee injuries are more common in female tennis players. These injuries tend to be 72% of the injuries reported in their case series of 39 players. Injuries to the knee included patellar tendinopathy, iliotibial band friction syndrome, quadriceps tendinopathy, Osgood-Schlatter's disease, patellofemoral pain syndrome, and an unspecified knee pain due to overuse. Others also describe patellofemoral pain and patellar tendonitis to be very common [7, 8].

R. C. Manske (✉)
Department of PT, Wichita State University,
Wichita, KS, USA
e-mail: Robert.Manske@wichita.edu

M. V. Paterno
Division of Occupational Therapy and Physical Therapy, Cincinnati Children's Hospital Medical Center, Cincinnati, OH, USA

Division of Sports Medicine, Cincinnati Children's Hospital Medical Center, Cincinnati, OH, USA
e-mail: Mark.Paterno@cchmc.org

Although as tennis players age the risk of osteoarthritis increases, an association with tennis has not [9] been highly correlated, at least in Swedish male tennis players. The purpose of this chapter is to describe knee injuries in competitive and recreational tennis. The chapter will start with a review of anatomy and biomechanics of the knee. This will be followed by a discussion of the various injuries and how they will be managed by sports medicine professionals. Finally a return to sports program for a player with a tennis injury will be described.

27.2 Anatomy and Biomechanics of the Knee

The anatomy and biomechanics section of the knee is presented as a foundation to better understand clinical decision-making regarding knee injuries. The knee joint proper consists of several joints and articulations including the tibiofemoral joint and the patellofemoral joint. The bones that are inherent to these joints include the femur, tibia, and patella. At first glance this seemingly simple synovial structure looks relatively nondescript; however upon a closer look, one will see that the knee is one of the more complex diarthrodial joints in the human body. As the knee sits at the confluence of the two longest bones in the human body, tremendous forces are placed upon this articulation. The knee is also expected to operate in both an open kinetic chain (OKC) and closed kinetic chain (CKC) functions.

27.3 Tibiofemoral Joint

The tibiofemoral joint is comprised of the distal femur and the proximal tibia. Each of these bones has unique characteristics. The distal femur includes the femoral condyles and the intercondylar notch. This portion of the femur is covered with hyaline articular cartilage which, when healthy, can tolerate large shear and compressive forces that are placed upon the knee. Two condyles, one lateral and one medial, are rounded protuberances that are centrally divided the intercondylar notch or fossa, which is the attachment site for the cruciate ligaments. Each of the condyles is cam shaped with a smaller curvature posterior that of the anterior. The lateral femoral condyle is wider both anterior-posterior and medial-lateral when compared to the medial femoral condyle. The medial condyle extends further anterior than the lateral; however because the shaft of the femur angles in a medial direction, the two condyles sit relatively even in the horizontal plane. The proximal tibia articulates with the distal femur. The proximal tibia is formed by the medial and lateral tibial plateau which expand its proximal end over the smaller shaft. The medial tibial plateau is slightly concave to accept the convex medial femoral condyle. However, the lateral tibial plateau is either flat or slightly convex [10, 11], which may create a problem with a convex distal lateral femoral condyle. An important ridge runs down the center of the tibia. This ridge, the intercondylar eminence, is the attachment of the anterior cruciate and posterior cruciate ligaments. Several other important landmarks on the tibia are the tibial tubercle and the Gerdy's tubercle. The tibial tubercle is situated on the anterior surface of the tibia and is the attachment site of the patellar tendon. Gerdy's tubercle is on the anterior lateral tibial flare and is the attachment site of the iliotibial band.

27.4 Patellofemoral Joint

The patellofemoral joint consists of the posterior patella and the anterior femoral trochlea. The patella is the largest sesamoid bone in the body. The patella is engulfed within the extensor mechanism which includes the quadriceps tendon and the patellar tendon. The patella has both a base (proximal) and an apex (distal). The anterior surface of the patella is very palpable due to its superficial location on the anterior knee. The patella is convex anteriorly in both superior-inferior and medial-lateral direction. The thickest cartilage in the body (up to 6 mm) is found on the posterior patella and is thought to distribute very large compressive and shear forces that occur at the patellofemoral joint during dynamic activities.

A vertical ridge runs down the center of the patella dividing it into almost equal medial and lateral halves. However, there is a second smaller vertical ridge that runs along the medial facet that separates the medial facet from the odd facet. Most of the posterior patella, except the distal inferior pole, is articular. The patellofemoral joint is a relatively unstable joint as the sulcus is shallow and patella does not fit deeply into the sulcus. As the intercondylar notch continues anteriorly, it becomes the trochlear grove also known as the femoral sulcus. This sulcus is bordered both medially and laterally by the patellar facets of the distal femur.

27.5 Ligaments and Knee Capsule

Because the knee has little inherent osseous stability, it relies on strong ligamentous restraint and dynamic muscular stability. The four major ligaments contributing support to the knee include the anterior cruciate (ACL), posterior cruciate (PCL), medial collateral (MCL), and lateral collateral (LCL) ligaments. Together these ligaments each individually and collectively provide both primary and secondary restraints to single-plane instability and multidirectional instability, respectively.

The ACL emerges from a position anterior and medial to the tibial eminence of the tibial plateau. It runs superiorly, laterally, and posteriorly to insert on the posterior margin of the medial wall of the lateral femoral condyle. The ACL is one ligament; however it is composed of two separate bundles, an anteromedial bundle and a posterolateral bundle. The anteromedial bundle is taut in 60° or more of knee flexion, while the posteromedial bundle is taut in extension and rotations. The PCL arises from the posterior tibia just below the tibial plateau. The PCL runs superiorly, anteriorly, and medially from the tibia to the femur. Very similar to the ACL, the PCL has two bands: the anterolateral band and the posteromedial band. The anterolateral band is taut in knee flexion, while the posteromedial band is taut in extension. The LCL is more chord-like or pencil shaped and runs from the lateral epicondyle of the femur to the fibular head. Between the LCL and the bony structures runs the popliteus tendon. This ligament restrains a varus stress placed on the knee. The MCL is a large, broad, flatter ligament that runs from the medial epicondyle of the femur to the tibia below the joint line. The MCL is divided into a deep and superficial portion. The deep portion attaches to medial meniscus and includes a meniscofemoral and meniscotibial portion. The superficial band inserts at the femoral epicondyle and the tibial plateau. (Fig. 27.1).

27.6 Meniscus

Due to the significant amount of movement around the tennis court, twisting, pivoting, and change of direction both medial-lateral and anterior-posterior are commonplace. It is exactly these movements, in which torsional rotation with the knee loaded in various degrees of flexion, which are a recipe for knee meniscal injuries. Meniscal injuries are so commonplace in athletics that arthroscopic treatment of meniscal tears has become the most common knee surgical procedure in the United States.

The medial meniscus is shaped similar to a C with the open end toward midline. Each meniscus has horns which are the attachments of the meniscus to the tibial eminence. The medial meniscus has a posterior horn which is larger (anteroposterior dimensions) than the anterior horns. A large portion of the medial meniscus is attached to the knee capsule and to the deep fibers of the medial collateral ligament. The meniscus is seen in the image in Fig. 27.2.

The lateral meniscus is almost a complete circle. Its anterior and posterior horns are much similar in size and much closer in proximity to each other than the medial meniscus. The lateral meniscus covers a larger % of total surface area than that of the medial meniscus. In about 3–5% of cases, known as lateral discoid meniscus, the structure covers the entire surface of the tibial plateau [12]. The lateral meniscus has two vestiges that run to the PCL. The ligament of Wrisberg comes from the PCL and is also known as the posterior meniscofemoral ligament. The

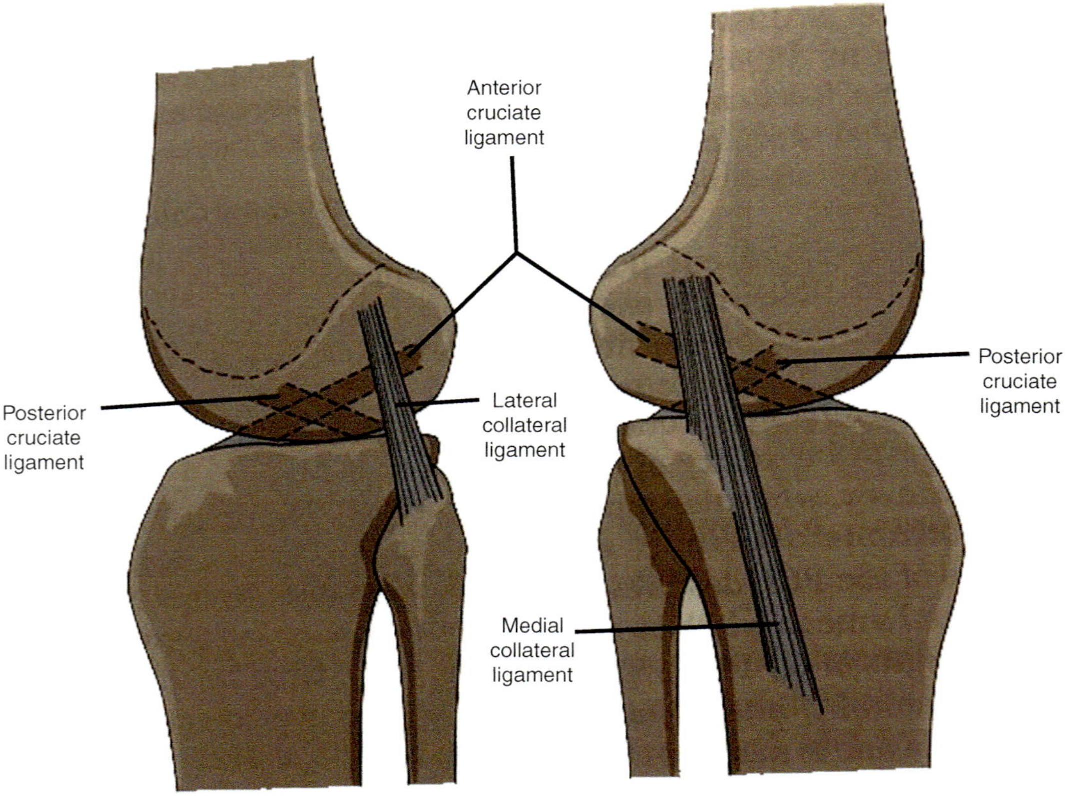

Fig. 27.1 Lateral and medial collateral ligaments. (Image taken from Loudon, Manske and Reiman. Clinical Mechanics and Kinesiology. Human Kinetics, 2013. Page 286, Figure 14.7)

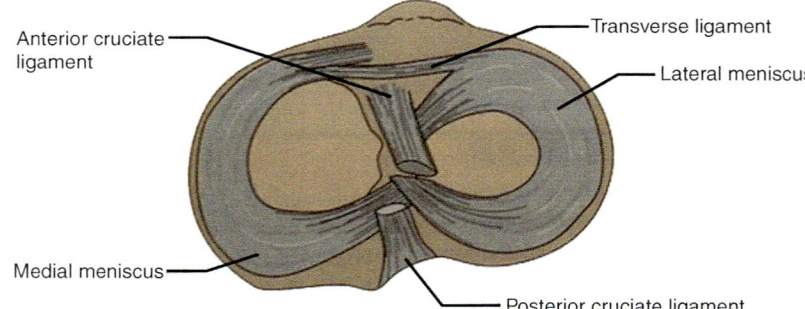

Fig. 27.2 Lateral and medial meniscus. (Image taken from Loudon, Manske and Reiman. Clinical Mechanics and Kinesiology. Human Kinetics, 2013. Page 288, Figure 14.8)

ligament of Humphrey is known as the anterior meniscofemoral ligament and runs from the PCL to the lateral meniscus.

Both menisci in the cross section are pie shaped or wedged. The outer periphery is thicker, while the inner portion is thinner. The vascular supply to the meniscus is from the superior and inferior branches of the medial and lateral genicular arteries. This blood supply reaches approximately 25% and 10–30% of the thicker periphery of the lateral and medial meniscus, respectively [13]. This is problematic for adequate healing if an injury to the meniscus occurs in the inner thinner portion of the meniscus. Due to the arrangement of the blood supply to the menisci, an injury to the periphery has a chance to heal, while injury to the inner 1/3 to 2/3 has minimal chance to heal intrinsically if at all.

27.7 Articular Cartilage

Hyaline articular cartilage is the material that covers the ends of long bones in synovial joints. Articular cartilage is primarily composed of water contributing up to 80% of its weight. It is water that gives the cartilage its ability to absorb stress and compressive forces that occur during normal activities of daily living such as walking, running, and jumping. The remaining components of cartilage include proteoglycans and non-collagenous proteins and collagen. Because cartilage covers the ends of long bones, it is especially important in knee function. This is especially true since the area of cartilage that is injured in the knee makes contact with the patella or femur around 30–70° of knee flexion [14]. This is even further problematic that following injury to articular cartilage, healing is often compromised due to cell apoptosis and the presence of catabolic enzymes. Due to these issues, articular cartilage cannot form a fibrin scaffold or mobilize cells to repair the defect.

27.8 Ligament Injuries

Ligament injuries may occur as the result of a non-contact mechanism during tennis. Frequent pivoting and cutting place the knee ligamentous structure at risk. Epidemiologic data suggests the knee ligaments at greatest risk while playing tennis are the anterior cruciate ligament, representing 11–13% of all knee injuries in tennis [2–4], the medial collateral ligament, and lateral collateral ligament [2].

27.9 Anterior Cruciate Ligament Injury

The ACL provides stability to the knee during pivoting, cutting, and rotational activities. Injury may occur when landing from a jump or planting/cutting activity. Classically, ACL injury was described as a hyperextension injury [15], but more recent evidence suggests that if the knee is positioned with excessive valgus and femoral/tibial rotation, it becomes vulnerable to injury as well [16]. Athletes who present with ligament dominance (reliance on ligamentous structures rather than neuromuscular contributions to control dynamic knee movement), quadriceps dominance (high quadriceps-to-hamstring strength ratio), limb dominance (tendency to favor one limb with dynamic activity) [17], and trunk dominance (excessive trunk movement) [16] often demonstrate high-risk movements during athletic activity and are, subsequently, at increased risk for ACL injury. Injury to the ACL results in mechanical instability of the knee as there is an increase in anterior tibial translation of the knee as well as excessive tibial rotations. If the ACL injury is coupled with other ligamentous injuries, this mechanical instability may be even greater. In addition to mechanical instability, the athlete may present with functional instability or a sensation that the knee is "giving way" after ACL injury. This sensation of giving way may be reported only with higher-level pivoting and cutting activities, such as tennis, or it may be reported with lower-level activities of daily living [18]. The level of activity, at which time the patient reports functional instability, often factors into the decision to undergo surgical management of the ACL injury.

Injury to the ACL can be medically treated both non-operatively and operatively. Non-operative treatment following ACL injury requires an immediate focus on the management of acute impairments as well as a systematic assessment of ability to safely participate in pivoting and cutting activities without the athlete reporting a sensation of "giving way." Repeated giving way at the knee results in high vulnerability to sustaining further meniscal and articular cartilage injury and necessitates surgical management to restore knee stability. Once the acute impairments of knee joint effusion and loss of motion and strength are managed, the athlete can be assessed to determine if they are a candidate to pursue non-operative management of ACL injury. In a body of work by

Fitzgerald, Snyder-Mackler, and colleagues from the University of Delaware [19, 20], a screening tool was developed to determine if a patient is a "coper" indicating potential to function in the absence of an ACL or a "non-coper" indicating an individual who likely would not function well with ACL deficiency. The screening tool includes assessment on four single-leg hop tests, reported number of giving way episodes, the Knee Outcome Survey, and a global rating of knee function [20]. Patients who are classified as "non-copers" are often recommended for surgical intervention. If the patient is determined to be a "coper," they participate in rehabilitation designed to enhance strength and mobility as well as a specialized "perturbation" rehabilitation program which focuses on balance and reactive neuromuscular control designed to maximally challenge and train the proprioceptive system as a means to enhance dynamic functional stability of the knee. Once rehabilitation is complete, the patient is able to successfully pass all return to sports assessments, and a functional progression back to tennis is complete; these athletes may attempt a return to sport. Although some athletes are successful with non-operative management of ACL injury, a 10-year outcome study of patients with ACL injury suggests a relatively low percentage of athletes are able to resume prior levels of function in the presence of ACL deficiency [21]. Further, a case report specific to tennis players with ACL deficiency noted that in a cohort that was able to return to recreational tennis, they continued to report lower level of tennis function as well as difficulty with higher-level movements [22]. Collectively, these data suggest return to high-level tennis with an ACL-deficient knee may be a challenge for many athletes, and a systematic evaluation of potential ability to succeed with this treatment course is required prior to attempting a non-operative course.

27.10 ACL Reconstruction Rehabilitation

If the athlete's goal is to return to high-level tennis, which requires fast-paced pivoting and cutting, surgical reconstruction may be necessary. The goal of the ACL reconstruction would be to provide mechanical and functional stability in the knee and allow for an attempt to return to pre-injury level of activity. Variation in surgical reconstruction technique as well as graft-type selection may result in necessary modification to the rehabilitation process. Despite these variables, rehabilitation after surgical reconstruction is guided by a criteria-based progression from immediate postoperative management to functional transition back to sport. Table 27.1 will outline this rehabilitation.

27.10.1 Phase I: Preoperative Phase

The preoperative phase is seen in Table 27.1 and is followed prior to surgery. Goals of this phase are to restore motility, increase quadriceps activation and decrease pain and effusion. Ambulation at this time is weight bearing as tolerated with crutches and a brace locked in full extension.

Gentle range of motion (ROM) as tolerated and a progression of exercises as patient is able to tolerate is utilized in this early preoperative period. Exercise progression should not increase symptoms, pain, or effusion.

27.10.2 Phase II: Immediate PO Phase

Acute phase rehabilitation after ACL reconstruction is focused on managing acute, postoperative swelling, range of motion (ROM), and initiation of quadriceps activation. Postoperative effusion is prevalent after ACL reconstruction and inhibits quadriceps activation [23] and mobility. Acute phase rehabilitation includes use of modalities such as cryotherapy and compression dressings to assist in swelling reduction. In addition, the patient is advised in frequent elevation and home use of compression and cryotherapy to assist in reduction of effusion. Early resolution of postoperative effusion assists in restoring the patient's ability to actively contract the quadriceps and slows postoperative disuse atrophy.

Weight bearing after ACL reconstruction is typically progressed over 3–6 weeks. Patients may initiate touch-down weight bearing immediately after ACL reconstruction and progress as

Table 27.1 ACLR table

Phase	Days–weeks	Goals	Restrictions	Treatment	Clinical milestones
Phase I: Preoperative	Pre-operative	Restore ROM both active and passive Quadriceps activation Decreased effusion Pain reduction	WBAT with bilateral axillary crutches Brace locked at 0°	RICE Electrical stimulation Extension ROM Passive flexion ROM Glute/Quad/Ham sets Hip abduction/adduction Leg presses Minisquats Step-downs	Surgical reconstruction Full knee extension Restoration of strength Minimal effusion No increased pain
Phase II: Immediate PO Phase	Post-operative Wks 0–2	WBAT bilateral axillary crutches locked in extension Full knee extension Quadriceps control Pain reduction Normal patellar mobility	Full WBAT brace locked in full extension × 1 week After week 1 PROM flexion can be started Brace still locked in extension for weight bearing until SLR with no extensor lag	Patellar mobilization Scar tissue mobilization PROM flexion and extension PROM flexion progressed to 110° week 1 130° week 2 Quadriceps sets Straight leg raise × 4 Ankle pumps CPM Weight shifts Cryotherapy	Previous milestones Clean incisions Good quadriceps recruitment SLR with minimal lag Normalized patellar mobility Weight bearing progressed without symptoms Minimal pain and effusion
Phase III: Intermediate PO Phase	Post-operative Wks 2–4	Normalized quadriceps recruitment Normal patellar mobility No pain or effusion Restoration of motion Maintain full weight bearing Improve balance	Braced unlocked for weight bearing as tolerated Crutches discontinued at approximately 2 weeks	Progression of previous isometric quad sets at 0°, 60°, and 90° Squats and leg press 0–60° Stationary bike Step-downs Calf raises Minisquats Balance drills Band exercises	Previous milestones Satisfactory clinical exam ROM 0–130° Improved stability with unilateral stance No pain Normal gait
Phase IV: Strengthening Phase	Post-operative Wks 4–12	Full bilateral ROM Increase strength and endurance No pain No swelling Preparation for activities	None	Previous strengthening Progress bilateral loading to single limb loading exercises Lunges 0–60° Advanced balance activities Hip extension progressing to isolated hamstring exercises in 12 weeks	Previous milestones Full motion: 0–130° Single leg stance × 30 s Squat 60° with equal weight bearing No pain or effusion

(continued)

Table 27.1 (continued)

Phase	Days–weeks	Goals	Restrictions	Treatment	Clinical milestones
Phase V: Return to Activity Phase	Post-operative Wks 12+	Restoration of full motion No swelling No pain Return of full activities	None	Previous strengthening Unilateral calf raises Progress CKC exercises Advance hamstring exercises Agility drills Advanced balance drills Sports specific drills	Previous milestones Full motion Full confidence in knee Function testing >90% of uninvolved Isokinetic testing >90% of uninvolved

CKC closed kinetic chain, *CPM* continuous passive motion, *PO* postoperative, *RICE* rest, ice, compression, elevation, *ROM* range of motion, *SLR* straight leg raise, *WBAT* weight bearing as tolerated, *Wks* weeks
Rehabilitation following anterior cruciate ligament reconstruction. (Taken from: From Manske RC, Lehecka BJ, DeCarlo M, McDivitt R. Rehabilitation of the Knee. In: Hoogenboom BJ, Voight ML, Prentice WE, (eds). *Musculoskeletal Interventions: Techniques for Therapeutic Exercise, 3rd ed.* Table 24-1 page 751: McGraw Hill Education, New York, 2014

effusion resolves and motion and quadriceps activation improve. The use of a postoperative brace such as an immobilizer or a postoperative ROM brace can provide additional support in the acute phase and may allow a more rapid progression of weight bearing but will require gait retraining to insure a normal gait pattern once the brace is discontinued. Patients are permitted to discontinue crutch use once they have resolution of postoperative effusion, full extension, and sufficient knee flexion to demonstrate a normal gait pattern and adequate quadriceps control to demonstrate a single-leg squat to 30° of knee flexion. Once these criteria are met, they can progress off of crutches.

Early exercise in the acute phase of ACL reconstruction rehabilitation is focused on muscle activation and ROM. Prior to progression to the subacute phase of rehabilitation, the patients must demonstrate full knee extension, flexion to 120–135°, sufficient quad activation to execute a straight leg raise without an extensor lag, and normal patellar mobility. Once these criteria are met, the patient is prepared to progress to the subacute phase of rehabilitation.

27.10.3 Phase III: Intermediate PO Phase

The intermediate PO phase of rehabilitation is focused and initiated when the initial acute impairments are resolved and focus turns to the advancement of foundational strength and neuromuscular control. While the return of quadriceps strength remains the primary focus after ACL reconstruction, progressive resistive exercises to address hamstring strength deficits, as well as hip and core strength, are critical.

Quadriceps strength training requires a dynamic incorporation of both open kinetic chain strengthening to address isolated quadriceps weakness often seen after ACL surgery and closed kinetic chain strengthening to encourage dynamic incorporation of quad activity while executing functional tasks. Open kinetic chain knee extension should be executed in protected ranges initially, avoiding full extension, to limit anterior translation stress on the healing graft.

Hamstring contraction provides dynamic resistance to anterior tibial translation. Return of hamstring strength after ACL reconstruction helps protect the healing graft as it reduces the underlying risk factor of quad dominance. Initiation of hamstring strengthening early after ACL reconstruction with a hamstring graft is contraindicated; however as the patient progresses to the neuromuscular reeducation phase of rehabilitation, hamstring strengthening can be progressed.

Proximal hip and core strengthening is critical after ACL reconstruction. Evidence has demonstrated the importance in hip strength and muscle activation [24], in reducing the risk of future injury as well as normalizing movement patterns postoperatively. Further, the ability to control trunk movement and maintain trunk position over the base of support during dynamic movement can help to reduce stress on the knee joint. Trunk strengthening as well as dynamic proprioception activities are critical during this phase of rehabilitation to prepare the athlete to participate in the final phase of rehabilitation.

27.10.4 Phase IV: Strengthening Phase

The final phase before release to return to tennis is the Strengthening and Return to sport phase. This phase is focused on introducing and reintegrating the athlete back into dynamic activity which will be experienced on the court. Prior to entering this phase of rehabilitation, the patient must demonstrate sufficient lower extremity strength and functional performance. The athlete who is ready to initiate the Return to Activity phase must demonstrate a solid foundation of strength as well as a baseline proficiency with the initiation of dynamic movement. Isokinetic quadriceps and hamstring strength deficits of less than 15% of the contralateral limb are necessary to enter this phase of rehabilitation. Similarly, functional hop test performance should be less than a 15% deficit, and patient-reported function on the IKDC should be a minimum of 85 prior to entry to this phase [25]. The focus of this phase should be on integration back to tennis-specific activity, beginning with activities at sub-max speed, followed by a progression to higher-level activity at max effort and full speed. Prior to full release to tennis activity, the patient should pass a return to sports assessment as outlined at the end of this chapter.

27.11 Medial Collateral Ligament Injury

Medial collateral ligament (MCL) injury occurs less frequently in tennis; however the pivoting and cutting stress of the sport do place the MCL at risk. Valgus stress to the knee, either through contact or non-contact mechanisms, can result in MCL injury. Injury to the MCL is diagnosed along a continuum with Grade I injuries representing the least structural damage to the ligament while Grade III injuries representing complete disruption of the MCL. Injuries can occur either at the attachment site or in the mid-substance of the ligament. As the MCL is an extra-articular ligament structure, there is potential for healing, and, as a result, the majority of these injuries are successfully managed nonoperatively.

Initial management of an acute MCL injury will be dependent on the extent of tissue injury and the expected time needed to allow tissue healing to occur. The focus of acute rehabilitation of MCL injury is pain and effusion management coupled with progression of ROM and strength. Grade I injuries may be permitted to initiate weight bearing and ROM activity without restriction in the early phases of rehabilitation if stability is good and pain is minimal. Grade III injuries may require a period of restricted ROM with a brace, which can protect against valgus stress, while limiting full extension as the MCL is at greatest tension in full extension. With respect to strengthening exercises, activity to focus on core, hip, and lower extremity strength can be initiated as tolerated by the patient as long as all valgus stress to the knee is avoided. Due to the wide continuum in the extent of MCL injuries, the length of time spent in the acute phase of rehabilitation after MCL injury is highly variable.

Once sufficient healing has occurred and the patient has regained full ROM, focus turns to advancing strength and neuromuscular control. Strengthening continues to be advanced with a continued focus on core, hip, quadriceps, and hamstring strengthening. Prior limitations with lateral movements and valgus stress may start to be slowly initiated at sub-max speeds and intensities and slowly progressed over time as tolerated. In addition to strengthening, balance and proprioception exercises should be progressed at this time. Advancement from double-leg to single-leg tasks and progression for sagittal plane to more tri-planer movement is indicated at this time. Once sufficient strength and neuromuscular control are gained, the patient must successfully progress through a transition to function phase, similar to the end of ACL reconstruction rehabilitation prior to progression back to sport. If residual laxity is a concern, the use of a brace may be considered prior to return to sport, but this is not typical in tennis.

27.12 Patellofemoral Pain

Patellofemoral pain syndrome (PFPS) is the most prevalent disorder involving the knee [26] and is the second most common musculoskeletal symptom presenting to physical therapists [26]. Despite this high prevalence, the potential etiology of and risk factors for developing PFPS are widespread and remain unclear [27], and a variety of theories about its etiology and appropriate rehabilitation exist. The presence of impaired anatomic morphology and/or altered dynamic neuromuscular function can result in an increased potential to experience anterior knee pain with overuse. Frequent participation in tennis has the potential to place repetitive stress on the anterior knee resulting in pain.

Once an accurate diagnosis highlights the underlying mechanism contributing to the overuse syndrome, appropriate rehabilitation can be initiated to target the underlying mechanisms. Rehabilitative and etiologic investigations have focused on three areas of dynamic neuromuscular function and their associated effect on PFPS: the proximal area at the trunk and pelvis, the distal area at the foot and ankle, and the local area at the quadriceps and the patellofemoral joint (PFJ) itself.

Proximal interventions for PFPS focus on enhancing proximal stability to serve as a stable base for distal extremity movements. Excessive trunk and pelvis movements as a result of core and hip weakness can translate into inefficient movement patterns and potentially placement of the lower extremity in at risk positions. Proximal interventions should be initiated when these deficits are identified in the presence of anterior knee pain.

Distal interventions at the foot and ankle in patients with patellofemoral pain are initiated when the patient presents with abnormal foot and ankle alignment which may alter stress on the knee joint. Typically, a more pronated or supinated foot may result in dynamic changes at the extensor mechanism, increasing susceptibility to anterior knee pain in the presence of overuse. Interventions may focus on orthotic stabilization to improve lower extremity alignment and reduce stress on the extensor mechanism.

Local interventions at the knee joint in patients with PFPS are utilized when the patient presents with knee-specific impairments contributing to anterior knee pain. This may include strength deficits, altered proprioception, or patellofemoral instability to name a few. Attempts have been made to classify types of anterior knee pain, in the hopes of guiding interventions [28]. In the tennis player, the most typical forms of local impairments contributing to anterior knee pain result from repetitive microtrauma and/or malalignment at the knee joint. These types of patellofemoral pain mechanisms are best managed with flexibility intervention in the presence of tightness and strengthening interventions in the presence of isolated weakness or weakness through the kinetic chain. The key in successful management of anterior knee pain in this population is proper identification of the underlying mechanism and an appropriate intervention plan to target these interventions. This should then be followed by a progressive return to tennis activity.

27.13 Meniscus

In any sports that requires running, twisting, and pivoting, meniscus and articular cartilage injuries are common. Meniscal and cartilage injuries can be treated both conservatively and surgically. The goal of treatment that is followed will depend on the athlete's ability to play without pain or symptoms. It is not uncommon to first attempt conservative treatment before jumping into surgical considerations.

27.14 Meniscus Tears

Meniscal tear types are numerous and include oblique, vertical longitudinal, radial (or transverse), horizontal cleavage, or complex (Fig. 27.3). The majority of meniscal tears are

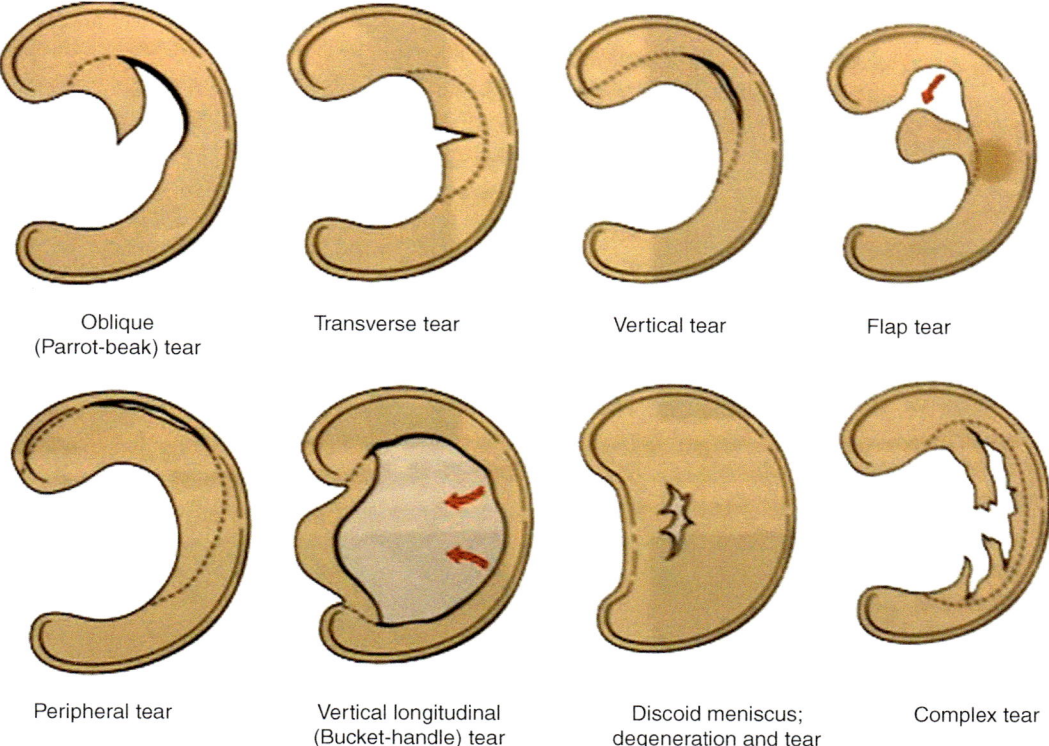

Fig. 27.3 Various types of meniscus tears. (Image taken from Magee D, Zachazewski JE, Quillen WS, Manske RC. Pathology and Intervention in Musculoskeletal Rehabilitation. Elsevier, 2016. Figure 21-6; page 779)

oblique or vertical longitudinal; however as one ages the risk of complex degenerative tears increases [29]. Vertical longitudinal tears are also known as the "bucket-handle" tear which occur more often in younger individuals and are associated with concomitant ACL injuries. If the bucket handle tear is large enough, it can be unstable and dislocate into the intercondylar area causing a mechanical "locking" of the knee. The complex or degenerative tear is one that occurs in multiple planes and is usually associated with an older athlete. These are more commonly in the medial side of the joint and may also be associated with degenerative arthritis. A radial tear is very problematic as it creates a total disruption of the meniscal tissue from the inner surface to the periphery. Lastly the horizontal cleavage tear begins near the inner margin and extends outward horizontally. This injury pattern creates a complete separation of the horizontally oriented collagen fibers of the meniscus.

Treatment of meniscal tears is predicated on the type and classification of the tear. Some tears are able to be treated conservatively, while others require surgical intervention. Many tears are not even symptomatic. Prevalence of asymptomatic tears is found in 5–36% of knees [30, 31]. Small stable asymptomatic tears certainly do not need acute treatment surgically. However if healing does not occur and these are left alone, they can progress eventually to degradation of hyaline cartilage.

Many forms of treatment exist for those tears that need surgery. Treatment includes total meniscectomy, partial meniscectomy, meniscal repair, and more recently meniscal allograft replacement. Total meniscectomy rarely results in positive long-term outcomes due to the increased joint stress that occurs when the meniscus is removed. Even small amounts of resection of meniscal tissue result in substantial increase in joint contact pressure and loads [32–34].

Therefore, total meniscectomy should be a last resort, while meniscal repair or partial meniscectomy with preservation of as much tissue as possible should be the treatment goal. Meniscus repair is an option if the tear is in the peripheral area where the meniscus still has an adequate blood supply. This blood supply is imperative for biologic healing of the torn meniscus. Surgical repairs historically have been repaired via an open procedure; however presently these repairs are done through a small incision or totally arthroscopically.

27.15 Meniscectomy Rehabilitation

Rehabilitation following meniscectomy is based on symptoms. Because there is nothing repaired or sutured together that requires soft tissue healing constraints, progression is fairly smooth. Most patients following meniscectomy respond well without problems. Evidence exists that demonstrate in some instances a home exercise program or medication following meniscectomy is equal to supervised therapy [35–37]. These studies are in contrast with those that have shown supervised therapy demonstrates increased strength deficit in the training group [38], significant extensor strength deficits for up to 6 months in those following meniscectomy [39], and both knee flexor and extensor strength deficits that would indicate a need for supervised therapy [40].

Table 27.2 from Manske RC, Lehecka BJ, DeCarlo M, McDivitt R. Rehabilitation of the Knee. In: Hoogenboom BJ, Voight ML, Prentice WE, (eds). *Musculoskeletal Interventions: Techniques for Therapeutic Exercise, 3rd ed.* outlines rehabilitation following a partial meniscectomy. Goals of phase I are to control swelling and edema, increase range of motion, normalize gait, and improve quadriceps control.

Phase I: (Days 1–7) Cryotherapy will be performed early either constantly or 6–8 times per day to control pain and swelling. Use of compressive garments is also beneficial to decrease edema control in the lower leg. Usually with a meniscectomy, a postoperative knee brace is not necessary. The leg should be elevated as much as possible to allow gravity to help decrease swelling in the first few days following surgery. The patient should restrict the amount of time standing with the lower leg in a dependent position which will also help decreased edema.

The ability to regain full knee extension is critical for almost all knee surgeries. Immediate extension should be the priority with flexion as tolerated. Towel extensions, prone hangs, and heel props all help to gain passive extension, while wall slides help with knee flexion range of motion. Extension can also be facilitated by weight shifting and locking out the knee in weight bearing.

Weight bearing following meniscectomy is as full as tolerated. Ambulation should be with bilateral axillary crutches, and these should be discontinued once the athlete is able to ambulate with normal gait. By 2 weeks the athlete should be independently weight bearing with no antalgia or limp.

Quadriceps, hamstring, and total leg strengthening exercises can begin and progress as tolerated. Straight leg raises (Fig. 27.4), quadriceps and hamstring sets, and calf raises can begin as tolerated.

Phase II: (Weeks 1–3) Goals of this phase are a complete return to full ROM equal to the uninvolved side, normalization of gait and improvement of strength and control, and return to controlled agility and sports-specific activities.

Cryotherapy can be continued as needed, especially following exercises and activities. If ROM is not yet symmetrical to the uninvolved side, exercises to facilitate it should continue. This may include manual therapy and joint mobilization techniques to continue progression until full. Weight-bearing exercises such as squats, lunges, and step-downs can all begin as long as pain and swelling do not return, sure signs of too fast of progression. Cardiovascular exercises such as stationary bike and elliptical or stair climber can begin at easy levels of 10–15 min progressing to moderate to high for 30 min or more.

Balance and proprioceptive exercises can begin to improve neuromuscular limb control. These forms of exercise should be performed bilaterally initially with simple weight shifting

Table 27.2 Rehab after partial meniscectomy

Phase	Days–weeks	Goals	Restrictions	Treatment	Clinical milestones
Phase I: Immediate PO Phase	PO Week 1	Independent ambulation Quadriceps activation Decreased effusion Wound healing Pain reduction	WBAT with bilateral axillary crutches as needed	RICE Glute sets Quad sets AAROM flexion to 60°	Full extension No limp No increased effusion No increased pain
Phase II: Intermediate PO Phase	PO Wks 1–3	Quadriceps control Pain reduction Normal patellar mobility Increased ROM Begin proximal strengthening	Full WBAT Discontinue crutches as tolerated	Exercises as previous Patellar mobilization Scar tissue mobilization Minisquats Step-ups Flexibility exercises Balance and proprioception	Previous milestones Full ROM Good quadriceps recruitment Normalized patellar mobility Full passive knee extension Full weight bearing without symptoms
Phase III: Advanced Strengthening Phase	PO Wks 3–6	Normalized quadriceps recruitment Normal patellar mobility Full active ROM No pain No effusion	None at this time	Progression of previous Advanced balance training Leg presses Endurance exercises	Previous milestones Satisfactory clinical exam Improved stability with unilateral stance No pain Equal hip strength bilaterally
Phase IV: Return to Activity Phase	PO Wks 6–8+	Return to sports and ADLs	None at this time	Previous strengthening Endurance drills Agility drills Plyometrics Initiation of running progression Sport-specific drills	Previous milestones Functional testing >90% of uninvolved Isokinetic testing >90% of uninvolved

ADLs activities of daily living, *AAROM* active assisted range of motion, *PO* postoperative, *RICE* rest, ice, compression, elevation, *ROM* range of motion, *WBAT* weight bearing as tolerated

Rehabilitation following meniscectomy. (Taken from: From Manske RC, Lehecka BJ, DeCarlo M, McDivitt R. Rehabilitation of the Knee. In: Hoogenboom BJ, Voight ML, Prentice WE, (eds). *Musculoskeletal Interventions: Techniques for Therapeutic Exercise, 3rd ed.* Table 24-4 page 764: McGraw Hill Education, New York, 2014)

progressing to unilateral as tolerated. All exercises should start out simple progressing to more complex as the athlete has demonstrated mastery of the easier exercise.

As strength and control start to return in these weeks, more traditional exercises can be included to try to incorporate the principle of muscle overload to allow gaining quadriceps and hamstring strength. Squats, leg presses, and hamstring curls can begin bilaterally and progress too unilaterally.

Phase II: (Weeks 3–6+) The focus of the final phase is on functional return. More detail on a functional return to sports will be presented near the end of this chapter. Suffice it to say that the athlete should have full ROM and strength at minimum. A gradual implementation of sports-specific activities includes running, agility, hopping, and jumping activities.

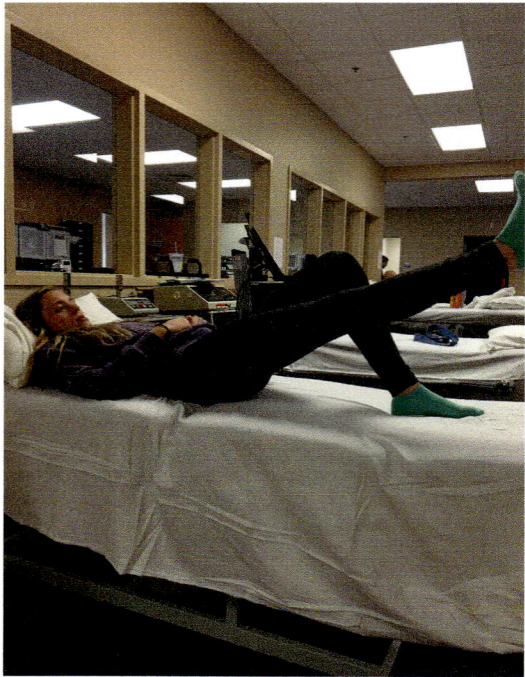

Fig. 27.4 Straight leg raise

27.16 Meniscus Repair Rehabilitation

Following a meniscus repair (Table 27.3), rehabilitation is more guarded than during meniscectomy. Weight-bearing status will depend on the type of tear that is repaired. With a peripheral tear, weight bearing in extension is protective [41]. Due to the shape of the meniscus, the compressive loads while weight bearing in full extension actually approximate the tear margins. However, with a radial tear or complex tear repairs, axial loading may actually disrupt the repair by creating separation at the tear margins. In this case weight bearing will be progressed more slowly and may even begin without weight bearing [42].

Phase I: (Weeks 0–4) Goals for phase 1 of the meniscus repair protocol include maintenance of meniscus repair, decreasing pain and swelling, increasing quadriceps activation, and start work on proximal and distal strengthening exercises for the lower limb. Weight bearing will be dependent on type of repair performed. If weight bearing is limited, bilateral axillary crutches should be utilized. ROM is limited to 0–60° of flexion for the first several weeks. Full symmetrical knee extension is achieved as soon as possible.

General exercises are tolerated at this time and include quadriceps sets, gluteal sets, and active assistive ROM from 0° to 60° flexion, ankle pumps, and straight leg raise. Modalities such as electrical stimulation can be used to decrease pain and decrease swelling. After about 2 weeks, soft tissue techniques can begin on or along portal incision sites to decrease risk of scar tissue formation creating pain and symptoms.

Phase II: (Weeks 4–6) Goals for this phase should be more geared toward continuing to increase quadriceps recruitment and normalizing ROM and gait. Additionally patellofemoral mobility should be normal by the end of this phase. After the 4 week time frame, the brace can be opened to 90° of flexion. If the athlete is able to walk without a limp and has good quadriceps activation, the postoperative brace can be discontinued.

Closed kinetic chain exercises can be progressed to include squats, step-ups, and lunges. If proximal strength is an issue, the leg press can be used with weight that is equal to less than the body weight. Leg press should begin bilaterally and progress unilaterally. Once weight bearing is full, the athlete can begin balance and proprioception exercises. Balance should begin bilaterally and progressing to unilateral. Tilt boards, foam pads, and BAPS boards can be used to facilitate return of neuromuscular control.

Phase III: (Weeks 6–10) Goals for phase III include more aggressive work on strength and power and endurance. This phase prepares the athlete for preparation to advanced sports activities.

After 6 weeks, as long as strength is adequate and swelling is resolving, the athletes brace is opened to 130° of flexion. ROM should be progressed to 130 either active or active assisted. PROM however should not be forced if it is

Table 27.3 Rehab after meniscus repair

Phase	Days–weeks	Goals	Restrictions	Treatment	Clinical milestones
Phase I: Immediate PO Phase	PO Wks 0–4	Quadriceps activation Decreased effusion Wound healing Pain reduction Begin proximal strengthening	WBAT with bilateral axillary crutches Brace locked at 0° ROM 0–60° flexion × 4 weeks	RICE Electrical stimulation Glute sets Quad sets AAROM flexion to 60° Hip abduction/adduction	Full knee extension ROM 0–60° knee flexion Minimal effusion No increased pain Single limb stance
Phase II: Intermediate PO Phase	PO Wks 4–6	WBAT bilateral axillary crutches Quadriceps control Pain reduction Normal patellar mobility Progress to CKC exercises	Full WBAT brace opened to 0–90° Discontinue crutches as tolerated	Exercises as previous Patellar mobilization Scar tissue mobilization AROM progressed to 90° Heel raises Minisquats Step-ups Flexibility exercises Balance and proprioception	Previous milestones Good quadriceps recruitment Normalized patellar mobility Full weight bearing without symptoms Normal gait
Phase III: Advanced Strengthening Phase	PO Wks 6–10	Increase strength, power and endurance Normalized quadriceps recruitment Normal patellar mobility No pain or effusion Preparation for advanced activities	Knee flexion motion not greater than 130° No pivoting	Progression of previous Advanced balance training Leg presses Endurance exercises Swimming and cycling	Previous milestones Satisfactory clinical exam Full ROM Improved stability with unilateral stance No pain Equal hip strength and bilaterally
Phase IV:	PO Wks 11–16+	Increase power and endurance Return to sports and ADLs Return to unrestricted activities	Avoidance of loaded full hyperflexion	Previous strengthening Endurance drills Agility drills Plyometrics Initiation of running progression Sports specific drills	Previous milestones Full confidence in knee Functional testing >90% of uninvolved Isokinetic testing >90% of uninvolved

ADLs activities of daily living, *AAROM* active assistive range of motion, *CKC* closed kinetic chain, *PO* postoperative, *RICE* rest, ice, compression, elevation, *ROM* range of motion, *WBAT* weight bearing as tolerated, *Wks* weeks Rehabilitation following meniscus repair. (Taken from: From Manske RC, Lehecka BJ, DeCarlo M, McDivitt R. Rehabilitation of the Knee. In: Hoogenboom BJ, Voight ML, Prentice WE, (eds). *Musculoskeletal Interventions: Techniques for Therapeutic Exercise, 3rd ed.* Table 24-3 page 761: McGraw Hill Education, New York, 2014)

painful at end range into full hyperflexion. Also even though ROM is increased, cutting and pivoting are still restricted. Because ROM is now past 90°, cycling is added to the exercise routine. No loading exercises should be performed in ranges past 60–80° before 12 weeks postoperatively [42].

At this time advanced balance and proprioception drills can begin. These include single-leg balance and perturbation-type exercises. If the athlete's balance is improved enough, they can perform balance drills also with eyes closed. Weight bearing and loaded exercises can continue to progress by adding weight or resistance.

Phase IV: (Weeks 11–16+) Goals for phase IV are increased strength, power, and endurance and sports-specific drills to return the athlete back to full activity. Restrictions of agility and pivoting are lifted at this time but should begin in a safe and controlled manner.

Exercises in this phase include advanced strengthening drills and initiation of sports-specific exercises that mimic or simulate sports activity. Agility drills are very important for tennis-specific training. Plyometric exercises can begin at this time starting bilaterally progressing to unilateral. Usually jogging can commence at 12–16 weeks if strength deficits of the quadriceps are less than 20%.

27.17 Articular Cartilage

27.17.1 Articular Cartilage Rehabilitation

In general there are two broad methods of surgery of articular cartilage defects: bone marrow stimulating procedures and replacement techniques. Bone marrow stimulation procedures include abrasion arthroplasty, drilling, and microfracture. These techniques utilize the athletes own pluripotent marrow stem cells to create reparative tissue consisting of fibrocartilage, primarily type I which has different wear characteristics of normal type II cartilage [43]. Replacement techniques include osteochondral autologous or allograft transplant surgery (OATS) and autologous chondrocyte implantation (ACI). Each of these procedures has their own specific rehabilitation guidelines with most including some degree of limited weight bearing and restricted controlled early ROM (Table 27.4).

Rehabilitation following articular cartilage surgery continues to evolve. As we begin to understand the biomechanics of cartilage and its response to injury and surgery to allow healing comes better understanding of how to handle these injuries postoperatively. Like many other knee procedures, early motion and a gradual progression to full weight bearing are important. However, exact time frames for when these should occur vary on pending surgeons and their particular preference or philosophies of cartilage healing. Until more specific guidelines can be agreed upon, communication between therapist and surgeon is paramount to achieving a successful rehabilitation. It is important to have a full understanding of the extent of damage, durability of the surgical procedure, size and location of the defect, and specific restrictions placed upon the athlete [44]. When possible a diagram of the lesion site is also helpful as it will enable the treating therapist to know where ROM limitations are and to ensure that the lesion is not engaged during exercises.

For general purposes of this chapter we will describe postoperative rehabilitation for both microfracture and ACI procedures that can be seen in Table 27.5.

27.17.2 Phase I: Weeks 1–6

The early postoperative phase is also known as the proliferation phase. Goals for this phase include independent ambulation, quadriceps activation, limiting effusion, wound healing, and pain reduction. During this phase there is a significant amount of constraint placed upon the athlete in an effort to protect the repair [45, 46]. In most instances weight bearing at this point is non-weight bearing or a controlled partial weight bearing. Communication is important at this time to ensure appropriate weight-bearing status. If you are unsure, it is better to error on the conservative side and begin non-weight bearing until status is confirmed.

Passive range of motion (PROM) of the tibiofemoral joint is performed by the therapist and the patient themselves (Fig. 27.5) or with assistance of a continuous passive motion (CPM)

Table 27.4 Rehab after microfracture and ACI

Phase	Weeks	Goals	Restrictions	Treatment	Clinical milestones
Phase I: Early PO Phase	PO 0–6	Independent ambulation Quadriceps activation Decreased effusion Wound healing Pain reduction	NWB or TTWB with bilateral axillary crutches	RICE Glute sets Quad sets in ROM that does not engage lesion PROM and AAROM in range restriction that does not engage lesion site per surgeon orders Full extension × 1 week Full flexion × 6 weeks OKC exercises light resistance in ROM that does not engage lesion × 4 weeks Patellar mobilization No CKC exercises	Full extension Independent use of ambulatory device No increased effusion No increased pain
Phase II: Intermediate PO Phase	PO 6–12	Quadriceps control Pain reduction Normal patellar mobility Increased ROM Begin CKC exercises Begin proximal strengthening Increased balance	DC crutches gradually as tolerated at 8 weeks May use pool or unweighting devices to transition to full weight bearing	Exercises as previous Begin CKC exercises Restrict range that does not engage lesion Minisquats Step-ups Flexibility exercises Balance and proprioception	Previous milestones Full ROM extension and flexion Good quadriceps recruitment Normalized patellar mobility Full passive knee extension Full weight bearing without symptoms
Phase III: Return to Activity Phase	PO 12+	Normalized quadriceps recruitment Normal patellar mobility Full active ROM No pain No effusion	Continue to increase tolerance to OKC, CKC exercises as tolerated limiting to ranges that do not engage lesion or cause symptoms	Progression of previous Advanced balance training Leg presses Endurance exercises Agility and sports specific exercises should begin at 50% effort progressing to full as tolerated Running delayed until 6 months	Previous milestones Satisfactory clinical exam Improved stability with unilateral stance No pain Equal hip strength bilaterally Quadriceps and hamstring strength to within 90% bilaterally

ADLs activities of daily living, *AAROM* active assisted range of motion, *CKC* closed kinetic chain, *NWB* non-weight bearing, *OKC* open kinetic chain, *PO* postoperative, *PROM* passive range of motion, *RICE* rest, ice, compression, elevation, *ROM* range of motion, *TTWB* touch-toe weight bearing

device. PROM is done to create movement or diffusion of synovial fluid to stimulate reparative cell production [47, 48]. Gentle movement of the knee is started immediately following surgery to help nourish articular cartilage. It also provides the additional benefit of preventing deleterious intra-articular scar tissue formation. Movement should not only occur at the tibiofemoral joint but also at the patellofemoral joint. Patellar mobilization and passive movement in all planes should occur, as limitations of patellar mobility can be disastrous for knee function.

Table 27.5 Post-operative rehabilitation for articular cartilage surgery (microfracture and autologous chondral implantation)

Phase	Weeks/months	Goals	Restrictions	Treatment	Clinical milestones
Phase I: Early PO phase	PO 0–6 weeks	Independent ambulation with assistive devices Quadriceps activation Decreased effusion Wound healing Pain reduction	NWB or TTWB with assistive device	RICE Gluteal sets SLR × 4 Quad sets in range that does not engage lesion PROM and AAROM Patellar mobilization Scar tissue mobilization No CKC exercises	Full extension × 1 week Full flexion × 6 weeks Independent use of ambulatory device No increased pain No increased effusion
Phase II: Intermediate/transition phase	PO 6–12 weeks	Quadriceps control Normal patellar mobility Increase ROM Begin CKC activities Proximal strengthening Begin balance and proprioception Pain reduction	DC assistive device as tolerated by 8 weeks My use pool or unweighting device to transition to FWB	Exercises as previous Begin CKC exercise Restrict ROM that does not engage lesion Mini-squats Step-ups Flexibility exercises Balance and proprioception	Previous milestones Full ROM extension and flexion Good quadriceps control Normal patellar mobility FWB without symptoms
Phase III: Remodeling phase	PO 3–6 months	Normalize quadriceps recruitment Normal patellar mobility Full AROM/PROM No pain No effusion	No cutting No deep squatting No running or jogging	Exercise as previous Progressive balance exercise challenging proprioceptive system Leg press Lunges Agility drills at 50% effort progressing to full after 6 months	Previous milestones Good balance and proprioception Ability to jump and land bilaterally without symptoms
Phase IV: Maturation and Return to activity phase	PO 6–9 months	Same as previous Return to full activity	No restrictions	Agility exercise Strength and power exercises Jumping progressing Hopping progression Running progression	Previous milestones Full confidence in knee Excellent clinical exam Pass functional testing measures

CKC closed kinetic chain, *FWB* full weight bearing, *NWB* non weight bearing, *PO* post-operative, *RICE* rest, ice, compression, elevation, *ROM* range of motion, *SLR* straight leg raises

Rehabilitation following microfracture and autologous chondral implantation. (Taken from: Manske RC, Lehecka BJ, DeCarlo M, McDivitt R. Rehabilitation of the Knee. In: Hoogenboom BJ, Voight ML, Prentice WE, (eds). *Musculoskeletal Interventions: Techniques for Therapeutic Exercise, 3rd ed.* Table 24-5 page 767: McGraw Hill Education, New York, 2014)

Due to weight-bearing limitations, exercises for the knee initially will be non-weight bearing. Quadriceps neuromuscular control will be used rather than pure strengthening. Exercises include quadriceps setting and straight leg raises (Fig. 27.4). If there is a lack of motor control with a volitional quadriceps contraction, the quadriceps can be supplemented with electrical stimulation.

27.17.3 Phase II: Weeks 6–12

Goals for this phase include improving quadriceps control, pain reduction, increasing range of motion, beginning closed kinetic chain exercises, beginning proximal strengthening, and increasing balance.

This phase is known as the transitional phase. At this time frame postoperatively, the lesion has

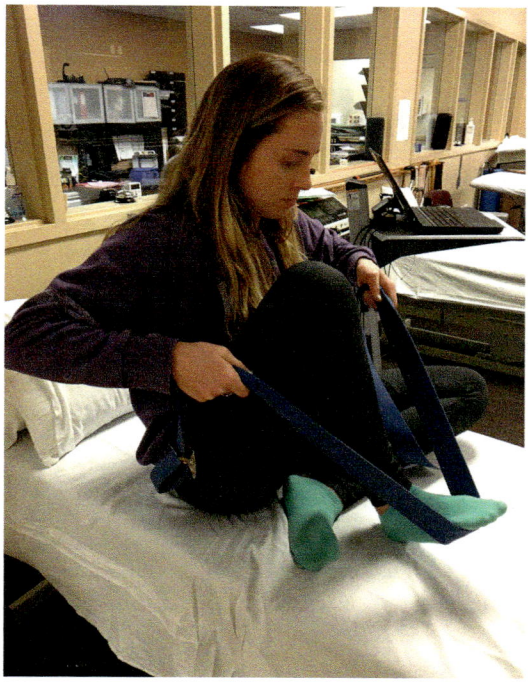

Fig. 27.5 Active assistive knee flexion range of motion

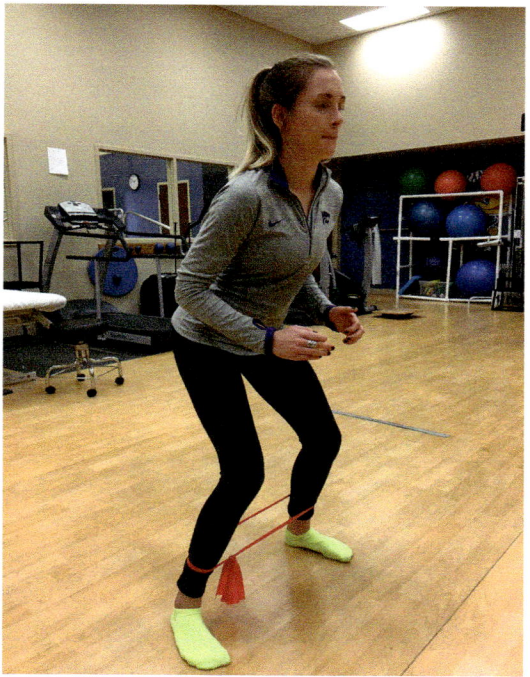

Fig. 27.6 Lateral stepping with bands

begun to fill with immature cartilage cells and is now able to tolerate some degree of progressive weight bearing. Controversy exists as too aggressive of weight bearing may risk cartilage delamination, while too conservative of approach may not provide adequate cartilage tissue stimulation [49, 50]. Weight bearing is usually progressed from non-weight bearing to partial and then to full. Increased knee pain, increased swelling, or decreased quadriceps volitional recruitment and motor control are indications that the weight-bearing progression is too fast. These signs and symptoms should be watched for closely during weight-bearing progressions and if seen may require alteration of normal progression to one more slowly in nature.

Exercise stresses can be gradually increased through increased loads and reps. Stresses should always begin bilaterally and in cardinal planes and progressing unilaterally and in multiple planes. Squats, lunges, and step-ups should begin in the cardinal planes moving anterior to posterior and medial and lateral (Fig. 27.6) directions before addition multiple plane rotational type movements or perturbation devices, which place greater stress to the articular surface due to increased shear forces (Fig. 27.7). Balance exercises are initiated bilaterally on level ground then progressing to single leg and on labile surfaces as the athlete improves (Fig. 27.8). Using this approach will ensure a gradual progression of applied loads and increased demands that will decrease the risk of damaging the healing articular cartilage.

27.17.4 Phase III: Months 3–6

Goals of the remodeling phase are to continue to work on quadriceps control, maintain ROM, progress weight-bearing ability, and increase balance. These goals are achieved through increasing difficulty of exercise in the progression.

Due to the ongoing remodeling during phase III, exercises are able to be applied with gradual increased load and intensity without harming the cartilage tissue that is becoming increasingly tolerant. Light functional activities can

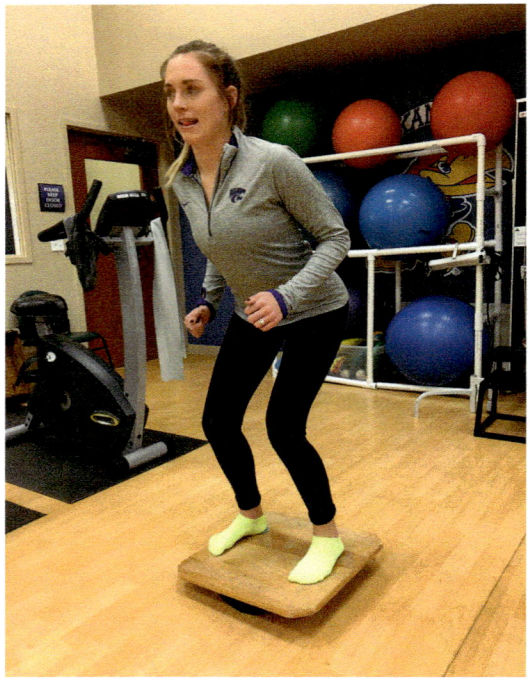

Fig. 27.7 Squats on a balance board for enhancing proprioception

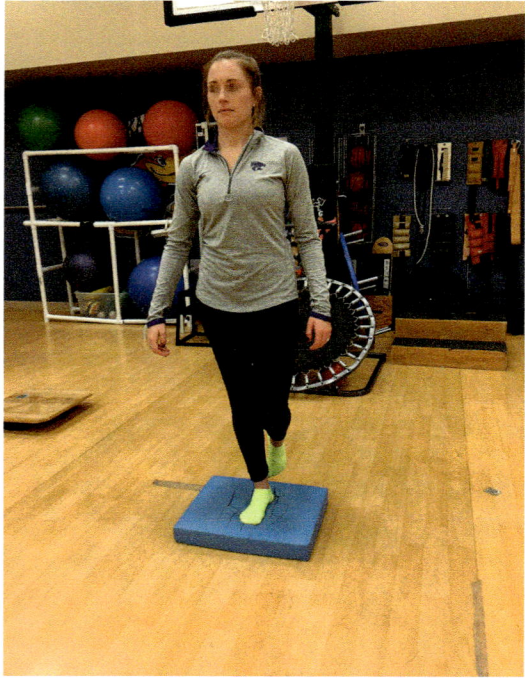

Fig. 27.8 Single-leg balance on a foam pad

begin including more sports-specific motions like ladder drills, carioca, etc. As in the previous phase, too fast of progression will be noted by symptoms listed above. Low to moderate impact functional and recreational activities can commence as long as symptoms remain resolved. These activities can include walking, cycling, and golfing. This is an excellent time with physician approval to begin adapted higher-level activities via unloading devices. Jogging in a pool or with an Alter G Antigravity Treadmill (Fremont, CA) or unweighting device may be permitted.

27.17.5 Phase IV: Months 6–18

Goals of the last phase, the maturation phase, include return to pain-free activities of daily living (ADL), full strength of the leg, full balance and proprioception, and tolerance for return to sport. Return to sports information will be discussed in more detail near the end of this chapter.

Many factors are determined when articular cartilage is fully matured and when it is safe to return to full activity. Factors include patient overall health and condition, patient age and expectations, location and size of the articular cartilage defect that was repaired, and the surgical procedure that was performed and its historical outcomes. Exercise load and intensity can continue to be progressed in an objective and systematic manner. Advanced strengthening and endurance exercise can continue to be progressed. Continued standard strengthening can be supplemented with more sports-specific drills including jumping, hopping, and directional changes.

27.18 Return to Sports: Tennis

The return to sports plan after any lower extremity injury should not be initiated until the patients have demonstrated a foundation of strength, balance, proprioception, and functional movements. Schmitt et al. [25] outlined these key foundational milestones which should be achieved prior to initiating a return to sports program. Specifically, the athlete should demonstrate a minimum of 85% limb symmetry with quadriceps and hamstring strength as well as performance on functional hop testing. Further, the athlete should present with a patient-reported outcome score on the IKDC of 85/100. Once these criteria are met, the patient is ready to initiate a return to sports program. The goal of this program is to integrate the athlete back to the prior intensity and magnitude of participation in tennis.

Initiation of a tennis-specific return to sports program begins with an understanding of the necessary movements to successfully resume activity. Tennis requires quick pivoting and cutting, reactionary activities, jumping and landing on a single limb, and rapid acceleration and deceleration. A successful return to sports program will include a dynamic progression to a point of proficiency at full speed for all these activities. The return to sports phase of rehabilitation should include a focus on advancement of residual strength and power deficits, transition to high-speed pivoting and cutting activities, and integration into sports-specific activities.

Maintenance of foundational strength and power or resolution of mild residual deficits in this area is a key component of the end phase of rehabilitation. Necessary strength criteria to enter this final phase of rehabilitation are sufficient to participate in these activities, but not sufficient to return to sport. Strengthening interventions at this phase are focused on a progression of closed kinetic chain and functional strengthening activities. Often, activities such as double-limb and single-limb squatting exercises initially on a stable surface but then progressing to unstable surfaces are examples of opportunities to advance functional strength. During all of these exercises, attention should be on maintaining good trunk and lower extremity alignment to insure normal movement patterns are engrained in the patients as they return to sport [16, 51].

Beyond the resolution of residual strength deficits, the return to sports phase must initiate and progress dynamic, sports-specific movements. The initiation of this process often begins in the end stages of traditional rehabilitation and translates into the return to sports phase. Plyometric activities are ideal interventions at this phase as they provide an opportunity to enhance functional strength and power while introducing sports-specific movements. Sub-maximum effort and plyometrics in a single plane of movement represent an ideal starting point. Plyometrics such as wall jumps and broad jumps helps to introduce the movement patterns while providing an opportunity to evaluate technique. Once technique is mastered, progression of plyometric activity can continue to more explosive movements, single-leg activities, and triplanar movement. Activities such as 180° jumps, single-limb maximum effort jumps, and single-limb lateral jumping are appropriate progressions. Tennis athletes should follow a continual progression of plyometric activities that align with sports-specific movements. Participation in tennis activities requires single-leg pivoting and cutting in all planes, single-limb jumping, and quick reactions. End-stage plyometrics for tennis players should mimic these movement patterns.

The final aspect of the return to sports phase is a reintegration to sports-specific movements. Agility drills, on the tennis court, which replicate tennis activities such as approaching the net, lateral movement, and diagonal cutting may begin at sub-maximal speed, in a planned pattern of movement, and progress toward full-speed, unanticipated movements. These activities may begin without a tennis racquet and the progress toward replicating these movements with ball and request involvement. Once the patient has demonstrated ability to successfully execute all necessary activities to participate in tennis, a return to play progression should begin. Based on the injury, the length of time in this phase may vary but should begin with an abbreviated time and intensity of participation and sequentially progress as indicated. At the culmination of the return to sports phase of rehabilitation, the athlete should present with a strength and functional performance deficit of less than 10% on the involved limb, as well as a successful completion of a progressive return to high-level pivoting and cutting as well as integration back to sport.

Conclusions

Tennis, when played at a high level, is a physically demanding sport. The quick pivoting and cutting maneuvers as well as repetitive acceleration and deceleration movements place the knee at risk for both acute, traumatic injuries and overuse injuries. The presentation of these injuries may vary greatly. Successful management from the acute phase through the return to sports integration requires an in-depth knowledge of knee anatomy and pathology, knee biomechanics, and appropriate rehabilitation progression after injury and surgery. Finally, understanding an appropriate progression through the return to sports phase which introduces stressors experienced on the tennis court and ultimately a transition back to tennis play will help facilitate an optimal outcome.

References

1. Chard MD, Lachmann SM. Racquet sports—patterns of injury presenting to a sports injury clinic. Br J Sports Med. 1987;21(4):150–3.
2. Majewski M, Susanne H, Klaus S. Epidemiology of athletic knee injuries: a 10-year study. Knee. 2006;13(3):184–8.
3. Kuhne CA, Zettl RP, Nast-Kolb D. Injuries- and frequency of complaints in competitive tennis- and leisure sports. Sportverletz Sportschaden. 2004;18(2):85–9.
4. Powell JM, Kavanagh TG, Kennedy DK, Marans HJ, Wright TA. Intra-articular knee injuries in racquet sports. A review of 128 arthroscopies. Surg Endosc. 1988;2(1):39–43.
5. Hjelm N, Werner S, Renstrom P. Injury profile in junior tennis players: a prospective two year study. Knee Surg Sports Traumatol Arthrosc. 2010;18(6):845–50.
6. Sell K, Hainline B, Yorio M, Kovacs M. Injury trend analysis from the US Open Tennis Championships between 1994 and 2009. Br J Sports Med. 2014;48(7):546.
7. Gecha SR, Torg E. Knee injuries in tennis. Clin Sports Med. 1988;7(2):435–52.
8. Perkins RH, Davis D. Musculoskeletal injuries in tennis. Phys Med Rehabil Clin N Am. 2006;17(3):609–31.
9. Thelin N, Holmberg S, Thelin A. Knee injuries account for the sports-related increased risk of knee osteoarthritis. Scand J Med Sci Sports. 2006;16(5):329–33.
10. Ateshian GA, Soslowsky LJ, Mow VC. Quantitation of articular surface-topography and cartilage thickness in knee joints using stereophotogrammetry. J Biomech. 1991;24(8):761–76.
11. Freeman MA, Pinskerova V. The movement of the normal tibio-femoral joint. J Biomech. 2005;38(2):197–208.
12. Vandermeer RD, Cunningham FK. Arthroscopic treatment of the discoid lateral meniscus: results of long-term follow-up. Arthroscopy. 1989;5(2):101–9.
13. Arnoczky SP, Warren RF. Microvasculature of the human meniscus. Am J Sports Med. 1982;10(2):90–5.
14. Rosenberg TD, Paulos LE, Parker RD, Coward DB, Scott SM. The forty-five-degree posteroanterior flexion weight-bearing radiograph of the knee. J Bone Joint Surg Am. 1988;70(10):1479–83.
15. King S, Butterwick DJ, Cuerrier JP. The anterior cruciate ligament: a review of recent concepts. J Orthop Sports Phys Ther. 1986;8(3):110–22.
16. Hewett TE, Myer GD, Ford KR, Paterno MV, Quatman CE. The 2012 ABJS Nicolas Andry Award: the sequence of prevention: a systematic approach to prevent anterior cruciate ligament injury. Clin Orthop Relat Res. 2012;470(10):2930–40.
17. Hewett TE, Paterno MV, Myer GD. Strategies for enhancing proprioception and neuromuscular control of the knee. Clin Orthop Relat Res. 2002;402:76–94.
18. Noyes FR, Mooar PA, Matthews DS, Butler DL. The symptomatic anterior cruciate-deficient knee. Part I: The long-term functional disability in athletically active individuals. J Bone Joint Surg Am. 1983;65(2):154–62.
19. Fitzgerald GK, Axe MJ, Snyder-Mackler L. A decision-making scheme for returning patients to high-level activity with nonoperative treatment after anterior cruciate ligament rupture. Knee Surg Sports Traumatol Arthrosc. 2000;8(2):76–82.
20. Fitzgerald GK, Axe MJ, Snyder-Mackler L. Proposed practice guidelines for nonoperative anterior cruciate ligament rehabilitation of physically active individuals. J Orthop Sports Phys Ther. 2000;30(4):194–203.
21. Hurd WJ, Axe MJ, Snyder-Mackler L. A 10-year prospective trial of a patient management algorithm and screening examination for highly active individuals with anterior cruciate ligament injury part 2, determinants of dynamic knee stability. Am J Sports Med. 2008;36(1):48–56.
22. Maquirriain J, Megey PJ. Tennis specific limitations in players with an ACL deficient knee. Br J Sports Med. 2006;40(5):451–3.
23. Kennedy JC, Alexander IJ, Hayes KC. Nerve supply of the human knee and its functional importance. Am J Sports Med. 1982;10(6):329–35.
24. Paterno MV, Schmitt LC, Ford KR, et al. Biomechanical measures during landing and postural stability predict second anterior cruciate ligament injury after anterior cruciate ligament

24. reconstruction and return to sport. Am J Sports Med. 2010;38(10):1968–78.
25. Schmitt LC, Byrnes R, Cherny C, et al. Evidence-based clinical care guideline for return to activity after lower extremity injury. http://www.cincinnatichildrens.org/svc/alpha/h/health-policy/otpt.htm, 2010; Guideline 38. p. 1–13.
26. Davis IS, Powers CM. Patellofemoral pain syndrome: proximal, distal, and local factors, an international retreat, April 30–May 2, 2009, Fells Point, Baltimore, MD. J Orthop Sports Phys Ther. 2010;40(3):A1–16.
27. Wilson T, Carter N, Thomas G. A multicenter, single-masked study of medial, neutral, and lateral patellar taping in individuals with patellofemoral pain syndrome. J Orthop Sports Phys Ther. 2003;33(8):437–43. discussion 444–8
28. Wilk KE, Davies GJ, Mangine RE, Malone TR. Patellofemoral disorders: a classification system and clinical guidelines for nonoperative rehabilitation. J Orthop Sports Phys Ther. 1998;28(5):307–22.
29. Metcalf R, Burks R, Metcalf M, McGinty J. Arthroscopic meniscectomy. In: Operative arthroscopy. 2nd ed. Philadelphia: Lippincott-Raven; 1996. p. 263–97.
30. LaPrade RF, Burnett QM 2nd, Veenstra MA, Hodgman CG. The prevalence of abnormal magnetic resonance imaging findings in asymptomatic knees. With correlation of magnetic resonance imaging to arthroscopic findings in symptomatic knees. Am J Sports Med. 1994;22(6):739–45.
31. Zanetti M, Pfirrmann CW, Schmid MR, Romero J, Seifert B, Hodler J. Patients with suspected meniscal tears: prevalence of abnormalities seen on MRI of 100 symptomatic and 100 contralateral asymptomatic knees. AJR Am J Roentgenol. 2003;181(3):635–41.
32. Atmaca H, Kesemenli CC, Memisoglu K, Ozkan A, Celik Y. Changes in the loading of tibial articular cartilage following medial meniscectomy: a finite element analysis study. Knee Surg Sports Traumatol Arthrosc. 2013;21(12):2667–73.
33. Seedhom B. Transmission of the load in the knee joint with special reference to the role of the menisci. Part I: Anatomy, analysis and apparatus. Eng Med. 1979;8(4):207–19.
34. Seedhom BB, Hargreaves DJ. Transmission of the load in the knee joint with special reference to the role of the menisci. Eng Med. 1979;8(4):220–8.
35. Birch NC, Sly C, Brooks S, Powles DP. Anti-inflammatory drug therapy after arthroscopy of the knee. A prospective, randomised, controlled trial of diclofenac or physiotherapy. J Bone Joint Surg Br. 1993;75(4):650–2.
36. Goodwin PC, Morrissey MC, Omar RZ, Brown M, Southall K, McAuliffe TB. Effectiveness of supervised physical therapy in the early period after arthroscopic partial meniscectomy. Phys Ther. 2003;83(6):520–35.
37. Jokl P, Stull PA, Lynch JK, Vaughan V. Independent home versus supervised rehabilitation following arthroscopic knee surgery—a prospective randomized trial. Arthroscopy. 1989;5(4):298–305.
38. Moffet H, Richards CL, Malouin F, Bravo G, Paradis G. Early and intensive physiotherapy accelerates recovery postarthroscopic meniscectomy: results of a randomized controlled study. Arch Phys Med Rehabil. 1994;75(4):415–26.
39. Gapeyeva H, Paasuke M, Ereline J, Pintsaar A, Eller A. Isokinetic torque deficit of the knee extensor muscles after arthroscopic partial meniscectomy. Knee Surg Sports Traumatol Arthrosc. 2000;8(5):301–4.
40. St-Pierre DM, Laforest S, Paradis S, et al. Isokinetic rehabilitation after arthroscopic meniscectomy. Eur J Appl Physiol Occup Physiol. 1992;64(5):437–43.
41. Heckmann TP, Barber-Westin SD, Noyes FR. Meniscal repair and transplantation: indications, techniques, rehabilitation, and clinical outcome. J Orthop Sports Phys Ther. 2006;36(10):795–814.
42. Starke C, Kopf S, Petersen W, Becker R. Meniscal repair. Arthroscopy. 2009;25(9):1033–44.
43. Moyad TF. Cartilage injuries in the adult knee: evaluation and management. Cartilage. 2011;2(3):226–36.
44. McAdams TR, Mithoefer K, Scopp JM, Mandelbaum BR. Articular Cartilage Injury in Athletes. Cartilage. 2010;1(3):165–79.
45. Brittberg M, Lindahl A, Nilsson A, Ohlsson C, Isaksson O, Peterson L. Treatment of deep cartilage defects in the knee with autologous chondrocyte transplantation. N Engl J Med. 1994;331(14):889–95.
46. Wilk KE, Macrina LC, Reinold MM. Rehabilitation following microfracture of the knee. Cartilage. 2010;1(2):96–107.
47. Buckwalter JA. Articular cartilage: injuries and potential for healing. J Orthop Sports Phys Ther. 1998;28(4):192–202.
48. Buckwalter JA, Mankin HJ. Articular cartilage: tissue design and chondrocyte-matrix interactions. Instr Course Lect. 1998;47:477–86.
49. Ebert JR, Fallon M, Robertson WB, et al. Radiological assessment of accelerated versus traditional approaches to postoperative rehabilitation following matrix-induced autologous chondrocyte implantation. Cartilage. 2011;2(1):60–72.
50. Ebert JR, Robertson WB, Lloyd DG, Zheng MH, Wood DJ, Ackland T. A prospective, randomized comparison of traditional and accelerated approaches to postoperative rehabilitation following autologous chondrocyte implantation: 2-year clinical outcomes. Cartilage. 2010;1(3):180–7.
51. Myer GD, Paterno MV, Ford KR, Quatman CE, Hewett TE. Rehabilitation after anterior cruciate ligament reconstruction: criteria-based progression through the return-to-sport phase. J Orthop Sports Phys Ther. 2006;36(6):385–402.

The Foot and Ankle at Risk of Injury in Tennis Players

28

Luca Avagnina

"Rehabilitation of foot and ankle injuries including orthotic management for the prevention and treatment of the lower extremity injuries in tennis players"

28.1 Role and Importance of the Foot in Tennis

An Italian ex-tennis player, trainer, and sport commentator said: "Tennis is not biomechanical it is ballistic, the height and point of impact is from where I get my trajectory" (Laura Golarsa).

But we know already that tennis is a multidirectional and asymmetric sport characterized by jumps, accelerations, decelerations, and frequent, fast, and aggressive changes in direction—forcing the foot to accelerate and decelerate which can be very demanding on the *functions of the foot*.

It is also a sport requiring coordination, needing fluidity of the body's movements, and with a complex balance of forces that often act in contrast excessive stress and serious physical problems, either on the musculoskeletal structures or on the structure of the foot and ankle specifically. It is always a sport "dependent on the foot functions."

In fact, we need to know that any movements either from simple walking to running or even jumping our body weight multiplies, loading up to 12 times our own body weight per centimeter squared! Taking this into account, in a run for 1 km the foot is loaded 500 times. It is easy to imagine to what effort it is subject to during a tennis match that can last for hours, while asking the foot to move 360° in every direction [1].

There are pathobiomechanical symptoms that should be noted and considered to prevent injury; however even in the best of circumstances the foot at a certain point can lose its "efficacy"; this is influenced by many different variables such as ground surface conditions, stress, fatigue or poor physical condition, and not the least type of shoes or type of orthotics.

Today the professional tennis athlete requires a lot of time for practice with irregular conditions and no ability to make an annual program. Even with a rigidly structured program, the more you win the more you will be "obligated" to compete more in a week.

Therefore it is even more important to manage the physiological side of the tennis players' performance to reduce the risk of injuries. Even the smallest sign may later become the starting point of any

L. Avagnina
Biomechanical and Postural Center,
Foot and Ankle Sport Clinic,
San Remo, Italy
e-mail: avagnina@podosport.it

possible injury. Feet are the "single point" on the ground for the whole body, and they are always the foundation of every possible athletic movement.

Until recently in tennis, the focus was mainly on the tennis racket, and new research was always made for improving its optimum length, weight, and size. Now the interest has shifted to the ball and also mainly on the kind of ground surface. The ground surface can be the determining factor for the possible injuries or accidents.

Perfect timing on the ball and the proper muscle balance and its functional impact on the distribution of forces due to the contact with the ball and the ground reaction on the body are important in tennis. For this reason we should seriously consider the function of the tennis player's foot: the first ground-body contact point [2].

Although it is impossible to avoid all acute injuries, in an attempt to do this, athletes mainly concentrate on stretching and strengthening routine and rarely consider their postural alignment of the foot and consequently the balance of the body.

Especially in an era where tennis is played often on hard surfaces and with various conditions, it becomes important to pay special attention to foot and ankle as athletes suffer mostly with injury when there are many changes to playing surfaces [3].

28.2 Podiatric Clinical Premises

When examining a tennis player, as in many of our clinical examinations, to arrive at an accurate diagnosis it is critical not only to examine and palpate the site of pain but also:

- Differentiating *how* the pain is manifested, if it is of postural, static, dynamic, neurological, inflammatory, metabolic, localized, or systemic origin (e.g., specific structure or general area, superficial or deep)
- Locating structure is the cause of pain, if it is a type of connective tissue, is it a bursa, cartilaginous, ligamentous, bone, nerve, fascia, tendinous, or a muscle. This is important in order not to trivialize with a "zone" diagnosis of a "simple spatial discrimination," for example, "sesamoiditis" or worse "metatarsalgia"
- Identifying the pain is manifested, for example, in the athletic tennis movements may occur when running forward, running side to side, on jumps, only with forehand strikes, or just in reverses

Of course to have a clear diagnosis, we have to use these variables in inductive reasoning to make an accurate diagnosis or its origin and etiological nature. A strict clinical protocol of clinical tests for muscle and postural examination along with assessment equipment like baropodometric platforms and electronic dinobaropodomeric insoles is necessary for the diagnosis.

However in tennis any athletic movement before reaching the hand and arm that is holding the racket is executed through the foot and is transmitted from the foot or in reverse, then is discharged to the ground through the feet. Therefore the foot has the task of creating and absorbing the "ground reaction forces" increased exponentially by the asymmetry of tennis.

Also if the athlete has some structural abnormalities, then there is a greater risk for injury. So the sports podiatrist will make a clinical diagnosis with the use of advanced equipment and study the surrounding environmental factors of the tennis player to gain a better understanding of the possible causes of injury and make a plan for prevention. This biomechanical and environmental analysis will also be important in the discovery of risk of injury to athletes [4].

28.2.1 What Are the Foot Mechanisms that Influence the Athletic Performance and How?

In sports, the "antigravity podo-mechanisms" are exacerbated.

The balance of power between the body and the environmental conditions has from time to time specific characteristics.

At an athletic level the muscular system strength is enhanced thus intensifying the acceleration of the body or parts of it. The foot, thus, has the task of creating and absorbing all the reaction forces of the ground, increased exponentially from "the asymmetry of tennis." The foot is rigid caused by the rotation of the limb causing supination of the foot locking the subtalar joint.

External rotation of the talus is accompanied with pronation of the calcaneus in rotation and supination of the heel; the hindfoot is "verticalized" (the forefoot resists and rotates in eversion), and the midtarsal is locked (the foot stiffens).

The relationship of the rearfoot and forefoot is fundamental for the speed and fluidity of the movement of the gradual transfer of rotation.

It is therefore logical that the function of the foot should be considered as important as other equipment required for tennis. Your feet have to adapt and respond to dynamic forces to ensure optimal movement; they heavily influence the mechanical function of the knee, hip, and the spine.

In tennis, a lot of musculoskeletal diseases that affect the joints of the knees, hips, back, and even the shoulder and arm may be caused by foot problems. When it comes to foot in tennis, however, most people think that this is due only to:

(a) The impact originating from the weight of the body, which, through the feet, strikes a hard surface
(b) Acceleration and continuous changes of direction
(c) Technique in play
(d) Type of court surface

All factors mentioned above load the forces, pressures, and tensions on all the joints, causing trauma and injuries of different entities. But few people know that even the most important factors of risk are:

(a) The static structure of the foot and of the lower limbs
(b) The dynamic function of the foot and of the lower limbs
(c) An altered biomechanical structure of the foot
(d) Abnormal postural alignment of the foot

In fact, changing the position of each foot in each individual area, we can change kinetic chains (joint and muscle) of the entire body to the arm [5].

28.3 The Most Common Injuries Associated with the Type of Structure of the Foot: Causes and Mechanisms

The foot that presents with anatomical abnormalities or biopathological problems will be more prone to injuries; not having the best biomechanical structure will lead to a fast or unexpected injury.

It's important to identify intrinsic factors such as axial defects (which have variations from the norm due to the type force applied to the structure), dysmetria of the lower limbs, muscle imbalances between agonists and antagonists, and hypotonia of one or more groups of muscle and the extrinsic factors such as incorrect training (e.g., workload, training techniques), ground surfaces, environmental conditions (cold or too humid climate), and inappropriate footwear for tennis, orthotics, insoles, or inadequate strapping of the foot or ankle.

For example, one intrinsic factor is the excessive pronation of the forefoot or the presence of an excessive pes cavus foot structure; this can be suggestive of asymmetry of the limbs with differences as little as 5–10 mm (excessive pronation of the rearfoot and ankle occurs with the longest limb) that can cause Achilles tendonitis and other forms of tendinopathies [6].

28.3.1 Preconceived Ideas

1. Orthopedic view under 1 cm it is not important.
2. Osteopathic/physiotherapy view; leg length discrepancies are always from muscular origin and never a boney discrepancy.

3. A misconception in all allied health fields; a leg length discrepancy can be measured in a clinic using a measuring tape only (no need for radiographic diagnosis).

28.3.2 Excessive Pronation Influence: Stability of the Foot and Knee and the Flexibility of the Joints of the Foot

We must always be able to distinguish between the rearfoot pronation and forefoot pronation especially if the forefoot has first ray joint hypermobility, because it creates a number of conflicting movements between the patellofemoral joint, the tibiofemoral joint, and subtalar joint, therefore reducing muscle efficiency.

With ankle hyperpronation syndrome, both the forefoot and rearfoot can develop Achilles tendonitis, tibial pain, and stress fractures.

On the contrary excessive supination could also be caused either in the forefoot and rearfoot and can be related to an increased risk of inversion and plantar flexion sprains, metatarsalgia, stress fractures, ankle sprains, heel pain, lower back pain, and patellofemoral pain.

The foot with excessive pronation (rearfoot) is characterized by a low medial arch height, medial protrusion of the talar head and body of the scaphoid, eversion of the calcaneus, and abduction of the forefoot.

This is the first category of an at-risk foot in tennis players [7].

Normally the foot pronation starts after the impact of the heel on the ground (heel contact phase) during the contact phase of gait and ends approximately in the middle of midstance, at the period of the central support of the foot. This is the period in which the other limb starts the swing phase of gait. If this fails a dysfunction occurs of hyperpronation of the forefoot creating delay.

The physiological pronation causes an internal rotation of the leg and eversion of the heel.

If the pronation persists beyond the propulsion phase, the foot will have an increased risk of injury.

Furthermore, with excessive and abnormal motion, this creates a number of conflicting movements not only with the foot but also between the knee and the subtalar joint.

The final result is the reduction of joint stability of the knee and the alteration of the normal articular and functional alignment of the foot, ankle, knee, hip, pelvis, and spine.

It also creates also an abnormal functional load on muscles and tendons and joints involved. Among other effects podiatric excessive pronation alters the function of the peroneus longus muscle, because it changes the forefoot position with respect to the rearfoot altering the force vector created by the peroneus longus muscle, which is no longer able to generate a stabilizing force on the hallux and transmitting hypermobility of the first ray with consequent instability, muscular activity not only creates movement but also creates stability.

The prone position of the foot creates excessive mobility at the Chopart's joint.

This reduces muscle efficiency and facilitates lateral ankle sprains.

Symptoms related to excessive pronation at the level of the foot are inflammation, toe deformities, metatarsalgia, and plantar fasciitis.

Above the ankle, symptoms that can manifest are Achilles tendonitis, shin pain, stress fractures, and knee pain.

The second category of risk is excessive supination.

A foot normally starts supination halfway between the midstance phase of gait and continues to supinate up to toe offstage.

The supination the foot makes a rigid structure; this makes it capable of transmitting the oscillating limb load. In general, a foot with excessive supination has a high medial arch. The talar head is aligned with the navicular bone and normally cannot be palpated medially, and the excessive height of the arc creates tension on the extensor mechanism, which alters the digital alignment and lesser toe deformities, e.g., hammer toes.

The Chopart is hypomobile and the foot is very stable.

Two causes that can create a foot in excessive supination are plantarflexed first ray and forefoot valgus. Both of these conditions create excessive subtalar joint supination and subsequent inversion of the hindfoot.

All this makes a particularly rigid foot during the different stages of contact, thus reducing its natural capacity to absorb the kinetic energy [8].

This type of gait is characterized by a sudden excessive heel impact, followed by a consequent difficult medial transfer of the load with limited ability to absorb shock.

This increased shockwave is then transferred to the knee, hip, and lower back.

Even the peroneal tendon function is impaired, and this creates lateral ankle instability, especially during the second half of midstance, when the body weight is transferred to the forefoot.

Symptoms due to excessive supination can be summarized as heel pain, metatarsal stress fractures of the fifth metatarsal, ankle sprains, patellar pain, and back pain.

The feet with excessive pronation or supination can be detected before injury by a biomechanical examination by a good podiatrist with advanced biomechanical assessment equipment.

These tools allow us to evaluate the biomechanical function of the athlete's foot and lower limb on a force platform, which reveals quantitatively the distribution and progression force over time.

This dynamic examination describes the what, the when, and the how of the functions of athlete's foot during walking or during specific athletic movement.

When you gain a basic understanding of the athlete's biomechanics, the study can be continued in the field under natural conditions of the game, using computerized insoles.

These insoles allow the athlete to move freely allowing the evaluation of the shoe and the foot during sports performance, under actual playing conditions.

This is then uploaded to the computer and synchronized with the data obtained in the static and single leg stance with knee flexed and extended [9].

28.4 Feet at Risk in Tennis

One of the most common injuries in the lower limb is the ankle sprain. This type of injury is the most common cause of prolonged interruption in sports. This injury can often cause chronic pain thereby reducing the tennis playing ability, making it a difficult path in returning to the same level of play.

The acute injury interrupts the competitions and training which becomes a serious problem for the athlete, interrupts training plans and tournaments, and often can become a major problem for the athlete.

Due to this, there is a team of specialists including a sports podiatrist, an orthopedic therapist, and an athletic trainer assisting in the recovery to achieve maximum results in the shortest possible time for the athlete.

The injury to soft tissue and bone cartilage is often overlooked, not taken seriously, or misdiagnosed.

This is due to the fact that the damage is often invisible through radiography.

Radiography, for this reason, 20–40% of all ankle sprains develop into chronic symptoms such as pain, swelling, and instability.

Some types of feet are more subject to these symptoms than others.

A lot of research has gone into how to treat an ankle sprain; however little research has been done on how to prevent it. Some types of feet may have abnormalities of the opposing ankle.

The functional biomechanical analysis will give us valuable information on the feet, which should be protected and prevented [10].

The lateral distortion is the most common type. This occurs when the foot is turned laterally past its end range of motion with respect to the leg, the foot rotates internally.

The muscles that oppose an opposing force are the long and short peroneus muscles.

Alterations in the biomechanical function in the foot will affect the function of these muscles.

The tennis movements during the game take place predominantly on the forefoot.

To exert greater driving force, the athlete tends to stay on toes while saving the stance time on the heel and midfoot which would require more time to execute the move.

This tendency leads to an overload to the metatarsal area of the foot, often due to acute or chronic conditions.

An uneven distribution of forefoot loading can lead to different consequences such as hyperkeratosis, periostitis, bursitis, and the subluxation of toes.

If we add to the excessive load to a particular deformity of the foot, for example, a failure of the first ray, we will find ourselves with sesamoiditis or hallux limitus.

Hallux limitus, or a foot with excessive pronation (pes planus valgus), especially during the drive period of the step, which is to alter the function of the peroneal. These feet are characterized by a lower median height of the arch, a medial protrusion of the talar head and the navicular bone body, the heel eversion, and abduction of the digits (often associated with a bunion or with a toe valgus).

A foot pronation will have an altered axis between forefoot and hindfoot. For this reason we need to evaluate this foot in subtalar neutral position with respect to the forefoot varus hindfoot. Normally the short peroneal creates a force of pronation and the posterior tibial muscle stabilizes the ankle. The peroneus longus creates an eversion force that flexes the first beam, stabilizing it in order to produce a propulsion force.

However, the foot is pronated excessively so that the short peroneal reduces its activity and the peroneus longus, no longer capable of creating a stabilizing force, results in hypermobility of the first ray. The pronated foot position biomechanically creates excessive mobility of the Chopart's joint line. Thus the activity of the muscle must not only create movement but must also make the foot stable. This reduces muscle efficiency and facilitates the lateral ankle sprains. Other feet at risk, strange as it may seem, are certain types of high-arched feet (cavus foot varus) [11].

Generally, 1 foot with excessive supination has a high medial arch, and the head of the talus is aligned with the navicular bone; therefore normally you do not notice, the hindfoot varus and hammer toes are often present. The Chopart is hypomobile and the foot is very stable. However, there are two types of supinated foot types which biomechanically make the foot at risk of injury.

These are:

1. Plantar flexion of the first ray
2. Forefoot valgus

Both standing creates excessive supination of the subtalar joint, consequently inversion of the hindfoot. This stretches the tendons of the peroneus that reduce the ability to react when the ankle joint passes the lateral movement.

Computer analysis often will highlight the sudden rupture of the heel, the forefoot load that begins along the mid column, and a rapid supination during the end of the contact. The curve of the force vector can also reveal subtalar instability indirectly due to poor control of the peroneal and tibial muscle. So the computer analysis can dynamically evaluate the biomechanical function and provide quantitative data that are repeated over time.

Ankle sprains in athletes often turn into chronic pain. Not all of this unfortunately can be avoided, but many can be prevented considering the biomechanical function of the foot. There are feet that are more prone to trauma and can be identified and protected through the use of the orthosis.

The proper foot function through Specialized Biomechanical Orthotics can reduce the trauma and improve the stability and muscle efficiency, which in turn will improve the athletic performance [12].

28.5 Specific Pathologies

(a) Dermatological pathologies

Corns, calluses, ingrown nails, hyperhidrosis, blisters, intertrigo mycotica, and hematoma under nail.

(b) Pathologies musculo-tendon and osteoarticular.

The Foot and Ankle
- Syndrome of the medial sesamoid
- Syndrome or entrapment of the tibial nerve specifically the lateral calcaneal branch
- Enthesopathy of the abductor hallux muscle
- Plantar fasciitis
- Heel pain from enthesopathy of flexor digitorum
- Bursitis of the second ray of the metatarsals

- Posterior and anterior tibial muscle, achilles and peroneal tendinopathy
- Sever's disease osteochondrosis

Lower Leg and Knee
- Tibial periostitis
- Ankle sprains
- Patellofemoral pain syndrome
- Pes anserinus tendonitis (goose foot tendonitis)
- Osgood-Schlatter's osteochondrosis
- Injuries of the meniscal cartilage in the knee joint

Hip and Pelvis
- Groin pain
- Coccydynia
- Lower back pain
- Abductor rectus syndrome
- Average gluteal and hamstring injuries [13]

28.6 What Innovative Diagnostic Tools Allow the Study of the Specific Signs of Improved Performance?

Next to the classic postural screening of baropodometric and stabilometric exams, I conducted a preliminary study aimed at the functional evaluation of the feet through the use of insole pressure sensors during various technical movements of tennis.

During the match, the insoles were attached with Velcro suitable to fix to the leg of the athlete allowing to hook cables connected to a data recorder that was later connected to the computer through a serial cable connection.

All subjects were evaluated barefoot with a baropodometer and with their tennis shoes with these electronic insoles.

The subjects were allowed to freely practice for a few minutes, while insoles were calibrated and checked.

The calibration was performed before each evaluation.

The subjects were asked to perform their tennis skill several times to make an average of foot pressure readings; a skill was performed and recorded bilaterally for each subject.

Plantar pressure was assessed during a forehand stroke and a backhand, taking into account the service.

This preliminary study has shown that one can obtain quantitative information using insole pressure sensors in athletic footwear.

Much has been done to protect the foot from multiple forces and optimize athletic performance.

The information obtained from this preliminary study can be used to compare how different shoes react on a given athlete, provide more knowledge about the construction and design of athletic footwear, and thus improve performance [14].

28.7 Orthotic Therapy: Our Experience

The fundamental role in preventing these types of injuries is choosing appropriate footwear to accommodate orthotic therapy.

More than 30 years of study and clinical trials, I have had success in the effectiveness of special custom orthotic therapy (Podiatric Orthotics) which through a postural and biomechanical integrated rebalancing, and thanks also to the use of specific technical hi-tech materials, they have three main actions:

1. Injury prevention
2. Performance optimization
3. Therapy in case of pathology or injury

A good insole, preferably designed and fabricated from the athlete's foot impression, ensures an ideal distribution of the loads and the forces, in the various phases of motor activity, this helps the athlete in the prevention of injuries or functional disorders. Some examples of this are reduced fatigue, cramps, tendinopathies, the formation of blisters and calluses, and nail deformities from pressure.

The sport footwear alone is often not enough plantar support especially if the foot is hypermobile.

Normally a plantar support must be applied to give adequate support especially if you use shoes with excessive flexibility.

For this reason research determines the correct support for the foot that reduces fatigue and allows for better distribution of loads and forces transmitted. Unforgettable shoes are produced with structures and standard insoles which do not adapt to the morphology of the foot in most cases.

28.8 Orthotics and Sport

Footwear, ground surface, and athletic skill are the elements that characterize each skill.

To optimize the foot-sport relationship with such unnatural elements and movements, we have "specialized" the Podiatric Orthotics with special application thermoformed layer by layer from different exclusive materials, highly innovative, based for the specific sport.

28.9 The Podiatric Orthotic

A plantar surface positive impression of the foot can be made by a technique of taking a negative impression in neutral static stance position and at a controlled dynamic stance. This allows a good neutral position impression (and not an impression of the pathological position that derives from the simple stand up without the foot being pushed in a neutral location) and then further corrections are made in a laboratory to rebalance depending on what the clinical examination concluded.

No orthotic is suitable for a specific sport if it is only designed through the examination of:

1. A simple visit static podoscopic
2. A trivial outlet of measurement of the contours on the sheet of paper
3. Or made from outdated materials such as leather, cork, and other rigid and not thermoformable

Basic prerequisites for effective sports orthoses are:

1. A clinic visit podiatric biomechanical and postural assessment combined with a dynamic assessment
2. A series of electronic computerized tests with kinematic baropodometric platforms and insoles
3. A multilayer differentiated orthotic designed specifically between right and left, between hindfoot and forefoot, for difference phases of the sport skill and with different kinetic wedging and thermoformable materials

This Podiatric Orthotic not only needs to be specifically designed for the sport of the athlete; we then realized it also should meet the following essential requirements:

- Space saving as much as possible can be inserted in your shoe
- Light weight (50 g)
- Flexible in all planes of motion—comfort and harmony with the foot
- Maximum stability—thanks to the flat bottom
- Hypoallergenic
- Washable—with any detergent
- Long duration—at least 1 year
- Transferability—ability to put from one shoe to another (same type)
- Selection in appropriate materials—for all types of foot pathology and for the individual (more or less, soft or rigid, self-modeling, insulation, shock absorber, viscoelastic, etc.)

28.10 Clinical Case Study Summary of Pathologies Treated in Tennis Players

In particular, with our experience we have treated the following podiatric pathologies in tennis players. Often they have more than one of these conditions with a relationship between each other:

- Heel pain (all types)—medial, lateral, plantar, posterior
- Plantar fasciitis
- Ankle sprains
- Anterior and posterior tendonitis
- Peroneus muscle tendonitis
- Achilles tendonitis
- Hallux adductor valgus
- Metatarsalgia single and multiple
- Intermetatarsal bursitis
- Digital subluxation
- Morton's neuromas
- Plantar hyperkeratosis
- Hyperkeratosis first plantar metatarsal area
- Sesamoiditis

Or these diseases were often in association with other diseases above the foot including the knees, hips, or back:

Knee pain
Patellofemoral pain syndrome
Tibial femoral pain
ITB or lateral knee pain
Tibial periostitis
Pubic, abductor retinaculum syndromes
Lower back pain

Clinical cases
Treatment and case and their solutions

References

1. Herbaut A, Chavet P, Roux M, Guéguen N, Gillet C, Barbier F, Simoneau-Buessinger E. The influence of shoe drop on the kinematics and kinetics of children tennis players. Eur J Sport Sci. 2016;16(8):1121–9. https://doi.org/10.1080/17461391.2016.1185163. Epub 2016 May 22
2. Iwamoto S, Fukubayashi T, Hume P. Pelvic rotation and lower extremity motion with two different front foot directions in the tennis backhand groundstroke. Sports Sci Med. 2013;12(2):339–45. eCollection 2013
3. Fong DT, Ha SC, Mok KM, Chan CW, Chan KM. Kinematics analysis of ankle inversion ligamentous sprain injuries in sports: five cases from televised tennis competitions. Am J Sports Med. 2012;40(11):2627–32. https://doi.org/10.1177/0363546512458259. Epub 2012 Sep 11
4. Sell K, Hainline B, Yorio M, Kovacs M. Injury trend analysis from the US Open Tennis Championships between 1994 and 2009. Br J Sports Med. 2014;48(7):546–51. https://doi.org/10.1136/bjsports-2012-091175. Epub 2012 Aug 25
5. Sacco IC, Sartor CD, Cacciari LP, Onodera AN, Dinato RC, Pantaleão E Jr, Matias AB, Cezário FG, Tonicelli LM, Martins MC, Yokota M, Marques PE, Costa PH. Effect of a rocker non-heeled shoe on EMG and ground reaction forces during gait without previous training. Gait Posture. 2012;36(2):312–5. https://doi.org/10.1016/j.gaitpost.2012.02.018. Epub 2012 Mar 17
6. Feit EM, Berenter R. Lower extremity tennis injuries: prevalence, etiology, and mechanism. J Am Podiatric Med Assoc. 1993;83:509–14.
7. Kulund DN, McCue FC, Rockwell DA, et al. Tennis injuries: prevention and treatment. Am J Sports Med. 1979;7:249.
8. Murphy RJ. Heat problems in the tennis player. Clin Sports Med. 1988;7:429.
9. Balduini FC. Abdominal and groin injuries in tennis. Clin Sports Med. 1988;7:349.
10. Wolgin M, Cook C, Graham C, et al. Conservative treatment of plantar heel pain: long term follow-up. Foot Ankle. 1994;15:97–102.
11. Davis P, Severud E, Baxter E. Painful heel syndrome: results of nonoperative treatment. Foot Ankle. 1994;15:531–5.
12. Powell M, Post WR, Keener J, et al. Effective treatment of chronic plantar fasciitis with dorsiflexion night splints: a crossover prospective randomized outcome study. Foot Ankle. 1998;19:10–8.
13. Hyer C, VanCourt R, Block A. Evaluation of ultrasound-guided extracorporeal shock wave therapy (ESWT) in the treatment of chronic plantar fasciitis. J Foot Ankle Surg. 2005;44:137–43.
14. Wang C, Chen H, Huang T. Shockwave therapy for patients with plantar fasciitis: a one-year follow up study. Foot Ankle. 2002;23:204–7.

Acute Management of Common Foot and Ankle Injuries

29

Clay Sniteman and Shuhei Suzuki

29.1 Introduction

Injuries to the foot and ankle region in elite male professional tennis players are common. Injury statistics from the ATP World Tour show foot and ankle injuries to comprise 12% of all injuries evaluated by physiotherapists and tournament physicians during the course of the 2014 and 2015 seasons. The most commonly encountered ankle injury is the plantar flexion/inversion ankle sprain, which accounted for 35–45% of all foot and ankle injuries on tour in the 2014 and 2015 seasons, respectively. In a survey study of over 800 elite junior tennis players by Kovacs et al. [1], ankle injuries ranked 3rd behind lower back and shoulder injuries among male and female players. Reece et al. [2] reported that 59% of all tennis injuries at the Australian Institute of Sport in elite junior players were lower extremity injuries, with an equal representation of trunk and upper extremity injury forming the remaining 41% of injuries.

In addition to this finding of the high incidence of ankle sprains in the elite male professional tennis player, data from the ATP's injury and illness recording system also shows a high incidence of blisters to the foot. Given the multi-directional movement patterning requiring up to 4.2 directional changes per point [3], friction imparted between the shoe and sock/skin interface can produce blisters on the plantar surface of the foot and toes. Blisters (foot and hand) account for 7% of all injuries reported in male professional tennis players in the calendar years 2014 and 2015, with foot blisters accounting for 57–59% of all blisters. Given this high incidence and the severe performance barrier that a foot blister imparts to the elite tennis player, several unique and key tennis-specific techniques for management and prevention of foot blisters will be covered in this chapter.

29.2 Plantar Flexion/Inversion Ankle Sprain

Ankle sprain is the most common lower extremity injury among tennis players. Most commonly, they occur while performing movements such as landing after smash or serve, quick change of directions, or a foot getting stuck on the playing surface (more common in grass and clay court). The force that is often placed on the ankle includes forefoot adduction, hindfoot internal rotation, leg external rotation, plantar flexion, and inversion [4].

C. Sniteman (✉)
ATP World Tour, Ponte Vedra Beach, FL, USA

Sundance Physical Therapy, Ogden, UT, USA
e-mail: csniteman@atpworldtour.com

S. Suzuki
ATP World Tour, Ponte Vedra Beach, FL, USA

TRIA Orthopaedic Center, Bloomington, MN, USA
e-mail: ssuzuki@atpworldtour.com

29.2.1 Anatomy

There are multiple structures that can be involved with lateral ankle sprain. The most commonly involved structures are the lateral ankle ligaments. It has been shown that 73% of the lateral ankle sprain involves anterior talofibular ligament, followed by calcaneofibular ligament, posterior talofibular ligament, and lateral subtalar ligament. In addition, soft tissue structures such as fibularis longus and brevis, extensor digitorum longus and brevis, tibialis anterior, and extensor and fibular retinacula can also be involved. In more severe cases, injuries involving osseous structures including osteochondral lesions and fractures are also possible [4, 5].

29.2.2 Clinical Presentation

After sustaining lateral ankle sprain, symptoms including ecchymosis and loss of ROM, strength, and function are commonly seen. The severity of ankle sprain can be categorized using the grading system (I, II, III) with grade I being the mild with no structural injury, to grade III being the most severe and complete rupture of the ligaments [5]. As part of acute management, early progressive weight bearing with the use of ankle brace and assistive device has been shown to be beneficial. Furthermore, compression, ice, and anti-inflammatory medication can be utilized in attempt to reduce swelling and pain and reduce secondary injury and hypoxic-related injury in the acute stage of this injury [5].

In a study examining 765 high school football and soccer players (523 girls and 242 boys), the athletes with previous history of an ankle sprain demonstrated a twofold increase in the risk of sustaining another sprain [6]. In addition, lack of use of external ankle support in sports including basketball and soccer increased the probability of athletes sustaining inversion ankle sprain in the group with or without previous history of ankle sprain [5, 7, 8]. This data may suggest that the players with previous ankle injury should have external ankle brace or taping when participating in sports. Furthermore, it may also be beneficial for those without any history of ankle sprain to reduce the risk of sustaining ankle injury. Both external ankle brace and ankle tape are commonly utilized by the elite tennis players.

After the player is determined to be fit to continue playing, it is important to protect the involved structures and to prevent the ankle from getting into the position of stress. Following is one example of the ankle tape technique commonly utilized on the professional tour. The primary movement that needs to be prevented is the calcaneal inversion and plantar flexion/dorsiflexion.

Materials needed:

Two heel and lace pads
Skin lube lubrication
Adhesive spray
One rigid athletic tape
Lightplast stretch tape

(Step by step)

1. The ankle is first prepared by positioning at neutral position and sprayed with the adhesives.
2. Heel and lace pads with the lubrication under the pad are placed for protection (see Fig. 29.1 below).

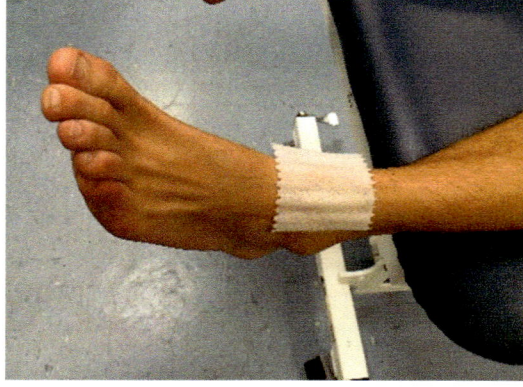

Fig. 29.1 Heel and lace pads

29 Acute Management of Common Foot and Ankle Injuries

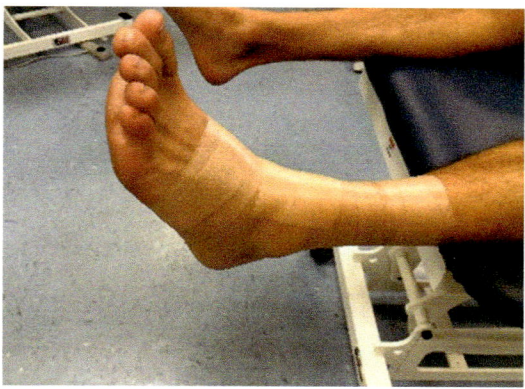

Fig. 29.2 Pre-wrap

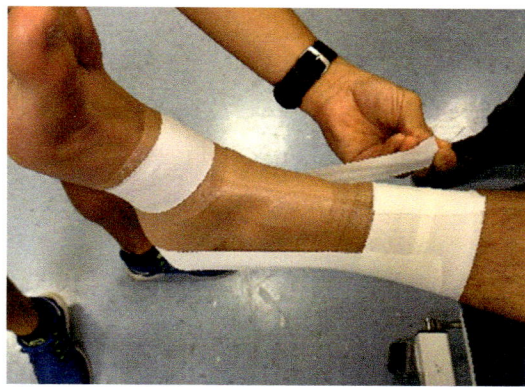

Fig. 29.4 Teardrops

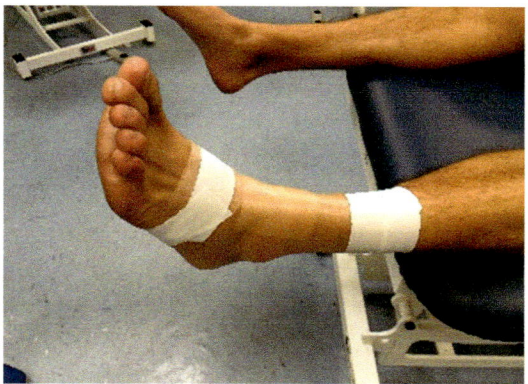

Fig. 29.3 Anchors

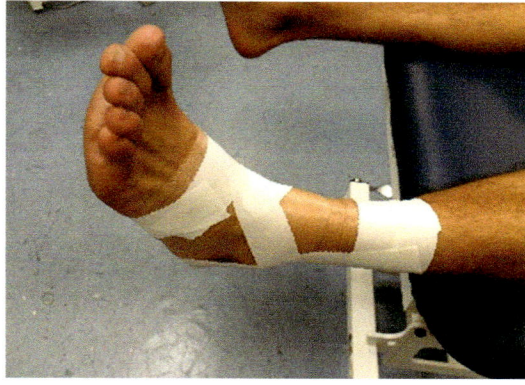

Fig. 29.5 Horseshoe

3. Nonadhesive prewrap is applied from distal 1/3 lower leg to just proximal to fifth metatarsal (see Fig. 29.2 below).
4. Two anchors proximally and one anchor distally are applied using rigid athletic tape (see Fig. 29.3 below).
5. Teardrop tape from medial portion of tibia to lateral portion of fibula is applied. This tape is applied to pull the calcaneus into eversion (see Fig. 29.4 below).
6. Horseshoe tape is applied to cover the ankle posteriorly (see Fig. 29.5 below).
7. Step 5 and 6 is repeated three times for reinforcement (see Fig. 29.6 below).

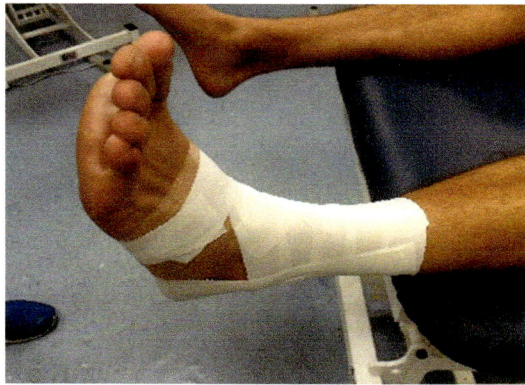

Fig. 29.6 Teardrop and horseshoe tape repeated

8. Heel lock is applied medially and laterally to further stabilize the hindfoot (see Figs. 29.7, 29.8, 29.9, and 29.10 below).
9. Figures 29.11 and 29.12 tape is applied by taping around the midfoot and distal tibiofibular joint.
10. Lightplast stretch tape is used to close off the ankle. One strip of rigid white tape is also applied to anchor the end of the Lightplast stretch tape (see Fig. 29.13 below).

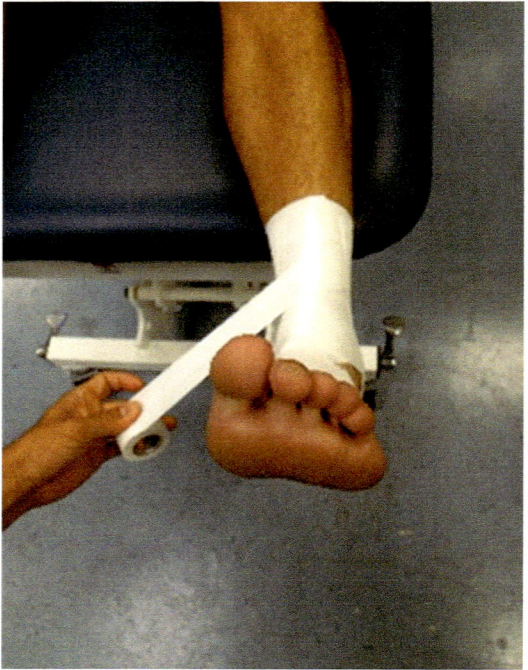

Fig. 29.7 Heel lock: medial to lateral

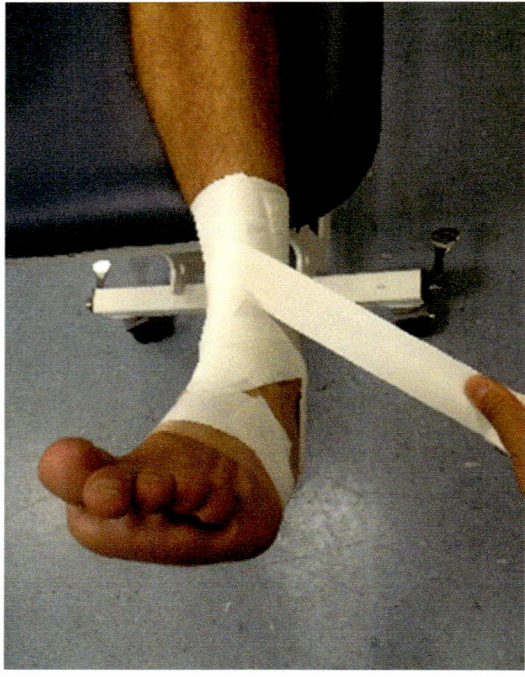

Fig. 29.9 Heel lock: lateral to medial

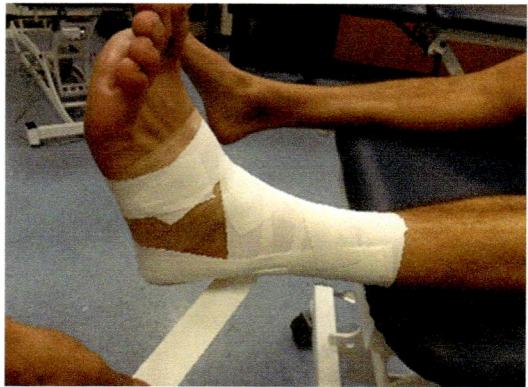

Fig. 29.8 Heel lock: medial to lateral

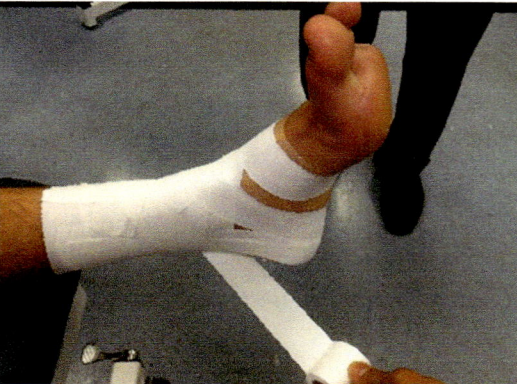

Fig. 29.10 Heel lock: lateral to medial

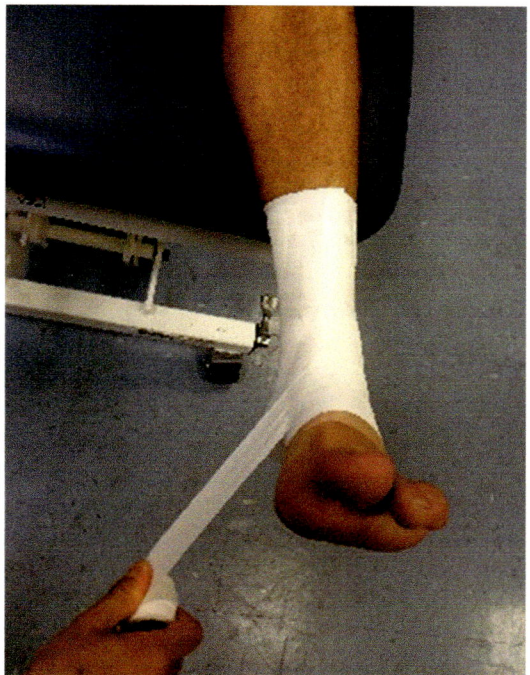

Fig. 29.11 Figure 29.8 around midfoot

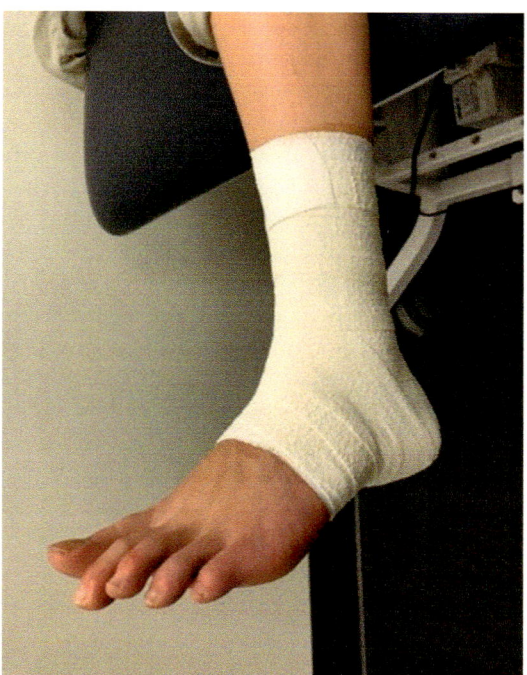

Fig. 29.13 Closing using Lightplast stretch tape

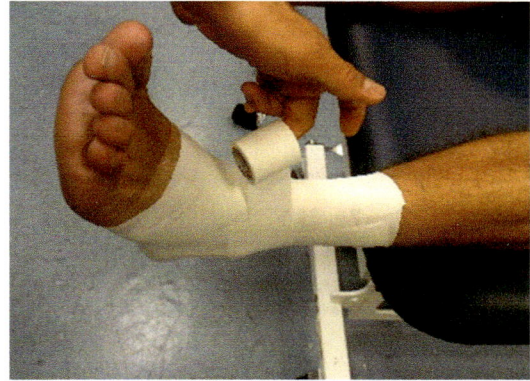

Fig. 29.12 Figure 29.8 around distal Tibiofibular joint

29.3 Syndesmotic Complex Injury

29.3.1 Anatomy

Syndesmotic complex consists of osseous structures involving the tibia and fibula and the ligamentous structures including anterior tibiofibular ligament, posterior tibiofibular ligament, interosseous membrane, and inferior transverse ligament. Together, these structures provide the passive stability to the ankle [9].

29.3.2 Clinical Presentation

The syndesmotic ankle sprain can occur with or without fractures, and it only consists 10–20% of all ankle sprains in general athletic population [10]. However, this injury is reported to have more prolonged recovery course compared to inversion ankle sprain. Hopkinson et al. [11] have reported that the syndesmotic sprain recovery time was 55 days compared to 28 days for the severe ankle sprain. Due to the complexity of this injury, it is important to understand the mechanism of injury and structures that are involved to manage the injury accurately.

The injury often occurs with the foot forced into dorsiflexion and external rotation with the foot planted on the ground, which pushes the distal tibia and fibula to spread and stress the ligamentous and/or osseous structures. Clinical features including tenderness directly over anterior part of syndesmosis and lack of pain over lateral ligaments are present. Clinical tests such as squeeze test and external rotation test can also be useful in assessing the involvement of syndesmosis. In addition to the clinical examination, radiographic images can be helpful in assessing the structures involved with the injury and formulating appropriate plan of care for the athletes. The biomechanical studies have suggested that the injury of deltoid ligament in conjunction with the syndesmotic sprain increases the ankle instability [9].

29.3.3 Treatment

Following the syndesmotic injury, conservative management including ice, rest, and period of casting can be beneficial. In severe cases with the sign of ankle instability, diastasis of syndesmosis, and/or fractures, surgical treatment may be recommended by the physicians.

For less severe injuries, taping may be helpful in augmenting the pain while continuing with play. The taping technique utilized for syndesmotic ankle sprain is similar to the taping technique for Achilles tendinopathy. The key component of the taping technique is to avoid end-range dorsiflexion and external rotation. In addition to the dorsiflexion-restricting tape, ankle tape demonstrated in Figs. 29.1, 29.2, 29.3, 29.4, 29.5, 29.6, 29.7, 29.8, 29.9, 29.10, 29.11, 29.12 and 29.13 is often applied to further support the ankle.

29.4 Heel Pain/Plantar Fasciopathy

Injury to the foot region has been suggested to be 10.6–26.4% among various population. Among the foot injuries, plantar fasciopathy has been shown to be one of the most common injuries among athletic population [12]. Due to the repetitive load placed on the foot, tennis players can often develop plantar heel pain involving plantar fascia. Anecdotally, development of the heel pain is often seen with recent changes of shoe type, recent increase in load placed on the foot after a period of rest, and repetitive loading placed on the foot.

29.4.1 Anatomy

Plantar fascia is a thick fibrous band located on the plantar surface of the foot which gives arch support. It serves an important function during gait to provide foot stability via "windlass mechanism" [13]. It originates from the medial process of calcaneus where it creates the fibrocartilaginous attachment. The plantar fascia shares the attachment with flexor digitorum brevis, abductor hallucis, and medial part of quadratus plantae. The band spreads into five bands and makes distal attachment to distal phalanges via plantar plate, metatarsal joints via collateral ligaments, and transverse metatarsal ligaments [14].

29.4.2 Clinical Presentation

The player will often describe the localized pain in the plantar medial aspect of calcaneus with initial weight bearing after a period of inactivity. Activities usually lessen their symptoms, but they often complain of increase in their symptom afterward. It is tender to palpation of medial process of calcaneus. The pain can also be elicited with extension of the toes and dorsiflexion.
Despite the typical labeling of "fasciitis," recent studies have suggested the thickening of plantar fascia without true inflammatory process, much like tendinopathy and pathoanatomy. Other studies have also suggested that the thickness of plantar fascia has been associated with the pain level reported in the people with plantar heel pain [15, 16].

29.4.3 Treatment

There has been number of studies investigating the effectiveness of taping in management of heel pain.

Radford et al. [13] have shown that participants with plantar fasciitis who received the low-dye tape reported with statistically significant reduction in "first-step" pain compared to those who received sham treatment alone 1-week post intervention. Furthermore, Abd El Salam and Abd ELhafz [17] have also demonstrated the use of either foot orthoses and augmented low-dye tape with conventional physical therapy resulted in a clinically significant improvement in foot pain and disability scores. These studies have suggested that in an early management of plantar heel pain, it is beneficial to incorporate taping into the treatment plan.

The taping technique demonstrated below combines the low-dye tape with additional support of medial longitudinal arch. Lightplast stretch tape is used to allow improved comfort for the athletes.

Materials needed:

Adhesive spray
5 cm cover-roll stretch tape
1 rigid athletic tape (split in half)
Lightplast stretch tape

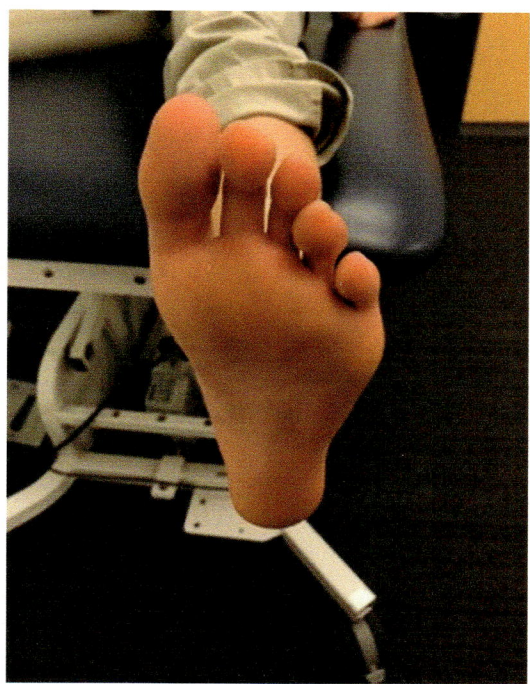

Fig. 29.14 Starting position

1. The foot is prepared by positioning the foot in a neutral position or with slight plantar flexion (see Fig. 29.14 below).
2. The tape adhesive is applied on the plantar and dorsal surface of the foot as well as posterior ankle.
3. One anchor is applied across the metatarsal heads and from medial aspect of first metatarsal head around the heel and to the lateral aspect of fifth metatarsal head. 5 cm cover-roll is used for the anchor (see Fig. 29.15 below).
4. The white rigid tape is split into half.
5. The tape is anchored at first metatarsal head, then around posterior heel, and back to first metatarsal head (see Fig. 29.16 below).
6. Step 5 is repeated for second to fifth metatarsals (see Fig. 29.17 below).
7. The white rigid tape is applied from lateral to medial aspect of the foot with the force pulling up on the foot (see Fig. 29.18 below).
8. The Lightplast stretch tape is taped in the same direction from the forefoot to midfoot just proximal to the plantar fascia origin (see Fig. 29.19 below).

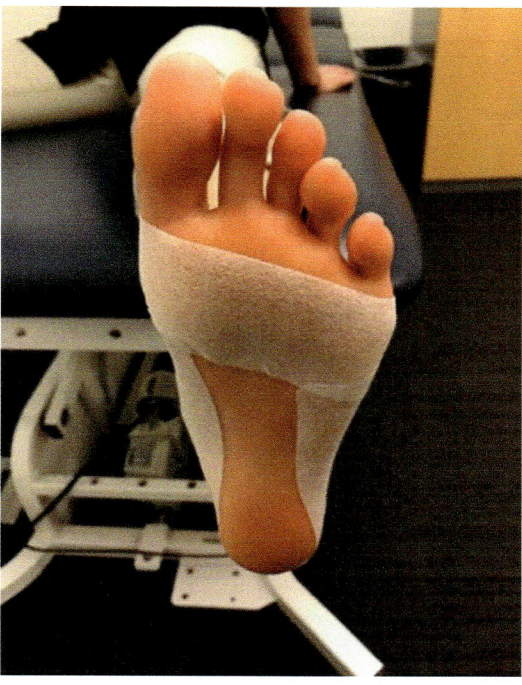

Fig. 29.15 Anchor strip—cover-roll

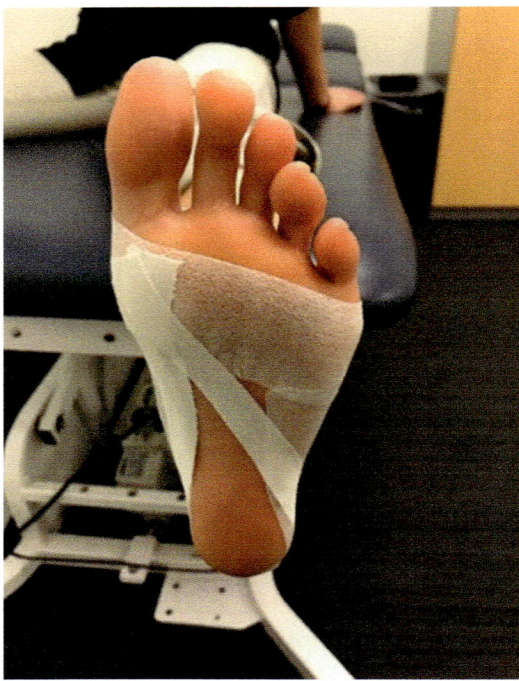

Fig. 29.16 Rigid tape—starting medial

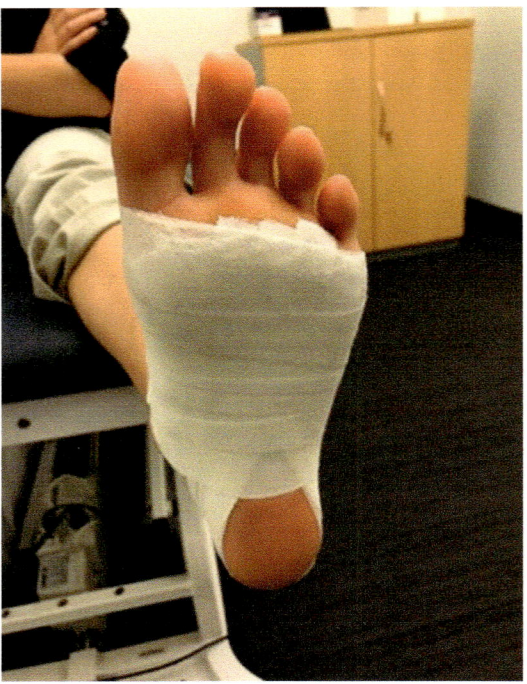

Fig. 29.18 Rigid tape—pulling lateral to medial

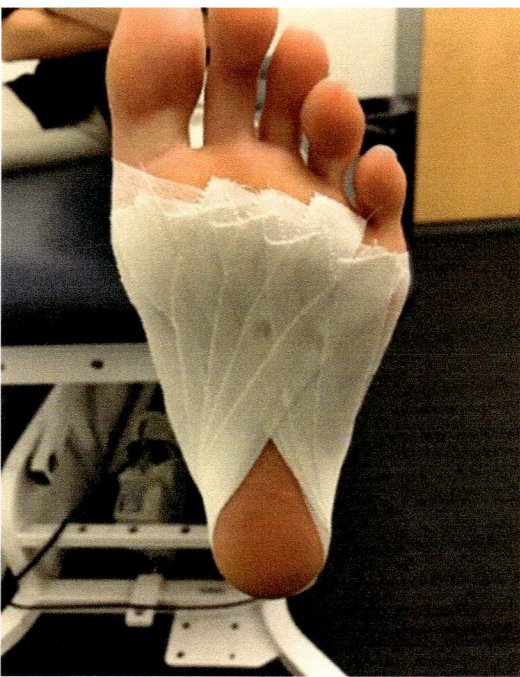

Fig. 29.17 Continue with rigid tape moving lateral

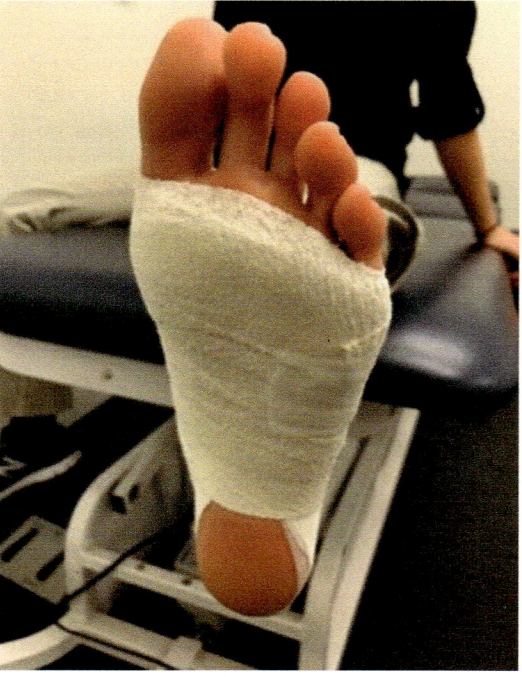

Fig. 29.19 Closing with Lightplast stretch tape

29.5 Sesamoiditis

Due to the amount of sliding and push-off required, players can develop the plantar forefoot injuries. Pathologies in the medial forefoot including sesamoiditis and turf toe are common injuries we see among the elite tennis players.

29.5.1 Anatomy

There are two sesamoid bones (medial and lateral), which sit on the plantar facets of the first metatarsal head. The sesamoid bones are positioned within the tendon of flexor hallucis brevis, and it formulates the part of plantar plate. The extension of this plantar plate makes distal connections with the proximal phalanx. The sesamoid bones have fibrous attachment with the adductor hallucis and abductor hallucis. In addition, respective sesamoid bones have additional ligamentous support on each side. The functions of sesamoid bones are to give the mechanical advantage to the short flexor tendon and to stabilize the first ray during push-off phase of the gait. Most of the weight bearing during the push-off is placed on the tibial sesamoid bone [18].

29.5.2 Clinical Presentation

Players with this condition often report symptom with direct palpation of the sesamoid bone as well as passive and active great toe extension. The athletes will most often report symptoms with toe-off phase of gait cycle and activities such as jumping during serve/smash and quick acceleration on the court. Upon clinical examination, it is tender to palpation and will have pain with passive/active great toe extension.

29.5.3 Treatment

Similar to turf toe management, acute management including rest, ice, and immobilization of first metatarsophalangeal joint can be beneficial in reducing the sesamoid irritation. Walking boot and stiff shoes/insole can be also helpful in limiting stress placed on the sesamoids. Addressing hindfoot, midfoot, and first ray mobility to reduce the stress over the first MTP joint is also critical in an early management of this injury.

In addition to those treatments, the taping technique shown below can be used to aid the symptom management when players go on court to hit. It is a similar taping technique compared to the forefoot blister preventative taping using the pads. The difference is the cutoff of the first MTP region to take the pressure off of the sesamoid bone. In addition to the padding, tape to restrict great toe extension, similar to turf toe tape, can be utilized prior to padding to manage the symptom.

Materials needed:

Adhesive spray
Foam pad (precut)
10 cm cover-roll stretch tape (precut)
Lightplast stretch tape

1. The foam pad is cut into the shape demonstrated in the photo below. The padding is shaped into a position with the cuff off around the first metatarsal and the sesamoid bones.
2. Cover-roll stretch tape (10 cm) is cut to conform the forefoot. The photo below is one example of how the tape can be cut.
3. The foot is prepared by positioning it in the neutral position (see Fig. 29.20 below).
4. The plantar and dorsal surface of the forefoot is sprayed with the adhesive spray. In a hot and humid condition, benzoin compound solution can also be applied to avoid sliding of the padding while playing.
5. The precut padding is applied on the plantar surface of the foot (see Fig. 29.21 below).
6. The cover-roll stretch tape is applied over the foam (see Figs. 29.22 and 29.23 below).
7. The forefoot is covered using Lightplast stretch tape to close off the padding (see Fig. 29.24 below).

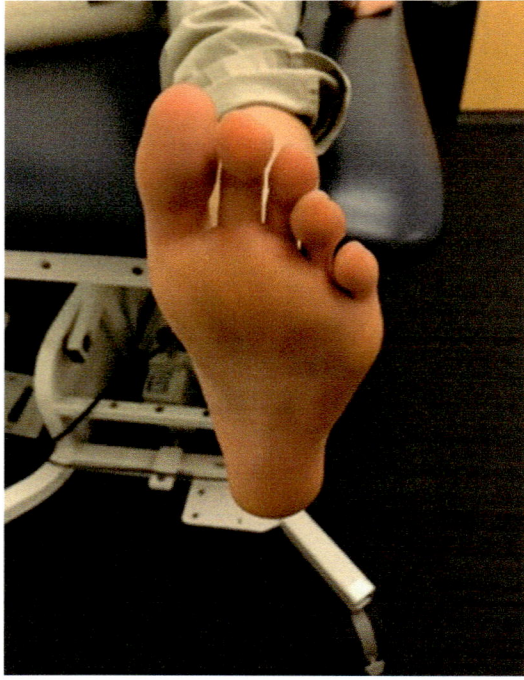

Fig. 29.20 Starting position

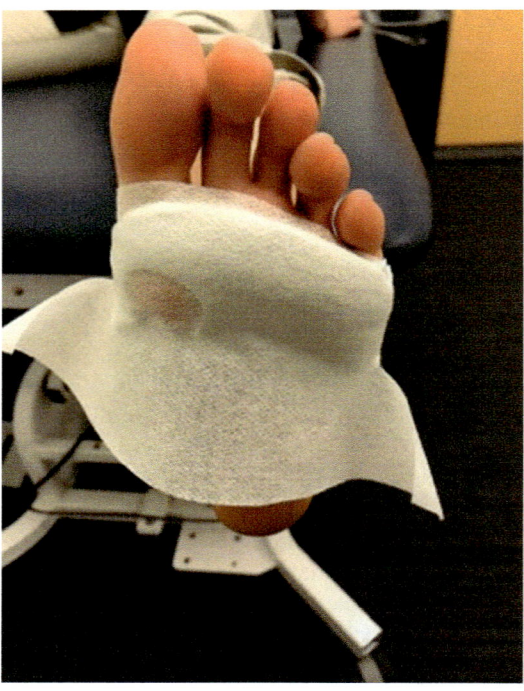

Fig. 29.22 Cover-roll placement on top portion of padding

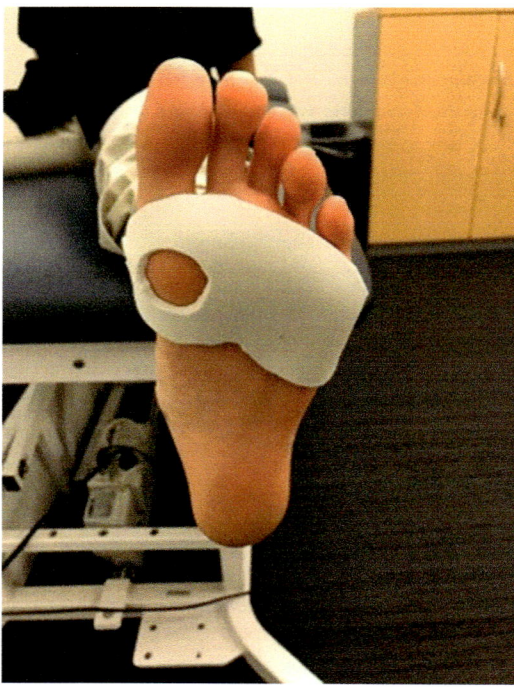

Fig. 29.21 Precut padding

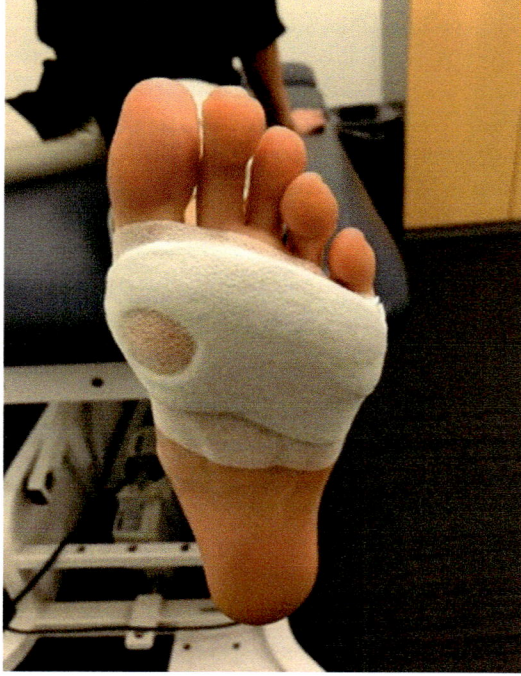

Fig. 29.23 Cover-roll stretch tape placed on bottom portion of padding

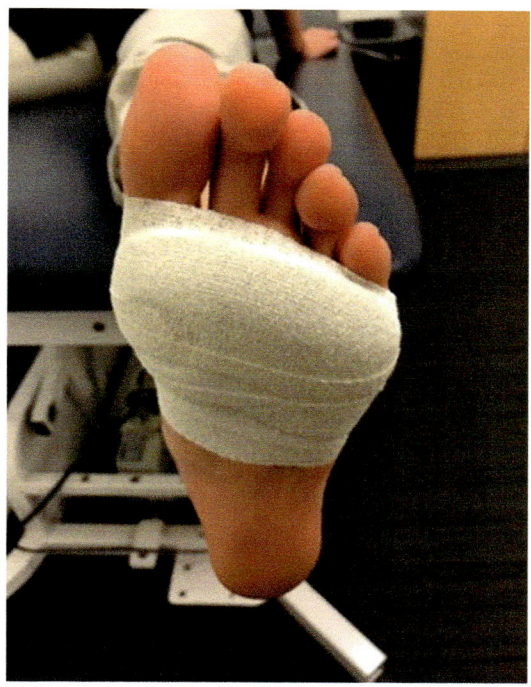

Fig. 29.24 Closing with Lightplast stretch tape

Taping Tips
- In order to ensure that the tape does not slide during play, especially in a hot and humid environment, the area where the tape is applied should be clean, dry, and oil-free. Rubbing alcohol can be used to whip any oil on the skin, and adhesive agents such as taping spray and benzoin compound solution should be used to secure the taping materials.
- After the tape is applied, foot powder can be applied to eliminate excess adhesive remaining on the skin and also to avoid the tape from sliding when the players put on the socks.
- To avoid the skin irritation, tape remover solution/whip should be used to take the tape off. This is especially important when taking the blister tape off to avoid ripping of the sensitive skin.

29.6 Blisters

Professional athletes must constantly deal with the problem of blisters. Repetitive maximal intensity movements combined with short intense bursts and directional changes often result in the skin breaking down.

While blistering of the skin is not as exotic as tendon tears or injuries that require surgery, a blister can have disastrous consequences. In one of the most celebrated US Open Tournaments (2016), the match between Rafael Nadal and Novak Djokovic had to be stopped twice as Nadal had to be attended to twice for a particularly severe foot blister. It therefore is no surprise that ATP tour physiotherapists are extremely attentive and vigilant to any sign of impending blister formation, particularly on the feet and toes.

On the ATP tour, players are constantly changing shoes. Minute differences in shoe brands combined with different court surfaces, wet socks, humidity levels, and lack of prevention are ready-made causes for blisters. Unfortunately, without being attentive and left untreated, significant problems may develop.

29.6.1 Prevention

To avoid friction areas that could result blister formation, ATP physiotherapists constantly stress the need for preventive care. Coaches are often enlisted in this effort as they are with players during practice and between tournaments. To combat blister problems, the ATP ships to all the training facilities, Friar's Balsam + Q-Tips™ (Unilever), Hypafix™ (BSN Medical) 10 cm wide roll, Leukoplast™ (BSN Medical), adhesive foam 3 or 4 mm thick, and Tuf-Skin Spray™ (Cramer or Muller) (Fig. 29.25).

29.6.2 Metatarsal Taping

Padding and attentive application are critical components in the prevention regimen. Even with shoes that are specifically sized for players by the shoe manufacturers, proper padding is needed to avoid blister and associated skin problems. Unfortunately, even with the best fit, the long and arduous tournament season simply plays havoc on the friction-prone skin areas of the foot.

Fig. 29.25 Materials needed

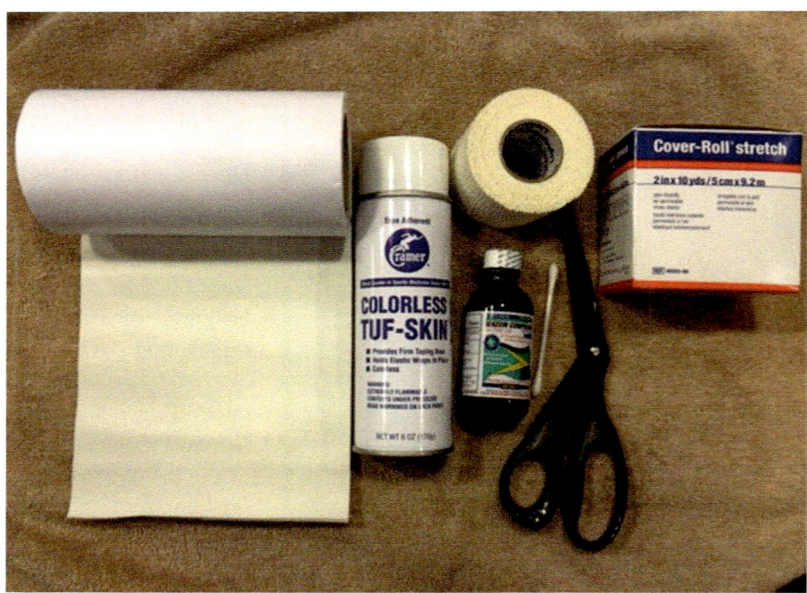

The following discussion with associated photos is included to emphasize and articulate many of the techniques used on the tour. These techniques are also used in myriad training facilities around the world to treat athletes that experience a great deal of lateral movements.

The following discussion with associated photos is included to emphasize and articulate many of the techniques used on the tour. These techniques are also used in myriad training facilities around the world to treat athletes that experience a great deal of lateral movements.

1. Preparation of the Skin Prior to Pad Application

   With Friar's Balsam™ and Tuf-Skin™, begin the treatment process.

   A Q-Tip™ is used to spread Friar's Balsam™ on the entire forefoot from the base of the toes to the middle of the foot (Fig. 29.2). It is essential to first make the skin sticky. Having the skin sticky allows the padding to remain in place (see Fig. 29.26 below).

   Once dry (and only when dried), Tuf-Skin™ should be sprayed over the same areas. The Tuf-Skin™ must also be dry before padding is applied (see Fig. 29.27 below).

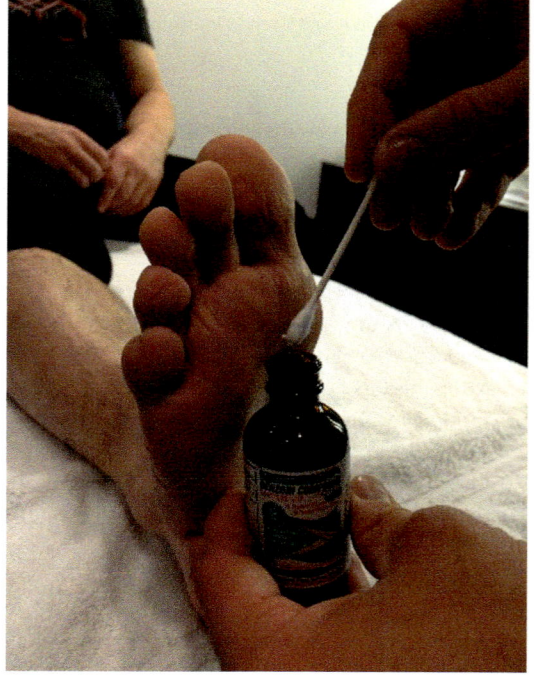

Fig. 29.26 Skin preparation

29 Acute Management of Common Foot and Ankle Injuries

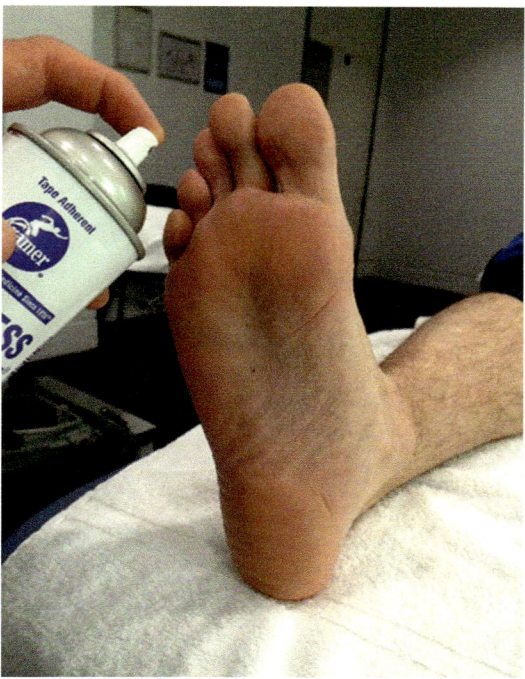

Fig. 29.27 Tuff skin applied to forefoot

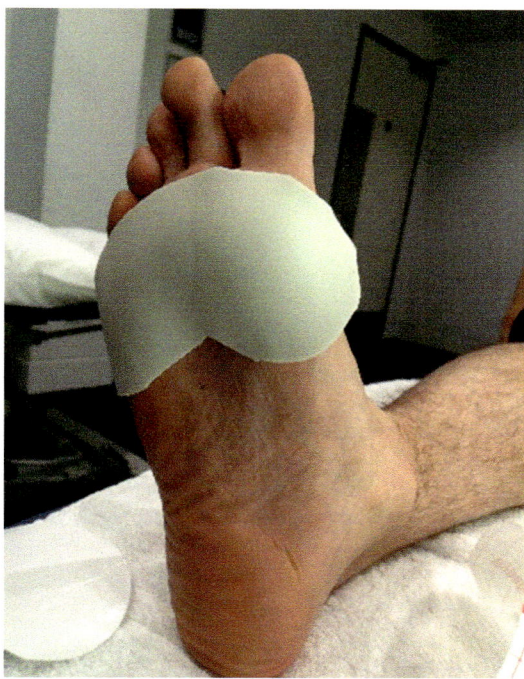

Fig. 29.29 Pre-cut padding applied to forefoot

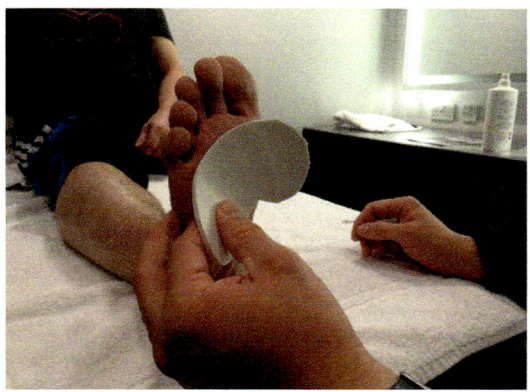

Fig. 29.28 Precut padding placement applied to forefoot

2. Pad Application

The pad should be cut in an "L" shape to conform to the shape of the foot (see Fig. 29.28 below).

It should be spread across the plantar surface of the foot and cover the sides of the dorsal surfaces to avoid the pad from sliding. If the padding is improperly wrapped, the foot can become extremely uncomfortable and affect the player's performance. In a tournament that may last for hours, it is critical that the pad be comfortable and secure.

3. Wrapping the Pad

Remove the protection from the foam, and place the padding on the foot as shown. It is very important to avoid wrinkles so as to not create additional problems (see Fig. 29.29 below).

Precut the Hypafix™ in the shape of an "H." The length should be approximately 10 cm longer than the width of the plantar service of the foot. Remove the protection or the backing of the tape to apply the central part of the "H" beginning with the base of the toes to cover the padding. Complete the application of the padding by applying the "ends" of the "H" on the sides of the foot, finishing on the dorsal surface of the foot. Additionally, it is important not to compress the big toe and the fifth toe by applying too much compression on the forefoot during the final Hypafix™ application (Figs. 29.30 and 29.31).

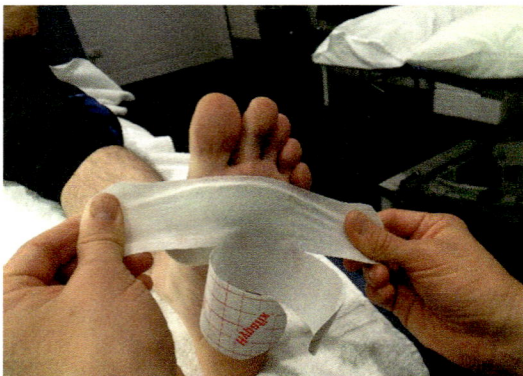

Fig. 29.30 Cover-roll placement on top portion of padding

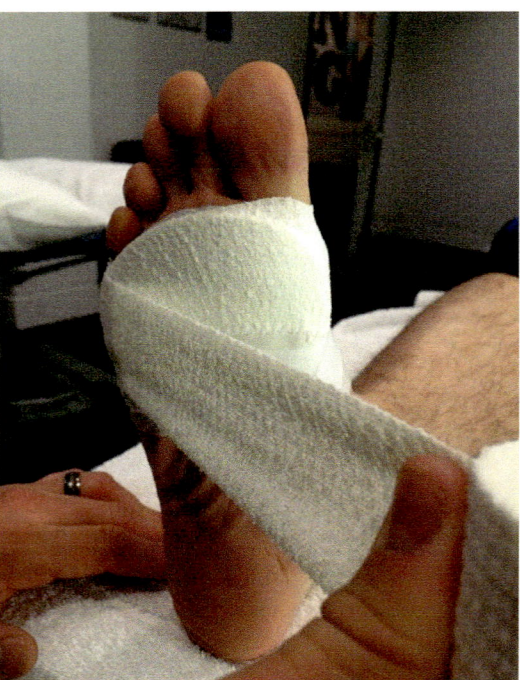

Fig. 29.32 Closing with Lightplast stretch tape

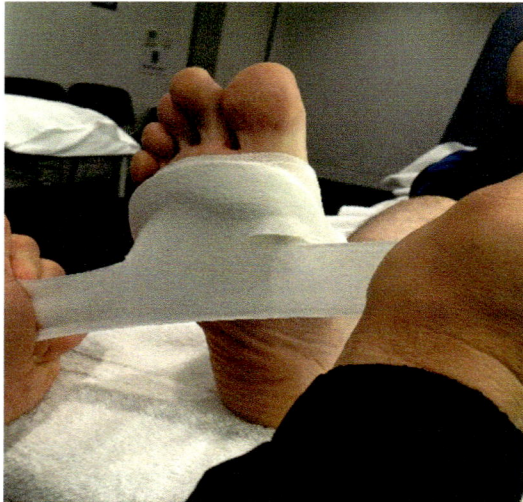

Fig. 29.31 Cover-roll stretch tape placed on bottom portion of padding

Finally, once the Hypafix™ is in place, Leukoplast™ is used to cover the complete tape and padding.

It is again important to point out that during the application of the Leukoplast™, great care should be taken not to compress the big toe and the fifth toe (Figs. 29.32 and 29.33). Do not use too much tension on the band, and finish again with these strips on the dorsal surface of the foot. Baby powder can then be applied over the tape to allow the tape to slide in the socks.

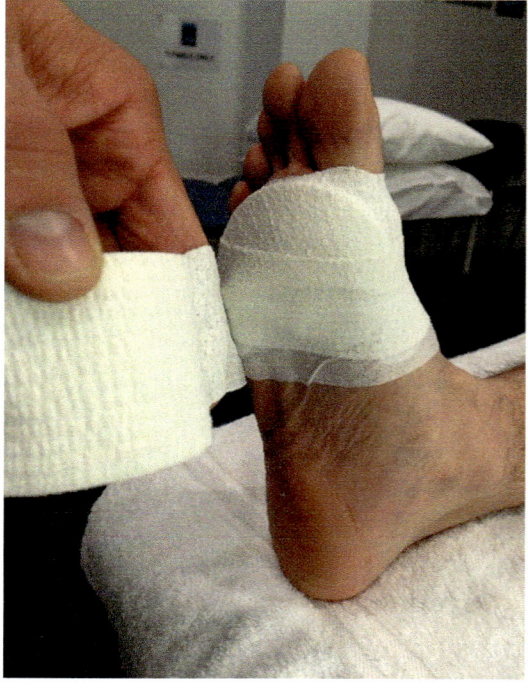

Fig. 29.33 Closing with Lightplast stretch tape

Fig. 29.34 Materials needed

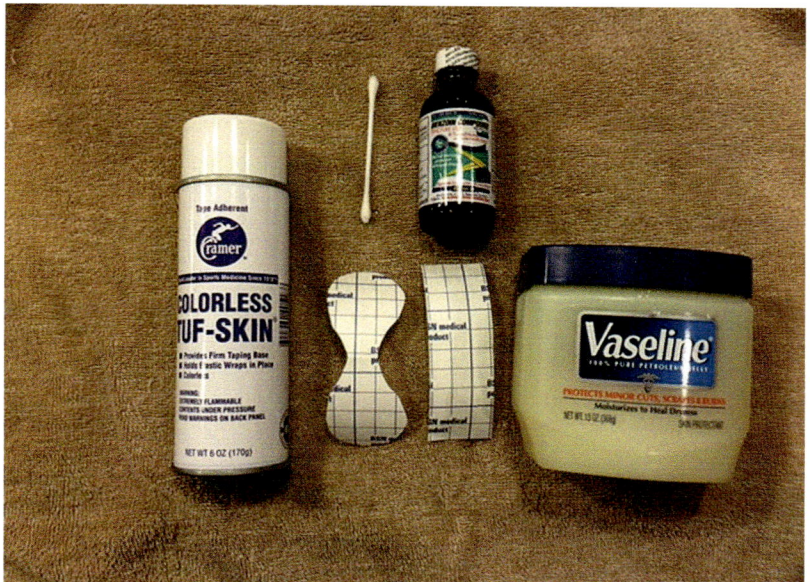

29.6.3 Taping of the Toes

Hypafix™ 3 × 10 cm (10 or 15 strips), Friar's Balsam™ and a Q-Tip™ along with Hypafix 3 × 8 cm (2 "special-shaped" strips), and Vaseline™ or skin lube are needed (see Fig. 29.34 below).

The preparation of the skin is similar to the procedures used into pad the foot. Friar's Balsam is used first; then Tuf-Skin™ spray is applied (see Fig. 29.35 below).

It is important to spray the foot from the bottom to the top to ensure all areas have been covered; otherwise, there will be places that the tape will not adhere.

Once completely dry (and not before), remove the protection, and apply the first special-shaped Hypafix™ strip to the top of the toe (Figs. 29.36, 29.37, 29.38, 29.39, 29.40, and 29.41). Then apply the second special-shaped strip of Hypafix™ perpendicular to the previous one on both inside and outside services of the toe. Finally, apply the rectangular strips sequentially to the other affected toes.

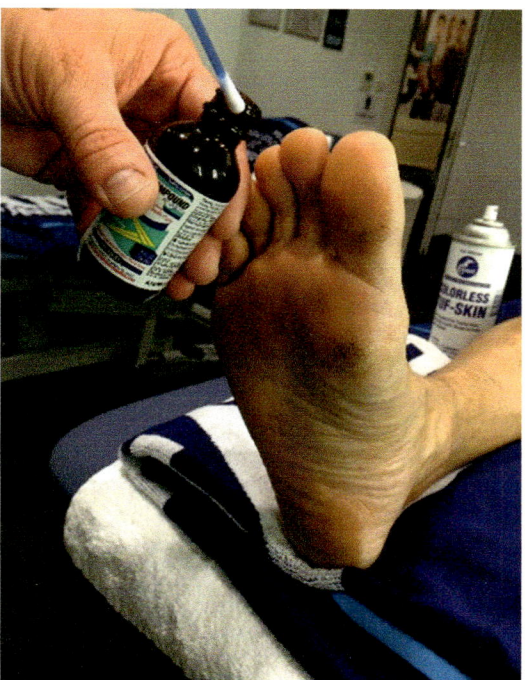

Fig. 29.35 Toe preparation

29.6.4 Additional Blister Information

While Friar's Balsam and Tuf-Skin spray and proper taping tend to be sufficient for most players, additional steps are often used over the course of the tournament season. ATP physios are particularly attentive to any hotspot formation or areas that are extremely tender due to palpitation. If

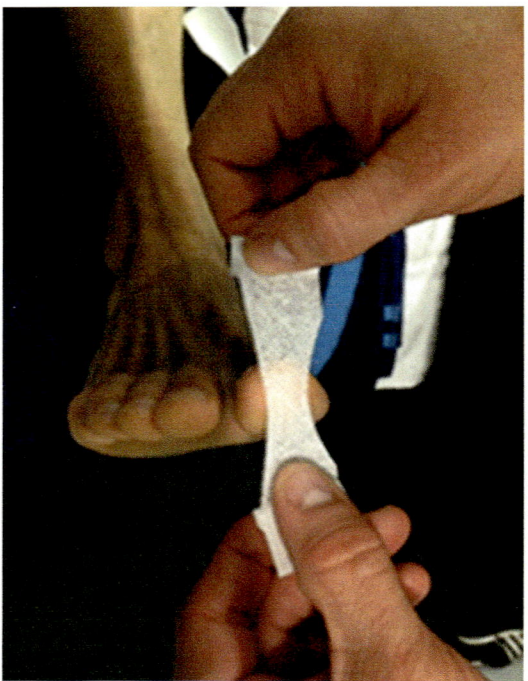

Fig. 29.36 Place the special shaped strip over the top of the toe

Fig. 29.38 Place the special shaped strip over the top of the toe in the opposite direction

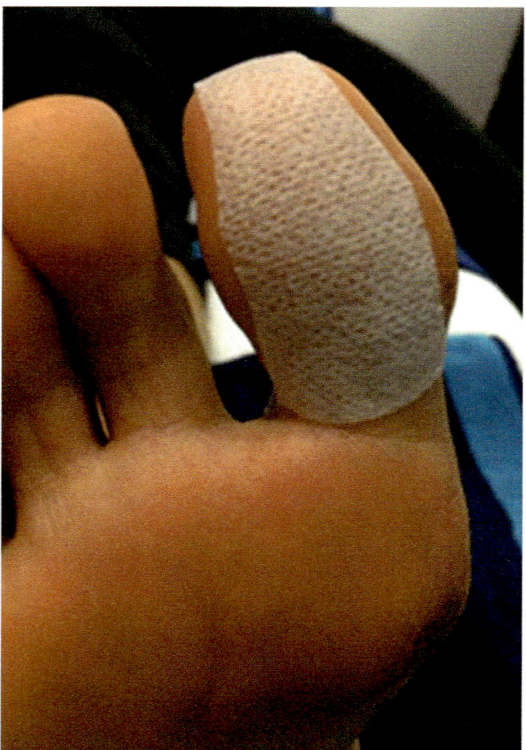

Fig. 29.37 Where the cover-roll tape should end

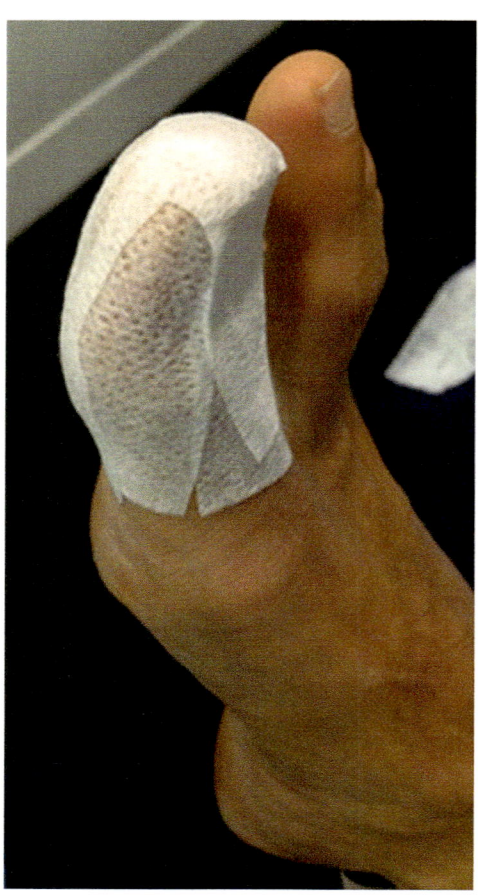

Fig. 29.39 How the cover-roll should be placed

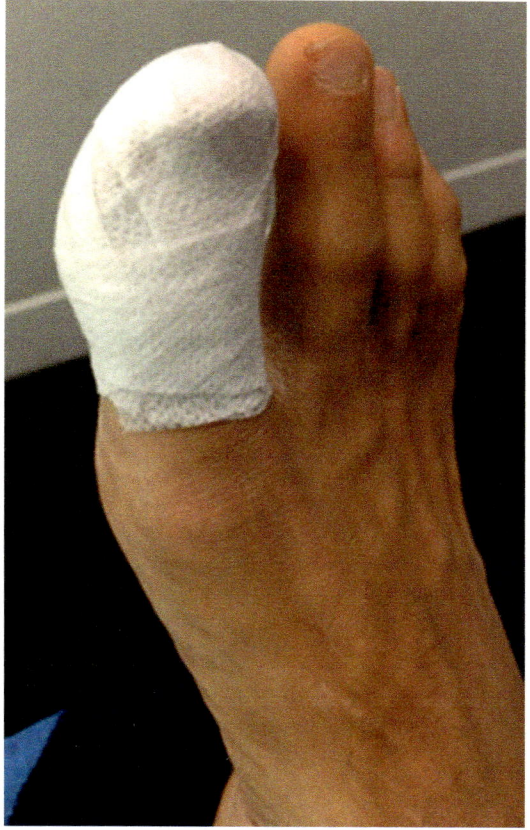

Fig. 29.40 Final presentation—front view

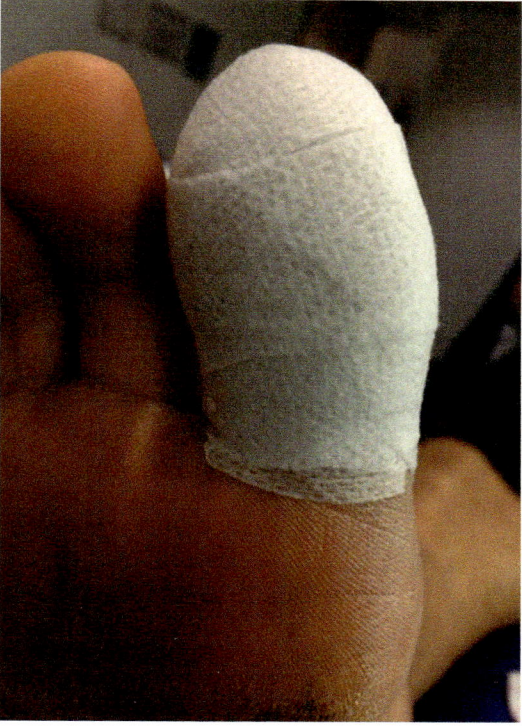

Fig. 29.41 Final presentation—back view

these occur, a foam doughnut (1/8 to 1/4 in thickness) is normally applied to the surrounding areas.

Many players desire the doughnut to be filled in with a Second Skin™ that often provides additional comfort. A small layer of Hypafix™ is used above and below the padding to ensure that the doughnut adheres to the skin. Baby powder completes the process.

29.7 Treating a Blister

Players shower and use locker rooms in different areas of the world. While all the facilities are thoroughly cleaned, infection potential that can occur with a ruptured blister is always present, and therefore every effort should be made to keep the blister intact.

If an open blister is found, it is essential that the wound and surrounding areas must be cleaned thoroughly. Once cleaned, Eosine™ is applied followed by Homeoplasmine™ cream. It is extremely important to avoid the tendency to remove loose skin as any remaining skin can be a good barrier to infection. A Second Skin™ on top of the loose skin can be applied to prevent potential tearing of any loose skin upon removal.

Depending upon the size of the blister, a simple Band-Aid or a larger pad that allows oxygen flow can suffice.

29.7.1 Aspiration of a Blister

Severe blisters will often require aspiration. If this occurs, the skin must be cleaned thoroughly. The application process must begin from the corner, not from the center. Once the blister has been aspirated thoroughly, a syringe filled with Eosine™ is injected back into the blister. (Eosine™ helps dry the skin inside the blister.) This procedure must often be repeated the following day, especially if the blister begins to refill. If this happens, the tissue inside the blister will be very soft and tender and a doughnut consisting of foam padding will be applied.

29.7.2 Court Calls

During the long ATP tournament season, there are times that the best proactive plans are overtaken by events that require immediate attention. If a court call is required to treat a blister, the goal becomes short term—doing what is necessary to keep the player competing. Time becomes critical as the clock is not the therapist's friend.

ATP therapists must quickly clean the blister thoroughly and remove any debris or tape that may have become imbedded. Triple antibiotic cream is then applied to avoid infection. A quick re-padding and re-taping then occur.

29.7.3 Final Comments

Blisters are an occupational hazard for professional athletes. It is therefore critical that therapists, athletes, and coaches be attentive to any skin aberration and take immediate steps to attend to potential problems.

29.8 Turf Toe

When excessive hyperextension force is applied to the metatarsophalangeal (MTP) joint, the plantar surface of the MTP joint is at risk to be injured and possibly severely damaged. The common name for this injury is called turf toe.

Turf toe occurs for myriad reasons. Sudden acceleration, improper shoe fitting, using the wrong type of shoe for a particular sport, artificial turf, and excessive hypertension of the big toe caused by aggressive running and jumping are the typical areas that result in turf toe problems.

In sports that require an athlete to immediately accelerate, such as professional tennis, football running backs, and track sprinters, turf toe is all too common. Acceleration in these sports often results in large force through the metatarsophalangeal joint [19].

The type and fitting of shoes may also contribute to a greater incidence of turf toe. As shoes become lighter and more flexible, there can be a great deal of pressure applied to the metatarsophalangeal region [20].

Artificial turf is another issue that shows up time and again in turf toe injuries. Artificial turf was first installed in 1964 and was heralded as a breakthrough that would eliminate uneven surfaces, water problems, and the problem of growing grass in indoor stadiums. However, it was quickly found that artificial turf was not without its problems. The incidence of increased damage to the metatarsophalangeal joint was a by-product of the hard surface as athletes could accelerate more quickly off of the hard surface than regular grass. While artificial turfs have undergone dramatic refinement, therapists that deal with athletes that continually play on artificial surfaces must still be attentive to the potential MTP problems.

Jumping is taken for granted as a normal activity; however, what is not appreciated is that the capsular ligamentous complex at the MTP undergoes additional pressure. Under normal activities, the pressure associated with jumping may vary from two to three times a person's body weight, but pressures could reach up to eight times a person's body weight when jumping [21]. During jumping, the big toe can be hyperextended as the heel raises. In tennis, lunges or pushing aggressively with one leg exacerbates the problems.

Once an athlete complains of toe issues, it is imperative that therapists ascertain the severity immediately. Point tenderness, swelling, malalignment, and an ecchymosis are all used in diagnosing and treating turf toe. Another determining factor is assessing active flexion to determine if there is a disruption of the plantar plate or flexor hallucis brevis (FHB). If a plantar plate rupture occurs, movement of the sesamoid in a proximal direction may occur [22].

Turf toe is typically diagnosed into three grades. Grade 1 is defined by a sprain of the plantar capsular ligamentous complex of the hallux MTP joint. Normally, with a grade 1 sprint, an athlete will still receive treatment but usually will continue with their playing regimen.

Grade II is more severe, as the plantar soft tissue of the hallux MTP joint evidences a partial rupture. If the plantar soft tissue completely ruptures at the hallux MTP joint, the injury is classified as a grade III. Surgery most likely will be the result [23].

If turf toe is suspected, three major areas are assessed in making the proper turf toe diagnosis: ankle dorsiflexion, ankle plantarflexion, and MTP extension [24].

Once an assessment is made, it is important to convey to an athlete and coach the necessity to take the necessary time to heal the injury. Often, an athlete may play down the severity to avoid restricting their activity because of a "simple" toe problem. However, a simple problem of the toe can become a major one if left untreated or if the athlete does not understand how quickly the problem can be exacerbated. If the diagnosis is a grade I injury, resting, icing, and medication may often reduce the swelling, and the athlete may return to competition and practice without restriction. Depending upon the severity, however, a walking boot can help to take the pressure off of the toe. If a boot is not required, a stiff-soled shoe with an insert plate or with a Morton's extension can limit the amount of hallux motion thereby also reducing pressure [25].

While most professional athletes' ankles are taped before every practice and match, the toes do not often get taped unless there is damage. It is important to stress the necessity to tape the toes even for a grade I incidence of turf toe in order to restrict motion. The goal is to decrease the inflammation along the MTP joint, and as long as continually pressure is applied, inflammation will not be significantly reduced.

The following is a step-by-step taping instruction:

The athlete should lay supine. Apply Tuf-Skin™ around the entire great toe.

Spray the plantar surface of the foot around the first metatarsal to the distal part of the arch.

Use (normally) a 1½-in. roll of tape. Tear in half (see Fig. 29.42 below).

Place the ¾" tape around just distal and proximal to the IP joint (which will create an anchor, distally and proximally).

Place another piece of tape (1½"w) proximal to the metatarsal heads that will create an anchor. The tape should be wrapped loosely around the entire foot while trying not to press the metatarsal heads together (see Fig. 29.43 below).

Have the athlete place the IP joint into 5–10° of plantar flexion. With the ¾" width tape, place first strip until it reaches the tape which has been placed around the metatarsal heads. The strips will run parallel to the foot. The ¾" width tape will move in a fanlike direction covering slight medial plantar and slight lateral portion of the great toe. Each one of the strips will connect onto both previously anchors (see Fig. 29.44 below).

After approximately seven to ten strips placed in a fanlike direction, place one additional proximal and distal anchor to seal the loose ends (see Fig. 29.45 below).

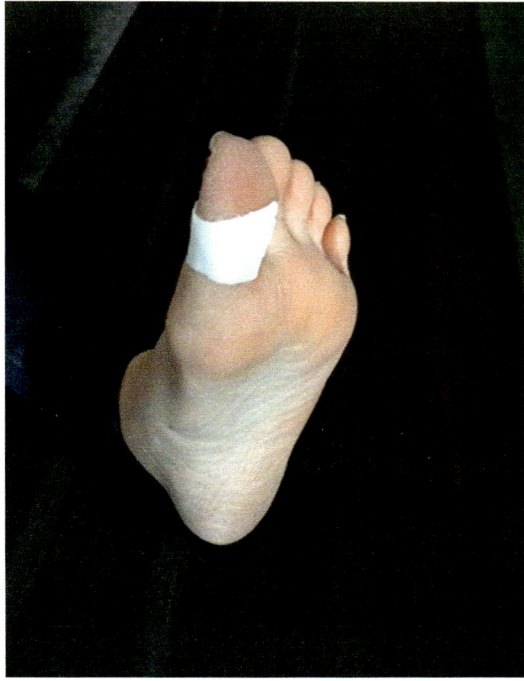

Fig. 29.42 Anchor tape around great toe

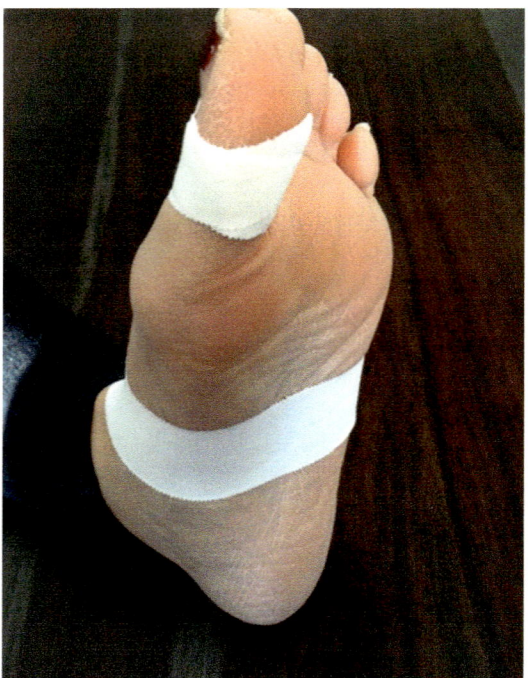

Fig. 29.43 Anchor placed around midfoot

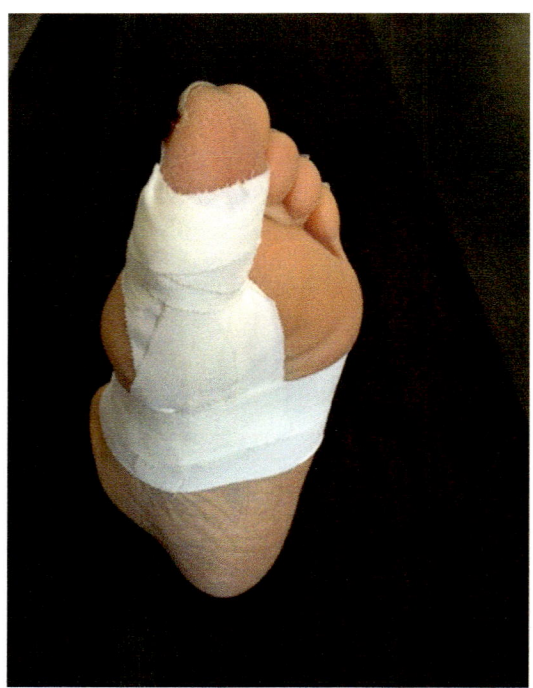

Fig. 29.45 Closing the tape with anchors on each end

Then place a strip starting by the toe wrap around the entire foot using Lightplast Pro™ tape until it reaches the proximal anchor.

Complete the procedure by using baby powder to prevent any rolling that can occur when putting on the sock.

References

1. Kovacs MA, Ellenbecker TS, Kibler WB, Roetert EP, Lubbers P. Injury trends in American competitive junior tennis players. J Sci Tennis Med. 2014;19(1):19–23.
2. Reece LA, Fricker PA, Maguire KF. Injuries to elite young tennis players at the Australian Institute of Sport. Aust J Sci Med Sport. 1986;18:11–5.
3. Kovacs MA, Roetert EP, Ellenbecker TS. Complete conditioning for tennis, vol. 2. Champaign, IL: Human Kinetics Publishers; 2016.
4. Martin RL, Davenport TE, Paulseth S, Wukich DK, Godges JJ. Clinical Practice Guidelines: Ankle stability and movement coordination impairments: ankle ligament sprains. J Orthop Sports Phys Ther. 2013;43(9):A1–A40. https://doi.org/10.2519/jospt.2013.0305.

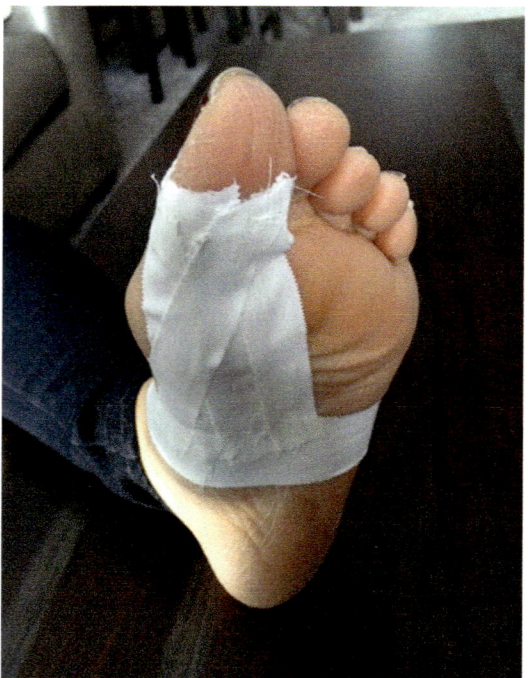

Fig. 29.44 Attaching tape to each end of the anchor

5. Kaminski TW, Hertel J, Amendola N, et al. National Athletic Trainers' Association Positional Statement: conservative management and prevention of ankle sprains in athletes. J Athl Train. 2013;48(4):528–45. https://doi.org/10.4085/1062-6050-48.4.02.
6. McGuine TA, Keene JS. The effect of a balance training program on the risk of ankle sprains in high school athletes. Am J Sports Med. 2006;34:1103–11. https://doi.org/10.1177/0363546505284191.
7. McGuine TA, Hetzel S, Wilson J, Brooks A. The effect of lace-up ankle braces on injury rates in high school football players. Am J Sports Med. 2012;40(1):49–57. https://doi.org/10.1177/0363546511422332.
8. McGuine TA, Brooks A, Hetzel S. The effect of lace-up ankle braces on injury rates in high school basketball players. Am J Sports Med. 2011;39(9):1840–8. https://doi.org/10.1177/0363546511406242.
9. Zalavras C, Thordarson D. Ankle syndesmotic injury. J Am Acad Orthop Surg. 2007;15:330–9.
10. Gerber JP, Williams GN, Scoville CR, Arciero RA, Taylor DC. Persistent disability associated with ankle sprains: a prospective examination of an athletic population. Foot Ankle Int. 1998;19:653–6.
11. Hopkinson WJ, St Pierre P, Ryan JB, Wheeler JH. Syndesmosis sprain of the ankle. Foot Ankle. 1990;10(6):325–30.
12. Cole C, Seto C, Gazewood J. Plantar fasciitis: evidence-based review of diagnosis and therapy. Am Fam Physician. 2005;72:2237–342.
13. Radford JA, Landorf KB, Buchbinder R, Cook C. Effectriveness of low-Dye taping for the short-term treatment of plantar heel pain: a randomised trial. BMC Musculoskelet Disord. 2006;7:64. https://doi.org/10.1186/1471-2474-7-64.
14. Tahririan MA, Motififard M, Tahmasebi MN, Siavashi B. Plantar fasciitis. J Res Med Sci. 2012;17(8):799–804.
15. Martin RL, Davenport TE, Reischl SF, McPoil TG, Matheson JW, Wukich DK, McDonough CM. Clinical Practice Guidelines: heel pain—plantar fasciitis: revision 2014. J Orthop Sports Phys Ther. 2014;44(11):A1–A23. https://doi.org/10.2519/jospt.2014.0303.
16. Lemont H, Ammirati KM, Usen N. Plantar fasciitis: a degenerative process (fasciosis) without inflammation. J Am Podiatr Med Assoc. 2003;93(3):234–7.
17. Abd El Salam MS, Abd ELhafz YN. Low-dye taping versus medial arch support in managing pain and pain-related disability in patients with plantar fasciitis. Foot Ankle Spec. 2011;4(2):86–91. https://doi.org/10.1177/1938640010387416.
18. Sims AL, Kurup HV. Painful sesamoid of the great toe. World J Orthop. 2014;5(2):146–50. https://doi.org/10.5312/wjo.v5.i2.146.
19. Coker TC, Arnold JA, Weber DL. Traumatic lesions of the great toe in athletes. Am J Sports Med. 1978;6:326–34.
20. Rodeo SA, O'brien S, Warren RF, Barnes R, Wichiewicz TL, Dillingham MF. Turf-toe: an analysis of metatarsophalangeal joint sprains in professional football players. Am J Sports Med. 1990;18:280–5.
21. Nigg BM. Biomechanical aspects of running. In: Nigg BM, editor. Biomechanics of running shoes. Champaign, IL: Human Kinetics; 1986. p. 1–25.
22. Prieskorn D, Graves SC, Smith RA. Morphometric analysis of the plantar plate apparatus of the first metatarsophalangeal joint. Foot Ankle. 1993;14(4):204–7.
23. Drago JJ, Oloff L, Jacobs AM. A comprehensive review of hallux limitus. J Foot Surg. 1984;23(3):213–22.
24. McCormick JJ, Anderson RB. Turf toe. Anatomy, Diagnosis, and Treatment. Sports Health. 2010;2(6):487–94.
25. Williams GN, Jones MH, Amendola A. Syndesmotic ankle sprains in athletes. Am J Sports Med. 2007;35:1197–207.

Part VI

Spinal Injury

Spondylolysis

30

Carles Pedret, Ramon Balius, and Angel Ruiz-Cotorro

Spondylolysis is a bone defect that affects the pars interarticularis of a vertebra (Fig. 30.1). The pars interarticularis is a small isthmus located between the facet joints of the vertebrae above and below. This usually occurs on a bilateral basis, affecting the L5 (85–95%) and on rarer occasions affecting the proximal lumbar vertebrae [1–3], the affectation of which is usually unilateral. An isthmic unilateral lesion is observed in 14–30% of cases [4–6]. It may be associated with injuries at other levels or with lysis on the contralateral side, which develops over time. Although it is rare, it may affect several levels simultaneously [7].

Spondylolisthesis is understood as the displacement of a vertebra on the one immediately below (Fig. 30.2). Said displacement will occur more frequently in the lumbosacral junction.

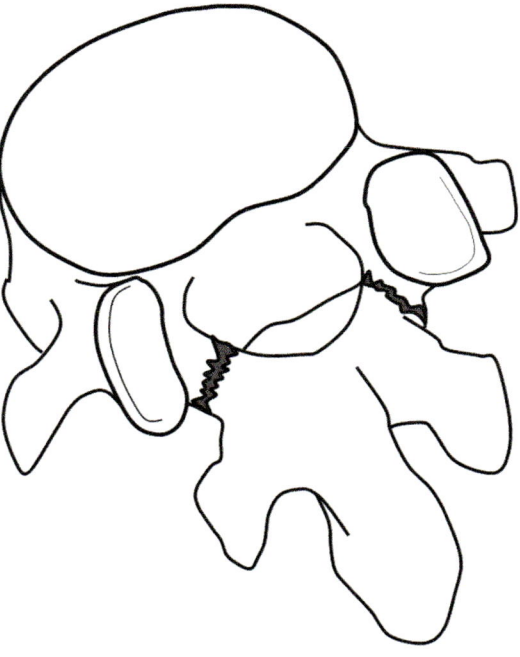

Fig. 30.1 Spondylolysis. Defect in the pars interarticularis

C. Pedret (✉)
Clínica Mapfre de Medicina del Tenis, Barcelona, Spain

Clínica Diagonal, Barcelona, Spain

R. Balius
Consell Català de l'Esport, Generalitat de Catalunya, Barcelona, Spain

Clínica Diagonal, Barcelona, Spain

A. Ruiz-Cotorro
Clínica Mapfre de Medicina del Tenis, Barcelona, Spain

Real Federación Española de Tenis, Barcelona, Spain
e-mail: aruizcotorro@clinicammtenis.com

Spondylolisthesis in the adolescent population can be developmental, with dysplastic pars or other posterior elements, isthmic (related to pars fracture) or secondary to tumour or trauma of the posterior elements [8]. Its prevalence in the Caucasian population is around 5%, while the isthmic spondylolisthesis appears in 25–30% of the first [1, 9].

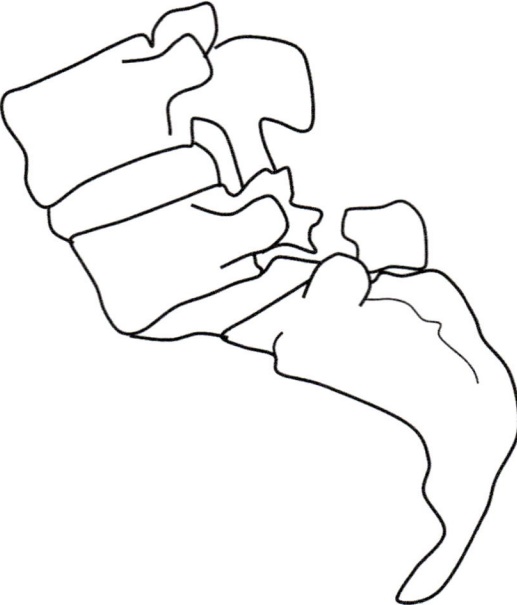

Fig. 30.2 Spondylolisthesis. Anterior displacement of a spinal body

30.1 Epidemiology

Spondylolysis is considered to be a stress fracture [10, 11], appearing in approximately 3–13% [1, 4, 12, 13] of the Caucasian population, with an increase in this prevalence in certain ethnic [14], sports [15, 16] and family groups [17]. The defect in the pars interarticularis is an entity that appears during childhood and does not increase significantly in adulthood [9]. The isthmic lesion affects men more than women [9, 17], although it seems that the latter develop greater olisthesis [18].

In a study conducted by the Royal Spanish Tennis Federation, retrospective analyses were carried out on 66 young tennis players in whom spondylolysis with or without spondylolisthesis was diagnosed between 2002 and 2004 [19].

A total of 66 cases of spondylolysis were studied, 42 men and 24 women, with a mean age of 14.8 years (range 12–21): 53 (80%) cases were at L5, 8 cases (12%) were at L4, 2 cases (3%) were at L3, and 1 (1%) bilateral case was at L2. Two more two-level cases were found (bilateral L5 and unilateral L4 and L3 on the right side).

The injured tennis players with pathological entities were classified on the basis of their performance in supplementary tests: 27 (mean age of 15.1 years (range 12–21); 17 men and 10 women) had developing spondylolysis (negative radiography, positive PBS/SPECT), 20 (mean age of 14.8 years (range 12–18); 12 men and eight women) had active lysis (positive radiography, positive PBS/SPECT) and 19 (mean age of 16.6 years (range 14–20); 13 men and six women) had established spondylolysis (positive radiography, negative PBS/SPECT).

The results of this study show a higher incidence rate of spondylolysis of what is seen in most current literature. This may be due to spondylolysis being so much more common in adolescents because the spine is still undergoing growth and remodelling, and the pars interarticularis does not reach bone maturity until an approximate age of 25 years [20].

30.2 Etiopathogenesis

In relation to spondylolysis, there are certain general predisposing factors which are widely described in the literature such as genetics [21, 22], age and gender [12, 13, 23], race [9, 12] and the structure of the pars [24] and of the rachis, of which the triggering factor is mechanical overload, especially the one that occurs during hyperextension and lumbar rotation [20, 25].

In the world of tennis, the combined movement of extension with forced rotation during the forehand stroke may be a contributing factor in the onset of isthmic lesions in young tennis players. Although introduction of a stance facing the trajectory of the ball seems to have increased the speed of the stroke, it has also increased overloading of the posterior arch [19]. Also, specific actions that cause overloading of the posterior arch of the vertebra are hyperextension when serving and the combined movement of extension with forced rotation during the forehand [19].

In recent years there has been a change in the characteristics of playing tennis. The change of materials involving rackets, strings, courts or event balls leads to an increase in speed and power of the shots, which require greater approximation to the ball and a much faster exit after hitting the shot. This leads to more abrupt lumbar rotation (with an associated flexo-extension) and more powerful impact in forehand and backhand.

It has been discussed whether this increase in rotation load to the spine is due more to the mechanism of the serve (where a forced hyperextension—lumbar flexion—takes place with a greater or lesser rotational component depending on the type of serve used) or in the forehand or backhand. In our experience in the Spanish Federation, we believe that at present, the forehand or backhand shots are more aggressive than the serve for a possible injury in the form of spondylolysis.

These mechanisms and movements of the game along with a weakness of the abdominal muscles and excessive rigidity of the hamstring muscles cause this stress reaction affecting the lumbar spine with a higher percentage among the sporting community [26].

In fact, the prevalence of isthmic injuries among the sporting community increases in comparison to the Caucasian population that does not play sports by about 10–20% [19, 20, 25]. Isthmic injuries are seen in sports with a predominance of flexo-extension (gymnastics [23], butterfly-style swimming [27]) sometimes associated to rotations (tennis [19], high jumping [28] and/or sports with simultaneous loading such as weight-lifting, diving or taekwondo) [20, 29].

One of the main complications of spondylolysis with an evolution over time is the appearance of spondylolisthesis. These are classified based on the Wiltse, Newman and MacNab's classification (1976) [30] which distributes spondylolisthesis into five different types. In sports we generally come across isthmic spondylolisthesis (type II) and, sometimes, dysplastic spondylolisthesis (type I).

30.3 Clinical Findings

Clinically, there are three types of pain associated with the isthmic and/or olisthesic injuries: lumbar pain caused by isthmic injury, lumbar pain related to an alteration to small joints and radicular pain associated to a lesion to the pars [19, 20].

Pain resulting from isthmic lesion (with or without olisthesis). Isthmic injuries often progress without symptoms [31]. It is calculated that up to 80% of cases are asymptomatic [32]. In this case, individuals who submit the rachis to repetitive extension or rotation are those who most often develop pain. This fact would be related to the biomechanical mechanisms producing the lesion mentioned above and evidently, among the sports community, in which a precise diagnosis will be essential [33].

The beginning of the pain is normally progressive and mechanical, although there are also references to sudden appearance or acute worsening of the picture after a fortuitous accident [8, 19].

It presents itself as a lower lumbar pain, with irradiation to buttocks and sometimes to the thighs, often disabling [8, 9, 16, 19, 20]. For Standaert and Herring [16], the only pathognomonic manoeuvre is possibly the one that involves a combined hyperextension of the hip and lumbar spine, keeping the individual on the other leg. This test is useful in unilateral spondylolysis, given that the pain appears when the patient puts weight on the healthy side. The pain is often associated to a reflected contracture of the hamstrings, a lumbar position in hyperlordosis [34] and a certain degree of scoliotic posture [35].

The reflected contracture of the hamstring has been associated to an irradiation of the nerve root or to an attempt to control the stability of the lumbosacral junction.

Lumbar pain related to alteration of the small posterior joints (facet syndrome). It is characteristic, but not inherent to spondylolysis already present or spondylolisthesis. It is related to a certain degree of lumbar instability or with a defective function of the olisthesic segment. Some authors consider the instability as responsible for the majority of lumbar pains in segments with isthmic lesion [36]. These would be false sciatica or pseudo-sciatica.

Lumbar pain of root type. The patient more rarely suffers radicular or root pain in one or both lower limbs associated to lower lumbar pain. These symptoms are found more frequently in frank spondylolisthesis. Young people, unlike adults, rarely show objective signs of nerve compression, such as motor weakness, alterations in any deep tendon reflexes or sensory deficits [37].

30.4 Diagnosis

The correct evolution of spondylolysis in teenage sports people depends to a great extent on early diagnosis. Therefore, when a sports person suffers acute lumbar pain or lasting pain, with greater or lesser radiculopathy, while also suffering pain with lateral moves and lumbar rotations and during one-legged lumbar hyperextension test and with reduced flexibility of the isquiosural muscles, the presence of spondylolysis must be ruled out.

For this, regardless of the clinic, there are four complementary tests each of which with different properties and characteristics. At all times, the combination of the clinical history with one or more of these tests will give a very accurate idea of the moment of the natural history of the lesion.

(1) *Conventional radiology.* This is a very specific yet hardly sensitive test [38]. These limitations are partly due to the spatial orientation of the defect. It is advisable to perform the A/P view with a 30° of axial deviation [19, 20, 38].

The most objective image of the lesion is provided via an oblique view (Fig. 30.3). This is provided through a 45° obliquity of the ray. The lesion is typically described as a puppy with a collar or "decapitated", according to the state of mind of the observer. It is recommended that the X-rays are taken while standing, given that an apparent spondylolysis in supine position can be revealed as a spondylolisthesis when standing. Between 16% and 20% of X-rayed spondylolysis are only seen through a conventional oblique view [39].

A side view (Fig. 30.4) is capable of objectifying a large number of spondylolyses and is ideal in the diagnosis of olisthesis. Equally, functional views are important given that in spondylolisthesis these will objectify any possible instabilities [40, 41], while its use is more limited in the case of spondylolysis.

(2) *Bone scan and SPECT.* Becoming aware of the physiopathology of injuries caused by overloads is due to a great extent to bone scans with technetium^{99m}-MDP combined with a tomographic technique (SPECT). A bone scan (Fig. 30.5a) is highly sensitive but not very specific [42]. The bone scintigraphic study provides an idea of the metabolic activity of the injury and whether it is a recent or old injury. Bone scan with or without SPECT technique is the only test that assesses, with great sensitivity, whether the bone injury is metabolically active [20, 38, 42, 43].

The SPECT technique (Fig. 30.5b) improves both the sensitivity and specificity of the bone scan and simple X-ray study [16, 19, 20, 30,

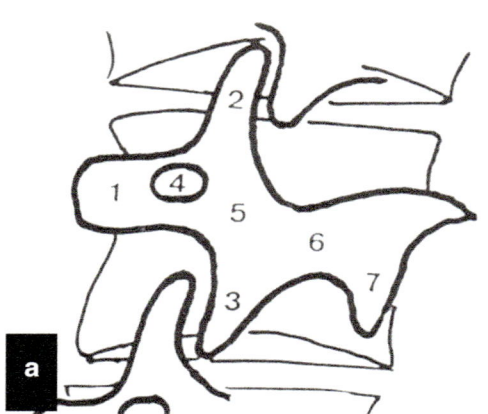 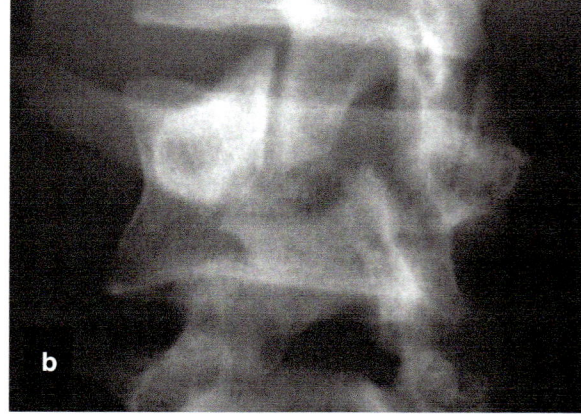

Fig. 30.3 (a) Oblique view of spondylolysis. 1, transverse process; 2, upper articular facet; 3, lower articular facet; 4, pedicle; 5, isthmus; 6, lamina; 7, spinous process. (b) 45° oblique projection of an isthmus injury

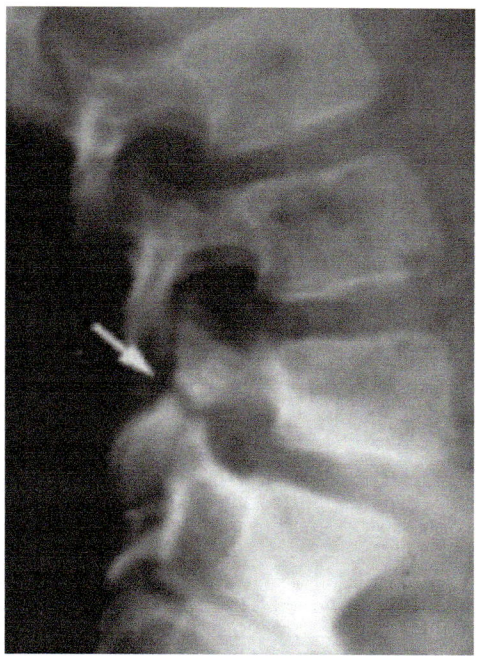

Fig. 30.4 Lumbar spine lateral view. Spondylolysis image (*arrow*) with a mild displacement of the L5 vertebra over the sacrum

42–45]. It provides information of when the injury occurred and, with this, the treatment to be followed [16, 19, 20]. The sensitivity of the bone scan for detecting spine injuries, especially in the posterior elements of the vertebrae, is significantly increased when using in combination with SPECT [44, 45]. In the lumbosacral spine, the bone SPECT increases the sensitivity by 20–50% in comparison to the planar study.

3. *Computed tomography (CT)*. The CT (Fig. 30.6) is considered to be of greater sensitivity than conventional radiology and more specific than the SPECT [44, 45]. Regardless of the cut performed, the CT will provide information on the status of the defect (acute fracture, nonconsolidated defect with geodes and sclerosis, consolidation or repair process of the pars) [46].

The *reverse gantry* view, perpendicular to the conventional, provides a greater view of the injury. It provides us with valuable information on the characteristics of the edges of the isthmic defect.

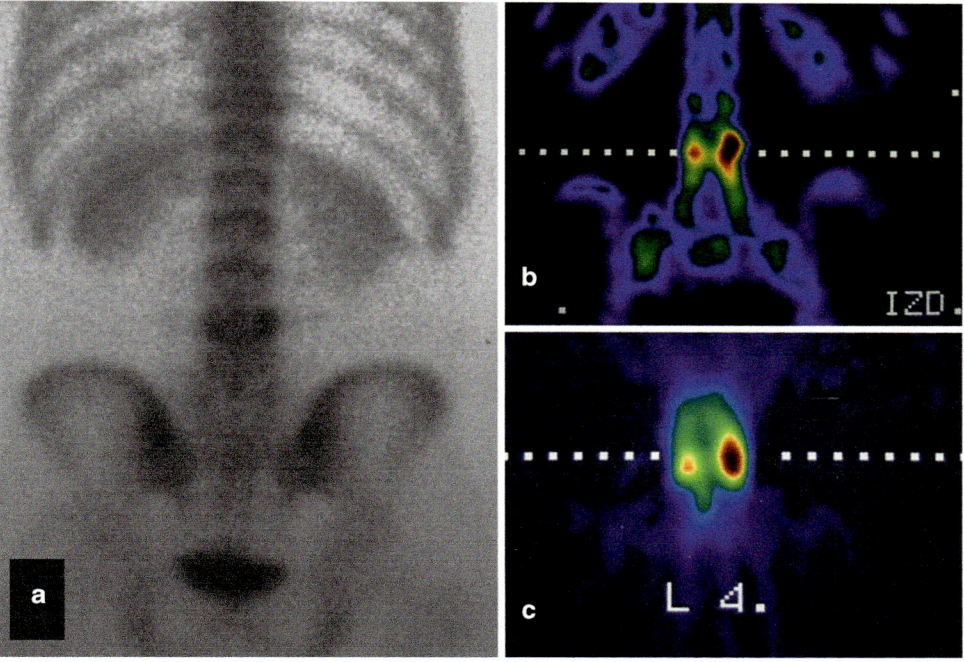

Fig. 30.5 (a) Planar bone scintigraphy image with increased uptake of the left L4 spinal bone comparing with right. SPECT bone examination coronal (b) and axial (c) image with the same increased uptake

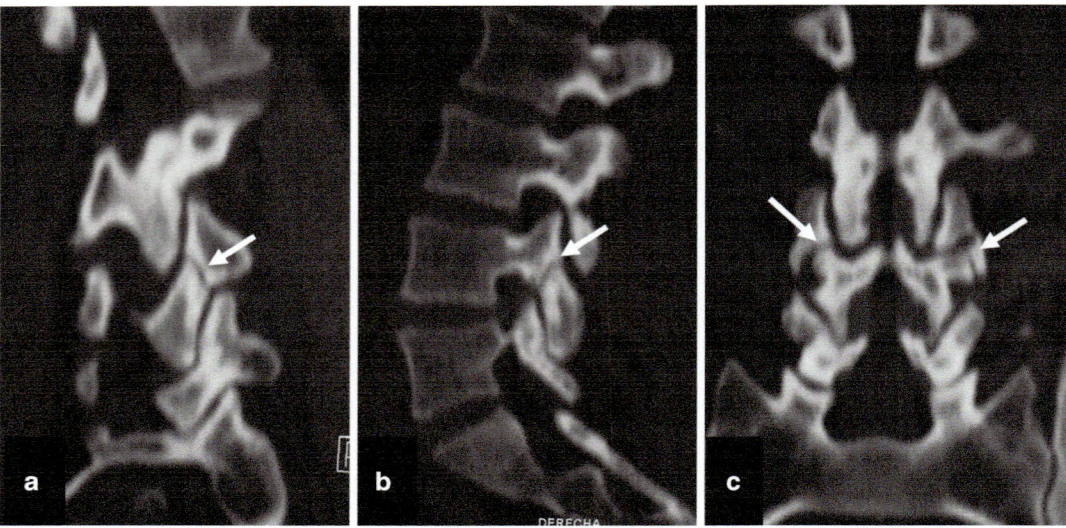

Fig. 30.6 Obliquely (**a**), sagittally (**b**) and coronally (**c**) reconstructed CT of the lumbar spine shows a defect of the pars interarticularis on the L4 (arrows). In coronal view is visible bilateral injury

4. *Magnetic resonance.* **It** allows to assess the injuries which are also associated to objectifying the isthmic injury [46]. The normal *pars* is viewed better in the T1 sequence than in T2 sequence. This technique objectifies that only three quarters of the *pars* are strictly normal [23, 47]. The MRI is also useful for assessing the fibrocartilaginous mass which develops at *pars* defect level (Gill's module).

The MRI is capable of detecting spondylolysis early on (Fig. 30.7). MRI allows for early objectivation of signal changes at *pars* level which are catalogued as "stress responsive" of the same and can be classified into different degrees of activity [48].

As discussed above, early diagnosis of the pathology is essential. Thus, in light of clinical suspicion of a spondylolysis, it is recommended to first request a bone scan with SPECT to obtain or rule out the diagnosis and, then, carry out follow-up MRI studies (except in specific cases in which it is believed that control should be carried out by means of bone scan with SPECT to assess the metabolic activity of the lesion). The use of CT is reserved for cases in which the exact pars defect is to be determined.

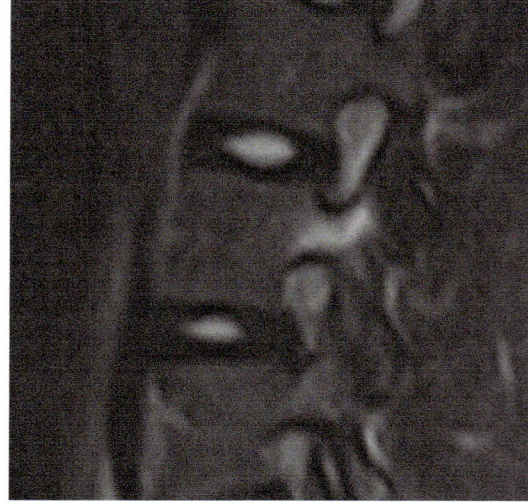

Fig. 30.7 Sagittal MRI image shows well-limited stress reaction in the pars interarticularis

30.5 Prognostic Factors

One of the main concerns is the progression to spondylolisthesis. In general, in sports, the risk of a spondylolysis, either with or without a low-grade spondylolisthesis, progressing to greater slipping is low [16, 19, 20]. The progression of the slippage can be seen in teenagers during growth spurts, and it seems that the initial slippage is greater in females [49].

Different factors have been proposed as prognostic factors: dysplastic alterations associated to the isthmic injury, degree of associated disc degeneration and instability. These last two concepts are closely related to each other given that disc degeneration involves instability, and this instability can be assessed by means of an MRI study of dynamic functional radiology.

Associated dysplastic alterations. The olisthesis that is typically from practising sports is the isthmic variation. However, the physician must identify whether the olisthesis is of a dysplastic origin, given that by definition the olisthesis may be greater. Having spina bifida occulta (SBO) is a prognostic factor for suffering a *pars* lesion or greater olisthesis [12, 16, 20, 50]. Equally, the dysplastic lumbosacral morphology is a predisposing factor to suffering spondylolysis with or without olisthesis. These are two alterations to be considered: the trapezoidal aspect of the fifth lumbar vertebra and the console shape of the upper surface of the sacrum. Observing these two alterations provide a simple way of assessing the possible progression or lack of (Fig. 30.8).

Associated disc degeneration. It has been proven that there is correlation between disc degeneration and spondylolysis and spondylolisthesis. Disc degeneration could facilitate olisthesis [37].

The disc degeneration process that occurs in parallel to the listhesic phenomenon goes through three stages [51]. First is *dysfunction*, in which there are minimum pathological changes in the disc, without causing alteration in its functionality. Second is *instability*, in which the height of the disc decreases and all the fibrous rings distend around the circumference transversally drawn by the disc. Third is *re-stabilisation*, the stage presided by the fibrous and osteophytic stabilisation of the segment.

Currently, by performing MRI the control and/or diagnosis of spondylolysis in young ath-

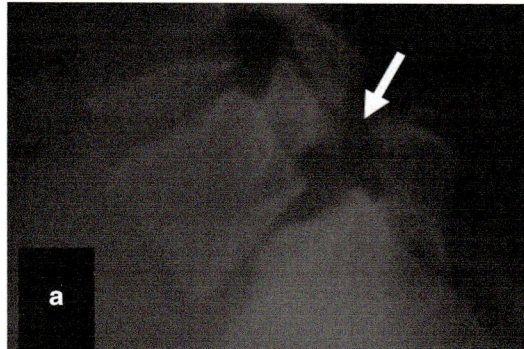
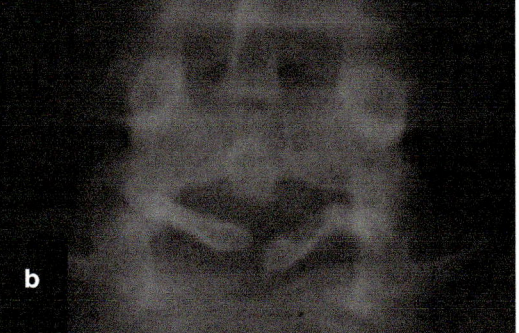
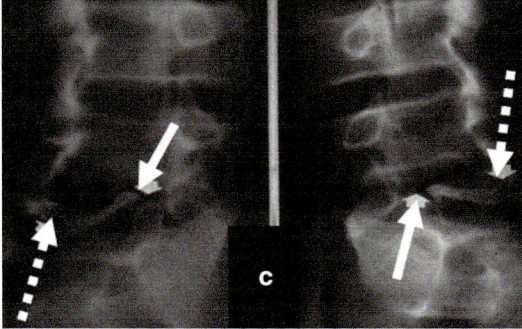

Fig. 30.8 Radiographic study of the lumbar spine shows spondylolysis at L5 (arrows) in lumbosacral dysplasia. (**a**) Sagittal view shows trapezoidal spinal bone with sacral promontory in S italic. (**b**) Frontal view shows spina bifida occulta at L5 related to injury. (**c**) Bilateral oblique view shows "floating sheet" limited by spondylolysis and spina bifida occulta (discontinuous arrows)

letes leads to more and more examples of these small disc degenerations at earlier ages.

Instability. The instability from a clinical point of view is the loss of the capacity of the rachis, due to physiological overload, to maintain its position between vertebrae, in such a way that

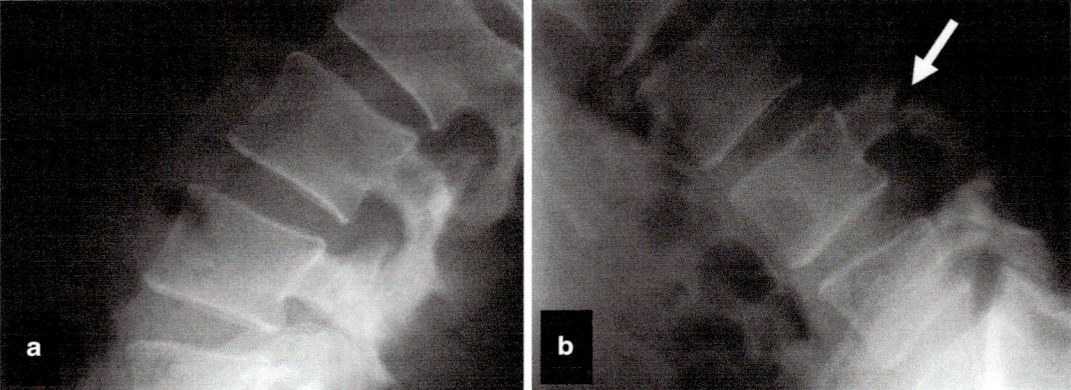

Fig. 30.9 Lateral view—extension (**a**) and flexion (**b**). A mild instability is observed that allows objectifying the isthmic defect during the flexion

there will be a lesion due to the instability itself and the subsequent irritation of the spinal canal or of the nerve roots. This disc functionalism is widely variable depending on age, gender, flexibility (obesity-thinness) or even in the same individual in different radiological examinations [38, 52]. The functional radiological examination must be performed under solely clinical criteria, observing the uniform closure of the discs to obtain a harmonious and regular lumbar curve [38, 52].

When performing radiological studies of the lumbar spine in maximum flexion and extension or with different types of loads, this often confirms, especially in the early stage of slippage, the presence of exaggerated mobility of the olisthesic vertebrae [52].

A dynamic study can be very useful for detecting some cases of lysis, of unnoticeable displacements in conventional standing examinations, and especially in the case of isthmic lesions in athletes (Fig. 30.9) [38].

As a criterion of instability, one assesses an abnormal movement exceeding a 12° dynamic angulation or an 8% intervertebral movement [53].

Another prognostic factor that should be considered, especially in tennis players, is that the pathology affects L5 and/or appears between the ages of 12 and 16 years as this is when athletes are undergoing their development process.

30.6 Treatment

Except for advanced cases and those with associated complications, the treatment of spondylolysis in tennis players is conservative. The reconstruction of the *pars* can be done using different types of support braces [16, 19, 20]. These may be rigid or soft and can exert on the rachis an anti-lordotic action or simply limiting lumbar extension [19].

The major discussions are in relation to the length of time this support brace should be worn for. In this sense, there are works that recommend 2 or 3 months' immobilisation or less and other recommend up to 6 months. We must also take into consideration that in many cases, excellent clinical results are obtained without the reconstruction of the pars, which is visible in X-rays, while isotopic or MRI tests show no activity [19, 20, 26, 54].

It must be noted that an isthmic lesion can be classified as *lysis in formation* (with osteogenesis activity objectified through SPECT and negative radiology), *active lysis* (with increased uptake SPECT and lesion visible through conventional radiology) or *silent or terminal lysis* (positive radiology with negative isotope study) [55]. Adapting this classification to the various studies consulted, the isthmic reconstruction of these has been seen in *forming* lesions and has been virtually non-existent in *silent or terminal lysis* and sometimes possible in *active lysis*. On the other hand, it seems that reconstructions are more likely to occur in cases involving unilateral lesion.

It is clear that when faced with an isthmic lesion that produces symptoms, the steps to follow will include athletic rest and avoiding associated activities that increase lumbar pain.

This treatment by means of wearing a support brace and athletic rest must be associated to carrying out lumbar recovery exercises that will be incorporated gradually as of the third or fourth week of wearing the support brace.

When conservative treatment fails, the recommendation would be to undergo surgical treatment, which becomes necessary in 9–15% of the cases of spondylolysis and/or low-grade spondylolisthesis. These are cases in which the slippage is progressive, the pain is untreatable or the lumbar pain is associated to neurological deficit or spinal instability [16, 20, 56].

30.7 Pathological Situations to be Considered

To determine the conduct to be implemented, we must take into account the biological age of the athlete, his/her growth potential and the symptoms suffered. All this is considered along with the results of the different complementary tests, to find out which stage the isthmic injury is at. In teenage tennis players, there are two possible situations based on their age and the existing injury:

- Child or teenager with spondylolysis
- Child or teenager with spondylolisthesis

30.8 Child or Teenager with Spondylolysis (Algorithm 1)

In a child or a teenager, faced with the suspicion of isthmic injury, we would initially carry out a radiographic study with postero-anterior, lateral and oblique projections at 45° associated to a SPECT bone scan. Based on these results, if necessary, the study may be complemented by a scan. There are three pathological situations which we may have to face.

30.9 Spondylolysis in Formation

It is very important that the pathology is diagnosed during this stage, as the prognosis improves considerably and the necessary treatment tends to

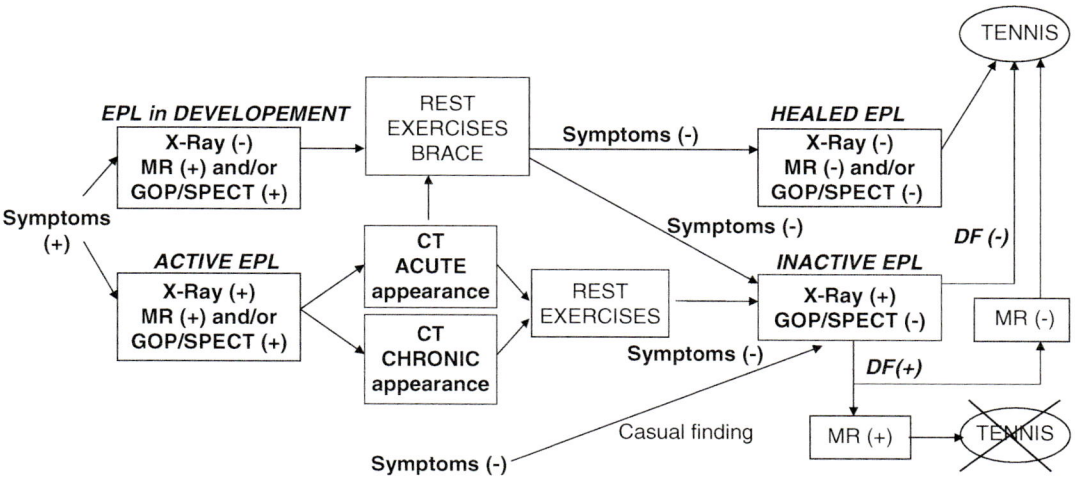

Algorithm 1 Algorithm to follow in an EPL in a child or adolescent

be less. Spondylolysis is suspected in an athlete that is seen due to suggestive lumbar pain and with reaction to stress observed in MRI or uptake bone scan with SPECT at isthmic level, even though the X-ray does not show lytic image. The corresponding formula will be:

clinic (+) + X-ray (−) + MRI (+) and/or bone scan/SPECT (+)

Faced with this situation, athletic rest is recommended. The patient may use a support brace until reaching negative tendency of the clinic and evident reduction in the sign shown in the MRI or the bone scan SPECT. The type of support brace, flexible or not, rigid or soft, must be optional and will ultimately depend on the physician responsible for the athlete. The objectives of the immobilisation are to repair the *pars* deffect and to reduce the pain. The time which the brace should be worn and the type of brace is highly variable. Within the Spanish Tennis Federation, as these are young individuals practising sports, often at a very high level, we consider that the brace should be worn for a minimum of 6 weeks. Thanks to which we will at least manage to eliminate the symptoms and in some cases the stabilisation and fusion of the pars.

It must be noted that if SPECT technique has been used; the negative tendency is hard to assess, as the great sensitivity of this method must be taken into consideration, given that it can capture minimum osteoblastic activities. Therefore, in many cases, we must consider the sharp decline in the uptake, associated to a total clinical improvement. The formula for this situation would be:

clinic (−) + X-ray (−) + MRI (−) and/or bone scan/SPECT (−)

In principle, when seeing a negative tendency, the athlete will be allowed to return to sports activities in a very progressive manner and not without previously implementing an in-depth stabilisation guideline at vertebral and lumbopelvic regions. On the occasions when the clinic is reactivated with pain and MRI (+) and/or bone scan/SPECT (+), the protocol will be applied again.

30.10 Active Spondylolysis

This situation is the one generally diagnoses either due to late consultation of the athlete or due to a lack of early diagnosis. This occurs when the studied clinic coincides with the existence of a radiologically verified lysis and a positive MRI and/or bone scan with SPECT. The corresponding formula will be:

clinic (+) + X-ray (+) + MRI (+) and/or bone scan/SPECT (+)

In light of this clinical picture and image, athletic rest is essential until seeing a clear reduction in the stress reaction shown by the MRI and/or reduction in uptake of the bone scan/SPECT. The use of a support brace will depend on whether an MRI or CT are performed, as these offer an image of the bone structure of the pars.

If the CT scan or MRI shows an image of continuity solution with sclerosis on the edges, periosteal reaction in the recent defect, geodes and irregular periosteal reaction, the use of a flexible support brace will be discouraged. The simple observation of the separation between the edges of the defect may lead us to think of greater difficulty for consolidation.

In the event of the edges of the fracture being clean and of recent appearance, using an immobilising support brace can be of great help and also optional.

The formula to consider for assessing the inactivation will be:

clinic (−) + X-ray (+/−) + MRI (−) and/or bone scan/SPECT (−)

In this case it can be seen that the isthmic lesion will be repaired or not in X-ray imaging, mainly depending on the condition of the pars when subjected to CT scan and the conduct to be followed. This would allow to reach the healing that could be summed up in this formula:

[clinic (−), X-ray (−), MRI (−) and/or bone scan/SPECT (−)]

or to the last diagnostic possibility, inactive spondylolysis.

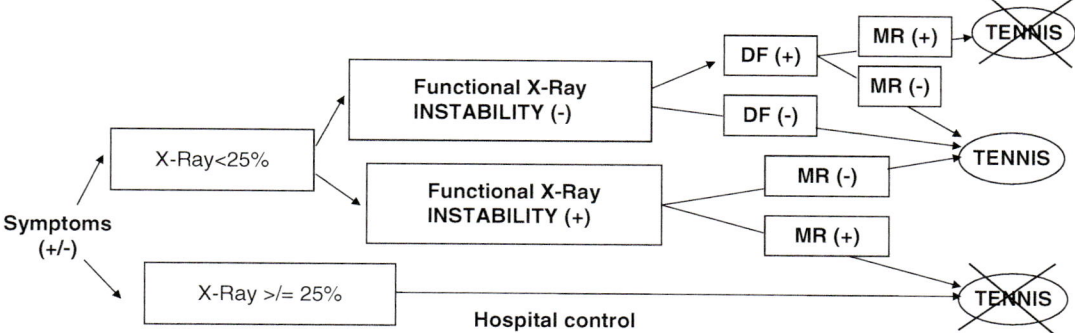

Algorithm 2 Algorithm in EPLT in a child or adolescent

30.11 Inactive Spondylolysis

This situation can be reached as of a case of active lysis or as a result of a casual finding in the course of a routine examination of the spine. The formula will be:

clinic (−) + X-ray (+) + MRI (−) and/or bone scan/SPECT (−)

When faced with this clinical picture, it is necessary to qualify according to the characteristics of the different cases. If the tennis player has a single dysplastic factor, or none, the athlete will be allowed to return to sports, regardless of the type and intensity of said sports.

On the other hand, if the tennis player is recreational and has more than one dysplastic factor (DF) associated to a marked disc alteration objectified by MRI, the athlete will be advised as a preventive measure to abandon tennis and turn physical activities that are less harmful to the lumbar spine.

In a tennis player with high-level growth, the latter will be allowed to continue playing the sport but reducing its intensity to avoid collateral exercises to tennis that could harm the lumbar spine.

30.12 Child or Teenager with Spondylolisthesis (Algorithm 2)

The conduct to be followed in the case of a child or teenager with spondylolisthesis is not only subject to the severity of the clinical picture. Whether there is lumbar pain or not and whether it irradiates or not, the conduct to be followed must be based on the existence of vertebral instability and the degree of disc degeneration. As a criterion of instability, we will assess an abnormal movement exceeding a 12° dynamic angulation or an 8% intervertebral movement.

30.13 Grade I Spondylolisthesis

In cases of spondylolisthesis with less than 25% displacement (grade I), we must assess the degree of instability this entails, as well as the associated disc degeneration. Therefore, a functional X-ray study and MRI must be carried out. As a criterion of instability, we will assess an abnormal movement exceeding a 12° dynamic angulation or an 8% intervertebral movement. In the event of not objectifying instability, the formula will be:

X-ray < 25%, instability (−)

In these cases, all sports may be practices, except when there is more than one dysplastic factor, situation in which an MRI must be carried out. If this shows signs of disc degeneration, the athlete will be advised to not play tennis.

If instability is objectified, an MRI must be carried out to assess the disc degeneration. When faced with a spine with grade I spondylolisthesis which is stable, without disc degeneration, the formula will be:

X-ray < or = 25% instability (+) MRI (−)

In this case the athlete will be allowed to play tennis at any level, regardless of the dysplastic factors.

When faced with lumbosacral instability with disc degeneration, the athlete will be advised to abandon playing tennis of any intensity.

X-ray < or = 25% instability (+) MRI (+)

30.14 Grade II or above Spondylolisthesis

When a teenage tennis player suffers from grade II spondylolisthesis, which corresponds to a percentage of 25% or above, this will force the athlete from abandoning all tennis regardless of its intensity. Equally, it is highly recommended that the evolution of the olisthesis is monitored at a hospital.

References

1. Amato ME, Totty WG, Gilula LA. Spondylolysis of the lumbar spine: demonstration of defects and laminal fragmentation. Radiology. 1984;153:627–9.
2. Danielson BI, Frennered AK, Irstam LK. Radiologic progression of isthmic lumbar spondylolisthesis in young patients. Spine. 1991;16:422–5.
3. Lee J, Ehara S, Tamakawa Y, et al. Spondylolysis of the upper lumbar spine: radiological features. Clin Imaging. 1999;23:389–93.
4. Roche MB, Rowe GG. The incidence of separate neural arch and coincident bone variations. J Bone Joint Surg. 1952;34:491–4.
5. Rossi F. Spondylolysis, spondylolisthesis and sports. J Sport Med Phys Fit. 1978;18:317–40.
6. Rossi F, Dragoni S. Lumbar spondylolysis: occurrence in competitive athletes. Updated achievements in a series of 390 cases. J Sport Med Phys Fit. 1990;30:450–3.
7. Sairyo K, Katoh S, Sasa T, et al. Athletes with unilateral spondylolysis are at risk of stress fracture at the contralateral pedicle and pars interarticularis. A clinical and biomechanical study. Am J Sports Med. 2005;33(4):583–90.
8. Randall R, Silverstein M, Goodwin R. Review of pediatric spondylolysis and spondylolisthesis. Sports Med Arthrosc Rev. 2016;24:184–7.
9. Fredrickson BE, Baker D, McHollick WJ, Yuan HA, Lubicky JP. The natural history of spondylolysis and spondylolisthesis. J Bone Joint Surg. 1984;66:699–707.
10. Morita T, Ikata T, Katoh S, Miyake R. Lumbar spondylolysis in children and adolescents. J Bone Joint Surg. 1995;77B:620–5.
11. Nozawa S, Shimizu K, Miyamoto K, et al. Repair of pars interarticularis defect by segmental wire fixation in young athletes with spondylolysis. Am J Sports Med. 2003;31(3):359–64.
12. Lawrence JP, Greene HS, Grauer JN. Back pain in athletes. J Am Acad Orthop Surg. 2006;14:726–35.
13. Jones GT, Macfarlane GJ. Epidemiology of low back pain in children and adolescents. Arch Dis Child. 2005;90:312–6.
14. Simper LB. Spondylolysis in eskimo skeletons. Acta Orthop Scand. 1986;57:78–80.
15. Cassidy RC, Shaffer WO, Johnson DL. Spondylolysis and spondylolisthesis in the athlete. Sports Med Update. 2005;28(11):1331.
16. Standaert CJ, Herring SA. Expert opinion and controversies in sports and musculoskeletal medicine: the diagnosis and treatment of spondylolysis in adolescent athletes. Arch Phys Med Rehabil. 2007;88(4):537–40.
17. Micheli LJ, Wood R. Back pain in young athletes: significant differences from adults in causes and patterns. Arch Pediatr Adolesc Med. 1995;149:15–8.
18. Hensinger RN. Spondylolysis and spondylolisthesis in children. Instr Course Lect. 1983;32:132–51.
19. Ruiz-Cotorro A, Balius Matas R, Estruch Massana A, Vilaro Angulo J. Spondylolysis in young tennis players. Br J Sports Med. 2006;40:441–6.
20. McCleary MD, Congeni JA. Current concepts in the diagnosis and treatment of spondylolysis in young athletes. Curr Sports Med Rep. 2007;6(1):62–6.
21. Wynne-Davies R, Scots JHS. Inheritance and spondylolisthesis. J Bone Joint Surg Am. 1979;61:301–5.
22. Albanese M, Pizzutillo P. Family study of spondylolysis and spondylolisthesis. J Pediatr Orthop. 1982;2:464–99.
23. Bennett DL, Nassar L, DeLano MC. Lumbar spine MRI in the elite-level female gymnast with low back pain. Skelet Radiol. 2006;35:503–9.
24. Sagi HC, Jarvis JG, Uhthoff HK. Histomorphic analysis of the development of the pars interarticularis and its association with isthmic spondylolysis. Spine. 1998;23:1635–40.
25. Miller SF, Congeni J, Swanson K. Long-term functional and anatomical follow up of early detected spondylolysis in young athletes. Am J Sports Med. 2004;32:928–33.
26. Kim HJ, Green DW. Spondylolysis in the adolescent athlete. Curr Opin Pediatr. 2011;23:68–72.
27. Nyska M, Constantini N, Cale-Benzoor M, Back Z, Kahn G, Mann G. Spondylolysis as a cause of low back pain in swimmers. Int J Sports Med. 2000;21:375–9.
28. Soler T, Calderon C. The prevalence of spondylolysis in the Spanish elite athlete. Am J Sports Med. 2000;28:57–62.
29. Sakai T, Sairyo K, Suzue N, Kosaka H, Yasui N. Incidence and etiology of lumbar spondylolysis: review of the literature. J Orthop Sci. 2010;15(3):281–8.

30. Wiltse LL, Newman PH, MacNab J. Classification of spondylolysis and spondylolisthesis. Clin Orthop Relat Res. 1976;117:23–9.
31. Hasler C, Dick W. Spondylolysis and spondylolisthesis during growth. Orthopade. 2002;31:78–87.
32. Logroscino G, Mazza O, Aulisa G, Pitta L, Pola E, Aulisa L. Spondylolysis and spondylolisthesis in the pediatric and adolescent population. Childs Nerv Syst. 2001;17(11):644–55.
33. Bhatia NN, Chow G, Timon SJ, Watts HG. Diagnostic modalities for the evaluation of pediatric back pain: a prospective study. J Pediatr Orthop. 2008;28:230–3.
34. Tallarico RA, Madom IA, Palumbo MA. Spondylolysis and spondylolisthesis in the athlete. Sports Med Arthrosc. 2008;16:32–8.
35. Masci L, Pike J, Malara F, Phillips B, Bennell K, Brukner P. Use of the one-legged hyperextension test and magnetic resonance imaging in the diagnosis of active spondylolysis. Br J Sports Med. 2006;40(11):940–6.
36. Hu SS, Tribus CB, Diab M, Ghanayem AJ. Spondylolisthesis and spondylolysis. J Bone Joint Surg Am. 2008;90:656–71.
37. Salminen JJ, Erkintalo MO, Pentti J, Oksanen A. Recurrent low back pain and early disc degeneration in the young. Spine. 1999;24:1316–21.
38. Ward CV, Latimer B, Alander DH, et al. Radiographic assessment of lumbar facet distance spacing and spondylolysis. Spine. 2007;32:E85–8.
39. Libson E, Bloom RA, Dinari G, Robin G. Oblique lumbar spine radiographs importance in young patients. Spine. 1984;151:89–90.
40. Friberg O. Lumbar instability: a dynamic approach by traction-compression radiography. Spine. 1987;12:119–29.
41. Beck NA, Miller R, Baldwin K, et al. Do oblique views add value in the diagnosis of spondylolysis in adolescents? J Bone Joint Surg Am. 2013;95:e65.
42. Van der Wall H, Storey G, Magnussen J, et al. Distinguishing scintigraphic features of spondylolysis. J Pediatr Orthop. 2002;22:308–11.
43. Takemitsu M, El Rassi G, Woratanarat P, Shah SA. Low back pain in pediatric athletes with unilateral tracer uptake at the pars interarticularis on single photon emission computed tomography. Spine. 2006;31:909–14.
44. Gregory PL, Batt ME. SPECT and rg-CT findings in patients with back pain investigated for spondylolysis. Clin J Sport Med. 2005;15(2):79–86.
45. Trout AT, Sharp SE, Anton CG, et al. Spondylolysis and beyond: value of SPECT/CT in evaluation of low back pain in children and young adults. Radiographics. 2015;35:819–34.
46. Campbell RS, Grainger AJ, Hide IG, Papastefanou S, Greenough CG. Juvenile spondylolysis: a comparative analysis of CT, SPECT and MRI. Skelet Radiol. 2005;34(2):63–73.
47. Rush JK, Astur N, Scott S, et al. Use of magnetic resonance imaging in the evaluation of spondylolysis. J Pediatr Orthop. 2015;35:271–5.
48. Major NM, Helms CA, Richardson WJ. MR imaging of fibrocartilaginous masses arising on the margins of spondylolysis defects. AJR. 1999;173:673–6.
49. Muschik M, Hahnel H, Robinson PN, et al. Competitive sports and the progression of spondylolisthesis. J Pediatr Orthop. 1996;16:364–9.
50. Urrutia J, Cuellar J, Zamora T. Spondylolysis and spina bifida occulta in pediatric patients: prevalence study using computed tomography as a screening method. Eur Spine J. 2016;25:590–5.
51. Hammerberg KW. New concepts on the pathogenesis and classification of spondylolisthesis. Spine (Phila Pa 1976). 2005;30(Suppl):S4–11.
52. Li Y, Hresko MT. Radiographic analysis of spondylolisthesis and sagittal spinopelvic deformity. J Am Acad Orthop Surg. 2012;20:194–205.
53. Wood KB, Popp CA, Transfeldt EE, Geissele AE. Radiographic evaluation of instability in spondylolisthesis. Spine. 1994;19:1697–703.
54. Sairyo K, Sakai T, Yasui N. Conservative treatment of lumbar spondylolysis in childhood and adolescence: the radiological signs which predict healing. J Bone Joint Surg Br. 2009;91(2):206–9.
55. Balius Matas R. Espondilólisis y espondilolistesis en el deporte. Factores pronóstico y estudio longitudinal (Spondylolysis and spondylolisthesis in sports. Prognosis factors and longitudinal study). Doctoral thesis. Universitat Autònoma de Barcelona, Barcelona, 1996.
56. Lundine KM, Lewis SJ, Al-Aubaidi Z, et al. Patient outcomes in the operative and nonoperative management of high-grade spondylolisthesis in children. J Pediatr Orthop. 2014;34:483–9.

Spinal Rehabilitation Strategies for the Elite Tennis Player

Hugo Gravil and Luke Fuller

31.1 Introduction

Due to the demands of the sport of tennis, the spine has one of the highest incidences of injury within the body [1–3]. Injuries are prevalent in the spine in elite junior players [2] as well as in both male and female professional players [3].

Data from the ATP World Tour shows the region of spinal injury treated in male professional tennis players. This figure shows the most frequent spinal region injured which is the lumbar, followed by cervical. This frequency of spinal injury region has proven consistent during year over year analysis. Fewer thoracic and SI joint injuries are reported in this professional population. These injuries include facet joint involvement, muscle strains, and discal pathology.

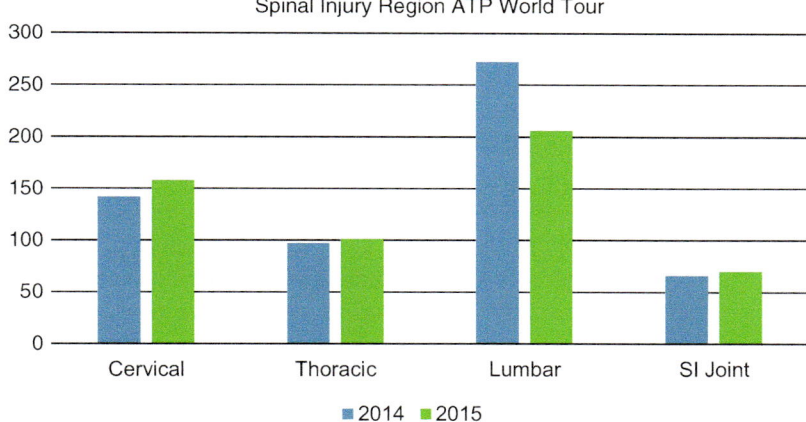

H. Gravil · L. Fuller (✉)
Ace Sports Clinic and ATP World Tour,
Toronto, ON, Canada
e-mail: lfuller@atpworldtour.com

Tennis involves multidirectional movements across multiple joints of the spine and upper and lower body [4]. These movements need to be synchronized and are often explosive, rapidly changing between concentric/eccentric and acceleration/deceleration, which requires a high level of neuromuscular control, flexibility, and spinal coordination.

Good spinal motion is an integral part of maximizing an elite tennis player's performance. The *cervical* spine is important for the ball toss, anticipation, and hand-eye coordination. The *thoracic* spine permits rotation that helps deliver elastic energy to the ball during ground strokes. The *lumbar* spine along with the surrounding "core" muscles acts as an important link and crucial zone of power for good kinetic chain motion related to the serve. The *pelvis* is the stable base on which the lower limbs can move and perform repeated directional changes. All of these distinct spinal areas then need to function in a fluid, segmental way that enables coordination and multidirectional movement.

31.2 Rehabilitation Considerations

When deciding on any specific rehabilitative or performance enhancing interventions, the practitioner should first consider a number of factors. These factors, along with others, should form part of your rationale behind your intervention selection.

31.2.1 Anatomy of the Spine

A thorough understanding of spinal anatomy and biomechanics is crucial to implement a successful, tennis-specific rehabilitation program. Basic anatomy like spinal curvatures, facet joint orientation, and regional vertebral characteristics should all be considered. Looking in a simplistic way, we can identify areas that may be taking too much load, not moving enough due to stiffness, or compensating for a concurrent injury.

While not exhaustive, some examples may include:

(a) Lack of thoracic rotation leading to lumbar disc overload
(b) Hyperextension and overload/pain of the lumbar facet joints secondary to tight hip flexors and anterior pelvic tilt
(c) Thoracic extension dysfunction caused by an upper costovertebral sprain leading to shoulder injury

31.2.2 Clinical Reasoning Behind Your Selection

A thorough clinical history and physical examination should underlie your working hypothesis. Static tests can be useful but should be carefully considered with functional tests. Especially at the elite level, athletes may only exhibit subtle asymmetries or weaknesses when challenged. One example of this may be subtle gluteal abduction weakness that is allowing energy to "leak" out of the human kinetic system. A player may have perfect balance with a Stork test or single leg balance test, but when observing landing on court and/or after ten explosive, hops may demonstrate an entirely different picture of lumbopelvic stability with a positive Trendelenburg sign.

Clinical reasoning can be developed through using a systematic approach to examination, by staying current on scientific literature, keeping an open mind and testing your working hypothesis, regular professional development and reflection, and through ongoing experience. In tennis, considering the incidence of spinal injury, surface and mechanism of injury may all be important factors in your clinical reasoning process.

31.2.3 Biomechanics of the Sport

The sport of tennis relies on fluid segmental motion and control of the spine. Some areas are relatively fixed when others are mobile, and this can change depending on the stroke and position of the player. The spine plays a key role in force generation and absorption. Understanding that the trunk and surrounding musculature form part of the kinetic system that allows the buildup of elastic energy to be recoiled and released onto the ball and ground reaction forces to be dissipated will help you build a good spinal strengthening or rehabilitation program.

Does a player lack lumbopelvic control and need enhancement of this via deep abdominal and multifidi recruitment?

Do they need more rotational power around the thoracic spine and obliques when challenged in an unbalanced position for optimal stroke mechanics?

Or can they achieve better reach and prevent back, hip, knee, and shoulder injuries by achieving better neutral zone alignment through balancing overactive hip flexor and weak extensor muscles?

These are a few questions that may need answering as part of your spinal program.

31.2.4 Player Preference

Experienced players know their bodies and have often tried many different spinal rehabilitation strategies. Listening to their opinion, what has worked in the past, can give you valuable direction.

31.2.5 Cultural Factors

Recognizing that what is practiced in one culture may not be as popular or encouraged at all in another culture may be crucial in obtaining best outcomes. Training and treatment methods, responses to pain/injury, and over- or under-training can be some factors that can vary widely between different cultures. Practicing empathy, good communication, and taking a collaborative team approach can enhance your program's success. Always involving your player in decisions and helping them understand why a particular exercise is important, benefits and helps build trust.

31.2.6 Equipment Available

While all tournaments on the ATP World Tour have a minimum standard of gym equipment available onsite, considering when and where your player will train, can influence exercises prescribed. Try to maximize what players can do when traveling easily and factor in what equipment they personally enjoy working with. An example may be that some players love to use a Pilates reformer during the off-season at home but find a Swiss ball more functional and available when traveling during the season.

31.2.7 Involvement of Coach/Fitness Trainer/Supportive Staff

Sometimes you need to offer alternatives or come to mutual agreement between different parties. Coaches, fitness trainers, and other therapists should all be considered and included. This leads to best outcomes and enables mutual respect and a team approach to be utilized in the best interest of the player.

31.2.8 Past Experience

Like anything, experience can be valuable. Calling on past experiences and successful spinal rehabilitative strategies may be beneficial in devising the best, most comprehensive spinal rehab program. Blending your individual experience and knowledge can assist in making the right calls on safe return to play, injury prevention and performance enhancement. We recommend talking to various experts not only in tennis but also in other sports to glean further ideas and build your spinal care repertoire.

31.2.9 Injury History

A player's injury history should always be considered. Have they had ongoing issues? If so, where have these been and when do they occur? Being prevention focused and open to changing when something may not be working for a particular player is recommended.

The remainder of this chapter will provide specific examples of techniques used by physiotherapists on the ATP World Tour and will provide practical application for clinicians who treat players at all levels of the game.

31.3 Dynamic Warm-Up

We recommend the use of a dynamic warm-up prior to any exercise program. A good warm-up can help increase performance and decrease injury potential, through enhancement of the cardiovascular and neuromuscular systems. In tennis, it is suggested that any dynamic warm-up program targets the shoulder, hips, and spine to prepare the athlete for the demands of the sport.

31.4 Practical Considerations of Dynamic Warm-up

Perform a general body aerobic warm-up prior to performing dynamic flexibility movements (i.e., jog around the court or do light calisthenics until a light sweat is developed).

Practice dynamic movements with one body part moving in relation to another.

Perform controlled regional segmental dynamic patterns, prior to tennis specificity.

Apply tennis-specific movement patterns.

Incorporate entire body movements and emphasize rotational movement patterns.

31.5 Examples of Dynamic Warm-Up Exercises Used on the ATP World Tour

31.5.1 Hip External Rotation Moving into Arabesque

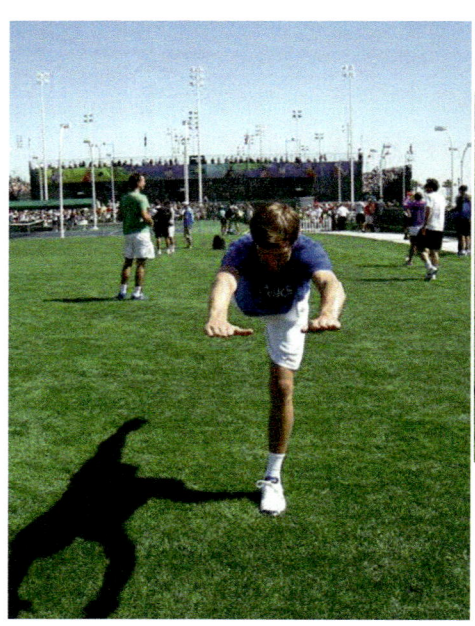
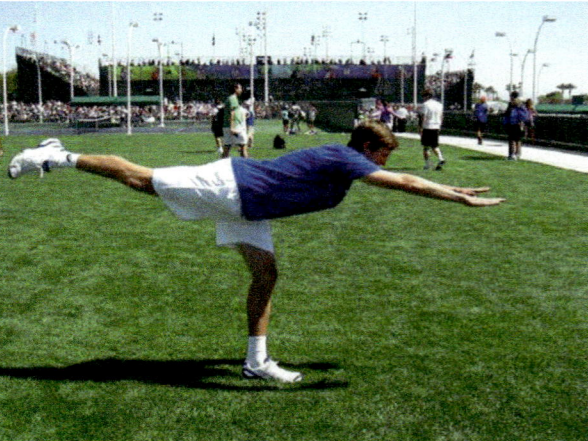

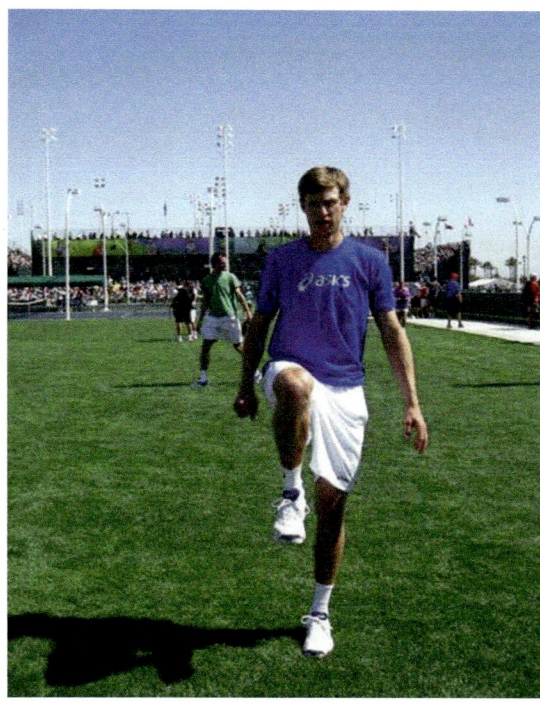
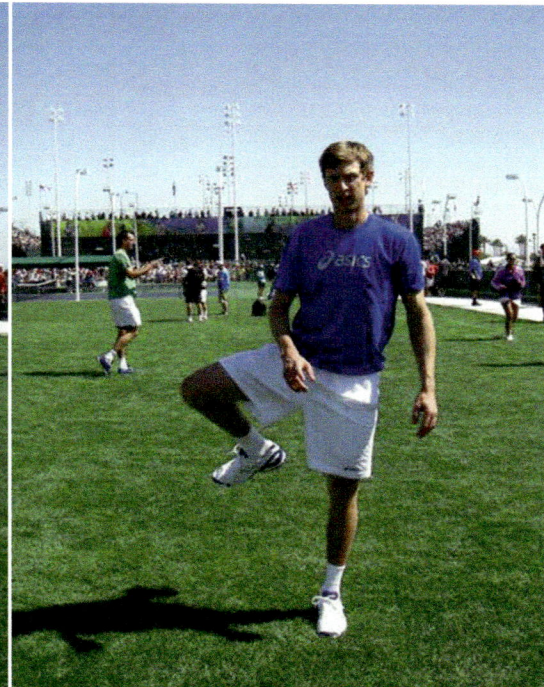

This exercise promotes balance, hip mobility, and trunk control.

Player starts standing on one leg. He then moves the knee back promoting hip external rotation before reaching out tall, lengthening the spine over the fixed foot. This helps lengthen and strengthen the hamstring and posterior chain.

31.5.2 Walking Lunge with Trunk Rotation

This exercise promotes trunk rotation with hip and knee flexion/extension.

The player walks along while lunging forward and then twisting to one side and then the other with the next step forward.

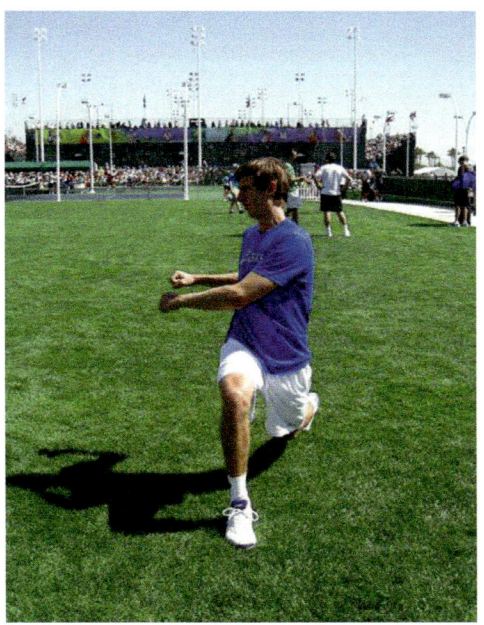

31.6 Walking Lunge with Side Reach

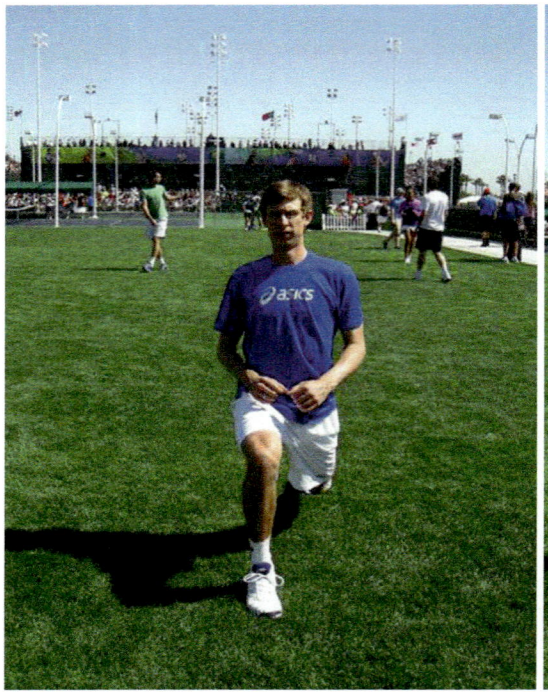 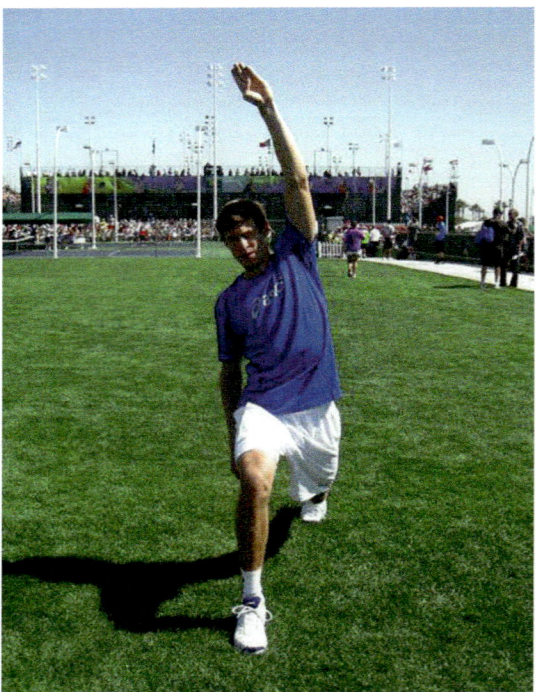

This exercise promotes trunk lateral flexion/ sidebending with hip and knee flexion/ extension.

The player walks along while lunging forward and then reaching up to one side and then the other with the next step forward.

31.6.1 Dynamic Arm Opener

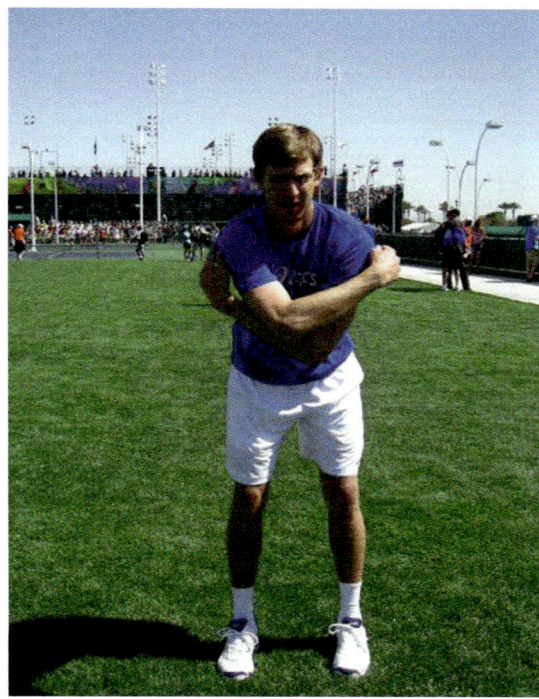
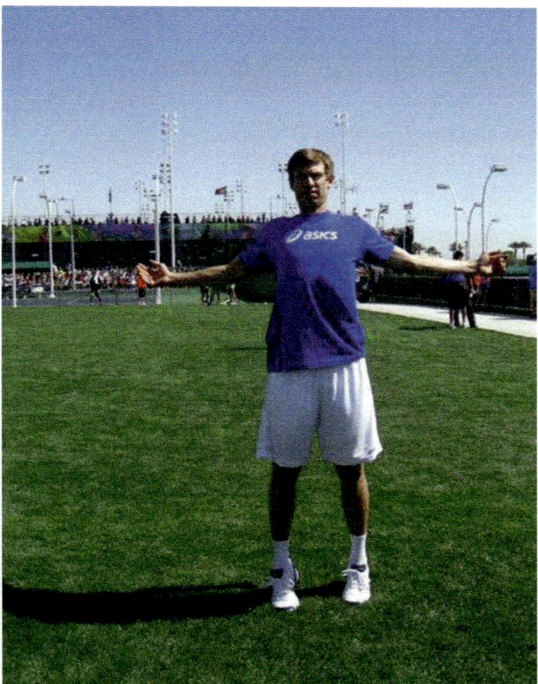

This exercise promotes hip and trunk flexion/extension while assisting to warm up the shoulders.

The player simultaneously squats down and brings his hands across his chest before explosively extending and opening his chest.

31.6.2 Downward to Upward Dog (Yoga Flow Pose)

This exercise promotes trunk flexion/extension while lengthening out the hamstrings.

31.7 Practical Aspects of Spinal Rehabilitation

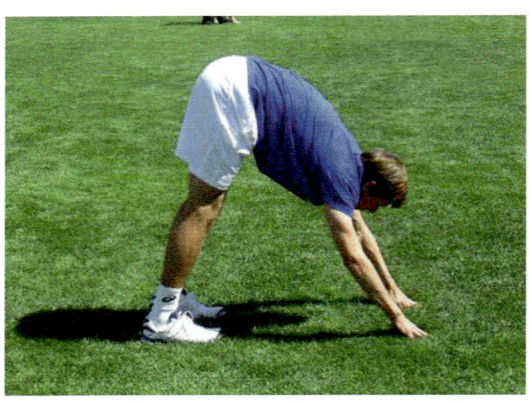
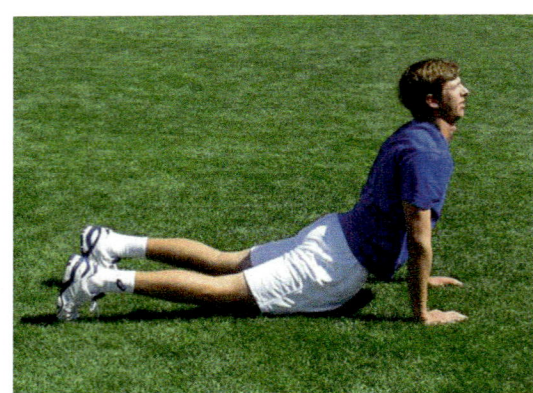

We have provided below some practical ideas and techniques to use in your spinal rehabilitation of the tennis player. While not exhaustive, we have structured these in a systematic way to include examples in different positions. We have made this component as visual and user friendly as possible, so these strategies can be applied in your practice immediately.

31.8 Supine

31.8.1 Low Spine Twist

The low spine twist is a great exercise to encourage lower spinal segmental rotation and counter-rotation of the pelvis on a relatively fixed thoracic spine. It can open tight lateral hip structures and enhance lower abdominal rotational control. This should be performed in a fluid, controlled fashion.

Player is on his back, with both hips and knees flexed and feet together on the table. The player then brings both the knees toward the table on the left side and then comes back to a neutral position, before rotating down to the right side and back again.

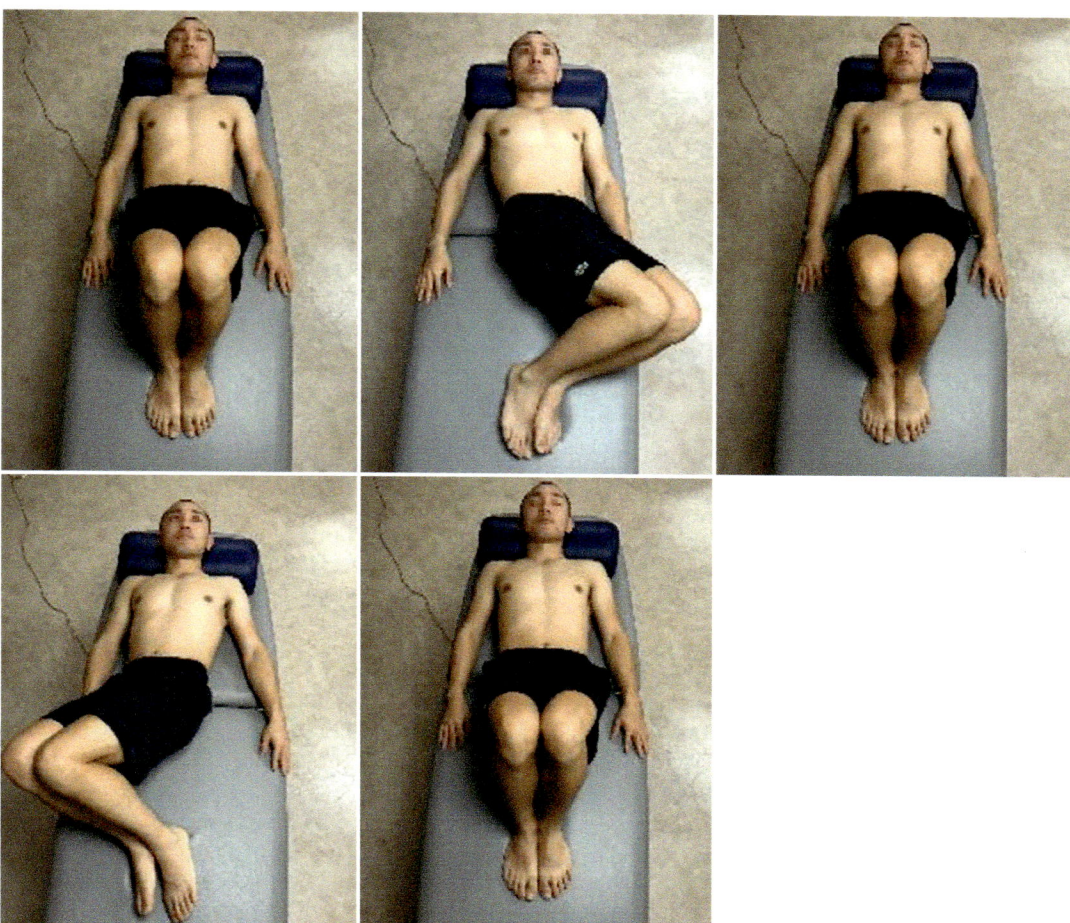

31.8.1.1 Progression

Player on his back crosses the right leg on top of the left one and rotates toward his right side and back to neutral for a predetermined number of repetitions. He then changes and crosses his left leg on top of the right one and rotates toward the left and back neutral.

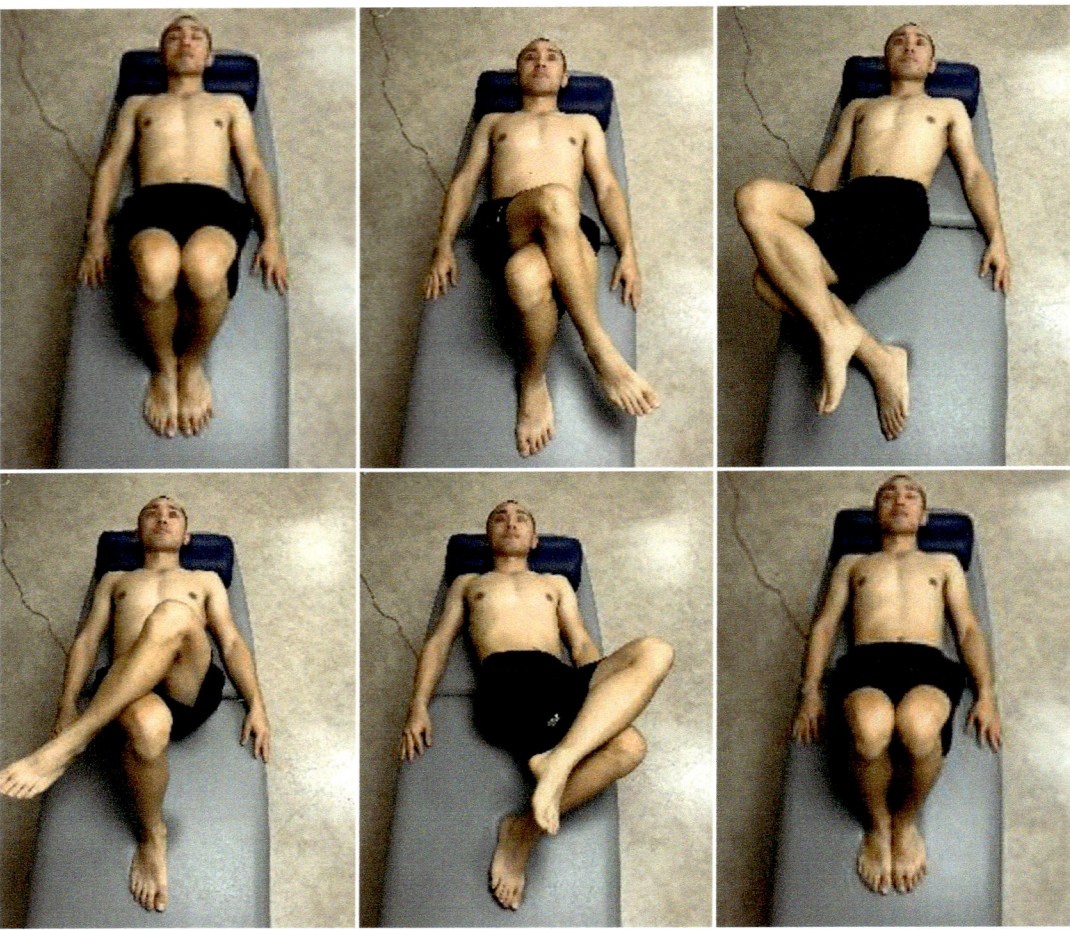

31.8.2 Pelvic Tilt

The pelvis is the foundation of the spine which influences all other spinal curves at rest and during exercise. Pelvic tilt in both directions is important for good spinal segmental motion. Too much or too little pelvic tilt in either direction can lead to spinal pain and dysfunction. Identifying a player's resting and optimal neutral pelvis before prescribing any mobility or stability exercises should guide your choice.

Player is on his back, with both hips and knees flexed and feet relaxed on the table. Player brings his pelvis backward in a *posterior pelvic tilt* (squeezes his abs and gluts) and then back to neutral and then forward in an *anterior pelvic tilt* (pushes his pelvis forward to increase distance between his low back and the table) and then back to neutral.

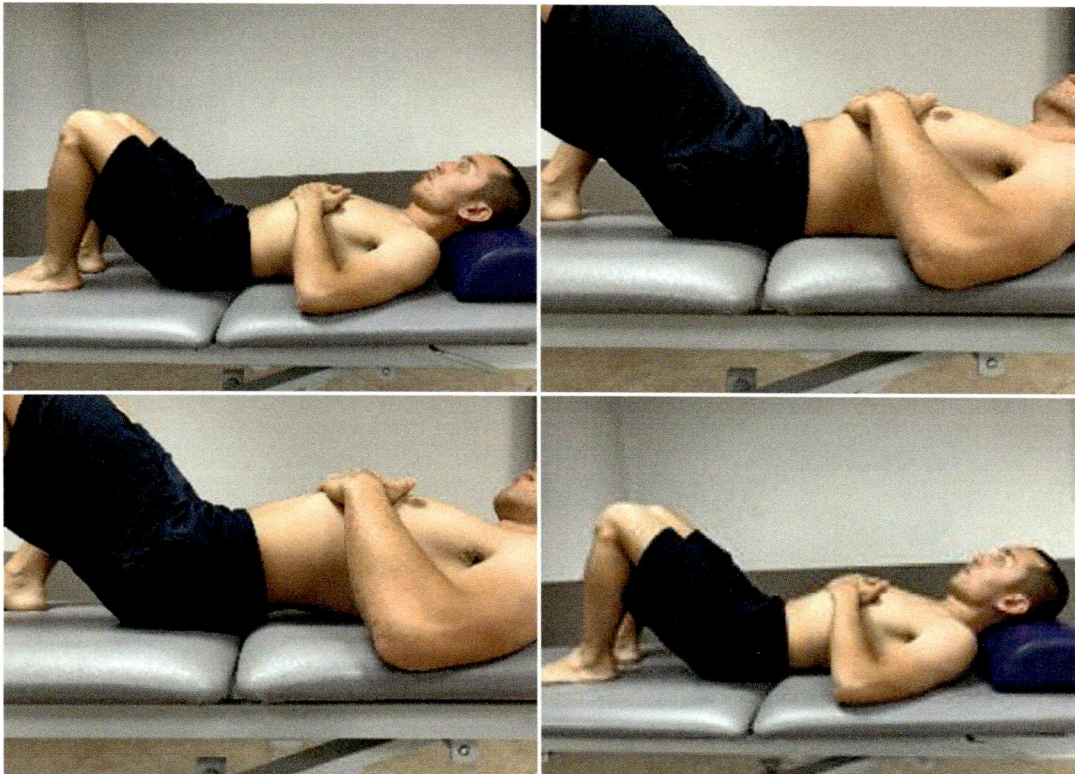

31.8.3 Enhancing Lateral Pelvic Tilt

Pelvic tilt in the coronal plane is just as important as above in the sagittal plane. Lateral pelvic tilt assists gait, the serve and on-court directional changes.

Player on his back tries to make one leg longer and one shorter and then alternates before coming back to neutral. This exercise can be used to enhance lateral pelvic tilt mobility or isometrically strengthen the pelvic stabilizers such as hip abductors.

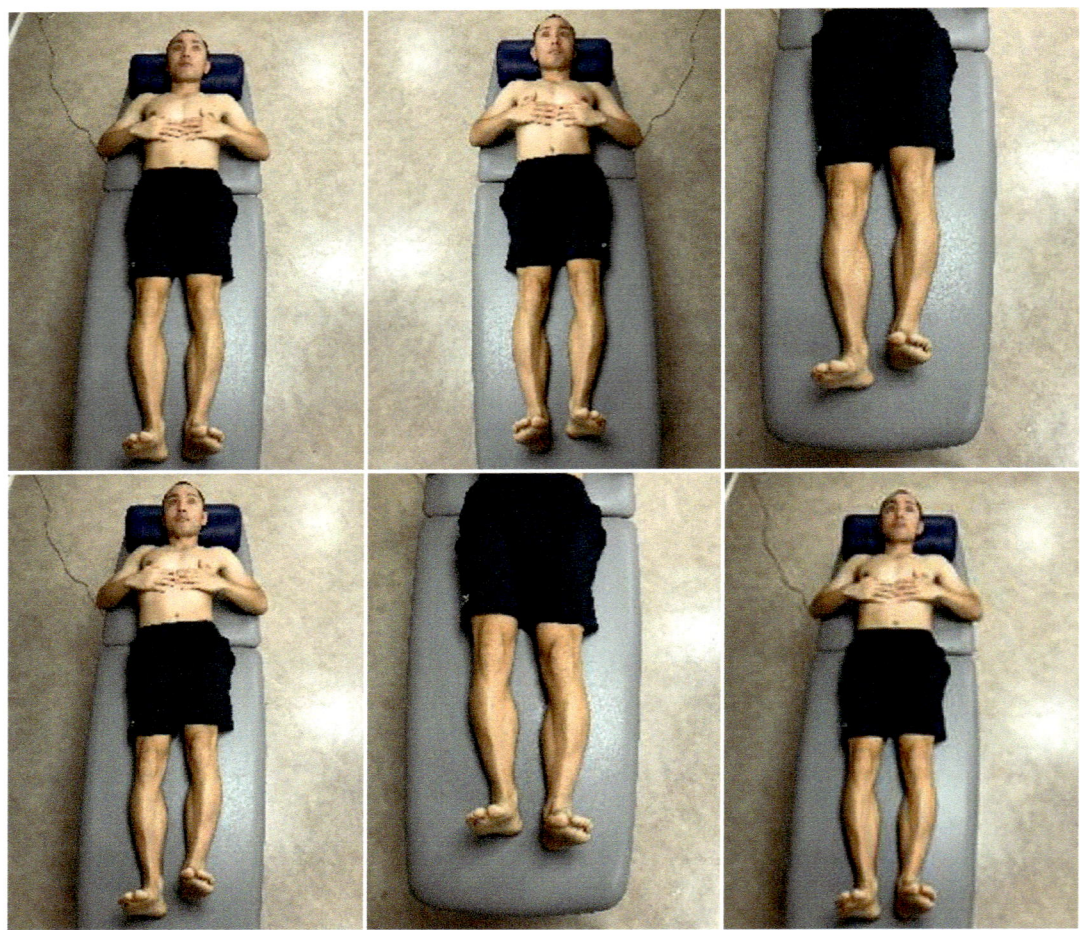

As a *progression*, the player's therapist can put manual resistance on the plantar aspect of 1 foot and on the back of the other one as he matches the resistance. The therapist then alternates his hand position, so the player can put manual resistance in the opposite direction before coming back to neutral.

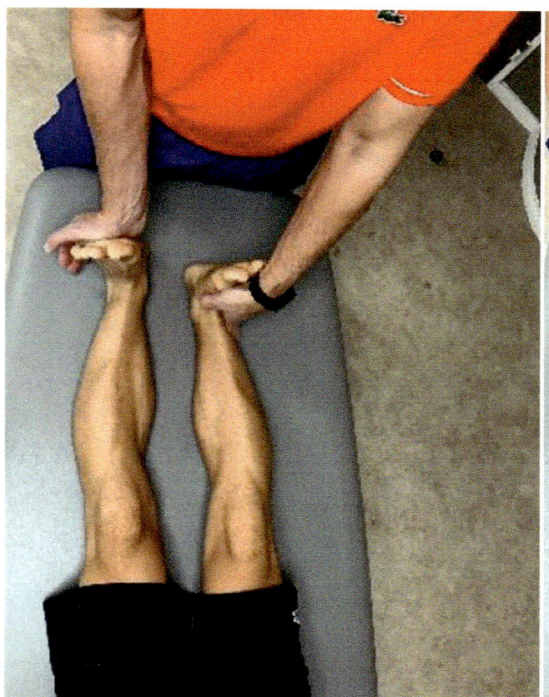 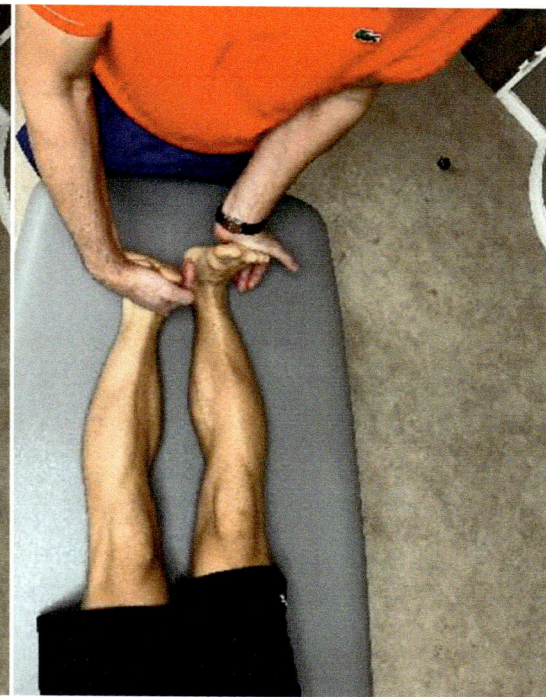

31.8.4 Strengthening Abdominal Obliques

A classical abdominal exercise is used to strengthen the oblique muscles and enhance trunk rotation.

Player is on his back, with both hips and knees flexed and feet joined together on the table. He crosses his arms on his chest and raises his trunk from the table to shoulder blade level before bringing his right shoulder close to his left knee. An isometric hold may be added, or the player can control his body back to the starting position in a concentric/eccentric fashion. Continual free flowing breathing is recommended. Repeat to the opposite side.

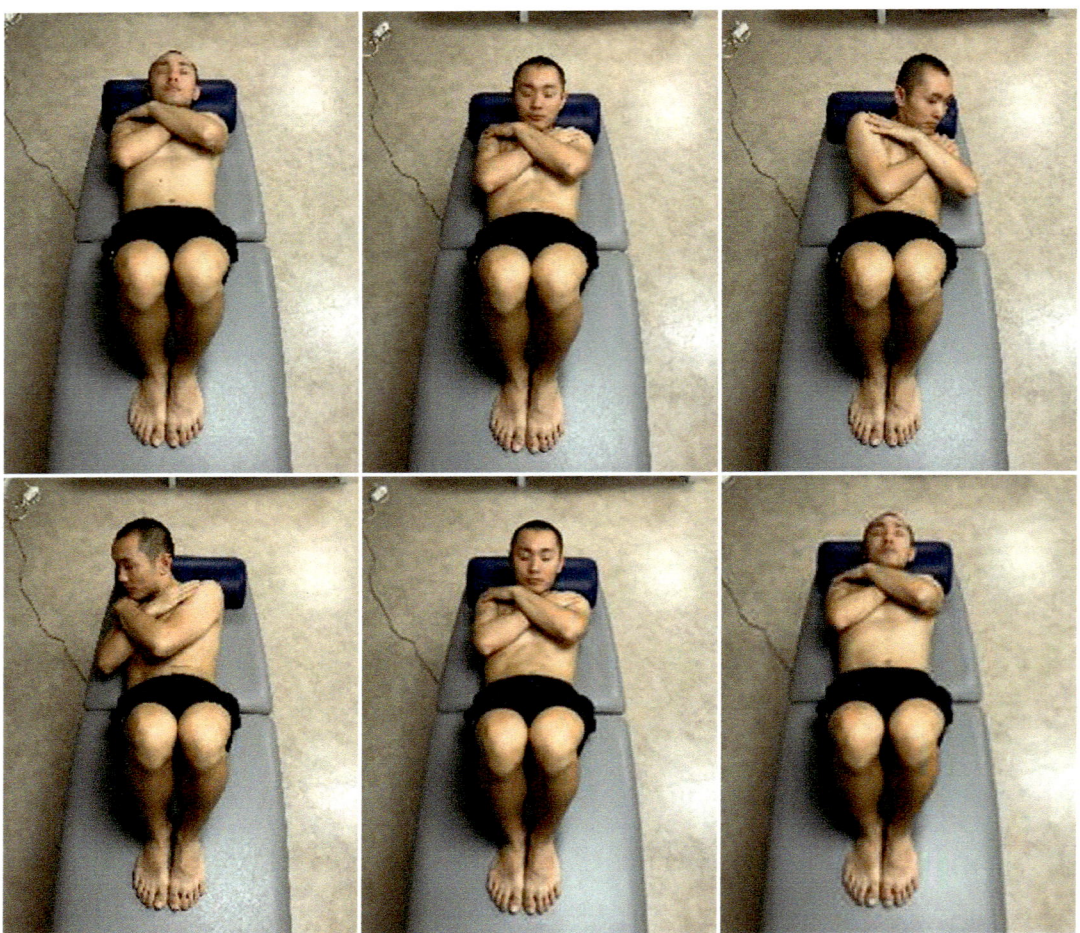

As a *progression*, the player can use a slightly longer lever and puts his hands behind his ears.

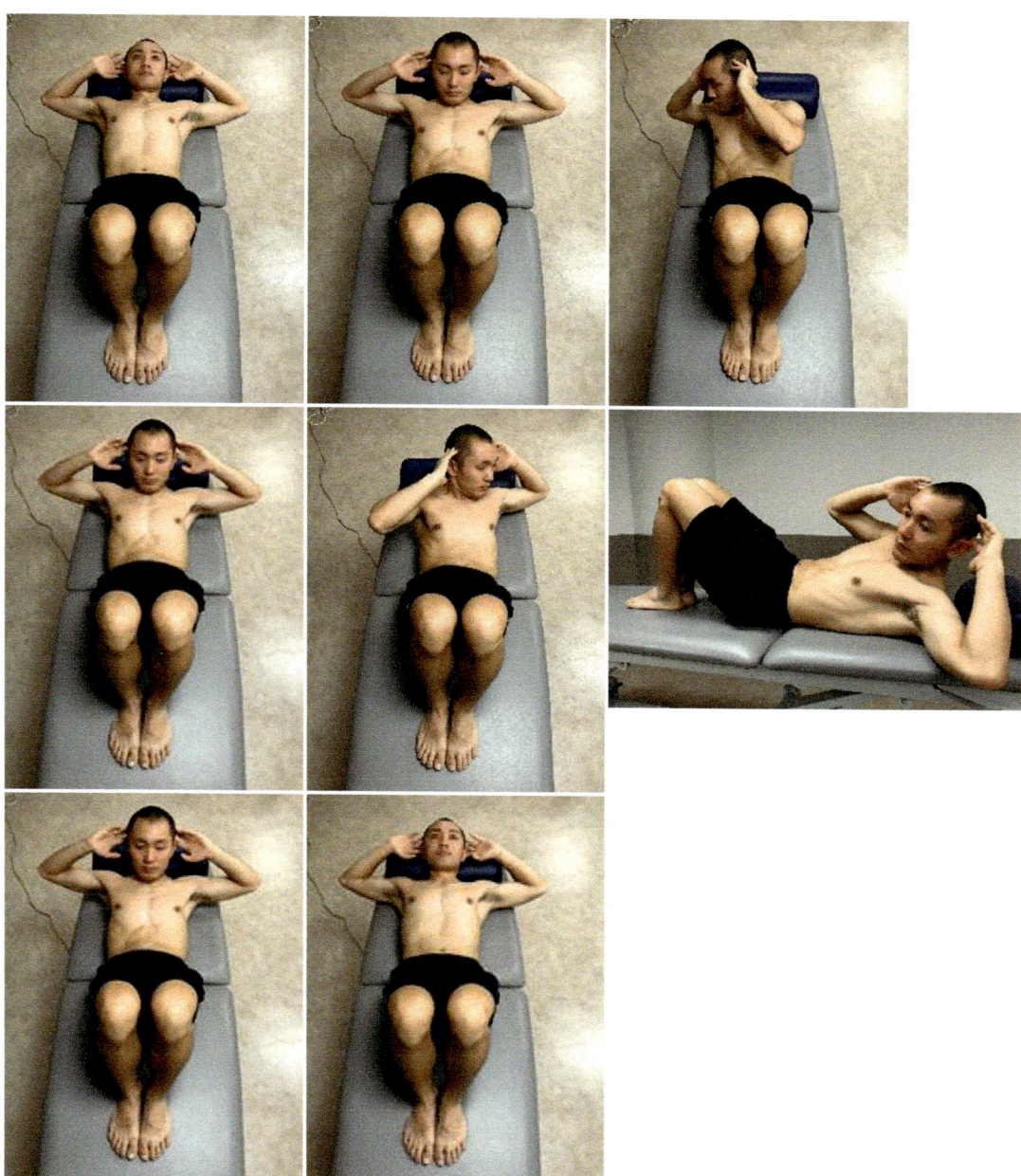

Progression 2: Raise one leg and keep it raised during the whole movement to decrease the base of support and increase the challenge to the oblique muscles.

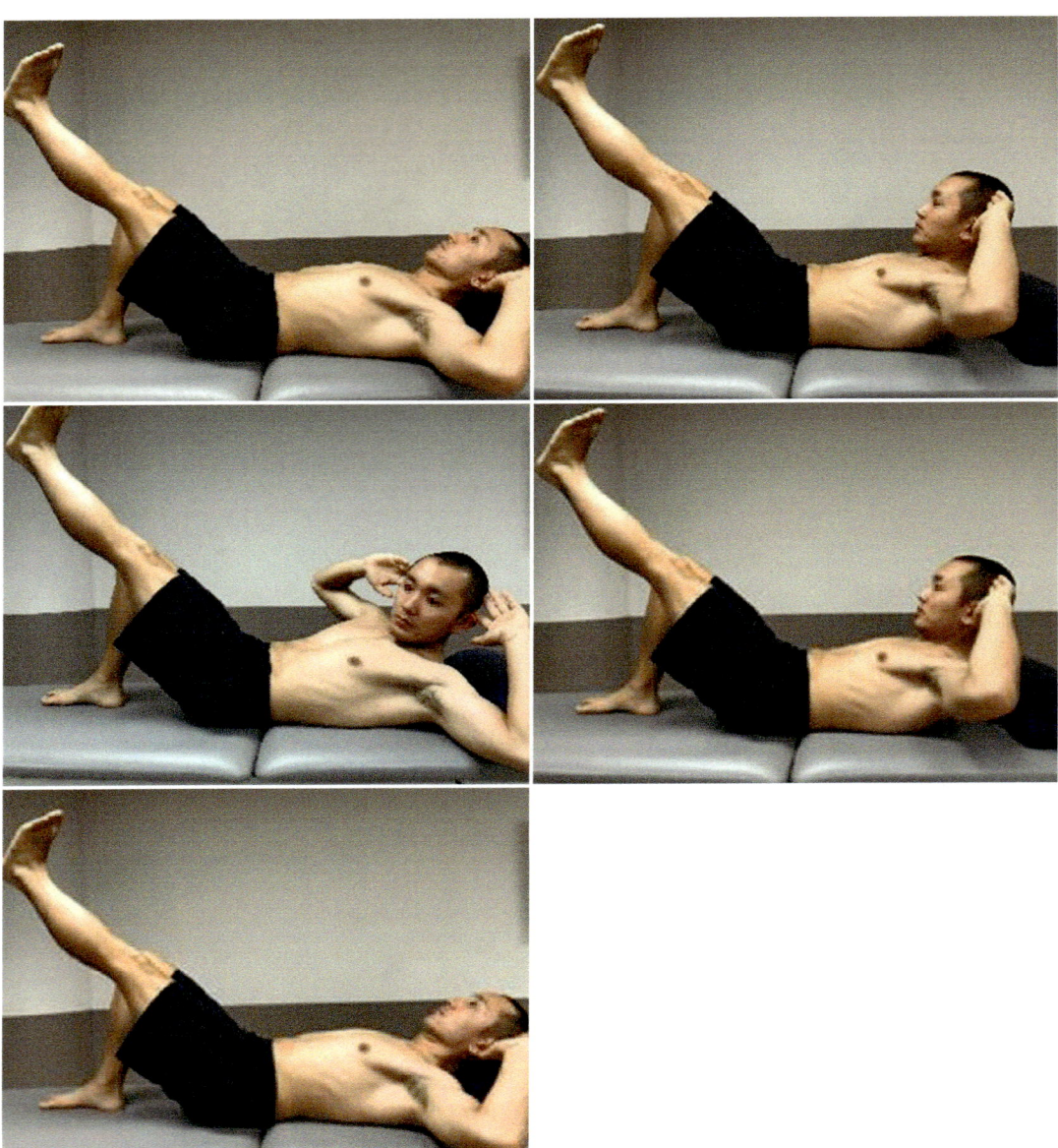

31.8.5 Enhancing Lateral Flexion/ Sidebending of the Trunk

The ability to laterally flex or sidebend toward a player's dominant side is an important element of the serve.

Player on his back slides one hand along his body as far as he can and then back to the neutral position before sliding to the other side and then coming back to the starting position.

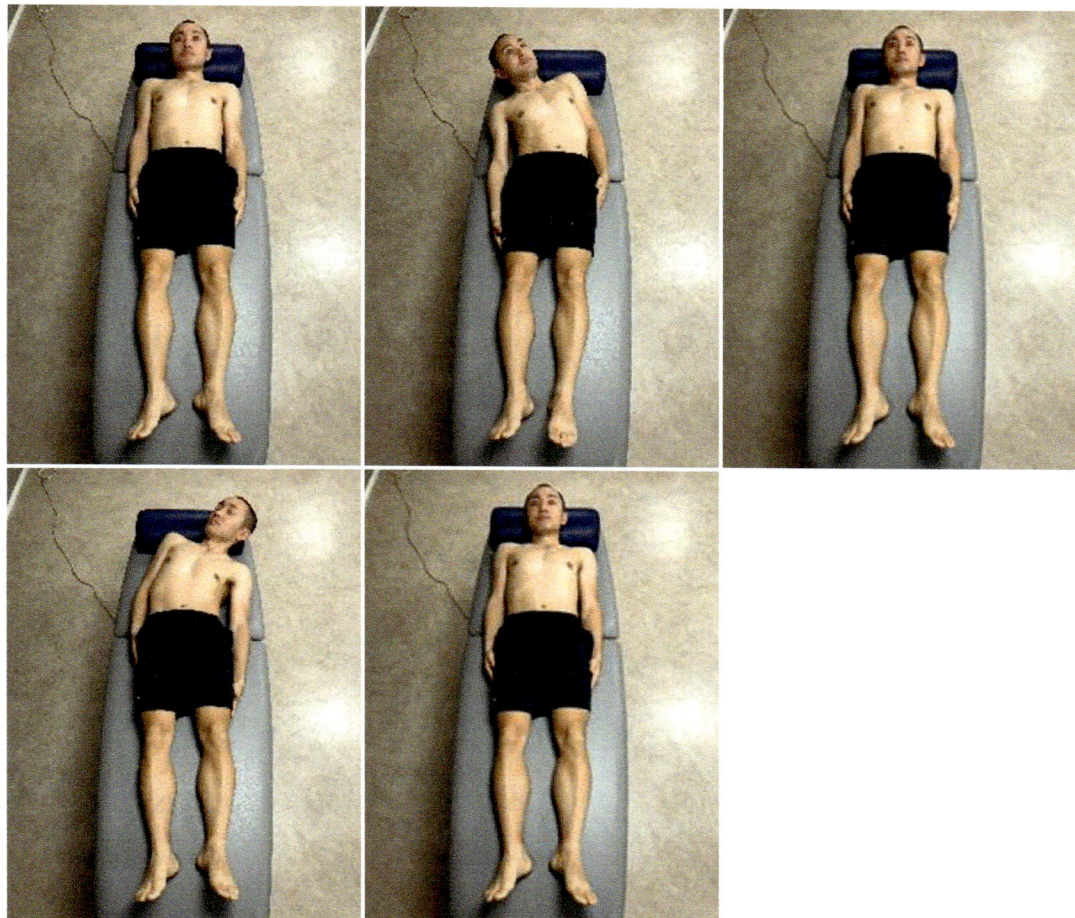

31.8.6 Dead Bug/Strengthening Abdominal Muscles

Player is on his back, with hips and knees 90° flexed and arms raised. The player can initially focus on lumbopelvic control maintaining a neutral spine while moving the *lower limb only*.

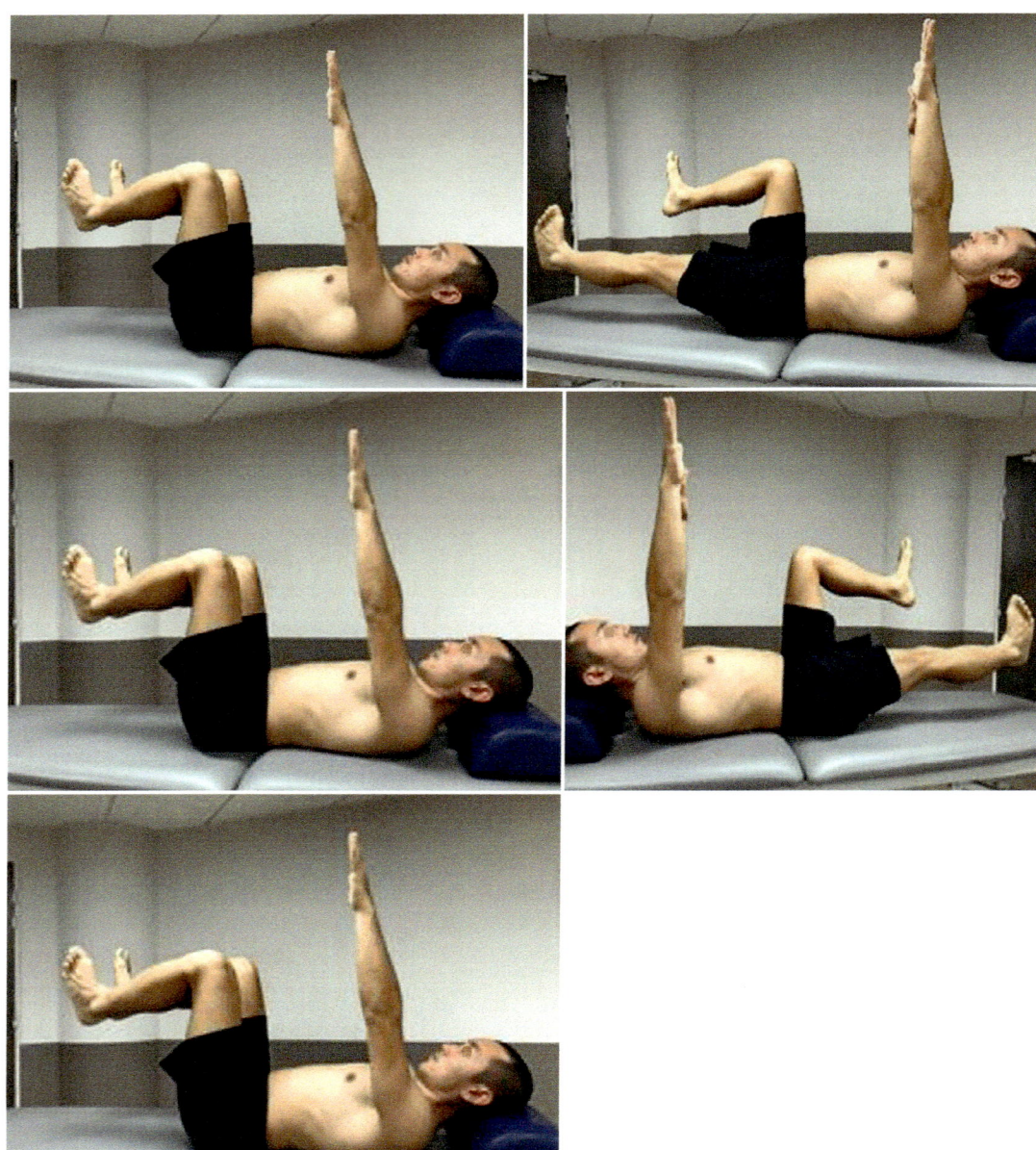

As a *progression*, the player can then move into a full "dead bug" exercise with alternate opposite arm and leg movement.

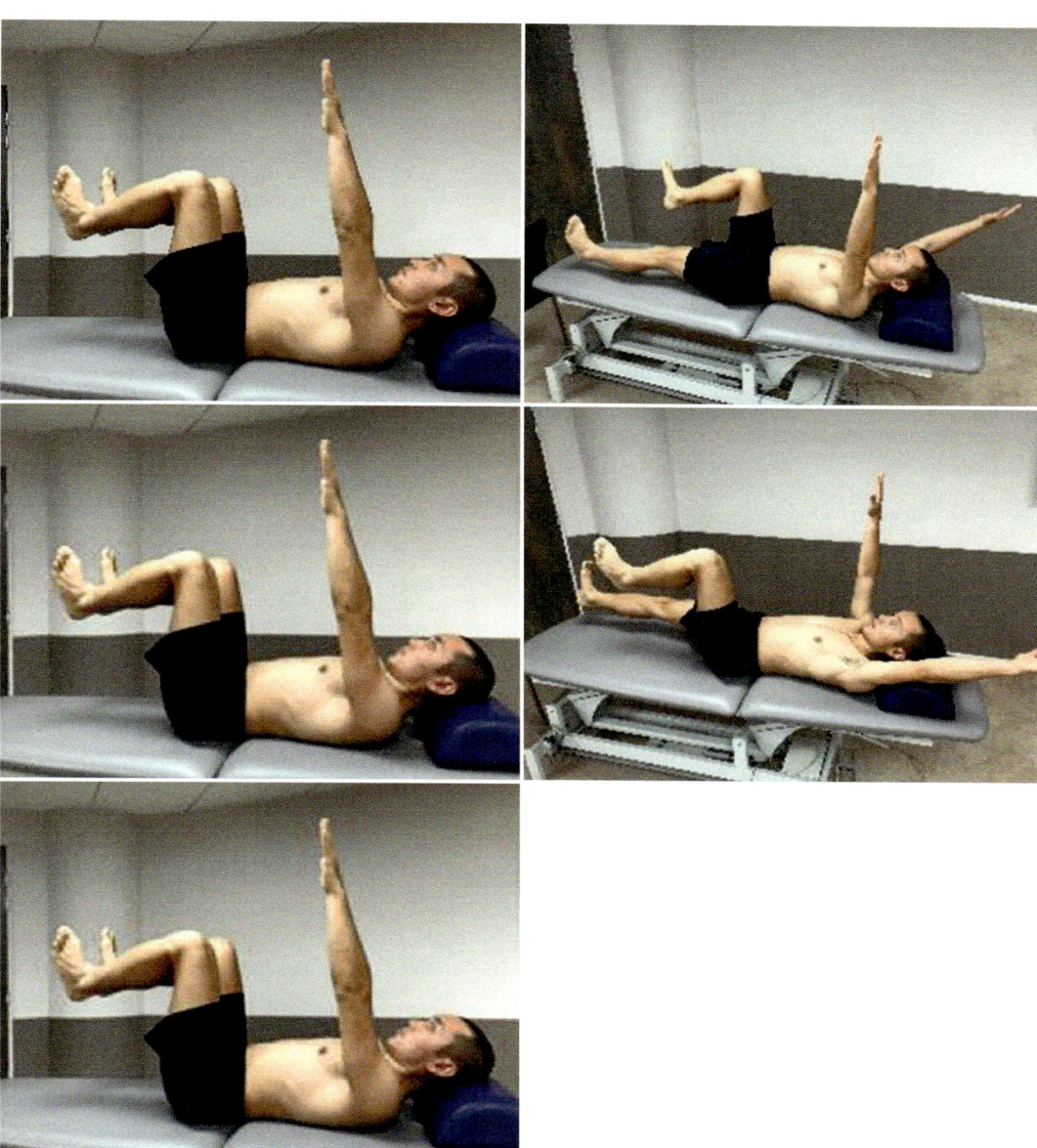

An added challenge can then involve using an elastic band.

Player holds the elastic band in one hand and passes his opposite foot in the loop. He then alternates movement to connect the core and contralateral side.

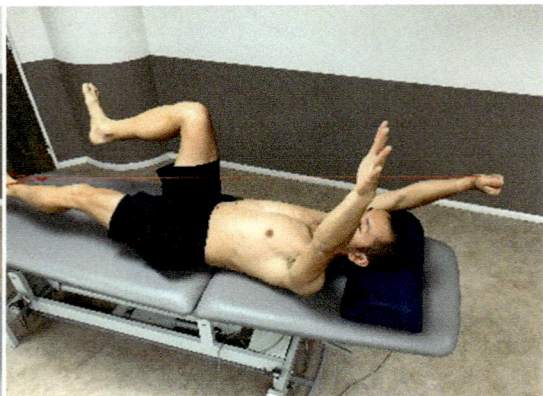
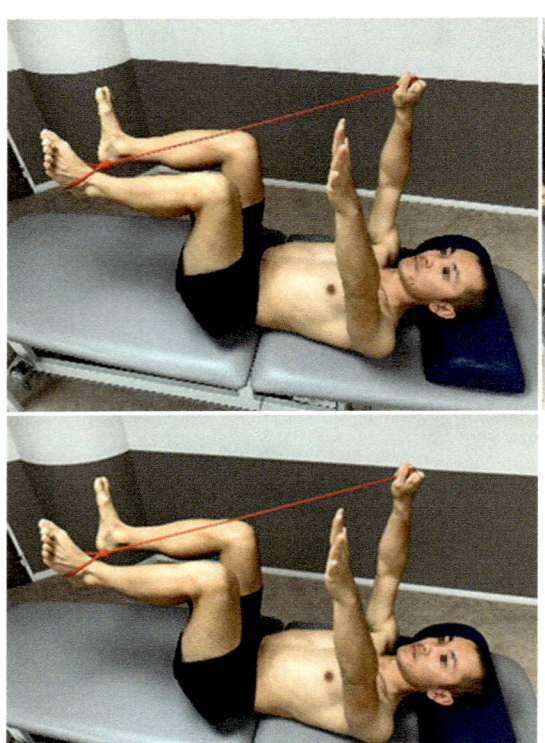

31.8.7 Double Leg Bridge

This encourages hip extension and can be used as either a mobility or strengthening exercise depending on the length of time in isometric hold.

It is useful in tennis as a warm-up also to balance the hips and pelvis (given the amount of time the hips are in a partially flexed position on-court).

Player is on his back, with both hips and knees flexed and feet comfortable hip distance apart on the table. The player lifts his hips and holds for a few seconds before going back down to the starting position.

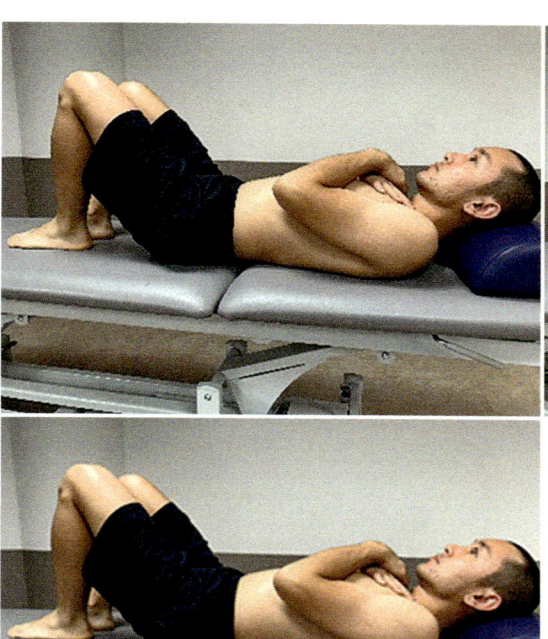
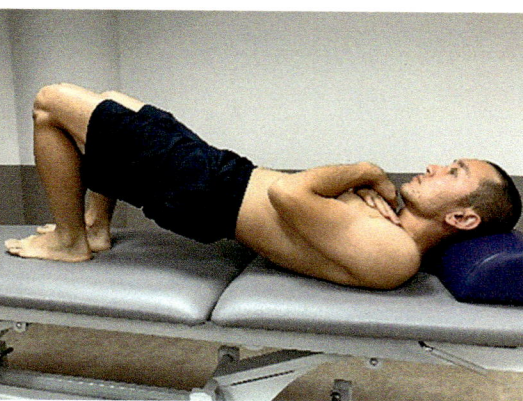
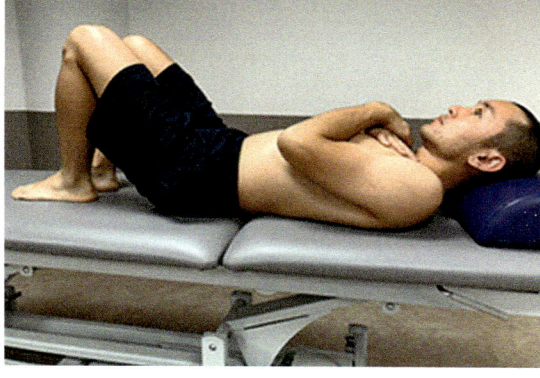

Progression 1: In same starting position, the player lifts his hips pushing through both his feet. Then he lifts 1 foot from the table and holds. The length of time can be increased as the player's strength improves.

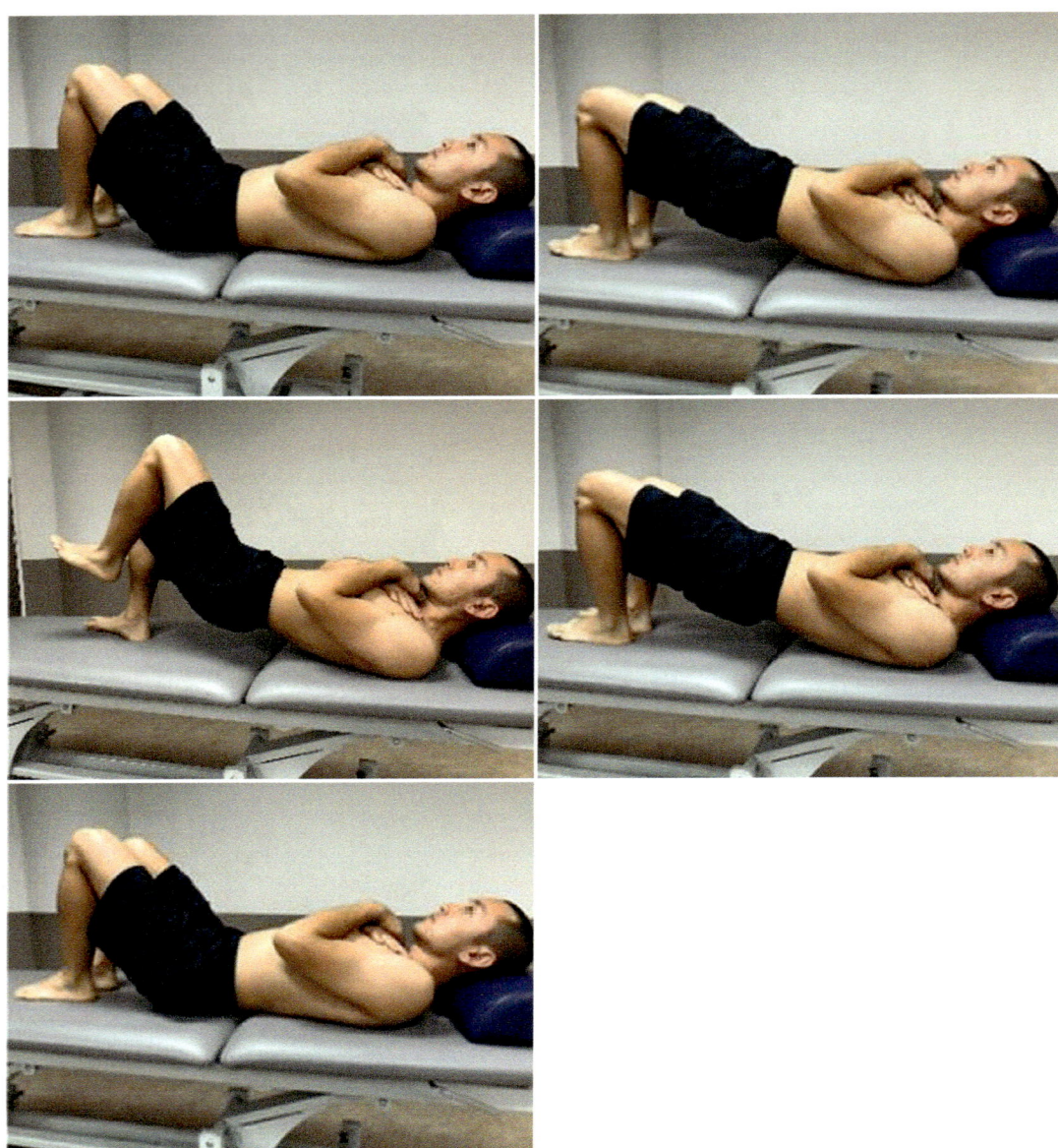

Progression 2: In same starting position, the player lifts his hips pushing through both his feet. He then lifts 1 foot from the table and lengthens, holding the position for a few seconds before returning to the starting position. This is a more advanced position using a longer lever hence challenging the unilateral gluteal muscle strength more.

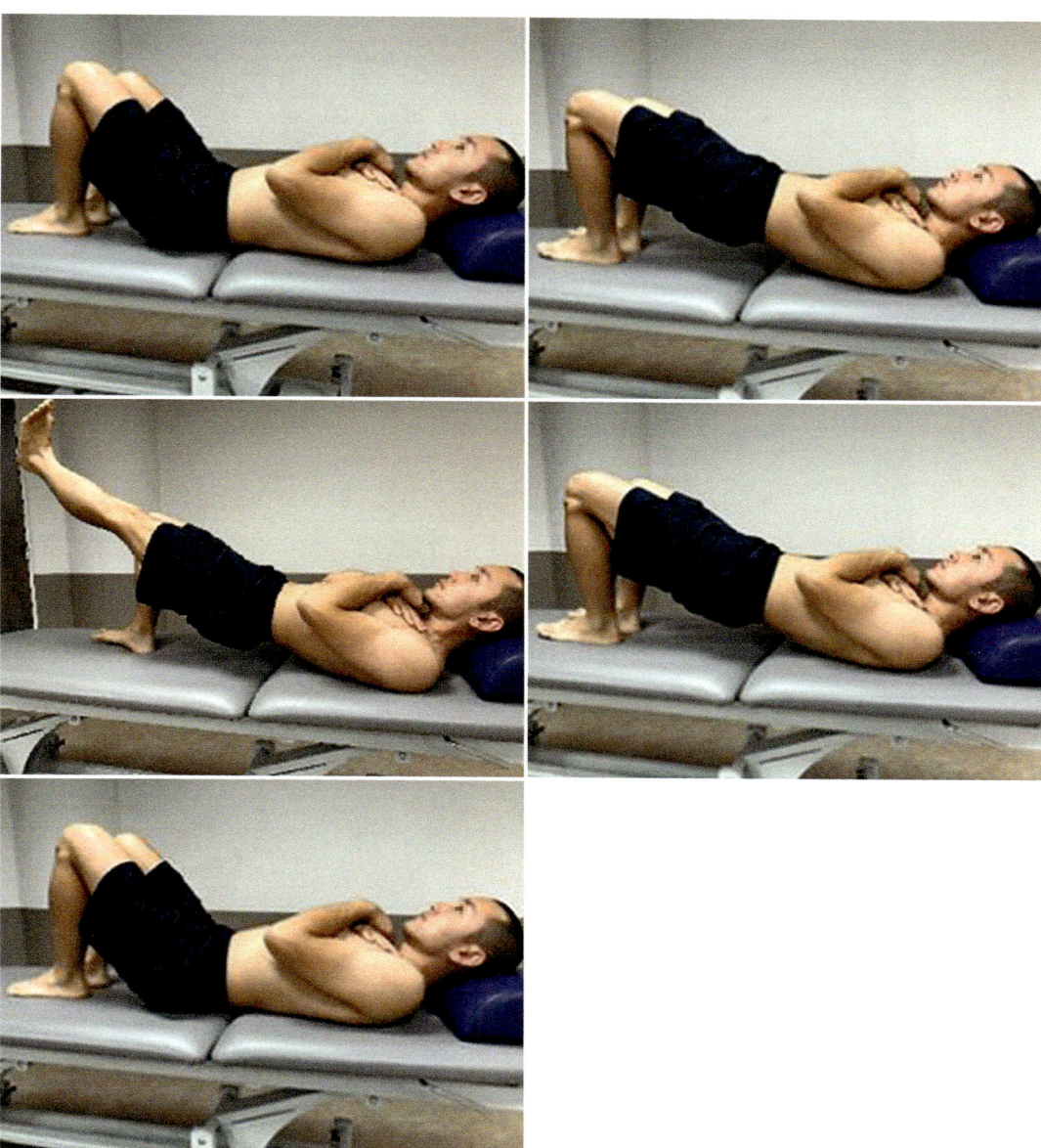

31.9 Side Lying

31.9.1 Coordinating Shoulder and Hip Motion

Player is lying on his right side with the right (lower) leg in hip and knee flexion to be more stable. The player then raises his left arm and fully extends the left leg, before changing and flexing his hip and shoulder to bring his left knee to his chest. This movement can be performed 5–10 times before changing to lie on the left side and doing the same series of movements with his right arm and leg.

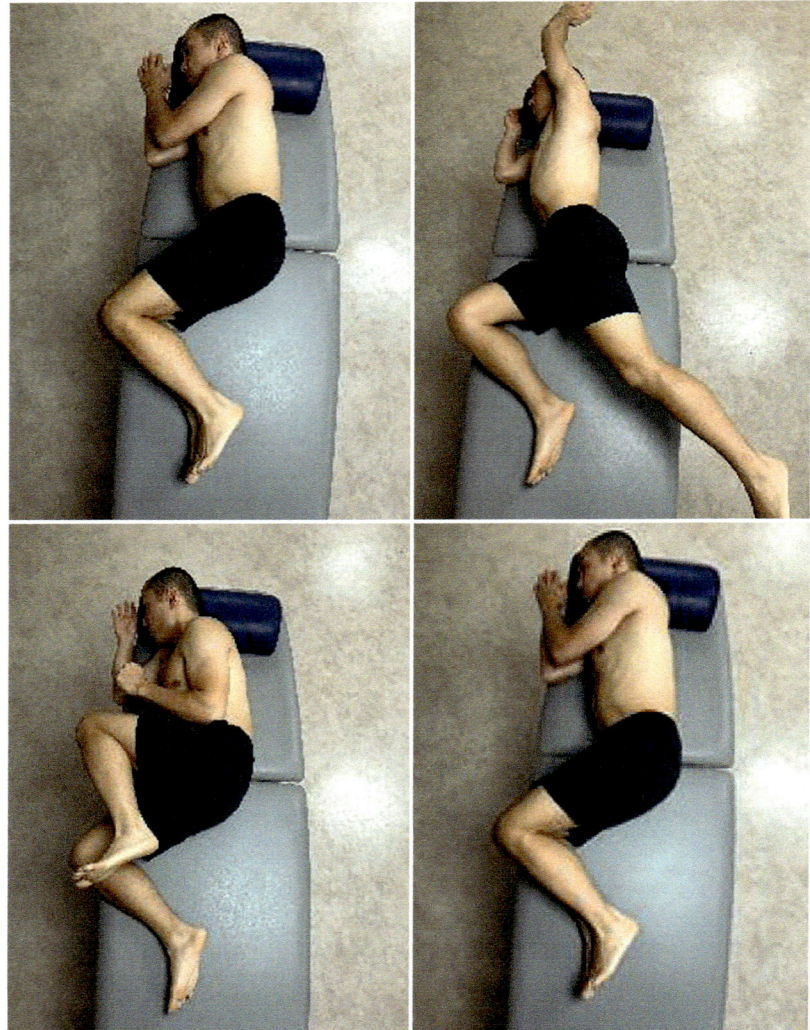

31.9.2 Arm Opener

This is a great exercise to enhance trunk rotation for ground strokes.

Player is lying on his left side with legs joined and hips and knees in slight flexion. Arms are stretched in front with palms together.

Breathing in to initiate the movement, the player starts to rotate and brings the top hand along the bottom arm before lengthening the top arm back.

The main focus of the exercise is to enhance thoracic/trunk rotation while keeping the pelvis stable. It can be repeated on the opposite side.

One consideration with this exercise is to balance out thoracic rotation. A right-handed player will always present with a slight thoracic rotation to the right given the dominance of the forehand and serve in tennis; therefore, in this example, this exercise could be given unilaterally to favor left rotation and balance the trunk.

31 Spinal Rehabilitation Strategies for the Elite Tennis Player

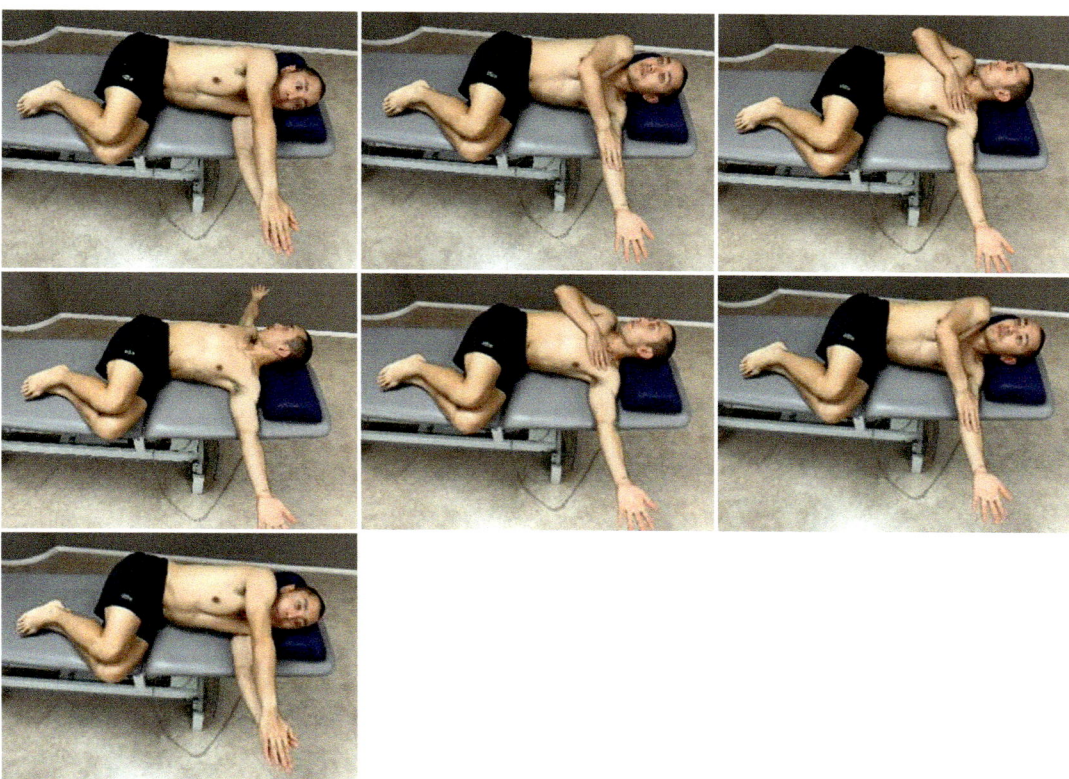

Progression 1: It is same movement except player keeps arm straight with elbow extended.

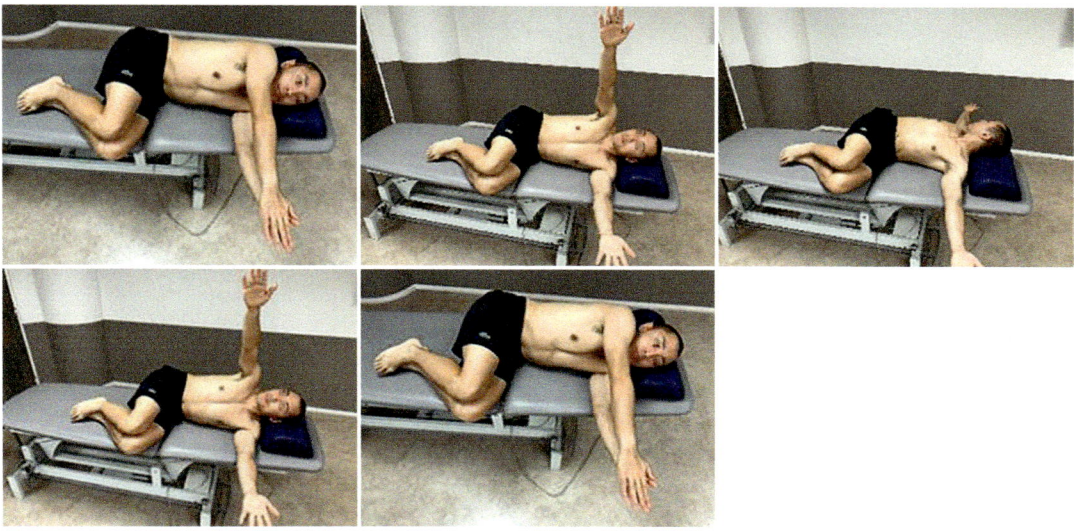

Progression 2: It is same movement using an elastic band for resistance with elbow initially bent.

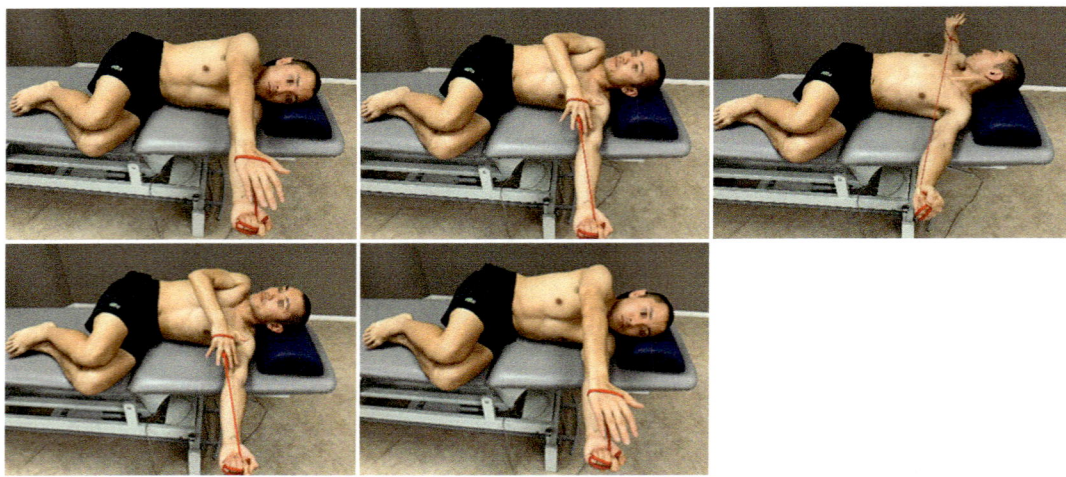

Then arms are opened and the elbow is extended. Using the band increases the work of the trunk rotators and posterior shoulder muscles turning the arm opener from a pure mobility exercise to a strength and control exercise.

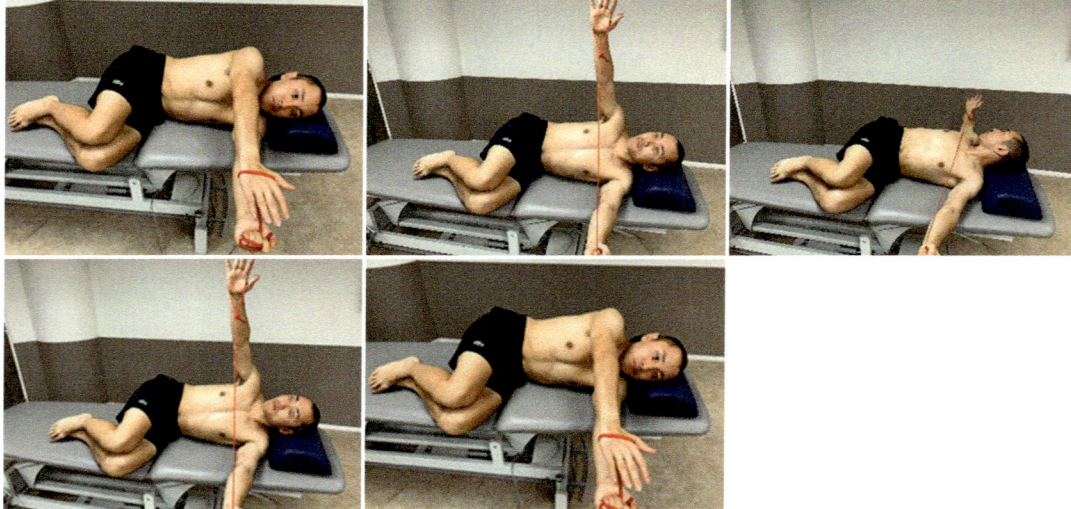

31.9.3 Ipsilateral Hip and Shoulder Control/Strengthening

Player is lying on the table on his right side with the right arm, hip, and knee flexed to 90° to enhance stability.

A slight diagonal position is useful as one leg will finish off the table.

The player raises one arm above his head and fully extends his left hip, so the left foot is now off the table. He will elevate and push his arm to reach as far up, while he lowers his left foot toward the ground. With this movement he will stretch and open his left lateral side. From this position he will then contract this left lateral side as if he wanted to bring his left shoulder close to his left hip.

He can then change sides to work on the opposite side.

This exercise promotes spinal, hip, and shoulder mobility, strength, and control. It is useful for reach and lateral flexion needed during the serve.

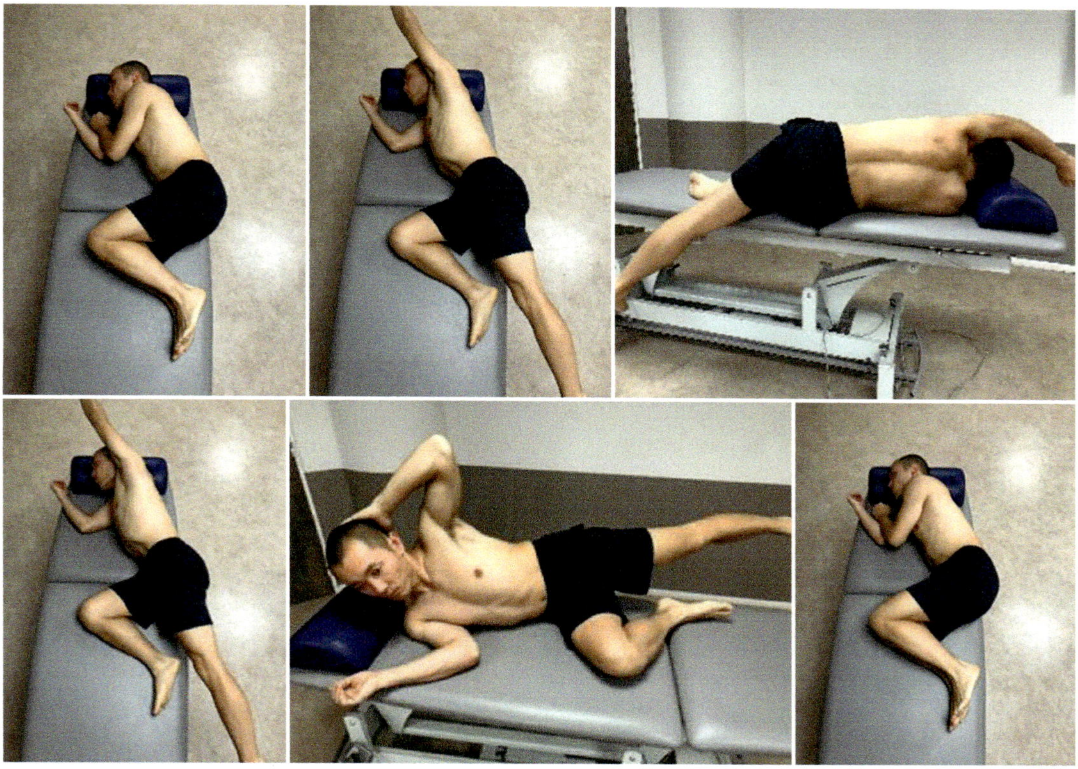

Progression 1: The therapist can put one hand on the left hip and his other hand on the player's left lower ribs. During the first phase (lowering), the therapist gently increases the stretch, and during the second phase (contraction) he creates a resistance which the player can match.

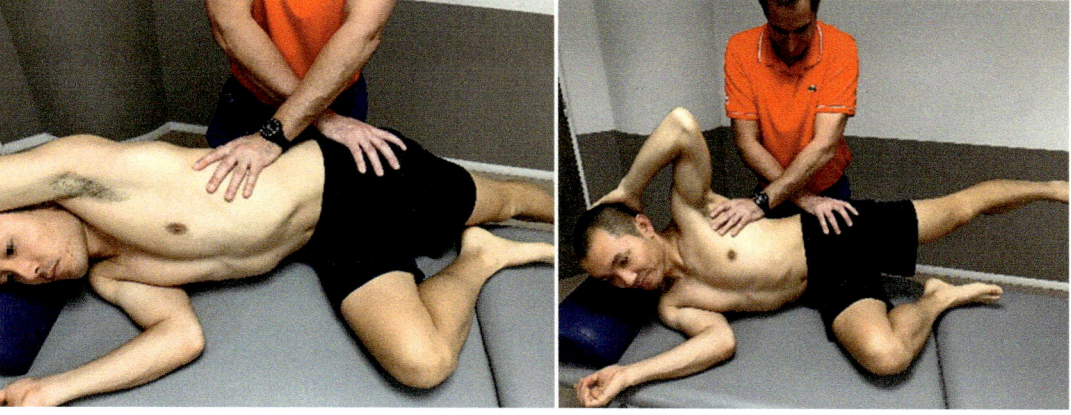

Progression 2: The therapist puts his hands further up on the player's shoulder and below near the player's ankle to firstly increase the lateral stretch and then challenge the returning lateral contraction.

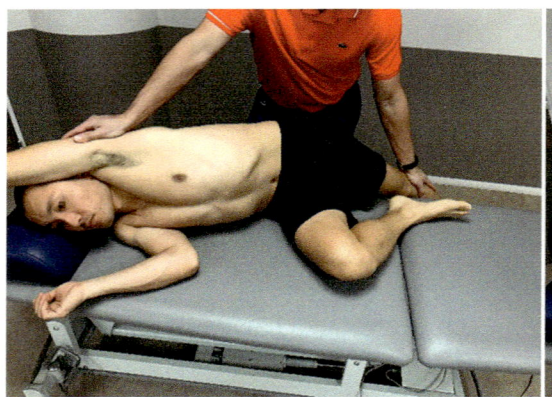
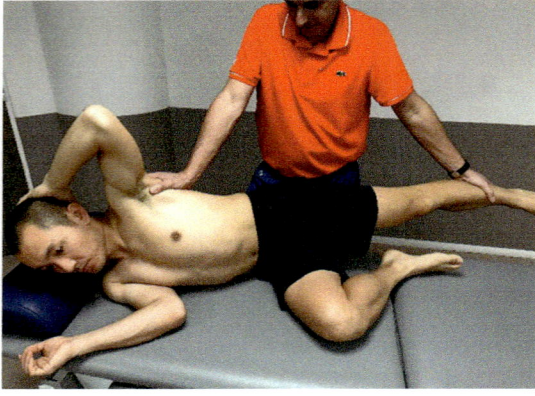

31.9.4 Lateral Flexion/Sidebending Mobilization of the Lumbar Spine

Player on his side, the therapist puts his thumbs on the lumbar spine and will gently push toward the table to mobilize the spine. Remember to do both sides to enhance general mobility or use more as a treatment technique if/when one side is restricted.

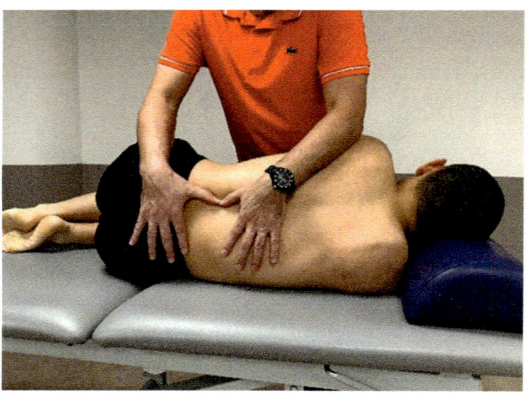

31.10 All 4's

31.10.1 Hump (Flexion) and Hollow (Extension)

Player on his hands and knees (all 4's) with his back in a neutral position. He will then increase his low back curve as much as he can (extend), before passing back through the neutral position and try to make his back as round (flexed) as he can.

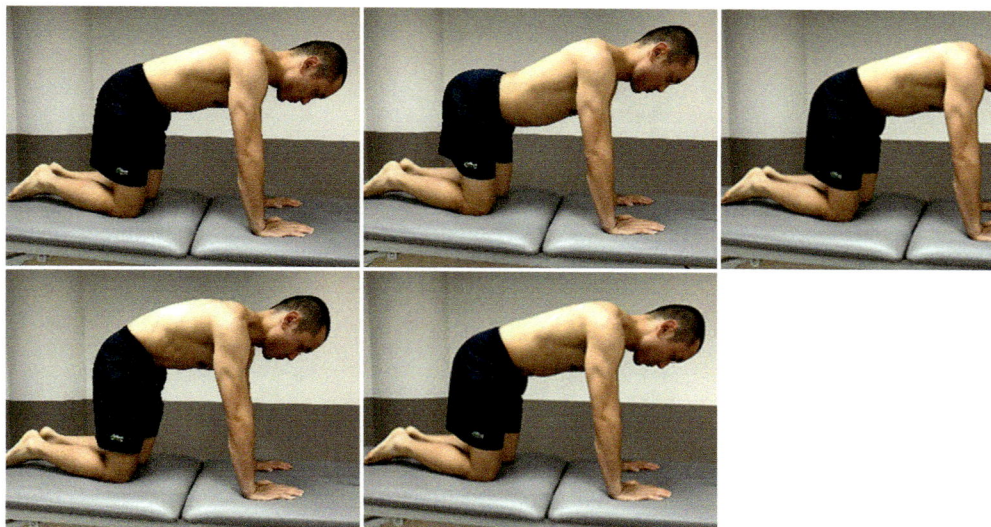

31.10.2 Bird Dog Variations

Player on all 4's maintaining a neutral spine and slowly extending one leg back before returning to the starting position. Perform alternate sides.

This exercise can be used to strengthen the posterior chain in particular the gluts and spinal erectors.

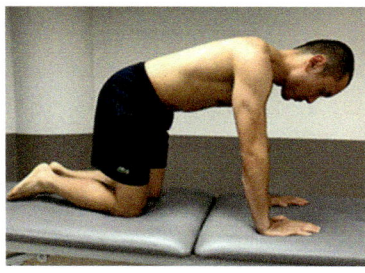 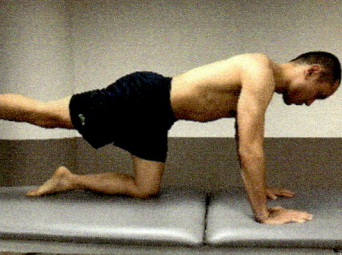 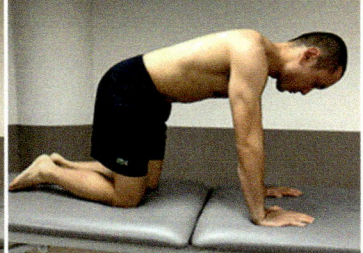

Progression 1: Player extends the opposite (contralateral) leg and arm out maintaining a neutral spine and fluid breathing pattern throughout (demonstrated below).

This can be further challenged with ipsilateral arm and leg motion.

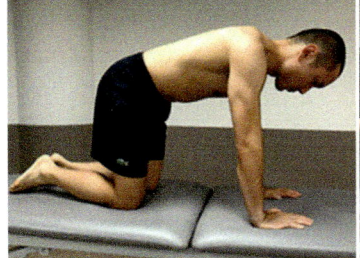 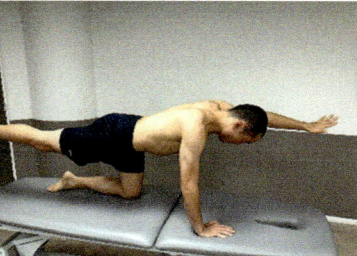 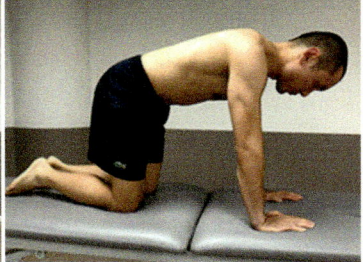

Progression 2: It is same exercise as above but including an elastic band to increase resistance.

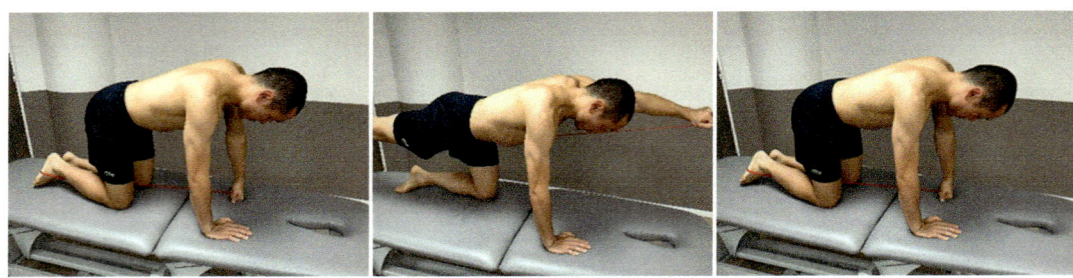

31.10.3 Bird Dog with Trunk Flexion Emphasis

Player on all 4's extends the opposite (contralateral) leg and arm out maintaining a neutral spine before moving into flexion attempting to touch his knee with his elbow before moving back into the starting position. Perform alternate sides.

This modification adds more abdominal strengthening.

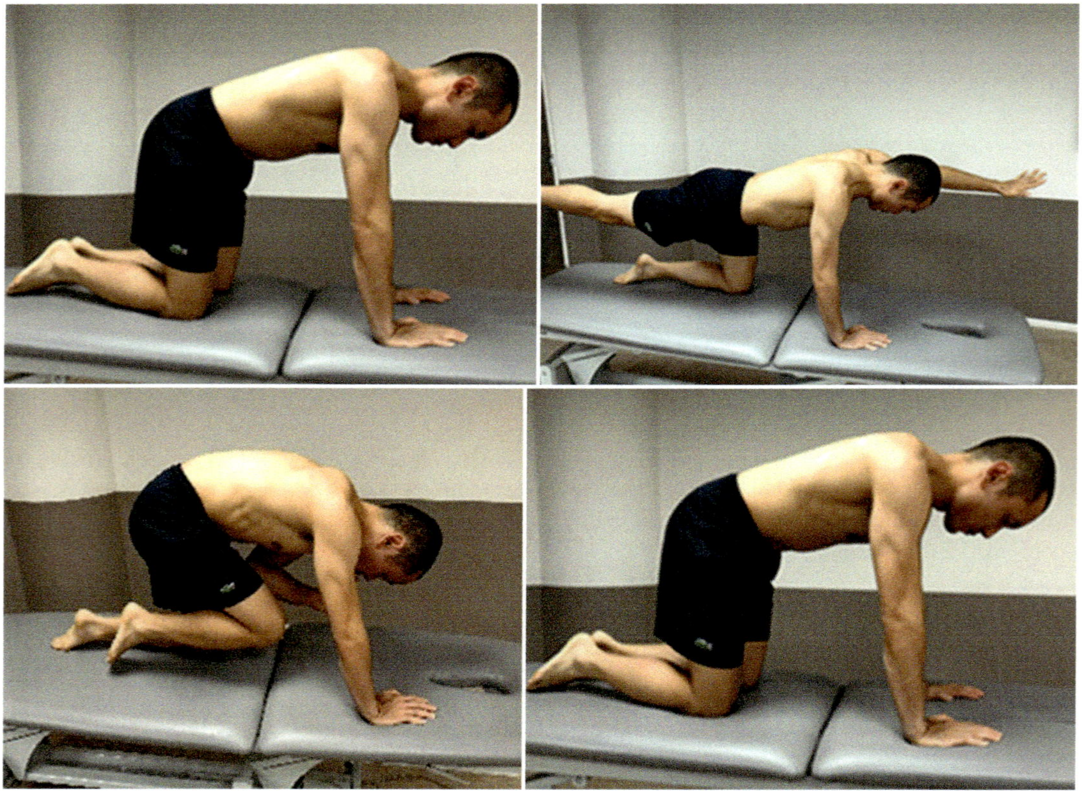

31.10.4 Thread the Needle

It combines trunk rotation with shoulder horizontal extension and flexion. This is great for lengthening the lat and pec muscles while stretching the thoracolumbar fascia.

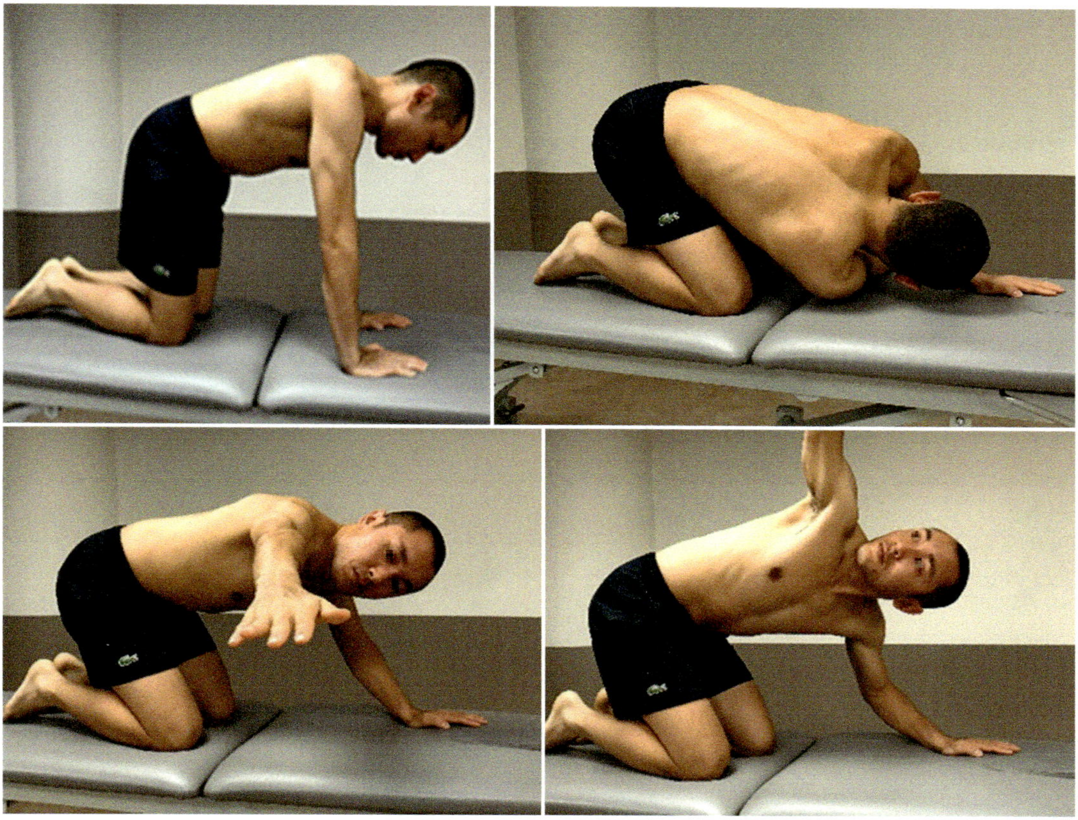

Progression: It is same movement with an elastic band.

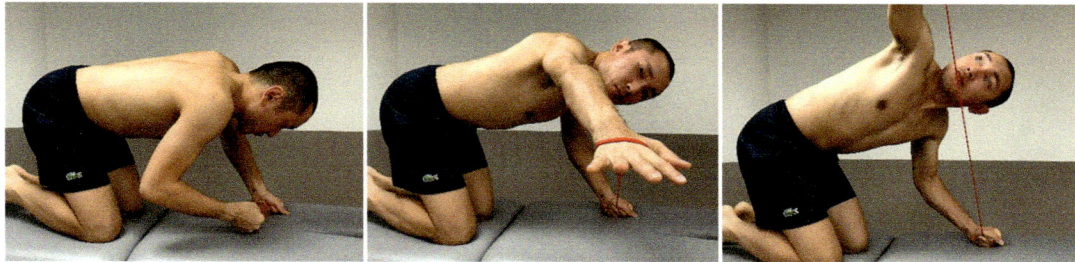

31.10.5 Thread the Needle plus Overpressure

Therapist can provide overpressure to the trunk near scapula to encourage trunk rotation and stretch the posterior shoulder capsule.

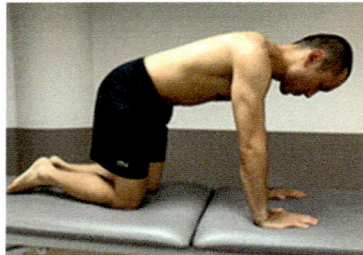 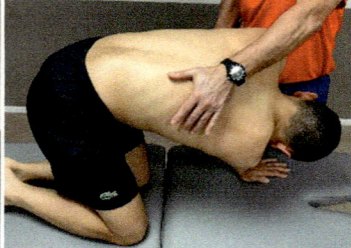 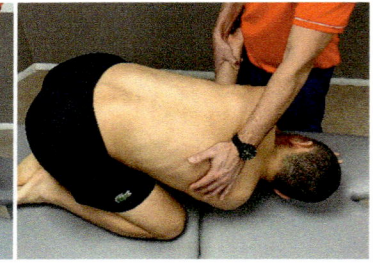

31.10.6 Child's Pose

Player on all 4's will move his hips toward his feet in order to lengthen out and flex his spine. It is recommended to go slowly and respect the front of the hips being aware of any discomfort or impingement.

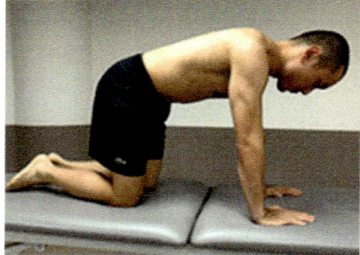 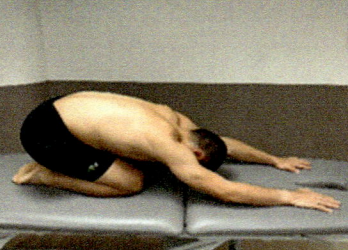 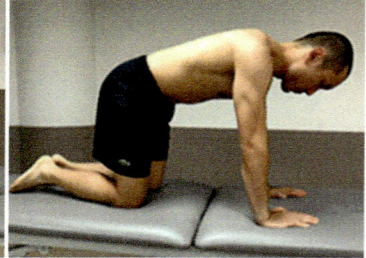

Progression: Therapist can apply a pressure on the player's back, so it increases the low back/lat stretch and mobilizes the spine.

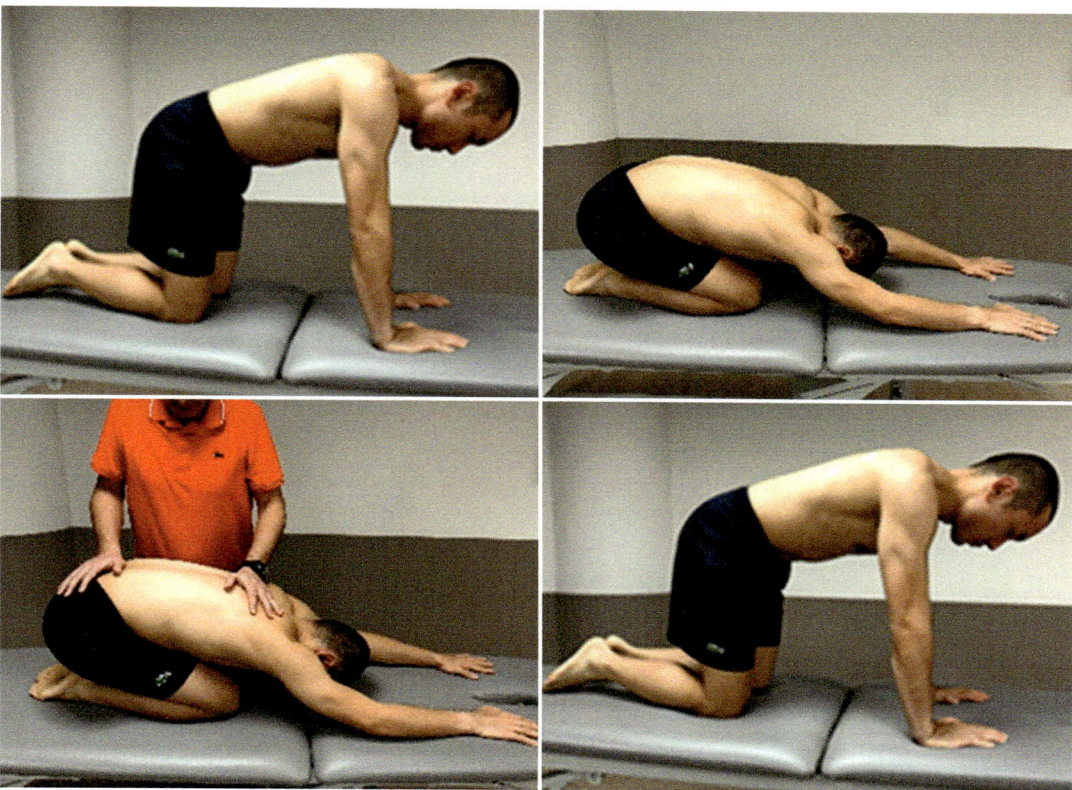

31.11 On the Knees

31.11.1 Encouraging Spinal Flexion and Extension

Player is on his knees in an upright position. He crosses the arms on the chest and starts to bend forward until maximum flexion is obtained. He then moves back to the starting position before going into extension and arching the back. This motion should be segmentally controlled to help lubricate the spine and relieve any stiffness.

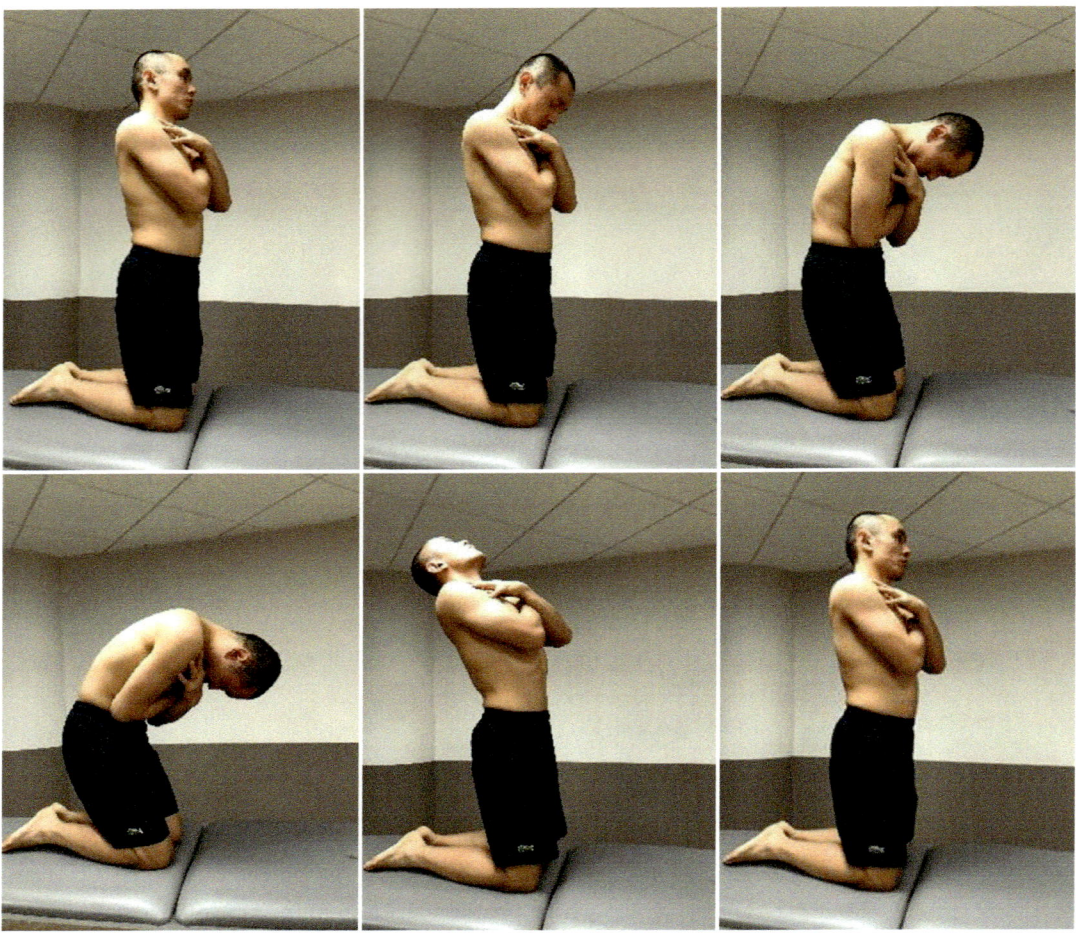

31.11.2 Encouraging Spinal Rotation

Player is on his knees in an upright position. He crosses his arms on his chest and starts to bend forward until maximum flexion is reached. Once in this position, the player will rotate to one side and then to the other before moving back to the starting position.

31 Spinal Rehabilitation Strategies for the Elite Tennis Player

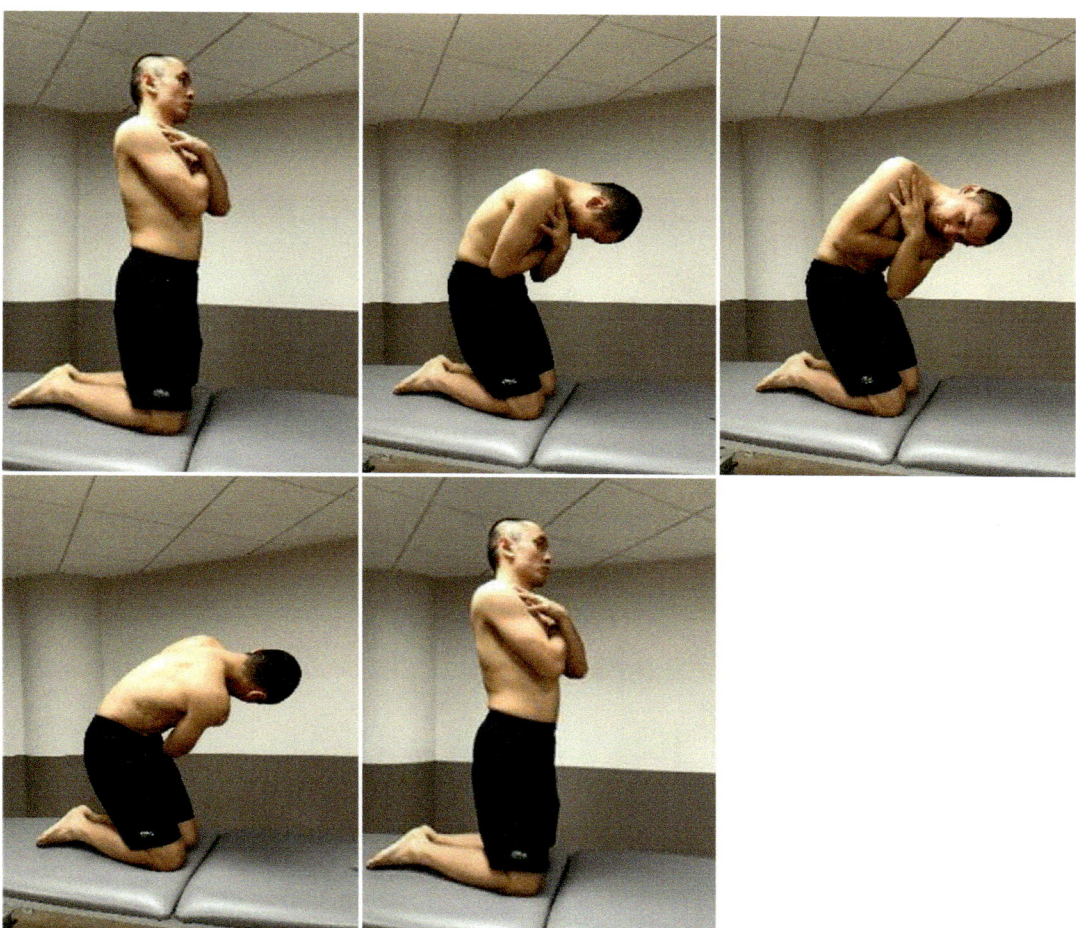

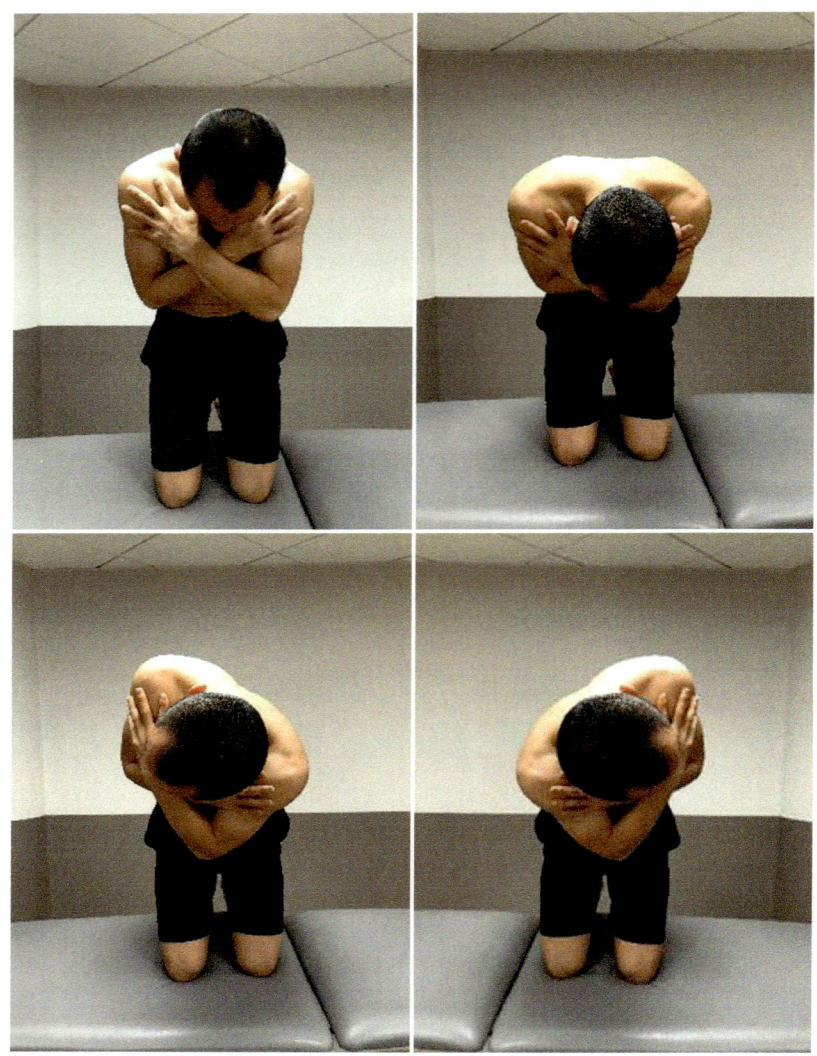

31.11.3 Encouraging Lateral Flexion/Sidebending

Player on his knees in an upright position. Crosses his arms on his chest and starts to sidebend as much as possible to one side before coming back to neutral. Repeat to the opposite side focusing on fluid motion.

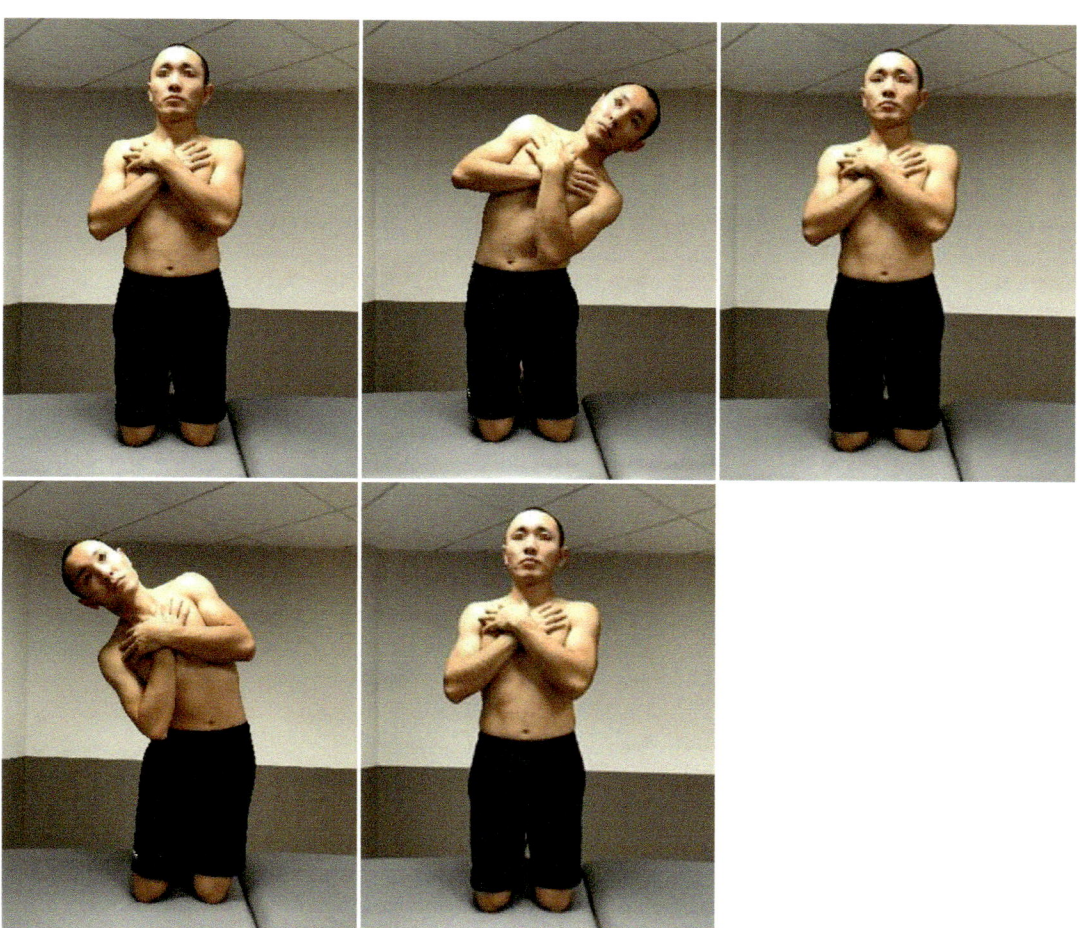

31.12 Prone

31.12.1 Strengthening Hip and Back Extension/Superman Variations

Player is lying flat facedown with hands behind ears. He activates deep abdominal muscles and maintains fluid breathing pattern. He extends one leg and arms together before controlling body slowly back down.

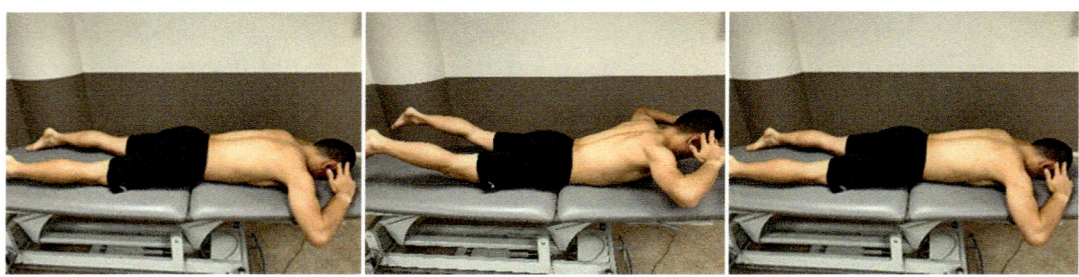

Progression 1: In same starting position, the player will stretch out and extend his arms and pause before coming back to the starting position.

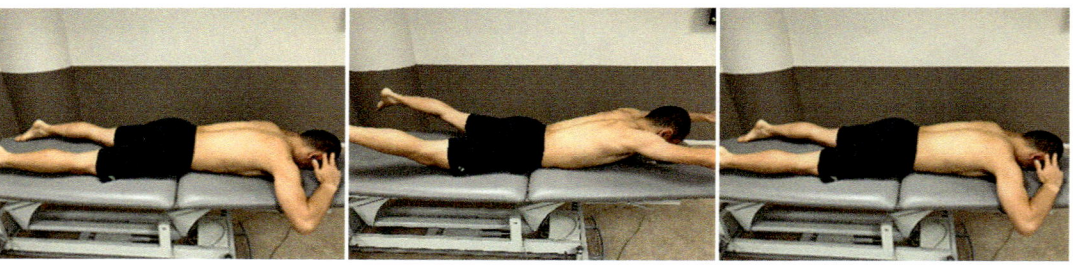

Progression 2: In same starting position, the player raises one stretched arm and the opposite leg before coming back to the starting position. Perform alternate sides.

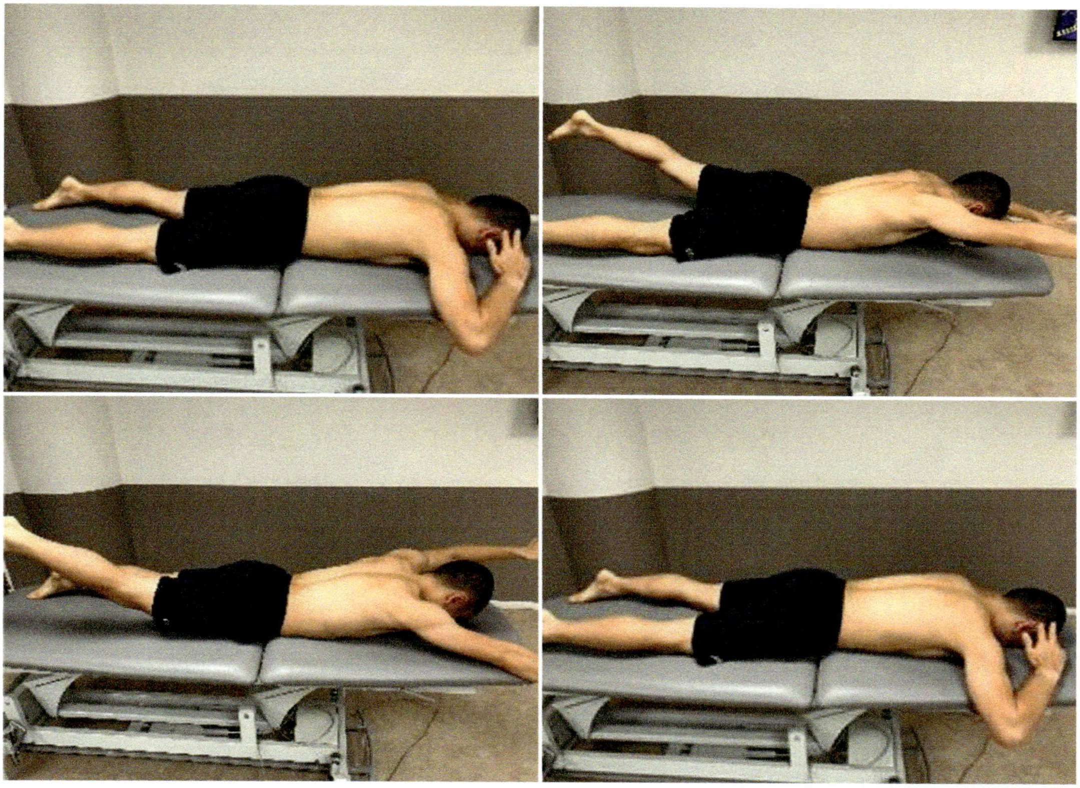

31.12.2 Spine Rotation Mobilization

To encourage rotation the player can have his therapist help to mobilize the spine.

The therapist can place one hand on the player's lower ribs as the other hand pulls up on the front of the player's pelvis. This technique can be modified to focus on specific stiff spinal segments and converted into a contract/relax muscle energy technique.

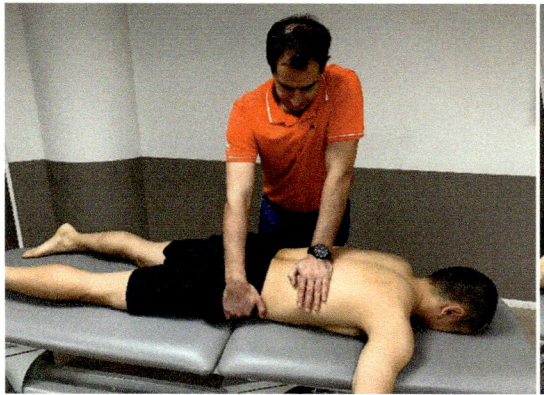
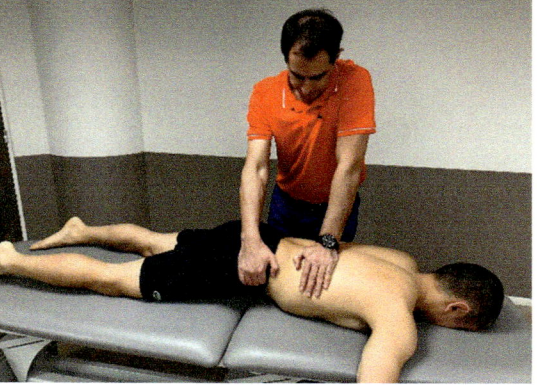

31.12.3 Scorpion

Player on his stomach with arms out at 90°. He lifts one leg into hip extension before crossing to the other side. Once he reaches his maximal range of motion, he returns to the starting position and does the same toward the other side.

This is a full body exercise that can be either used as part of a dynamic warm-up or to address spinal stiffness into extension and rotation.

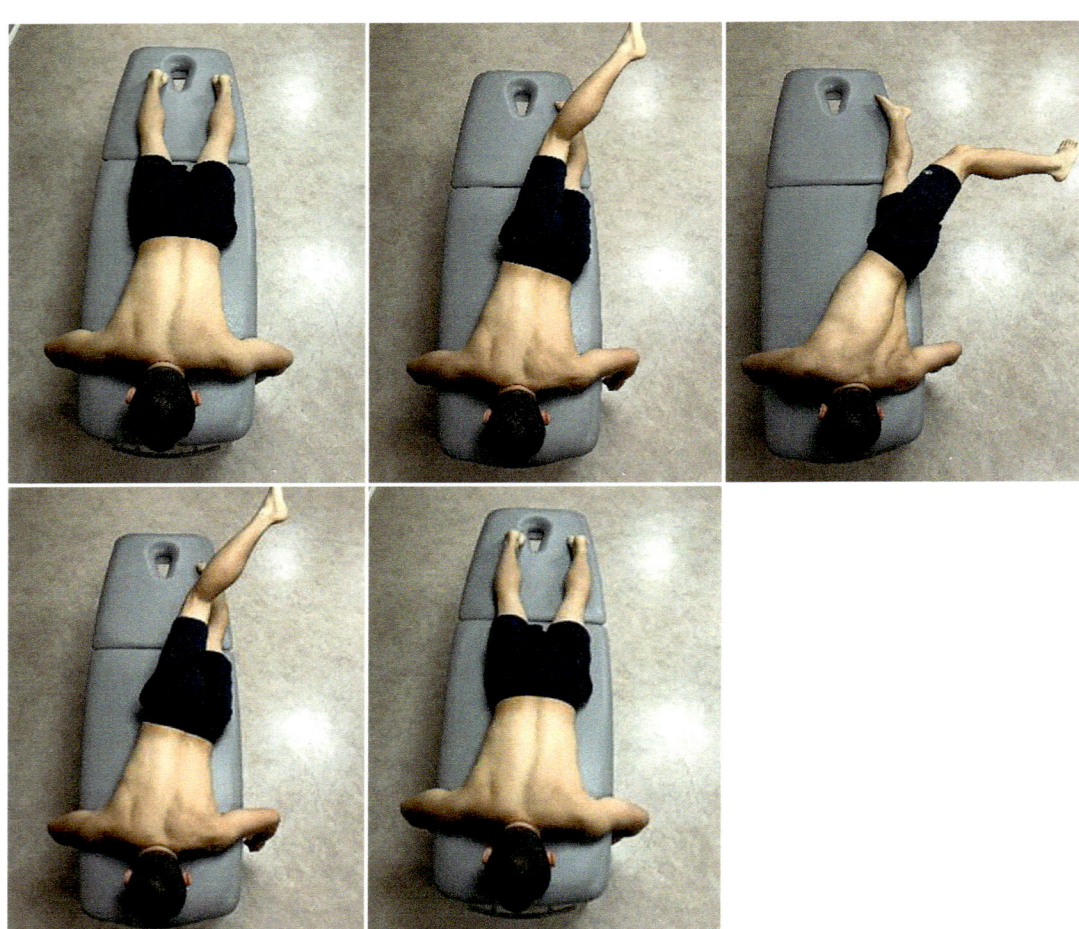

31.13 Sitting

31.13.1 Encouraging Spinal Rotation

Player is sitting on the table with his arms crossed on his chest. He starts to rotate to one side and then rotates to the other side before coming back to the starting position.

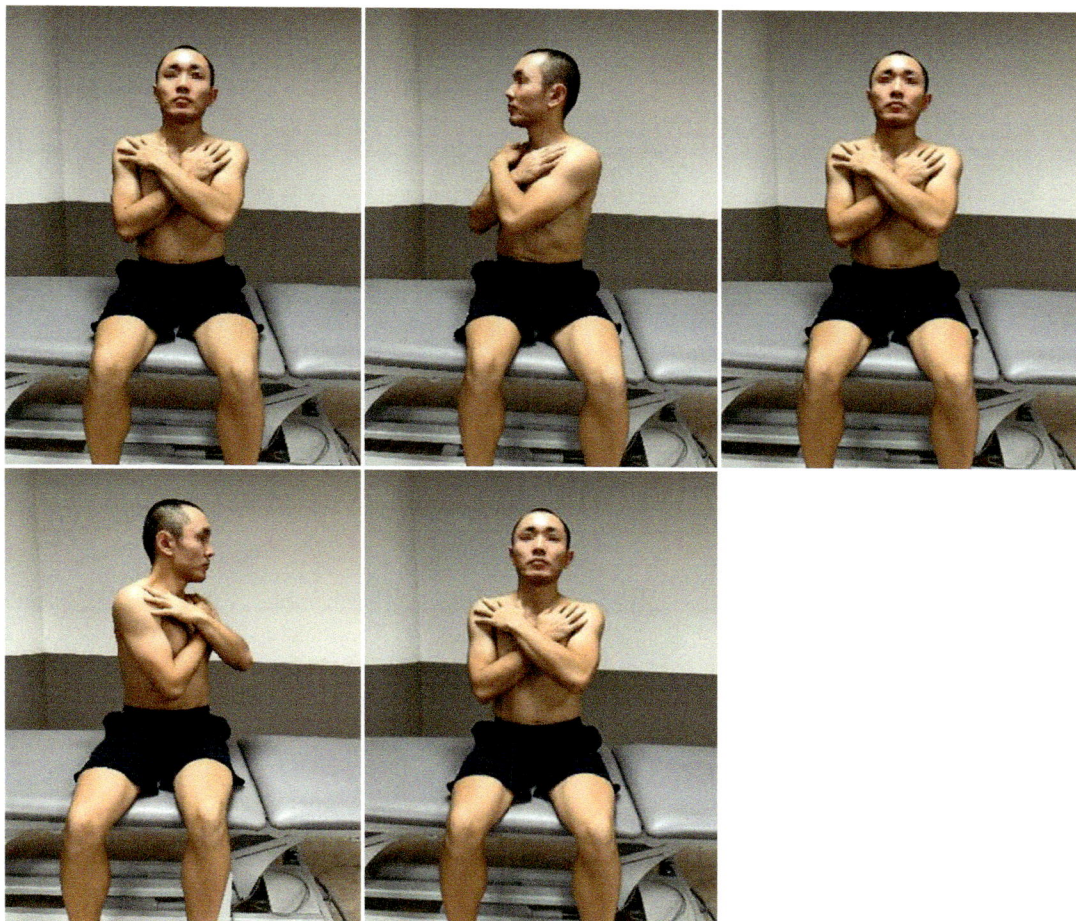

Progression: Therapist is behind the player with the heel of one of his hands along the player's spine, while his other hand grabs the lower elbow of the player. The therapist pulls the elbow back while simultaneously pushing the player's thorax forward to increase rotation, moving toward the end of the range and then back to the neutral position. The player then changes his arm position (places his upper arm below the other). The therapist also changes hands and does the same motion toward the other side before coming back to the starting position.

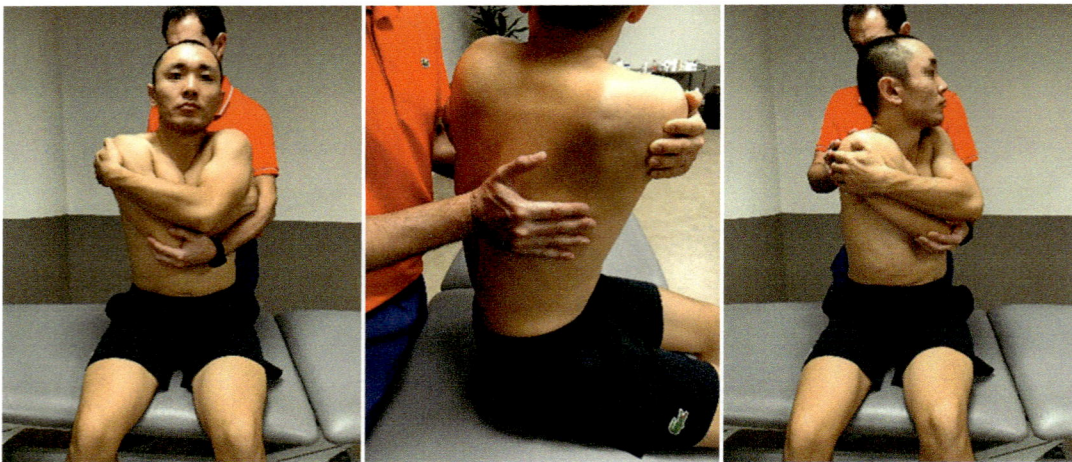

31.13.2 Encouraging Spinal Extension

Player sitting on the table crosses his arms in front of his forehead. The therapist who is positioned on the side, holds the player's arm with one hand and places his other hand on the back of the player. The therapist then brings the player forward and simultaneously will push on his back to increase thoracic extension. The therapist will modify his hand placement in order to mobilize all or specific spinal segments.

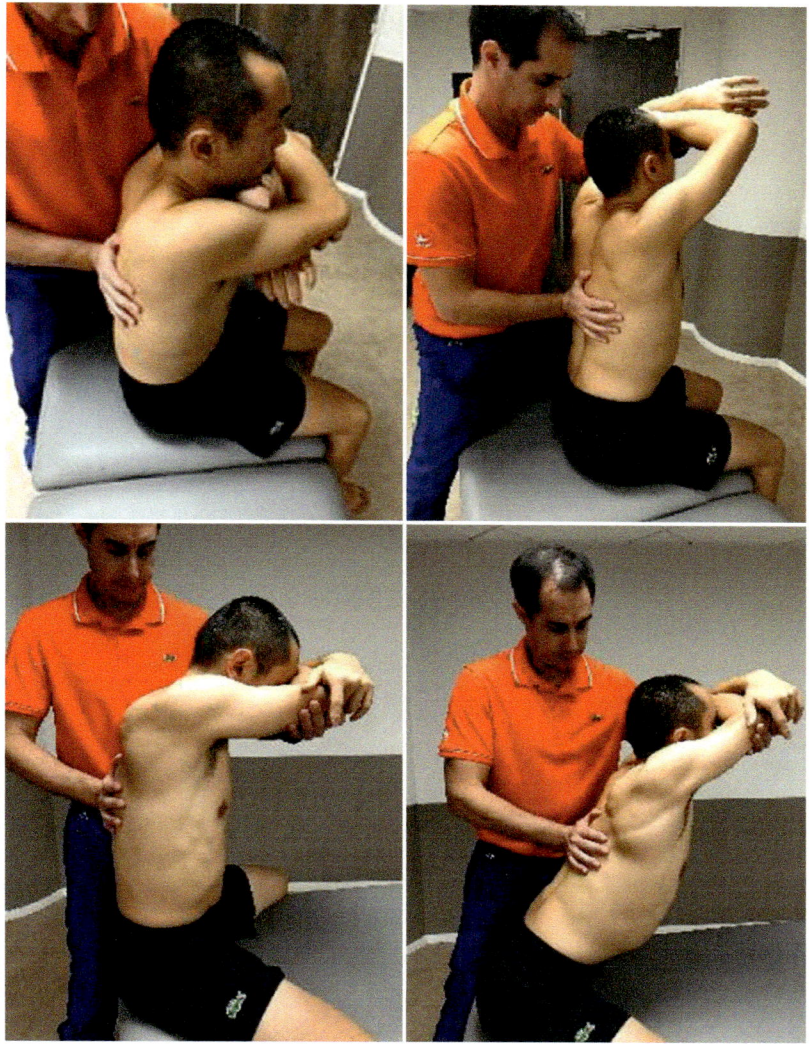

31.13.3 Encouraging Lateral Flexion/Sidebending

Player sitting on the table with his arms crossed on his chest. He starts to bend to one side gently toward the end of the range and then goes back and bends to the opposite side before coming back to the starting position.

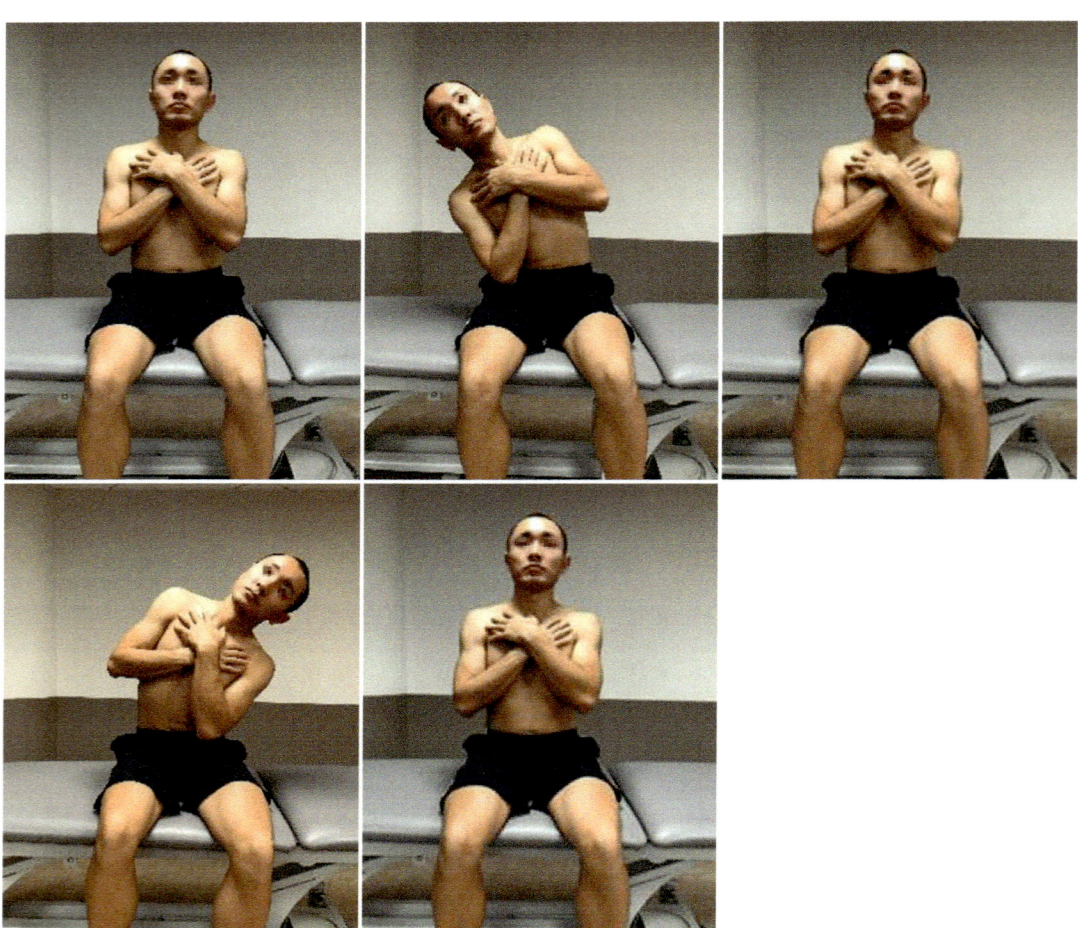

References

1. Pluim BM, Staal JB, Windler GE, Jayanthi N. Tennis injuries: occurrence, aetiology, and prevention. Br J Sports Med. 2006;40(5):415–23.
2. Kovacs M, Ellenbecker TS, Kibler WB, Roetert EP, Lubbers P. Injury trends in American competitive junior tennis players. J Sci Med Tennis. 2012;17(3):91–117.
3. Okholm Kryger K, Dor F, Guillaume M, Haida A, Noirez P, Montalvan B, et al. Medical reasons behind player departures from male and female professional tennis competitions. Am J Sports Med. 2015;43:34–40.
4. Kovacs M, Roetert EP, Ellenbecker TS. Complete conditioning for tennis, vol. 2. Champaign IL: Human Kinetics Publishers; 2017.

Core Stability in Tennis Players

Natalie L. Myers and W. Ben Kibler

32.1 Introduction

The musculoskeletal core of the body includes the lumbar spine, the muscles of the abdominal wall, the back extensors, the quadratus lumborum, the diaphragm, and the pelvic floor [1, 2]. The core has been conceptually described as a muscular box [3]. The abdominal wall creates the anterior and lateral walls, the extensors form the posterior wall, and the top and the bottom of the box are formed by the diaphragm and pelvic floor, respectively. The muscles of the hip help to reinforce the bottom of the box and are essential for force generation and energy transfer to distal extremities. The core serves as the center of functional kinetic chain movement. It has been described as a corset that works as a unit to stabilize the body and spine, with and without limb movement [4]. It is particularly important in sports requiring overhead motion as it provides proximal stability for distal mobility [5].

32.2 Anatomy of the Core

The abdominal muscles consist of the transverse abdominus, the internal and external obliques, and the rectus abdominus. Contracting the transverse abdominus increases intra-abdominal pressure and tensions the thoracolumbar fascia. The transverse abdominus have been shown to be critical in the stabilization of the lumbar spine [6, 7]. Abdominal muscle contractions help create a rigid cylinder, enhancing stiffness of the lumbar spine [8]. It is important to note that the rectus abdominus and oblique abdominals are activated in direction-specific patterns with respect to limb movements, thus providing postural support before limb movements [9–11]. Contractions that increase intra-abdominal pressure occur before initiation of large segment movement of the upper limbs [12, 13]. In this manner, the spine (and core of the body) is stabilized before limb movements occur to allow the limbs to have a stable base for motion and muscle activation [14]. Clinically, it has been shown that only a very small increase in activation of the multifidi and abdominal muscles is required to stiffen the spinal segments (5% of maximal voluntary contraction for activities of daily living and 10% of maximal voluntary contraction for rigorous activity) [15].

Core stability requires control of trunk motion in all three planes. In order to provide stability in all planes of motions, muscles may be activated in patterns that are different from their primary

N. L. Myers (✉)
Department of Health and Human Performance,
Texas State University, Austin, TX, USA
e-mail: natalie.myers@txstate.edu

W. B. Kibler
Shoulder Center of Kentucky, Lexington Clinic Orthopedics, Lexington, KY, USA

functions. For example, the quadratus lumborum (QL) muscle functions mainly as a stabilizer of frontal plane flexion and extension activities. However, the QL is attached from the transverse processes of the spine and the 12th rib to the iliac crests. This orientation allows QL muscle activation that occurs in association with flexion, extension, and lateral bending activities to buttress shearing of the spine in the plane of movement, making it more than just a frontal plane stabilizing muscle [16].

The roof of the core muscle structures is the diaphragm. Simultaneous contraction of the diaphragm, the pelvic floor muscles, and the abdominal muscles is required to increase intra-abdominal pressure, providing a more rigid cylinder for trunk support, decreasing the load on the spine muscles, and allowing increased trunk stability [13, 15, 17]. The diaphragm contributes to intra-abdominal pressure before the initiation of limb movements, thereby assisting spine/trunk stability. This activation occurs independently of the respiratory actions [18].

At the opposite end of the trunk component of the core muscles are the pelvic floor muscles. Because of the difficulty in directly assessing these muscles, they are often neglected or ignored with respect to musculoskeletal rehabilitation. Synergistic activation patterns exist involving the transverse abdominus, abdominals, multifidi, and pelvic floor muscles that provide a base of support for all the trunk and spinal muscles [13].

The hips and pelvis and their associated structures are the base of support for the core structures. Critical to functioning of the hip and pelvis are the many major muscle groups in this area. These muscles have large cross-sectional areas and, in addition to their stabilizing role, can generate a great deal of force and power for athletic activities.

32.3 Core Stability

Core stability is an important component maximizing efficient athletic function. Function is most often produced by the kinetic chain, the coordinated, sequenced activation of body segments that places the distal segment in the optimum position at the optimum velocity with the optimum timing to produce the desired athletic task [19]. The core is important to provide local strength and balance and to decrease injury. In addition, since the core is central to almost all kinetic chains of sports activities, control of core strength, balance, and motion will maximize all kinetic chains of upper and lower extremity function.

There is no single universally accepted definition of core stability. A general definition of core stability that will be used in this chapter is the ability to control the position and motion of the trunk over the pelvis and leg to allow optimum production, transfer and control of force, and motion to the terminal segment in integrated kinetic chain activities.

Developing core stability should not be isolated to one muscle; in fact McGill et al. suggest that spinal stability results from highly coordinated muscle activation patterns involving many muscles [20]. Athletes participating in sports must be able to withstand external loads or unanticipated movements. When an external load is applied to the human body, the stability of the system is mitigated by the stiffness of the musculature. According to Lee [21]:

> Insufficient stiffness via muscular activation may cause the system to buckle or not return to its initial state, which in terms of the spine may lead to injury. If muscular activation is trained and sufficient stiffness is present, then no buckling should occur, and stability should be preserved.

All core musculature must work together to create a balance in stiffness needed to ensure stability of the spine [20].

Core stability is a prerequisite for distal extremity movement. In a sport such as tennis, the rotational demands about the pelvis and trunk are imperative to generate distal forces. Therefore, proximal control and muscular activity is essential in multiple planes of movement. The ipsilateral external oblique has been shown to activate almost at foot strike during overhead throwing tasks [22]. Similarly, the external oblique and rectus abdominus exhibit high activations during the descending windup phase of the tennis serve [23]. The co-contraction of bilateral external and internal obliques during the serve provide a stabilizing force to the lumbar spine [23, 24].

32.4 Measures of Core Stability

There is no standard way that has been described to measure core stability. Electromyography (EMG) activity has been recorded in several different core stability maneuvers providing a level of validity to certain tests [25, 26]. Different investigators have used different techniques to try to gauge core stability through functional and multi-planar movement patterns and [5, 27–29] sustained isometric muscular holds and dynamic movement [30–35]. These data can give an approximate estimate of core stability. Often, to assess all the different muscles that function together to provide core stability, evaluation of specific motion patterns, and quality of movement may be done.

One option to assess core stability that incorporates many of these variables is to look at one-leg standing balance ability and a one-leg squat. In a standing balance test, the patient is asked to stand on one leg with no other verbal cue. Deviations such as a Trendelenburg posture or internally or externally rotating the weight-bearing limb indicate inability to control the posture and suggest proximal core deficits [5]. A more objective measure of single-leg standing balance has been described by Radwan et al. [36]. Overhead athletes with shoulder dysfunction were asked to maintain appropriate balance for 45 s or until failure of the task occurred. Failure was defined as opening of the eyes, uncrossed arms, shifted weight, elevated foot contacting the floor, or the stance leg being no longer in the starting position. Overhead athletes with shoulder dysfunction had a 9-s deficit when performing the single-leg balance test compared to healthy athletes. The results of the study indicated that overhead athletes with shoulder dysfunction had less balance compared to healthy athletes [36].

If the standing balance test is done well, a one-leg squat would be the next progressive evaluation. Assuming the same starting point as the standing balance test, the patient is asked to do repetitive partial quarter to half squats with no other verbal cues. Similar deviations in the quality of the movement are assessed as in the standing balance test. A Trendelenburg posture, which may not be noted on standing balance, may be brought out with a single leg squat. The patient may use their arms for balance or may go into an exaggerated flexed or rotated posture in order to put the gluteal or short rotator muscles on greater tension to compensate for other muscular weakness. The single-leg squat test was shown to have moderate reliability when using a four-point grading scale [28]; however, the use of a three-point grading scale improved reliability to substantial agreement [37].

Several studies have attempted to quantify muscular activity during stabilization exercises. A series of studies have shown that three forms of exercise produced stabilizing patterns while challenging the core muscles to an appropriate level using the curl up [38], side bridge [16], and birddog [39]. These exercises are commonly referred to as the big three [39]. In addition to the big three exercises, the bridge, unilateral bridge, and prone bridge exercises (plank on the elbows) provide safe levels of muscle activation without harmful external loading making these exercises excellent for core stabilization [40].

Clinical tests used to measure core stability are on the rise as clinicians become more aware of the important role proximal stabilizers play in overhead movement patterns. However, these clinical tests are most often performed on healthy participants with investigations aimed toward establishing the test's reliability and normative values. The majority of the tests presented in this section have no validity data to fully understand their clinical utility. Table 32.1 includes a summary of core stabilization tests that may be implemented in order to quantify stability.

In addition to these tests, some researchers have tried to identify the association between core stability control and athletic injuries. Chaudhari et al. [46] found that poor lumbopelvic

Table 32.1 Summary of core stability tests

Author	Participants	Clinical test of stability	Equipment and instruction	Outcome
O'Connor et al. [33]	15 healthy male athletes	Alternative trunk stability push-up test	Strip of athletic tape Lie prone with tape at the forehead, feet together, and shoulder and elbow at 90/90° Lift right leg slightly off the ground and press up while lifting the body as a unit Rating scale: 0–4	ICC intra-tester reliability range: 0.73–0.90 ICC inter-tester reliability: 0.97 Average score: 3.57 ± 0.65
Krause et al. [41]	Healthy volunteers 50 men 50 women	Double-leg lowering test	Requires two examiners Examiner 1: Lie supine with legs in vertical position with the knees extended Instruct participants to keep the lumbar spine in contact with the table while lowering the legs Examiner 1 monitors the position of the lower back with the hand between the lower back and table and signal examiner 2 when participant begins to lift back off table Examiner 2: At the signal to end the test, use inclinometer to record the position of the leg Inclinometer placed along the long axis of the femur	ICC intra-tester reliability: 0.98 Men lower legs on average 15 ± 2° from a horizontal reference and women on average 37 ± 4°
Radwan et al. [36]	48 healthy overhead (OH) athletes 14 OH athletes with shoulder dysfunction	Single-leg balance test	Eyes closed, arms crossed at the chest, contralateral leg slightly flexed Measured until failure or 45 s is reached "Refer to body of text for errors"	Right leg (significant difference) OH athletes with shoulder dysfunction 10 ± 7 s OH healthy athletes 19 ± 15 s Left leg (no difference) OH athletes with shoulder dysfunction 10 ± 7 s OH healthy athletes 17 ± 14 s
Butowicz et al. [35]	20 healthy males and females	Unilateral hip bridge endurance test (UHBE)	Participants lie supine with arms across the chest, the knees in flexion, and the feet flat on the floor Instruct participants to extend the hips, and once the spine and pelvis are neutral, the subject extends one knee Test is terminated when participants are no longer able to maintain neutral pelvic position as noted by 10° change in transverse or sagittal plane movement Pelvic position in the transverse plane monitor with inclinometer Pelvic position in the sagittal plane assess visually	Concurrent validity: Moderate significant relationship between UHBE and biomechanical measures of core neuromuscular control (−0.49 to 0.056)

Study	Participants	Test	Description	Results/Notes
Stanton et al. [29]	22 healthy male athletes	Sahrmann core stability	Participant lie supine. An inflatable pad of a stabilizer pressure biofeedback unit (PBU) is placed under the lumbar curve and inflated to 40 mm Hg. The test consists of five levels, with each level increasing in difficulty. Level 1: Begin in supine, crook-lying position during abdominal pre-setting (activation). Slowly raise 1 leg to 100° of hip flexion with comfortable knee flexion. The opposite leg is then brought to same position. Level 2: From hip-flexed position, slowly lower one leg until the heel contacts the ground, fully extend the knee, return to starting flexed position. Level 3: From hip-flexed position, slowly lower one leg until the heel is 12 cm above the ground, fully extend the knee, return to starting flexed position. Level 4: From the hip-flexed position, slowly lower both legs until heels contact the ground, fully extend both knees, return to starting position. Level 5: From the hip-flexed position, slowly lower both legs until heels are 12 cm above the ground, fully extend both knees, return to starting position. In order to attain each new level of the Sahrmann test, the lumbar spine position should be maintained as indicated by a change of no more than 10 mm Hg in pressure on the PBU	Reliability: 0.95
McGill and Karpowicz [42]	8 healthy men	Curl up	Participants lie supine with one leg straight and the other bent. One hand behind the lumbar spine and raise chest up to ceiling with shoulder blades removed from ground	While stiffening the torso with an abdominal brace, both external and internal obliques increased activation, with the internal oblique approaching 50% of maximal voluntary contraction
McGill and Karpowicz [42]	8 healthy men	Birddog	Participants in quadruped position. Initially, participant lifts only the left arm and then progresses to the right leg only. Next, the left arm and right leg are lifted. Draw squares with opposite hand/foot to increase difficulty	Drawing squares with the hand/foot while in the birddog position posture enhances activation of many muscle groups
McGill et al. [32]	Healthy volunteers 31 men 44 women	Extensor endurance test	Participants lie prone with the lower body fixed at ankles, knees, and hips, upper body cantilevered over test bench, arms crossed, lift upper body until torso is horizontal to the floor. Maintain position as long as possible	Average time Men: 146 ± 51 s Women: 189 ± 60 s
McGill et al. [32]	Healthy volunteers 31 men 44 women	Flexor endurance test	Sit on test bench with back rested against 60° support, knees and hips both at 90°, arms crossed across chest. Maintain body position while support is moved back. Ends when torso falls below 60°	Average Time Men: 144 ± 76 s Women: 149 ± 99 s

(continued)

Table 32.1 (continued)

Author	Participants	Clinical test of stability	Equipment and instruction	Outcome
McGill et al. [32]	Healthy volunteers 31 men 44 women	Side bridge test	Lie on mat, legs extended, top foot on top of lower foot, support on one elbow, uninvolved arm across the chest Lift hips off mat so body is a straight line Continue until hips fall to the mat	Average time Right side: Men: 94 ± 34 s Women: 72 ± 31 s Left side: Men: 97 ± 35 s Women: 77 ± 35 s
Pontillo et al. [43]	26 healthy collegiate varsity football players	Closed kinetic chain upper extremity stability test	Two pieces of tape, shoulder width apart Push-up position, move one hand to the opposite tape line, and return to starting position; repeat with opposite hand Repeat as many times as possible in 15 s	Number of touches: 22 ± 4
Garrison et al. [44]	Baseball players 30 with UCL tear 30 healthy	Y balance test	Perform single-limb stance while reaching with the opposite leg to designated indicator box (anterior, posteromedial, or posterolateral directions) Balance measurements recorded as a % of leg length	ICC intra-tester reliability range: 0.86–0.95 Y balance test composite score Lead limb, % (significant difference) Healthy: 96 ± 6 UCL: 89 ± 7 Y balance test composite score Stance limb, % (significant difference) Healthy: 95 ± 6 UCL: 88 ± 8
Strand et al. [45]	Healthy volunteers 194 males 277 females	Forearm plank	Assume forearm plank position with only toes and forearms supporting the body Hold as long as possible	Time holding position Males: 124 ± 72 s Females: 83 ± 6 s

control, as measured using the single-leg raise test, was associated with days missed due to an injury in baseball pitchers. Pitchers with less lumbopelvic control were three times more likely to miss at least 30 days than pitchers demonstrating more lumbopelvic control. The closed kinetic chain upper extremity stability test (CKCUEST) has also demonstrated predictive characteristics in football athletes. Football players demonstrating 21 touches or below were 18 times more likely to sustain a shoulder injury than those reaching more than 21 touches. Swimmers aged 12–14 years without shoulder pain were able to hold a side bridge 8 s longer than those who reported shoulder pain in the same age group [47]. While not statistically significant, trends of reduced core stability were seen in symptomatic swimmers at the high school and master level undergoing the side bridge and prone bridge [47]. Competitive high school and college baseball players with a diagnosed ulnar collateral ligament (UCL) tear demonstrated decreased Y balance composite scores on both limbs compared to healthy age-matched controls [44]. While this study cannot conclude that decreased balance was a cause of elbow injury, authors do suggest a potential association between poor core control as measured by the Y balance test and upper extremity injury to the elbow.

32.5 Evidence-Based Methods for Training the Core

There is no universally accepted program for the promotion of core training. Currently, dynamic core exercises incorporating both proximal and distal segments are recommended to improve performance and strength, but the specific exercises and at what training regime (number of sets and repetitions) are limited in the literature. According to Kibler et al. [48], strengthening and stability of the core and lower extremity musculature are critical because of their contributions to the overhead motion. The athlete should engage in lower extremity and core exercises such as the rotational chop-and-lift activities that simulate the rotational demands like those seen in tennis [49].

The core is a popular target for athletic development and training when trying to improve performance. There are studies that have implemented core-focused interventions within an athletic population; however, the outcomes among these studies are quite variable (Table 32.2).

Several studies incorporate functional tests assessing balance [51, 53, 54, 57, 58], core stability [29, 52, 55], core strength [50, 58], and core power [56]. However only a few report actual sport performance measures. Palmer et al. [56] are the only authors to our knowledge that implemented two sport-specific trunk

Table 32.2 Core-focused training protocols in different athletic populations

Author	Participants	Intervention	Outcome measure	Results
Stanton et al. [29]	22 male athletes	6 weeks Control or Swiss ball training	Sahrmann core stability test Swiss ball prone stabilization core stability test	Swiss ball training significantly improved core stability compared to control
Patil et al. [50]	60 male and female competitive swimmers	6 weeks Control or core training group	Core muscle strength performance Stroke rate Stroke length Stroke index 50 m freestyle	Core training significantly improved 50 m freestyle time and core muscle strength performance compared to control
Sandry et al. [51]	13 track and field athletes	6 weeks Core stabilization training	Star excursion balance test (SEBT) Abdominal fatigue test (AFT) Back extensor test (BET) Side bridge test (SBT)	Core stabilization training improved SEBT, AFT, BET, and SBT measures

(continued)

Table 32.2 (continued)

Author	Participants	Intervention	Outcome measure	Results
Kim et al. [52]	16 females basketball players	8 weeks Control or unilateral core training	Trunk angular displacement	Trunk angular displacement reduced in both rotational directions in the core training group
Romero-Franco et al. [53]	33 male sprinters	6 weeks Control or proprioceptive exercise program including core stability exercises	Stability test with eyes open and closed Postural stability Gravity center of control	Stability in the mediolateral plane with eyes open, gravity center of control in the right and posterior direction improved following proprioceptive exercise training
Filipa et al. [54]	20 female soccer players	8 weeks Control or neuromuscular training program focused on core stability	SEBT	Neuromuscular training program significantly improved SEBT composite score on both limbs compared to the control group
Lust et al. [55]	6 weeks 25 college baseball players	6 weeks Control or open kinetic chain/closed kinetic chain (OKC/CKC) or OKC/CKC/core stability (CS)	CKCUEST Functional throwing performance index (FTPI) Back extensor test (BET) AFT SBT	Increase in all measures from pre to post No group differences
Palmer et al. [56]	46 college male and female softball and baseball players	7 weeks Traditional endurance training or power stability training *Both regimes with an emphasis on core rotation*	Throwing velocity Chop and left Test Endurance planks	Significant improvements in peak-throwing velocity and the chop-and-lift test following power stability training compared to endurance training
Samson et al. [57]	Tennis players	5 weeks Core stabilization training program	SEBT	SEBT improved from pre to post following core stabilization training program
Lephart et al. [58]	15 healthy male golfers	8 weeks Golf-specific exercise program *Incorporated rotational stretching, rotational strengthening, and balance exercises*	Swing mechanics Torso, shoulder, and hip strength testing Balance assessment Shoulder and hip range of motion	Significant improvement in bilateral torso rotation strength, bilateral hip abduction strength, shoulder and hip range of motion, and anterior-posterior and mediolateral sway in balance and swing mechanics following training program
Tse et al. [59]	45 college rowers	8 weeks Control or core training group	BET AFT SBT	SBT significantly improved in core training group compared to control
Fernandez-Fernandez et al. [60]	30 male competitive tennis players	6 weeks Control or multimodal training *Incorporated upper/lower extremity and core training*	Serve velocity Serve accuracy	Significant difference from pre to post in multimodal training group

stability training regimes, one with an emphasis on endurance with the other emphasizing power stability. Overhead athletes in the power stability group had a 56% increase in mean throwing velocity compared to the endurance training group. Another study that assessed serve velocity used multimodal training, incorporating upper and lower extremity and core/trunk exercises into an exercise protocol [60]. Nationally ranked junior tennis players were shown to have improvements in serve velocity following a 6-week intervention. In fact, it has been suggested that isolated training of the core should not be the primary emphasis for programs with the goal of enhancing overhead velocity. The results of a meta-analysis revealed that an effective 6-week intervention aimed toward improving velocity should incorporate multimodal training [61].

While the majority of the interventions presented in Table 32.2 were not implemented on tennis-specific populations, we do believe tennis players may see benefits in performance and core stability following one or more of these exercise programs. Following core stability exercises, the core should be challenged to withstand the demands of sport. Therefore, the authors have provided a series of exercises based off literature reviews and clinical experience that may be used on healthy players to improve performance, core strength, endurance, and power and possibility diminish the risk of injury.

32.5.1 Single-Leg Balance with Hip Extension and Trunk Rotation

Description: Standing on one leg, the athlete is instructed to extend the free limb while rotating the torso away from the stance leg while maintaining a stable core. This exercise can be progressed with therabands placed around the lower leg of the free limb and/or the torso. The athlete can also perform this exercise with a racket in hand to mimic the backhand or forehand motions (Fig. 32.1).

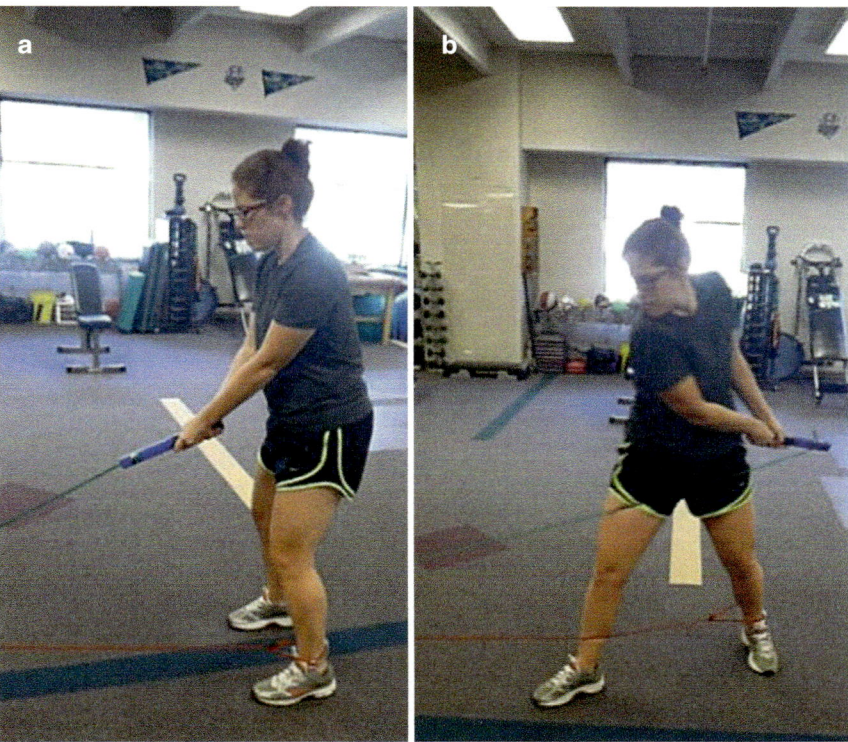

Fig. 32.1 Single-leg balance with hip extension and rotation. (**a**) Starting position. (**b**) Ending position

32.5.2 Single-Leg Step-Up with Ball/Racket Separation

Description: Standing parallel to a step, the athlete is instructed to step up with the dominant leg (ipsilateral to racket arm) onto the platform while performing ball/racket separation. Hold top position for 5 s (Fig. 32.2). Resistance can also be added to the torso.

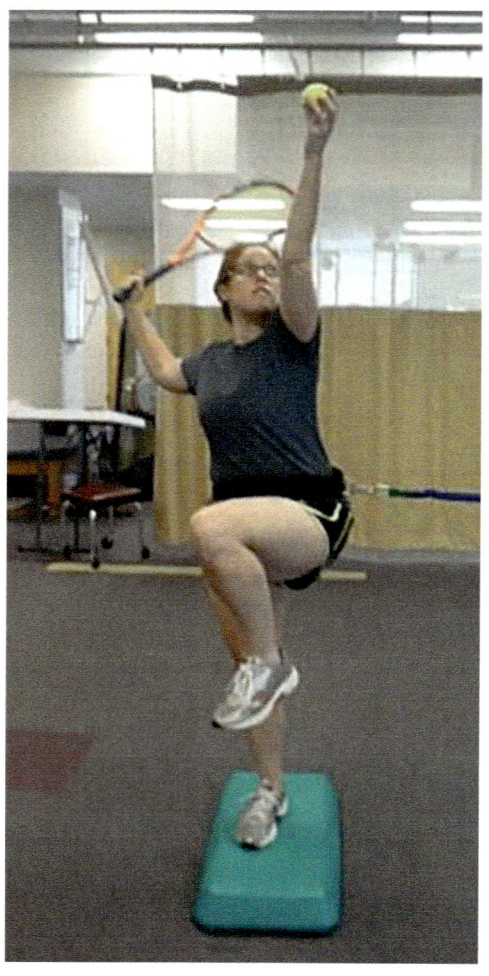

Fig. 32.2 Single-leg step-up with ball/racket separation

32.5.3 Lateral-Band Walking with Torso Rotation

Description: Place a theraband distally around both ankles. The athlete is instructed to perform a mini squat and to step laterally while keeping tension in the theraband. As the athlete steps laterally, they are instructed to rotate the torso to the same side as the step and then to the opposite side. To progress this exercise, a medicine ball can be held. This exercise should be performed in both directions (Fig. 32.3).

32.5.4 Trunk Rotation Abdominal Throw

Description: With a medicine ball, the athlete is instructed to assume a v-sit position with the arms reaching out. The athlete rotates the torso away from the rebounder and performs a rotational toss and catch, allowing trunk rotation to occur in a controlled midrange of motion. The emphasis should not only be put on the toss phase but also control the eccentric movement during the catching phase. This exercise should be performed bilaterally (Fig. 32.4).

32.5.5 Diagonal Chop-and-Lift Theraband Pulls

Description: Athlete is instructed to keep the core stable while performing diagonal chop-and-lift patterns. The athlete can be placed on an Airex pad, foam roller, BOSU ball, or dyna disk and undergo different stance positions (double-limb, single-limb, tandem, lunge, or squat position). Note: External perturbation may be provided by the healthcare professional to push on the athlete's pelvis or torso during the maneuver (Fig. 32.5).

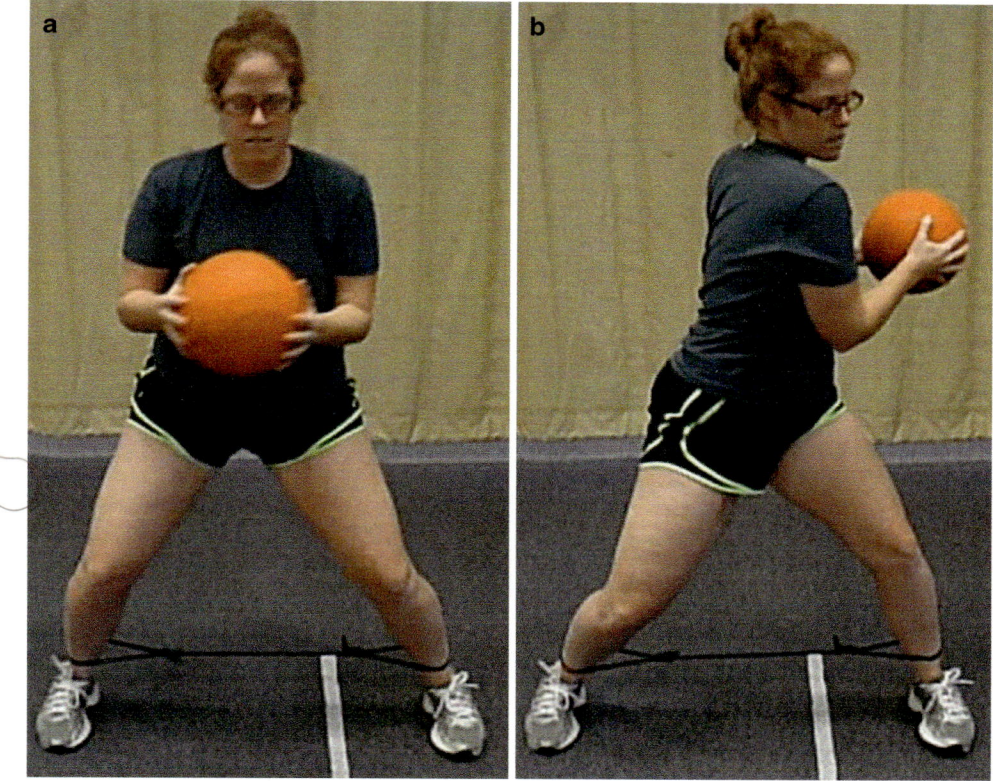

Fig. 32.3 Lateral-band walking with torso rotation. (**a**) Starting position. (**b**) Ending position

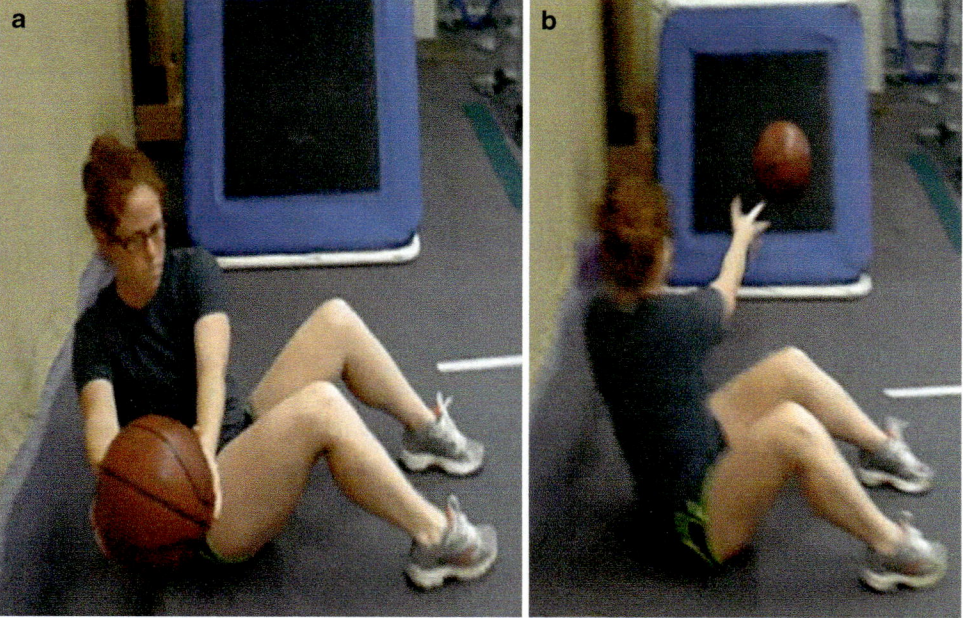

Fig. 32.4 Trunk rotation abdominal throw. (**a**) Starting position. (**b**) Ending position

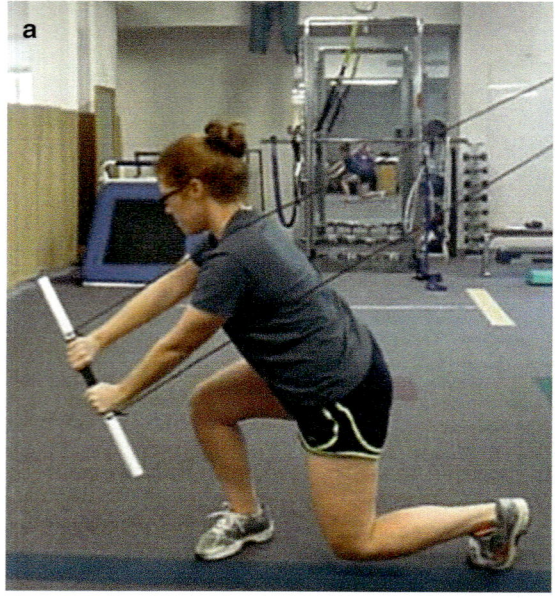
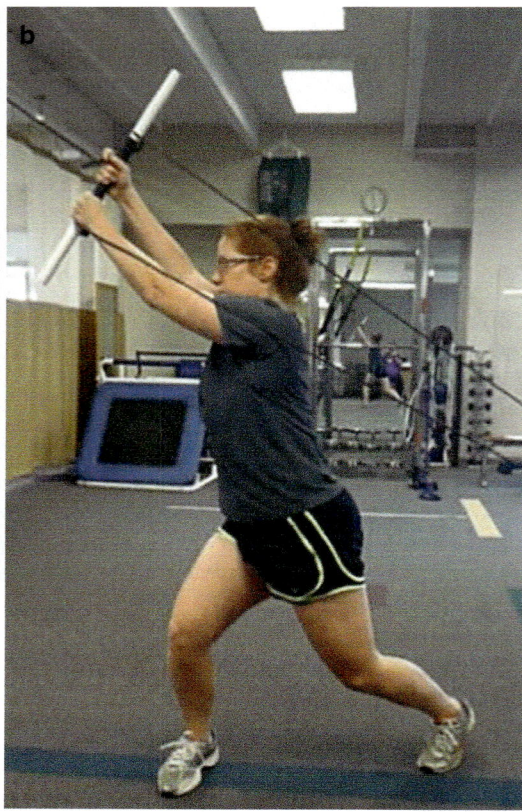

Fig. 32.5 Diagonal chop-and-lift pulls. (**a**) The chop maneuver. (**b**) The lift maneuver

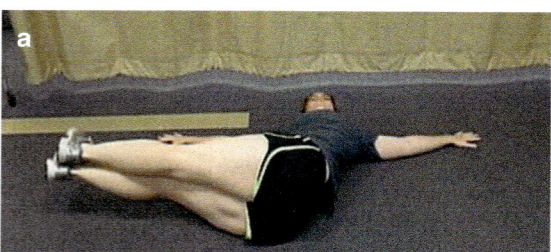
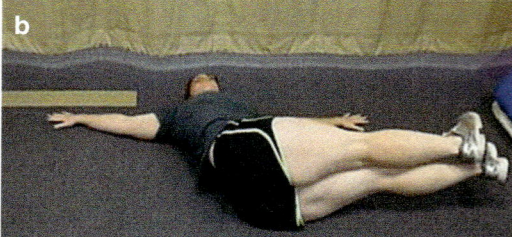

Fig. 32.6 Windshield Wiper. (**a**) Rotation to the right. (**b**) Rotation to the left

32.5.6 Windshield Wiper

Description: Athlete is in supine position and is instructed to spread the arms to the side in a "T" position and bring the hips to 90°. The athlete will let the legs slowly drop to the right side until parallel with the arms, and before the legs touch the ground, the athlete with reverse the movement using the core to pull the legs to the left side (Fig. 32.6).

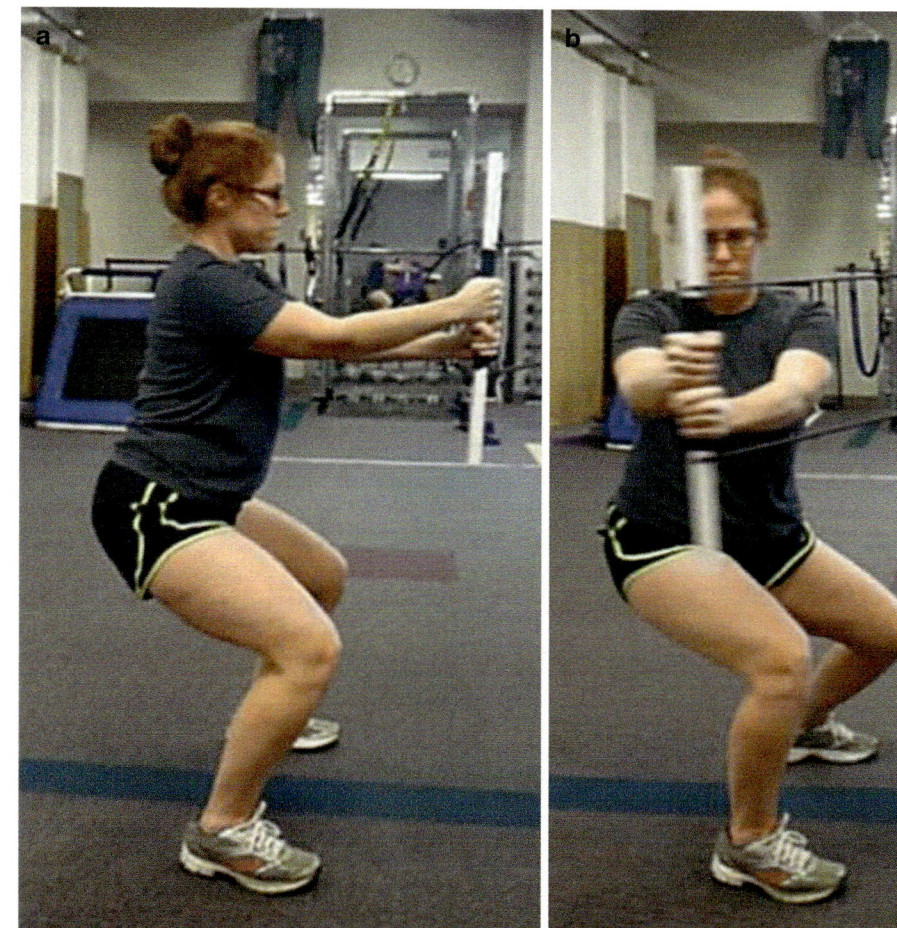

Fig. 32.7 Squat with torso rotation. (**a**) Starting position. (**b**) Ending position

32.5.7 Squat with Torso Rotation

Description: Athlete will assume a double-leg or single-leg mini squat with the arm reaching out in front of them holding a tensed theraband. The athlete is instructed to rotate the trunk to the left side and then to right side (Fig. 32.7).

32.5.8 Supine Straight-Leg Torso Twists

Description: Athlete will lie supine with the hip flexed to 90° and the knees at 0°. The athlete is instructed to touch the palm of the hand to the outside of the opposite foot and to repeat on the other side (Fig. 32.8).

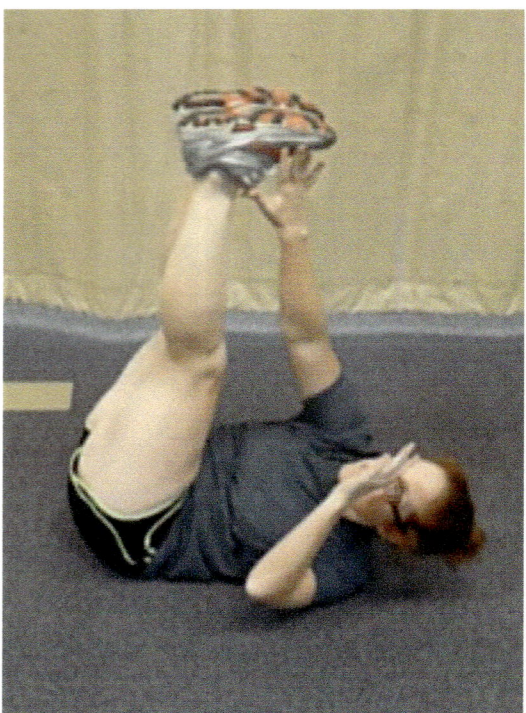

Fig. 32.8 Supine straight-leg torso twists

Conclusion

Core stability is a pivotal component in normal athletic function and activity. It is best understood as a highly integrated activation of multiple segments that provides force generation, proximal stability for distal mobility, and generates interactive movement. Core stability can be measured reliably with a limited amount of equipment using a variety of different tests. Core stability deficits have been shown to have relationships to injury in a variety of different sports. Few studies have investigated performance enhancement in sporting activities despite observing improvement in core stability and core strength following a core training program. The core should be trained in a progressive fashion, beginning with neuromuscular recruitment in a variety of different positions and then transition to total dynamic and sport specific movement patterns.

References

1. Barr KP, Griggs M, Cadby T. Lumbar stabilization: core concepts and current literature, part 1. Am J Phys Med Rehabil. 2005;84(6):473–80.
2. McGill S. Core training: evidence translating to better performance and injury prevention. Strength Cond J. 2010;32(3):33–46.
3. Richardson CA, Hodges P. Therapeutic exercise for spinal segmental stabilization in low back pain: scientific basis and clinical approach. Edinburgh, NY: Churchill Livingstone; 1999.
4. Akuthota V, Nadler SF. Core strengthening. Arch Phys Med Rehabil. 2004;85:86–92.
5. Kibler WB, Press J, Sciascia A. The role of core stability in athletic function. Sports Med. 2006;36(3):189–98.
6. Cresswell A, Oddsson L, Thorstensson A. The influence of sudden perturbations on trunk muscle activity and intra-abdominal pressure while standing. Exp Brain Res. 1994;98(2):336–41.
7. Oddsson LI. Control of voluntary trunk movements in man: mechanisms for postural equilibrium during standing. Acta Physiol Scand Suppl. 1990;595:1–60.
8. McGill S, Norman RW. Reassessment of the role of intra-abdominal pressure in spinal compression. Ergonomics. 1987;30(11):1565–88.
9. Aruin AS, Latash ML. Directional specificity of postural muscles in feed-forward postural reactions during fast voluntary arm movements. Exp Brain Res. 1995;103(2):323–32.
10. Hodges PW, Richardson CA. Feedforward contraction of transversus abdominus is not influenced by the direction of arm movement. Exp Brain Res. 1997;114:362–70.
11. Cordo PJ, Nashner LM. Properties of postural adjustments associated with rapid arm movements. J Neurophysiol. 1982;47(2):287–308.
12. Hodges P, Butler J, McKenzie D, et al. Contraction of the human diaphragm during rapid postural adjustments. J Physiol. 1997;505(2):539–48.
13. Hodges PW. Core stability exercise in chronic low back pain. Orthop Clin North Am. 2003;34(2):245–54.
14. Jensen BR, Laursen B, Sjogaard G. Aspects of shoulder function in relation to exposure demands and fatigue – a mini review. Clin Biomech. 2000;15(Suppl 1):S17–20.
15. Cholewicki J, Juluru K, McGill SM. Intra-abdominal pressure mechanism for stabilizing the lumbar spine. J Biomech. 1999;32(1):13–7.
16. McGill SM. Low back stability: from formal description to issues for performance and rehabilitation. Exerc Sport Sci Rev. 2001;29(1):26–31.
17. Daggfeldt K, Thorstensson A. The role of intra-abdominal pressure in spinal unloading. J Biomech. 1997;30(11):1149–55.

18. Ebenbichler GR, Oddsson LI, Kollmitzer J, et al. Sensory-motor control of the lower back: implications for rehabilitation. Med Sci Sports Exerc. 2001;33(11):1889–98.
19. Putnam CA. Sequential motions of body segments in striking and throwing skills: description and explanations. J Biomech. 1993;26:125–35.
20. McGill SM, Grenier S, Kavcic N, et al. Coordination of muscle activity to assure stability of the lumbar spine. J Electromyogr Kinesiol. 2003;13(4):353–9.
21. Lee B. Trainability of core stiffness: studies of core training methods on naive and savvy populations. Master of Science, University of Waterloo; 2013.
22. Hirashima M, Kadota H, Sakurai S. Sequential muscle activity and its function role in the upper extremity and trunk during overarm throwing. J Sports Sci. 2002;20:301–10.
23. Chow JW, Park S-A, Tillman MD. Lower trunk kinematics and muscle activity during different types of tennis serves. Sports Med Rehabil Ther Technol. 2009;1(1):24.
24. Chow JW, Shim JH, Lim YT. Lower trunk muscle activity during the tennis serve. J Sci Med Sport. 2003;6(4):512–8.
25. Schellenberg KL, Lang JM, Chan KM, Burnham RS. A clinical tool for office assessment of lumbar spine stabilization endurance: prone and supine bridge maneuvers. Am J Phys Med Rehabil. 2007;86(5):380–6.
26. Kim CR, Park DK, Lee ST, Ryu JS. Electromyographic Changes in Trunk Muscles During Graded Lumbar Stabilization Exercises. PM R. 2016;8(10):979–89.
27. Cowley PM, Swensen TC. Development and reliability of two core stability field tests. J Strength Cond Res. 2008;22(2):619–24.
28. Weir A, Darby J, Inklaar H, Koes B, Bakker E, Tol JL. Core stability: inter- and intraobserver reliability of 6 clinical tests. Clin J Sport Med. 2010;20(1):34–8.
29. Stanton R, Reaburn PR, Humphries B. The effect of short-term Swiss ball training on core stability and running economy. J Strength Cond Res. 2004;18(3):522–8.
30. Leetun DT, Ireland ML, Willson JD, Ballantyne BT, Davis IM. Core stability measures as risk factors for lower extremity injury in athletes. Med Sci Sports Exerc. 2004;36(6):926–34.
31. Faries MD, Greenwood M. Core training: stabilizing the confusion. Strength Cond J. 2007;29(2):10–25.
32. McGill SM, Childs A, Liebenson C. Endurance times for low back stabilization exercises: clinical targets for testing and training from a normal database. Arch Phys Med Rehabil Aug. 1999;80(8):941–4.
33. O'Connor S, McCaffrey N, Whyte E, Moran K. The development and reliability of a simple field based screening tool to assess core stability in athletes. Phys Ther Sport. 2016;20:40–4.
34. Nesser TW, Huxel KC, Tincher JL, et al. The relationship between core stability and performance in division I football players. J Strength Cond Res. 2008;22(6):1750–4.
35. Butowicz CM, Ebaugh DD, Noehren B, Silfies SP. Validation of two clinical measures of core stability. Int J Sports Phys Ther. 2016;11(1):15–23.
36. Radwan A, Francis J, Green A, et al. Is there a relation between shoulder dysfunction and core instability? Int J Sports Phys Ther. 2014;9(1):8–13.
37. Crossley KM, Zhang WJ, Schache AG, et al. Performance on the single-leg squat task indicates hip abductor muscle function. Am J Sports Med. 2011;39(4):866–73.
38. Axler CT, McGill SM. Low back loads over a variety of abdominal exercises: searching for the safest abdominal challenge. Med Sci Sports Exerc. 1997;29(6):804–11.
39. Callaghan JP, Gunning JL, McGill SM. The relationship between lumbar spine load and muscle activity during extensor exercises. Phys Ther. 1998;78(1):8–18.
40. Ekstrom RA, Donatelli RA, Carp KC. Electromyographic analysis of core trunk, hip, and thigh muscles during 9 rehabilitation exercises. J Orthop Sports Phys Ther. 2007;37(12):754–62.
41. Krause DA, Youdas JW, Hollman JH, Smith J. Abdominal muscle performance as measured by the double leg-lowering test. Arch Phys Med Rehabil. 2005;86(7):1345–8.
42. McGill SM, Karpowicz A. Exercises for spine stabilization: motion/motor patterns, stability progressions, and clinical technique. Arch Phys Med Rehabil. 2009;90(1):118–26.
43. Pontillo M, Spinelli BA, Sennett BJ. Prediction of In-Season Shoulder Injury From Preseason Testing in Division I Collegiate Football Players. Sports Health. 2014;6(6):497–503. https://doi.org/10.1177/1941738114523239.
44. Garrison JC, Arnold A, Macko MJ, Conway JE. Baseball players diagnosed with ulnar collateral ligament tears demonstrate decreased balance compared to healthy controls. J Orthop Sports Phys Ther. 2013;43(10):752–8.
45. Strand SL, Hjelm J, Shoepe TC, Fajardo MA. Norms for an isometric muscle endurance test. J Hum Kinet. 2014;40(1):93–102.
46. Chaudhari AM, McKenzie CS, Pan X, Oñate JA. Lumbopelvic control and days missed because of injury in professional baseball pitchers. Am J Sports Med. 2014;42(11):2734–40. https://doi.org/10.1177/0363546514545861.
47. Tate A, Turner GN, Knab SE, Jorgensen C, Strittmatter A, Michener LA. Risk factors associated with shoulder pain and disability across the lifespan of competitive swimmers. J Athl Train. 2012;47(2):149–58.

48. Kibler WB, Kuhn JE, Wilk K, et al. The disabled throwing shoulder: spectrum of pathology-10-year update. Arthroscopy. 2013;29(1):141–61. e126
49. Voight ML, Hoogenboom BJ, Cook G. The chop and lift reconsidered: integrating neuromuscular principles into orthopedic and sports rehabilitation. N Am J Sports Phys Ther. 2008;3(3):151–9.
50. Patil D, Salian SC, Yardi S. The effect of core strengthening on performance of young competitive swimmers. Int J Sci Res. 2014;3(6):2470–7.
51. Sandrey MA, Mitzel JG. Improvement in dynamic balance and core endurance after a 6-week core-stability-training program in high school track and field athletes. J Sport Rehab. 2013;22(4):264–71.
52. Kim Y, Kim J, Yoon B. Intensive unilateral core training improves trunk stability without preference for trunk left or right rotation. J Back Musculoskelet Rehabil. 2015;28(1):191–6.
53. Romero-Franco N, MartÍNez-LÓPez E, Lomas-Vega R, Hita-Contreras F, MartÍNez-Amat A. Effects of proprioceptive training program on core stability and center of gravity control in sprinters. J Strength Cond Res. 2012;26(8):2071–7.
54. Filipa A, Byrnes R, Paterno MV, Myer GD, Hewett TE. Neuromuscular training improves performance on the star excursion balance test in young female athletes. J Orthop Sports Phys Ther. 2010;40(9):551–8.
55. Lust KR, Sandrey MA, Bulger SM, Wilder N. The effects of 6-week training programs on throwing accuracy, proprioception, and core endurance in baseball. J Sport Rehab. 2009;18(3):407–26.
56. Palmer T, Uhl TL, Howell D, Hewett TE, Viele K, Mattacola CG. Sport-specific training targeting the proximal segments and throwing velocity in collegiate throwing athletes. J Athl Train. 2015;50(6):567–77.
57. Samson KM, Sandrey MA. A core stabilization training program for tennis athletes. Athletic Ther Today. 2007;12(3):41–6.
58. Lephart SM, Smoliga JM, Myers JB, Sell TC, Tsai Y-S. An eight-week golf-specific exercise program improves physical characteristics, swing mechanics, and golf performance in recreational golfers. J Strength Cond Res. 2007;21(3):860–9.
59. Tse MA, McManus AM, Masters RS. Development and validation of a core endurance intervention program: implications for performance in college-age rowers. J Strength Cond Res. 2005;19(3):547–52.
60. Fernandez-Fernandez J, Ellenbecker T, Sanz-Rivas D, Ulbricht A, Ferrautia L. Effects of a 6-week junior tennis conditioning program on service velocity. J Sports Sci Med. 2013;12(2):232–9.
61. Myers NL, Sciascia AD, Westgate PM, Kibler WB, Uhl TL. Increasing ball velocity in the overhead athlete: a meta-analysis of randomized controlled trials. J Strength Cond Res. 2015;29(10):2964–79.

Part VII

Medical Issues

Key Medical Issues for Tennis Players

33

Bradley G. Changstrom, Babette M. Pluim, and Neeru Jayanthi

33.1 Introduction

The aim of this chapter is to review key medical issues for tennis players and review key health benefits. Across all levels of play, tennis provides positive health benefits including improved aerobic fitness, reduced risk of cardiovascular disease, improvements in bone health, and a favorable lipid profile [1]. Racket sports, including tennis, had the most favorable health profile when evaluating morbidities compared to many other sports [2]. Other countries have used tennis clubs as a medium to address medical public health concerns including exercise, safety, and nutrition [3].

To start, the chapter will review exercise physiology of the tennis athlete and discuss the key medical issues for adult recreational tennis players with specific impacts on chronic medical conditions. It will then focus on the competitive tennis player, encompassing elite junior players, collegiate players, and tennis professionals. The highest-level tennis players can often tolerate higher loads of training. However, these elite players are at risk for illness and musculoskeletal injuries including overtraining syndrome and the female athlete triad and may even have some potential detrimental quality of life health issues. Some elite players are exposed to international travel and year-round environmental exposure, which may result in travel-related illness and impact sleep and mood. Efforts have been made by the Women's Tennis Association (WTA) and the Association of Tennis Professionals (ATP) World Tours to help improve the transition into these challenging professional environments. Specifically, the WTA has had long-term follow-up on the effects of the Age Eligibility Rule and its player development programs. Finally, the chapter will review special medical considerations in the tennis athlete including bone health, the female athlete triad, and risks of non-accidental violence in sport.

In summary, while other chapters will review specific issues related to musculoskeletal screening (Chap. 10), pre-participation evaluation (Chap. 11), sports nutrition (Chap. 36), heat-related issues (Chap. 37), and dermatologic conditions (Chap. 39), this chapter will in essence discuss the comprehensive medical care of the tennis athlete.

B. G. Changstrom
Division of General Internal Medicine, Department of Medicine, CU Sports Medicine, University of Colorado Hospital, Aurora, CO, USA
e-mail: Bradley.changstrom@ucdenver.edu

B. M. Pluim (✉)
Royal Netherlands Lawn Tennis Association, Amersfoort, The Netherlands
e-mail: b.pluim@knltb.nl

N. Jayanthi
Orthopedics and Family Medicine, Tennis Medicine, Emory Sports Medicine Center, Society for Tennis Medicine and Science (STMS),
Atlanta, GA, USA

33.2 Physical Fitness

33.2.1 Case #1

"An 18-year-old competitive tennis player is training to prepare for college tennis. What are the physiological characteristics of tennis to help guide his training?"

33.2.1.1 Exercise Intensity and Aerobic Capacity

The American College of Cardiology and American Heart Association consider tennis to be a moderate static and high dynamic activity [4]. This is an update from previous guidelines, including the 36th Bethesda Conference, where tennis was listed as a low static and high dynamic activity [5]. Newer data suggests that tennis may even be considered a high dynamic and high static strength sport in some athletes as echocardiograms of male professional tennis players demonstrated both concentric and eccentric left ventricular hypertrophy [6]. Typical points last an average of ~6-7s s in high-level collegiate players, and work-to-rest intervals vary between 1:2 and 1:5 [7]. The level of intensity of tennis play varies mostly by level of play and in singles versus doubles [7].

Moderate to vigorous activity is thought to be of the greatest health benefit for reduced morbidity and mortality [8]. Generally, tennis is considered a mixed aerobic and anaerobic activity in recreational players. However, elite tennis players may be considered highly aerobically trained as VO_2 max ranges between 44 and 69 mL/kg/min [7].

33.3 Health Benefits of Tennis in Adults

33.3.1 Case #2

"A 50-year-old female former multisport high school athlete is trying to become active again. She is debating which activity would give her the greatest health benefit between tennis, swimming, and running."

33.3.1.1 General Health Benefits of Tennis

This section will largely address specific health benefits in the adult recreational tennis player with skill levels 2.5–5.0 US National Tennis Rating Program (NTRP) [9, 10]. The health benefits of tennis have been outlined in several reviews [1, 11–14]. The benefits include many medical, physical, psychological, and cognitive benefits. Studies have demonstrated a risk reduction in mortality related to physical activity. In a prospective study of nearly 10,000 men, starting a physical activity program with moderate to vigorous intensity, such as tennis, demonstrated a risk reduction in mortality of 44% compared to unfit men [15]. Another study showed similar benefits with decreases of 27–32% in overall mortality [16]. In these studies, the distinction in health benefit was between being fit versus being unfit rather than mode of exercise by sport; however, tennis met the physical activity guidelines for fitness that would demonstrate a mortality benefit.

In a review by Kovacs et al., it was suggested that the intensity of exercise, more than the duration of exercise alone, may be more beneficial for overall health [14]. Therefore, those elite adult tennis players who are more vigorously active are more likely to get greater health benefits and mortality risk reduction than those who don't play tennis. More specifically, in a recent large prospective epidemiologic study, mortality risk reduction of tennis was the greatest out of all sports. Over 80,000 British adults were followed for up to 9 years while adjusting for other cardiovascular risk factors. This study found a 9-year mortality risk reduction of 47% for racket sports while the next closest sport of swimming had only a 28% risk reduction [2]. This is the strongest data to date regarding the sport-specific health benefit of racket sports, including tennis. Other specific health benefits including cholesterol, diabetes, bone health, and hypertension will be presented later in this chapter and in Table 33.1.

Table 33.1 Health benefits of consistent participation in tennis

Increased aerobic capacity
Lower resting heart rate and blood pressure
Increased bone density
Improved reaction time
Lower body fat
Improved muscle tone, strength, and flexibility
Reduced stress
Lower cardiovascular risk
Lower mortality rate

Adapted from Kovacs et al. 2016, Journal Medicine and Science in Tennis [14]

33.3.2 Case #3

"A 45-year-old male NTRP 4.0 tennis player presents for evaluation of hypertension. What advice can you provide this recreational tennis player about the health benefits of tennis for his chronic medical condition?"

33.3.2.1 Hypertension

Generally speaking, blood pressure increases acutely with exercise, though the long-term effect of exercise is to lower blood pressure. A small study of middle-aged and older men reported an average increase in blood pressure from 130/90 to 170/80 mmHg during singles play with heart rate ranging from 140 to 180 beats per minute [17]. Adult recreational players in a study of 25 males and 25 females who played regular tennis (average 9.7–11.1 h/week), but did not regularly participate in other exercise programs, demonstrated an average blood pressure 117/75 mmHg for males and 107/68 mmHg for females [18].

In another study of 28 senior male tennis players (NTRP 3.5 and above) with 18 moderately active controls, there was no difference in blood pressure between the two groups. Average blood pressure in the 40- to 59-year-old tennis player group was 121/78 mmHg compared to 124/79 mmHg in the moderately active control group. In the 60 and above age group, the average was 136/82 and 135/81 mmHg, respectively. There was no mention of whether the study controlled for those on antihypertensive medications [19].

33.3.3 Case #4

"A 51-year-old female NTRP 3.5 tennis player presents for evaluation of hyperlipidemia. What advice can you provide this recreational tennis player about the health benefits of tennis for her chronic medical condition?"

33.3.3.1 Cholesterol

Several studies have focused on the effects of tennis participation on lipid profiles in the adult recreational player. Vodak et al. evaluated 25 men and women in a cross-sectional study whose exclusive mode of regular exercise was tennis play compared to a sedentary group matched for age, sex, and education. Most notably, when controlled for weight, cigarette smoking, alcohol intake, and oral contraceptive use (in females), the high-density lipoprotein (HDL) cholesterol concentration was higher in females compared to sedentary controls (73.9 ± 12.3 versus 61.7 ± 13.3 mg/100 ml), though not statistically different in males (57.8 ± 13.9 versus 46.2 ± 12.0 mg/100 ml) [20].

With a running intensive tennis training program (Cardio Tennis) as an intervention ($N = 30$), Ferrauti et al. evaluated 11 men and 11 women—after excluding eight players due to failure to maintain nutritional habits—compared to 16 control subjects as part of a longitudinal study. The tennis intervention group participated in three 90-min sessions over 6 weeks. On average, the running intensive tennis group lost 1.4 kg; however, despite some trends toward a more favorable lipid profile, there were no statistically significant differences in total cholesterol, low-density lipoprotein (LDL), HDL, or triglycerides [21]. After one 120-min session of running intensive tennis compared to a traditional 120-min session of technically oriented tennis training, the authors found that HDL levels increased acutely [21].

33.3.4 Case #5

"A 60-year-old female NTRP 3.0 has been managing her type II diabetes mellitus with diet and exercise. What advice can you provide this recreational tennis player about the health benefits of tennis for her chronic medical condition?"

33.3.4.1 Diabetes

Diabetes is a common medical condition in the adult patient. One large study on the effect of exercise on diabetes included tennis players as part of the study population; this demonstrated a reduced risk of non-insulin-dependent diabetes in patients with moderate to vigorous intensity physical activity [22]. A small interventional study of 12 patients with type II diabetes evaluated tennis as an intervention for diabetes. Untrained beginners played tennis twice a week with 90-min training sessions; after 6 weeks, there were no significant changes in hemoglobin A1C, though there were small but statistically significant increases in plasma insulin and c-peptide production [23].

33.3.5 Case #6

"A 47-year-old male NTRP 3.5 recently underwent coronary revascularization. What advice can you provide this recreational tennis player about the health benefits of tennis for his chronic medical condition?"

33.3.5.1 Cardiovascular Disease

Although exercise poses risk for sudden cardiac death in the acute setting [24], several studies demonstrate that tennis benefits cardiovascular health. Houston et al. evaluated medical students between 1948 and 1964 and followed them for 22 and 40 years for risk of cardiovascular events. Those students who rated themselves as having a "high" level of ability with tennis had a relative risk of 0.56 (95% confidence interval (CI), 0.35–0.89) for cardiovascular events compared to 0.67 (CI, 0.47–0.96) in the "low" level of ability and the "no" level of ability [25].

A study of 80,306 Scottish and English patients in a polled population-based cohort demonstrated that athletes who participated in racket sports (tennis, badminton, and squash) had the lowest all-cause mortality compared to other sports with a hazard ratio of 0.53 (95% CI 0.40–0.69) and decreased cardiovascular mortality with a hazard ratio of 0.44 (95% CI 0.24–0.83) [2].

Finally, as a pilot study, Garcia et al. demonstrated improvements in lipid profiles compared to baseline with tennis as an intervention for post myocardial infarction [26]. In a larger randomized follow-up study, as an intervention for post myocardial infarction in low-risk patients, a modified tennis program compared similarly to a traditional bicycling program for rehabilitation on several physiologic and metabolic parameters. After a 3-month training program, lipid profiles, quality of life measurements, and METs improved in the intervention groups (both tennis and biking) compared to the control group [27].

In summary, although the studies on tennis and its specific effect on blood pressure, lipid profiles, and diabetes are small, we know that regular physical activity can benefit these chronic medical conditions and that tennis meets the guidelines for regular physical activity. More impressively, however, is that there are large studies on the relationship between tennis and cardiovascular risk with clear reduction in cardiovascular disease with regular tennis play.

33.4 Junior Tennis

33.4.1 Case #7

"A 13-year-old elite single-sport junior female tennis player with a national ranking is now wondering if she wants to continue on with a tennis career. What advice should you consider?"

33.4.1.1 Sport Specialization

The data on intensive training and sport specialization in young athletes is still evolving. Multiple organizations including the American Academy of Pediatrics, the International Olympic Committee, the American Medical Society for Sports Medicine, and the American Orthopedic Society for Sports Medicine (AOSSM) have all advised against early sports specialization and recommended modifying intense training to limit burnout and injury risk [28–33]. While there are inherent risks of single-sport specialization related to overuse and serious injury, the burnout risks are also being acknowledged [28, 30, 34]. Specifically, tennis seems to have the highest rate of single-sport specialization [34]. For example, nearly 70% of >500 US midwest elite junior players specialize at a mean age of 10.4 years old. In this population, the mean enjoyment and satisfaction ratings were lower in >14-year-olds than in those <14-year-olds, where there were the highest rates of specialization [34].

Attrition rates of junior tennis players have not been determined; we have little data on the long-term effects of quality of life on tennis players specifically. However, two studies suggest that quality of life ratings of former college athletes may be lower than nonathletes despite no difference in rates of physical activity [35, 36]. This data was not sport-specific. A preliminary analysis of the quality of life of competitive and specialized child athletes showed equally high quality of life to those who were less competitive and specialized [37].

33.4.1.2 Medical Withdrawals and Recommendations for Time Off

Junior tennis players are at risk of overtraining, especially those players who specialize in tennis as the only sport. Players who specialized in tennis were 1.5 times more likely to report an injury [38]. Of those players who had reported an injury, they were at 5.4 times greater risk for a subsequent medical withdrawal from a tournament [38]. In addition, risk of medical withdrawal from a tournament increased in players competing in more than 40 USTA matches annually [38]. Within a single tournament, players were more likely to have a medical withdrawal when playing beyond a fourth match [38]. Players with 1 day off or less per week were more likely to suffer an injury compared to those with 2 or more days off per week [38]. Based on these findings and others, the AOSSM and Society for Tennis Medicne and Science (STMS) released training

Table 33.2 Recommendations to reduce injury risk in junior tournament tennis players

Recommendation	Sort level
Exercise caution in junior tournament players competing in their fifth match and beyond, particularly in older age divisions	B
Consider having at least 1–2 h between same-day matches to allow sufficient recovery	B
Caution when playing >10 h per week with a history of prior injury, particularly in the low back, and before a tournament	B
Participate in fewer tennis hours per week than the player's age to prevent overuse injury – Consider regular screening of pain or injury in higher risk areas (low back, shoulder, elbow) in junior tennis players to limit re-injury risk	B
Consider delaying specialization in tennis until middle or late adolescence for injury prevention as well as for successful performance – There may be a risk of early specialization in tennis Consider delaying specialization beyond prepubescent development	B
Consider 1–2 tournaments per month	C
Consider age-appropriate play with low-compression balls for most players younger than 10 years old	C

Adapted from AOSSM eBook "Let's Discuss Adolescent Sports Injuries" [38, 39]

recommendations for junior players that are reviewed in Table 33.2.

33.4.1.3 Tennis in the Family

Despite these risks associated with early sport specialization, tennis is positioned as a unique sport in that it can have positive health benefits throughout an individual's lifetime and also within a single family. While there are other potential risks of single-sport specialization and intense training in young athletes particularly in tennis players [28, 34], one small study of the health of parent and child athletes of specialized versus multisport tennis players found that all the children (aged 8–18) met the American College of Sports Medicine activity guidelines [8, 40]. Interestingly, the tennis-only parents and tennis-only children had more moderate-vigorous exercise than their multisport counterparts, whereas the multisport parents were much more likely to exercise with their children [40].

33.5 Elite Tennis Players

33.5.1 Case #8

"A 23-year-old female professional tennis player develops abdominal pain prior to the start of the United States (US) Open. She would like to be evaluated for this condition by the tournament physician. What is the prevalence of medical illness in professional tennis tournaments?"

Published studies have demonstrated a significant number of medical illnesses affecting players in professional tournament play. A study of medical withdrawal in ATP and WTA tournaments from 2001 to 2012, other than the four major tournaments, found that medical illness was the reason for withdrawal in 20.3% of women (10.53/1000 match exposures [ME]) and 18.7% in men (8.10/1000 ME) [41]. Withdrawal due to medical illness did not vary by court surface [41]. A smaller study of medical withdrawal at 2013 USTA pro-circuit tournaments reported medical illness as a reason for withdrawal in only 0.92/1000 ME in men and 0.33/1000 ME in women [42]. Finally, one retrospective study of Davis Cup World Group matches evaluated medical withdrawals from 2006 to 2013. Perhaps not surprisingly, rates of medical withdrawal (for either injury or illness) were higher in matches once the outcome of the competition had been decided ("residual matches") at 6.41% compared to matches where the decision of the tie was in question ("effective matches") at 1.66%. For statistical analysis, the authors excluded the residual matches. Of the 906 total matches, only 12 of the 24 retirements occurred during 719 effective matches. Only two of those withdrawals involved medical illness [43]. The reasons for the approximately tenfold difference in incidence in medical withdrawal due to illness in these studies are unclear.

Sell at el. evaluated rates of medical illness by organ system in the United States (US) Open from 1994 to 2009. In this study, the authors looked at cases that had been evaluated by a medical staff member during the US open, rather than rates of medical withdrawal. Women were evaluated for medical illness at a rate of 35.74/1000 ME at the US open while men were evaluated at a rate of 37.73/1000 ME [44]. Ear, nose and throat (ENT) and dermatological conditions were the most likely reason for evaluation of medical illness between 1994 and 2009 at the US Open [44]. Interestingly, at this Grand Slam tournament, only 1.07 cases/1000 match exposures results in a medical withdrawal. Compared to the rates of medical withdrawal described above, the data suggests that many players continue to play despite these medical illnesses.

Finally, the International Tennis Federation (ITF) facilitated a meeting of medical experts to produce a consensus statement regarding epidemiologic studies in tennis players. This study outlined how future studies may also be able to record more detail about medical illness during both match and training environments, as the above studies in tennis professionals are currently limited to only match exposures and do not capture any medical illness that occurred during training periods [45].

33.5.2 Case #9

"A 15-year-old highly ranked junior ITF player feels she can compete fully on the women's professional tour. What should she be aware of as she transitions to professional tennis?"

33.5.2.1 WTA (Women's Tennis Association) Age Eligibility Rule

With the evolution of the sport of women's tennis, a women's league-the WTA- was founded in 1973 and with it came some very talented and successful young female tennis players. However, it became apparent that there was a potential issue with the appropriate transition into women's professional tennis for younger players. After recognizing this potential problem and forming a player development advisory panel of sports sciences and memdicine experts, the WTA revised its existing Age Eligibility Rule (AER) [46] and concurrently introduced Player Development Programs for both athletes and the members of their support teams. The intent of this was to address concerns about the health, well-being, and safety of adolescent players, increase career longevity, and reduce premature

Table 33.3 Tournament Eligibility Chart

Age	WTA	ITF Women's Circuit	Wild cards	Fed cup	Olympics	Exhibition/non-WTA events
18	Unlimited	Unlimited	According to WTA and ITF rules	Yes	Yes	Unlimited, subject to exhibition/non-WTA event rule
17	16+ WTA Finals or WTA Elite Trophy		According to WTA and ITF Rules	Yes	Yes	Unlimited, subject to exhibition/non-WTA event rule
16	12+ WTA Finals or WTA Elite Trophy		4	Yes	Yes	Unlimited, subject to exhibition/non-WTA event rule
15	10+ WTA Finals or WTA Elite Trophy		3 (maximum of 1 for premier tournaments and remaining for international tournaments, WTA 125 Ks and/or ITF Women's Circuit)	Yes	Yes	Unlimited, subject to exhibition/non-WTA event rule
14	0, except by wild card	8	3 (maximum of 1 for international tournaments, maximum of 2 for WTA 125 Ks and remaining for ITF Women's Circuit)	Yes	No	Unlimited, subject to Exhibition/non-WTA event rule
13	0	0	0	0	0	0

Adapted from WTA 2018 Official Rulebook [47]

retirements. The components of this included a phased-in approach to professional tennis between 14 and 18 years old (Table 33.3), with potential merit-based exceptions, and player development programs geared toward assisting with the transition to the woman's professional tour. The WTA emphasized health, safety, and player welfare, and performed a 10-year AER review [46] to identify impact. This initial review demonstrated reduction of premature retirements from 7% to 1% and median career longevity increased by 24% (3 years) [46]. The WTA reviews its AER and Player Development Programs annually and revises them when necessary to keep consistent with the latest research in sports sciences and player development. There has been no other published long-term evaluation of an Age Eligibility Rule in any other sport.

33.5.3 Case #10

"A 25-year-old male professional tennis player presents for evaluation prior to his upcoming season on the ATP World Tour. He plans on traveling to Australia, Europe, North America, and China throughout the year and will participate in Davis Cup play. What medical aspects of travel should be considered?"

33.5.3.1 Travel Considerations

Due to the international tournament schedule, most professional tennis players will need to consider travelers' health as part of their medical care [48]. In addition to securing travel documents (e.g., passports, visas, etc.), travel tickets, and lodging, tennis players will need to review travel vaccinations and emergency plans. Several websites review appropriate vaccinations and safety concerns including the Centers for Disease Control and Prevention [49]. At a minimum, players should consider vaccination against tetanus, diphtheria, pertussis, influenza, hepatitis A and B, measles, mumps, poliomyelitis, and varicella [48].

In addition, players should review whether there are any travel advisories for the destination. The authors recommend travel insurance in the event an athlete may need to be evacuated to their home country in case of an emergency.

Jet lag and acclimatization are common problems with tournament scheduling. Both eating and sleeping habits are commonly disrupted with international travel. Changes in ambient temperature and humidity place players at risk for heat illness. Players should quickly attempt to set regular daily routines to the local schedule and attempt to arrive early to tournaments to adjust. To address jet lag, athletes should keep regular bedtimes and regular mealtimes. Recent data suggests that injury risk increases 1.7 times with <8 h sleep for high school athletes compared to athletes who slept for ≥8 h [50]. Sleep is increasingly important with travel in a tennis player. In addition, the body needs more adjustment when traveling eastwards (adjustment typically takes 1 day per hour time zone difference) compared to westward travel (adjustment typically takes ½ day per hour time zone difference). Naps longer than 1 hour should be avoided to avoid disruptions in natural sleep patterns. If needed, melatonin can be used to help readjust the body's circadian rhythm (sleep-wake cycle) [48]. Adequate hydration can help avoid heat illness; however, general advice is to arrive at least 1–2 weeks before competition in order to properly adjust to heat as the body can adapt sweat production and core temperature with proper time [48].

Traveler's diarrhea is a common occurrence for travelers, and the dehydration associated with this may limit participation in tournaments. Thirty to 70% of travelers may experience traveler's diarrhea, depending on the destination and season of travel [49]. Tournament participants should be encouraged to consider the source of drinking water and food preparation in pre-match planning. If players develop traveler's diarrhea, medical staff should restrict play if fever or signs of dehydration are present. Regular use of bismuth salicylate may reduce incidence of traveler's diarrhea but is not practical for most travelers and should be avoided in children <12, aspirin allergy or those at risk for renal insufficiency [51]. Prophylactic antibiotics are not currently recommended. Treatment varies between 1 and 3 days with fluoroquinolone and macrolide antibiotics [49].

For both male and female athletes, contraception should be discussed and offered prior to travel as adequate contraceptive measures can be difficult to obtain in some foreign countries.

33.6 Special Considerations

33.6.1 Case #11

"A 19-year-old female collegiate tennis player presents for evaluation of a metatarsal stress fracture. She reports one previous stress fracture in her tibia. What additional medical history do you need to consider in this athlete?"

33.6.1.1 Female Athlete Triad

The female athlete triad describes the relationship between energy availability, bone health, and menstrual regularity that can become disordered in sporting women [52]. Female athletes present with abnormalities of any one of the three triad components; early recognition is critical to prevent progression to more serious illness like clinical eating disorders, amenorrhea, and osteoporosis [52].

There are limited epidemiological studies on tennis players and the female athlete triad across all levels of participation. Overall, rates of the female athlete triad are lower in ball game sports like tennis compared to aesthetic sports; however, the prevalence of eating disorders in female ball sport athletes increased from 11% in 1990 to 16% in 1997 [53–56], and there are two studies that suggest this risk could be underestimated. A 1999 NCAA study using a 133-item questionnaire of 1445 student athletes reported that 8% of collegiate women tennis players have disordered eating, and 50–60% are at risk due to poor body image, a "drive for thinness," and experimentation with disordered eating practices [57]. In contrast, a 2000 NCAA study using questionnaires of women's tennis players and women's tennis coaches concluded that tennis players were not at a greater risk of eating disorders than other young women. In addition, this study also concluded that college coaches did not appear to be encouraging abnormal eating behaviors [58]. A more recent study looked specifically at adolescent female tennis players in Rio de Janeiro. This study of 24 female tennis athletes and 21 female controls at some pubertal developmental stage found that 91.7%, 33.3%, and 25% of athletes and 71.4%, 9.5%, and 33.3% of controls met criteria for disordered eating and/or low energy availability, menstrual irregularities, and low bone mass, respectively. A greater percentage of athletes than controls presented with one or two of the female athlete triad components, and 4.2% of tennis athletes presented with the full syndrome [59].

Generally speaking, tennis players have improved bone health compared to peers [1]. However, subtle disruptions in energy availability can have significant impacts on overall bone health. Athletes with oligomenorrhea and subclinical menstrual disturbances (e.g., anovulation and luteal phase defects) were found to have mild to moderate low bone mineral density (BMD) [52, 60, 61]. This is especially important in the younger tennis player as 90% of peak bone mass is attained by 18 years of age [62]. The WTA Professional Development Advisory Panel recognized that the female athlete triad was a risk for athletes for when evaluating the Age Eligibility Rule [46].

Tennis-specific guidelines on screening for the female athlete triad do not currently exist at the professional level. Recommendations at the collegiate and high school level are variable. The 2014 Female Athlete Triad Coalition Consensus Statement on Treatment and Return to Play of the Female Athlete Triad recommended that female athletes should undergo annual screening with the triad-specific self-report questionnaire and that finding any one of the triad component should prompt more thorough investigation for the others [52].

Athletes can be assessed using the Female Athlete Triad Cumulative Risk Assessment Tool provided by the Triad Consensus Panel [52]. This provides an objective method of determining an athlete's risk of triad-related sequelae. This can then be used in conjunction with the clearance and return-to-play guidelines [52]. The self-report questionnaire, risk assessment tool, and clearance guidelines are summarized in Fig. 33.1.

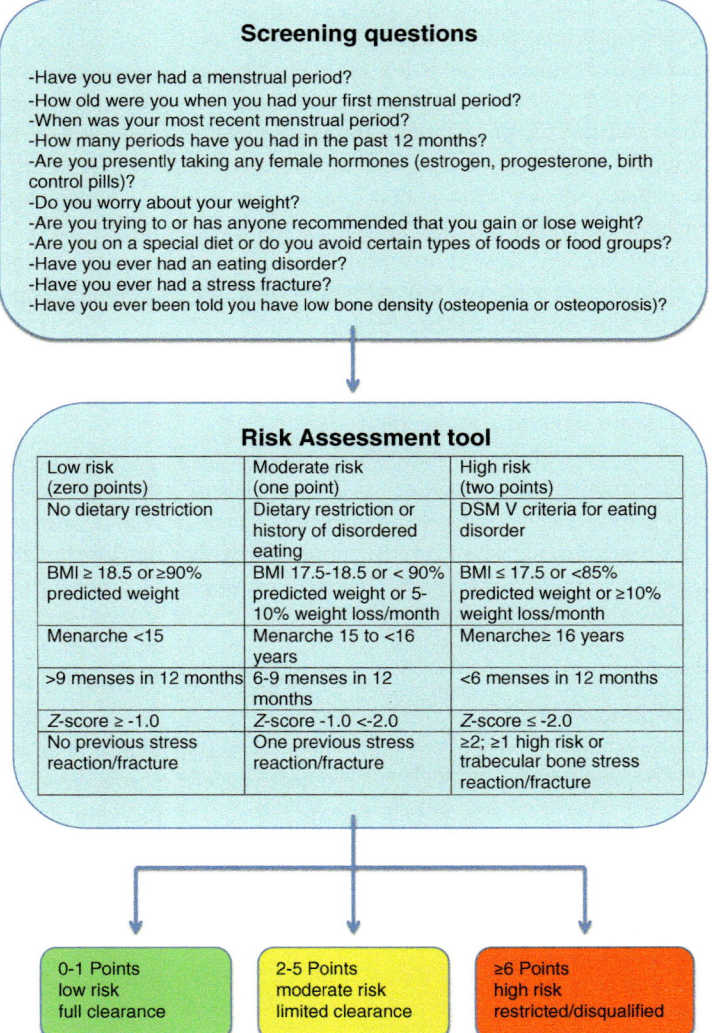

Fig. 33.1 Female athlete triad risk assessment, clearance, and return to play (adapted from DeSouza et al. 2014, British Journal of Sports Medicine) [52]

Treatment of the female athlete triad often requires a multidisciplinary approach including the athlete, coaches, athletic trainers, physicians, physical therapists, sports nutritionists, and sports psychologists [52, 63]. The treatment goal is to improve energy availability through increasing caloric intake or restricting energy expenditure. Return-to-play decisions should be made with the athletes' short-term health and long-term health in mind. Despite these consequences, the American College of Sports Medicine encourages all girls and women to participate in physical activities because the benefits of exercise outweigh the risks [1, 64].

Finally, there are some emerging data about the effects of low energy availability on male athletes [63]. The International Olympic Committee released a consensus statement describing this spectrum of disease inclusive of male athletes and termed this *Relative Energy Deficiency in Sport* (RED-S) [63]. Although the risk of stress fractures may not be as high in men because of the effects of estrogen on bone, men with low energy availability are also at risk for low bone mineral density, low testosterone levels, and decreased performance [63]. Although there are early studies in male athletes, this risk is not well studied in male tennis players. Future research studies are needed to further evaluate and define RED-S for both men and women.

Providers unfamiliar with the female athlete triad or relative energy deficiency in sport should review these two consensus statements when caring for athletes at risk or refer to a provider with experience in treating these illnesses if these resources are available [52, 63].

33.6.2 Case #12

"A 66-year-old female NTRP 4.0 tennis player with a history of osteoporosis presents for follow-up of her bone density scan (dual-energy x-ray absorptiometry—DEXA). She has played tennis 2–3 times weekly for the last 30 years. Due to a history of lumbar fusion surgery in the past year, you have obtained images of the distal radius in addition to the hips. What changes would you expect in the distal radius?"

33.6.2.1 Bone Health

Tennis players are asymmetric athletes. Muscular and bony hypertrophy of the dominant upper extremity and non-dominant lower extremity and trunk has been well documented [1, 65, 66].

Increases in both bone mineral density and bone mineral content are consistently found in the dominant arm of the tennis athlete compared to the non-dominant arm [1]. In general, these asymmetries in bone mineral density and bone mineral content are found across all levels with junior, elite, and recreational level players, though are more pronounced with younger starters compared to older starters and with length of participation in tennis [1]. When compared to non-tennis controls, tennis players have improved bone mass and bone mineral density in the hip and lumbar spine. Exercise-induced bone gain was greater in young than in old starters [1].

In this athlete, the DEXA should be interpreted with an understanding of whether the images obtained were from the dominant or non-dominant upper extremity.

33.6.3 Case #13

"A 20-year-old female collegiate tennis player presents with complaints of burnout. Her coach recently began yelling at her for performance and has threatened to remove her scholarship. He has also begun to make comments about her weight. What steps can you take to help this athlete?"

33.6.3.1 Non-accidental Violence in Sport

Tennis is an international sport with professional competitions played throughout the world. As an individual sport and as a sport with limited centralized resources, tennis players are at risk for exploitation and non-accidental violence. Non-accidental violence ranges from discrimination to harassment and abuse [67]. At the most severe end, several incidents highlight these risks of abuse in professional tennis. On April 30, 1993, Monica Seles, the world's #1 player at the time, was stabbed in the back with a knife during an on-court attack. It took Seles more than 2 years before she returned to the court and struggled to perform at the same level. More commonly, abuse originates from interpersonal violence like coaches, parents, or managers. Isabelle Demongeot, former number two tennis player in France, wrote a book detailing years of sexual abuse by her coach [68]. Unfortunately, coaches have been implicated and prosecuted in several other cases of sexual abuse toward players.

Psychological or emotional harassment impacts athletes at all levels [67]. Athletes report belittling, shouting, humiliating, scapegoating, and isolating behaviors from a variety of sources. Online abuse has become more common and the Tennis Integrity Unit (TIU) has been working with players and governing bodies to address these concerns [69]. Coaches, athletes, managers, fans, medical staff, friends, or family members can all bring about this form of interpersonal violence. Typically, power differentials in sex, gender, sexual orientation, race, ethnicity, athletic ability, faith, or other traits underlie the cultural context that can lead to non-accidental violence [67]. Unfortunately, the risk of experiencing psychological, physical, and sexual violence rises as the athlete's performance progresses upward [70, 71]. Lesbian, gay, bisexual, transgender, and queer (LGBTQ) athletes, athletes with disability, and children/adolescents are at the highest risk for non-accidental violence [32, 67, 71, 72].

The individual cost of non-accidental violence can be severe and long lasting with negative impacts on the athlete's physical, social, and psychological health [73]. For example, athletes may develop eating disorders, post-traumatic stress disorder, depression, and anxiety or participate in self-harm behaviors like suicide, and they may experience social exclusion and economic losses [67, 73]. In addition, non-accidental violence may impair performance, be associated with doping, and increase willingness to cheat or lead to athlete dropout. Finally, non-accidental violence can impact organizations as well. Reputational damage may result in loss of players, fans, sponsorship, and asset depreciation [67].

Sports medicine providers should be trained to recognize the signs and indicators of non-accidental violence, effectively and appropriately respond to disclosures of non-accidental violence, ensure access to a multidisciplinary professional support team prior to initiating any treatment plan for athletes, and, finally, know where and how to refer disclosures or suspicions [67].

References

1. Pluim BM, Staal JB, Marks BL, et al. Health benefits of tennis. Br J Sports Med. 2007;41:760–8.
2. Oja P, Kelly P, Pedisic Z, et al. Associations of specific types of sports and exercise with all-cause and cardiovascular-disease mortality: a cohort study of 80 306 British adults. Br J Sports Med. 2017;51:812–7. https://doi.org/10.1136/bjsports-2016-096822.
3. Pluim BM, Earland J, Pluim NE. The development of healthy tennis clubs in the Netherlands. Br J Sports Med. 2014;48:898–904.
4. Levine BD, Baggish AL, Kovacs RJ, et al. Eligibility and disqualification recommendations for competitive athletes with cardiovascular abnormalities: task force 1: classification of sports: dynamic, static, and impact. J Am Coll Cardiol. 2015;66:2350–5.
5. Maron B, Zipes D, Ackerman M. 36th Bethesda conference: eligibility recommendations for competitive athletes with cardiovascular abnormalities. J Am Coll Cardiol. 2005;45:1312.
6. Osborn RQ, Taylor WC, Oken K, et al. Echocardiographic characterisation of left ventricular geometry of professional male tennis players. Br J Sports Med. 2007;41:789–92. discussion 792
7. Kovacs MS. Applied physiology of tennis performance. Br J Sports Med. 2006;40:381–5. discussion 386
8. Haskell WL, Lee I-M, Pate RR, et al. Physical activity and public health: updated recommendation for adults from the American College of Sports Medicine and the American Heart Association. Circulation. 2007;116:1081–93.
9. Jayanthi N, Sallay P, Hunker P, Przybylski M. Skill-level related injuries in recreational competition tennis players. Med Sci Tennis. 2005;10:12–5.
10. Changstrom B, Jayanthi N. Clinical evaluation of the adult recreational tennis player. Curr Sports Med Rep. 2016;15:437–45.
11. Marks BL. Health benefits for veteran (senior) tennis players. Br J Sports Med. 2006;40:469–76. discussion 476

12. Groppel J, DiNubile N. Tennis: for the health of it! Phys Sportsmed. 2009;37:40–50.
13. Pluim BM, Staal JB, Marks BL, et al. Health benefits of tennis. J Med Sci Tennis. 2014;19:55–68.
14. Kovacs M, Pluim B, Groppel J, et al. Health, wellness and cognitive performance benefits of tennis. J Med Sci Tennis. 2016;21:14–21.
15. Blair SN, Kohl HW, Barlow CE, et al. Changes in physical fitness and all-cause mortality. A prospective study of healthy and unhealthy men. JAMA. 1995;273:1093–8.
16. Leitzmann MF, Park Y, Blair A, et al. Physical activity recommendations and decreased risk of mortality. Arch Intern Med. 2007;167:2453.
17. Jetté M, Landry F, Tiemann B, Blümchen G. Ambulatory blood pressure and Holter monitoring during tennis play. Can J Sport Sci. 1991;16:40–4.
18. Vodak PA, Savin WM, Haskell WL, Wood PD. Physiological profile of middle-aged male and female tennis players. Med Sci Sports Exerc. 1980;12:159–63.
19. Swank AM, Condra S, Yates JW. Effect of long term tennis participation on aerobic power, body composition, muscular strength, flexibility and serum lipids. Sport Med Train Rehabil. 1998;8:99–112.
20. Vodak PA, Wood PD, Haskell WL, Williams PT. HDL-cholesterol and other plasma lipid and lipoprotein concentrations in middle-aged male and female tennis players. Metabolism. 1980;29:745–52.
21. Ferrauti A, Weber K, Strüder HK. Effects of tennis training on lipid metabolism and lipoproteins in recreational players. Br J Sports Med. 1997;31:322–7.
22. Helmrich SP, Ragland DR, Leung RW, Paffenbarger RS. Physical activity and reduced occurrence of non-insulin-dependent diabetes mellitus. N Engl J Med. 1991;325:147–52.
23. Nessler A. Sportmedizinische Befunde und Sportpraktische Erfahrungen zum Tennisunterricht in der Bewegungstherapie von Typ-2-Diabetikern. Cologne: Deutsche Sporthochschule; 2001.
24. Marijon E, Uy-Evanado A, Reinier K, et al. Sudden cardiac arrest during sports activity in middle age. Circulation. 2015;131:1384–91.
25. Houston TK, Meoni LA, Ford DE, et al. Sports ability in young men and the incidence of cardiovascular disease. Am J Med. 2002;112:689–95.
26. García JPF, Barrado JG, Durán JB, et al. A cardiac rehabilitation program in a tennis training session. Rev Int Med y Ciencias la Act Fis y del Deport. 2009;9:454–65.
27. García JPF, Giraldo VMA, Barrado JJG, Casasola CD. Tennis training sessions as a rehabilitation instrument for patients after acute myocardial infarction. J Sports Sci Med. 2013;12:316–22.
28. Jayanthi N, Pinkham C, Dugas L, et al. Sports specialization in young athletes: evidence-based recommendations. Sport Health. 2013;5:251–7.
29. LaPrade RF, Agel J, Baker J, et al. AOSSM early sport specialization consensus statement. Orthop J Sports Med. 2016;4:2325967116644241.
30. Jayanthi NA, LaBella CR, Fischer D, et al. Sports-specialized intensive training and the risk of injury in young athletes: a clinical case-control study. Am J Sports Med. 2015;43:794–801.
31. Brenner JS, Council on Sports Medicine and Fitness. Sports specialization and intensive training in young athletes. Pediatrics. 2016;138:e20162148.
32. Bergeron MF, Mountjoy M, Armstrong N, et al. International Olympic Committee consensus statement on youth athletic development. Br J Sports Med. 2015;49:843–51.
33. Difiori JP, Benjamin HJ, Brenner J, et al. Overuse injuries and burnout in youth sports: a position statement from the American Medical Society for Sports Medicine. Clin J Sport Med. 2014;24:3–20.
34. Jayanthi N, Dechert A, Durazo R, Luke A. Training and specialization risks in junior elite tennis players. J Med Sci Tennis. 2011;16:14–20.
35. Sorenson SC, Romano R, Azen SP, et al. Life span exercise among elite intercollegiate student athletes. Sports Health. 2015;7:80–6.
36. Simon JE, Docherty CL. Current health-related quality of life is lower in former division I collegiate athletes than in non-collegiate athletes. Am J Sports Med. 2014;42:423–9.
37. Patel T, Jayanthi N. Health-related quality of life of child athletes. 3rd annual pediatric medicine student research forum; 2016.
38. Jayanthi N, Feller E, Smith A. Junior competitive tennis: ideal tournament and training recommendations. J Med Sci Tennis. 2013;18:30–5.
39. LaPrade RF, Kocher MS. Let's discuss adolescent sports injuries. Rosemont, IL: American Academy of Orthopedic Surgeons; 2016.
40. Schneider A, Jayanthi N, Luke A, et al. Health and fitness status of parent-child dyads: tennis-only athletes versus multisport athletes in the competitive adolescent population. J Med Sci Tennis. 2016;21:6–13.
41. Okholm Kryger K, Dor F, Guillaume M, et al. Medical reasons behind player departures from male and female professional tennis competitions. Am J Sports Med. 2015;43:34–40.
42. Hartwell MJ, Fong SM, Colvin AC. Withdrawals and retirements in professional tennis players: an analysis of 2013 United States Tennis Association Pro Circuit Tournaments. Sport Health. 2017;9(2):154–61.
43. Maquirriain J, Baglione R. Epidemiology of tennis injuries: an eight-year review of Davis Cup retirements. Eur J Sport Sci. 2016;16:266–70.
44. Sell K, Hainline B, Yorio M, Kovacs M. Illness data from the US Open Tennis Championships From 1994 to 2009. Clin J Sport Med. 2013;23:25–32.
45. Pluim BM, Fuller CW, Batt ME, et al. Consensus statement on epidemiological studies of medical conditions in tennis, April 2009. Br J Sports Med. 2009;43:893–7.
46. Otis CL, Crespo M, Flygare CT, et al. The Sony Ericsson WTA Tour 10 year age eligibility and professional development review. Br J Sports Med. 2006;40:464–8. discussion 468

47. WTA Tour (2018) Women's Tennis Association-2018 Official Rulebook. http://wtafiles.wtatennis.com/pdf/publications/2018WTARulebook.pdf. Accessed 13 June 2018.
48. Hainline B, Pluim B, Bullock M, et al. Australian Open, Roland Garros, Wimbledon, US Open, Shanghai Masters and Back: winning out of a suitcase. Aspetar Sport Med J. 2016;5:22–7.
49. Chen LH, Hochberg NS, Magill AJ. The pre-travel consultation. In: Centers for Disease Control and Prevention, editor. CDC yellow book. Atlanta, GA: Centers for Disease Control and Prevention; 2016. https://wwwnc.cdc.gov/travel/yellowbook/2016/the-pre-travel-consultation/the-pre-travel-consultation. Accessed 1 May 2017.
50. Milewski MD, Skaggs DL, Bishop GA, et al. Chronic lack of sleep is associated with increased sports injuries in adolescent athletes. J Pediatr Orthop. 2014;34:129–33.
51. Diemert DJ. Prevention and self-treatment of traveler's diarrhea. Clin Microbiol Rev. 2006;19:583–94.
52. De Souza MJ, Nattiv A, Joy E, et al. 2014 female athlete triad coalition consensus statement on treatment and return to play of the female athlete triad: 1st international conference held in San Francisco, California, May 2012 and 2nd international conference held in Indianapolis, Indiana, May 2013. Br J Sports Med. 2014;48:289.
53. Irion J, Irion G. Women's health in physical therapy. Baltimore, MA: Lippincott, Williams & Wilkins; 2010.
54. Sundgot-Borgen J. Risk and trigger factors for the development of eating disorders in female elite athletes. Med Sci Sports Exerc. 1994;26:414–9.
55. Sundgot-Borgen J, Torstveit MK. Prevalence of eating disorders in elite athletes is higher than in the general population. Clin J Sport Med. 2004;14:25–32.
56. Rathod R, Hess JL, Graham M, et al. Specific health issues in female athletes. J Med Sci Tennis. 2014;19:69–77.
57. Johnson C, Powers PS, Dick R. Athletes and eating disorders: the National Collegiate Athletic Association study. Int J Eat Disord. 1999;26:179–88.
58. Harris MB. Weight concern, body image, and abnormal eating in college women tennis players and their coaches. Int J Sport Nutr Exerc Metab. 2000;10:1–15.
59. Coelho GM de O, de Farias MLF, de Mendonça LMC, et al. The prevalence of disordered eating and possible health consequences in adolescent female tennis players from Rio de Janeiro, Brazil. Appetite. 2013;64:39–47.
60. Tomten SE, Falch JA, Birkeland KI, et al. Bone mineral density and menstrual irregularities. A comparative study on cortical and trabecular bone structures in runners with alleged normal eating behavior. Int J Sports Med. 1998;19:92–7.
61. Sowers M, Randolph JF, Crutchfield M, et al. Urinary ovarian and gonadotropin hormone levels in premenopausal women with low bone mass. J Bone Miner Res. 1998;13:1191–202.
62. Matkovic V, Jelic T, Wardlaw GM, et al. Timing of peak bone mass in Caucasian females and its implication for the prevention of osteoporosis. Inference from a cross-sectional model. J Clin Invest. 1994;93:799–808.
63. Mountjoy M, Sundgot-Borgen J, Burke L, et al. The IOC consensus statement: beyond the Female Athlete Triad—Relative Energy Deficiency in Sport (RED-S). Br J Sports Med. 2014;48(7):491.
64. Nattiv A, Loucks AB, Manore MM, et al. American College of Sports Medicine position stand. The female athlete triad. Med Sci Sports Exerc. 2007;39:1867–82.
65. Jayanthi N, Esser S. Racket sports. Curr Sports Med Rep. 2013;12:329–36.
66. Sanchis-Moysi J, Dorado C, Vicente-Rodríguez G, et al. Inter-arm asymmetry in bone mineral content and bone area in postmenopausal recreational tennis players. Maturitas. 2004;48:289–98.
67. Mountjoy M, Brackenridge C, Arrington M, et al. International Olympic Committee consensus statement: harassment and abuse (non-accidental violence) in sport. Br J Sports Med. 2016;50:1019–29.
68. Demongeot I. Service volé-Une championne rompt le silence. Neuilly-sur-Seine: Michel Lafon; 2007.
69. Brook P. Tennis integrity unit annual review 2016. London: TIU; 2017. http://www.tennisintegrityunit.com/annual-review/2016/. Accessed 17 Jan 2017
70. Fasting K, Brackenridge C, Knorre N. Performance level and sexual harassment prevalence among female athletes in the Czech Republic. Women Sport Phys Act. 2010;19:26–32.
71. Vertommen T, Schipper-van Veldhoven NH, Hartill MJ, Van Den Eede F. Sexual harassment and abuse in sport: the NOC*NSF helpline. Int Rev Sociol Sport. 2015;50:822–39.
72. Denison E, Kitchen A. Out on the fields: the first international study on homophobia in sport. 2015. http://www.outonthefields.com/. Accessed 2 Feb 2017.
73. Tofler IR, Morse ED. The interface between sport psychiatry and sports medicine. Clin Sports Med. 2005;24(4):745–998.

Sports Nutrition for Tennis Players

34

Susie Parker-Simmons and Page Love

34.1 Introduction

Tennis is a sport that can be played both indoors and outdoors; on a variety of court services from grass, clay, and synthetic materials; and is intermittent in nature with the work to rest ratio depending on the playing style and court surface. Tennis involves both the upper and lower body, requires speed and agility with short sprints ranging from 1 to 12 per point, and rallies generally lasting 2–10 s [1, 2].

Professional tennis is played year long, and in 33 countries around the world, which introduces the players to constant international travel, different cultures, and cuisines. In major events, Grand Slam tournaments, the title is won over seven matches spread over a fortnight of competition. Players therefore play matches every second day ranging from best of 3 sets for women and 5 sets for men. Some players may play every day due to rain delays, or competing in more than one competition (singles, doubles, mixed doubles) [2]. In general, professional tennis players' training exceeds 6 h a day either on court competing, training on court, and/or performing off-court conditioning [3].

Playing surface, playing style, environmental conditions, constant travel, growth and maturation, and frequency of competition are some of the factors that influence the physiological demands and nutritional needs of the tennis player. Due to the lack of nutrition-related research on professional tennis players, the experience from the authors of this chapter who are the sport dietitians working with the Women's Tennis Association (WTA) and the Association of Tennis Professionals (ATP) is utilized.

34.2 Nutrition Assessment

An athlete nutrition assessment is an in-depth evaluation of both objective and subjective data related to an individual's food and nutrient intake, training, and medical history. Once the data on an individual is collected and analyzed, the sport dietitian sets the athlete goals, intervention strategies, and treatment plans to help optimize the athlete's health, performance, and if relevant growth and maturation. Common data collected in the nutrition assessment are identified below.

(a) Dietary Assessment

Each player should have an initial dietary assessment every 1–2 years and it should be completed by sport dietitians who are educated to provide sport-specific and clinical nutrition evaluation. This screening can then form the foundation of nutrition monitoring, treatment, and education throughout the annual year. The dietary assessment includes assessing the athlete's energy,

S. Parker-Simmons
Womens Tennis Association and United States Olympic Committee, St. Petersburg, FL, USA

P. Love (✉)
Nutrifit, Sport, Therapy, Inc., Atlanta, GA, USA
e-mail: pagelove@nutrifitga.com

macronutrient, micronutrient, and fluid intake which is then compared to the athlete's tennis requirements. The dietary assessment should also include the collection of social, cultural, medical, and psychological influences on food choices [4]. It can also gather medical, biochemical, training, and anthropometric data.

(b) Bloods

A blood test is a laboratory procedure that can determine a person's medical and nutritional status. Dietary biomarkers are frequently used in the athletic population to determine if the individual has what they need for optimal health and performance. These tests are objective and beneficial in identifying small imbalances to larger problems which reflect insufficient dietary intake, defective absorption, and/or increased utilization or excretion [4]. Population reference ranges for biomarkers are generally used except for certain nutrients where athlete performance ranges are adopted.

(c) Body Composition

The sport of tennis has allowed a range of physiques to be successful at the game. Over the last two decades as tennis has moved to a more power-based sport, the typical player is generally taller than the average population, as stature can provide a benefit through the execution of the service, volley, and on-court reach.

Professional tennis players are often in the public eye through the sporting media. This has allowed unforgiving comments from the media and fellow players on body composition to become public. This has led to increased pressure for tennis players to achieve an "ideal" physique. Evaluating the player's body composition and prescribing an appropriate meal plan intervention to manipulate body composition is recommended. Extreme methods of weight control and unrealistic time frames can be detrimental to the athlete's health and performance [5].

Recommended techniques to assess body composition include dual energy X-ray absorptiometry (DXA) and anthropometry assessment [5]. DXA was originally designed to measure the bone mineral density of the hip and spine of older adults. More recently DXA has become a popular tool to determine body composition in athletes and is used for the analysis of fat-free soft tissue mass and fat mass gain/loss in response to exercise or nutritional interventions. It is also recognized as having the lowest standard error of estimate [5]. The International Society for the Advancement of Kinanthropometry (ISAK) has developed international standards for anthropometric assessment. This field test includes the measurement of height, weight, skinfolds, girths, lever lengths, and bone breadths to enable the monitoring of health and growth variables.

(d) Fluid Balance and Sweat Analysis

A wide range of sweat rates have been reported among athletes, and it is due to differences in genetics, maturation, body size, exercise intensity, environmental conditions, and heat acclimatization status [6, 7]. Fluid balance studies that assess body mass changes can be used to estimate sweat loss during training and competition. For tennis, this helps determine the volume of fluids players need per hour on court for a specific temperature and humidity. An analysis of sweat sodium concentrations will help estimate the requirements of salt during exercise. The aim of salt intake during exercise is to partially replace the amount of sodium and chloride lost by sweat and to enhance maintenance of body water and electrolyte homeostasis [7]. High losses of fluid and sodium can cause cramping and heat stress. Newer techniques are also being used on site to assess hydration status and body composition analyses in ATP players and may be a future direction for practical analyses on site with such tools as the SECA BIA analyses with results showing positive hydration trends before/after play.

Identifying individual needs is important for prevention of dehydration and optimizing performance.

The outcomes of the nutrition assessment will help set individual-specific dietary goals and structure a plan that helps optimize the player's health and tennis performance. Nutrition goals and requirements are not static and a periodized program which prepares an athlete for peak performance is required [5].

34.3 Energy Requirements of Tennis Players and Macronutrient Requirements

(a) Caloric needs

Tennis players have most recently been shown to expend 30–45 kJ/min or 7.5–11 kcal/min [1] and total caloric expenditure during match play range reported between 649 kcal ± 105 and ≤3244 kcal ± 524 [8]. However, most research shows that total energy intakes fall short of recommended intakes in studies (1815 kcal ± 916) and (1664 kcal ± 515) [9]. One study shows that adolescent male players (aged 14–18 yrs.) reported estimated total energy intake to be 2967 kcal and found that 63% of the athletes consumed >1.5 g/kg$^-$/d$^-$ protein [10]. Protein needs are often met through normal dietary intake; however, current guidelines to recommend protein quickly in the 15–45 min following match play. Players often choose protein recovery beverages or chocolate milk to help supplement these needs [11]. At female pro camps for US tennis players average caloric intakes of 2203 kcal for female pros and 2567 kcal for male pros vs projected needs of 3025 kcal for females and 4200 kcal estimated daily needs were measured through metabolic testing. Players also reported high use of sport beverage (100%) and energy bars (50%). Breakdown of dietary macronutrients averaged 58% carbohydrate, 19% protein, and 23% fat [12]. The International Tennis Federation recommends that most players consume at least 2500 calories a day. Some players may need over 3000 calories, and professionals should take in from 3500 to 5000 calories [13].

(b) Energy Needs

- Carbohydrate

Because of the short point play in tennis, point averaging 10 s and required 300–500 bursts of energy needed over the average course of a match, tennis is considered a high level of anaerobic power fueled by carbohydrate [3]. In fact, in a study on blood glucose levels taken during tournament play in elite players found that glycogen stores were enough to provide energy for 100 min of exercise [14]. Because of the highly anaerobic nature of the sport, it is recommended to follow a high carbohydrate diet between 6 and 10 g/kg/day to allow for adequate muscle glycogen energy stores. It is also recommended that players consume 30–60 g/h$^-$ during matches to maintain energy homeostasis and meet muscle glycogen need as well as 1.5 g/kg after matches when glycogen synthesis is highest to facilitate repletion [2, 15]. Current recommendations support intakes of 50–70% of calories in the diet coming from carbohydrate food sources including complex carbohydrate foods such as breads, starchy vegetables, and pastas, as well as fruit and vegetables. In practical terms this means 1–2 cups of complex carbohydrate foods at each meal during the day.

- Protein

Protein needs for tennis players range from 1.2 to 2.0 g/kg/day and newer recommendations suggest consuming .3 g/kg after play and strength training and every 3–5 h thereafter [3]. High-quality proteins in animal protein form or complete protein sources are recommended for consumption. Current tennis nutrition recommendations also suggest consuming a quick protein recovery source such as in the form of chocolate milk as players are leaving the court, these sources also help to hydrate and provide some sodium and carbohydrate.

In practical terms, most tennis players will need between 3 and 5 ounces (20–35 g) of lean proteins in meat form or vegetable protein equivalents such as tofu, beans, and meat analogs. As well, dairy protein or vegetarian dairy alternatives should be consumed in the range of 3–4 servings per day at major meals to meet these anabolic and recovery needs of tennis players.

- Fat

Fat has also been shown to contribute to a significant part of the energy expenditure especially in longer matches, for example, one record-breaking match lasting 11 h 5 min at Wimbledon in 2010; endurance becomes an important component of tennis play. One study reported 70% of male players consuming >30% of total energy per day from fat, so fat needs for male players may be higher than current general sport guidelines [11]. Conversely, players should be discouraged from consuming less than 20% of their energy from fat as they may not meet their essential fatty acid needs and may suffer from fat deficiency issues such as underweight, fatigue, suppressed hormones, and poor recovery and healing [3].

34.4 Micronutrient Requirements of Tennis Players

The demands of a year-long competitive season, international travel, and the importance of the ranking system make nutrition planning and the maintenance of optimal nutrition status difficult. Blood testing is often recommended yearly or biannually to help determine the status of the at-risk micronutrients for tennis players. Micronutrients at risk of depletion and deficiency are iron and vitamin D. Multivitamin and mineral supplements are often used by professional players to help support the demands of performance and international travel.

(a) Iron

Iron depletion and deficiency are a common problem seen in athletic populations, including professional tennis players. The causes are seen to be multifactorial and the exercise-mediated processes include gastrointestinal bleeding, hematuria, sweating, and hemolysis [16, 17]. A gender influence includes the menstrual cycle of female athletes which increases iron lost through menses. A dietary stimulus includes vegetarian athletes who consume the less efficiently absorbed non-heme iron sources. Recent research however suggests that there may also be a hormonal link to the development of an iron deficiency in athletic populations. A liver-produced hormone Hepcidin appears to influence the regulation of iron absorption in the gut. Hepcidin functions by binding to the iron exporter channels of the body known as Ferroportin, effectively shutting them down and not allowing iron to enter the system [18]. In athletes exercise-induced inflammation may upregulate hepcidin, thus reducing iron absorption and thereby causing iron deficiency [16, 17].

Dietary recommendations include:

- Test iron status of professional tennis players every 3 months to gain insight into the individual's specific iron demands.
- Test iron status through a complete blood count (hemoglobin, hematocrit, and red cell count and indices), ferritin (iron stores), serum iron, and transferrin saturation (circulates iron in the body) [16].
- Prescribe oral iron supplementation (i.e., ferrous sulfate) or high iron containing meals at a time when hepcidin levels should be at their lowest. This might occur prior to training sessions, 8–12 h after a training session, or periodized on rest days. The second approach might be to bypass the gut entirely through intravenous or intramuscular iron supplementation [16].
- Oral iron supplement for at least 3 months as total iron body stores take 3–6 months to be restored [19].
- Consume foods that include both types of iron: heme iron (animal foods) and non-heme iron (plant foods). As non-heme iron is poorly absorbed, combine with foods rich in vitamin C (e.g., pineapple, orange, grapefruit and their juices; strawberries, peppers, broccoli, tomato, kiwis) or heme iron food sources. Reduce the intake of calcium-rich foods, certain types of fiber (e.g., phytates and oxalates), tea, coffee, and cocoa around the time of eating iron-rich foods as they can all inhibit iron absorption.

(b) Vitamin D

Vitamin D plays an important role in a tennis player's health, training, and performance. Vitamin D is a fat-soluble vitamin that regulates calcium and phosphorus absorption, and it plays a key role in maintaining bone health [4, 5]. Emerging research suggests vitamin D's role in immune function, protein synthesis, cellular growth, inflammatory response, hormone synthesis, and even optimal muscle performance and injury prevention [4]. Further research is needed to support these claims. The term "vitamin D" refers to several different forms of this vitamin. Two forms are important in humans: vitamin D2, which is made by plants, and vitamin D3, which is made by human skin when exposed to sunlight. Foods and supplements may be fortified with vitamin D2 or D3.

The risk factors for poor vitamin D status in tennis players include:

- Players who live at latitudes >35th parallel
- Training indoors or early morning or late in the evening
- Dark or extremely fair skin
- Sunscreen use and UVB blocking clothing
- Low dietary vitamin D intake
- Low or high body fat levels [5]

Yearly or biannual blood tests (spring and autumn) should be performed to help determine vitamin D status and correct any deficiencies. Circulating 25-hydroxyvitamin D (25(OH)D) concentration is currently considered the best indicator of vitamin D status [4]. Education on sun exposure, diet, and supplement use should occur after each test. Sun exposure can be an important contributing source to build vitamin D stores. On average, the skin can synthesize about 10,000–20,000 IU of vitamin D in less than 30 min of exposure. Tennis players are recommended to have 5–20 min of sun exposure per day (without sunscreen) to help build up vitamin D stores. Sunlight should reach arms, legs, and trunk for greatest benefit. Unprotected sun exposure is contraindicated for tennis players with a history of skin cancer.

34.5 Fluid Requirements for Tennis

Environmental conditions, intensity of play, genetics, acclimatization to heat, fitness, age, and fluid intake on- and off-court can all impair temperature regulation, hydration status, and therefore tennis performance [3, 15]. Sweat rates increase as the environment gets hotter and more humid, intensity of play increases, and when a player becomes more aerobically fit and acclimatized to heat.

A study showing the impact of ingesting specifically formulated pre-exercise, endurance, and recovery sport drinks on glycemia and tennis performance highlighted a higher stroke frequency during play with decreased rates of perceived exertion [20].

One early study on hydration showed most adult tennis players will lose between 1.0 and 2.5 L of water each hour of competition singles [14]. Although sweat rates of 3.5 L per hour have been observed during play in very hot (above 95 F, 35 °C) conditions. Sodium losses of 0.5–1.8 g have been recorded in tennis players [1].

If the tennis player commences the match hydrated, carbohydrate stores replenished, and the match is short (approximately 1 h), then water consumption is suitable to consume. For matches longer than 1 h the player is recommended to consume a carbohydrate-electrolyte drink [14]. Electrolyte and carbohydrate-electrolyte solutions promote fluid absorption better than water while commercially made carbohydrate-electrolyte sport drinks delay the onset of both fatigue and dehydration.

Fluid intake should be individualized through fluid balance testing and sweat analysis, but general recommendations include a fluid intake of 200 ml should be consumed at every change of ends in temperatures <27 °C. For temperatures above 27 °C, players should aim for >400 ml per change of ends to help maintain fluid balance [1]. A body mass change of 1 kg (2.2 lb.) represents approximately 1 L (32 oz) of water loss. As little as a 2% body water deficit can lead to performance decrements. This can affect aerobic performance, balance, cognition, mood, and mental readiness [6]. A low level of hydration also impairs the body's heat dissipating mechanism and puts the athlete at risk of heat illness.

The effects of inadequate sodium replacement may include incomplete rehydration between matches as well as muscle cramps or increased heat exhaustion [21]. When competing in hot environments, increased sweat rates occur which also causes an increase mineral loss. Electrolyte balance is necessary to decrease the chance of fatigue, heat stress, and cramping. Sodium in the drink will help restore sodium lost in sweat, increase drink palatability, and restore body water content.

It is important for tennis players to train their body to drink, be educated on their body's needs, and not to rely on thirst as a mechanism to base your fluid requirements on. When competing on the professional circuit in hot environments, maintaining fluid, mineral, and glycogen balance should be a priority [15].

34.6 Preparation for Competition

The competition nutrition strategies include obtaining adequate substrate stores to meet fuel and hydration demands of the match and support cognitive function [5]. Preparing for a tournament match can also be challenged by the unpredictability of starting time of a match. Unless you are first court on, your starting time will be determined by the length of the match/s previously held on that day.

(a) Pre-tournament and Match:

Anything consumed before a match needs to provide fuel for tennis play for hours, and it is important that a variety of all macronutrients be present in the pre-match meal but particularly a meal with a higher carbohydrate profile to fuel the energy needs of the match, pre-match meals and snacks should be:

- familiar to you and known to settle hunger
- high in carbohydrates so that your muscles will have adequate energy
- moderate in protein
- low in fat
- quickly digested (not high in fiber or fat)
- Meals and snacks that meet all these criteria include pasta, bread, fresh fruit, granola bars, energy bars, and sports drinks. You probably don't want to load up simply on the energy bars, however

Here is a sample ideal tennis nutrition lunch to consume about 2–3 h before a match: a lean meat such as chicken, plentiful starch in bread, pasta or rice, fresh fruit apple, 8–24 oz. water, and sports drink. According to the Academy of Nutrition and Dietetics, appropriate pre-fueling should range between 1 and 4 g/kg of carbohydrate 1–4 h before competition [5].

A pre-match snack may still be needed and should be consumed about 1–2 h before the big match; eat bland fruit such as a banana, water, energy bar, 8–24 oz. of water, and sports drink.

(b) During Training and Matches:

Carbohydrates, electrolytes, and water are the principal nutrients that need to be consumed while playing tennis. During tennis training and matches that last more than 60 min, it is recommended to consume between 30 and 60 g of carbohydrates per hour [4]. This is to ensure a delay in the onset of fatigue. The carbohydrates can come in different forms but generally a combination of glucose, sucrose, fructose, and/or dextrose is recommended. Taking the carbohydrates in a liquid form ensures quicker digestion than solid foods. Recommended carbohydrate products include sport drink, gels, chews, chomps, and sport beans.

Taking small amounts of protein and fat during training and competition has not been shown to improve performance and may delay digestion and/or cause digestive discomfort [4]. Protein is not a major fuel source for tennis and fats which is a fuel source takes longer to break down.

The specific fluid requirements a player needs to consume will depend on sweat rate and the average number of changeovers per hour. On average, one cup of fluid (about eight gulps) during the changeover is required. The later stages of tournaments are the time when athletes are more susceptible to dehydration, glycogen depletion, mineral losses, and heat-related declines in performance [22].

(c) Recovery:

Recovery techniques aim to limit the severity of fatigue and/or speed recovery from fatigue [15]. Due to the time between matches being insufficient for complete recovery, players often start the next match with suboptimal fueling and hydration status. The international nature of the sport and the need to accrue points toward the overall player ranking cause athletes to travel around the world and frequently cross several time zones. This causes extra demands on the body and can prevent the player from recovering from the last tournament before competing in the next one. Optimum recovery methods need to be adopted including nutrition and sports medicine strategies so a high level of performance can occur over a match, tournament, season, and career.

The main components of nutrition-related recovery include water-electrolyte intake for rehydration, restoration of carbohydrate stores, and protein ingestion for muscle recovery.

(d) Rehydration:

In tennis fluid losses through sweating occur to dissipate body heat and regulate core temperature. To ensure complete rehydration tennis players should drink 1–1.5 L (32–48 oz) of fluids for each 1 kg (2.2 lb.) of body mass lost. Consuming sodium in the fluid replacement beverage helps stimulate fluid uptake into the cells and it encourages more drinking behavior. The addition of sodium also helps reduce the risk of hyponatremia [4].

(e) Replacement of Glycogen (Carbohydrate) Stores:

Carbohydrates are the important substrates for tennis in contracting skeletal muscle and aiding central nervous system function [6]. Due to the repetitive anaerobic nature of tennis and the limited capacity of the body of store carbohydrates, a decrease in glycogen stores and blood glucose is commonly seen. The outcome is fatigue, slowing down of the player on court, decreased ability to concentrate and make correct decision on court. It also puts the athlete at risk of injury and illness.

If the player has two practices per day or a match and practice session, the recovery period available to the player is short. If they have less than 8 h of recovery, then the player should digest 1 g/kg of body weight of carbohydrates in the first 30 min post the first session. If they have 24 h between training sessions or matches, then there is less urgency to replace carbohydrate stores immediately. It is important to provide enough carbohydrates in the diet during the next 24 h.

(f) Replacement of Protein:

Protein should be consumed in the recovery diet to stimulate muscle protein resynthesis and decrease the rate of muscle protein breakdown. Twenty to twenty-five grams of protein is recommended post exercise as higher rates of protein intake have not been shown to provide greater benefits [4]. A high-quality protein that provides all the essential amino acids especially leucine is needed for recovery.

34.7 Nutrition Issues for the Traveling Tennis Player

The nutrition planning phase before departing for a tournament is crucial for the performance of the tennis player. To prepare for tournaments, it is important to be proactive and develop travel nutrition plans of time. When away from home, often the foods offered are unfamiliar or may not be available. This can lead to suboptimal or under-fueling, decreased performance, and other complications.

(a) Before travel

Research what restaurants and shops are available at your airport terminal and near and at your hotel. Determine if the hotel you plan to stay at has a mini fridge and cooking facilities. Plan to take specialized food that you need but may not be able to purchase at your destination (e.g., gluten-free grains, lactose-free milk products, sports food products). Some players may choose to carry travel nutrition equipment which allows them to prepare suitable athletic meals anywhere in the world. This can include a hot pot travel cooker, travel blender, travel power converter, measuring cups, spoons, a smoothie mixer container (shaker bottle), and a selection of the following foods:

Food to pack for the plane:

- Bottled water and sport beverages
- Powdered sports drink (individual sachets)
- Low fat muesli bars
- High carbohydrate sports bars
- Home-made sandwiches

Food to pack for trips abroad or bring for onsite or send ahead:

- Protein—nuts and nut butters, pouch chicken, salmon, tuna, tofu, dried jerky
- Carbohydrates—instant noodles, rice and couscous, breakfast cereal, oatmeal, granola, pretzels Sports Products-approved sports drink, gels, chews, sports bars, and recovery drink

Nutrition Supplementation:

- Travel with your supplements in extra plastic sealable bags or vitamin storage container and keep them sealed.
- Take enough vitamins and other sport food supplements with you to get through your entire trip.
- Check with customs about what you can carry with you to your destination. Be aware of travel rules and limitations: some countries have strict quarantine laws about bringing food and beverages into the country. You may need to ship your supplements and food directly to your destination.

(b) During Travel

At airports, familiarize yourself with healthier restaurant options that meet training diet recommendations for higher complex carbohydrate and lower fat content

During your flight:

- Choose tomato juices, soups, and salty snack such as pretzels in flight to help maintain fluid status.
- Buy a sport beverage in the airport and drink it on the flight.
- Take a drink bottle onboard and refill frequently and drink extra fluids (water and/or electrolyte drinks) at each meal. Drinking an extra 15–20 mL/h has been shown to minimize jet lag [23]
- Choose either the regular meal option or, to meet any special dietary needs, order your special meal, such as a vegetarian or low-cholesterol in advance to obtain a meal more suitable for sport performance.
- If airline meals are too small for you, ask for extra bread and fruit.
- Carry additional snacks onboard for the flight and layovers, such as bars, crackers, and pretzels that are high in carbohydrates.
- Do remember that if you are inactive for long periods of time, you may not require as many additional snacks as you would when training or playing matches.
- Eat more iron-rich foods before flights but avoid iron supplements on the day you fly because of risk of constipation.
- Eat foods that help prevent constipation (e.g., black European licorice; prunes; dried figs; wholegrain dried cereal).

(c) Once at destination

Go shopping as soon as you arrive to buy foods and fluids you need to optimize health and performance. It is important to incorporate adequate fruits and vegetables into your nutrition plan during travel. Fruits and vegetables contain antioxidants which are known to reduce respiratory illness and asthma symptoms and are beneficial to your health. Obtaining safe, fresh, and readily available produce can be a challenge. Make sure that you wash (using clean bottled water) any fruit and vegetables that have skins. It may be safer to consume bottled juices and cooked vegetables if you are uncertain about the safety of the water.

34.8 Ergogenic Aids

Ergogenic aids are commonly used by professional players to prepare for competition. According to one recent study, 81% of professional players (from top 100 ranked players; 62 males and 9 females) use at least one nutritional supplement or ergogenic aid [24]. The most common products used were caffeine, creatine, iron, and carbohydrate and protein mixtures. Additionally, in another more recent publication, bicarbonate and B-alanine and nitric oxide are being used due to reported ergogenic benefits [25]. But, according to the USTA Player Development, a review about ergogenic aid use suggests more research needs to be done to prove the efficacy of these products. Often players are encouraged to try these products before the scientific literature supports the proven safety, and supplement companies may conduct their own research which is often not peer reviewed. For example, in the case of creatine, increased stress on the thermoregulatory system may be a risk and ergogenic benefit in tennis has not been proven [26]. Hormone-like compounds including plant sterols and stimulant plant herbs may cause positive doping, may cause negative health consequences as well as positive doping test results. Currently supplement manufacturers can put some unproven claims on their packaging. Players should proceed with caution as they may be putting themselves at risk for positive doping tests and should check with their governing sport bodies as well as the World Anti-Doping Agency (WADA) and NSF—Dietary Supplement Safety certification to check about sport food and ergogenic aid safety.

Conclusions

The tennis players' nutritional goals are to ensure enough nutrient-dense fueling to maximize health, performance, and growth and development. Having a personalized plan for training and competition is important for all players. Key nutritional components for all tennis players whose specific needs may vary slightly include:

(a) Ensure enough and consistent calories dispersed throughout the day.
(b) Fuel adequately before, during, and after training and matches.
(c) Hydrate sufficiently on-, off-court, and during travel days and times of heat acclimatization. An individually customized strategy should be adopted.
(d) Time consumption of foods and fluids appropriately before matches.
(e) Try and keep up to date with sports nutrition and ensure you have the highest quality sports medicine and science professionals around you.

An individual-specific athlete-based diet is the first step in optimizing the nutritional status of tennis players. If the diet is lacking supplements, pills and potions will not have an impact.

References

1. Ranchordeas MK, Rogersion D, Ruddock A, Killer SC, Winter EM. Nutrition for tennis: practical recommendations. J Sports Sci Med. 2013;12(2):211–24.
2. Burke L. Racket sports. In: Practical ports nutrition. Champaign, IL: Human Kinetics; 2007. p. 241–52.
3. Karpinski C, Rosenbloom C. Sports nutrition: a handbook for professionals, vol. 466-481. Chicago: The Academy of Nutrition and Dietetics; 2017. p. 572–3.
4. Burke L, Deakin V. Clinical sports nutrition. 5th ed. Australia: McGraw Hill Education Pty Ltd; 2015.
5. Thomas DT, Erdman KA, Burke LM. Position of the academy of nutrition and dietetics, dieticians of Canada, and The American college of sports medicine: nutrition and athletic performance. J Acad Nutr Diet. 116(3):501–28.. http://www.eatrightpro.org/~/media/eatrightpro files/practice/position and practice papers/position papers/nutritionathleticperf.ashx.
6. Maughan R. Water and electrolyte loss and replacement. In: Sports nutrition. UK: Wiley and Sons, Ltd.; 2014. p. 174–84.
7. Beatriz L, Gallo-Salazar C, Puente C, Areces F, Salinero JJ, Del Coso J. Interindividual variability in sweat electrolyte concentration in marathoners. J Int Soc Sports Nutr. 2016;13:31.
8. Christmass MA, Richmond SE, Cable NT, Arthur PG, Hartmann PE. Exercise intensity and metabolic response in singles tennis. J Sports Sci. 1998;16(8):739–47.

9. Gropper SS, Sorrels LM, Blessing D. Copper state of collegiate female athletes involved in different sports. Int J Sport Nutr Exerc Metab. 2003;13:343–57.
10. Nutter J. Seasonal changes in female athlete's diets. Int J Sport Nutr. 1991;1:395–407.
11. Juzwiak CR, Amancio OM, Vitalle MS, Pinheiro MM, Szejnfeld VL. Body composition and nutritional profile of male adolescent tennis players. J Sports Sci. 2008;26:1209–17.
12. Love P. US tennis players average caloric intakes and sport food use, presented at USPTA Tennis Symposium. 2010.
13. International Tennis Federation. Retrieved from: https://www.itftennis.com/scienceandmedicine/nutrition/eating-right.
14. Bergeron MF. Heat cramps: fluid and electrolyte challenges during tennis in the heat. J Sci Med Sport. 2003;6:19–27.
15. Kovacs MS, Baker LB. Recovery interventions and strategies for improved tennis performance. Br J Sports Med. 2014;48:118–21.
16. Burden RJ, Morton K, Richards T, Whyte GP, Pedlar CR. Is iron treatment beneficial in, iron-deficient but non-anemic endurance athletes? A systematic review and meta-analysis. Br J Sports Med. 2015;49:1389–97.
17. Malczewska J, Raczynski G, Stupnicki R. Iron status in female endurance athletes and in non-athletes. Int J Sport Nutr Exerc Metab. 2000;10(3):260–76.
18. Peeling P, Dawson B, Goodman C, Landers G, Trinder D. Athletic induced iron deficiency: new insights into the role of inflammation, cytokines and hormones. Eur J Appl Physiol. 2008;103:381–91.
19. Garvican LA, Lobigs L, Telford R, Fallon K, Gore CJ. Haemoglobin mass in an anemic female endurance runner before and after iron supplementation. Int J Sports Physiol Perform. 2011;6:137–40.
20. Brink-Effegoun T, Ratel S, Lepretre P-M, Metz L, et al. Effects of sport drinks on the maintenance of physical performance during 3 tennis matches: a randomized controlled study. J Int Soc Sports Nutr. 2014;11:46.
21. Bergeron MF, Armstrong LE, Maresh CM. Fluid and electrolyte losses during tennis in the heat. Clin Sports Med. 1995;14:23–32.
22. Kovacs M. Hydration and temperature in tennis–a practical review. J Sports Sci Med. 2006;5(1):1–9.
23. Ferrauti A, Pluim BM, Busch T, Weber K. Blood glucose responses and incidence of hypoglycaemia in elite tennis under practice and tournament conditions. J Sci Med Sport. 2003;6:28–39.
24. Lopez-Samanes A. Nutritional ergogenic aids in tennis: a brief review. Strength Cond J. 2015;37(3):1–11. https://doi.org/10.1519/SSC41.
25. Lopez-Samanes A. Use of nutritional supplements and ergogenic aids in professional tennis players. Nutr Hosp. 2017;34(5):1463–8. https://doi.org/10.20960/nh.1404.
26. Love P. Nutrition: sport supplements: do they enhance your game? http://www.playerdevelopment.usta.com/Improve-Your-Game/Sport-Science/114733_2018.

Heat Stress, Hydration, and Heat Illness in Elite Tennis Players

35

Julien D. Périard and Olivier Girard

35.1 Introduction

In recent years, several heat-related incidents have occurred in major tennis tournaments, highlighting the health and performance issues associated with playing in extreme heat. In January 2014, play was suspended for several hours during the Australian Open when the Extreme Heat Policy was invoked following days of hot weather and air temperatures exceeding 40 °C. This entailed a stoppage in play; however, only after a plastic bottle had reportedly started melting on court, a ball boy and a male player fainted, a female player experienced cramping and vomiting, and several notable players voiced their concerns regarding the appropriateness and safety of continuing to compete in such conditions [1]. In 2016, with air temperatures reaching 42 °C, play was again suspended as officials enforced the Extreme Heat Policy. This transpired after a player fainted during a match, commenting afterward that it was hazardous to be playing in such dangerously hot conditions [2]. In the previous season, the 2015 US Open saw a record number of withdrawals due to heat complaints, with a male player experiencing cramping and eventually collapsing due to the heat

J. D. Périard (✉)
Research Institute for Sport and Exercise, University of Canberra, Bruce, Australia
e-mail: julien.periard@canberra.edu.au

O. Girard
School of Psychology and Exercise Science, Murdoch University, Perth, Australia

[3]. These sequences of events were played out on the international stage but are mirrored each year in numerous lower-profile events around the world, consistently demonstrating the challenges and consequences of competing under severe heat stress.

Match-play tennis requires the combination of physical attributes such as speed, agility, power, muscular and aerobic endurance, as well as the capacity to anticipate, react, and make split second decisions. During prolonged matches under environmental heat stress (i.e., elevated air temperature and humidity), these attributes may be compromised relative to when play is undertaken in cooler conditions. Indeed, physiological (e.g., heart rate) and perceptual (e.g., perceived exertion and thermal discomfort) responses are exacerbated during play in the heat, as are strength losses in the lower limbs (e.g., maximal isometric force production capacity) following play [4–6]. These alterations relate to the development of thermal strain, which is characterized by a rise in whole-body temperature (i.e., core, skin, and muscle temperature). The rise in thermal strain during match-play tennis initiates both behavioral and autonomic thermoregulatory responses. Behavioral thermoregulation is a psychological response associated with a drive to achieve thermal satisfaction or minimize thermal discomfort. It elicits behaviors such as seeking shade, wearing light-colored clothing, and reducing physical exertion. The autonomic response involves an increase in blood flow to peripheral vascular beds and the initiation of sweating. This occurs so that metabolically generated heat may be dissipated to the environment via convection and evaporation. The increase in sweating during exercise in the heat is often accompanied by progressive dehydration if fluids are not sufficiently consumed [7, 8]. During match-play tennis, sweat rates vary based on ambient temperature and humidity but can reach 2.5 L h^{-1} in certain individuals [9, 10]. Severe levels of dehydration (>3%) exacerbate the development of hyperthermia, which contributes to impair prolonged exercise performance [11, 12]. Moreover, the loss of total body water often accompanies the occurrence of exertional heat illness [13].

Heat illness during sport and exercise can develop from relatively mild symptoms such as muscle cramps, to heat exhaustion, to heat injury, and to the more serious and life-threatening condition of exertional heatstroke. Although hyperthermia and dehydration can influence aerobic performance and lead to exertional heat illness, strategies and countermeasures can be utilized prior to and during match-play tennis that can alleviate the influence of heat stress. These include adopting an individualized hydration regimen, cooling strategies, and heat acclimation [14]. In addition to these strategies, event organizers can also help in reducing the impact of heat stress on health and performance by implementing various initiatives.

The aim of this chapter is to outline the influence of heat stress and hydration status on adjustments in match-play tennis performance and describe the underlying mechanisms mediating these modifications. The impact of playing tennis in the heat will also be examined in relation to the development of exertional heat illness, while strategies and countermeasures for preventing and treating heat illness, and optimizing performance, will be examined.

35.2 Heat Stress and Performance

The development of hyperthermia during exercise in the heat relates to the intensity of exercise and the prevailing environmental conditions. Tennis is characterized as high-intensity intermittent exercise. Its overall metabolic response, however, is similar to that of prolonged moderate-intensity exercise such as running or cycling [15]. This stems from work periods performed at 60–75% of maximal aerobic capacity (VO$_{2max}$), interspersed with periods of light activity or rest with work-to-rest ratios of 1:2–1:5 [16]. Consequently, mean relative exercise intensity for a match hovers around 55% VO$_{2max}$ [4, 17, 18] with duration ranging from 1 to 6 h, depending on the number of sets played [18–20]. The overall energetic demands of match-play tennis and the rate of rise in core temperature are therefore strongly influenced by the work-to-rest ratio, as longer rallies result in greater metabolic loads [6, 18, 21].

35.2.1 Aerobic Performance

When conducted under heat stress, prolonged self-paced exercise performance (e.g., cycling) has been shown to be progressively impaired (e.g., power output decreases) relative to when undertaken in cooler conditions [22]. This impairment has been suggested to stem from a narrowing of the core-to-skin temperature gradient reflexively increasing cutaneous blood flow [23] and from a rise in heart rate mediated by an elevated core temperature and sympathetic nervous activity [24]. The thermoregulatory redistribution of blood toward peripheral vascular beds, in combination with the exacerbated heart rate response, contributes to reduce central blood volume and compromise the maintenance of cardiac output. These adjustments have been shown to decrease VO$_{2max}$, causing an increase in relative exercise intensity (i.e., %VO$_{2max}$) when exercising at a given absolute workload, or decrease sustainable power output during self-paced efforts [25].

Match-play tennis in hot ambient conditions elicits a similar rise in thermal and physiological strain to that of continuous aerobic exercise. In tennis, core temperature has been shown to increase and stabilize around 38.5 °C during matches undertaken within a wide range of air temperatures (14.5–43.1 °C) [4, 21, 26–30]. However, core temperatures exceeding 39.5 °C have been reported during play [4, 6, 21, 26, 29].

For example, end-match rectal temperature (~39.4 °C vs. ~38.7 °C) increased to a greater extent in hot relative to cool conditions during simulated play (Fig. 35.1) [6]. This was also accompanied by elevated physiological and perceptual strain (Figs. 35.1 and 35.2). The attainment of higher levels of strain has been identified as a challenge to sustained performance proficiency during competitive match-play tennis [31].

Match characteristics during play in the heat fall within the wide range of those recorded during actual and simulated three set matches in various environmental conditions: match duration (80–120 min), point duration (6–10 s), between point duration (17–25 s), work-to-rest ratios (1:2–1:5), and effective playing percentage (17–28%) [16, 21, 31, 32]. Effective playing percentage represents the time spent with the ball in play relative to total match time. It has been shown to decrease in the heat and to be strongly associated with thermal sensation (i.e., afferent feedback regarding the thermal environment). Indeed, Morante et al. [29] suggested that behav-

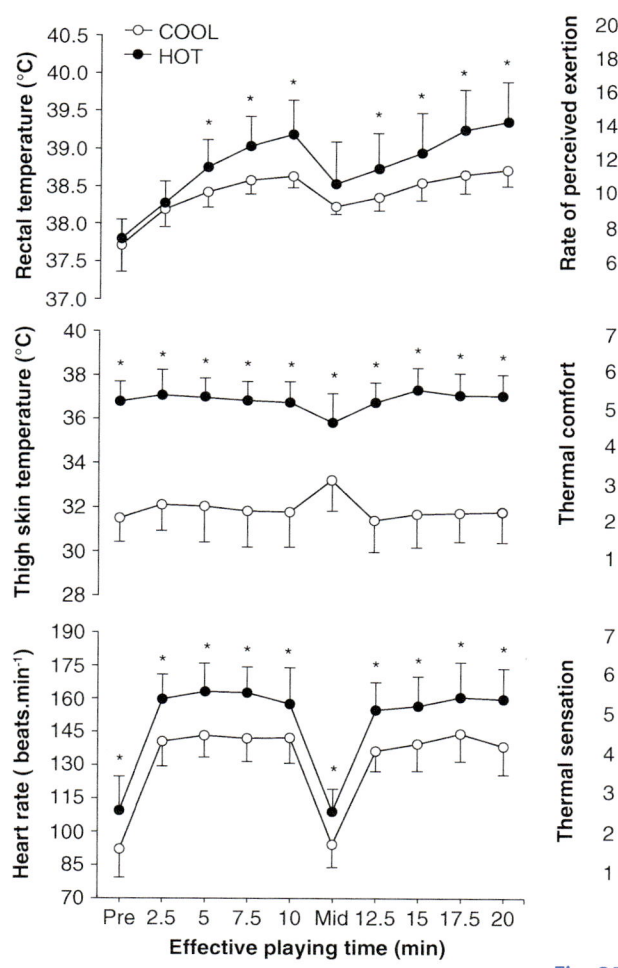

Fig. 35.1 Rectal temperature, thigh skin temperature, and heart rate during 20 min of effective match-play tennis (2 × 10 min) in COOL (22 °C) and HOT (37 °C) conditions. *Significantly different from COOL, $P < 0.05$. Reproduced with permission from Périard et al. [6]

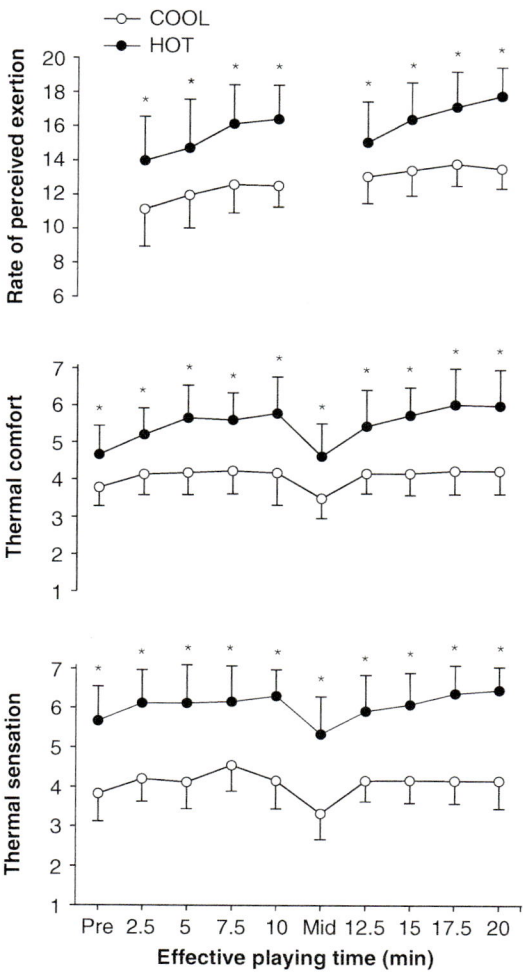

Fig. 35.2 Ratings of perceived exertion, thermal comfort, and thermal sensation during 20 min of effective match-play tennis (2 × 10 min) in COOL (22 °C) and HOT (37 °C) conditions. *Significantly different from COOL, $P < 0.01$. Reproduced with permission from Périard et al. [6]

ioral thermoregulation occurs during match-play tennis via a decrease in mean point duration when the environmental conditions are rated as uncomfortably hot (i.e., high rating of thermal sensation). It has since been shown that increasing the time between points also contributes to normalize thermal sensation by decreasing effective playing percentage [6]. This represents two strategies by which high-level players may behaviorally decrease their workload and concomitantly metabolic heat production.

Alternatively, during prolonged matches the development of hyperthermia is accompanied by an elevated heart rate (Fig. 35.1), which is characteristic of sustained aerobic exercise in the heat [22]. As match-play becomes protracted and hyperthermia develops, a progressive reduction in VO_{2max} is likely to occur. As a result, relative exercise intensity would increase during long or intense rallies, possibly leading to lengthier recovery periods between points [6], or the conscious decision to reduce point duration [29]. Future research should examine match characteristics more closely to determine whether decreasing point duration and/or increasing between point duration during play in the heat are behavioral strategies regularly adopted by players of all levels, age groups, and gender.

35.2.2 Sprint Performance

Improvements in single-sprint performance (i.e., mean and/or peak running speed or cycling power output) can be achieved following an increase in muscle temperature via passive heating (e.g., warm baths and/or heated blankets) or via increases in whole-body temperature after an active warm-up [33]. Enhanced single-sprint performance resulting from transient heat exposure can be attributed to improved muscle contractility [34] and accelerated muscle fiber conduction velocity, as individual sarcomeres become more rapidly activated at higher muscle temperatures [35].

Repeated-sprint ability tests are commonly used to assess the ability of racquet sport athletes to reproduce efforts at maximal intensity with limited recovery [36]. Elevations in thermal strain during match-play tennis in the heat are associated with increased cardiovascular and metabolic loads, in addition to decreased voluntary muscle activation in large muscle groups (e.g., knee extensors) [5]. There is compelling evidence to suggest that important performance decrements occur when repeated-sprint exercise (brief recovery periods, usually <60 s) is performed in hot compared with cool conditions (Table 35.1) [33]. For example, earlier and larger reductions in power output occurred during 5 × 15 s maximal efforts on a cycle ergometer when core and muscle temperature were elevated before a repeated sprint ability test, following the completion of a 40-min intermittent exercise bout in the heat [37]. Poorer intermittent-sprint performances (recovery periods long enough to allow near complete recovery, usually 60–300 s) have also been observed following exercise heat stress (core temperature >39 °C) [33].

Over the course of a tennis match, players repeatedly execute forceful lower-limb actions to produce explosive strokes and rapid on-court movements (e.g., accelerations, decelerations, and multidirectional displacements).

Table 35.1 Impact of increasing skin, muscle, and core temperature on performance of a single sprint, repeated, and intermittent sprints as well as the consequences associated with the implementation of countermeasures to mitigate the influence of heat stress

	Increase in temperature			Countermeasures		
	Skin temperature	Muscle temperature	Core temperature	Cooling methods	Acclimation	Hydration
Single sprint	+	+++	+/−	− − −	+	+/−
Repeated sprints	− −	+	− − −	+/−	++	++
Intermittent sprints	−	+/−	− −	++	++	++

The number of + or − symbols refers to possible (1), likely (2) and very likely (3) positive or negative effects

Consequently, technical proficiency has been suggested to suffer during closely contested or extended 3- to 5-set matches, with this effect being mostly visible in challenging ambient conditions [31]. However, when assessing the time course of changes in physical performance, it was shown that jumping ability (i.e., squat and countermovement jumps) and leg stiffness (i.e., mechanical index associated with explosive-type movements) are not further impaired during (mid-match) and following (24 h post-match) match-play under heat stress, despite the attainment of greater levels of thermal strain than during play in cool conditions [38]. Concurrently, similarly slower initial and longer cumulated sprint times were noted in hot and cool conditions when performing a repeated-sprint ability test (3 × 15 m, 15 s rest) after ~2 h of match-play. A decreased ability to sprint repeatedly when fatigued may lengthen the time required to achieve whole-body stability and control during stroke execution, which may be expected to cause less accurate or powerful strokes and/or enhance error rate [39]. With match-related fatigue impairments primarily occurring at mid-match (~60 min) and recovery (24 h post-match) responses displaying similar patterns between hot and cool conditions [38], it would appear that the typical match-induced reductions in the ability to tolerate impact forces or stretch load after repetitive short exhaustive runs [40] were not exacerbated under heat stress. Notwithstanding, neuromuscular system integrity in the lower limbs (i.e., knee extensors and plantar flexors) has been shown to be compromised immediately following match-play tennis in hot and cool conditions [5]. The compromise was attributed the development of peripheral fatigue, with larger and persistent (24 h) strength losses observed in the knee extensors following play in the heat associated with greater levels of central fatigue. Interestingly, Kraemer et al. [41] reported that 24 h of recovery allowed for neuromuscular performance characteristics to fully recover following successive days of indoor tournament play. However, the authors also suggested that mental and physical perceptions of fatigue persisted, which may explain the sustained reduction in voluntary muscle activation noted in the knee extensor after play in the heat.

35.2.3 Summary

The rise in thermal, physiological, and perceptual strain during match-play tennis in the heat elicits a cascade of responses, including the initiation of autonomic and behavioral thermoregulatory responses. The former leads to increases in skin blood flow and sweating, the latter to conscious decreases in point duration and/or increases in time between points, diminishing metabolic heat production. Heat stress does not appear to exacerbate match-related fatigue impairments in repeated-sprint ability, explosive power and leg stiffness, or neuromuscular system integrity. However, an element of central or mental fatigue associated with playing in the heat may lead to larger and persistent strength losses in larger muscle groups.

35.3 Hydration Status During Match-Play Tennis

Being euhydrated contributes not only to optimize athletic performance and cognitive function, but also to reduce the risk of exertional heat illness [42]. Euhydration, the state of being in body water balance, is a dynamic continuum represented by degrees of negative and positive water balance induced by dehydration and rehydration. During exercise in hot ambient conditions, the development of hyperthermia induces a rise in sweat rate that can lead to progressive dehydration if whole-body fluid losses are not offset by increasing fluid consumption. Exercise-induced dehydration is associated with a decrease in plasma volume and an increase in plasma osmolality that are proportional to the reduction in total body water [42]. This plasma hyperosmolality reduces sweat rate for any given core temperature and decreases evaporative heat loss [43]. The rate of heat storage and cardiovascular strain are therefore exacerbated, and the capacity to tolerate exercise in the heat is reduced. This is also due to decreases in cardiac filling and arterial blood pressure regulation, which lead to a decrease in VO_{2max} and aerobic performance impairments.

It has been suggested that drinking to thirst in ecologically valid settings (e.g., outdoor cycling time trial) allows athletes to compensate for elevated sweat rates and meet their fluid needs [44]. However, thirst has historically not been considered a good indicator of body water needs during exercise heat stress since ad libitum water consumption often results in incomplete fluid replacement or voluntary dehydration [45]. It has therefore been recommended that hydration regimens be individualized based on sweat rate, as well as composition (e.g., sodium) [31]. However, gastric emptying is related to exercise intensity, mode, duration, as well as the nature of the meal/fluid ingested [46], which may prevent some hydration regimens to fully offset fluid losses when sweating is profuse. It is thus further recommended to replace fluid losses to minimize dehydration (e.g., >3%) during prolonged exercise and that fluid consumption should not result in a gain of body mass; this may be irrelevant if an individual begins exercise in a severely dehydrated state [14].

The loss of total body water during match-play tennis has been identified as a limiting factor for performance [8, 31]. For example, a reduction in body mass of <3% was shown to negatively influence 5– and 10–m sprint times after competing for 120 min in warm conditions (31 °C and 75% RH) [47]. In a recent study, an individualized hydration regimen—6 mL kg body mass^{-1} of water with 185 mg L^{-1} of sodium every 2.5 h the day before a match and 70% of fluid losses replaced during play—was compared with the typical hydration habits of high-level players during a match in hot conditions (37 °C, 33% RH) [48]. The main difference conferred by the hydration regimen was that it allowed for undertaking the match in a euhydrated state, relative to when typical hydration habits were followed. This lead to an attenuation in thermal, physiological, and perceptual strain (Fig. 35.3). The elevated urine-specific gravity values (>1.020)

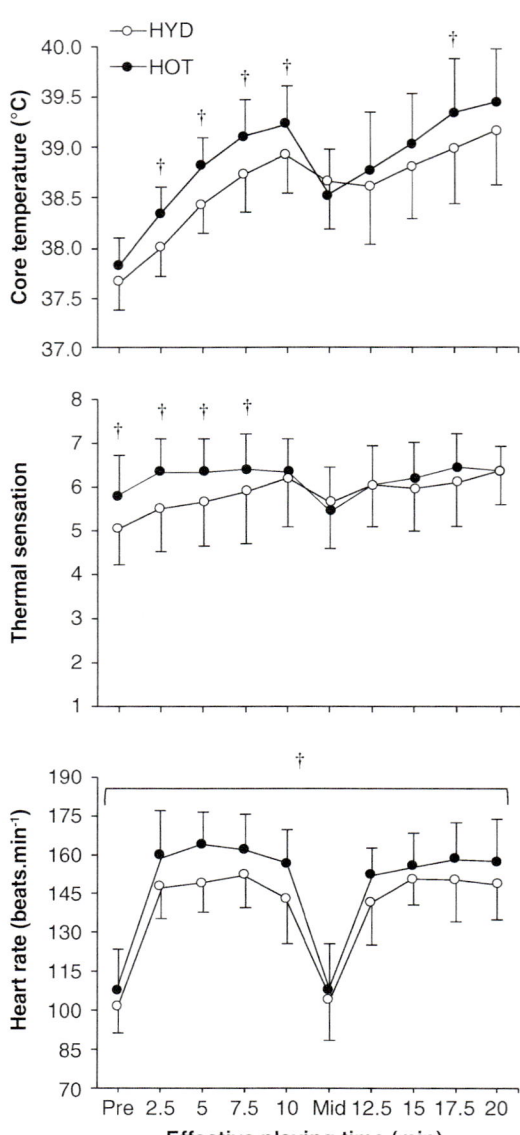

Fig. 35.3 Core temperature, thermal sensation, and heart rate during 20 min of effective match-play tennis in 37° C ambient air conditions with (HYD) and without (HOT) a hydration regimen. †Significant difference between HOT and HYD, $P < 0.05$. Amended with permission from Périard et al. [48]

noted prior to the match without a hydration strategy reinforced the notion that tennis players typically have poor match preparation hydration habits and start matches in a hypohydrated state. Notwithstanding, changes in body mass during play were similar between the hydration and normal habit regimens. This was due to similar sweat rates and fluid intake [48]. Furthermore, enough fluids were consumed to maintain body mass losses <1% even in the match condition without a predetermined hydration strategy. This is likely a reflection of the frequent breaks that occur during match-play tennis, which provide sufficient opportunities to rehydrate. Consequently, body mass losses rarely exceed 2% of pre-match values, even during play in the heat [4, 21, 26, 27, 29, 48, 49]. Interestingly, it has been shown during indoor play that fluid consumption can even surpass sweat losses [50].

35.3.1 Recommendations

35.3.1.1 Pre-exercise Hydration

When exposed to heat stress in the days preceding competition, tennis players should drink sufficiently and replace electrolyte losses to ensure that euhydration is maintained. Generally, drinking 5–6 mL of water per kg of body mass during this period, as well as 2–3 h before training or competition in the heat, is advisable but should be practiced. The most widely utilized methods to evaluate hydration status include monitoring body mass changes and measuring plasma osmolality and urine-specific gravity. Establishing a baseline body mass prior to competition is important as daily variations may occur during tournament play. This is best achieved by measuring post-void nude mass in the morning on consecutive days after consuming 1–2 L of fluid the prior evening. Moreover, since exercise, diet, and prior drinking influence urine concentration measurements, first morning urine is the preferred assessment time point to evaluate hydration status. If first morning urine cannot be obtained, urine collection should be preceded by several hours of minimal physical activity, fluid consumption, and eating.

35.3.1.2 Exercise Hydration

Sweat rates during match-play tennis in the heat vary dramatically depending on metabolic rate, environmental conditions, and heat acclimation status. As such, it is recommended during prolonged tennis matches in the heat to minimize body mass losses (without increasing body weight) in order to reduce physiological strain and preserve optimal performance. As sodium is the main electrolyte lost in sweat, heavy sweaters may deliberately increase sodium (i.e., salt) intake prior to, during, and following hot weather training and competition to maintain sodium balance (e.g., 300 mg of sodium added to 500 mL of a carbohydrate-electrolyte drink). During matches lasting longer than 1 h, players should aim to consume a solution containing 500–700 mg L^{-1} of sodium. In players experiencing muscle cramping, it is recommended to increase sodium intake to 1500 mg L^{-1} of water or sport drinks. Players should also aim to include 30–60 g h^{-1} of carbohydrates in their hydration regimen for training or matches lasting longer than 1 h and up to 90 g h^{-1} for events lasting over 2.5 h. This can be achieved through a combination of fluids and solid foods.

35.3.1.3 Post-exercise Rehydration

Following training or competing in the heat, rehydration is particularly important to optimize recovery. If fluid deficit needs to be urgently replenished, it is suggested to replace 150% of body mass losses within 1 h following the cessation of exercise, including electrolytes to maintain total body water. From a practical perspective, this may not be achievable for all players for various reasons (e.g., time, gastrointestinal discomfort). Thus, it may be more realistic to replace 100–120% of body mass losses over several hours. The preferred method of rehydration is through the consumption of fluids with foods, including salty food. Given that exercise in the heat increases carbohydrate metabolism, players spending long hours on the court should ensure that not only water and sodium losses are replenished, but carbohydrates stores as well. To ensure the highest rates of muscle glycogen resynthesis, carbohydrates should be consumed during the first hour after exercise. Moreover, drinks containing protein (e.g., milk) might allow to better restore fluid balance after exercise than a standard carbohydrate-electrolyte sports drink. Combining protein (0.2–0.4 g kg^{-1} h^{-1}) to carbohydrate (0.8 g kg^{-1} h^{-1}) has also been reported to maximize protein synthesis rates. Therefore, tennis players are encouraged to consume drinks such as chocolate milk, which has a carbohydrate-to-protein ratio (i.e., 4:1), as well as sodium following exercise.

35.4 Exertional Heat Illness During Match-Play Tennis

Exertional heat illness represents a continuum of medical conditions with potentially severe consequences that can affect physically active individuals in both hot and temperate environments (Table 35.2). The severity of exertional heat illness can escalate from relatively benign symptoms such as muscle cramping to heat exhaustion, heat injury, and heatstroke [13]. Heat exhaustion is considered a mild to moderate illness associated with a core temperature of 38.5–40 °C and an inability to maintain cardiac output. Heat injury is defined as a moderate to severe illness characterized by organ (e.g., liver and renal) and tissue (e.g., gut and muscle) damage with a high body temperature, typically >40 °C. Given that organ dysfunction is typically not observed during the early time course of heat injury, it is thus difficult to distinguish this condition from heat exhaustion. The most severe exertional heat illness, heatstroke, is characterized by high core temperatures (>40 °C), profound central nervous system dysfunction (e.g., combativeness, delirium, seizures, and coma), as well as organ and tissue damage and can lead to death. Unlike classic heatstroke, which is primarily observed in vulnerable and immunocompromised populations during seasonal heat waves, exertional heatstroke occurs in healthy young individuals performing strenuous physical activity. A further heat- and hydration-related illness is hyponatremia, which is a clinical condition associated with a serum sodium concentration below 135 mmol L^{-1}. Hyponatremia occurs when plasma is diluted, causing the movement of water from the extracellular fluid into intracellular spaces, resulting in the swelling of cells. This fluid shift can congest the lungs, swell the brain, and alter central nervous system function [52]. Given the clinical signs and symptoms of hyponatremia, including confusion, disorientation, altered consciousness, headache, nausea, vomiting, and muscle weak-

Table 35.2 Exertional heat illness signs/symptoms and management

Heat illness	Signs/symptoms	Management
Muscle cramping	Sudden, involuntary, and painful skeletal muscle spasms of brief duration	Rest, stretching, replacement of electrolytes Avoid salt tablets
Heat exhaustion	Mild to moderate illness associated with an inability to sustain cardiac output Moderate (>38.5 °C) to high (>40 °C) core temperature Often accompanied by dehydration	Move individual to a supine position in cool, shaded area, and elevate legs Loosen or remove clothing Actively cool skin Administer oral fluids
Heat injury	Moderate to severe condition characterized by tissue or organ damage Often accompanied by high (>40 °C) core temperature	Organ dysfunction is typically not observed during the early time course of heat injury Difficult to distinguish from heat exhaustion Heat injury may progress to heatstroke if the patient is not rapidly cooled
Heatstroke	Profound central nervous system dysfunction (e.g., agitation, delirium, stupor, coma) Accompanied with severe hyperthermia (>40 °C)	Ensure an open airway and move to a cool area Immediately cool to <39 °C using ice packs, water bath, wetting with water, and continuous fanning Administer IV fluid if hyponatremia is ruled out Reestablish normal central nervous system function Avoid antipyretics or drugs with liver toxicity

Table amended from Leon et al. [51]

ness, it is often confused with dehydration. The occurrence of exertional heat illness often arises in the presence of certain risk factors, such as extreme environmental conditions, medication and drug use, compromised health status, and underlying genetic conditions [13]. Heatstroke also often occurs in individuals considered low risk and performing routine physical activities in heat stress conditions [42]. Accordingly, it is difficult to identify individuals that may be at risk of exertional heat illness. Table 35.2 provides an overview of the signs/symptoms of exertional heat illnesses and the management of each illness.

The development of hyperthermia during match-play tennis is of particular concern when tournaments are played in hot and humid conditions, such as the US and Australian Opens where the wet-bulb globe temperature (WBGT) can surpass 30 °C [53]. The WBGT is an index that provides an estimate of the thermal load an environment imposes based on ambient temperature, humidity, wind speed, and solar radiation [54]. A WBGT >28 °C is considered an extreme risk for thermal injury [55], and the American College of Sports Medicine recommends to cancel competition due to the elevated level risk for exertional heat illness, namely, heatstroke [56]. Based on these recommendations, the International Tennis Federation (ITF) and Women's Tennis Association (WTA) have provided guidelines for optimizing player safety and health in the heat (Table 35.3).

Few data exist regarding the occurrence of heat illness during match-play tennis. In an epidemiological examination of the incidence of illnesses during the US Open between 1994 and 2009, Sell et al. [57] documented environmental (i.e., heat) illness occurrence rates of 2.84 and 1.42 per 1000-match exposures in men and women, respectively. More recently, the effect of environmental temperature on heat illness occurrence and changes in match-play characteristics were examined in males during Australian Open matches from 2014 to 2016 [58]. It was reported that a rise in WBGT increased total match doctor and trainer consults for heat stress, as well as post-match heat stress consults (WBGT > 32 °C) and calls for cooling devices (WBGT > 28 °C). Adjustments in match-play tactics included a reduction in net approaches and increased aces, reinforcing the notion that players behaviorally adapt during play in the heat.

Tennis as a sport appears to be at the forefront regarding the management of play in the heat by implementing firm cutoffs (Table 35.3). Notwithstanding, there remain concerns as to whether the current guidelines and practices for effectively and safely playing tennis in the heat, or the thresholds to suspend play, are adequate and sufficiently evidence based [59]. As per the rules and regulations of the ITF, 20 s are allocated between points, 90 s between game changeovers, and 120 s between sets. However, it appears that referees sometimes use discretion as Hornery et al. [21] demonstrated during an international tournament, with time between points increasing to ~25 s during matches undertaken in ~40 °C heat. These observations highlight the

Table 35.3 Examples of recommended actions by the International Tennis Federation (ITF) and Women's Tennis Association (WTA) based on the wet-bulb globe temperature (WBGT)

WBGT (°C)	Organization	Athlete concerned	Recommendation
32.2	ITF	Wheelchair tennis players	Immediate suspension of play
32.2	WTA	Women	Immediate suspension of play
30.1	ITF-WTA	Juniors and women	10-min break between second and third set
30.1	ITF	Wheelchair tennis players	Suspension of play at the end of the set in progress
28.0	ITF	Wheelchair tennis players	15-min break between second and third set
28.0	Australian Open	Tennis players	10-min break between second and third set

ITF International Tennis Federation, *WTA* Women's Tennis Association
http://www.itftennis.com/media/163398/163398.pdf, http://www.itftennis.com/media/166656/166656.pdf, http://www.wtatennis.com/SEWTATour-Archive/Archive/AboutTheTour/rules2014.pdf, http://www.ausopen.com/en_AU/event_guide/a_z_guide.html
Table amended with permission from Racinais et al. [14]

importance of allowing players the opportunity to self-regulate their effort through slightly protracted rest intervals between points, without affecting the continuity of play, to ensure their safety and avoid heat-related illness. A 10-min break in WBGT conditions of 30.3 °C was shown to decrease core temperature by ~0.25 °C [49], whereas a 25-min break at a WBGT of 34 °C led to a 0.4 °C reduction in core temperature [6]. As such, enforcing the ITF-WTA extreme weather condition rule whereby a 10-min break is allowed between the second and third sets in tournament play, not only at the professional level but for amateurs as well, may further reduce the risk of heat illness and encourage optimal performance (Table 35.2).

Most of the research regarding match-play tennis, whether in hot or cool conditions, is conducted on elite or high-level amateur male players. While most athletes are able to cope with various environmental conditions given adequate hydration and appropriate scheduling of training and matches (including recovery time), professional athletes typically possess a better ability to cope with high core temperatures due to their increased fitness level and partial acclimation to heat stress [60]. However, female, youth, and wheelchair tennis may be differently affected by the deleterious effects of heat stress. Indeed, males and females differ in their thermoregulatory responses to exercise heat stress, mostly due to a reduced sudomotor function in females, when a certain requirement for heat loss is exceeded [61]. When this requirement is matched for a given heat production, females incur a greater change in core temperature, likely due to physical differences in body mass and composition [62]. Females may thus reach greater core temperatures in a shorter time period, potentially putting them at greater risk of exertional heat illness. In infants, there appears to be an elevated risk for classic heatstroke because of their greater surface area to body mass ratio, which accelerates heat gain, their limited or suppressed thermoregulatory behavior, and predisposition for preexisting respiratory infections [13]. During adolescence, total body water and exchangeable sodium losses increase during exercise due to a rise in whole-body sweat rate [54, 63]. Maturing youth athletes may thus be more susceptible to reaching greater levels of thermal strain if fluid losses are not compensated, which could negatively impact on performance and increase the risk of exertional heat illness. In players with a spinal cord injury, there is a loss of vasomotor and sudomotor effector responses below the level of the lesion [64]. The risk of heat illness in wheelchair tennis is thus increased in warm conditions due to greater heat storage within the lower body and a reduction in whole-body sweat rate. Additional research is needed in these populations to enhance our understanding of their responses to match-play tennis in the heat.

35.4.1 Summary

The potential for exertional heat illness exists in tennis as with other outdoor sports sometimes played in extreme heat. This has been observed in professionals during the Australian and US Opens but is a scenario that can occur at all levels, including in youth and wheelchair players. The identification of specific heat illnesses is important to ensure proper treatment, as is their prevention through the implementation of evidence-based guidelines for suspending play in the heat. In order to reduce the risk and incidence of heat-related health issues at all levels, several countermeasures have been developed including more breathable clothing, improved hydration practices, and a variety of on-court cooling measures and strategies. The following section highlights some of these countermeasures.

35.5 Countermeasures to Optimize Performance and Health

35.5.1 Heat Acclimation

The most important intervention one can adopt to reduce physiological strain and optimize performance in hot ambient conditions is to heat acclimate [14]. Indeed, the chronic exposure to heat stress enhances thermoregulatory responses, improves submaximal exercise performance, increases VO_{2max}, and improves thermal comfort in the heat. The benefits of heat acclimation are achieved through enhanced sweating and skin blood flow responses, plasma volume expansion, better fluid balance and cardiovascular stability, a lowered metabolic rate, and acquired thermal tolerance [60, 65]. The time course of heat acclimation is remarkably rapid, with most of the improvements occurring during the first week of heat exposure, and the remaining thermoregulatory benefits generally being complete or optimized after 10–14 days (Fig. 35.4). The process of adaptation related to heat acclimation can occur in artificial/laboratory settings (i.e., heat acclimation) and from exposure to natural environments (i.e., heat acclimatization). It is recommended that athletes planning on competing in the heat prepare by heat acclimatizing, so as to be exposed to the precise conditions in which play will occur. The heat regimen should be 7–10 days in length with daily (60–90 min) exposure to heat sufficient enough to induce an increase in core and skin temperatures and stimulate sweating.

35.5.2 Cooling Strategies

A number of pre-exercise and in-play cooling strategies (i.e., cold water immersion, ice vests, applying ice onto the skin, ice slurry ingestion) have been employed in an attempt to mitigate the influence of exercise heat stress and the associated physiological alterations that impair the ability to compete in the heat. Although cold water immersion is effective at reducing core temperature, it also cools the muscles and consequently decreases nerve conduction and muscle contraction velocities, requiring athletes to rewarm up before competition. Using a mixed method approach and ice packs to precool the quadriceps has been shown to enhance repeated and intermittent-sprint capacity in the heat, with the cooling responses likely providing a volume (i.e., surface area coverage) and/or duration-dependent effect [66]. As with cold water immersion, however, this approach may be detrimental to the performance of single sprint or the first few repetitions of a multiple-sprint test protocol, due to lower muscle temperatures reducing short-term power output (Table 35.1). On the other

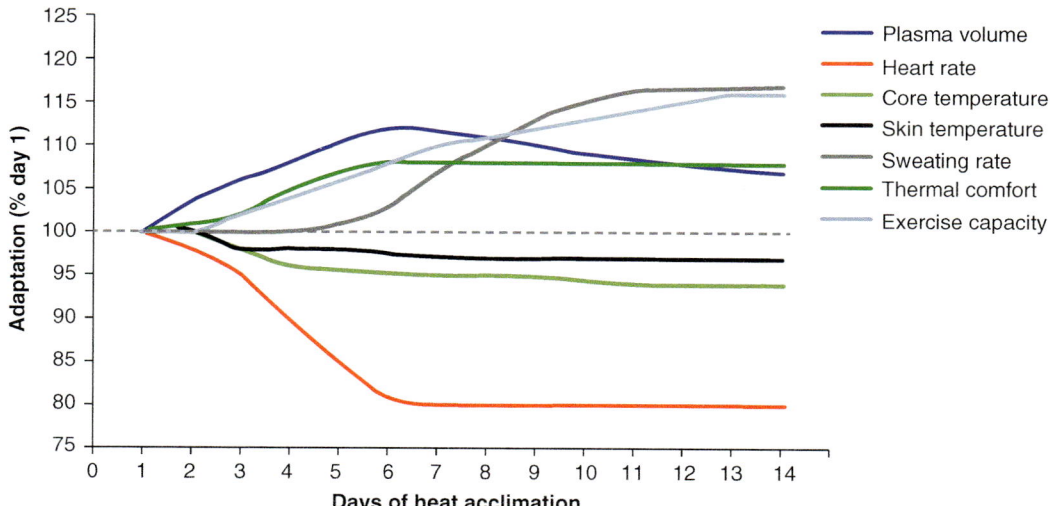

Fig. 35.4 The time course of adaptations to exercise-heat acclimation. Within a week of acclimation, plasma volume expansion occurs, and heart rate is reduced during exercise at a given work rate. Core and skin temperatures are also reduced when exercising at a given work rate, whereas sweat rate increases. Perceptually, the rating of thermal comfort is improved. As a result, aerobic exercise capacity is increased. Of note, the magnitude of these adaptations is dependent on the initial state of acclimation and the acclimation protocol (e.g., environmental conditions and exercise intensity). Reproduced with permission from Périard et al. [60]

hand, cooling-related improvements in effort perception may enhance the willingness to maintain maximal efforts during successive efforts/sprints.

Ingesting very cold or iced (slurry) drinks is a method being used more and more frequently in the field to optimize performance [67]. Based on the theory of enthalpy, ice requires substantially more heat energy (334 J/g) to cause a phase change from solid to liquid (at 0 °C) compared with the energy required to increase the temperature of water (4 J/g/°C). As such, ice slurry ingestion may be more effective than cold water ingestion in cooling athletes. Indeed, the combination of fluid ingestion and cooling via ice slurry ingestion can (1) lower pre-exercise core temperature, (2) attenuate the rate of rise of core temperature during exercise, and (3) extend the core temperature attained at the end of exercise [67]. Drinking should ideally be spread over the entirety of a match (i.e., during breaks in play) so as to maximize heat loss and maintain a larger heat sink. Individuals should experiment with ice slurry and large volumes of cold fluid ingestion prior to competition to ensure discomfort, or gastrointestinal issues do not occur. Moreover, despite the potential benefits of ice slurry ingestion, there are practical limitations associated with this practice, such as access to ice, the availability of large volumes of water, electricity to power the slurry machine, and disruption to warm-up activities.

35.5.3 Tennis-Specific Cooling

A practical approach for reducing whole-body temperature during exercise in hot/humid environments might be the use of electric fans and commercially available ice cooling vests, which can provide effective cooling without impairing muscle temperature [14]. The use of ice towels is currently recommended to provide on-court relief during play in the heat [68]. This involves the application of ice wrapped in a wet towel around the neck with damp, cold towels simultaneously placed on the head and thighs. The efficacy of this in-play cooling strategy for mitigating heat strain was recently evaluated during simulated four-set match-play activity (i.e., treadmill running) in 36 °C and 50% RH, which is similar to the most extreme conditions during the US Open [69]. This strategy was compared with a new cooling intervention purported to optimize evaporative heat loss by wetting the arms, neck, face, and lower legs with a sponge while sitting in front of a fan. Given that the evaporation of water from the skin surface liberates ~7 times more heat per gram (2427 J g^{-1}) than the melting of ice [70], the cooling strategy promoting evaporative heat loss was considered as potentially being a more efficacious alternative than ice towels [69]. The authors reported that relative to a control condition during which only cold water ingestion was permitted, the use of ice towels led to a smaller elevation in core temperature (~0.5 °C), lower rating of perceived exertion, cooler whole-body thermal sensation, and lower heart rate (~15 beats min^{-1}) during simulated match-play activity. The intervention promoting evaporative heat loss via wetting the skin in front of an electric fan decreased physiological and perceptual heat strain to similar levels as the ice towel strategy [69]. Despite these similar improvements, the strategy of reducing thermal strain though skin wetting and fanning may represent a more practical alternative in lower resource settings.

In a follow-up study, a hot/dry environment akin to the peak 2014 Australian Open conditions (44 °C, 10% RH, 475 W/m^2 simulated solar radiation) was simulated, and the strategies highlighted above, as well as one in which fanning was used without skin wetting, were evaluated [71]. The use of an electric fan with skin wetting was shown to be more effective at mitigating thermal and perceptual strain compared to the control and fanning without skin wetting conditions. Wetting the skin while sitting in front of a fan resulted in lower final core (~0.6 °C) and skin temperatures, along with cooler thermal sensations throughout simulated match-play activity. The use of ice towels yielded comparable core temperature and thermal sensation responses to that of fanning wet skin, although skin temperature was ~1.3 °C lower. Collectively, these observations suggest that using either the ice towel approach, or optimizing evaporative heat loss by wetting the skin with a sponge while sitting in front of a fan, helps elicit a cooler thermal sensation and reduces thermal strain during simulated tennis match-play activity in hot/wet and very hot/dry and sunny conditions [69, 71].

35.5.4 Event Organization

In order to reduce the risk to player health and increase safety during tournament play in hot conditions, event organizers can modify scheduling and start matches based on weather patterns (i.e., cooler parts of the day). They may also adapt the rules and refereeing to include extra breaks, as well as allow players the opportunity to slightly increase the rest interval between points, without affecting the continuity of play. Making cooling and rehydration options available during play (i.e., game and set breaks) are also positive steps toward the aim of reducing exertional heat illness incidence and optimizing performance.

> **Conclusion**
>
> Tennis is a popular sport predominately played in the summer on outdoor courts. Compared to cool conditions, playing tennis under heat stress leads to exacerbated thermal (i.e., core and skin temperatures), physiological (e.g., heart rate), and perceptual (e.g., perceived exertion and thermal comfort/sensation) strain, which in turn may influence physical performance and match tactics. While hyperthermia-induced dehydration contributes to impair aerobic capacity, as well as speed and power during match-play, it would appear that the nature of the game with its regular breaks allows for players to remain sufficiently hydrated when competing in the heat. However, players are advised to monitor their hydration status and endeavor to start matches in a well-hydrated state. Given the high-profile incidents occurring at the Australian and US Opens in recent years, emphasis should be placed in understanding the risk and incidence of heat illness during tennis play in the heat. Players should adequately prepare for competing in hot conditions by heat acclimatizing and utilizing individualized cooling strategies (e.g., ice towels and fanning) based on the type of environment they will encounter (e.g., hot/dry vs. hot/humid). Event organizers should also be prepared to implement transparent Extreme Heat Policies based on the specificities of match-play tennis in hot environmental conditions.

References

1. Bishop G. At the Australian Open, it's not the heat, it's the stupidity. https://www.nytimes.com/2014/01/18/sports/tennis/players-are-not-cool-with-australian-open-heat-policy.html?_r=0. Accessed 10 Oct 2016.
2. ESPN. Extreme heat stops play at the Australian Open. http://www.espn.com/tennis/story/_/id/14560568/extreme-heat-again-stops-play-australian-open. Accessed 10 Oct 2016.
3. Garber G. Jack Sock retires midmatch vs. Ruben Bemelmans http://www.espn.com/tennis/usopen15/story/_/id/13573860/american-jack-sock-withdraws-fourth-set-second-round-us-open. Accessed 10 Oct 2016.
4. Morante SM, Brotherhood JR. Air temperature and physiological and subjective responses during competitive singles tennis. Br J Sports Med. 2007;41:773–8.
5. Périard JD, Girard O, Racinais S. Neuromuscular adjustments of the knee extensors and plantar flexors following match-play tennis in the heat. Br J Sports Med. 2014;48:i45–51.
6. Périard JD, Racinais S, Knez WL, Herrera CP, Christian RJ, Girard O. Thermal, physiological and perceptual strain mediate alterations in match-play tennis under heat stress. Br J Sports Med. 2014;48:i32–8.
7. Kovacs MS. Hydration and temperature in tennis – a practical review. J Sports Sci Med. 2006;5:1–9.
8. Kovacs MS. A review of fluid and hydration in competitive tennis. Int J Sports Physiol Perform. 2008;3:413–23.
9. Bergeron MF, Armstrong LE, Maresh CM. Fluid and electrolyte losses during tennis in the heat. Clin Sports Med. 1995;14:23–32.
10. Bergeron MF, Maresh CM, Armstrong LE, Signorile JF, Castellani JW, Kenefick RW, LaGasse KE, Riebe DA. Fluid-electrolyte balance associated with tennis match play in a hot environment. Int J Sport Nutr. 1995;5:180–93.
11. Cheuvront SN, Carter RC, Sawka MN. Fluid balance and endurance exercise performance. Curr Sports Med Rep. 2003;2:202–8.
12. Sawka MN, Latzka WA, Matott RP, Montain SJ. Hydration effects on temperature regulation. Int J Sports Med. 1998;19:S108–10.

13. Leon LR, Bouchama A. Heat stroke. Compr Physiol. 2015;5:611–47.
14. Racinais S, Alonso J-M, Coutts AJ, Flouris AD, Girard O, Gonzalez-Alonso J, Hausswirth C, Jay O, Lee JKW, Mitchell N, Nassis GP, Nybo L, Pluim BM, Roelands B, Sawka MN, Wingo JE, Périard JD. Consensus recommendations on training and competing in the heat. Scand J Med Sci Sports. 2015;25:6–19.
15. Bergeron MF, Maresh CM, Kraemer WJ, Abraham A, Conroy B, Gabaree C. Tennis: a physiological profile during match play. Int J Sports Med. 1991;12:474–9.
16. Fernandez J, Mendez-Villanueva A, Pluim BM. Intensity of tennis match play. Br J Sports Med. 2006;40:387–91.
17. Ferrauti A, Bergeron MF, Pluim BM, Weber K. Physiological responses in tennis and running with similar oxygen uptake. Eur J Appl Physiol. 2001;85:27–33.
18. Smekal G, von Duvillard SP, Rihacek C, Pokan R, Hofmann P, Baron R, Tschan H, Bachl N. A physiological profile of tennis match play. Med Sci Sports Exerc. 2001;33:999–1005.
19. Christmass MA, Richmond SE, Cable NT, Arthur PG, Hartmann PE. Exercise intensity and metabolic response in singles tennis. J Sports Sci. 1998;16:739–47.
20. O' Donoghue P, Ingram B. A notational analysis of elite tennis strategy. J Sports Sci. 2001;19:107–15.
21. Hornery DJ, Farrow D, Mujika I, Young W. An integrated physiological and performance profile of professional tennis. Br J Sports Med. 2007;41:531–6.
22. Périard JD, Cramer MN, Chapman PG, Caillaud C, Thompson MW. Cardiovascular strain impairs prolonged self-paced exercise in the heat. Exp Physiol. 2011;96:134–44.
23. Rowell LB. Circulatory adjustments to dynamic exercise and heat stress: competing controls. In: Rowell LB, editor. Human circulation: regulation during physical stress. New York, NY: Oxford University Press; 1986. p. 363–406.
24. Coyle EF, Gonzalez-Alonso J. Cardiovascular drift during prolonged exercise: new perspectives. Exerc Sport Sci Rev. 2001;29:88–92.
25. Périard JD, Racinais S. Self-paced exercise in hot and cool conditions is associated with the maintenance of %VO2peak within a narrow range. J Appl Physiol. 2015;118:1258–65.
26. Bergeron MF, McLeod KS, Coyle JF. Core body temperature during competition in the heat: National Boys' 14s Junior Championships. Br J Sports Med. 2007;41:779–83.
27. Bergeron MF, Waller JL, Marinik EL. Voluntary fluid intake and core temperature responses in adolescent tennis players: sports beverage versus water. Br J Sports Med. 2006;40:406–10.
28. Elliott B, Dawson B, Pyke F. The energetics of singles tennis. J Hum Mov Stud. 1985;11:11–20.
29. Morante SM, Brotherhood JR. Autonomic and behavioural thermoregulation in tennis. Br J Sports Med. 2008;42:679–85.
30. Therminarias A, Dansou P, Chirpaz-Oddou MF, Gharib C, Quirion A. Hormonal and metabolic changes during a strenuous tennis match. Int J Sports Med. 1991;12:10–6.
31. Hornery DJ, Farrow D, Mujika I, Young W. Fatigue in tennis: mechanisms of fatigue and effect on performance. Sports Med. 2007;37:199–212.
32. Torres-Luque G, Sánchez-Pay A, Bazaco MJ, Moya M. Functional aspects of competitive tennis. J Hum Sport Exerc. 2011;6:528–39.
33. Girard O, Brocherie F, Bishop DJ. Sprint performance under heat stress: a review. Scand J Med Sci Sports. 2015;25:79–89.
34. Racinais S, Oksa J. Temperature and neuromuscular function. Scand J Med Sci Sports. 2010;20(Suppl 3):1–18.
35. Gray SR, De Vito G, Nimmo MA, Farina D, Ferguson RA. Skeletal muscle ATP turnover and muscle fiber conduction velocity are elevated at higher muscle temperatures during maximal power output development in humans. Am J Physiol Regul Integr Comp Physiol. 2006;290:R376–82.
36. Fernandez-Fernandez J, Zimek R, Wiewelhove T, Ferrauti A. High-intensity interval training vs. repeated-sprint training in tennis. J Strength Cond Res. 2012;26:53–62.
37. Drust B, Rasmussen P, Mohr M, Nielsen B, Nybo L. Elevations in core and muscle temperature impairs repeated sprint performance. Acta Physiol Scand. 2005;183:181–90.
38. Girard O, Christian RJ, Racinais S, Périard JD. Heat stress does not exacerbate tennis-induced alterations in physical performance. Br J Sports Med. 2014;48:i39–44.
39. Ferrauti A, Pluim BM, Weber K. The effect of recovery duration on running speed and stroke quality during intermittent training drills in elite tennis players. J Sports Sci. 2001;19:235–42.
40. Girard O, Micallef JP, Millet GP. Changes in spring-mass model characteristics during repeated running sprints. Eur J Appl Physiol. 2011;111:125–34.
41. Kraemer WJ, Piorkowski PA, Bush JA, Gomez AL, Loebel CC, Volek JS, Newton RU, Mazzetti SA, Etzweiler SW, Putukian M, Sebastianelli WJ. The effects of NCAA Division 1 intercollegiate competitive tennis match play on recovery of physical performance in women. J Strength Cond Res. 2000;14:265–72.
42. Sawka MN, Leon LR, Montain SJ, Sonna LA. Integrated physiological mechanisms of exercise performance, adaptation, and maladaptation to heat stress. Compr Physiol. 2011;1:1883–928.
43. Montain SJ, Latzka WA, Sawka MN. Control of thermoregulatory sweating is altered by hydration level and exercise intensity. J Appl Physiol. 1995;79:1434–9.

44. Goulet ED. Effect of exercise-induced dehydration on time-trial exercise performance: a meta-analysis. Br J Sports Med. 2011;45:1149–56.
45. Greenleaf JE. Problem: thirst, drinking behavior, and involuntary dehydration. Med Sci Sports Exerc. 1992;24:645–56.
46. Horner KM, Schubert MM, Desbrow B, Byrne NM, King NA. Acute exercise and gastric emptying: a meta-analysis and implications for appetite control. Sports Med. 2015;45:659–78.
47. Magal M, Webster MJ, Sistrunk LE, Whitehead MT, Evans RK, Boyd JC. Comparison of glycerol and water hydration regimens on tennis-related performance. Med Sci Sports Exerc. 2003;35:150–6.
48. Périard JD, Racinais S, Knez WL, Herrera CP, Christian RJ, Girard O. Coping with heat stress during match-play tennis: does an individualised hydration regimen enhance performance and recovery? Br J Sports Med. 2014;48:i64–70.
49. Tippet ML, Stofan JR, Lacambra M, Horswill CA. Core temperature and sweat responses in professional women's tennis players during tournament play in the heat. J Athl Train. 2011;46:55–60.
50. Lott MJ, Galloway SD. Fluid balance and sodium losses during indoor tennis match play. Int J Sport Nutr Exerc Metab. 2011;21:492–500.
51. Leon LR, Kenefick R. Pathophysiology of heat-related illness. In: Auerbach P, editor. Textbook of wilderness medicine. Philadelphia, PA: Mosby Elsevier; 2011. p. 215–31.
52. Montain SJ, Cheuvront SN, Sawka MN. Exercise associated hyponatraemia: quantitative analysis to understand the aetiology. Br J Sports Med. 2006;40:98–105.
53. Mountjoy M, Alonso JM, Bergeron MF, Dvorak J, Miller S, Migliorini S, Singh DG. Hyperthermic-related challenges in aquatics, athletics, football, tennis and triathlon. Br J Sports Med. 2012;46: 800–4.
54. Bergeron MF, Mountjoy M, Armstrong N, Chia M, Cote J, Emery CA, Faigenbaum A, Hall G Jr, Kriemler S, Leglise M, Malina RM, Pensgaard AM, Sanchez A, Soligard T, Sundgot-Borgen J, van Mechelen W, Weissensteiner JR, Engebretsen L. International Olympic Committee consensus statement on youth athletic development. Br J Sports Med. 2015;49:843–51.
55. Binkley HM, Beckett J, Casa DJ, Kleiner DM, Plummer PE. National Athletic Trainers' Association Position Statement: exertional heat illnesses. J Athl Train. 2002;37:329–43.
56. Armstrong LE, Casa DJ, Millard-Stafford M, Moran DS, Pyne SW, Roberts WO. American College of Sports Medicine position stand. Exertional heat illness during training and competition. Med Sci Sports Exerc. 2007;39:556–72.
57. Sell K, Hainline B, Yorio M, Kovacs M. Illness data from the US Open Tennis Championships from 1994 to 2009. Clin J Sport Med. 2013;23:25–32.
58. Smith TP, Reid M, Kovalchik S, Duffield R. The effect of environmental temperature on heat illness incidence and tennis match characteristics at the Australian Open. J Sci Med Sport. 2017;pii:S1440-2440(17)31763-2.
59. Périard JD, Bergeron MF. Competitive match-play tennis under heat stress: a challenge for all players. Br J Sports Med. 2014;48:i1–3.
60. Périard JD, Racinais S, Sawka MN. Adaptations and mechanisms of human heat acclimation: Applications for competitive athletes and sports. Scand J Med Sci Sports. 2015;25:20–38.
61. Gagnon D, Kenny GP. Sex differences in thermoeffector responses during exercise at fixed requirements for heat loss. J Appl Physiol. 2012;113:746–57.
62. Havenith G. Human surface to mass ratio and body core temperature in exercise heat stress – a concept revisited. J Therm Biol. 2001;26:387–93.
63. Bergeron MF. Training and competing in the heat in youth sports: no sweat? Br J Sports Med. 2015;49:837–9.
64. Price MJ. Thermoregulation during exercise in individuals with spinal cord injuries. Sports Med. 2006;36:863–79.
65. Périard JD, Travers GJS, Racinais S, Sawka MN. Cardiovascular adaptations supporting human exercise-heat acclimation. Auton Neurosci. 2016;196:52–62.
66. Minett GM, Duffield R, Marino F, Portus M. Volume-dependent response of precooling for intermittent-sprint exercise in the heat. Med Sci Sports Exerc. 2011;43:1760–9.
67. Tan PMS, Lee JKW. The role of fluid temperature and form on endurance performance in the heat. Scand J Med Sci Sports. 2015;25:39–51.
68. Ellenbecker TS, Stroia KA. Heat research guides current practices in professional tennis. Br J Sports Med. 2014;48:i5–6.
69. Schranner D, Scherer L, Lynch GP, Korder S, Brotherhood JR, Pluim BM, Périard JD, Jay O. In-play cooling interventions for simulated match-play tennis in US Open conditions. Med Sci Sports Exerc. 2017;49:991–8.
70. Wenger CB. Heat of evaporation of sweat: thermodynamic considerations. J Appl Physiol. 1972;32:456–9.
71. Lynch GP, Périard JD, Pluim BM, Brotherhood JR, Jay O. Optimal cooling strategies for players in Australian Tennis Open conditions. Br J Sports Med. 2017;21:232–7.

On-Site Management and Coverage for Tournament Physicians in Professional Tennis

36

Mark E. Batt, Philip A. Bell, and Ian M. McCurdie

The chapter is written from the perspective of three sport and exercise medicine physicians who have covered tennis events for 20 years including Wimbledon, Davis Cup, ATP World Tour Finals and Olympic Games. It covers what is expected of tournament physicians before, during and after events. It also addresses specific considerations of injury management in competition. The aim is to provide a practical resource for tournament medical staff.

The chapter is divided into sections addressing the pre-competition preparation and set-up, duties and awareness during practice and play and consideration of the clinical challenges arising at an event.

36.1 Tournament Preparation

The tournament physician's preparation for any event will need to cover a variety of aspects of medical care provision. These include staffing, equipment, care pathways, protocols and communication.

M. E. Batt (✉)
Centre forl Sports Medicine, Queens Medical Centre, Nottingham University Hospitals, Nottingham, UK
e-mail: Mark.batt@nottingham.ac.uk

P. A. Bell
BMI The Paddocks Clinic, Princes Risborough, UK

I. M. McCurdie
Defence Medical Rehabilitation Centre, Headley Court, Surrey, UK

Preparation for any tournament should start as soon as the previous year's tournament finishes. A formal tournament medical report will highlight any issues identified and actions to be taken during the year.

Certain aspects of an event will be 'fixed' and will not change from year to year, whilst others may be quite different. For instance, the draw size, playing surface and venue layout will usually remain unchanged (although it is good practice to check, rather than assume), allowing for some degree of confidence in estimating staffing and equipment levels and, arguably, predicting injury patterns. Other elements, such as the local environmental conditions, current local health issues and individual player fitness can be much more difficult to predict. These issues are illustrated by comparing the medical cover required for two high-profile but very different events—The Championships, Wimbledon and the ATP World Tour Finals, currently held at the O2 Arena in London. The former is an outdoor, grass court Grand Slam tournament, with up to 480 competitors in the main draw, playing 662 matches over a 2-week period, at a venue that has 19 competition courts and a further 22 practice courts. By contrast, the latter event is an indoor, hard court competition, with only 24 male players, held over an 8-day period, at a venue with one competition court and three practice courts.

36.1.1 Staffing

Staffing for medical cover should be determined by draw size and duration of the event and should ensure that a balanced skill mix is maintained throughout. This should ensure that primary care, emergency care and injury management are all provided for the 'target' population, usually the players and their entourage. Depending on the size of the event, there will be variable numbers of allied health professionals (AHP), such as physiotherapists, soft tissue therapists, strength and conditioning coaches, podiatrists and others who work alongside the medical team. Effective interdisciplinary teamwork is critical in this environment, and large clinical teams will need to be familiar with each other's practice and communicate closely in preparation for, and during, the event.

Emergency care support will often be provided by on-site paramedic services. It is vitally important that the event medical team communicates closely with the paramedic team and that each fully understands the nature and limitations of their role and responsibilities. Player evacuation from court may, for instance, be managed by the medical team but needs access to wheelchair or stretcher transport from the paramedic team. The paramedic team will often act as the link between the event medical team and local ambulance and hospital services.

Each event should have a nominated local hospital, with which contact has been established. Hospital-based specialists, such as radiologists, surgeons and physicians should be identified well in advance of the event, and links with laboratory services, emergency departments, local ambulance services and pharmacies should be established. These extended support services will come to understand the potential requirements of the event and deliver an improving service over time. Information about the forthcoming event should be communicated to appropriate personnel within each of these organisations, as well as to the event medical team, AHPs and ATP/WTA representatives, to ensure that every element of this large support team is aware of its roles and responsibilities.

The terms and conditions, under which tournament physicians work, should be established in advance of the event. These should include agreements on hours of work, remuneration (including any subsistence payments), codes of conduct and reporting lines.

It is also critically important to ensure that a tournament physician has the appropriate level of professional indemnity to cover all work during, and related to, the event.

36.1.2 Equipment

Equipment for an event is largely determined by its size and location. Medical rooms vary in size and complexity but should be equipped with the following as a minimum:

- Medical room diagnostic equipment should include stethoscope, sphygmomanometer, ophthalmoscope, otoscope, thermometers, glucometer and peak flow meter.
- Medical room consumables should include ice, intravenous fluids, cannulae, giving sets, drip stand, sterile packs and gloves, basic formulary of medicines, venepuncture and suture kits, wound care dressings, crutches and braces. An AED should be available.
- Office equipment should include stationary (including patient registration and imaging request forms), internet access, telephone, printer, copier and fax machine, fridge, plinth, chairs, desk, lockable drugs cupboard and a sharps disposal container.

Additional equipment might include a diagnostic ultrasound scanner and television monitoring of court activity during play.

36.1.3 Care Pathways and Protocols

Within the constraints of any elite sporting event, it should still be possible to deliver effective medical care that optimises the player's health and wellbeing and helps enable them to achieve their best performance. The medical care of injury and illness, which is extensively covered elsewhere in this book, should always aim to follow best practice guidelines. It is recommended that all event medical teams develop and disseminate their emergency care protocols. These should be rehearsed in advance and should include clear roles and responsibilities for doctors, paramedics, ambulance services, primary healthcare providers (PHCP), referees and umpires, event management, ground staff and venue security. Lines of communication should be clearly established to ensure a rapid response in the event of a medical emergency.

Tournament physicians should acquaint themselves with the current WADA Code, including the list of prohibited substances and methods, and the use of therapeutic use exemptions (TUE).

36.1.4 Communication

Communication between members of the multidisciplinary team is critical for the effective delivery of high-quality care. Meetings should be held in advance of the event to plan and prepare, and all outcomes and actions should be circulated appropriately. During the event, there should be daily 'briefings' among the lead clinicians to handover specific case details and discuss any emerging health issues. The former allows medical staff to monitor 'at-risk' players who may be on court that day, whilst the latter is especially important in relation to public health, where early awareness of emerging sickness trends among players and others can help prevent the spread of infectious illness.

Medical staff must always abide by their professional codes of conduct, especially in relation to confidentiality and the disclosure of sensitive information. There may be occasions when this becomes difficult, as either coaching staff, management or the media push for information about a player's health. All tournament physicians should desist from communicating any such information without first taking advice from their medicolegal experts, senior peers, press liaison officer, ATP/WTA representative and others following a full, frank and confidential discussion with the player.

All tournament physicians should complete a pre-event checklist and post-event report. The latter will take the form of a WTA or ATP feedback questionnaire, as well as a tournament medical report to help inform those preparing for the next year's event. The planning and preparation of medical care for any professional tennis event should be a cyclical process that ensures that lessons are learned, and quality improvement initiatives are implemented, to enhance the event each year.

36.2 Tournament Cover

36.2.1 The Venue

Tournament physicians should acquaint themselves with the tournament venue and on-site medical provision. This should include a formal walk around the venue to understand its complexity and foibles, as well as establishing the quickest routes from the medical rooms to each court when it is filled with spectators (Fig. 36.1). Medical staff should be familiar with the location of all AEDs and the access points for local ambulance services.

36.2.2 The Team

The size of the medical team at a tournament will depend on the size of the draw. At larger tournaments, in addition to ATP and WTA PHCPs, the medical team will be augmented by local physiotherapists, massage therapists, podiatrists, strength and conditioning coaches and locker room attendants. All of these team members play important roles, and making yourself known to them is good practice and courteous.

Tournament physicians should meet and acquaint themselves with the tournament supervisors and referee before the event starts. There is usually a referee's meeting, which is a good opportunity for the whole team to meet and discuss issues pertinent to the tournament. Many of

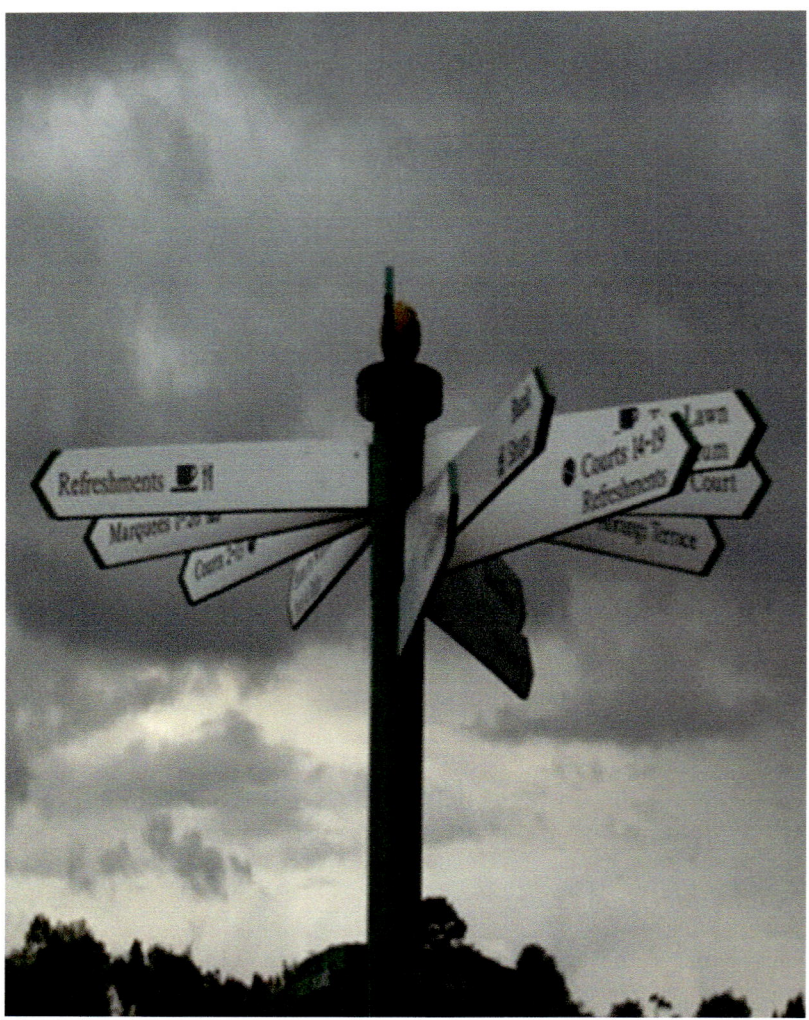

Fig. 36.1 "Know your way around the venue"

these will not be medical, but time is usually given to consider medical issues, such as the anticipated weather (including implementation of the heat rule), evacuation procedures and venue emergency planning.

Effective communication is critical for the safe and smooth running of any tournament. Do not assume that radios that worked during practice will work flawlessly once the tournament commences! Lists of important telephone numbers should be available to all medical staff, and appropriate radio and telephone etiquette should be discussed.

Continuity of care is a challenge in professional tennis, as it is with many other individual global sports. The Athlete Health and Medical System (AHMS) has helped in this regard, but some anxieties remain about the quality and consistency of medical care throughout the year. Only the top 100 ranked players can regularly access PHCPs. Tournament medical staff should appreciate that players are with them for 1 or 2 weeks of the year, whereas the ATP/WTA PHCP team provide year-round care. Players will also have relationships with their own medical, conditioning and commercial teams, as well as their national governing bodies. Consequently, it is important for tournament medical staff to appreciate the context of a player's presence in a given tournament and understand a player's priorities with regard to their season's objectives, ranking points and possible national commitments. Players may ask tournament physicians to interact with their wider healthcare and support team with regard to these issues.

36.2.3 During Play

For most tournaments the physician will be expected to be on site during play and also for 1 h before and after play starts and finishes. There may also be a requirement for out-of-hours 24-h cover, which needs to be discussed before the tournament commences.

The tournament physician will be expected to take care of illness and injury. The AHMS is used throughout the world by the ATP and WTA and is part of the communication system that supports athlete health, record keeping and governance. ATP and WTA staff will help tournament physicians to understand the system before the tournament begins. It is essential that entries onto the system are made in a timely manner, as this forms the backbone of the tennis player's medical record. In addition to recording all medical encounters on AHMS, tournament physicians may elect to keep local records of clinical activity to help inform service development initiatives, audit activities and ultimately improve future quality and service provision. At Wimbledon we have collected data over many years, dividing acute injury presentations into 'acute new', where the injury occurs at the tournament, and 'acute prior' where the injury presents at the tournament but occurred elsewhere. We also recognise recurrent injuries and differentiate these from chronic conditions [1].

36.2.4 Court Calls

Player presentations to the medical team may be through the locker room, medical offices or whilst on court. Players experiencing an injury or illness on court may seek help from the ATP/WTA PHCP through the chair umpire. Whilst current regulations deem that the PHCP is always the first responder, tournament physicians should make themselves available for medical support if needed. The only exception to this would be in the event of an obvious medical emergency (e.g. player collapse) when the physician would be expected to attend to the player as soon as possible. Tournament physicians must acquaint themselves with court call and medical timeout rules to avoid unnecessary delays in the match. Court call evaluations take place on court unless more privacy is required. Physicians should have previously ascertained potential examination facilities close to each court. Particular attention should be paid to show courts where the presence of television and the press add a further challenge. Should a player collapse, or be unable to stand and walk off court, there should be a plan in place for player extrication. This requires an extrication team (usually including paramedic support, security and venue stewards) and a predetermined route, appropriate for stretcher or wheelchair, from each court to the medical rooms or ambulance port.

Court calls require the tournament physician to have an appropriately equipped medical bag. The bag should be of a size that is easily transportable in a crowded area and contain medication and equipment that reflect the anticipated needs of court calls. In addition to any emergency equipment (including an eye and nosebleed kit, Epipen and asthma inhaler), the physician should carry a range of medications including analgesics, anti-inflammatories, anti-emetics and antidiarrheals, as well as drops and sprays for allergy and nasal congestion.

The range of medical problems encountered by physicians on court is broad and, at times, unexpected. Over 17 years at Wimbledon, we have encountered eye and laryngeal trauma, arrhythmia, collapse, cramping, fractures and significant knee and ankle ligament injuries.

36.2.5 Additional Challenges

Weather conditions are important in many sports and particularly so for tennis when played outdoors. Surface conditions, technique and injury risk are significantly affected by rain. Unpredictable rain delays can significantly disrupt players' preparation and performance during the tournament, through interrupted play and alterations in the competition schedule (Fig. 36.2). Wind seldom causes suspension of play but is of concern to players on court when ball position during serve changes and injury risk may be increased. The heat rule is instituted differently within the men's and women's game and aims to reduce the risk of heat illness. Medical staff should acquaint themselves with the rule and be alert to players who are suffering from heat illness at times of high temperature and/or humidity. Tournament physicians should be able to recognise the signs and symptoms of heat illness and heatstroke.

Tournament physicians will be asked to provide medical care for a wider population than just the players. Players travel with increasing numbers of support staff. This 'entourage' can include coaches, hitting partners, therapists, agents, family members and others. There will be members of the event organisation, and other groups, who will seek to access the on-site medical care. Whilst these groups may not be the primary focus of the tournament

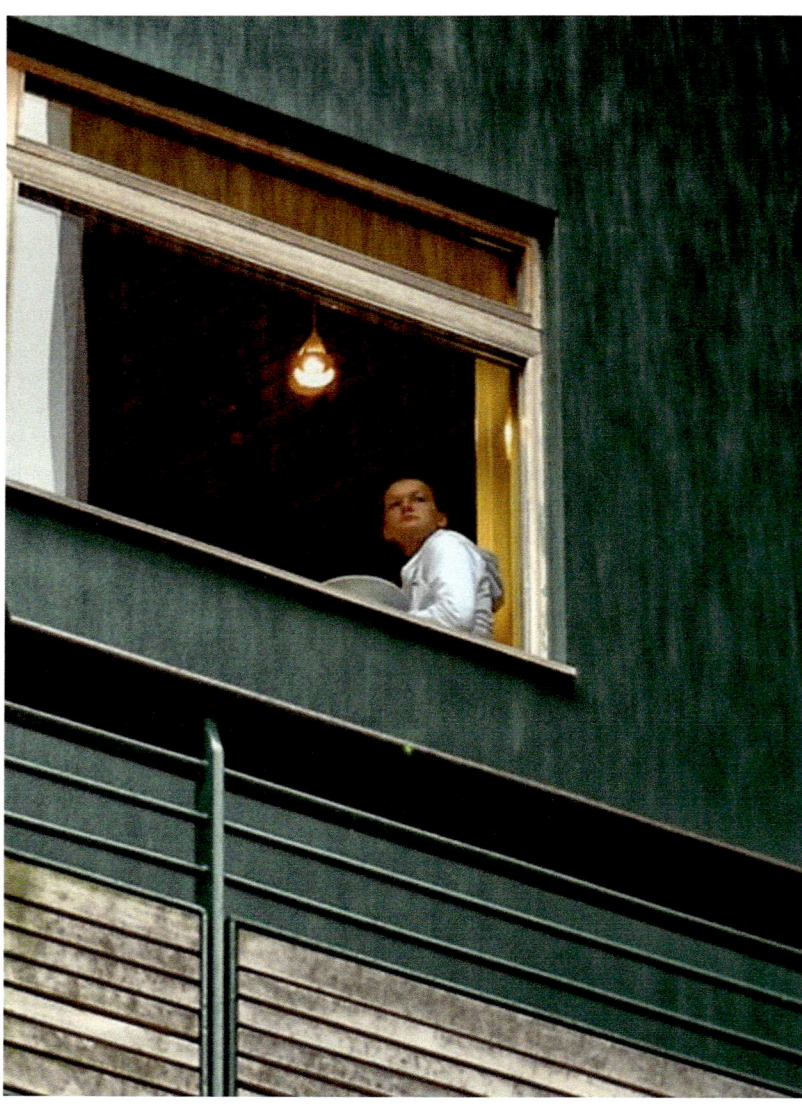

Fig. 36.2 Rain delay

physician's role—and at times can provide a significant and unwelcome distraction from player care—it should be noted that many of these non-player patients are important for the smooth running of the event and for the players' overall wellbeing. Effective time management is needed to ensure that any attention given to these nonplayers does not compromise player medical care.

Infectious illness can have a devastating effect on the health of any community and is a constant threat during large sporting events. The health and wellbeing of the players are the tournament physicians' highest priority and will be influenced by a wide range of factors, some of which are modifiable. Advice on hand hygiene, early reporting of symptoms and illness surveillance, to identify illness clusters at an early stage, can all help to reduce the risk. Any player (or other) with a potentially contagious illness should be discouraged from coming to the event venue, or visiting the medical rooms, and alternative arrangements should be made to assess them elsewhere.

The diversity of challenges facing a tournament physician is both unlimited and unpredictable. At almost any event, there will be occurrences for which no plan has been made and for which the medical team will be required to deliver a solution. It has been said in military circles that 'no battle plan survives first contact with the enemy'. Similarly, in the world of professional tennis medicine, there will always be surprises and unexpected challenges. Prior preparation and planning will help to mitigate the risk of these occurrences, but any planning must incorporate a degree of flexibility to deal with whatever might come the tournament physician's way. The final section of this chapter draws on many years of experience of tournament physician cover to help illustrate some of the challenges that are unique to this role.

36.3 Clinical Challenges for the Tournament Physician

Due to the very nature of the modern game of tennis, the tournament physician should expect to see injuries affecting virtually all anatomical sites of the upper and lower limbs and axial spine. The nature of the professional game has changed considerably over time with the advent of bigger, lighter racquet heads and longer strings, the western grip and open stance and the shorter backswing with huge power generation through the legs, hips and pelvis. In addition injuries will be influenced by court surface, change of surface, environmental conditions and time of the tennis season. Grass court wear patterns reflect the changing game as baseline play predominates and the traditional serve and volley disappear. Grass courts can be slippery producing their share of muscle strains and tears to the gluteal, adductor and calf muscles, and acute impingements anteriorly at the knee, and posteriorly at the ankle, as players slip into knee hyperextension. Players brought up on hard and clay courts may find grass an alien surface and the switch from one surface to another challenging. Andre Agassi, in his autobiography *Open*, describes the challenge perfectly: "The sudden change from one surface to another changes everything. Clay is a different game, so your game must become different, and so must your body. Instead of sprinting from side to side, stopping short and starting, you must slide and lean and dance. Familiar muscles now playing support roles, dormant muscles dominate".

36.3.1 Imaging Support

At the Championships two MSK radiologists support the medical team. At a major championship, the players will expect rapid access to imaging, and image-guided procedures, where appropriate. Stand-alone and portable ultrasound machines, which provide excellent image quality, are available on-site within the medical centre. Players requiring other imaging such as x-ray, CT or MRI are scanned in a local private hospital within easy reach of the venue by tournament transport, on the same day, after communication with the radiologist. At least one radiologist attends the medical centre on each day of the Championship to conduct a formal diagnostic ultrasound list, usually attended by the case managing tournament physician, the PHCP and the player's own physical therapist and coach, if appropriate. This is immediately followed by a case management review. The radiologist will discuss any other imaging that may have been performed that day off-site and review any scans pertinent to cases that are ongoing or under review.

Over 9 years at the Championships, 527 diagnostic ultrasound scans (average 59 per Championship) and 76 MRI scans (average 8 per Championship) have been performed. This reflects the preponderance of soft-tissue lesions, such as rectus abdominis tears, calf and hamstring strains and patella tendinopathy. Rectus abdominis tears are relatively common at the Championships, and we have used ultrasound to assess the severity of these injuries and assist us in counselling the player on the benefits and risks of a return to play in the tournament. Our experience suggests that players with low-grade injuries on ultrasound can compete effectively and win but with some risk of exacerbating the lesion, but those with partial tears, and demonstrable separation of rectus abdominis muscle fibres on resisted testing on ultrasound, are most unlikely to do so.

The tournament physicians have MSK ultrasound training and use it within the limits of their competencies. The medical centre is fully equipped to provide a comprehensive injection service on-site, and tournament physicians can readily access spinal steroid injections (SSIs) off-site, under specialist care, should the need arise. Clinicians should be familiar with, and be able to discuss the respective merits of novel, alternative or unproven injection therapies, such as Traumeel, Actovegin, stem cells and platelet-rich plasma. Requests for these therapies are not uncommon during the Championships.

At the Championships the radiologist and tournament physicians perform injections, mostly using ultrasound guidance or location. These include both therapeutic injections and local anaesthetic (L.A.) injections to enable a player to play, with an injury, without pain. The use of L.A. injections at the Championships by tournament physicians is minimal and judicious and requires them to use their knowledge and expertise to assist the player in making an informed decision. Accurate diagnosis is the firm foundation of any such decision, and involvement of all interested parties is considered essential. Examples of pathologies where L.A. has been used to enable a player to perform pain-free include tibialis anterior tenosynovitis (with normal tibialis anterior tendon on ultrasound and MRI), chronic posterior elbow impingement, intermetatarsal bursa/neuroma, first metatarsophalangeal joint osteoarthritis and dorsal wrist impingement lesions. It should be added that not all injured players present to the medical centre for treatment and that tournament physicians have no jurisdiction over the injection philosophy or techniques used by other clinicians. Injection timing, with respect to the order of play, can be problematic during a tournament played outdoors during inclement weather. Currently only Centre Court at the Championships has a retractable roof. Only the first match on court has a predictable start time, and rain delays are not uncommon. The medical centre has TV monitoring of all the competition courts, which assists in injection timing. If possible the clinician should trial the planned injection during practice to assess the efficacy of the local anaesthetic in reducing pain and to monitor any side effects such as paraesthesia or motor control loss. A mixture of short- and long-acting local anaesthetic is preferred to ensure rapid onset and long duration of action. A supply of insulin injection syringes is recommended for low volume injections, where accuracy of placement is required, such as wrist ligament or impingement lesions.

36.3.2 Retirements, Withdrawals and Fitness to Play

The Championships singles winner will earn around £2 million pounds in prize money, the winner of the doubles will share £350,000, and even first-round singles losers earn around £30,000 at the time of writing. For some the rewards in terms of prize money and ranking points are the difference between success and failure in their job as a tennis player. A young player, with a wild card entry, may earn as much money as a first-round loser as they do in the rest of the year.

In the event of a retirement during a match, or withdrawal from the tournament, a player is required to see the tournament physician for evaluation. The physician must then complete the appropriate retirement/withdrawal form, with an agreed problem description for the media, which is then signed by the physician, player, ATP/WTA PHCP and tour supervisor.

There are concerns that Grand Slam prize money encourages players to play, and collect a loser's cheque, when they are not fit to go on court. There has been a slight increase in first-round Grand Slam retirements overall in the last 20 years, but this may simply reflect the rise in injury rates and the increasing physicality of the sport. It should also be remembered that retirements after the first round are only slightly lower. It is interesting that the Championships injury data show that the majority (60%) of the injuries seen in the medical centre, whether acute prior, chronic or recurrent, were originally sustained prior to arrival at the tournament. Return to play criteria may not be as robust as they should be on a busy first morning of a Grand Slam tournament, with over 400 players in the main draw, when a player turns up with their coach and support team, shortly before practice, and asks to be signed off as 'fit to play'.

It is an unedifying spectacle for all concerned, not least the spectators, to watch a Show Court singles finish within minutes of it starting due to a player retiring with a pre-existing injury. Although this scenario is rare, tournament physicians should be mindful of their important role in return to play decisions and the benefits of close communication with the ATP/WTA medical support teams who know the players, and their retirement/withdrawal records, so much better than they do. Conversely, it may be difficult to persuade the player to come off court, and there have been incidences at the Championships where players have sustained an acute fracture and elected to continue to play (against medical advice) and been able to complete and win their match.

If a player is considered unable to compete, due to illness or injury, the tournament physician or PHCP should inform the tour supervisor, having first obtained the player's consent. If a player's participation puts their health at serious risk, the tour supervisor has the authority to rule a player ineligible to compete. If a player withdraws or retires from an event at a tournament, the player may subsequently compete in another event at the same tournament if the tournament physician determines that the player's condition has improved and they are fit to return to play and perform at the appropriate level.

36.3.3 Player Medical Emergencies

It should be remembered that player medical emergencies may occur just about anywhere in the tournament venue including the competition and practice courts, the gym facilities, the warm up and warm down areas, the ice bath facility and the changing rooms. It is important the tournament physicians know their way around and obtain accredited access to all areas. Staffing levels should ensure that the medical centre continues to function effectively when tournament physicians are attending to court calls and medical emergencies.

Both the ATP and WTA PHCPs have 'red flag' documents, which highlight players with medical conditions that could potentially give rise to a medical emergency, such as cardiac arrhythmias, allergies and history of heat illness. This knowledge can be matched with the order of play to highlight any potential medical problem, and its location, during the day.

It can be stressful evaluating and managing acute medical situations in front of large crowds, and larger television audiences. The tournament physician may have missed the incident or mechanism of injury, but someone courtside will have seen it, so ask them if you have time. Utilise the expertise of those around you, particularly the PHCPs, who typically have conducted their evaluation before you are called on to court. The purpose of the evaluation is to determine if the player has a treatable medical condition and should be performed within a reasonable length of time. However, the tournament physician must ensure adequate time is taken to assess the player and should remember that access to a suitable facility off-court is available if required. Once a decision is made to continue the match, the player should be reassured, and the tournament physician should be prepared to remain courtside to observe their response to treatment. When prescribing medication, the tournament physician should ascertain any allergies, tolerance of certain medications and medication taken on the day and be sure to tell the player how long it will take for the medicine to act. If blood or vomit has been spilled onto the court, or in its immediate vicinity, it must be cleared up before play resumes and soiled towels disposed of and replaced. Finally, the tournament physician should ensure the player and PHCP understand any arrangements for follow-up.

Tournament physicians should be prepared for any eventuality, such as cardiac arrhythmia, collapse of unknown cause, exercise-associated muscle cramp (EAMC) and laryngeal trauma (from a blow in the throat by a ball or racquet). Generalised body cramping, involving muscles of the face, trunk and upper and lower limbs, is a medical emergency and extremely distressing for player and medical team alike. Players may have experienced previous episodes, lasting many hours, and it is our practice to curtail these episodes as quickly as possible. We have experience of using I.V. benzodiazepines, with rapid relief, and have found accepted strategies, such as ice cooling and muscle massage, ineffective (probably due to the likely aetiology of central fatigue, rather than raised core temperature).

We have administered to, and extracted, players with ankle ligament tears, anterior cruciate ligament ruptures and fractures of the radial head and distal radius. We have fished out errant contact lenses and dealt with medication side effects, such as on-court drowsiness due to NSAIDs and paraesthesia due to proton-pump inhibitors. However well you prepare, there will usually be a 'curveball'.

Each tournament venue presents its unique challenges and no day is the same. It can be a fulfilling experience for the tournament physician to challenge their knowledge, skills and experience, within the wonderful sport of tennis.

Reference

1. McCurdie I, Smith S, Bell PA, Batt ME. Injury data from The Championships, Wimbledon from 2003 to 2012. BJSM. 2016;51(7):607–11. https://doi.org/10.1136/bjsports-2015-095552.

Dermatologic Conditions in Elite Tennis Players

37

Walter C. Taylor and Brian Adams

37.1 Introduction

Those who provide medical care for the elite tennis player will commonly encounter players with skin conditions. In this chapter we review the most common skin conditions that affect elite tennis players. We have divided these into four main causes: infectious, allergic, inflammatory, and traumatic. Each of these categories is further divided with specific skin conditions.

37.2 Infectious

The skin conditions that most commonly cause skin infection in the athlete can be further broken down into bacterial, fungal, and viral infections and are listed in Table 37.1. In the medical literature, tennis is not a sport that has had much attention, as most of the literature has dealt with sports that involve more skin to skin contact such as wrestling and football [1]. Sports medicine providers caring for tennis players need to be aware of these infectious conditions and the situations where the player would need to be restricted from competition.

Table 37.1 Common skin infections in the tennis player

Bacterial
   Staphylococcus aureus
      Methicillin sensitive
      Methicillin resistant
   Pitted keratolysis
      Kytococcus sedentarius
      Dermatophilus congolensis
      Corynebacterium spp.
Viral
   Varicella/zoster
   Wart(s)—*human papillomavirus*
Fungal
   Tinea pedis
   Tinea versicolor
   Onychomycosis

37.2.1 Bacterial

Staphylococcus aureus is a common cause of bacterial infection in athletes but not as common in tennis players as athletes who have more skin to skin contact during their sport. Athletes do have a higher incidence of community-acquired methicillin-resistant *Staphylococcus aureus* (CA-MRSA) compared to nonathletes [2]. Skin and soft tissue infection

W. C. Taylor (✉)
Department of Family Medicine, Mayo Clinic College of Medicine,
Jacksonville, FL, USA

Women's Tennis Association, St. Petersburg, FL, USA
e-mail: wtaylor@wtatennis.com

B. Adams
Women's Tennis Association, St. Petersburg, FL, USA

Department of Dermatology, University of Cincinnati College of Medicine, Cincinnati, OH, USA

VAMC, Cincinnati, OH, USA

with CA-MRSA can present as a variety of skin infectious conditions such as cellulitis, abscess, carbuncle, furuncles, and folliculitis. Treatment involves incision and drainage of any fluid collection which should be sent for culture and sensitivities which should direct antimicrobial therapy. If empiric antibiotic treatment is begun prior to available sensitivities, the following oral antibiotics can be used: trimethoprim-sulfamethoxazole, clindamycin, doxycycline, or minocycline [3]. Some patients however may develop photosensitive rash with use of doxycycline and sulfa-based medications, and this is important for tennis players who play outdoors and have significant sun exposure.

Pitted keratolysis (Fig. 37.1), a condition of the plantar surface of the feet caused by Kytococcus sedentarius (formerly Micrococcus spp.), *Dermatophylus congolensis*, and *Corynebacterium* spp., has been reported in tennis players [4]. Excessive moisture due to sweating on the plantar surface of the feet helps set up the environment for these infectious agents to cause infection. These appear as multiple eroded lesions of 0.5–7 mm in size that cause a very foul odor due to sulfur compounds produced by the infection. Use of synthetic socks and spending less time in occlusive shoes to reduce moisture is key. to prevention of pitted keratolysis. Treatment with topical agents includes clindamycin, benzoyl peroxide 5%, erythromycin, or mupirocin.

37.2.2 Viral

Varicella zoster virus (VZV) is one of the herpesviruses which cause an infection that rarely occurs in elite young tennis players. However due to differences in immunization practices between various countries, some young elite tennis players may not have been immunized or had varicella as a young child. Therefore, the clinician providing care at a tournament where players are present from various countries must be mindful to think of primary varicella infection, also known as chickenpox, if a player presents with a vesicular rash.

The clinical manifestations are a very pruritic generalized vesicular rash that usually occurs with fever and malaise. The rash has four stages, and lesions start as macules that progress to papules and then vesicles and finally crust over [5]. The characteristic finding is that there will be lesions in various stages all at the same time.

Because primary VZV is an extremely contagious infection and because the adolescent or adult compared to the young child has a greater risk for complications or more severe disease, any tennis player suspect of this illness must be isolated. The player must be restricted from competition and practice/training. They must avoid contact with anyone who is not immune to the virus or is unsure of their immunity. They should not be present at any tournament venue as the chances of infecting other persons without immunity or any immunocompromised persons are very high. Unfortunately individuals subsequently diagnosed with active primary VZV may be contagious up to 48 h prior to onset of the rash and until all lesions have crusted. The incubation period for the virus is up to 21 days. Therefore, if a person who is not immune has been exposed to a person with active VZV, they have up to 21 days to develop the infection from that exposure. Infected individuals may be contagious prior to the onset of the rash. The virus is spread through respiratory droplets or by skin to skin contact with the rash.

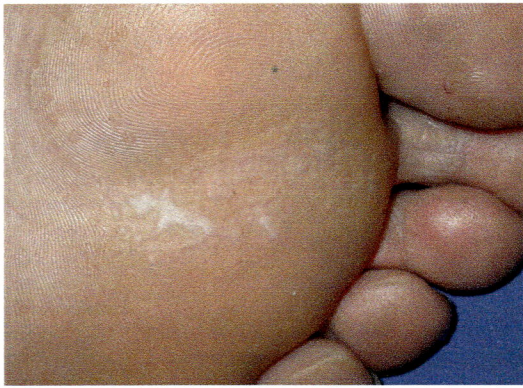

Fig. 37.1 Pitted keratolysis is characterized by clusters of multiple discrete white and sometimes yellow circular lesions with pitting of the lesions on the plantar surface of the foot, and this skin condition causes a characteristic foul odor

About 20% of persons who received one dose of VZV vaccine may still develop the illness if exposed to the virus, but the clinical manifestations and complications are much less severe [6].

Treatment is generally supportive with rest, adequate oral hydration, antipyretics with acetaminophen, and bathing in Oatmeal Aveeno to help with the pruritus. Antiviral medications such as acyclovir and valaciclovir can be used, but in order to be effective in reducing the length of illness, these are most effective when started within 24 h of the onset of the rash.

The other manifestation of VZV is zoster or shingles which is a reactivation of the virus in immunocompetent persons who previously had primary VZV infection. Zoster is characterized by a unilateral dermatomal rash that is described as multiple vesicles on an erythematous base (Fig. 37.2). This manifestation mostly commonly occurs in older individuals. However, in our experience, we have seen this occurs on rare occasion in young elite tennis players. The rash usually crusts over within 10 days. The clinician must distinguish this from herpes simplex infection which may look similar to a mild case of zoster. In any event, the player should be restricted from contact with other persons due to the risk of transmission of the VZV virus to persons who do not have immunity against VZV or those persons who are pregnant or immunocompromised.

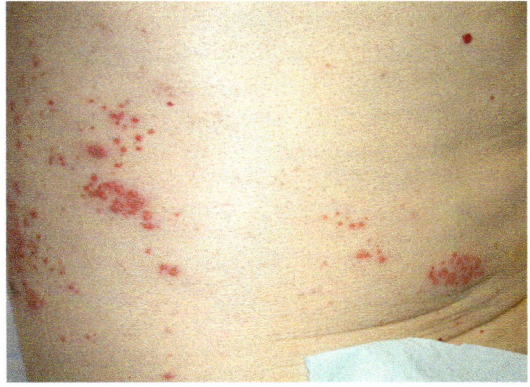

Fig. 37.2 Herpes zoster/shingles is characterized by multiple vesicles on an erythematous base in a dermatomal distribution

Initiating treatment with oral antivirals within 72 h of the onset of the rash may decrease the length of the illness. As with primary VZV, patients with zoster are contagious until all lesions have crusted over. In the young elite immunocompetent tennis player, complications such as postherpetic neuralgia are rare. However, as with primary VZV, secondary bacterial infection can occur.

Warts or verruca are caused by the *human papillomavirus* and for those affecting the skin can be divided into common warts (verruca vulgaris) that frequently affect the hand and plantar warts (verruca plantaris) that affect the plantar surface of the feet. Depending on the location and size of the wart on the hand, this may be painful when gripping the racquet. Likewise plantar warts can sometimes cause pain depending on their location and size. Sometimes a wart can be confused with a callus or corn, but if the top layers are shaved down, the wart has a typical appearance of multiple dots within the base that are loops of capillary vessels [7]. Warts should be distinguished from actinic keratosis, squamous cell carcinoma of the skin, and calluses. If the wart(s) are not causing any discomfort or symptoms, then treatment may not be necessary. Multiple types of treatments are available and have been assessed by the British Association of Dermatologists [7]. Topical salicylic acid preparations with concentrations of 10–26% have the highest level of evidence for treatment efficacy. However these must be applied daily after the thick keratin layer is removed for 3–6 months. Another common treatment option that is utilized is cryotherapy with liquid nitrogen. Several treatments may be necessary. If these methods fail to clear the wart and it remains symptomatic, then referral to a dermatologist is recommended for consideration of other treatments such as immunotherapy.

37.2.3 Fungal

The fungal infections most common among tennis players are tinea pedis and tinea versicolor. Tinea pedis or athlete's foot is caused by

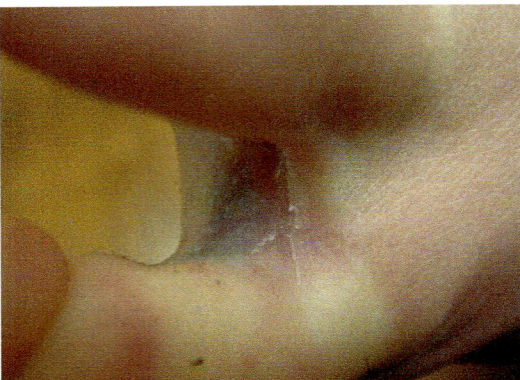

Fig. 37.3 Tinea pedis—interdigital configuration with scaling with some surrounding erythema in the web spaces between the toes

Trichophyton rubrum and *Trichophyton mentagrophytes*, and athletes are predisposed to these infections due to excessive sweating and occlusive footwear [8, 9]. The interdigital pattern of this is seen in Fig. 37.3. One large epidemiological study of European subjects found that athletes were 1.6–2.3 times at risk for developing tinea pedis compared to nonathletes [10]. When the diagnosis is suspected by physical examination, it can be confirmed with microscopic assessment of KOH scrapings from the affected area. Treatment is typically via topical antifungal medications. Prevention is the key and is achieved through trying to keep the feet dry, using moisture wicking socks, changing socks frequently, and using well-ventilated shoes and sandals in the shower and locker room [11].

Tinea versicolor also known as pityriasis versicolor is a very common superficial fungal infection of the skin caused by *Malassezia* species [12]. The tennis player is at risk for this infection as it occurs more frequently in warmer climates. The rash of tinea versicolor commonly occurs on the trunk and proximal arms and legs and is characterized by multiple slightly scaly hyper or hypopigmented oval macules. If there is any question about the diagnosis, a KOH skin scraping can be performed and viewed under the microscope. Treatment is usually topical with either lotion or shampoo containing ketoconazole, selenium sulfide, or zinc pyrithione to the affected area [13]. This should be left in place for 10 min and then washed off daily for 1–4 weeks. To prevent recurrence of the rash, this regiment can be performed 1 day per month.

Onychomycosis is a fungal infection of the nails. The toenail is also more commonly affected in athletes [10]. Athletes are thought to be more prone due to repetitive trauma to the nail and increased sweating with occlusive footwear that promotes moisture [11]. Onychomycosis must be distinguished from other nail disorders such as trauma, tennis toenail, psoriasis, malignant melanoma, and lichen planus [14]. In addition to the same preventative recommendations for tinea pedis, athletes should keep their nails shorter. As in other patients, if athletes are having discomfort related to the thickened toenail from onychomycosis, then they could be considered for medication therapy. In a recent meta-analysis of oral and topical treatment options, oral therapy was more effective than topical therapy [15]. Terbinafine 250 mg daily for 12–16 weeks or itraconazole 200 mg daily for 12 weeks was more efficacious than other oral treatments. Pulse therapy with itraconazole is only approved for fingernails. One of the possible side effects is liver dysfunction, and these medications can have significant interactions with other medications. Itraconazole can prolong the QT interval on the electrocardiogram (ECG) which can lead to serious ventricular arrhythmias, and therefore patients should have a baseline ECG to rule out baseline prolonged QT syndrome prior to starting therapy with this medication. Topical therapies including efinaconazole 10% nail solution, tavaborole 5% nail solution, ciclopirox 8% nail lacquer, and amorolfine 5% nail lacquer have all been shown to be better than placebo for treatment but have lower mycologic cure rates compared to oral therapies [15].

37.3 Allergic Disorders

Allergic disorders of the skin in the athlete can be further divided into exercise-related urticarial and anaphylaxis.

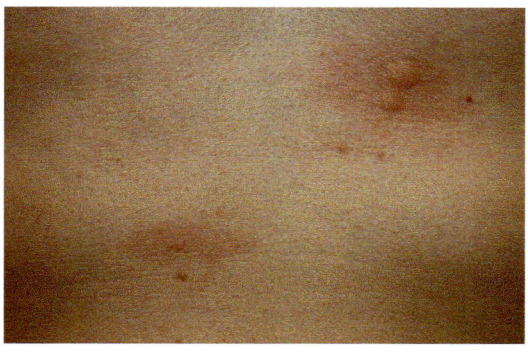

Fig. 37.4 Cholinergic urticaria are characterized by multiple small 2–5 mm raised lesions that sometimes coalesce

37.3.1 Exercise-Induced Urticaria

Urticaria related to exercise includes cholinergic, cold, pressure, solar, and aquatic. The tennis player is more likely to be affected by cholinergic or solar urticaria [16]. Urticaria characteristically involves raised plaques that are red with intense pruritus and resolves or fluctuates within 24 h. Cholinergic urticaria is characterized by multiple small 2–5 mm raised lesions that will sometimes coalesce (Fig. 37.4). These typically start on the trunk and spread to the extremities. These are triggered by increase of body temperature. For tennis players training, practicing, and playing in the heat, this can easily trigger urticaria.

The mainstay of treatment is antihistamines. Avoiding exercise especially in hot conditions is a preventative approach but one that will not be practical in the competitive tennis player.

Solar urticaria is another type of physical urticaria. It is estimated to be 0.5% of all urticaria and so is relatively rare [17, 18]. This condition develops rapidly within 10–15 min of sun exposure and typically resolves quickly within hours of removal from sun exposure. It is characterized by typical urticaria on sun-exposed areas, but if there is less exposure, some individuals will develop itching and erythema without typical wheals [16]. Treatment is with sunscreen, pre-exposure antihistamines, and desensitization with phototherapy.

37.3.2 Exercise-Induced Anaphylaxis

Exercise-induced anaphylaxis (EIA) is a potential life-threatening illness that can occur sporadically. Some patients with EIA may also require ingestion of a specific food prior to exercise in order to trigger the symptoms. This is known as food-dependent exercise-induced anaphylaxis [19]. The most common form of exercise reported as a trigger is running, but this has been reported in other sports including tennis [20].

Athletes will experience itching, urticaria, flushing of the skin, angioedema, laryngeal edema, and possible bronchospasm. They may also experience abdominal pain and nausea. The concern is that this progresses to vascular collapse and death.

Wheat products are the most common food that is known to be a factor in food-dependent exercise-induced anaphylaxis. But other foods associated with this are shellfish; seeds such as mustard and sesame; nuts; vegetables and fruits such as celery, onion, mushroom, soy, red beans, tomato, grape, and orange; meat like beef and pork; and others such as milk and wine [21].

If the diagnosis of FDEIA is established, then it is probably best to counsel the player to avoid that particular food identified as a trigger. However, if the athlete were to eat that food, they should avoid exercise for at least 3 h after that ingestion. For the athlete that has just completed exercise, they should avoid eating that food for at least 1 h. The authors again counsel players to try to avoid the inciting food all together. The medical team should provide the athlete with an emergency plan in case the player develops symptoms of anaphylaxis. This includes always carrying the appropriate injectable epinephrine kit which may be an auto-injector. The tennis medicine physician and player must be aware that use of injectable epinephrine is a doping violation unless the athlete has a valid TUE. Therefore, the physician prescribing this treatment should complete a TUE application, and if approved the player will be able to self-administer this medication should they have an anaphylactic reaction when medical care is not immediately accessible. However, in the case of an emergency in which the physician administers the epinephrine for anaphylaxis, a retroactive TUE application would be required. The player also needs education on when to seek medical care should they develop another episode of anaphylaxis.

37.4 Inflammatory Conditions

37.4.1 Acne Vulgaris

Acne vulgaris and acne mechanica both commonly occur in the elite tennis player [22, 23]. Acne vulgaris is characterized by comedones (closed or open), erythematous papules, pustules, and nodules. Genetically predisposed athletes develop these lesions typically on the face and upper trunk.

Acne vulgaris grading allows for a directed therapeutic approach. Grade 1 acne vulgaris consists of comedones, either closed or open. Tennis players with grade 2 acne vulgaris demonstrate not only comedones but erythematous papules, and those athletes with grade 3 acne vulgaris have pustules in addition to the aforementioned lesions. Nodules (along with comedones, erythematous papules, and pustules) typify grade 4 acne vulgaris. The main approach to early stage disease is to rid the athlete of comedones, the primary lesions of acne vulgaris. Comedolytic agents include topical benzoyl peroxide and retinoids (Table 37.2). Tennis players with grade 2 acne vulgaris will also need to apply topical antibiotics or in diffuse cases, to take oral antibiotics. While theses antibiotics have an effect on *P. acne* (an organism partially responsible for acne vulgaris), the main mechanism of the effectiveness of antibiotics is anti-inflammatory in origin. In general, athletes with grade 3 acne vulgaris will require topical retinoic acid, benzoyl peroxide, topical antibiotics, and an oral antibiotic. Grade 4 athletes are treated similarly to grade 3 acne vulgaris but may need oral isotretinoin for complete control.

Due to the extensive sun exposure received, elite tennis players need to carefully protect themselves with sunscreen when using doxycycline. Minocycline is less likely to cause a phototoxic eruption. Doxycycline not uncommonly causes stomach irritation especially if it is taken on an empty stomach. Tennis players should take the medication with food; the meal should not contain milk or dairy products as these items decrease the absorption of the medication. Both minocycline and doxycycline can cause pseudotumor cerebri in very rare instances. The retinoids and benzoyl peroxide can cause dryness, and when tennis players play or practice in arid conditions, this side effect can be enhanced. While quite effective at clearing and even curing acne vulgaris, many athletes and coaches fear the use of oral isotretinoin. In addition to extremely dry lips and dry skin, concerning issues for the elite tennis player include myalgias and arthralgias. Some athletes on this medication note that they feel sore as though they have done an intense workout. One small study, however, demonstrated little effect of isotretinoin on muscle strength, fatigue, and endurance [24].

Female athletes have two other options for their acne vulgaris: oral contraceptives and spironolactone. The latter agent may need a TUE.

37.4.1.1 Xerosis

Elite tennis players often play in arid conditions both in practice and in competition. Dry skin, otherwise known as xerosis, can appear anywhere on the body; however, athletes most often present with involvement of their trunk. Xerosis presents with flaky skin without erythema. Unfortunately, xerosis can be extremely pruritic and distracting to the elite tennis player. The treatment of xerosis includes regular application of topical moisturizers at least three times per day. Several approaches minimize the likelihood that an athlete will develop xerosis. First, athletes

Table 37.2 Specific common acne vulgaris medications

Topical retinoids (gels and cream)	Topical antibiotics (most often in a benzoyl peroxide product)	Oral antibiotics
Tretinoin	Clindamycin	Doxycycline
Adapalene	Erythromycin	Minocycline
Tazarotene		Trimethoprim-sulfamethoxazole

should not use soap except on their face, axilla, and groin. Water alone sufficiently cleans the rest of their skin without removing the oils necessary to keep their skin moist. Second, humidifiers in the bedroom can also add moisture to the athlete's skin. Last, athletes who apply moisturizer three times daily to their skin will ward off xerosis. Often, tennis players will note that they use moisturizers, but they do not apply them frequently enough. Applying a moisturizer only once per day is tantamount to using an umbrella for only one block on a three-block walk and then being surprised that one is wet.

37.4.1.2 Dermatitis

Eczema is a general term that refers to itchy red skin. Most often clinicians relate "eczema" to the genetic form of dermatitis, namely, atopic dermatitis. Dermatitis is a general clinical term that relates to morphologic features that typify three main forms. First, acute dermatitis exhibits blisters and redness but lacks scale. Subacute dermatitis, the most common of the dermatitis types, presents with erythema and scale but not with vesicles. Last, chronic dermatitis lacks erythema and blisters but has thick scale.

The morphologic descriptors of dermatitis suggest that duration of the eruption is integral to the naming of the condition. Unfortunately, the naming of the types of dermatitis relates *only* to the morphologic features of the eruption. Some of the most common subacute dermatitis conditions persist for very long periods, including lifelong. A prototypic subacute dermatitis is atopic dermatitis. This genetically based condition affects the athlete as a lifelong disease.

Atopic dermatitis typically affects the nape of the neck and the antecubital and popliteal fossa, although lesions can occur anywhere on the body. Many types of subacute dermatitis exist, so a correct diagnosis of atopic dermatitis is based on identifying the typical distribution in addition to noting the presence of classic associations. Clinicians who suspect atopic dermatitis should inquire about (1) personal or family history of asthma, (2) seasonal allergies, and (3) the presence of "sensitive" skin as a child.

The mainstay of therapy includes topical steroids; rarely will athletes require systemic steroids. The choice of topical steroids depends on both severity of the disease and the location of the eruption. Topical steroids are characterized by class. The class one steroids are the most potent, while class six steroids yield the least potent results.

37.5 Traumatic Conditions

37.5.1 Ultraviolet Related

Elite tennis players endure repeated assaults by ultraviolet radiation. Many risk factors exist that place them more at risk than nonathletes. First, they practice and compete during the peak hours of ultraviolet radiation, namely, between 10 am and 4 pm. Second, one study revealed that sweat enhances the effect of ultraviolet radiation, such that athletes who sweat will burn far more easily [25]. Third, the total duration of lifetime exposure is extraordinary; most players have been playing tennis since a very early age.

One of the most common untoward effects of excessive ultraviolet exposure is sunburn; these burns can be painful enough to interfere with playing ability. Altitude and latitude play a major role in the amount of ultraviolet radiation experienced [26]. Athletes who compete at tournaments at higher elevations will receive greater doses of sun exposure as there is less atmosphere to filter the ultraviolet radiation. Unfortunately, multiple studies have shown that no treatment effectively alleviates sunburn.

Another very common acute eruption directly related to excessive sun exposure is activation of herpes labialis [27]. Elite tennis players exhibit an increased risk for sunburn if they take photosensitizing oral antibiotics for their acne vulgaris as is discussed previously in the section on acne vulgaris.

In addition to the acute effects of ultraviolet radiation, tennis players also experience chronic effects. Elite tennis players, especially those with fair skin, develop precancerous lesions (actinic keratoses) far earlier in life than expected. The

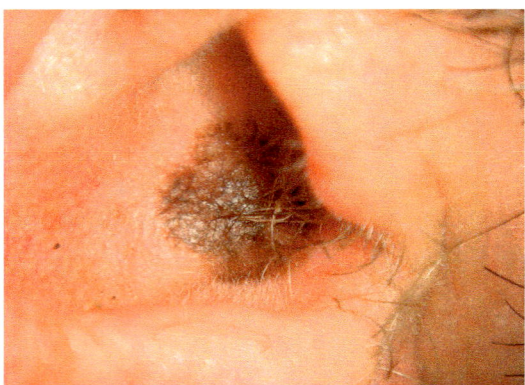

Fig. 37.5 Malignant melanoma showing a pigmented lesion with some irregular borders and varying shades of brown within the lesion

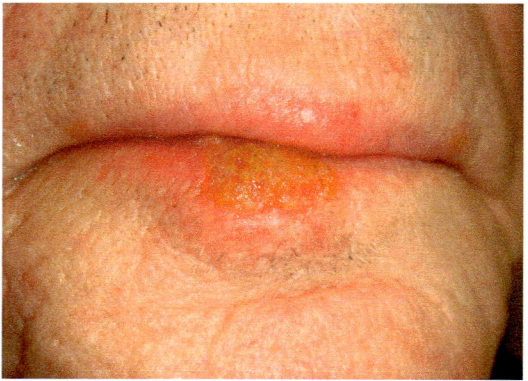

Fig. 37.6 Squamous cell carcinoma of the skin of the lower lip with a raised erythematous lesion with crusting

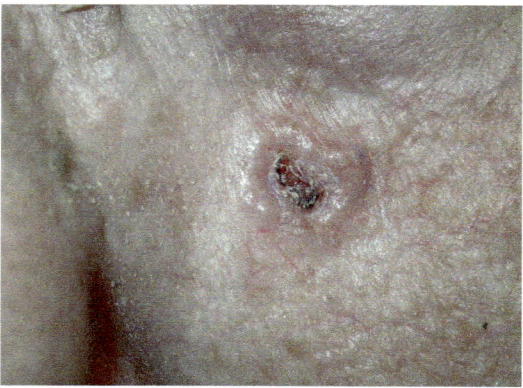

Fig. 37.7 Nodular basal cell carcinoma with classic features of a raised skin lesion that is pearly in appearance with central depression and rolled borders and some telangiectasias

intense and prolonged ultraviolet radiation exposure also puts the elite tennis player at risk for melanoma (Fig. 37.5), squamous cell carcinoma (Fig. 37.6), and basal cell carcinoma (Fig. 37.7) [28]. Clinicians should pay particular attention to the elite tennis player's skin at least once per year and ideally, twice per year, especially for those with increased risk factors. The six main risk factors that confer higher risk for the development of melanoma include (1) numerous nevi (>50), (2) fair skin, (3) personal history of melanoma, (4) family history of melanoma, (5) abnormal moles as defined under the microscope, and (6) blistering sunburns as a child.

Elite tennis players can prevent both the acute and chronic side effects by employing sun safe behaviors. First, athletes should apply sunscreen to all exposed areas, to specifically include the ears and hair parts in the scalp. Sprays are not only effective but allow the tennis player to apply and reapply without making their palms sticky or greasy. Hats and visors provide much needed shade for the face but fail to protect the ears. Darker-colored clothing provide the best UV protection but unfortunately can also retain heat [22]. As such, elite tennis players should always wear moisture wicking, dark-colored clothing, at least in practice, to keep them relatively cool and protected from ultraviolet radiation.

37.5.2 Heat Related

Elite tennis players also endure the heat-related effects of the sun which can rarely cause unusual skin conditions. One such eruption, miliaria crystallina, appears as several to many, tiny blisters [22]. This condition does not require therapy but indicates that the athlete needs to pay close attention to the extreme heat.

37.5.3 Friction

Among the most common skin ailments of the elite tennis player are friction blisters that occur on the hands and feet. As the skin cycles over the racquet handle or the footwear, redness (erythema) appears, and with continued friction, blisters form. Heat and moisture increase the likelihood of blister formation, so prevention techniques focus on keeping the skin dry and cool. Moisture wicking socks minimize risk, and application of Vaseline or aquaphor to high-risk areas decreases the coefficient of friction and ameliorates the risk for blister formation [22]. Athletes can also wear two layers of socks; friction will distribute over the socks instead on the skin.

Once an athlete develops a friction blister, the clinician should lance and drain the lesion in one focal area [22, 29]. It is critical to try to keep the blister roof intact as it represents an ideal biological dressing that will decrease infection and speed healing.

37.5.3.1 Pressure

The two most common pressure-related skin conditions in the elite tennis player are tennis toenail (Fig. 37.8) and talon noire. Clinicians often mistake talon noire for verruca (warts). Pinpoint black macules appear on the heel of affected tennis players. These lesions develop due to shearing forces between the athlete's foot and their footwear [30]. Talon noire does not need treatment but often results in misdiagnosis and mistreatment with destructive methods meant for warts. Heel pads prevent talon noire, but most often elite players are not concerned about these lesions once they learn that they are not warts.

Tennis toenail develops from constant slamming of the longest toe into the toe box of the shoe with sudden stops and starts [22, 31]. The pressure experienced by the nail, specifically the nail matrix (the factory of nail manufacturing), creates nail dystrophy. This dystrophy presents with thickened and discolored nails. Frequently, clinicians mistake these nail changes for onychomycosis (fungal nails) and inappropriately treat tennis athletes with topical or oral antifungal agents. The oral medications have potentially serious side effects and should only be used for confirmed onychomycosis. Clinicians should also know that once an elite tennis player develops nail dystrophy, they are more likely to develop secondary onychomycosis in that tennis toe.

References

1. Likness LP. Common dermatologic infections in athletes and return-to-play guidelines. J Am Osteopath Assoc. 2011;111(6):373–9.
2. Braun T, Kahanov L, Dannelly K, Lauber C. CA-MRSA infection incidence and care in high school and intercollegiate athletics. Med Sci Sports Exerc. 2016;48(8):1530–8.
3. Liu C, Bayer A, Cosgrove SE, Daum RS, Fridkin SK, Gorwitz RJ, Kaplan SL, Karchmer AW, Levine DP, Murray BE, J Rybak M, Talan DA, Chambers HF. Infectious Diseases Society of America. Clinical practice guidelines by the infectious diseases society of america for the treatment of methicillin-resistant Staphylococcus aureus infections in adults and children. Clin Infect Dis. 2011;52(3):e18.
4. Kantor GR, Bergfeld WF. Common and uncommon dermatologic diseases related to sports activities. Exerc Sports Sci Rev. 1988;16:215–53.
5. Heininger U, Seward J. Varicella. Lancet. 2006;368(9544):1365–76.
6. Chavess SS, Zhang J, Civen R, Watson BM, Carbajal T, Perella D, Seward JF. Varicella disease among vaccinated persons: clinical and epidemiological characteristics 1997-2005. J Infect Dis. 2008;197(Suppl 2):S127.
7. Sterling JC, Gibbs S, Hussain H, Mohd Mustapa M, Handfield-Jones SE. British Association of Dermatologists guidelines for the management of cutaneous warts 2014. Br J Dermatol. 2014;174:696–712.
8. Adams BB. Skin infections in athletes. Dermatol Nurs. 2008;20(1):39–44.

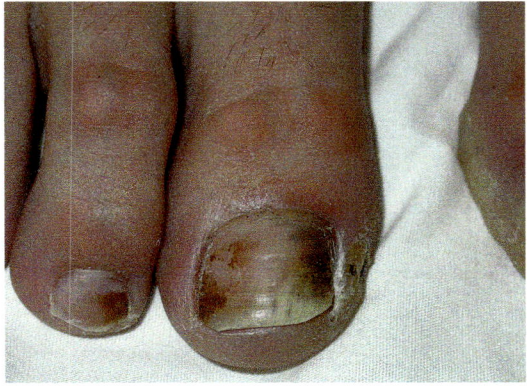

Fig. 37.8 Tennis toenail with brown or black discoloration of several toenails from repetitive striking of the toenails with the front of the tennis shoe

9. De Luca JF, Adams BB, Yosipovich G. Skin manifestations of athletes competing in the summer Olympic games. Sports Med. 2012;32(5):399–413.
10. Caputo R, De Boulle K, Del Rosso J, Nowicki R. Prevalence of superficial fungal infections among sport-active individuals: results from the Achilles survey, a review of the literature. J Eur Acad Dermatol Venereol. 2001;15:312–6.
11. Field LA, Adams BB. Tinea pedis in athletes. Int J Dermatol. 2008;47:485–92.
12. Prohic A, Sadikovic TJ, Krupalija-Fazlic M, Kuskunovic-Vlahovljak S. Malassezia species in healthy skin and in dermatological conditions. Int J Dermatol. 2016;55:494–504.
13. Renati S, Cukras A, Bigby M. Pityriasis versicolor. BMJ. 2015;h1394:350. https://doi.org/10.1136/bmj.h1394.
14. Ameen M, Lear JT, Madan V, Mohd Mustapa MF, Richardson M. British Association of Dermatologists' guidelines for the management of onychomycosis 2014. Br J Dermatol. 2014;171:937–58.
15. Gupta AK, Daigle D, Foley KA. Network meta-analysis of onychomycosis treatments. Skin Appendage Disord. 2015;1:74–81.
16. Dice JP. Physical urticaria. Imunol Allergy Clini North Am. 2004;24:225–46.
17. Champion RH. Urticaria: then and now. Br J Dermatol. 1988;119(4):427–36.
18. Humphreys F, Hunter JA. The characteristics of urticaria in 390 patients. Br J Dermatol. 1998;138(4):635–8.
19. Robson-Ansley P, Toit GD. Pathophysiology, diagnosis and management of exercised-induced anaphylaxis. Curr Opin Allergy Clin Immunol. 2010;10:312–7.
20. Castells MC, Horan RF, Sheffer AL. Exercise-induced anaphylaxis. Curr Allergy Asthma Rep. 2003;3:15–21.
21. Bonini M, Palange P. Anaphylaxis and sport. Curr Opin Allergy Clin Immunol. 2014;14:323–7.
22. Adams BB. Sports Dermatology. New York, NY: Springer; 2006.
23. Basler RSW. Acne vulgaris mechanica in athletes. Cutis. 1992;50:125–8.
24. Yıldızgören MT, Rifaioğlu EN, Demirkapı M, Ekiz T, Micooğulları A, Şen T, Turhanoğlu AD. Isotretinoin treatment in patients with acne vulgaris: does it impact muscle strength, fatigue, and endurance? Cutis. 2015;96:33–6.
25. Moehrle M, Koehle W, Dietz K, et al. Reduction of minimal erythema dose by sweating. Photodermatol Photoimmunol Photomed. 2000;16:260–2.
26. Rigel DS, Rigel EG, Rigel AC. Effects of altitude and latitude on ambient UVB radiation. J Am Acad Dermatol. 1999;40:114–6.
27. Rooney JF, Bryson Y, Mannix ML, et al. Prevention of ultraviolet-light-induced herpes labialis by sunscreen. Lancet. 1991;338:1419–22.
28. Adams BB. Dermatologic disorders of the athlete. Sports Med. 2002;32(5):309–21.
29. Cortese TA, Fukuyama K, Epstein W, et al. Treatment of friction blisters. Arch Dermatol. 1968;97:717–21.
30. Wilkinson DS. Black heel a minor hazard of sport. Cutis. 1977;20:393–6.
31. Basler RS, Garcia MA. Acing common skin problems in tennis players. Phys Sportsmed. 1998;26:37–44.

Part VIII
Special Topics

Strength and Conditioning in Developmental Tennis Players

38

Jaime Fernandez-Fernandez and Mark Kovacs

38.1 Introduction

In the last few years, it has been a significant change in the area of strength and conditioning, with a significant increase in terms of volume and intensity, especially in training programs focused in young athletes [1]. This coupled with the increase in sport-specific year-round training has led to a discussion around the possible negative effects provoked by the amount of training during the development process of these young athletes, at a time when they are experiencing a wide range of physical, physiological, and psychological changes as a result of growth and maturation [2, 3]. Young athletes can be considered as a "special" population [4]. Regarding young tennis players, they are routinely exposed to sport-specific training and extensive competitive schedules which can result in inadequate overall preparation, leading to suboptimal recovery, and a higher risk of injury [5]. In this regard, young athletes cannot merely be considered *adults in miniature* [1], and the physiological adaptations caused by training in children and adolescents are significantly different from that of mature adults [6]. Although competing in sport and strength and conditioning programs have many benefits, the training and competition schedules and program design should reflect the many differences in the young athlete compared to a fully developed adult athlete.

38.2 The Youth Athlete

When we mention the concept of "youth," it is important to clarify that it is a global term, including both children (from the age of 2 to 11 years old) and adolescents (from 11 to 19 years old) [7]. Also, the concepts of growth and maturation are very important here. *Growth* refers to a quantifiable change in body composition, body size, or dimensions of specific regions of the body. As children grow, they become taller and heavier, there is a change in the body composition, and experience increase in size of their various organs, along with other physiological changes. *Maturation* refers to the highly variable timing and tempo of progressive change within the human body from childhood to adulthood [8]. This process is specific to each body system, as various biological systems have differing rates of achieving maturity.

Physical performance during childhood seems to improve in a nonlinear fashion as a result of growth and maturation, and sometimes it is difficult to differentiate for coaches/parents if performance changes are attributed to these physiological processes (i.e., nervous system

J. Fernandez-Fernandez (✉)
Faculty of Physical Activity and Sports Sciences, University of Leon (Spain), Elche, Spain

M. Kovacs
International Tennis Performance Association (iTPA), Atlanta, GA, USA

development, cerebral maturation, cellular changes, etc.) or by training itself. Once the athletes reach the onset of puberty, they will experience what is defined as the adolescent growth spurt, a phase of physical development during which hormone concentrations (i.e., growth hormone and sex hormone) are significantly increased [6]. This "environment" will lead to natural adaptations in physical components such as speed, strength, aerobic endurance, and muscular power, and together with the supplementary training programs, youth athletes will be able to reach high-performance levels.

38.2.1 Chronological Age vs. Biological Age

Norm values and percentile table for junior tennis players which have been generated and used to assess a given performance are commonly based on chronological age [9–11]. Like most competitive sports, youth tennis competition is divided into age categories based on chronological age as defined by a player's date of birth [12]. Research in different sports has found that athletes born early within the selection year are more likely to be selected for elite teams and talent development programs than those born later in the same year [13]. This overrepresentation of relatively older athletes in youth sport has been labeled as the relative age effect (RAE) [12]. In tennis, several studies documented the existence of RAE, with a skewed birthdate distribution (e.g., favoring those born in the first half of the year) in top junior players as well as in senior players [14]. The existence of RAE has been associated with a loss of potential talent, and leading coaches mistakenly granting fewer opportunities (e.g., instruction, access to elite group or team) to relatively younger individuals than should be warranted by their latent ability or talent [15]. A maturational hypothesis has been suggested as a possible explanation for the RAE [16]. This hypothesis is based on the large interindividual biological differences within the same chronological age groups during childhood, assuming that players born close to the selection date profit from their advanced physical and cognitive maturation. A recent study [15] showed that although RAE exists in the selection of youth tennis players in Germany, being more pronounced with an increased competition level in youth players, players selected into the higher competitive groups (regional and national) were physically homogeneous regardless of relative age.

Thus, chronological age can differ markedly compared to biological age, sometimes by as much as 4 or 5 years [17]. Therefore, it seems that chronological age is not a good indicator on which to base athletes training programs. A practical approach to design optimal individual training programs which are related to certain periods of trainability during the process of maturation is the use of an athletes' peak height velocity (PHV) as a reference point (i.e., in males occurs between 12 and 14 years and in females between 11 and 13 years) [18]. The PHV is the fastest rate of growth during the adolescent growth spurt (which differs from total rate of growth) and can be a useful reference point providing valuable information about an individual's stage of maturation, enhancing the efficiency of development training, competition, and recovery programs. It is recommended that coaches longitudinally track (approximately every month) basic somatic measures, which can be used to predict biological age. For example, Mirwald et al. [19] developed a regression equation that can predict how far in years an individual is from PHV to within a standard error of approximately 6 months:

Girls
Maturity offset = $-16.364 + 0.0002309 \times$ leg length and sitting height interaction $+ 0.006277 \times$ age and sitting height interaction $+ 0.179 \times$ leg by height ratio $+ 0.0009428 \times$ age and weight interaction.

Boys
Maturity offset = $-29.769 + 0.0003007 \times$ leg length and sitting height interaction $- 0.01177 \times$ age and leg length interaction $+ 0.01639 \times$ age and sitting height interaction $+ 0.445 \times$ leg by height ratio.

Based on this information together with the normative data of physical fitness testing, coaches are able to establish percentiles based on biological age and to design individualized training programs considering the stage of maturation [20].

38.2.2 Risks of an Early Specialization in Tennis Players?

Early specialization in sport is typically characterized by a combination of intensive, year-round training in a specific sport, excluding other activities, from an early age [21]. In tennis, since early ages, players spend most of the training time mastering their individual sport-specific skills, with tennis-specific (i.e., technical and tactical) and physical training volumes often exceeding 15–20 h per week [22]. Moreover, match scheduling, participation in multiple draws (singles and doubles), and training demands require young high-level tennis players to often complete numerous training sessions and/or competitive matches on consecutive days. This environment leads to an "undertraining" situation as young players have not enough time to rest and recover and to enable normal growth and maturation processes to occur. Additionally, the preparation phases should be viewed as an opportunity to regain or improve on precompetition levels of fitness that would typically have decreased as a result of the demands of the competitive periods [23].

Analyzing the ages of the top 100 in the ATP and WTA rankings performed in 2014 data shows an average of 27.9 ± 3.55 and 25.21 ± 4.12 years for males and females, respectively [24]. Thus, we can suggest that, because of the technical requirements of the sport, tennis needs an early initiation, but not an early specialization. In this regard it is also important to highlight some recent research regarding injury risk, as increased years of play is also a factor in young tennis players. In a study analyzing 148 tennis players, it has been reported that those players who had "hips at risk" (i.e., risk of suffering femoroacetabular impingement) played tennis longer compared with those without hips at risk (9.5 years compared with 8.6 years) [25]. Thus, although some degree of sport specialization seems to be necessary to attain elite-level skill [26], research has shown that intense training specialized in a single sport leads to risks including overuse injuries, burnout, and social isolation [21, 27, 28] and should be delayed until late adolescence to optimize success while minimizing these risks.

38.3 The Development Plan

Based on the information presented earlier, the training organization seems to be fundamental at developmental ages because, as previously mentioned, the different systems (neural, hormonal, and cardiovascular) develop with advances in biological age, leading to corresponding changes in neuromuscular and athletic performance [5]. Moreover, levels of biological and physiological maturation can be markedly different between young athletes of the same chronological age. The long-term athlete development (LTAD) model [29, 30] has been adopted, in various forms, by a number of sports federations worldwide in an attempt to align training prescription with maturation as opposed to chronological age. This model proposes that there are some periods of accelerated adaptation offering *windows of opportunity* where training responses will be maximized [18], representing a time of increased sensitivity to training, although empirical evidence supporting this suggestion is lacking. In fact, research has shown that most fitness components are trainable throughout childhood and should not be restricted to these "windows" at various stages of development [31–33]. Moreover, another critic is the lack of a more holistic approach within the LTAD model, which only includes five physical qualities (i.e., stamina, suppleness, speed, strength, and skill) [18]. More recently, the youth physical development (YPD) has been proposed [3], comprising an overview of total physical development using existing empirical research from the development of individual components of fitness, while identifying when and why the training of each physical component should be emphasized. One of the improvements in this model over previous models is the increased focus and emphasis of training all physical qualities at all stages of development for both males and females. However, coaches should prioritize certain qualities depending on the maturational status, sex, and initial training level, which further emphasize the need for individualization of training prescription for any young athlete [30]. The YPD model also emphasizes on the development of muscular strength and movement competency (i.e., enhance of fundamental movement skills before sport-specific skills) since early ages. This is based on extensive research showing that early exposure to strength training leads to not only performance enhancement and reduction of injury risk but also improvement of health markers [34, 35]. Regarding movement skill competency, research has shown that it is associated with physical activity engagement and improved measures of health and well-being in both normal and overweight/obese youth [36–38].

38.4 Developing Physical Qualities

Once the development plan is defined and implemented, it is important to take into account that certain periods in an athlete's development require different focus and time contributions. Based on the information reported in previous research [30, 39, 40], in order to enhance performance, prevent injuries, and promote general health, muscular strength and motor skill development are basic qualities at all stages of development.

38.4.1 Fundamental Movement Skills (FMS)

FMS include locomotor (e.g., running and hopping), manipulative or object control (e.g., catching and throwing), and stability (e.g., balancing and twisting) skills [38]. In the development plan, these skills are considered to be the building blocks that lead to specialized movement or sport-specific skills required for adequate participation in any physical activities [30].

Research has shown that all these qualities can be enhanced when children follow age-appropriate training programs. Although the aim of this section is not to describe specific training approaches for every single skill, strength training [34], plyometric training [41], combined strength and power training, and integrative neuromuscular training (i.e., including balance and trunk control) [34, 42] have all resulted in significant improvements in the ability to perform various basic movement skills, such as running, jumping, or throwing.

Although basic skills are an important part in prepubertal stages (i.e., accounting for approximately 70% of the total training sessions), in order to prepare children for advanced training methods such as weightlifting, high-intensity plyometrics, and sport-specific speed and agility exercises, several authors recommended the integration of specific *athletic motor skill competencies* (AMSCs) [30, 40]. These AMSCs comprise movement patterns that will feature in most advanced training movements commonly used by elite-level athletes, such as lower-/upper-body bilateral competency, anti-rotation (i.e., core strength), or acceleration/deceleration. As children progress through adolescence, it is then recommended that a greater focus be placed on more complex exercises, although basic movement skills should also form part of the training sessions (~10–15% of the session) to reinforce correct movement mechanics [43]. The warm-up seems to be the most appropriate part of the session to reduce the risk of fatiguing effects on upper and lower extremities, as well as the number of injuries [43, 44]. In general it would be recommended to include these kinds of sessions 2 or 3 days per week on non-consecutive days. A sample warm-up session for prepubertal and post-pubertal tennis players can be found in the following tables.

38.4.2 Strength and Power

The benefits of youth strength training are well documented and are becoming accepted among sports and health professionals around the world

[34, 35]. Although there are still some misunderstandings and misconceptions related to the topic of strength training in youth, there is a general agreement that individualized strength training programs are safe and beneficial in youth when performed under qualified supervision [35]. In fact, it has been shown that strength training programs for children that were administered and supervised by qualified personnel reported very low incidence of injuries of any type [35]. Among the benefits which can be observed, there are improvements in several indices of health and fitness, including musculoskeletal strength, body composition, cardiovascular risk factors, movement competency, and psychosocial well-being [34].

One of the misconceptions regarding youth strength training in the past was that strength training prior to puberty was not viable or effective, based on the assumption that it is necessary a favorable hormonal environment with increases in circulating anabolic hormones, as it happens during puberty [6]. However, it now appears that prepubescents exhibit significant scope for strength gains, far beyond those attributable to normal growth and maturation, with relative gains in strength similar to those shown by adolescents [34]. Gains in strength and power during childhood are not typically a result of structural changes at a muscle-fiber level (i.e., hypertrophy) but are instead usually driven by improvements in both inter- and intramuscular coordination [45]. Thus, when children and adolescents are exposed to different forms of strength training, including manual strength, machine weights, plyometric training, elastic bands and medicine balls, and free-weight exercises, and following short- to medium-term strength training programs (8–20 weeks), enhancements of ~30% [34] in muscular strength can be expected. However, variability in terms of enhancements should be expected in youth populations.

Power, acknowledged as the product of force and velocity, is also another important part of the training models in youth, as it is well known that the ability to generate high levels of power is essential for sporting success [46]. This is especially true in tennis, where players are required to possess powerful strokes and also to move with short and explosive efforts around the court [41]. Thus, almost every explosive action in tennis involves a stretch-shortening cycle (SSC) [47]. The SSC describes an eccentric phase or stretch followed by an isometric transitional period (amortization phase), leading into an explosive concentric action, and is the muscle action that is central to successful plyometric performance [33].

It has been shown that there are periods of rapid development in muscular power before the PHV, between the ages of 5 and 10, with a secondary spurt in muscular power between the ages of 9 and 12 years in girls and between 12 and 14 in boys [48]. Plyometric training provides the required stimuli to train the SSC mechanism enhancing explosive contractions in both pubertal and prepubertal populations [33] and seems to be a specific training method in many sports, including tennis [41, 49], because of its emphasis on multidirectional jumping, hopping, and throwing. Moreover, examining the interaction of maturation and training responsiveness [32], it has been reported that children pre-PHV benefitted most from plyometric and then sprint training, supporting the idea that children who are pre-PHV benefit most from training that has a primarily neural basis. Thus, the inclusion of PT programs seems to be an important stimulus for enhancing explosive actions in young tennis players.

38.4.2.1 Strength/Power Training Program Design

When programming for muscular strength and power for young athletes, the primary consideration of the strength and conditioning coach should be training age and technical competency [48]. In tennis, apart from the performance enhancement, the reduction in the risk of injury in young players seems to be essential [50]. Research has shown that both the upper and lower body strength in a tennis player can be extremely useful not only in the enhancement of physical performance but also in the prevention and rehabilitation of injuries [51]. For example, muscular exertion in the upper extremity required during tennis strokes leads to the development of sport-specific muscular adaptations in tennis players (i.e., muscular imbalances in the rotator cuff and scapular musculature, loss of internal rotation range of motion (ROM) in the shoulder) which, in the long term, can lead to overuse injury in the glenohumeral joint [52]. Although research has been inconsistent regarding where the majority of tennis injuries occur in younger athletes, the shoulder and the back have been identified as the two major areas that need a greater focus in training and injury prevention programs [51], with overuse injuries representing the most common health problem in young players [53–55] and with a high rate of hip injuries which warrants further investigation [25]. It should be noted that injuries in young tennis players do differ somewhat to injuries seen in professional adult tennis players [56].

Based on the information presented, the number one reason for strength training in tennis seems to be injury prevention. However there is a lack of injury prevention interventions, and future research should focus on establishing the important role strength training plays in directly preventing injuries in tennis. Thus, the aim for tennis sport scientists and S&C coaches is to develop and establish injury prevention programs, such as the "FIFA 11+" in soccer, which was designed for soccer and has been shown not only to be effective in reducing soccer injuries in female and male players [57] but also a good warm-up with results comparable to those reported in the literature for other warm-up routines [58]. Again, as presented earlier (Tables 38.1 and 38.2), the warm-up seems to be the "perfect" moment of the training session for this kind of workout.

Once we identified the needs of the athletes, a "general" approach to strength training should be recommended, challenging all the major muscle groups and the joints around. Regarding the "dose response," there are several training guidelines based on international consensus [34, 35, 59], but programs should be individualized (i.e., identify the optimal power load for different exercises) and adapted to the demands of tennis, with safety as one basic condition for strength prescription. Table 38.3 summarizes the primary training variables that should be considered when designing strength programs for youth athletes.

Regarding plyometric training, training programs ranging from 4 weeks [62] up to 10 weeks [63] have reported positive effects on performance in different youth athletes. As previously mentioned for regular strength training programs, prior to starting structured plyometric training programs, it would be essential to determine the initial technical competency (i.e., trunk rotation, landing mechanics) of the athlete. From a general point of view, guidelines for plyometric training in young athletes include:

- At pre-PHV ages a range of low-intensity plyometrics should be introduced, ensuring that technical competency is mastered, prior to loading with any great intensity, volume and/or frequency [33].

Table 38.1 Examples of different warm-up routines for pre-pubertal tennis players

	Exercises	Volume (sets × repetitions)	Intensity	Rest
Pre-PHV	*Warm-up (basic movement skills)*			
	Foam roller complex	2–3 × 10 each site	NA	1 min
	Thoracic/hip mobilization	2 × 8–10	Body weight	1 min
	Shoulder complex (int/ext. rotation, scapula retraction…)	2 × 8–10	Light TheraBand/body weight	1 min
	Hip strength (band clamshells, band glute bridge, etc.)	2–3 × 10 each	Light band	1 min
	Plank variations	2 × 30 s each exercise	Body weight	1 min
	ABC of running	2 × 10 each exercise	NA	30 s
	Single-leg balance	2 × 30 s each leg	Body weight	1 min
	Jump to low box	3 × 6–8	Body weight	1 min
	CMJ (bilateral/unilateral)	2 × 6 each leg	Body weight	1 min
	Multidirectional jumps (bilateral/unilateral)	2 × 6 each leg	Body weight	1 min

Table 38.2 Examples of different warm-up routines for post-pubertal tennis players

	Exercises	Volume (sets × repetitions)	Intensity	Rest
Post-PHV	*Warm-up (basic movement skills)*			
	Foam roller complex	2–3 × 10 each site	NA	1 min
	Thoracic/hip mobilization	2 × 8–10	Body weight	1 min
	Mini-band monster walks	2 × 8 each leg	Medium resistance band	1 min
	Jump rope (with jump variations)	2 × 150 jumps	NA	1 min
	Box (30 cm) jumps (bilateral/unilateral)	2 × 8 each	Body weight	1 min
	DJ + acceleration + deceleration (multidirectional)	2 × 4 each	Body weight	1 min

Table 38.3 Basic training variables in the designing of strength programmes for youth athletes

Variables	Recommendations
Exercise modality	A logical order would be to begin with bodyweight exercises, medicine balls, elastic bands and fixed weight machines, and finally, when the skill competency is good enough, more complex free weight exercises can be introduced
Training frequency	Ideally, strength and power training should be performed 2–3 times per week on non-consecutive days, in periods of 9–12 weeks [34]. One session per week may be sufficient to maintain muscle strength gains following strength training for several weeks. However multiple sessions per week have shown to provide greater benefits
Training intensity	Lighter loads (45–60% of estimated one repetition maximum (1RM) [60] or using the optimum power [61]) should initially be used in an effort to emphasize correct exercise techniques at the expense of any higher-intensity loads. Players can increase loads as technique improves
Volume	Training using high volumes does not seem to be necessary in order to achieve optimal strength improvements. One to three sets of the same exercise most likely provide sufficient training stimulus [48] and number repetitions leading not to failure and that allow the maintenance of optimum power should be executed [60]. Rest periods can largely be dependent upon the individual, but rest periods of 30–120 s represent the norm

- Volume has previously been discussed in relation to the total number of foot contacts or throws performed during a single session [64]. Moderate volumes of 2–4 sets of 4–8 exercises, with ground contacts and throws ranging from 60 to 150 per session, depending on the age, level of experience, and the training intensity, can be found in the literature [33, 41, 46, 65–67]. Therefore, low-volume plyometrics is recommended as compared to higher-volume plyometrics.
- Intensity in these exercises refers to the amount of stress placed on the musculotendinous unit, which is normally related to the eccentric strain added to the selected exercise [68]. Therefore, at pre-PHV ages, the eccentric component of the plyometric exercises should be limited using exercises like multiple hops, jumps onto boxes, and repeated jumps over mini-hurdles and, gradually over time, introducing more demanding exercises (i.e., multiple box jumps, drop jumps (DJ) from excessive heights). Execution of these exercises should be always as fast as possible (if power development is the goal), and high repetition velocity should be maintained. Also, intermittent feedback from the coach could increase athlete motivation and subsequent performance outcome.
- Regarding training frequency, previous research has proposed that children can perform plyometric exercises twice weekly on non-consecutive days [65]. Power production requires a "fresh" or "rested" neuromuscular system.

Weightlifting in the Young Tennis Player

There is widespread acceptance by various scientific associations (i.e., National Strength and Conditioning Association (NSCA), Australian

Strength and Conditioning Association (ASCA), and American Academy of Pediatrics (AAP), among others) that advanced multi-joint exercises such as Olympic-style lifts and plyometrics can be incorporated into a youth strength training program [59]. Traditionally, weightlifting movements have been associated with potential injuries, although there is no evidence indicating that weightlifting has a direct correlation with injuries in young athletes, and also its injury rate is reportedly lower than other forms of resistance training and sports in general [69]. On the contrary, risk factors prevalent to weightlifting (and strength training in general) include unsafe environment and equipment, excessive load and volume of training, and limited rest intervals [48]. Although there is a lack of scientific research regarding the use of weightlifting programs in youth athletes, some previous studies recognized that a well-structured weightlifting program can elicit positive training adaptations in young athletes for strength and power [70, 71]. It seems interesting to highlight the study from Chaouachi et al. [70], showing that the training gains (i.e., jump height, balance, strength/power measures, and sprint time) from Olympic weightlifting training (i.e., with cleans, snatches, and shoulder push presses) and plyometrics were generally comparable or superior to traditional strength training program in children of 10–12 years old. Again, like for traditional strength training, children must progress from learning weightlifting through to performance weightlifting [72], meaning that the main aim until the age of 11–12 years old is to achieve the fundamental skills to be able to focus on more technical competency regarding the different lifts (i.e., snatch, clean, jerk), which can be done before the PHV. After the PHV, training program contents may fluctuate between technical competency and external loading [72].

Regarding the use of Olympic weightlifting in tennis players, although they can be very useful in their training programs, there are several concerns to pay attention to. First is the usefulness of using the complete movements (i.e., starting from the floor). Starting from the "hang" position is preferable for tennis athletes when working on explosive power, following the training principle of specificity, as there are no specific movements in tennis requiring these full squat positions. Second, the *catch position* is one area that many tennis players struggle with. The reason is typically lack of wrist, forearm, and shoulder flexibility. As the wrist is a common injury area in tennis [73], the full and power clean are both lifts that may not be appropriate for many tennis players, if they have not learned the movements at a young age and are appropriately flexible. Finally, as shoulder problems are a frequently reported injury in elite tennis players (i.e., shoulder impingement), overhead vertical pressing movements are limited in the tennis player, and for many players, it may not be suggested at all. However, the push press and power jerk, when performed correctly, are less of a slow, mechanical shoulder pressing movement and more of a power movement utilizing the lower body and core muscles to explosively propel the weight to arm's-length overhead [74].

38.4.3 Speed and Agility

In competitive tennis, the average point length is significantly less than 10 s [75, 76] with the recovery between points usually between 20 and 25 s depending on certain rules. After every two games (minimum of eight points), the athlete has a 90-s break before the next point is played. Although every tennis point is vastly different, tennis players make an average of four directional changes per point [77] but can range from a single movement to more than 15 directional changes on a very long point. In a competitive match, it is not uncommon for players to have more than 1000 direction changes. Ferrauti et al. [78] reported that 80% of all strokes were played with less than 2.5 m covered, and fewer than 5% of strokes were played requiring more than 4.5 m between strokes. Other similar studies have found movement distances on average to be approximately 4 m per change of direction [79]. Relatively short distances that a player covers on each stroke are typically less than 2.0 m, yet under higher time pressure (increased running demand), athletes can run on average about 4 m (maximum of between 8 and 12 m) [80]. It is interesting to note that tennis players can cover about 0.25–0.50 m more on their forehand side than their backhand side [80]. These are important findings, as most speed and quickness programs for other sports focus on distances that are longer where a full traditional acceleration position may be reached. In tennis, it is rare that distances are achieved where a traditional acceleration technique will be experienced by the athlete. Furthermore, the majority of tennis movements are lateral or multidirectional [80]. It is known that linear acceleration, linear maximum velocity, and agility are all separate and distinct biomotor skills that need to be trained separately [81], as training one will not directly impact the improvement of the other. Therefore, preferred training recommendations for tennis should be to focus training between 60% and 80% of the time on lateral and multidirectional movements, 10–30% of the time on linear forward movements, and only about 10% of the time on linear backward movement.

38.4.3.1 Tennis Speed

With lateral focused tennis-specific movements, the spinal reflex times of the following muscles improve (vastus medialis/lateral medialis due to anterior tibial translation), and the cortical response time improved in the gastrocnemius and medial hamstring (semimembranosus, semitendinosus) [82]. There are a multitude of movements that a tennis athlete performs during every match or practice (in a perfect scenario all possible movements and distances will be trained); however, three distinct initiating movements that are usually used by players during baseline movement—jab step, pivot step, and the gravity step—are described below.

- The *jab step* has been defined as stepping first with the lead foot in the direction of the oncoming ball [83].
- The *pivot step* involves pivoting on the lead foot while turning the hips toward the ball and making the first step actually toward the ball with the opposite leg [83].
- The *gravity step* involves bringing the lead foot in toward the body and away from the direction of the oncoming ball and ultimately away from the direction of the intended movement. This small step (unweighting) actually moves the center of gravity outside the base of support [83].

In a study that compared the jab, pivot, and gravity step on tennis movement, it was found that the fastest method to move laterally was by utilizing the gravity step [84]. The authors speculated that the greater speed to the ball and greater control were due to the fact that the gravity step produces an overall movement toward the ball after the initial movement of the lead leg in a direction away from the ball. Unlike the jab step (where the center of gravity remains between the base of support), the gravity step creates a "dynamic imbalance" [84]. This movement of the center of gravity outside the base of support actually assists in moving the body laterally to the ball. This is a similar principle to the back step (or drop step) seen when athletes attempt to break inertia in a forward direction [85].

Having a good understanding of the needs of the sport helps when designing effective tennis-specific speed and agility programs. Basic human movements are still important for tennis athletes, and it is important to understand and subsequently teach the basic movements. A jump involves a take-off from one or both feet and a landing on both feet simultaneously [86]. A leap (sometimes called a bound) occurs from taking off on one foot and landing on the other [86]. A hop is when the take-off and landing occur on the same single foot [86]. Other common athletic skills that need to be prioritized (especially before puberty) are the gallop, shuffle, and skip. Galloping and shuffling are a combination of a step and leap, whereas skipping requires combining a step with a hop [86]. Upper body actions are not as easy to distinguish as lower body actions.

To develop tennis-specific speed and agility, a relationship with strength and power is also required (see earlier section). Plyometric exercises alone can improve jumping ability [87–90]. Jumping is specifically related to tennis. Split step and improving jumping ability can impact first step speed and improve split-step ability. Research has shown that improvements of 12.7% in take-off velocity accounted for 71% of the observed improvement in jumping performance [91]. This highlights the importance of instruction for take-off technique and the ability to take off with maximal velocity. Therefore, landing and jumping mechanics should be viewed as separate motor skills and trained independently in the tennis athlete [86]. The combination of resistance and plyometric training caused greater improvements in vertical jump (i.e., power output) ability than either training modality alone [92]. It is important to understand that young athletes cannot increase power simply by becoming stronger and that utilizing any increase in strength at appropriate speeds is the key factor for performance enhancement and improved movement [93]. It is important to consider when developing elite-level tennis athletes that a close interplay exists between strength, speed, and power development to optimize training adaptations.

38.4.3.2 Tennis Agility

Changes in direction occur nearly every point in tennis and are one of the most important physical skills needed to be a successful tennis player at any level. Agility includes deceleration followed immediately by reacceleration of the entire body or individual body segment(s) [86, 94]. Agility has been described as an efficient, coordinated movement in multiple planes performed at multiple velocities [95, 96]. Although agility has been shown to be an independent athletic attribute [97], additional qualities are considered important, including dynamic balance, spatial awareness, rhythm, and visual processing [98]. As tennis is a reactionary sport, it is important to train agility utilizing drills, exercises, and progressions that involve the athlete responding to visual stimulus similar to what may be seen on a tennis court.

In the young tennis player, the development of agility requires appropriate movement patterns and the ability to integrate locomotor skills efficiently (e.g., running, jumping) with proprioceptive awareness. Their movement efficiency is often poor, however, and associated with awkward arm motion, overall unbalanced posture, and a general lack of timing and coordination. At the younger ages (prepuberty), kids should perform a large variety of general movement patterns in an effort to develop a foundation of motor skills. Adding resistance too early to an athlete will change the movement mechanics and have a negative effective on mechanics.

Young athletes will be able to move quickly as they mature if they maintain/improve technique. For reasons of safety and injury prevention, however, they should initially perform drills at submaximal speeds. More complexity and specificity are the focus of a progressive agility training. The same drill can be made more difficult simply by using different visual and proprioceptive conditions, including a partner, or implementing an area or time restriction. Once mastery of skills has been achieved, athletes should perform nearly all of the drills at high speeds, as slower movements have been shown to alter muscle activation patterns [99]. However, if muscle mechanics are compromised due to muscle imbalances or technique issues, then these areas should be improved in supplemental exercises at slower speeds or more controlled environments to ensure mastery. An example may be an athlete who struggles to change direction effectively after hitting a wide backhand groundstroke, has weak gluteus medius strength, and should therefore focus on developing gluteus medius strength in the gym while still working on agility movements close to (or at) match speed.

38.4.3.3 Recover Movement

Recovery movement occurs immediately after an athlete has completed their stroke and they are attempting to return to a position that will allow for efficient movement toward the next stroke. There are two typical movement positions used during the recovery movement—the lateral crossover or the lateral shuffle. The lateral crossover is more appropriate for movements that require quicker responses and greater distances. The lateral shuffle is more common when the athlete has a little extra time to get back in position before having to explosively move to the next shot. It is important to incorporate both of these when structuring tennis movement sessions.

38.4.4 Reaction Time

One other area which can have an immediate impact on how fast an athlete *appears* in short distances is the athlete's reaction time. *Reaction time* is defined as the time from a stimulus (visual awareness of the opponents stroke/ball) until the production of force [100]. For over 100 years, the accepted figures for simple reaction times for college-age individuals have been about 190 ms (0.19 s) for light stimuli and about 160 ms (0.16 s) for sound stimuli [101, 102]. However, the fastest athletes in the world consistently have reaction times less than 0.15 s [103, 104]. In identical events, women have been shown to have longer reaction times than men [105]. However, reaction time does not correlate well with sprints lasting longer than a few seconds [104], yet, it does correlate very well with distances typically seen in tennis play [104]. Therefore, training an athlete to improve reaction time should be a component of training tennis movement, alongside, technique, strength, and power. In the training drills, a visual stimulus needs to be used to help develop visual reaction time. An auditory stimulus (whistle, voice, hand clap) is less tennis specific than the visual cue. The average reaction times (from ball machine release to initial racket movement) in skilled tennis players' volleys were 0.226 s for the forehand and 0.205 s for the backhand according to a study [106].

As a practical application, Table 38.4 summarizes some of the main contents in tennis speed and agility training sessions depending on the biological age of the athletes [3, 43].

38.5 Flexibility

Flexibility has long been recognized as an essential physical ability to be developed in both youths and adults, especially in specific sports such as gymnastics or martial arts.

Since injuries in tennis can involve all the areas of the body, due to the repetitive demands and musculoskeletal stressors, the range of motion (ROM or the amount of movement a person has at each joint) and flexibility seem to be essential [52]. Flexibility could be defined as "the ability to move joints fluidly through a full range of motion." [107] Thus, in the case of a tennis player, the ability to move freely and effectively through an optimal range of motion will be an important performance goal. Prior research has identified sport-specific shoulder and hip ROMs and muscular strength patterns in elite junior and adult tennis players. In the shoulder, several anatomical and mechanical adaptations have been described,

Table 38.4 Basic characteristics of the speed and agility traning sessions in youth tennis players

	Pre-PHV	Around PHV	Post-PHV
Sprint training focus	Locomotor movement skills; technical development; change of direction speed	Technical development; maximal sprints; change of direction speed	Maximal sprints; change of direction speed
Complementary training	Physical literacy development plyometrics Coordination/movement skills; reactive agility training	Plyometrics; strength (hypertrophy: latter part of this stage); coordination (during growth spurts); reactive agility training	Reactive agility training; hypertrophy; strength Complex training
Volume intensity	100–250 m; sprint distances from 0 to 20 m; multidirectional exercises Submaximal-maximal	250–400 m; sprint distances from 0 to 30; multidirectional exercises Submaximal-maximal	Up to 600 m; sprint distances from 0 to 30; multidirectional exercises Maximal
Frequency (sessions/week)	1–2	2–3	2–3

Suggested ages (years): pre-peak height velocity (PHV), males 8–12 and females 8–11; around PHV, males 12–16 and females 11–15; post-PHV, males 16+ and females 15+

which may be associated with increased risk of shoulder injury in overhead athletes [108]. Among the most important ones, we can find a strength imbalance between the agonist and antagonist muscles of the glenohumeral joint [109], scapular dyskinesis [110], and asymmetries between the dominant and non-dominant shoulders in rotational passive ROM (i.e., higher external rotation (ER), lower internal rotation (IR)) and lower total arc of motion (TAM, the sum of IR and ER) of the dominant shoulder [111].

As previously mentioned, during tennis play, the lower extremities are also subjected to repetitive loading forces (e.g., cutting movements). However, research related to the lower extremity ROM is scarce, with only a few studies that have examined the tennis-related alterations on the lower extremity joints (i.e., hip internal and external rotation ROM profile) in elite or professional players [112, 113], showing no specific hip alterations in rotational ROM. More recently, in a group of 109 elite tennis players, Moreno-Perez et al. [114] showed no clinically significant differences between extremities in bilateral measurement of hip flexion, extension, abduction, and IR or ER ROM. However, restricted values of hip flexion, extension, and abduction were found in both limbs for males and females. Furthermore, male tennis players also had restricted passive and active hip internal rotation ROM values.

Based on the ROM impairments reported, it appears necessary, especially at young ages, to restore the tennis player's normal shoulder ROM before in between matches as well as to improve general flexibility. This can be done educating the players to use specific stretching routines, joint mobilization, and other short-term recovery strategies, such as self-myofascial release using a foam roller, in order to avoid overuse injuries and to maintain performance levels. Light joint mobilizations (i.e., for both the upper and lower body) together with stretching routines involving those overloaded joints (i.e., shoulder and hips) should be performed a minimum of twice a week for a total of 15–20 min per session [115]. For example, shoulder exercises like the cross body or the sleeper stretch should be performed to mild discomfort for five repetitions of 30 s and should be conducted daily after the training session. Moreover, the use of the foam roller (2–3 sets of 30 s to 1 min) may offer short-term benefits for increasing joint ROMs at the hip, knee, and/or ankle without affecting muscle performance [116].

Conclusion

The objectives of a structured strength and conditioning program for both a prepubertal and post-pubertal tennis athlete are firstly to reduce the likelihood of injury and secondly improve on-court tennis performance. The road to physical mastery requires appropriate progressions based on consistent analysis of where each athlete is currently performing on the process to their goals. The information provided in this chapter includes some specific areas of focus to help the coach, trainer, strength and conditioning professional, and sport scientist better plan strength and conditioning programs for the developmental and elite tennis player.

References

1. Malina RM, Bouchard C, Bar-Or O. Growth, maturation, and physical activity: human kinetics. Champaign, IL: Human Kinetics; 2004.
2. Wiersma LD. Risks and benefits of youth sport specialization: perspectives and recommendations. Pediatr Exerc Sci. 2000;12(1):13–22.
3. Lloyd RS, Oliver JL. The youth physical development model: a new approach to long-term athletic development. Strength Cond J. 2012;34(3):61–72.
4. Malina RM. Early sport specialization: roots, effectiveness, risks. Curr Sports Med Rep. 2010;9(6):364–71.
5. Lloyd RS, Cronin JB, Faigenbaum AD, et al. National Strength and Conditioning Association position statement on long-term athletic development. J Strength Cond Res. 2016;30(6):1491–509. https://doi.org/10.1519/JSC.0000000000001387.
6. Naughton G, Farpour-Lambert NJ, Carlson J, et al. Physiological issues surrounding the performance of adolescent athletes. Sports Med. 2000;30(5):309–25.
7. Capranica L, Millard-Stafford ML. Youth sport specialization: how to manage competition and training? Int J Sports Physiol Perform. 2011;6(4):572–9.
8. Beunen GP, Malina RM, Freitas DI, et al. Cross-validation of the Beunen-Malina method to predict adult height. Ann Hum Biol. 2010;37(4):593–7. https://doi.org/10.3109/03014460903393865.

9. Birrer R, Levine R, Gallippi L, et al. The correlation of performance variables in preadolescent tennis players. J Sports Med Phys Fitness. 1986;26(2):137.
10. Roetert EP, Garrett GE, Brown SW, et al. Performance profiles of nationally ranked junior tennis players. J Strength Cond Res. 1992;6(4):225–31.
11. Roetert P, Ellenbecker TS. Complete conditioning for tennis. Champaign, IL: Human Kinetics; 2007.
12. Mujika I, Vaeyens R, Matthys SP, et al. The relative age effect in a professional football club setting. J Sports Sci. 2009;27(11):1153–8.
13. Delorme N, Boiché J, Raspaud M. Relative age effect in elite sports: methodological bias or real discrimination? Eur J Sport Sci. 2010;10(2):91–6.
14. Musch J, Grondin S. Unequal competition as an impediment to personal development: a review of the relative age effect in sport. Dev Rev. 2001;21(2):147–67.
15. Ulbricht A, Fernandez-Fernandez J, Mendez-Villanueva A, et al. The relative age effect and physical fitness characteristics in german male tennis players. J Sports Sci Med. 2015;14(3):634.
16. Sherar LB, Baxter-Jones AD, Faulkner RA, et al. Do physical maturity and birth date predict talent in male youth ice hockey players? J Sports Sci. 2007;25(8):879–86.
17. Baxter-Jones AD, Sherar LB. Growth and maturation. In: Armstrong N, editor. Paediatric exercise physiology, advances in sport and exercise science series. Churchill Livingston: Elsevier; 2007. p. 1–26.
18. Balyi I, Way R, Higgs C. Long-term athlete development. Champaign, IL: Human Kinetics; 2013.
19. Mirwald RL, Baxter-Jones AD, Bailey DA, et al. An assessment of maturity from anthropometric measurements. Med Sci Sports Exerc. 2002;34(4):689–94.
20. Ulbricht A, Fernandez-Fernandez J, Ferrauti A. Conception for fitness testing and individualized training programs in the German Tennis Federation. Sports Orthopaed Traumatol. 2013;29(3):180–92.
21. Myer GD, Jayanthi N, Difiori JP, et al. Sport specialization, part I: does early sports specialization increase negative outcomes and reduce the opportunity for success in young athletes? Sports Health. 2015;7(5):437–42. https://doi.org/10.1177/1941738115598747.
22. Reid M, Crespo M, Lay B, et al. Skill acquisition in tennis: research and current practice. J Sci Med Sport. 2007;10(1):1–10.
23. Murphy A, Duffield R, Kellett A, et al. The effect of pre-departure training loads on post-tour physical capacities in high-performance junior tennis players. Int J Sports Physiol Perform. 2015;10(8):986–93.
24. Kovacs M, Mundie E, Eng D, et al. How did the top 100 professional tennis players (ATP) succeed: an analysis of ranking milestones. J Med Sci Tennis. 2015;20:50–7.
25. Cotorro A, Philippon M, Briggs K, et al. Hip screening in elite youth tennis players. Br J Sports Med. 2014;48(7):582.
26. Myer GD, Jayanthi N, DiFiori JP, et al. Sports specialization, Part II: alternative solutions to early sport specialization in youth athletes. Sports Health. 2016;8(1):65–73. https://doi.org/10.1177/1941738115614811.
27. LaPrade RF, Agel J, Baker J, et al. AOSSM early sport specialization consensus statement. Orthopaed J Sports Med. 2016;4(4):2325967116644241. https://doi.org/10.1177/2325967116644241.
28. Feeley BT, Agel J, LaPrade RF. When is it too early for single sport specialization? Am J Sports Med. 2016;44(1):234–41. https://doi.org/10.1177/0363546515576899.
29. Ford P, De Ste Croix M, Lloyd R, et al. The long-term athlete development model: physiological evidence and application. J Sports Sci. 2011;29(4):389–402. https://doi.org/10.1080/02640414.2010.536849.
30. Lloyd RS, Oliver JL, Faigenbaum AD, et al. Long-term athletic development – part 1: a pathway for all youth. J Strength Cond Res. 2015;29(5):1439–50. https://doi.org/10.1519/JSC.0000000000000756.
31. Baquet G, Van Praagh E, Berthoin S. Endurance training and aerobic fitness in young people. Sports Med. 2003;33(15):1127–43.
32. Rumpf MC, Cronin JB, Pinder SD, et al. Effect of different training methods on running sprint times in male youth. Pediatr Exerc Sci. 2012;24(2):170–86.
33. Lloyd RS, Meyers RW, Oliver JL. The natural development and trainability of plyometric ability during childhood. Strength Cond J. 2011;33(2):23–32.
34. Faigenbaum AD, Lloyd RS, MacDonald J, et al. Citius, altius, fortius: beneficial effects of resistance training for young athletes: narrative review. Br J Sports Med. 2016;50(1):3–7. https://doi.org/10.1136/bjsports-2015-094621.
35. Faigenbaum AD, Lloyd RS, Myer GD. Youth resistance training: past practices, new perspectives, and future directions. Pediatr Exerc Sci. 2013;25(4):591–604.
36. Jaakkola T, Yli-Piipari S, Huotari P, et al. Fundamental movement skills and physical fitness as predictors of physical activity: a 6-year follow-up study. Scand J Med Sci Sports. 2016;26(1):74–81. https://doi.org/10.1111/sms.12407.
37. Bryant ES, Duncan MJ, Birch SL. Fundamental movement skills and weight status in British primary school children. Eur J Sport Sci. 2014;14(7):730–6. https://doi.org/10.1080/17461391.2013.870232.
38. Lubans DR, Morgan PJ, Cliff DP, et al. Fundamental movement skills in children and adolescents: review of associated health benefits. Sports Med. 2010;40(12):1019–35. https://doi.org/10.2165/11536850-000000000-00000.
39. Lloyd RS, Oliver JL, Faigenbaum AD, et al. Long-term athletic development, part 2: barriers to success and potential solutions. J Strength Cond Res. 2015;29(5):1451–64. https://doi.org/10.1519/01.JSC.0000465424.75389.56.
40. Myer GD, Lloyd RS, Brent JL, et al. How young is "too young" to start training? ACSMs Health Fit J. 2013;17(5):14–23. https://doi.org/10.1249/FIT.0b013e3182a06c59.

41. Fernandez-Fernandez J, Sanz-Rivas D, Sáenz d-VE, et al. The effects of 8-week plyometric training on physical performance in young tennis players. Pediatr Exerc Sci. 28(1):2015, 77–86.
42. Faigenbaum AD, McFarland JE, Keiper FB, et al. Effects of a short-term plyometric and resistance training program on fitness performance in boys age 12 to 15 years. J Sports Sci Med. 2007;6(4):519.
43. Lloyd RS, Read P, Oliver JL, et al. Considerations for the development of agility during childhood and adolescence. Strength Cond J. 2013;35(3):2–11.
44. Mandelbaum BR, Silvers HJ, Watanabe DS, et al. Effectiveness of a neuromuscular and proprioceptive training program in preventing anterior cruciate ligament injuries in female athletes 2-year follow-up. Am J Sports Med. 2005;33(7):1003–10.
45. Behringer M, von Heede A, Yue Z, et al. Effects of resistance training in children and adolescents: a meta-analysis. Pediatrics. 2010;26(5): e1199–210.
46. Michailidis Y, Fatouros IG, Primpa E, et al. Plyometrics' trainability in preadolescent soccer athletes. J Strength Cond Res. 2013;27(1):38–49. https://doi.org/10.1519/JSC.0b013e3182541ec6.
47. Fernandez-Fernandez J, Ellenbecker T. Effects of a 6-week junior tennis conditioning program on service velocity. J Sports Sci Med. 2013;12(2):232.
48. Lloyd RS, Oliver JL. Strength and conditioning for young athletes: science and application. Abingdon: Routledge; 2013.
49. Salonikidis K, Zafeiridis A. The effects of plyometric, tennis-drills, and combined training on reaction, lateral and linear speed, power, and strength in novice tennis players. J Strength Cond Res. 2008;22(1):182–91. https://doi.org/10.1519/JSC.0b013e31815f57ad.
50. Kovacs MS. Strength and conditioning for the young tennis player. The young tennis player. New York, NY: Springer; 2016. p. 55–86.
51. Ellenbecker TS, Pluim B, Vivier S, et al. Common injuries in tennis players: exercises to address muscular imbalances and reduce injury risk. Strength Cond J. 2009;31(4):50–8.
52. Ellenbecker TS, Cools A. Rehabilitation of shoulder impingement syndrome and rotator cuff injuries: an evidence-based review. Br J Sports Med. 2010;44(5):319–27.
53. Hjelm N, Werner S, Renstrom P. Injury risk factors in junior tennis players: a prospective 2-year study. Scand J Med Sci Sports. 2012;22(1):40–8.
54. Pluim B, Loeffen F, Clarsen B, et al. A one-season prospective study of injuries and illness in elite junior tennis. Scand J Med Sci Sports. 2015;26(5):564–71.
55. Kovacs MS, Ellenbecker TS, Kibler WB, et al. Injury trends in american competitive junior tennis players. J Med Sci Tennis. 2014;19(1):19–24.
56. Sell K, Hainline B, Yorio M, et al. Injury trend analysis from the US Open Tennis Championships between 1994 and 2009. Br J Sports Med. 2014;48(7):546–51.
57. Barengo NC, Meneses-Echávez JF, Ramírez-Vélez R, et al. The impact of the FIFA 11+ training program on injury prevention in football players: a systematic review. Int J Environ Res Public Health. 2014;11(11):11986–2000.
58. Bizzini M, Impellizzeri FM, Dvorak J, et al. Physiological and performance responses to the "FIFA 11+" (part 1): is it an appropriate warm-up? J Sports Sci. 2013;31(13):1481–90. https://doi.org/10.1080/02640414.2013.802922.
59. Lloyd RS, Faigenbaum AD, Stone MH, et al. Position statement on youth resistance training: the 2014 International Consensus. Br J Sports Med. 2014;48(7):498–505. https://doi.org/10.1136/bjsports-2013-092952.
60. Pareja-Blanco F, Rodríguez-Rosell D, Sánchez-Medina L, et al. Effect of movement velocity during resistance training on neuromuscular performance. Int J Sports Med. 2014;35(11):916–24.
61. Legaz-Arrese A, Reverter-Masia J, Munguia-Izquierdo D, et al. An analysis of resistance training based on the maintenance of mechanical power. J Sports Med Phys Fitness. 2007;47(4):427–36.
62. Lloyd RS, Oliver JL, Hughes MG, et al. The effects of 4-weeks of plyometric training on reactive strength index and leg stiffness in male youths. J Strength Cond Res. 2012;26(10):2812–9. https://doi.org/10.1519/JSC.0b013e318242d2ec.
63. Kotzamanidis C. Effect of plyometric training on running performance and vertical jumping in prepubertal boys. J Strength Cond Res. 2006;20(2):441–5.
64. Saez-Saez de Villarreal E, Requena B, Newton RU. Does plyometric training improve strength performance? A meta-analysis. J Sci Med Sport. 2010;13(5):513–22. https://doi.org/10.1016/j.jsams.2009.08.005.
65. Johnson BA, Salzberg CL, Stevenson DA. A systematic review: plyometric training programs for young children. J Strength Cond Res. 2011;25(9):2623–33. https://doi.org/10.1519/JSC.0b013e318204caa0.
66. Ramirez-Campillo R, Andrade DC, Izquierdo M. Effects of plyometric training volume and training surface on explosive strength. J Strength Cond Res. 2013;27(10):2714–22. https://doi.org/10.1519/JSC.0b013e318280c9e9.
67. Ramirez-Campillo R, Meylan C, Alvarez C, et al. Effects of in-season low-volume high-intensity plyometric training on explosive actions and endurance of young soccer players. J Strength Cond Res. 2014;28(5):1335–42. https://doi.org/10.1519/jsc.0000000000000284.
68. Ramírez-Campillo R, Gallardo F, Henriquez-Olguín C, et al. Effect of vertical, horizontal and combined plyometric training on explosive, balance and endurance performance of young soccer players. J Strength Cond Res 2015 29(7):1784-1795.
69. Byrd R, Pierce K, Rielly L, et al. Strength and conditioning (michael stone sub-editor: young weightlifters' performance across time). Sports Biomech. 2003;2(1):133–40.
70. Chaouachi A, Hammami R, Kaabi S, et al. Olympic weightlifting and plyometric training with children

provides similar or greater performance improvements than traditional resistance training. J Strength Cond Res. 2014;28(6):1483–96.
71. Channell BT, Barfield J. Effect of olympic and traditional resistance training on vertical jump improvement in high school boys. J Strength Cond Res. 2008;22(5):1522–7.
72. Lloyd RS, Oliver JL, Meyers RW, et al. Long-term athletic development and its application to youth weightlifting. Strength Cond J. 2012;34(4):55–66.
73. Pluim BM, Staal J, Windler G, et al. Tennis injuries: occurrence, aetiology, and prevention. Br J Sports Med. 2006;40(5):415–23.
74. Harbili E, Alptekin A. Comparative kinematic analysis of the snatch lifts in elite male adolescent weightlifters. J Sports Sci Medicine. 2014;13(2):417.
75. Kovacs MS. A comparison of work/rest intervals in men's professional tennis. Med Sci Tennis. 2004;9(3):10–1.
76. Kovacs MS. Applied physiology of tennis performance. Br J Sports Med. 2006;40(5):381–6.
77. Kovacs M, Chandler WB, Chandler TJ. Tennis training: enhancing on-court performance. Vista, CA: Racquet Tech Publishing; 2007.
78. Ferrauti A, Maier P, Weber K. Schnelligkeitstraining. Leistung, Athletik, Gesundheit. In: Handbuch für Tennistraining. Meyer and Meyer Verlag, Aachen, Germany; 2014. p. 229–258.
79. Pieper S, Exler T, Weber K. Running speed loads on clay and hard courts in world class tennis. Med Sci Tennis. 2007;12(2):14–7.
80. Weber K, Pieper S, Exler T. Characteristics and significance of running speed at the Australian Open 2006 for training and injury prevention. Med Sci Tennis. 2007;12(1):14–7.
81. Young WB, McDowell MH, Scarlett BJ. Specificity of sprint and agility training methods. J Strength Cond Res. 2001;15(3):315–9.
82. Wojtys EM, Huston LJ, Taylor PD, et al. Neuromuscular adaptations in isokinetic, isotonic, and agility training programs. Am J Sports Med. 1996;24(2):187–92.
83. Kovacs MS. Movement for tennis: the importance of lateral training. Strength Cond J. 2009;31(4):77–85.
84. Bragg RW (2001) The lateral reaction step in tennis footwork. XIX international symposium on biomechanics in sports, San Francisco; 2001.
85. Kraan GA, van Veen J, Snijders CJ, et al. Starting from standing; why step backwards. J Biomech. 2001;34:211–5.
86. Kovacs M. Plyometric, speed and agility exercise prescription. In: Chandler TJ, Brown LE, editors. Conditioning for strength and human performance. 2nd ed. Philadelphia, PA: Lippincott, Williams & Wilkins; 2012. p. 383–420.
87. Brown ME, Mayhew JL, Boleach LW. Effect of plyometric training on vertical jump performance in high school basketball players. J Sports Med Phys Fit. 1986;26:1–4.
88. Fatouros IG, Jamurtas AZ, Leontsini D, et al. Evaluation of plyometric exercise training, weight training, and their combination on vertical jumping performance and leg strength. J Strength Cond Res. 2000;14:470–6.
89. Luebbers PE, Potteiger JA, Hulver MW, et al. Effects of plyometric training and recovery on vertical jump performance and anaerobic power. J Strength Cond Res. 2003;17:704–9.
90. Wilson GJ, Murphy AJ, Giorgi A. Weight and plyometric training: effects on eccentric and concentric force production. Can J Appl Physiol. 1996;21:301–15.
91. Ashby BM, Heegaard JH. Role of arm motion in the standing long jump. J Biomech. 2002;35:1631–7.
92. Adams K, O'Shea J, O'Shea K, et al. The effect of six weeks of squat, plyometric, and squat-plyometric training on power production. J Appl Sports Sci Res. 1992;6:36–41.
93. Bobbert MF, Van Soest AJ. Effects of muscle strengthening on vertical jump height: a simulation study. Med Sci Sports Exerc. 1994;26:1012–20.
94. Kovacs MS, Roetert EP, Ellenbecker TS. Efficient deceleration: the forgotten factor in tennis-specific training. Strength Cond J. 2008;30(6):58–69.
95. Drabik J. Children & sports training: how your future champions should exercise to be healthy, fit, and happy. Stadion: Island Pond, VT; 1996.
96. Verstegen M, Marcello B. Agility and coordination. In: Foran B, editor. High performance sports conditioning. Champaign, IL: Human Kinetics; 2001.
97. Little T, Williams AG. Specificity of acceleration, maximal speed and agility in professional soccer players. J Strength Cond Res. 2005;19(1):76–8.
98. Ellis L, Gastin P, Lawrence S, et al. Protocols for the physiological assessment of team sports players. In: Gore CJ, editor. Physiological tests for elite athletes. Champaign, IL: Human Kinetics; 2000.
99. Neptune RR, Wright IC, van der Bogert AJ. Muscle coordination and function during cutting movements. Med Sci Sports Exerc. 1999;31:294–302.
100. Schmidt RA, Lee TD. Motor control and learning: a behavioral emphasis. 3rd ed. Champaign, IL: Human Kinetics; 1999.
101. Galton F. On instruments for (1) testing perception of differences of tint and for (2) determining reaction time. J Anthropol Institute. 1899;19:27–9.
102. Brebner JT, Welford AT. Introduction and historical background sketch. In: Welford AT, editor. Reaction times. New York, NY: Academic; 1980. p. 1–23.
103. Gambetta V, Winckler G. Sport specific speed: the 3S system. Gambetta Sports Training Systems: Sarasota, FL; 2001.
104. Mero A, Komi PV. Reaction time and electromyographic activity during a sprint start. Eur J Appl Physiol. 1990;61:73–80.
105. Mero A, Komi PV, Gregor RJ. Biomechanics of sprint running. Sports Med. 1992;13(6):376–92.
106. Chow JW, Carlton LG, Chae WS, et al. Movement characteristics of the tennis volley. Med Sci Sports Exerc. 1999;31(6):855–63.
107. McNeal JR, Sands WA. Stretching for performance enhancement. Curr Sports Med Rep. 2006;5(3):141–6.

108. Moreno-Pérez V, Moreside J, Barbado D, et al. Comparison of shoulder rotation range of motion in professional tennis players with and without history of shoulder pain. Man Ther. 2015;20(2):313–8.
109. Saccol MF, Gracitelli GC, da Silva RT, et al. Shoulder functional ratio in elite junior tennis players. Phys Ther Sport. 2010;11(1):8–11.
110. Struyf F, Nijs J, Baeyens JP, et al. Scapular positioning and movement in unimpaired shoulders, shoulder impingement syndrome, and glenohumeral instability. Scand J Med Sci Sports. 2011;21(3):352–8.
111. Ellenbecker TS, Wilk K. Sport therapy for the shoulder: evaluation, rehabilitation, and return to sport. Champaign, IL: Human Kinetics; 2016.
112. Ellenbecker TS, Ellenbecker GA, Roetert EP, et al. Descriptive profile of hip rotation range of motion in elite tennis players and professional baseball pitchers. Am J Sports Med. 2007;35(8):1371–6.
113. Young SW, Dakic J, Stroia K, et al. Hip range of motion and association with injury in female professional tennis players. Am J Sports Med. 2014;42(11):2654–8.
114. Moreno-Pérez V, Ayala F, Fernandez-Fernandez J, et al. Descriptive profile of hip range of motion in elite tennis players. Phys Ther Sport. 2016;19:43–8.
115. Harshbarger ND, Eppelheimer BL, McLeod TCV, et al. The effectiveness of shoulder stretching and joint mobilizations on posterior shoulder tightness. J Sport Rehabil. 2013;22(4):313–9.
116. Cheatham SW, Kolber MJ, Cain M, et al. The effects of self-myofascial release using a foam roll or roller massager on joint range of motion, muscle recovery, and performance: a systematic review. Int J Sports Phys Ther. 2015;10(6):827–38.

Strength and Conditioning of the Hips and Core (Practical Applications)

Carl Petersen and Nina Nittinger

39.1 Introduction

Tennis is an explosive sport, requiring players to react to numerous emergencies with movement in multiple directions and through multiple planes of movement for short bursts of time. It has high demands in all of the physical components including hip and core strength and stability. Movements include sprinting, side-to-side running, cutting, twisting, sliding, and quick stops and starts [1]. These quick movements pass through many planes of motion and create rotational and torsional forces on numerous joints and muscles at the same time. In tennis players, the abdominal musculature plays a significant role in trunk and core stability providing a mechanical link between the lower and upper limbs [2]. If an athlete's alignment, balance control, connected core stability, deceleration strength, and extended hip stability required to carry out these maneuvers are not optimal, the player may be at risk of injury.

Historically many tennis players avoided traditional strength training methods fearing it would slow down court movements and make them too muscular interfering with the suppleness needed to perform. However, the changing nature and demands of the modern game means that players are bigger, more powerful, stronger, and faster than players of generations past. With these increased training demands and participation by ever-younger players, we must be proactive in our training of these developing athletes as well as with more mature players.

Over the last two decades, strength and stability training for tennis players has become increasingly common and is included in the yearly periodization plan which is discussed further in Chap. 43. Properly planned strength training of the upper core and arms and lower core and legs (hips) will enhance on-court performance and allow players to increase maximal force and power to optimize training and as well protect against injury. The goals of the program will be to increase stability in all three planes of motion with functional exercise progressions.

39.2 Planes of Motion

There are three primary planes of motion, transverse, sagittal, and frontal planes. All exercises are carried out in one or more of these planes. Multi-planar exercises utilize more than one plane of motion and more closely mimic the demands of tennis. An example would be any medicine ball throwing motions with involve several planes of movement.

C. Petersen (✉)
High Performance City Sports and Physiotherapy Clinic, Vancouver, Canada
e-mail: carl@citysportsphysio.com

N. Nittinger
St. Moritz, Switzerland

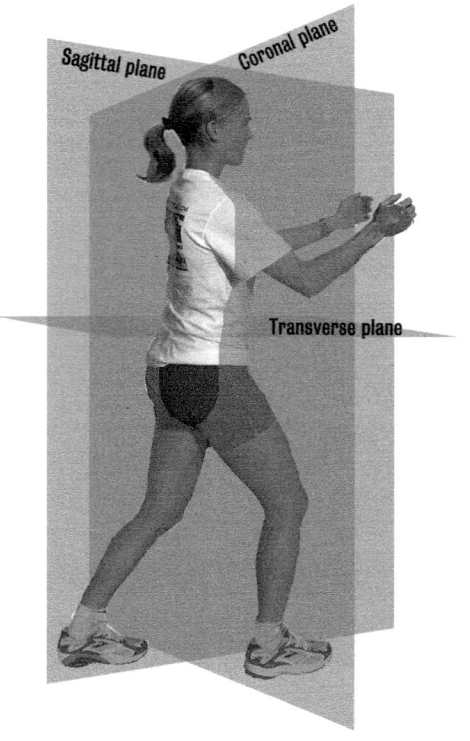

Three planes of motion. Courtesy of RaquetTECH publishers

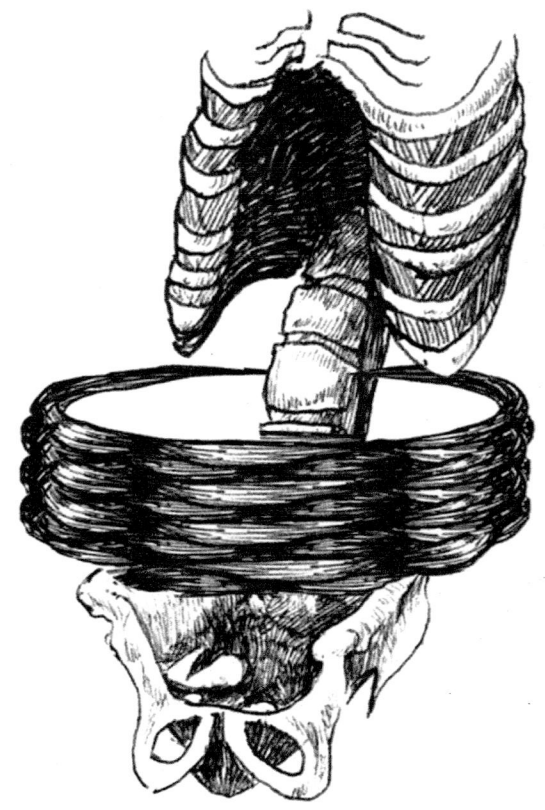

Inner core (adapted after Celebrini, 2002). Courtesy of RaquetTECH publishers

39.3 Importance of the Core

The core musculature includes muscles of the trunk and pelvis that are responsible for the maintenance of stability of the spine and pelvis and help in generation and transfer of energy from the large to small body parts during many sports activities [3, 4]. Bergmark and others have classified muscles into two systems: local and global. The local system pertains to those muscles essential for segmental or intrapelvic stabilization [5]. This "inner unit" [6] consists of four main muscles: the transversus abdominis, the multifidus, the pelvic floor muscles, and the diaphragm.

The first muscle to be recruited prior to any upper and/or lower body movements is the transversus abdominis. Normally it switches on in pre-anticipation of the movements required in tennis, but with dysfunction there is a timing delay, and players may not have the core stability needed for strokes. Studies have shown that without efficient and optimal recruitment, subsequent spinal dysfunction can occur [7] which may lead to injury.

The global muscle system appears to be more responsible for regional stabilization (between the thorax and pelvis or pelvis and legs) and motion [6, 8]. There are four commonly accepted global muscle slings that should be addressed when designing multi-planar exercises that mimic the acceleration, deceleration, diagonal patterns, rotational, and stability needs of tennis strokes. They are the posterior oblique sling, anterior oblique sling, longitudinal sling, and lateral sling [9, 10]. These slings are comprised of many muscles that attach the "lower core" lumbo-pelvic-hip complex and spine with the "upper core" spine, ribs, and scapular region.

These slings of muscles help transfer energy up the kinetic chain from the legs through the core (trunk) to the upper body and scapula funneling it to distal segments of the arm and hand. Past research has used a mathematical analysis to show the contributions of different segments of the body to the energy and force that move through the kinetic chain of sequential activation of body segments. It was determined that from the ground to the hand, 51% of the energy and 54% of the force are generated by the legs and trunk muscles [11]. When activated and recruited properly, the stability of the upper and lower core forms the stable base or foundation for other more distal movements. This is especially important in tennis due to the rotation, acceleration, and deceleration required during all strokes.

39.4 Concepts of Chain Exercises (Closed Chain vs. Open Chain vs. Partially Closed Chain)

Many commonly prescribed exercises are machine based and involve or isolate a single joint only allowing movement in one plane of motion without full kinetic chain involvement. They do not always address the finer aspects of postural awareness during weight bearing through the kinetic chain. A closed kinetic chain activity is defined as an activity in which the terminal joint meets considerable external resistance which prohibits or restrains free motion, whereas, an open kinetic chain activity is defined as an activity in which the terminal joint is free [12]. Examples of this would be a squat or lunge motion being a closed chain exercise for the lower extremity and an overhead raise with no resistance as an open chain exercise for the upper extremity. Closed kinetic chain activities may help improve dynamic stability through joint approximation and co-contraction [13] as well as have multiple-joint segments and groups of muscles involved. Another variation is a partially closed kinetic chain exercise where you would partially support your body weight or utilize other resistance requiring an integrated response from the muscles of the body; examples of this would be a push-up position where the hands and feet partially bear the weight or any activity that loads resistance through the hands and arms and into the torso, as when using resistance bands [14].

Closed chain exercise lower extremity

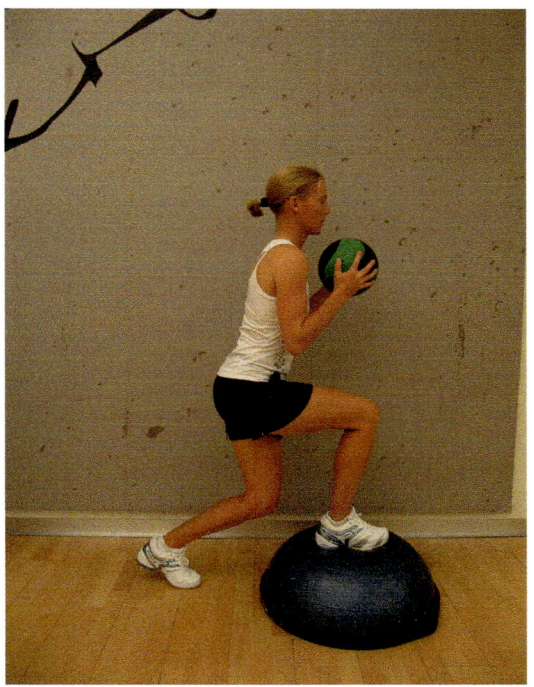

Open chain exercise upper extremity

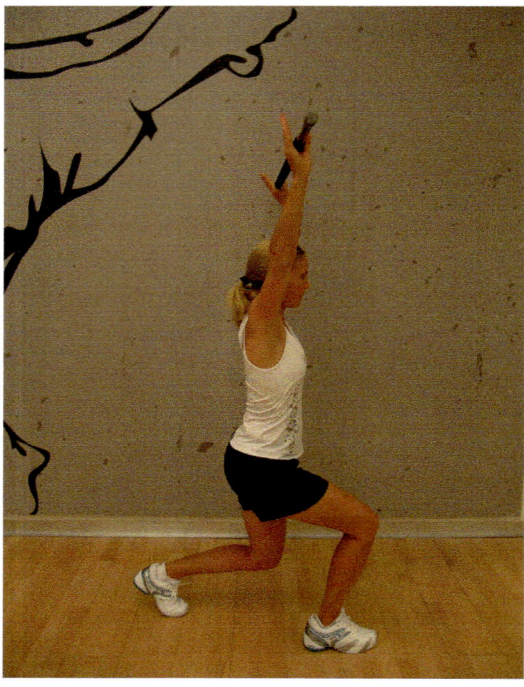

Partially closed chain upper extremity

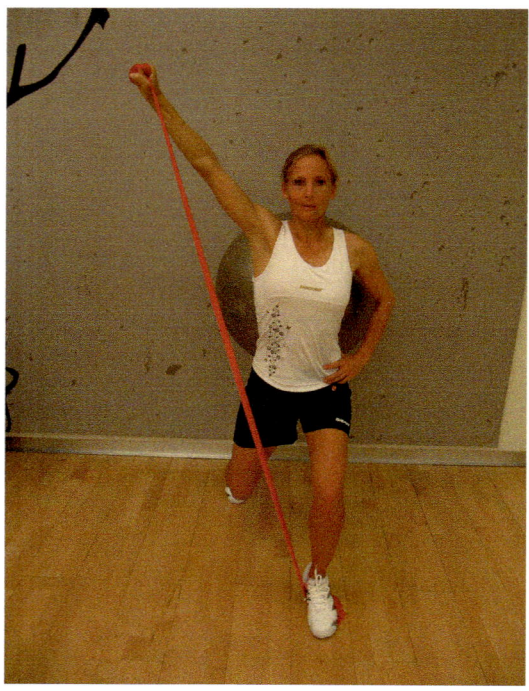

The challenge for busy clinicians and fitness coaches is how to effectively prescribe hip and core exercises that ensure optimal recruitment, balance, timing, and deceleration control that mimic the performance demands of tennis. Partially closed kinetic chain exercises allow for more variety and modes of resistance at faster speeds that utilize multiple joints and muscles involved in different planes of motion. These hip and core exercises that include multidirectional upper and lower core stability training provide smart training strategies that can be taught to players of all ages. The focus of connecting the core exercises should follow the ABCs of smart training.

Alignment: Stand tall with good posture, head and torso up, and shoulders square. When bending keep knees over toes to ensure proper tracking and knee alignment.

Balance: Challenge your balance daily to improve function and performance in all three dimensions. As well ensure a balanced approach to muscle development by choosing exercises that work the upper and lower body as well as the right and left sides and rotational movements.

Connect your core: You need a strong upper core and lower core to form a stable platform for the arms and legs to work off of during activities. Choose multi-planar exercises that involve several joints that utilize the functional slings and are combinations of closed, open, and partially closed kinetic chain movements.

Deceleration control: Is needed in both the upper and lower extremity musculature and core muscle to improve performance and protect against injury.

Extended hip strength: Stability and strength in this position is important for all tennis movement and strokes.

Fun: Your exercise program should be fun, stimulating, and varied regularly. If *not* why are you doing it?

39.5 Benefits of Connect the Core Stability Training [15]

- Improves postural set and helps maintain correct pelvic alignment

- Improves strength of functional muscle slings that connect the upper and lower core
- Improves joint and muscle position sense (kinesthetic awareness), helping to center the joint and absorb stress.
- Improves stability in a functional hip-extended position
- Improves ability to counter-rotate or dissociate the upper and lower torso and extremities
- Improves dynamic balance and movement efficiency
- Adds additional force vectors of resistance to traditional training methods
- Helps to improve athletic performance and helps the body to be able to react to unexpected events
- Provides exercises that are versatile, practical, transportable, and affordable

39.6 Individual Evaluation

To help address the individual needs of each player, a pre-participation evaluation should be performed that that includes relevant fitness and injury history as well as an objective evaluation of strength and stability. This is expanded in Chaps. 11 and 12. Any areas for improvement should be noted, and deficiencies should be addressed with a targeted program of exercises.

39.7 Movements in Tennis

To help design a tennis-specific hip and core strength and stability program, a needs analysis must be performed. Tennis is a ground-based sport requiring the lower core and legs to push into the ground and generate force up the kinetic chain through the core/torso to the upper body and arms. Many of the movements require a hip-extended position, lunging, and torso rotation at the same time. In the modern game, open stance forehand and the service motion comprise the majority of strokes. Players need to train in three dimensions and ensure the rotational, acceleration, and deceleration needs are addressed with a well-balanced approach to training.

The average point length in tennis is less than 10 s. On average, 3–5 directional changes are required per point, and it is not uncommon for players to perform more than 500 directional changes during a single match or practice [16]. As well, in "professional players," it was found that more than 70% of movements were side to side with less than 20% of movements in forward linear direction and less than 8% of movements in a backward linear direction [17]. Individuals designing training programs for tennis players must keep these time frames, directions of movement, and additional needs in mind when prescribing exercises for the different physical components.

39.8 Proper Form

When doing strength and stability training, proper form is important. Follow the instructions in the training tips section of each exercise. Proper form will ensure correct muscle sequencing and lead to better results and protect against injury. Movements should be controlled throughout the set. Don't sacrifice good form at the expense of completing the repetitions. It is better to do 10 reps with good form than 15 with poor form. Correct breathing patterns will have you inhaling at the start of the exercise and exhaling as you exert through the movement.

39.9 Repetitions (Reps), Sets, and Volume

Reps are the number of times a specific exercise is carried out per set. A set is the number of cycles of reps that are completed. The total volume of training is determined by the sets, repetitions, and weight (resistance):

$$\text{Total volume} = \text{sets} \times \text{reps} \times \text{weight (resistance)}.$$

39.10 Appropriate Resistance and Equipment

Not all of the exercises in this hip and core stability chapter require weights for resistance. Many rely on body weight and gravity to provide resistance. Others use elastic tubing and band resistance, weights, medicine balls, and different types of unstable bases to challenge the body. As well, gym-based weight machines or pulley machines can be utilized. The prescribed exercises should be individualized to the age, experience, and fitness level of the athlete. As a general rule, start with 1–2 sets of 5–10 repetitions and progress to 2–3 sets of 10–15 repetitions. If you are new to strength and stability training or have had a period of inactivity prior to returning to it, you will need to decide how much resistance to use as you complete the suggested number of repetitions and sets at the tempo outlined.

For the exercises described in this chapter, choose a resistance that allows you to complete the suggested reps with correct form while feeling like your muscles have worked hard but not to the point of failure. It should be a challenge to finish the set while maintaining correct form. Initially err on the side of caution to see how your body responds to the different challenges since you can always increase the resistance and complexity in future workouts.

39.11 Tempo

The tempo of the exercises is the cadence at which each repetition is performed [18]. In this chapter we use the following examples of tempo. A squat with a 3-0-1 tempo means 3 s down (lengthening/eccentric phase), 0 s hold (pause/isometric), and 1 s up (shortening/concentric). Another example would be a supine bridge exercise with a 1-4-1 tempo; it is 1 s up, 4 s pause, and 1 s down. If training explosive power which is important in tennis, the tempo for a lunge or a throw could be 1-0-*, 1 s down, 0 s hold, and * explosive up.

39.12 Rest Intervals

Rest is the amount of time between each set and depends on the training sessions goals. When training muscular endurance, rest of 1 min is usually adequate. However when training for explosive power or maximum strength, the rest period should be longer. The rest period following exhaustive anaerobic exercise may need to be up to 3 min to allow the ATP stores in the muscles to be replenished [19]. Regularly scheduling rest or recovery days (at least one per week) helps tissues adapt to the new stresses being placed on them through training and tennis and protect against staleness or overtraining.

39.13 Frequency

Frequency refers to how often the session is carried out. This will be determined by the individual goals of the athlete as well as their chronological age and training age. A general recommendation is to train the same muscle groups two to three times per week to get a training effect. For core muscles training harder every second day is recommended. As well light exercises for switching on the core should be included daily as part of the warm-up for all training including on-court sessions. During the competitive period, the frequency may need to be reduced, or alternative training may need to be implemented depending on the volume, density, and intensity of tournament play.

39.14 Overload

The training load must be high enough to tax the body's systems during a training session.

Overload encourages physical change and promotes adaptation. To achieve overload, the duration of the activity must be long enough to produce a training effect, and the intensity of the workouts must increase in a gradual and progressive manner. A good rule of thumb is to increase intensity 10% per week.

39.15 Diversity and Development

Diversity of training is important for athletes to develop strength and stability. Diversity includes variation in exercise and equipment selection, resistance used, tempo of the exercise, and rest period. Lack of diversity can lead to a plateau in the training effect and delay development by not optimizing stress on the tissues due to over- or under-training.

Exercise ball precautions

- For individuals new to exercise, check with your physician before starting this or any other exercise program.
- Check your ball for flaws before each use.
- Avoid placing ball near heat or in direct sunlight.
- Avoid sharp objects and jewelry.
- Start gradually and get a feel for the ball before progressing.

Resistance bands precautions:

- When using resistance tubing or bands, ensure they are of high quality.
- Avoid placing resistance bands near heat or in direct sunlight.
- Avoid sharp objects and jewelry
- Start gradually and get a feel for the resistance of the bands before progressing or increasing the tension.
- Regularly inspect the stretch band or tubing for wear and tear or weak spots and replace as appropriate.
- Ensure that it is securely attached before applying resistance.

39.16 Exercise Selection

It is outside the scope of this chapter to outline every single hip and core conditioning exercise devised for tennis. The exercises in this chapter work all of the important muscle groups of the hip and core by connecting the lower and upper core with exercises that focus on the functional anatomic slings. The exercises include concentric, eccentric, and isometric muscle actions in varying planes of motion using both single- and multiple-joint exercises. They will serve as a good starting point of safe, effective, easy-to-replicate, and easily transportable exercise programs that are suitable for athletes of varying training age and experience. They are described with specific training tips and a suggested number of repetitions, sets, and tempo which can be changed based on the experience of the athlete and the type of resistance used. All of the exercises or variations of them can add external resistance in the form of hand weights, dumbbells, barbells, or cuff weights to increase the number of motor units being recruited.

All exercise photos in this chapter courtesy of My Pocket Coach Fitness 1. www.my-pocket-coach.com

39.17 Always Begin with a Dynamic Warm-Up

Before starting this or any exercise routine, do some light dynamic warm-up. Doing assisted squats, leg swings, and sumo (plie) squats with arm raises and alternating lunges help to warm up the muscles of the lower core and legs and upper core and arms and also challenges balance and lubricates the joints.

Assisted squats

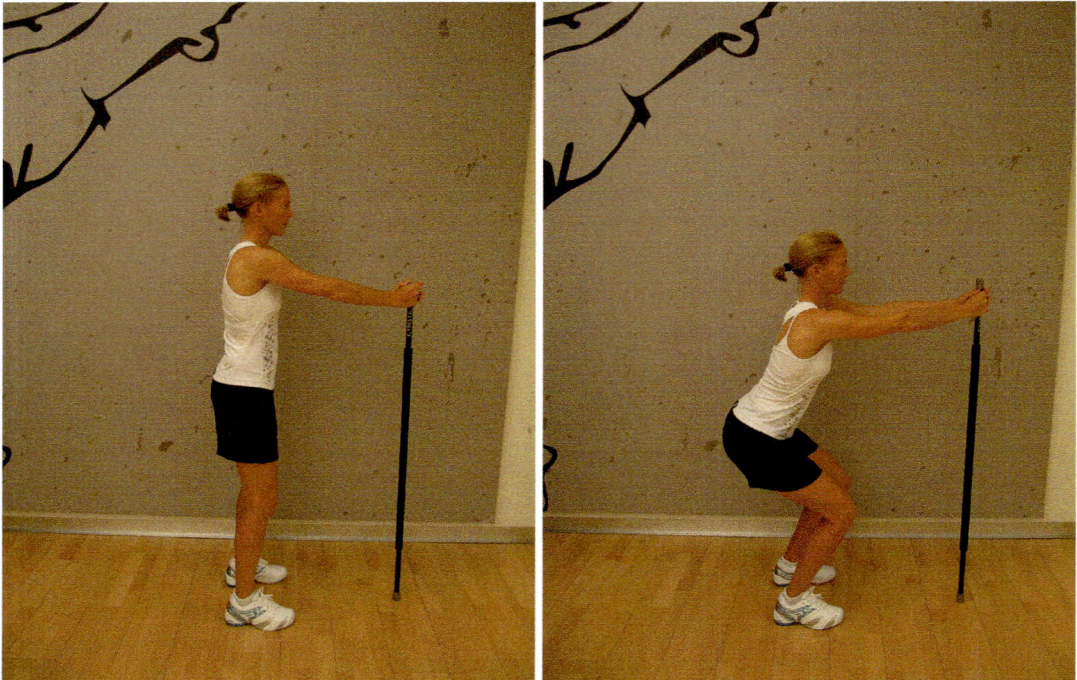

Training tips:

- Hang onto something for balance taking some weight through your arms.
- Switch on your core muscles.
- With feet pointing straight ahead, squat down slowly like sitting down in a chair.
- Keep knees aligned over toes but not going past them.

Reps, 10; sets, 1–2; tempo, 2-0-1.

Leg swings

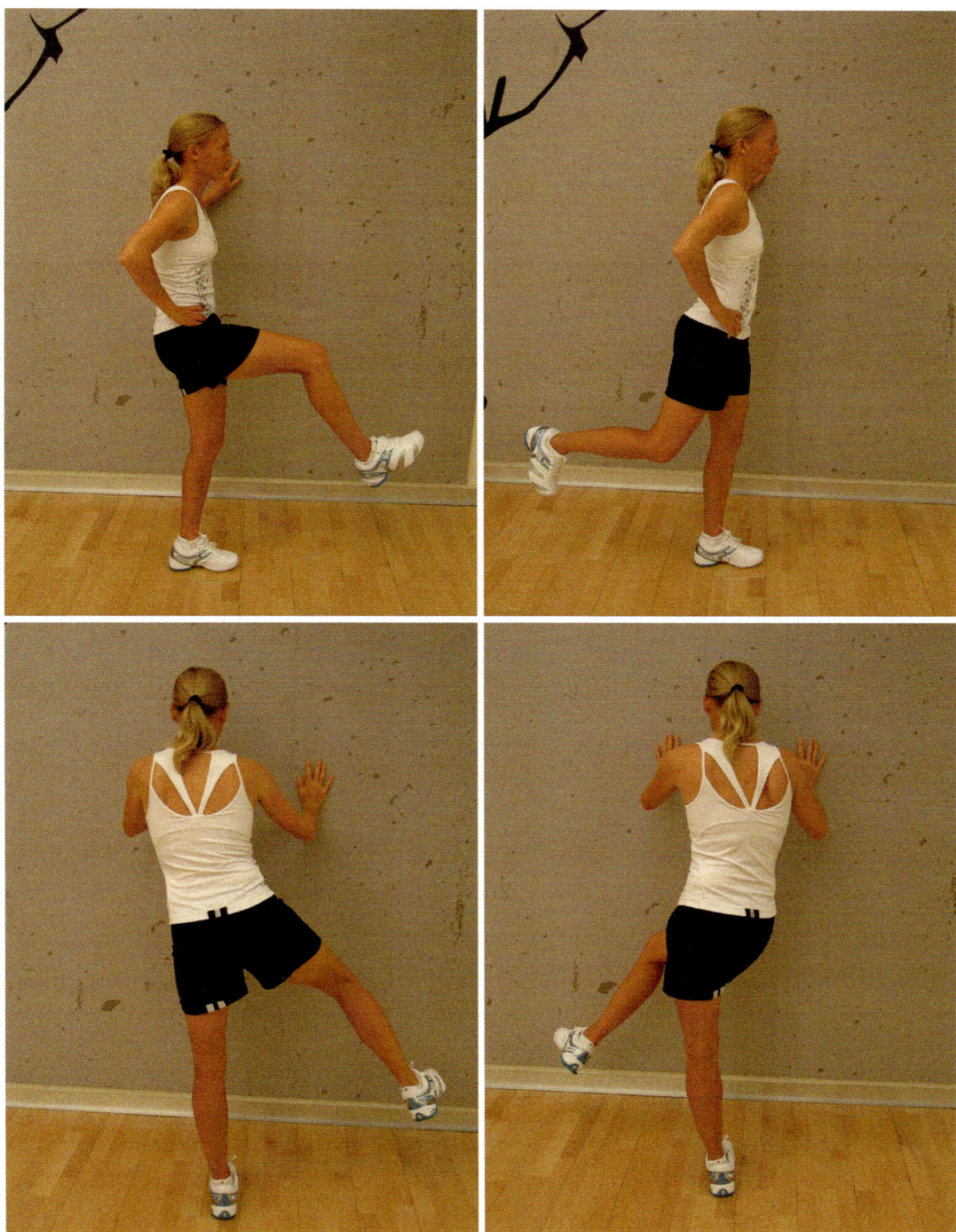

Training tips:

- Stand tall with soft knee (slightly bent) on stance leg.
- Switch on your core muscles and do leg swings.

Do three different ways (a and b shown)

(a) Swing leg front and back.
(b) Swing leg side to side.
(c) Swing leg in a figure of eight patterns.

Reps, 5–10; sets, 1–2; tempo, 1-0-1.

Sumo (Plie) squats with shoulder overhead press

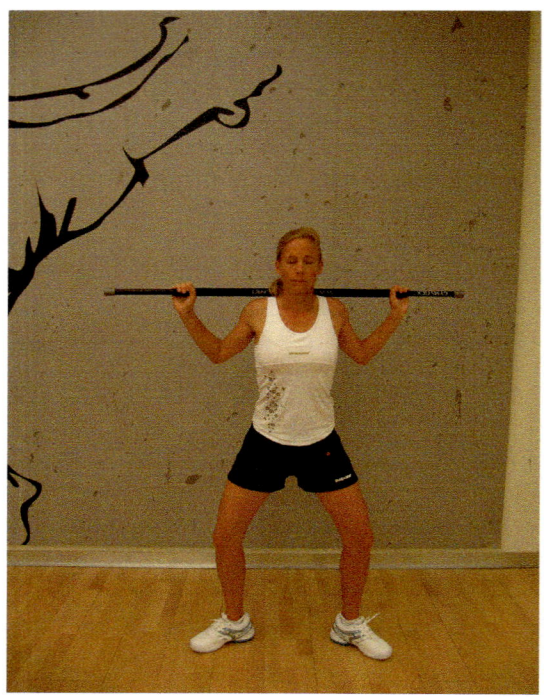 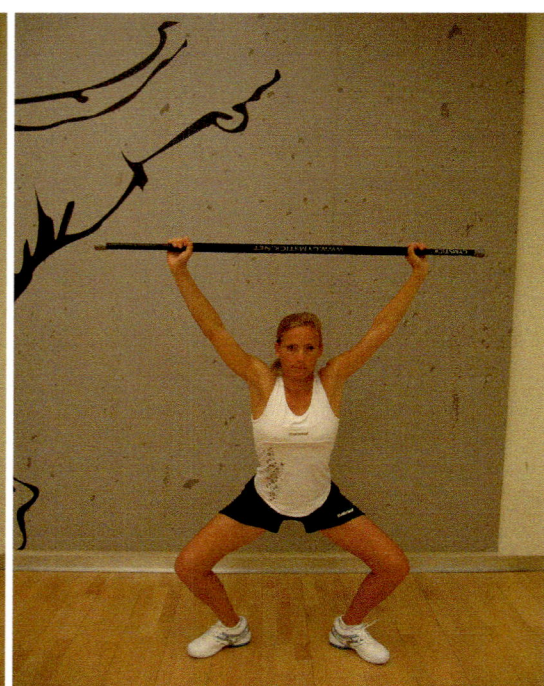

Training tips:

- Start standing in a sumo (plie) stance position with a stick held behind your shoulders.
- Switch on your core.
- Do a sumo (plie) squat keeping knees aligned with toes but not going past them.
- At the same time, press/raise the stick overhead.

Reps, 10; sets, 1–2: tempo, 2-0-1 or 3-0-1 core muscles.

Alternating lunges

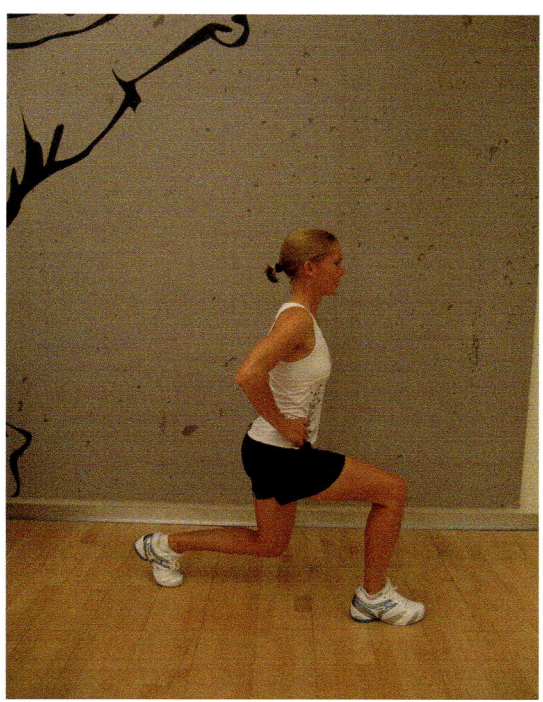

Training tips:

- Stand tall with soft knees.
- Switch on your core muscles.
- Do some alternating lunges ensuring knees aligned over toes but not going past them.
- The depth of the lunge should progress slowly.

Reps, 5–10; sets, 1–2; tempo, 1-0-1.

39.18 Core and Hip Base Work Series

While doing your core and hip exercises, you should always "switch on your core" (like turning up the dimmer switch on a light) [20]. Using this cue while doing these stability exercises will help connect the upper and lower core musculature through the central core "inner unit." Functional data suggests that elite adolescents possess poor proprioception, strength, and agility in key spine stabilizers, including multifidus, iliopsoas, and transversus abdominis [21]. Therefore starting with the core and hip base work series is important when working with developing athletes or after any injury or circumstance that prevents training for a period of time.

39.18.1 Tennis Relevance

Improves ability to activate and switch on core muscles during all sudden movements by creating a stable platform for the extremities to work off of as you counter-rotate or dissociate in preparation for all tennis strokes. Since weaknesses and imbalances of the core have been related to low back pain [22] and lower extremity injuries [23], doing base work helps protects against injury and aids in rehabilitation and pre-habilitation.

39.18.2 Core Base Work Series

(a) Core base work: tighten and leg slide

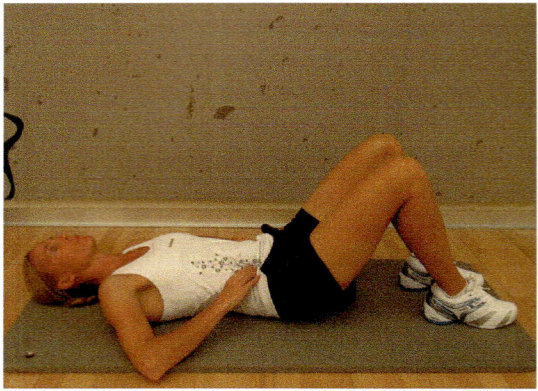
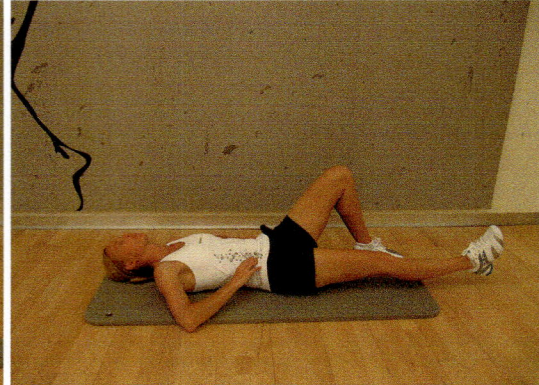

Training tips:

- Start lying on your back with both knees bent up.
- Switch on your core muscles.
- Do each of the exercises below.
- Slowly slide one heel out until leg straight and then back up again to the start position.

 Reps, 5–10; sets, 1–2; tempo, 5-0-5.

(b) Core base work: tighten and leg fall out

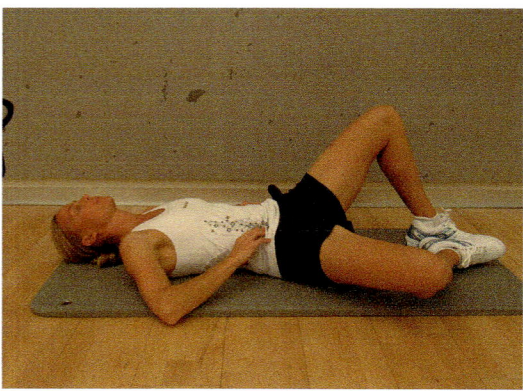

- Slowly let one leg fall out to the side and then back up again to start position.

(c) Base work supine/lying on your back: tighten and leg march

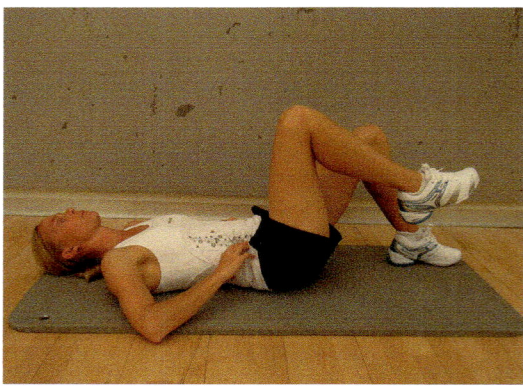

- Slowly march feet up and down.

(d) Core base work: tighten and arm/leg march

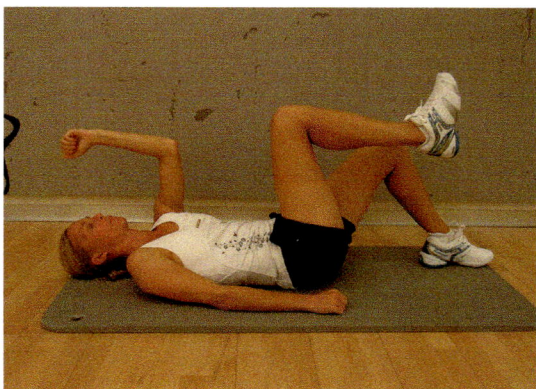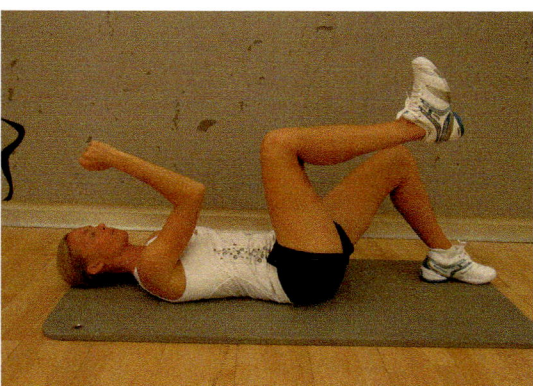

- Slowly move right arm and left leg toward each other (contralateral).
- Repeat with left arm and right leg.
- Try doing same side right arm and right leg/left arm and left leg (ipsilateral).

Reps, 5–10; sets, 1–2; tempo, 5-0-5.

39.19 Hip Base Work Series

39.19.1 Tennis Relevance

These exercises are important early progressions for improving general hip strength in non-weight-bearing positions. A longitudinal study looked at core stability parameters and found that weakness in hip external rotation was correlated with incidence of knee injury [24]. The literature indicates that decreased hip flexibility in rotation or decreased strength in abduction (positive Trendelenburg) was seen in 49% of athletes with arthroscopically proven posterior-superior labral tears [25]. Ensuring hip base work is carried out regularly will help augment hip and knee stability and improve kinetic chain function which helps protect against injury up and down the kinetic chain.

Clamshell hip abduction

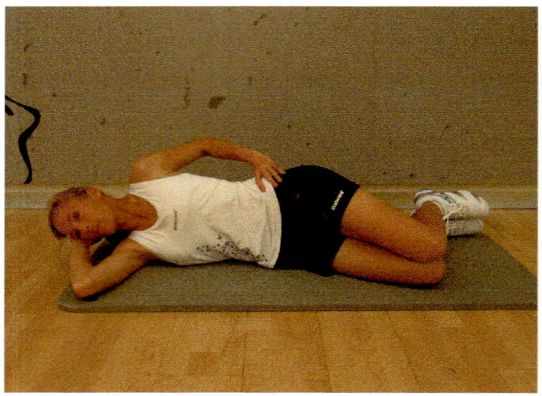
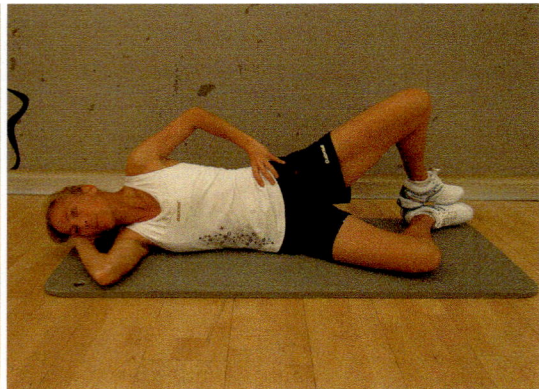

Training tips:

- Start lying on your side with both knees bent up.
- Switch on your core and raise one knee up keeping ankles together—like a clam opening its shell.
- Hold for 2 s and slowly return to start position for a 2-s count.

Reps, 5–10–15; sets, 1–3; tempo: 2-2-1.

Side lying hip adduction

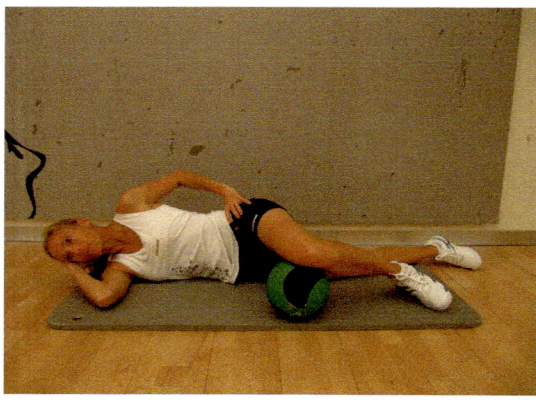
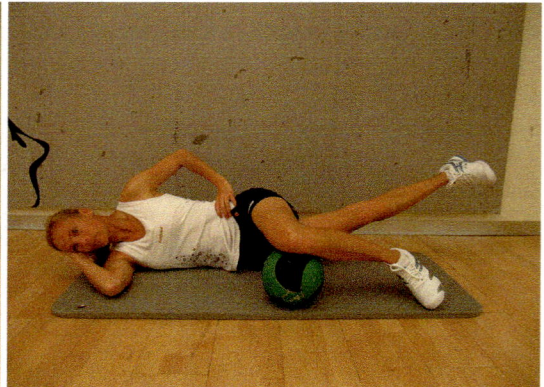

Training tips:

- Start lying on your side with top knee bent and placed a ball or small stool on the floor.
- Keep bottom knee straight.
- Switch on your core.
- Raise bottom leg up off the mat and hold for 2 s and lower to a count of 2 s.

Reps, 5–10–15; sets, 1–3; tempo, 2-2-1.

Side lying hip abduction

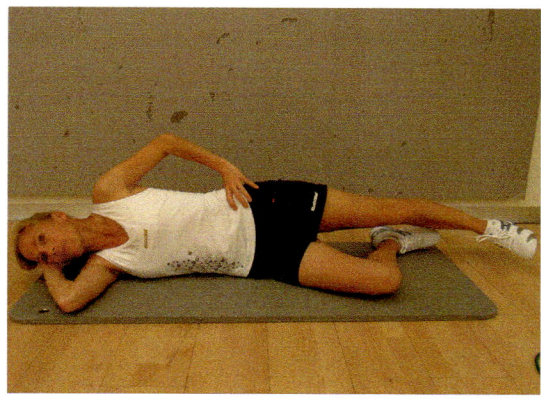 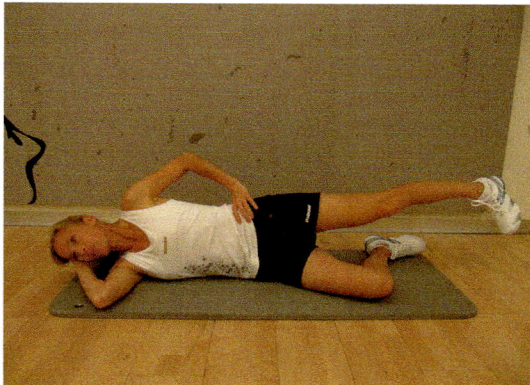

Training tips:

- Start lying on your side with bottom knee bent and top knee straight.
- Switch on your core.
- Point toes down to floor on top leg and raise leg up.
- Hold for 2 s and down slow for a 2-s count.

Reps, 5–10–15; sets, 1–3; tempo, 2-2-1.

Kneeling resisted hip rotation

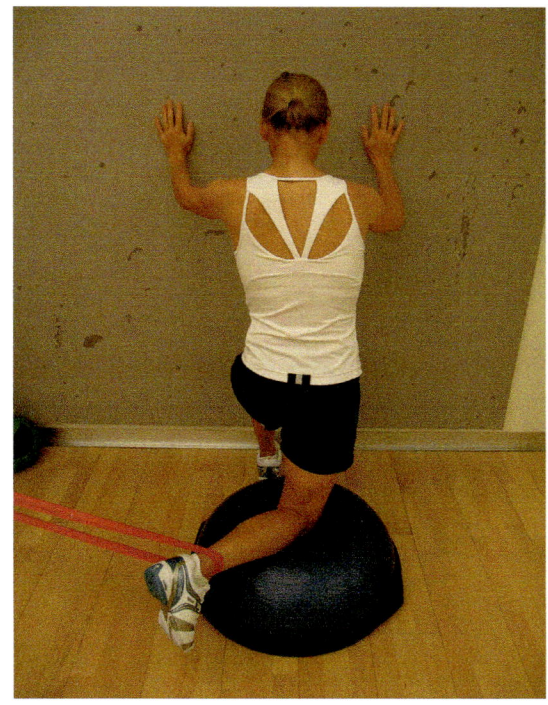 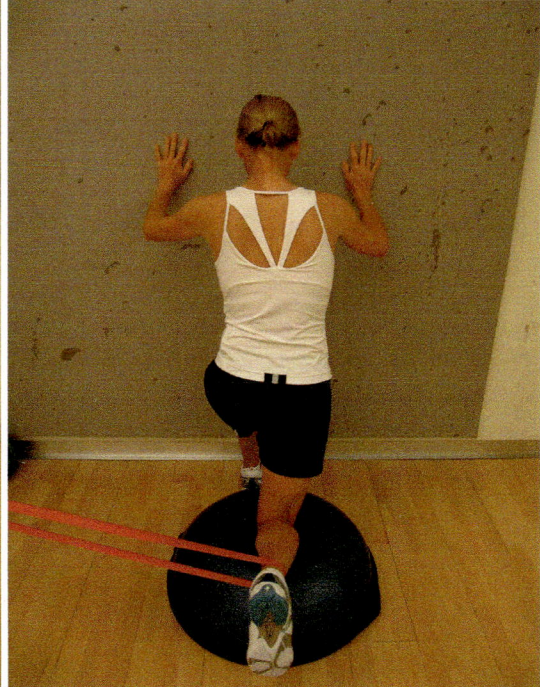

Training tips:

- Start in a kneeling lunge position with one knee on a BOSU® ball or other soft support with hands on the wall.
- Place a stretch band around the ankle and anchored to something stable.
- Switch on your core muscles.
- Now rotate hip internally or externally against stretch band resistance and back to start position.

Reps, 5–10–15; sets, 1–2; tempo, 1-2-1.

Seated hip rotations

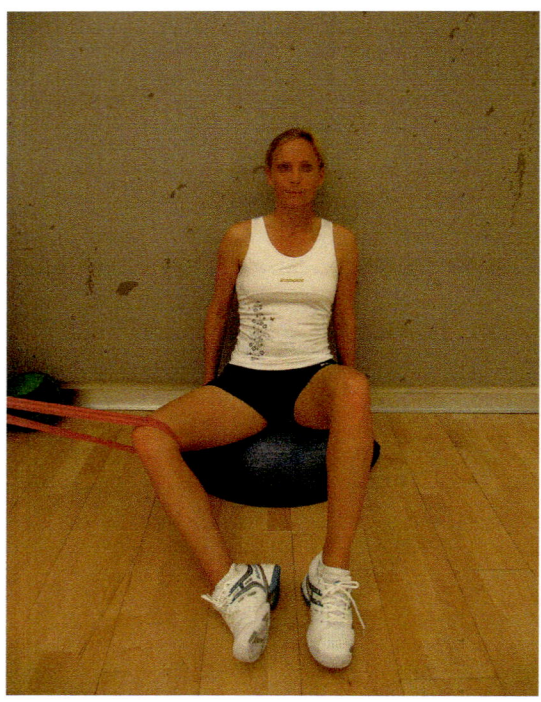 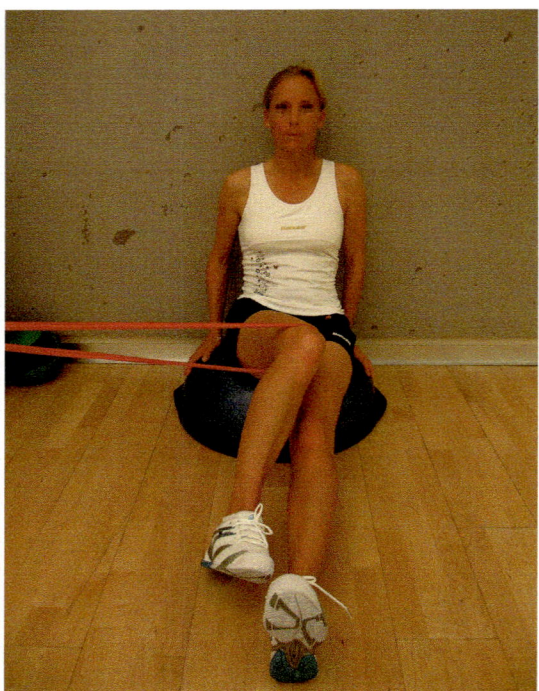

Training tips:

- Start seated on a BOSU® ball, other soft support, or a low bench.
- Place a stretch band around the knee and anchored to something stable.
- Switch on your core muscles.
- Now rotate hip against stretch band resistance and back to start position.
- Do for both internal and external hip rotation.

Reps, 5–10–15; sets, 1–2; tempo, 1-2-1.

39.20 Quadruped and Seated Bridging Series

39.21 Quadruped Bridge Series

(a) Quadruped bridge with rocking movements

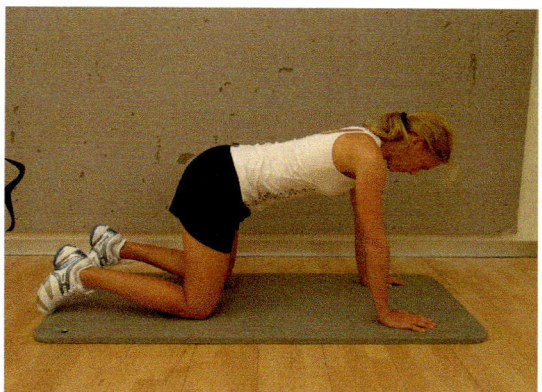
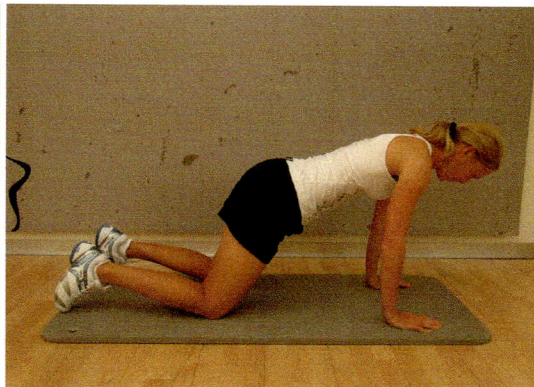

Training tips:

- Start kneeling on all fours and find your neutral position with back flat.
- Switch on your core muscles.
- Now rock back and forth in different motions.

Variations:

- Try front and back, side to side, diagonals, and circles

(b) Quadruped bridge and knee circles

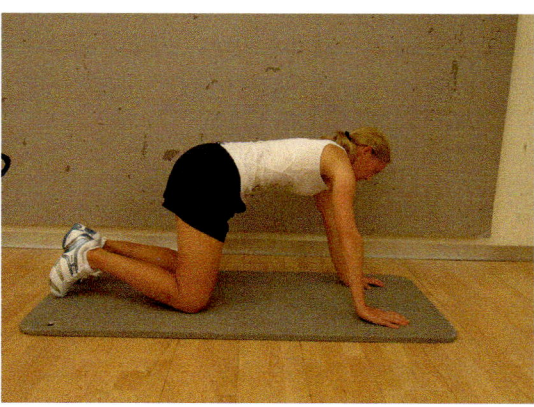
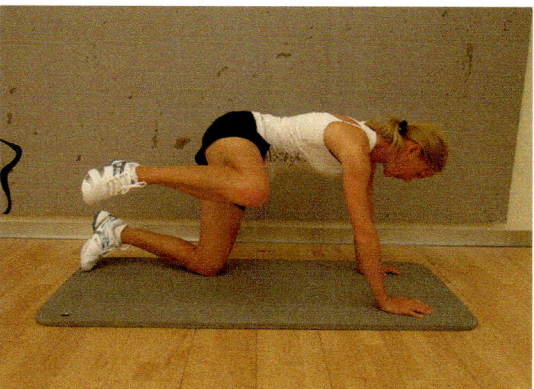

- Now raise one leg off the ground and do slow circles with your knee.

(c) Quadruped bridge single arm and leg raises

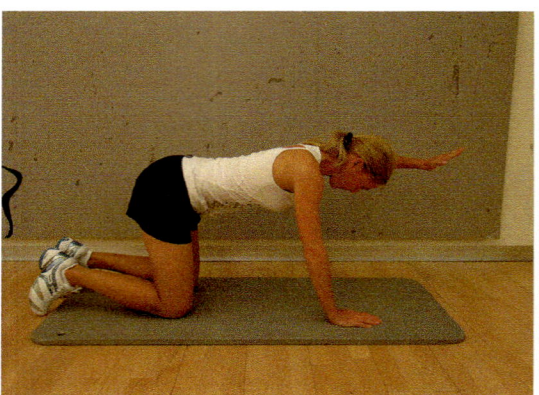
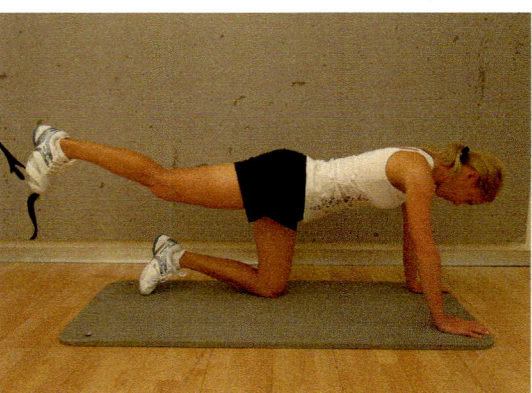

- Now raise one leg up and hold or one arm up and hold.
- Repeat on both sides.

(d) Quadruped bridge: opposite arm and leg raises

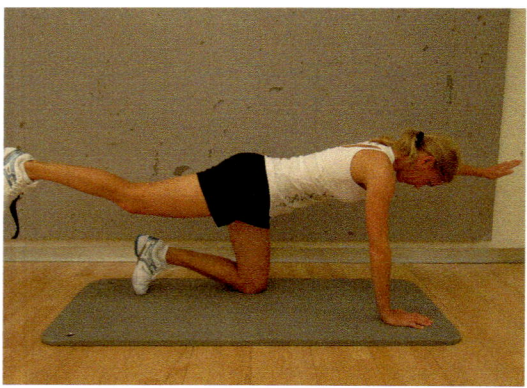

- Now raise one arm and opposite leg up and hold for 2 s.
- Repeat with opposite arm and leg.

Reps, 5–10; sets, 1–3; tempo, 1–1-1 or 1-2-1.

39.22 Connecting the Core Concepts

Connecting the core with upper and lower core stability training provides a stable three-dimensional power platform from which the extremities can work during multi-planar, multi-joint, and multi-muscle tennis strokes that involve acceleration and deceleration forces. Research has demonstrated that lower extremity position influences scapular muscle recruitment and muscle balance ratios in closed kinetic chain exercises [26]. As well, trunk and lower extremity position and movement influence scapular muscle recruitment and muscle balance ratios in open kinetic chain exercises [27]. By utilizing closed and partially closed chain exercises with varied resistance to increase stability of the different slings will help connect the core and improve the player's dynamic balance and athletic function. These exercises can be done in a variety of different body positions with additional force vectors added using elastic or other external resistance. Similar patterns have been well described in past literature on proprioceptive neuromuscular facilitation (PNF) patterns and techniques using spring systems [28].

Quadruped bridge and torso rotations with band resistance.

(a) Seated bridging with leg lift and diagonal pattern

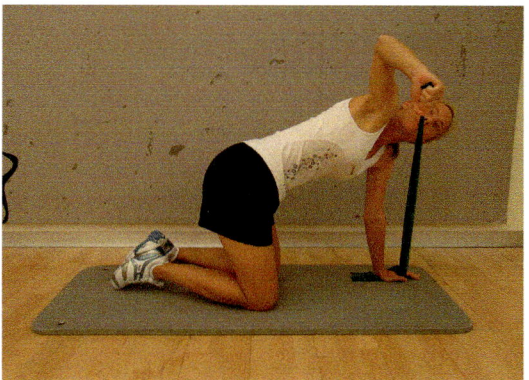

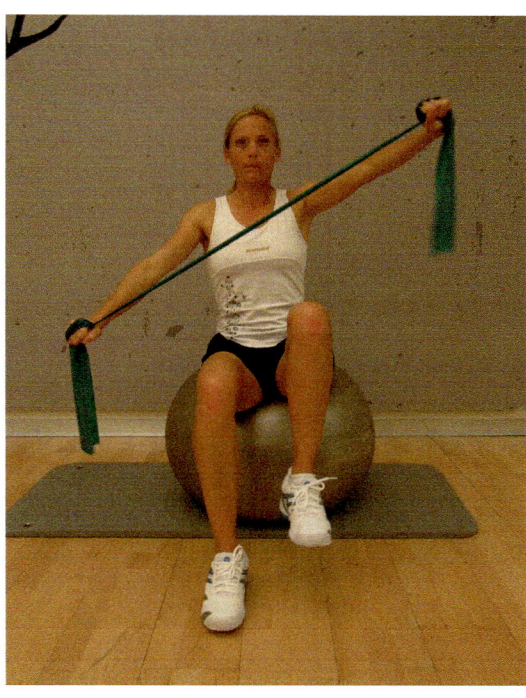

Training tips:

- Start kneeling on all fours and find your neutral position with back flat.
- Hold a stretch band in both hands.
- Switch on your core muscles.
- Now take one arm and thread through other arm rotating torso.
- Now rotate torso up raising arm with elbow bent retracting shoulder using stretch band for resistance.
- Repeat with opposite arm.

Reps, 10–15–20; sets, 2; tempo, 2-0-1.

Training tips:

- Start sitting on a physio/exercise ball with a stretch band in both hands.
- Switch on your core muscles and raise one foot off ground.
- Pull band in a diagonal pattern.

(b) Seated bridging with alternating bicep curls

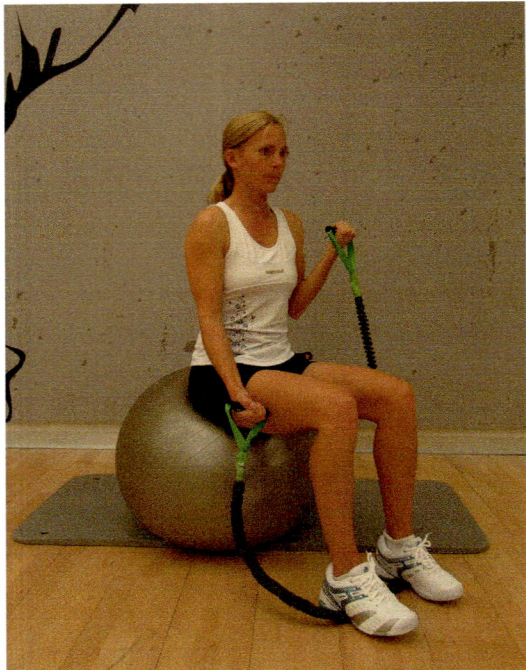

— Now raise one hand up doing a bicep curl with band elastic resistance or hand weights.

Reps, 5–10–15; sets 1–2; tempo, 1-2-1.

39.23 Supine Bridge (Hip/Hamstring Thrust) Series

39.23.1 Tennis Relevance

Hip extensor and hamstring stability and strength is required to decelerate the lower extremity during movements on court. It is especially important in hip-extended (open stance) groundstrokes and for low volleys (closed stance backhand). Female athletes rely more on their quadriceps muscles and respond to anterior (forward) tibial translation by activating their quadriceps first rather than their hamstrings [29]. Therefore hamstring-specific strength is needed to help overcome the quadriceps dominance seen in developing players especially females.

As well, gluteal and hamstring muscles are often weak and tight due to lifestyle factors including prolonged sitting.

Supine bridging/lying on your back

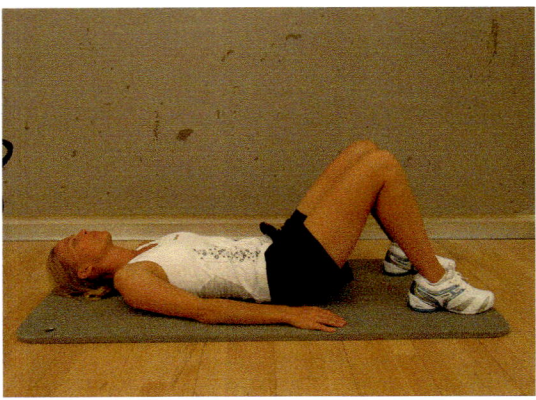
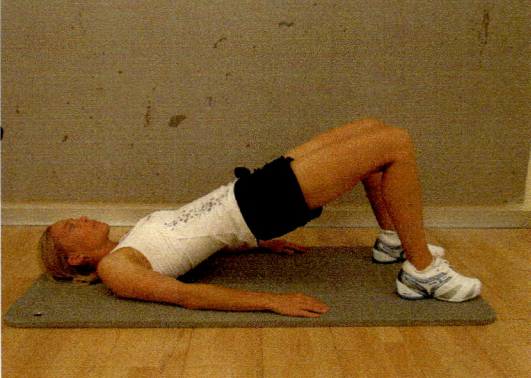

Training tips:

- Start lying on your back with both knees bent up.
- Switch on your core and raise hips off the mat.
- Hold for 4 s and lower back down to start position.
- Do with feet and knees hip width and feet and knees together.

Reps, 5–10; sets, 1–3; tempo, 1-4-1.

Supine bridging/lying on your back

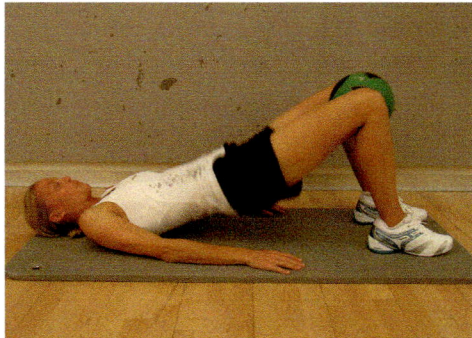

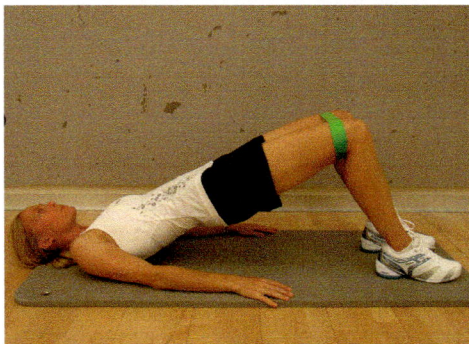

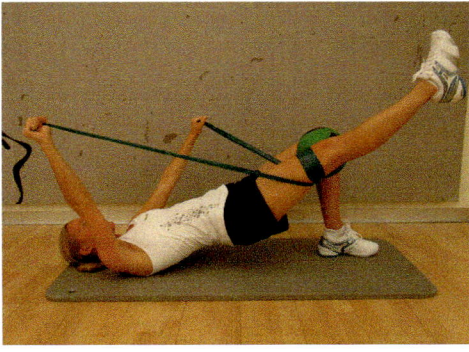

Training tips:

- Start lying on your back with both knees bent up.
- Switch on your core and raise hips off the mat while squeezing a small ball between knees or pulling a stretch band apart.
- Hold for 4 s and lower back down to start position.

Variations:

- Adding arm resistance will help stabilize the upper core.
- Squeezing a ball between knees and straightening one leg further challenge the lower core.

Reps, 5–10–15; sets, 1–3; tempo, 1-1-1 to 1-4-1.

Supine bridging and ball squeeze with single or double arm diagonal pull

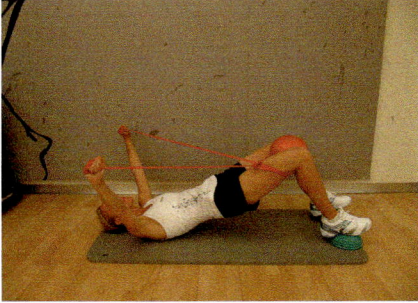

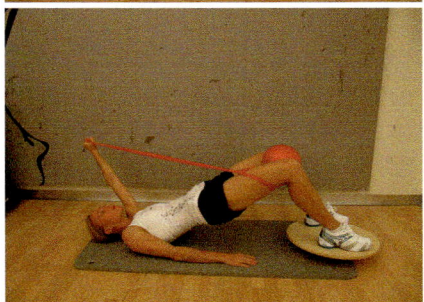

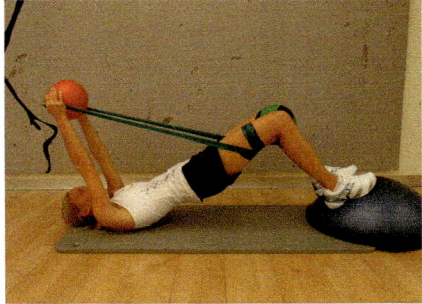

Training tips:

– Start in a supine bridge position with feet on a balance pod, wobble board, BOSU®, or other unstable base.
– Place a ball between your knees and squeeze gently.
– Hold a long stretch band anchored to legs.
– Switch on your core muscles.
– Raise hips up and pull one arm diagonally back with resistance from the stretch band.

Variations:

– Raise hips up and pull both arms diagonally back with resistance from the stretch band.
– Add a weighted ball; add to the core challenge.

Reps, 5–10; sets, 1–3; tempo, 3-1-1.

Supine bridge and hamstring thrust

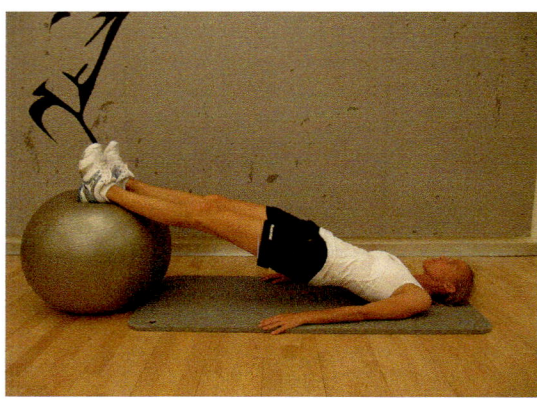
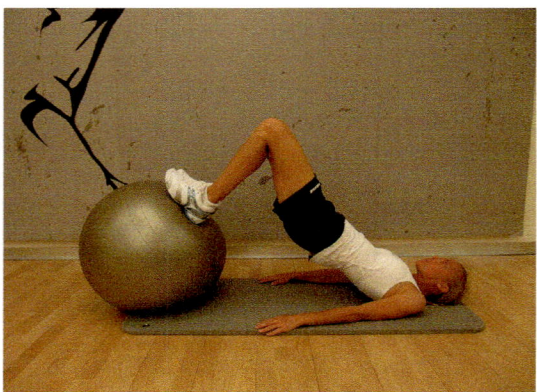

Training tips:

– Start lying on your back with lower leg and feet on a physio/exercise ball.
– Switch on your core muscles.

– Bridge/thrust hips up and pull ball toward the buttocks and hold for 2 s and return to start position.

Reps, 5–10; sets, 1–3; tempo, 1-2-1.

Supine bridge and hamstring pull ball between knees

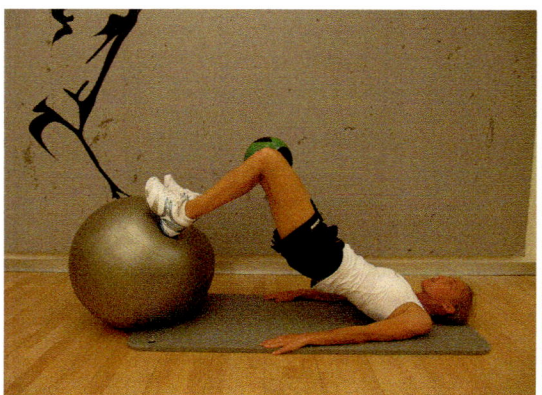
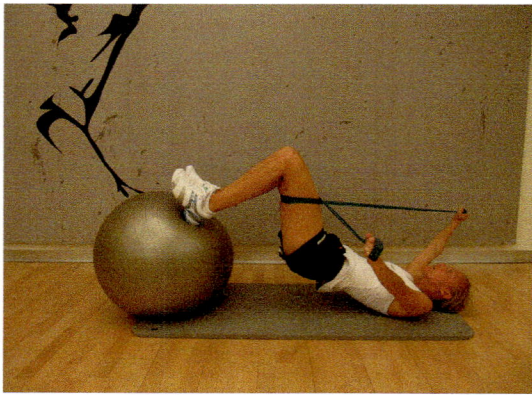

Training tips:

- Start lying on your back with lower leg and feet on a large physio/exercise ball.
- Place a small ball between knees and squeeze lightly.
- Switch on your core muscles.
- Bridge up hips and pull ball toward the buttocks and hold for 2 s and return to start position.
- This exercise can also be done pulling a stretch band for resistance.

Reps, 5–10; sets, 1–3; tempo, 1-2-1.

39.24 Prone and Lateral Bridging Series

39.24.1 Tennis Relevance

These bridging exercises are primarily isometric in nature with some use of stretch-shortening cycle as you move into position. They help provide a stable platform or base of support which provides proximal stability for distal mobility and control. They strengthen the combined upper and lower core by augmenting the functional slings helping to protect against injury.

Prone bridging on forearms and knees or toes

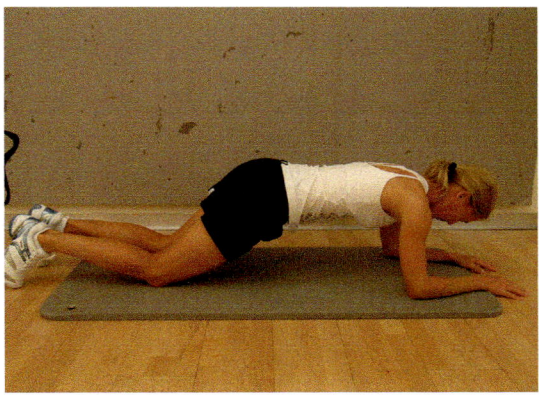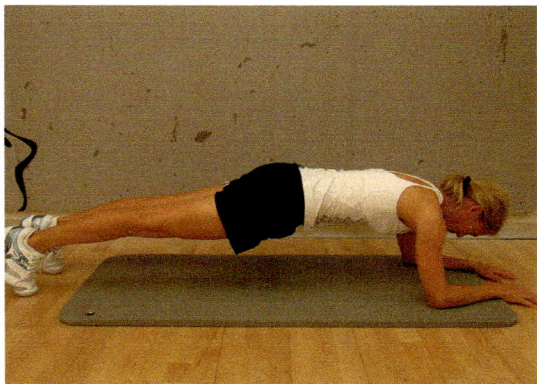

Training tips:

- Start lying in prone/on stomach.
- Now bridge up on to knees or toes (depending core strength) and forearms.
- Switch on your core muscles and find your neutral position with back flat and hold.
- Beginners should start off their knees and progress to off toes as strength improves.

Reps, 5–10; sets, 1–2; tempo, 1-5-1 to 1-10-1 to 1-20-1.

(a) Prone bridging and single limb raise

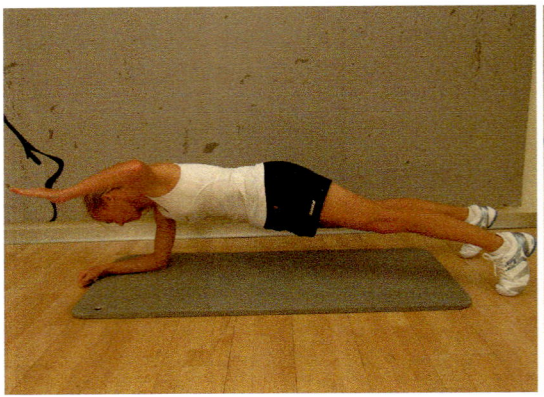
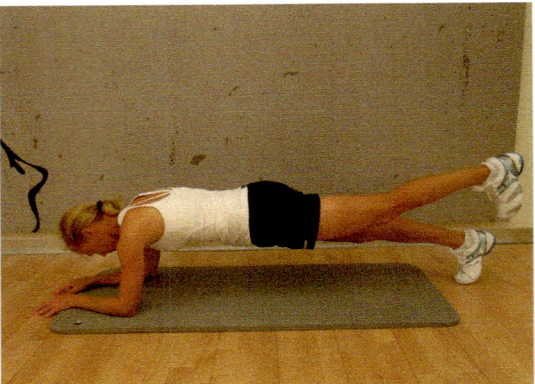

Training tips:

- Start in a prone bridge position on forearms and toes.
- Switch on your core muscles.
- Now raise up one leg or one arm and hold.

(b) Prone bridging with opposite arm and leg raise

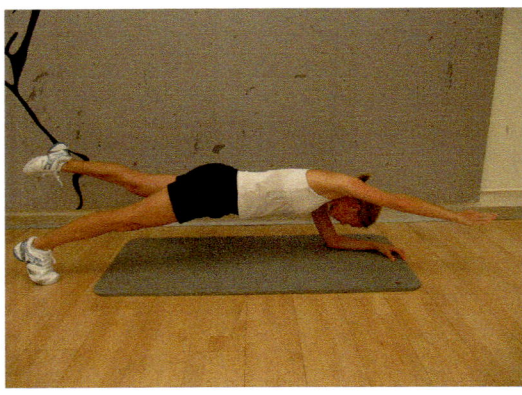

- Now raise up opposite arm and leg and hold.

Reps, 5–10; sets, 1–2; tempo, 1-3-1 to 1-5-1 to 1-10-1.

Prone bridge feet on ball and knee tuck

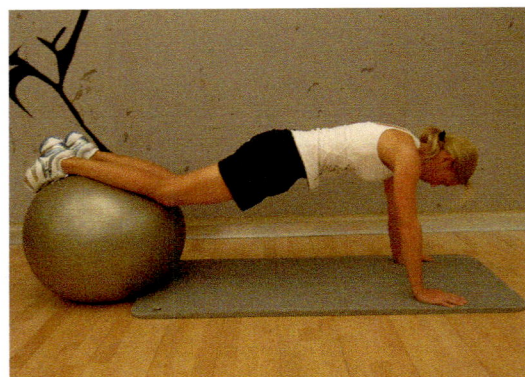
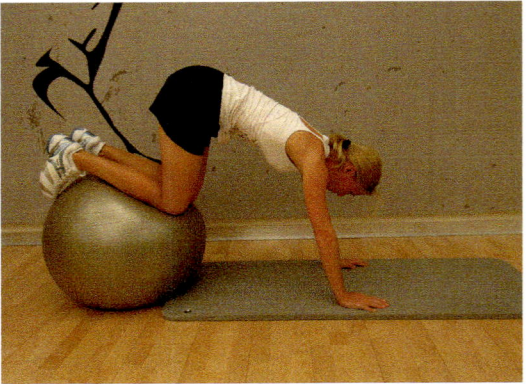

Training tips:

– Start in a prone push-up position with lower legs on a physio/exercise ball and extended out behind you.
– Switch on your core muscles.
– Pull ball up toward hips maintaining a stable core and keeping a neutral spine position.
– Then return to the start position.

Reps, 5–10; sets, 1–2; tempo, 3-0-1 or 1-0-1.

Lateral bridging with arm raise and knee drive

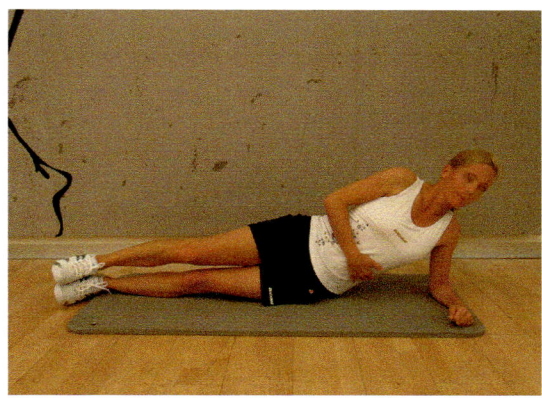 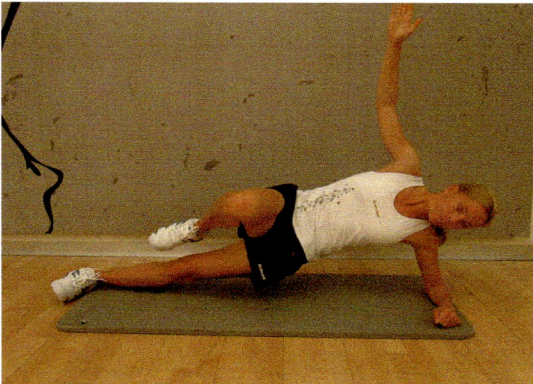

Training tips:

– Lying on your side with forearm on a mat.
– Switch on your core muscles.
– Bridge your hips up and then raise one arm and one leg up and hold.

Reps, 5–10; sets, 1–2; tempo, 1-5-1 to 1-10-1.

Lateral bridging on physio ball with leg raise

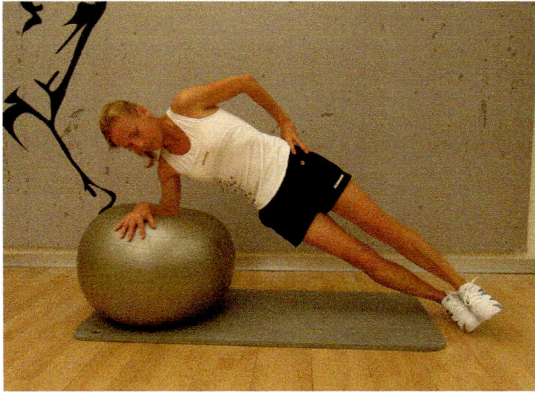 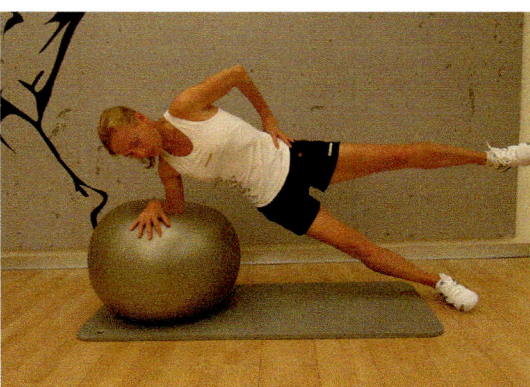

Training tips:

- Start in a lateral bridge position with feet on the floor and forearm and hand on a large
- physio/exercise ball.
- Switch on your core muscles.
- Place upper hand on hips and raise leg up and hold.

Reps, 5–10; sets, 1–2; tempo, 1-3-1 to 1-5-1.

39.25 Core Deceleration and Rotation Series

39.25.1 Tennis Relevance

The muscles comprising the cylindrical lower and upper core must contract and relax during all tennis strokes. There function and stability are important to allow for shoulder and hip separation during the service motion and other strokes. The obliques need to be trained for endurance, strength, and power during both concentric-acceleration and eccentric-deceleration phases of the strokes. This will improve performance and protect against injury when hitting a large number of balls during on-court training or in match play situations.

Supine ball handover four positions

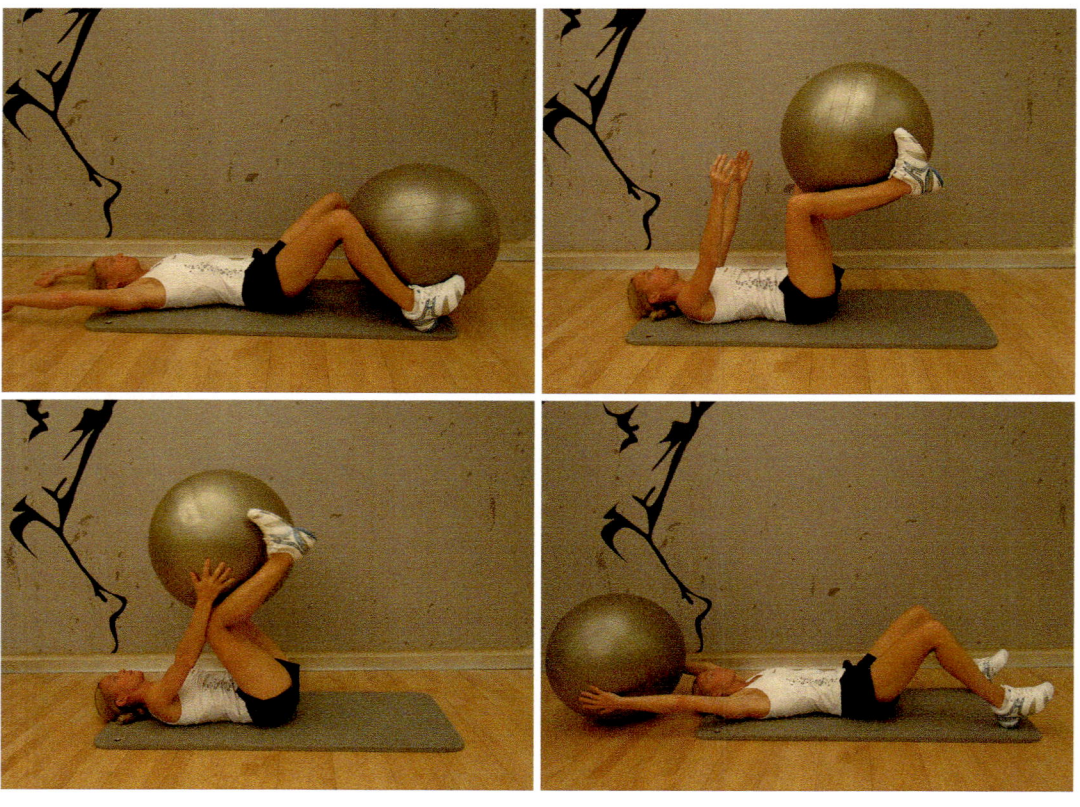

39 Strength and Conditioning of the Hips and Core (Practical Applications)

Training tips:

- Start lying on your back with a large physio/exercise ball between ankles.
- Switch on your core muscles.
- Now raise legs and arms up to exchange physio/exercise ball from ankles to hands and then lower overhead.

Reps, 10–15–20; sets, 1–2; tempo, 1-1-1.

Sit downs sitting on a ball

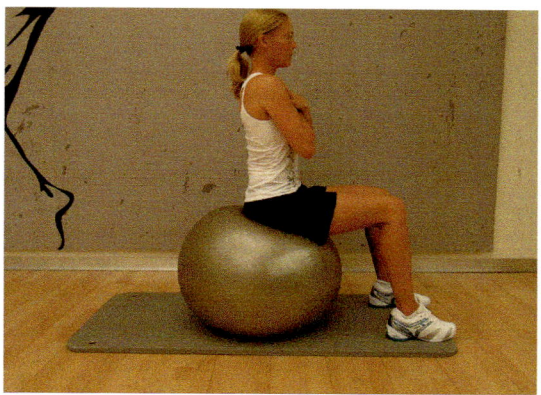
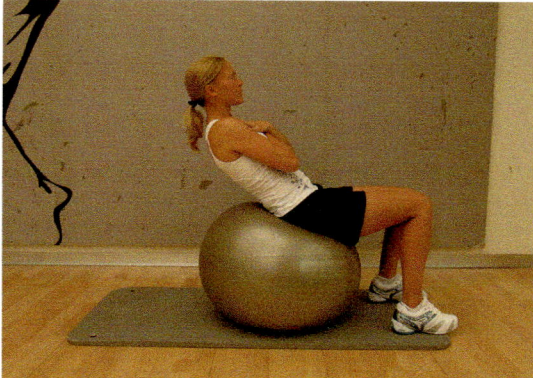

Training tips:

- Start sitting on a physio/exercise ball with knees together and feet apart.
- Switch on your core muscles.
- Lean back slowly working your abdominals as they lengthen and then return to start position.

Sit downs with medicine ball on chest

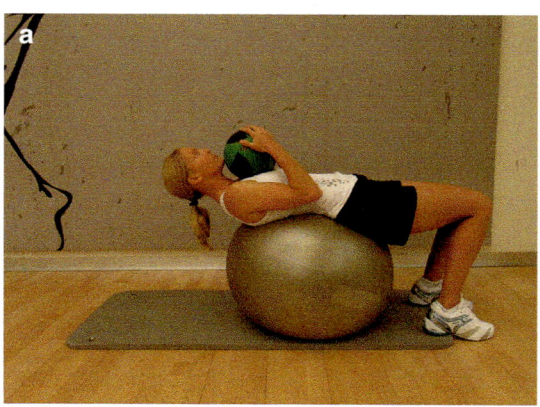
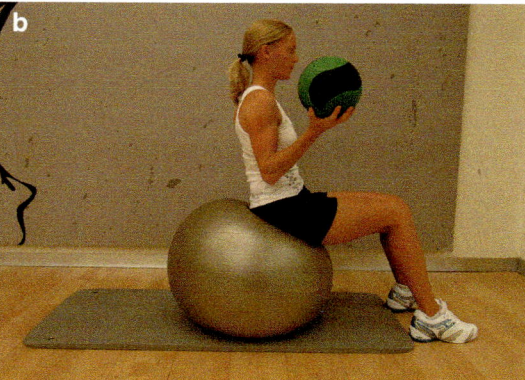

- Hold a medicine ball on chest.
- Switch on your core muscles.

Sit downs with medicine ball in hand

- Lean back slowly working your abdominals as they lengthen and then return to start position.

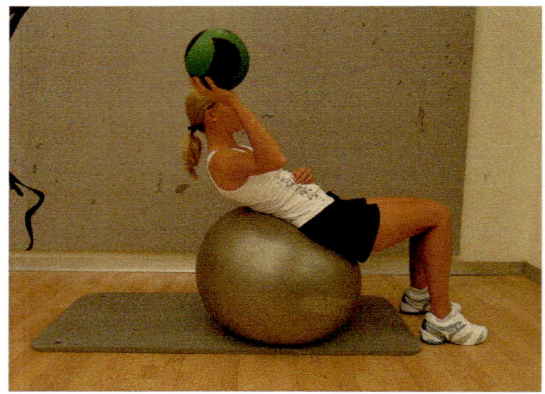
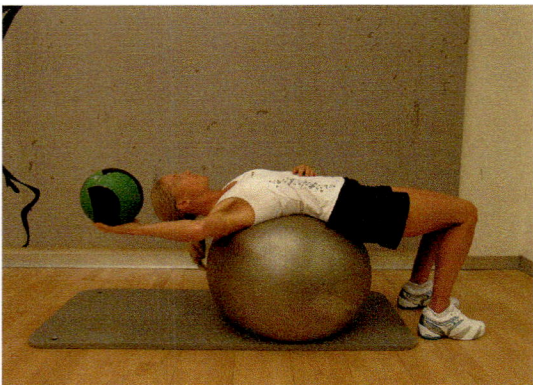

Training tips:

- Hold a medicine ball in one hand.
- Switch on your core muscles.

Seated diagonal torso twists

- Lean back slowly working your abdominals as they lengthen and then return to start position.
- Repeat on both sides.

Reps, 10–15–20; sets, 1–2; tempo, 1-1-1 or 1-0-*.

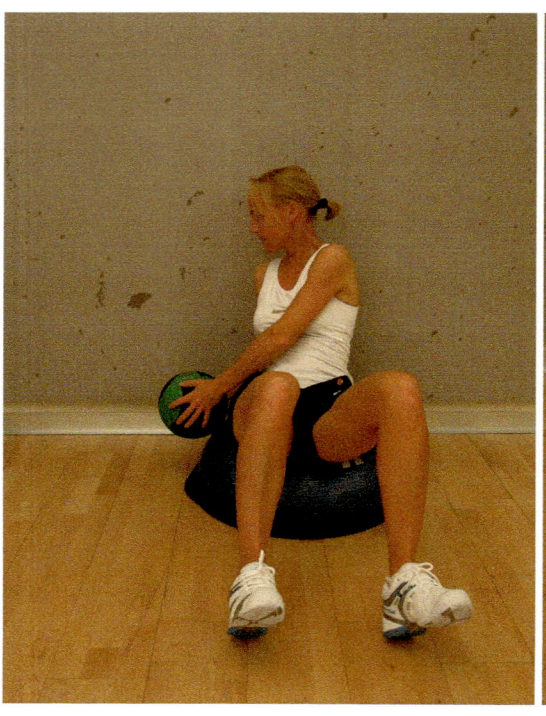
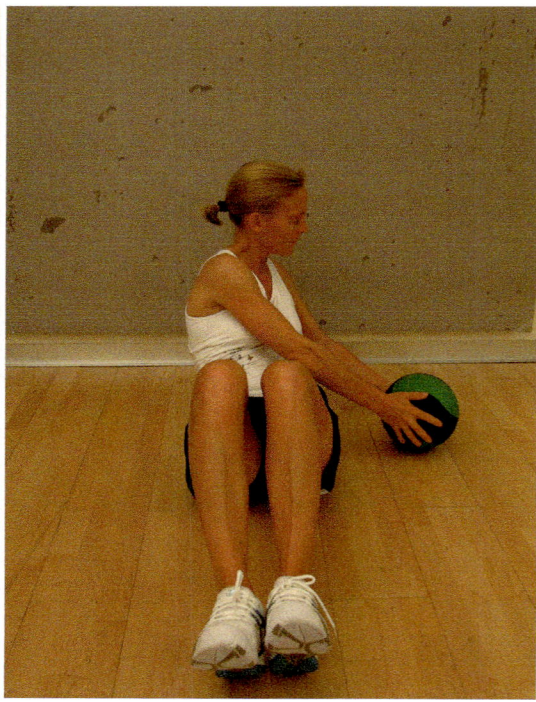

39 Strength and Conditioning of the Hips and Core (Practical Applications)

Training tips:

- Start sitting on the floor, on a BOSU® ball, or other unstable base.
- Hold a medicine ball in hands with arms straight.
- Switch on your core muscles.
- Now rotate torso and touch medicine ball close to the floor on each side of the hips and return back to start position.

Reps, 10–15–20; sets, 1–3; tempo, 1-1-1 or 1-0-*.

Seated horizontal torso twists

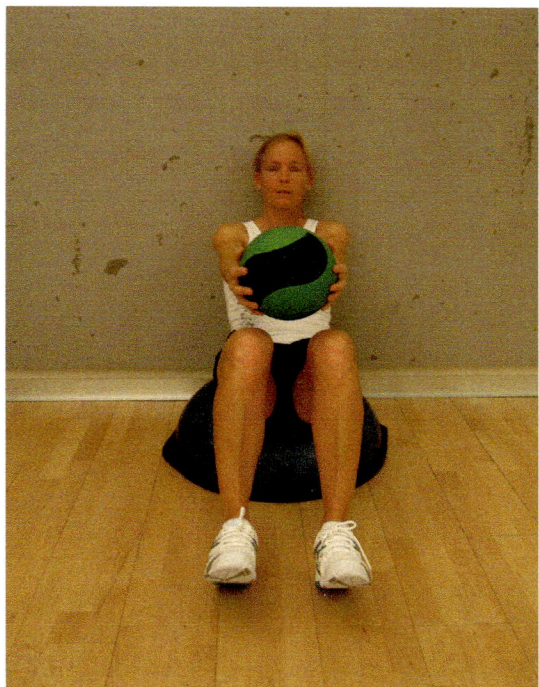
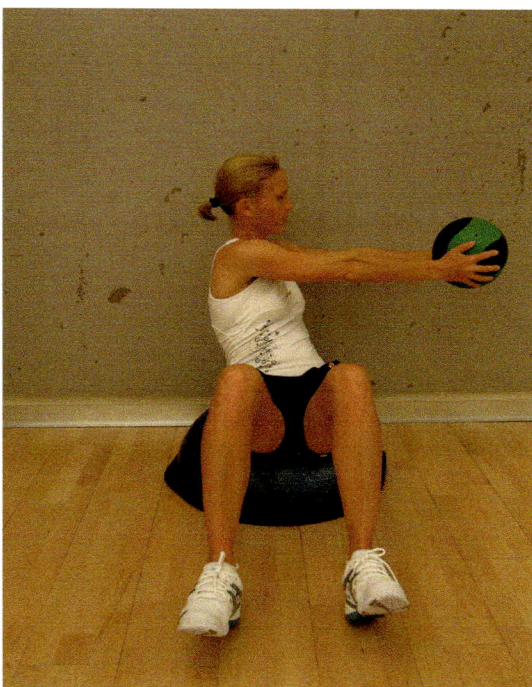

Training tips:

- Start sitting on the floor, on a BOSU® ball, or other unstable base.
- Hold a medicine ball in hands with arms straight.
- Switch on your core muscles.
- Now rotate torso and keeping arms horizontal to the floor and return back to start position.

Reps, 10–15–20; sets, 1–3; tempo, 1-1-1 or 1-0-*.

Supine bridging with balls, bands, and torso rotation

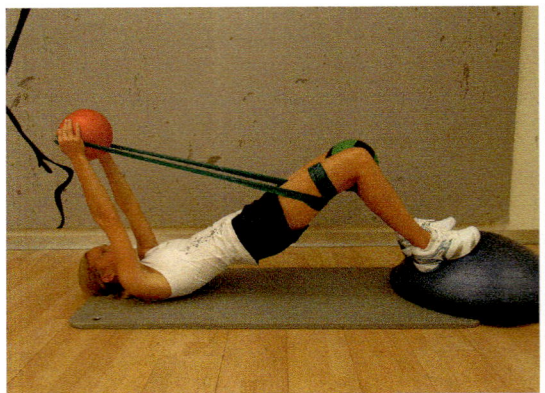
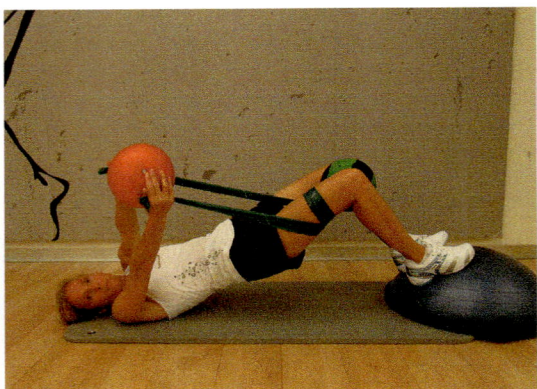

Training tips:

- Start in a supine bridge position with feet on a BOSU® ball or other unstable base.
- Place a ball in hands and between knees.
- Hold a long stretch band anchored to legs.
- Switch on your core muscles.
- Now squeeze the ball lightly between knees and raise hips up.
- Pull arms up and rotate torso with resistance from stretch band.

Reps, 5–10–15; sets, 1–3; tempo, 1-1-4, 1-1-2 or 1-1-*.

Supine bridge and torso rotation with ball squeeze

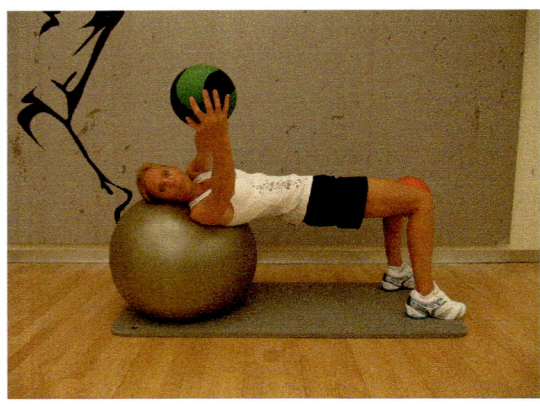
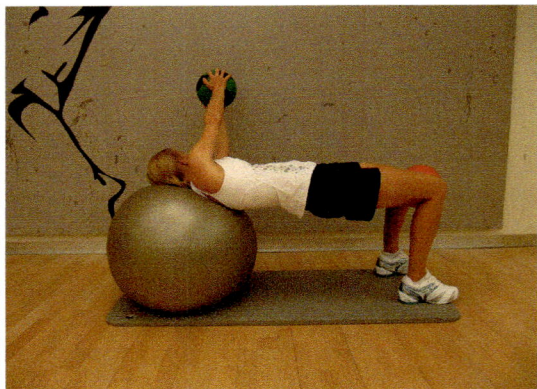

Training tips:

- Start lying with upper back over a large physio/exercise ball.
- Place a small ball between knees and squeeze lightly.
- Hold a medicine ball or lightweight overhead with arms straight.
- Switch on your core muscles.
- Rotate torso slowly from one side to the other.

Reps, 5–10–15; sets, 1–3; tempo, 1-1-4, 1-1-2 or 1-1-*.

39.26 Band Walk Series

39.26.1 Tennis Relevance

The unweighting required with the partial squats doing band walks increases coordination and timing required for effective first step movement in all directions. They as well help improve hip stability for single leg stance to transfer power from one leg to the other as the player moves into position. The drop and drive drills in lateral and diagonal directions emphasize the center of gravity (COG) over base of support (BOS) which helps to improve body posture and athletic balance.

Lateral band walks

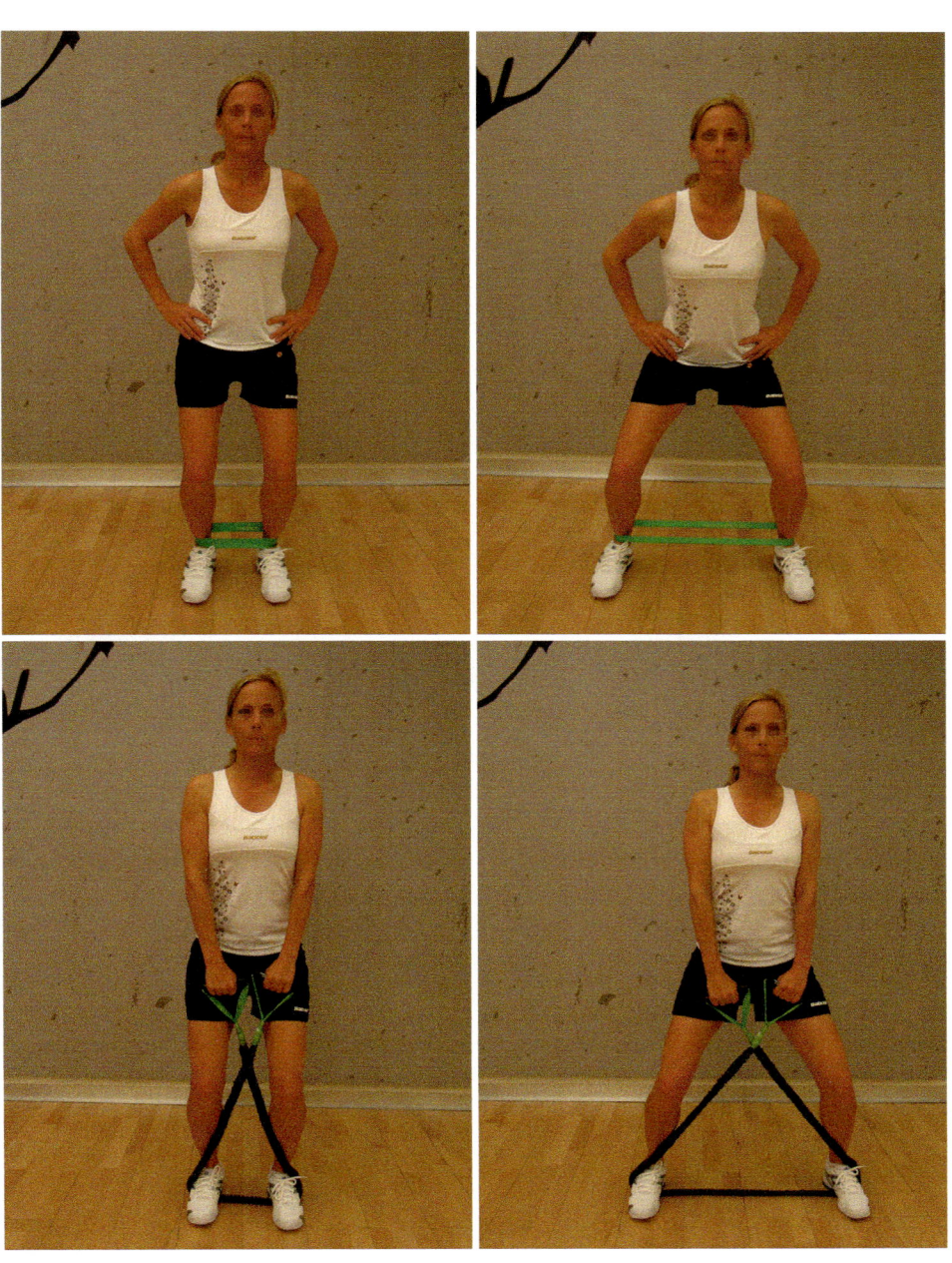

Training tips:

- Start standing in an athletic stance with a light stretch band around ankles or lower leg or a long cord under feet and anchored with hands.
- Switch on your core muscles.
- Squat or drop slightly and drive one leg laterally out with resistance from the elastic band.
- Can also be done holding a racket in your dominant hand.

Reps, 5–10; sets, 1–3; tempo, 1-1-2 or 1-1-1.

Diagonal band walks

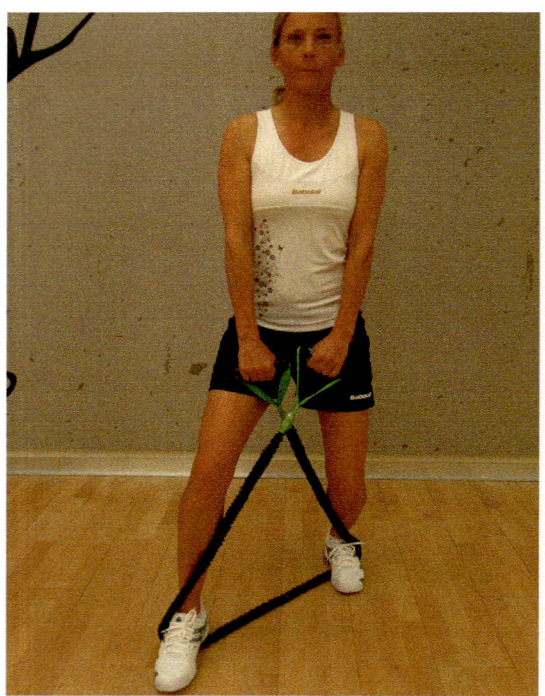 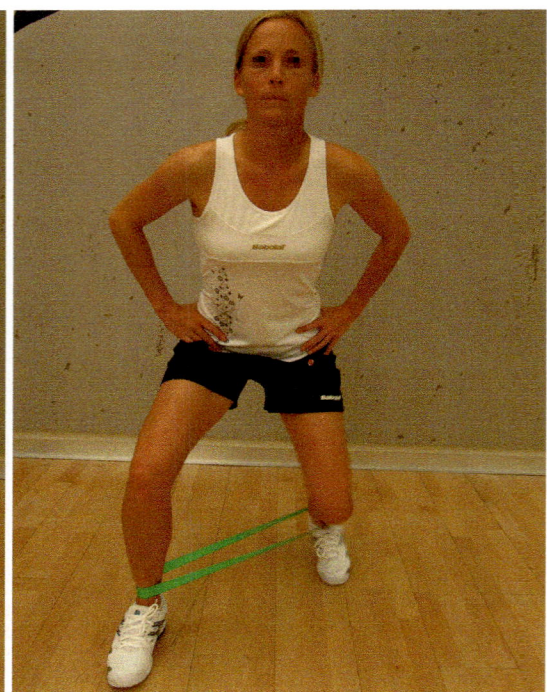

Training tips:

- Start standing in an athletic stance with a stretch band around ankles or lower leg or a long cord under feet and anchored with hands.
- Switch on your core muscles.
- Drop or squat slightly and drive one leg out on a diagonal with resistance from the elastic band.

Reps, 5–10; sets, 1–3; tempo, 1-1-2 or 1-1-1.

Diagonal band walks

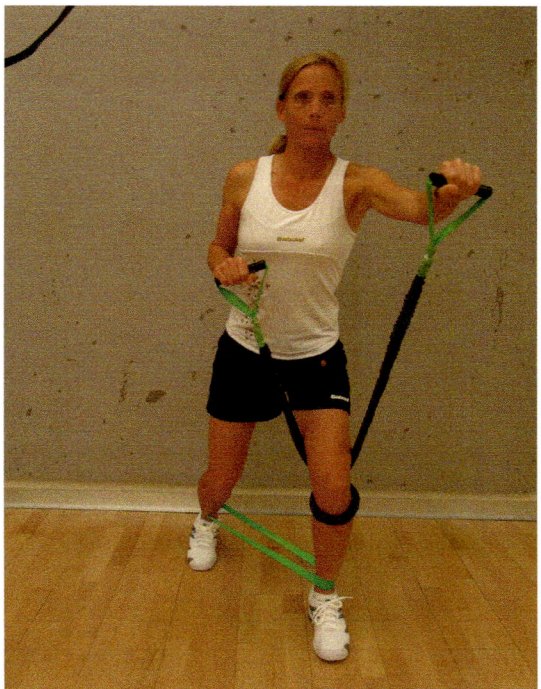
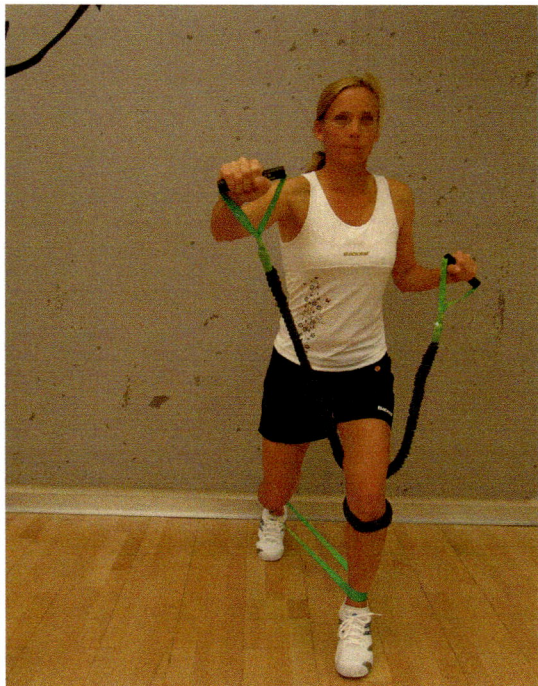

Training tips:

- Start standing in an athletic stance with a stretch band around ankles and a long cord attached to lower leg and held in hands.
- Switch on your core muscles.
- Drop or squat slightly and drive one leg back on a diagonal with resistance from the elastic band.
- At the same time, drive one arm forward on either the same (ipsilateral) or opposite (contralateral) side against the band resistance.

Reps, 5–10; sets, 1–3; tempo, 1-1-2 or 1-1-1.

39.27 Functional Squats and Step-Up Series

39.27.1 Tennis Relevance

All tennis strokes require weight-bearing movements that are initiated from the ground up and have strength and stability of the lower core and legs as a key factor. These exercises work on the large, strong prime movers and secondary muscles needed for push off and landing. They improve joint and muscle position sense (kinesthetic awareness), helping to center the joint and absorb stress. The athletic stance or ready position is improved on in preparation for first step speed and deceleration during direction changes. Squat movements provide a stable support base of the lower core and legs to hit all ground, and step-ups improve single leg stance stability.

(a) Wall squats: ball at back

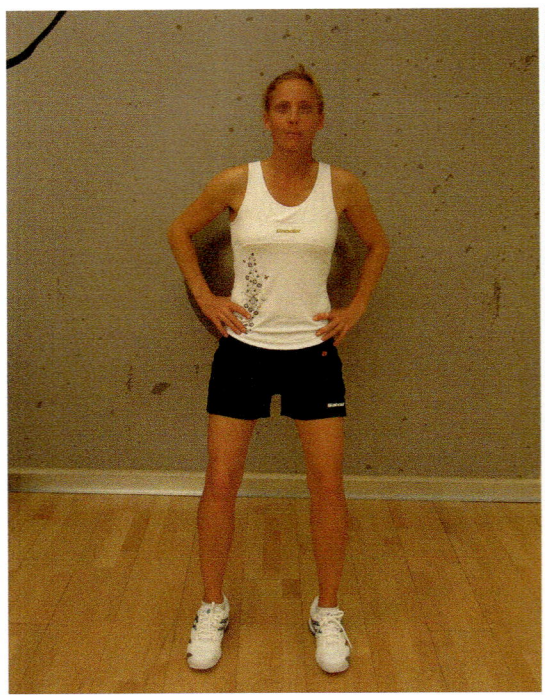 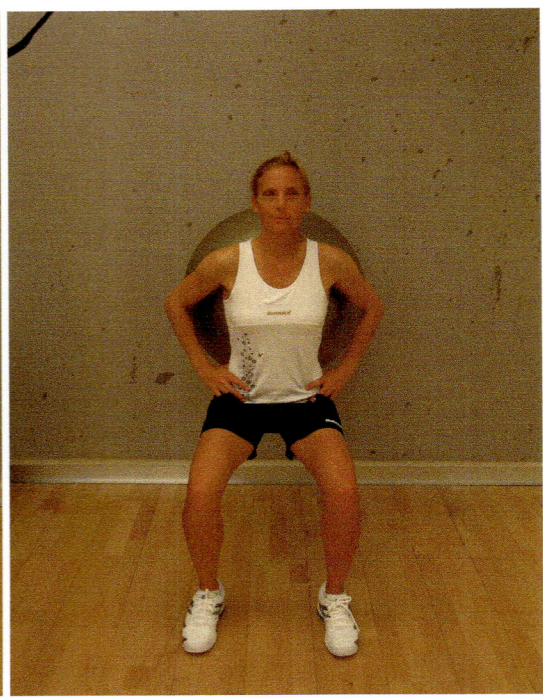

Training tips:

- Start standing tall with a physio ball at your back.
- Switch on your core muscles.
- Squat down slowly keeping knees aligned over toes and return to start position.

Variation:

- Can also be done with an unstable base under the feet

(b) Wall squats: ball at back with ball squeeze and band diagonal pull

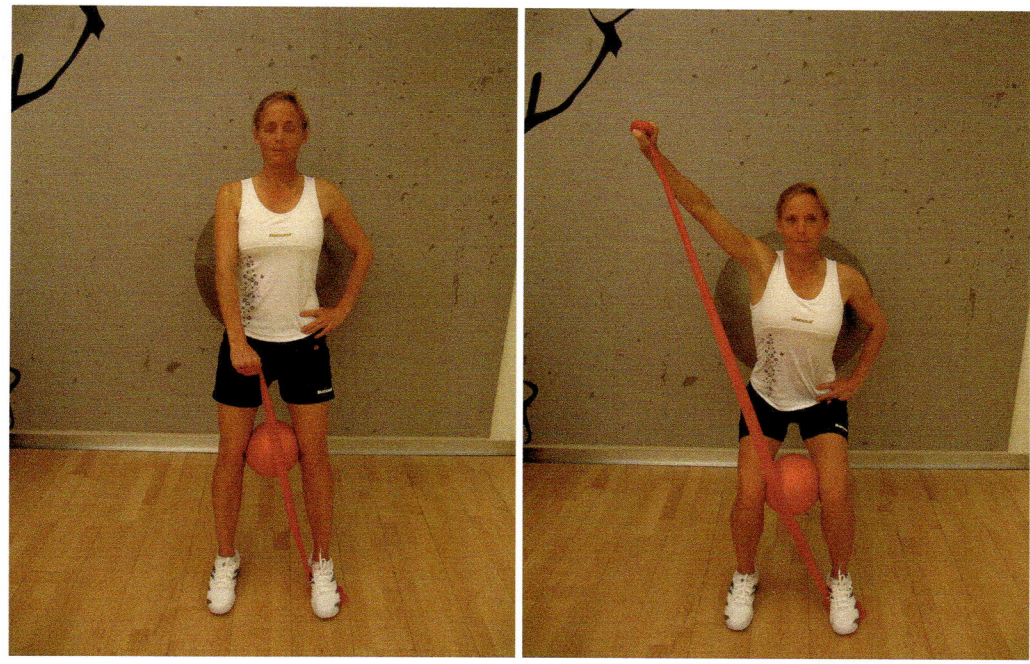

– Squeeze small ball lightly between your knees and do a diagonal pull with stretch cord anchored under foot.

Reps, 10–15–20; sets, 1–3; tempo, 2-0-1 or 3-0-1.

(a) Sumo squats: ball at back

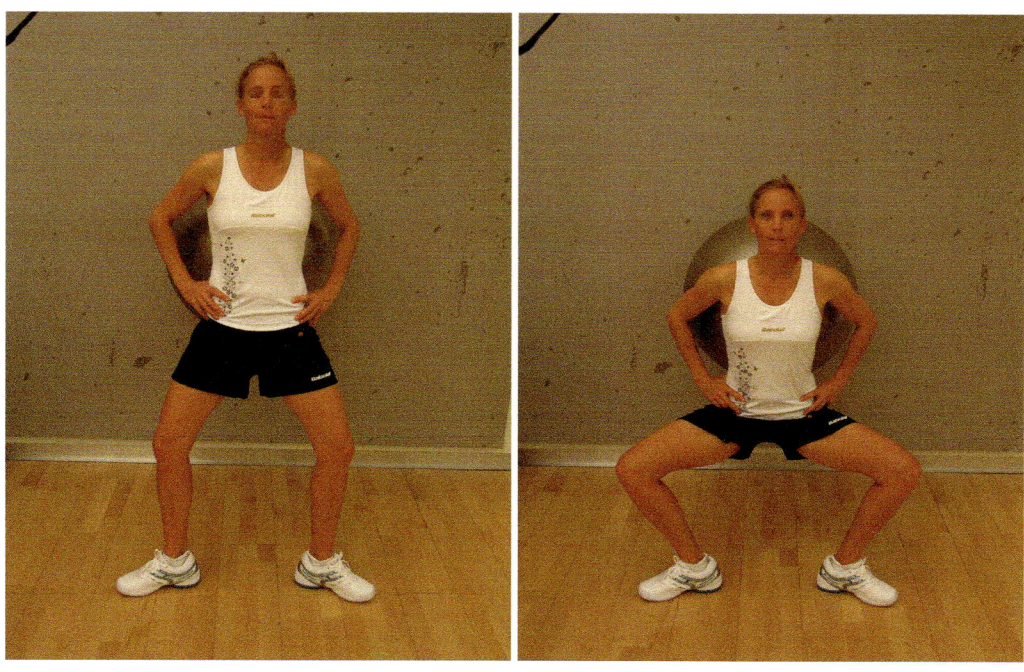

Training tips:

- Start standing tall in a sumo squat position with a physio ball at your back.
- Switch on your core muscles.
- Squat down slowly keeping knees aligned over toes and return to start position.

(b) Sumo squats with diagonal pull

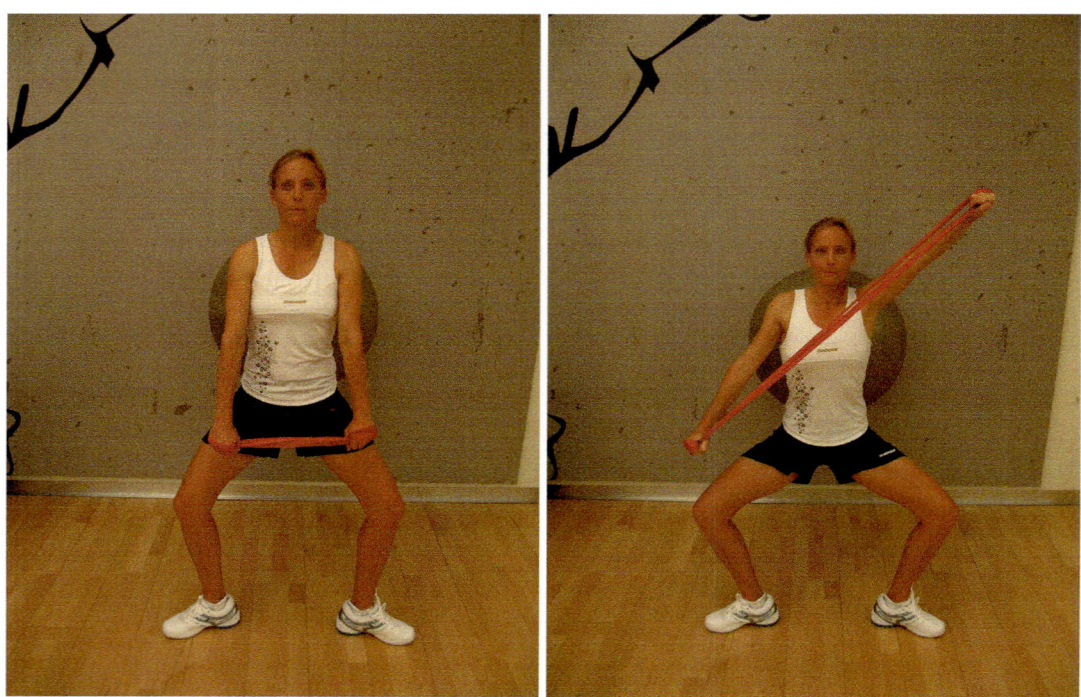

- Squat down slowly keeping knees aligned over toes and pull a stretch band in a diagonal then return to start position.

Reps, 10–15–20; sets, 1–3; tempo, 2-0-1 or 3-0-1.

Single leg ¼ squat: ball at side

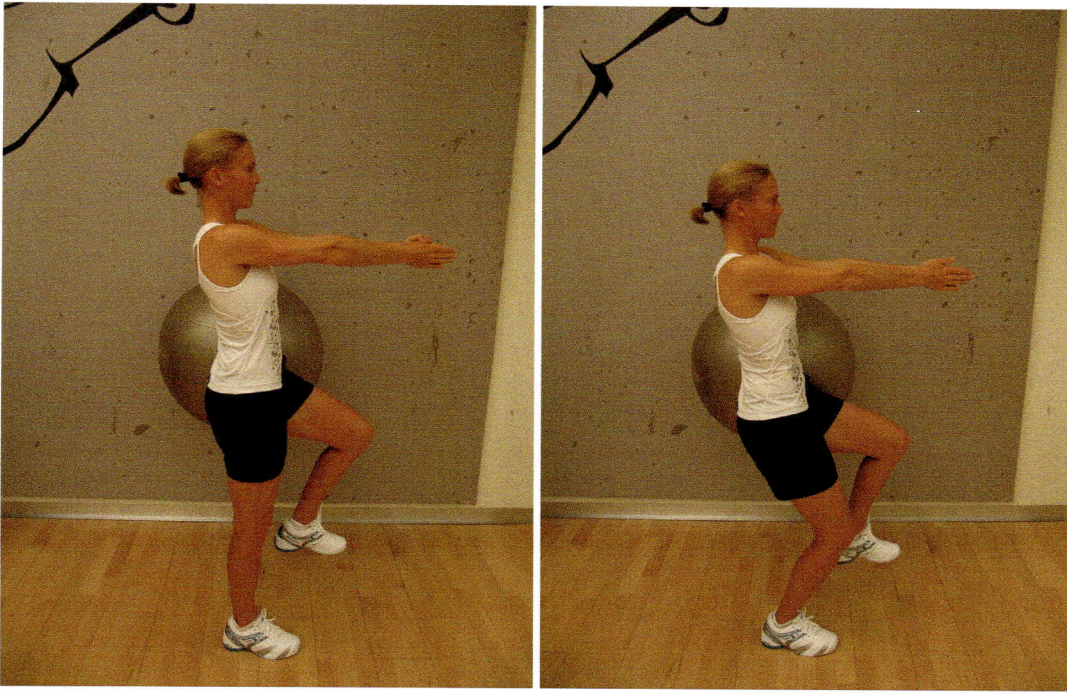

Training tips:

- Start standing on one leg with a physio ball at your side against a wall.
- Lift inside knee to hip height.
- Switch on your core muscles.
- Do a single leg ¼ squat down.
- Keep stance knee aligned over toes but not going past them.

Reps, 5–10; sets, 1–3; tempo. 2-0-1 or 1-0-*.

Step-ups with knee drive and diagonal ball raise

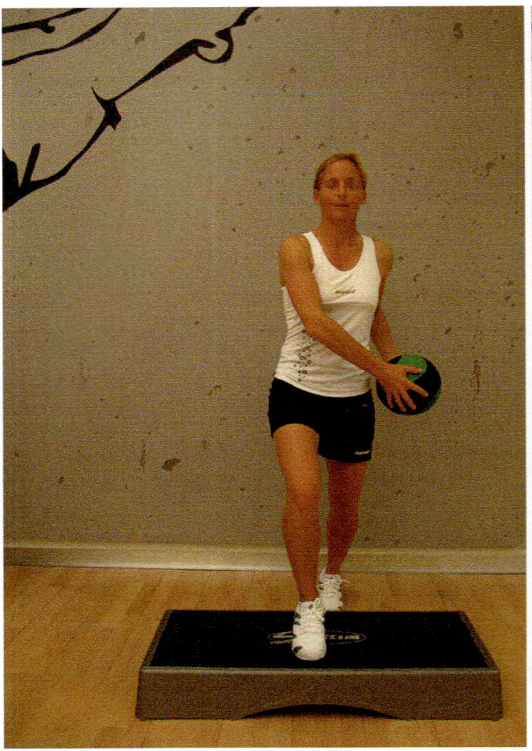 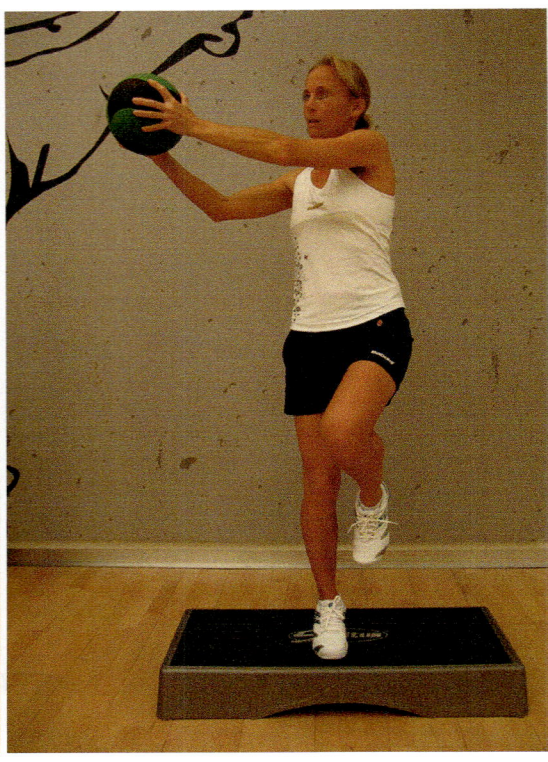

Training tips:

- Stand with one foot on a step.
- Switch on your core muscles.
- Do a 45-degree step-up.
- Resistance can be added with dumbbells or a barbell.

Reps, 10–15–20; sets, 1–3; tempo, 2-0-1 or 1-0-*.

Petersen (back lateral) step-ups

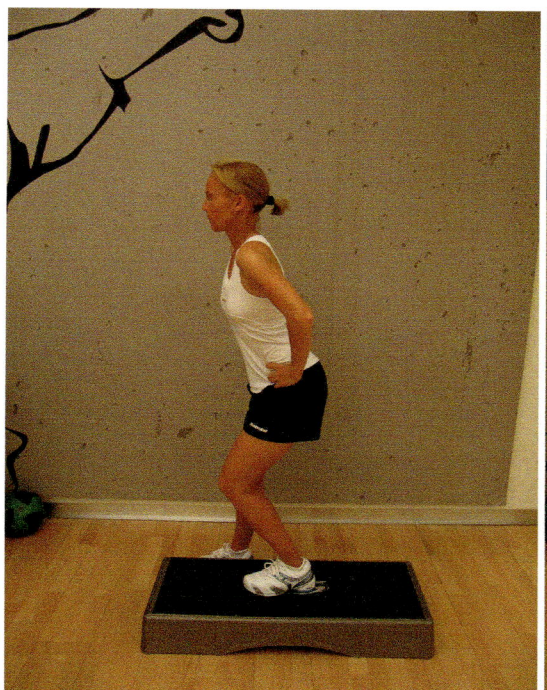
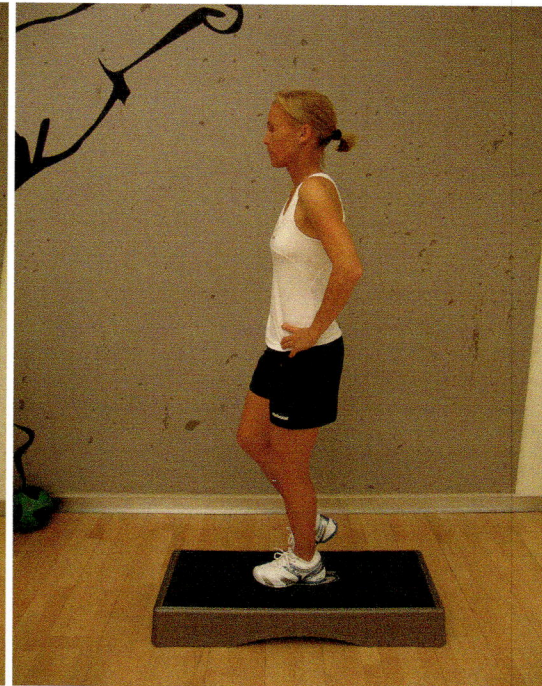

Training tips:

- Stand sideways to low step with one foot in a back lateral position (toe in line with heel).
- Switch on your core muscles and drive hip back at an angle until COG over back foot.
- Now do a back lateral step-up and return to start position.
- Resistance can be added with dumbbells or a barbell.

Reps, 10–15–20; sets, 1–3; tempo, 2-0-1 or 2-0-*.

Step-ups with knee drive and diagonal ball raise

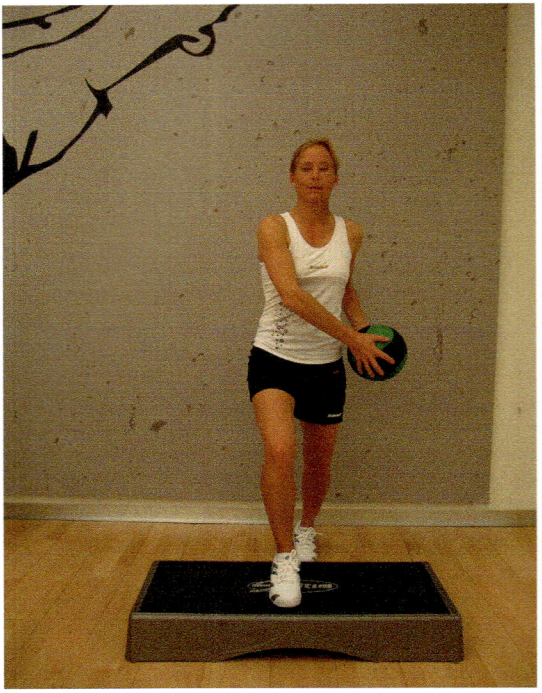 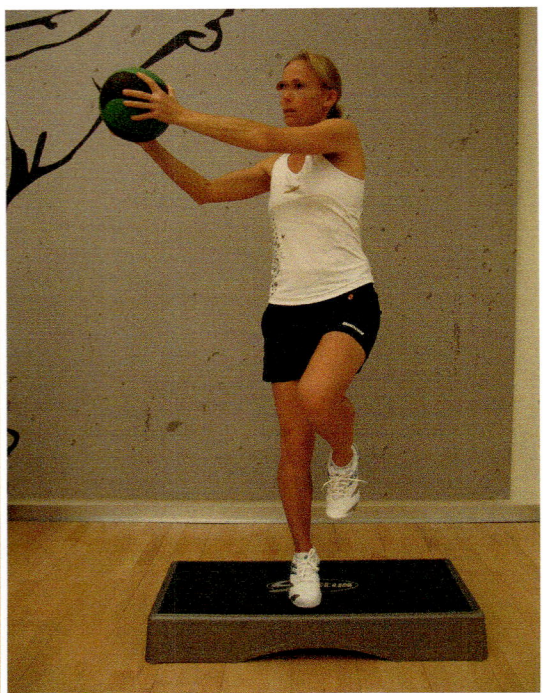

Training tips:

- Stand with one foot on a step holding a medicine ball at one side of your hips.
- Switch on your core muscles.
- Do a step-up and drive one knee up to hip height at the same time as moving the medicine ball in a diagonal pattern.

Reps, 10–15–20; sets, 1–3; tempo, 2-0-1 or 1-0-*.

Step-ups with knee drive and diagonal band pull

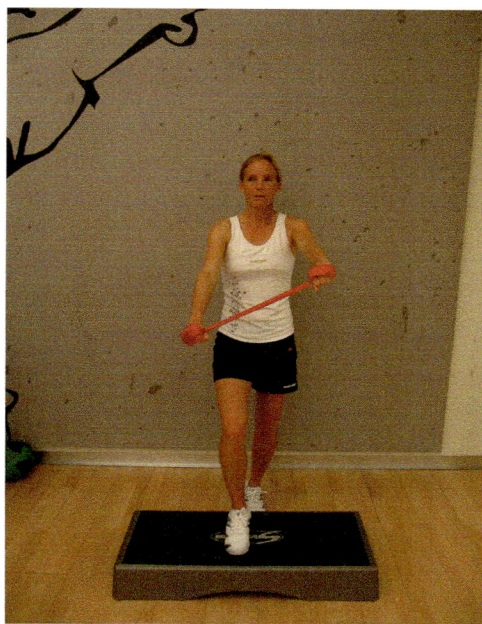 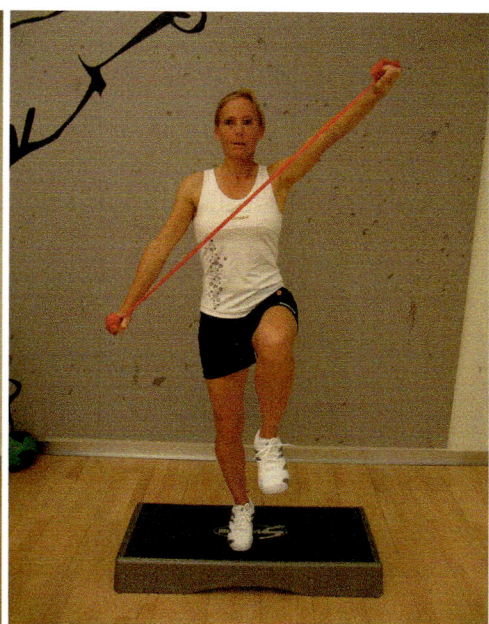

Training tips:

- Stand with one foot on a step holding a stretch band in both hands.
- Switch on your core muscles.
- Do a step-up and drive one knee up to hip height at the same time doing a diagonal pull with the stretch band.

Reps, 10–15–20; sets, 1–3, 2; tempo, 2-0-1 or 1-0-*.

Side step-ups with bicep curls

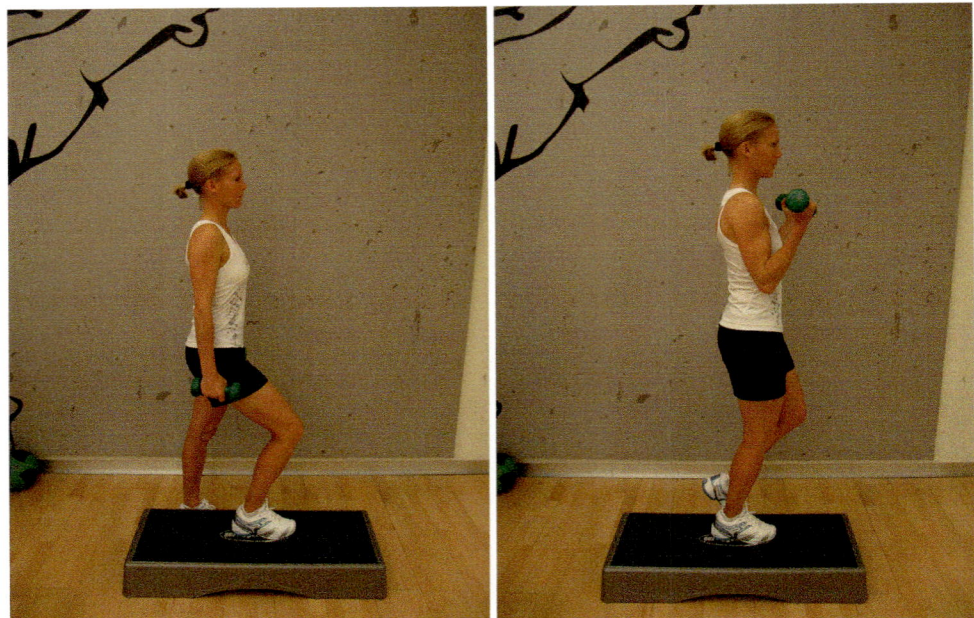

Training tips:

- Stand sideways to a step with one foot on holding dumbbells.
- Switch on your core muscles.
- Do a side step-up and alternating bicep curls at the same time.

Reps, 10–15–20; sets, 1–3; tempo, 2-0-1 or 1-0-*.

39.28 Split Squat and Lunge Series

39.28.1 Tennis Relevance

Tennis-specific motion gets torso and legs in the correct position to execute proper technique. Hip and core training must include exercises that promote both dynamic flexibility and strength in a hip-extended position that use multidimensional and multi-joint movement.

These exercises improve stability in the hip needed for forehand and backhand volleys as well as the dynamic lunging needed to reach wide on groundstrokes. Players often have to hit balls when out of position with poor balance and on one leg so training for this with a variety of split squat, lunge, and single leg squat activities will improve stability and protect against injury to the lower core and legs during acceleration and deceleration.

Split squat on ball with straight arm torso rotation

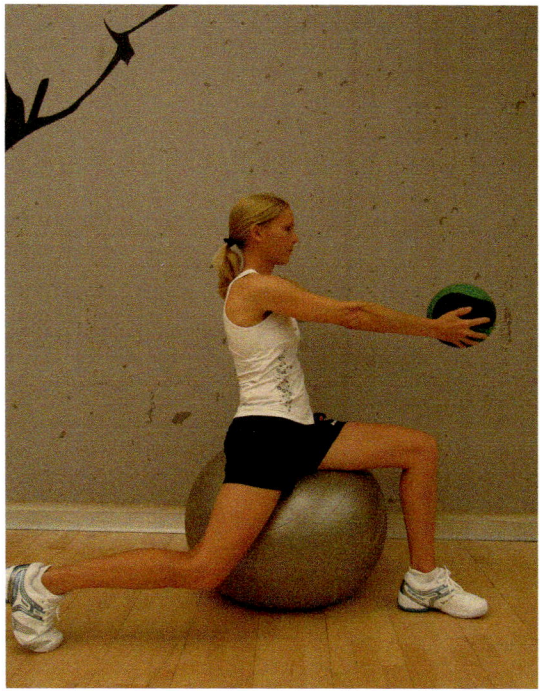 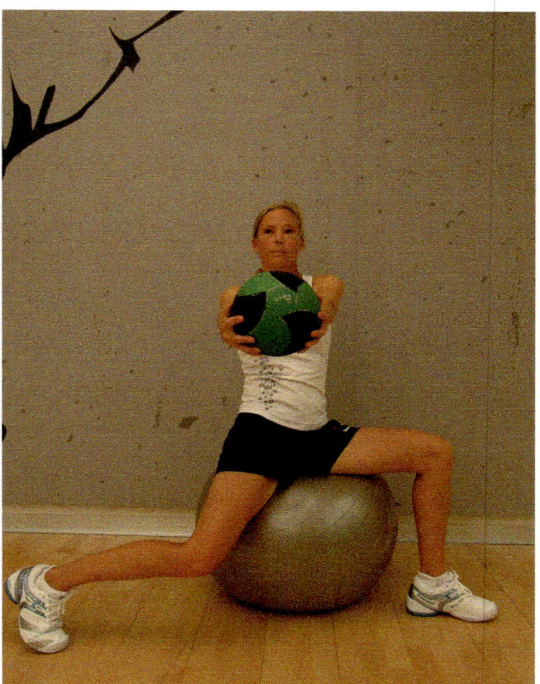

Training tips:

- Start sitting on a physio ball in a split squat position.
- Hold a medicine ball in hands with elbows straight.
- Switch on your core muscles.
- Rotate torso rotating the medicine ball back and forth.

Reps, 10–15; sets 1–2; tempo, 2-1-1 or 1-1-1.

Dynamic hip hikes ball pull down (anterior oblique sling drill)

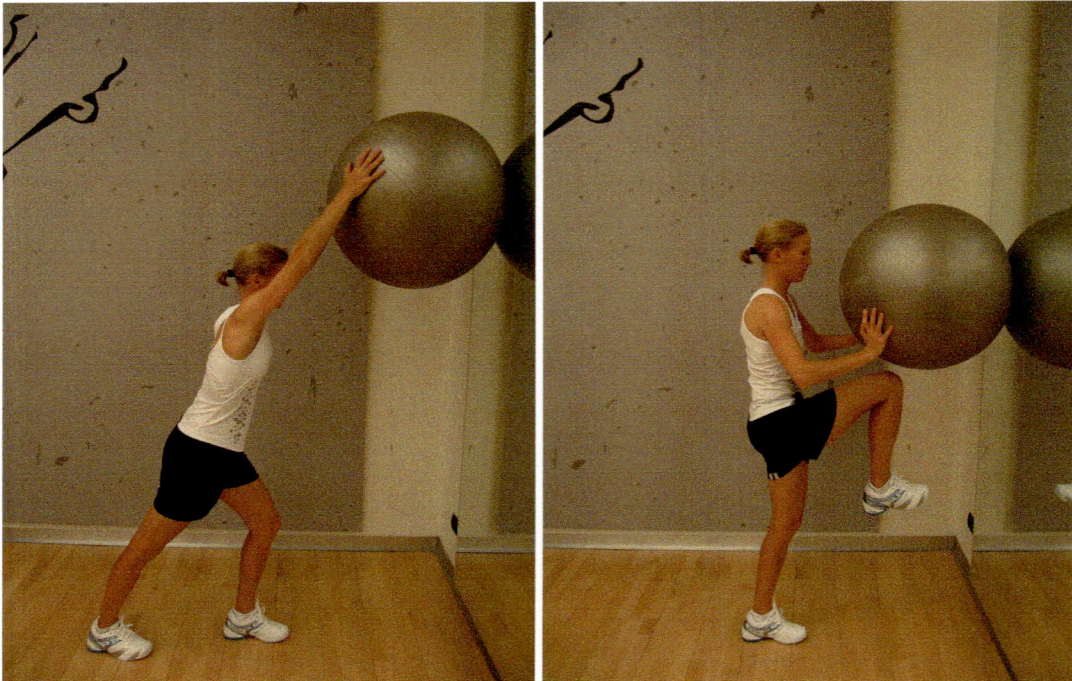

Training tips:

– Start in a split squat position facing a wall and grasping large physio/exercise ball overhead with your hands.
– Switch on your core muscles.
– Drive back knee up to the ball as you squeeze the ball between hands and pull down.
– Return to start position.

Reps, 10–15; sets 1–2; tempo, 2-0-1 or 1-0-1.

Hip extension and lat pulldown (posterior oblique sling drill)

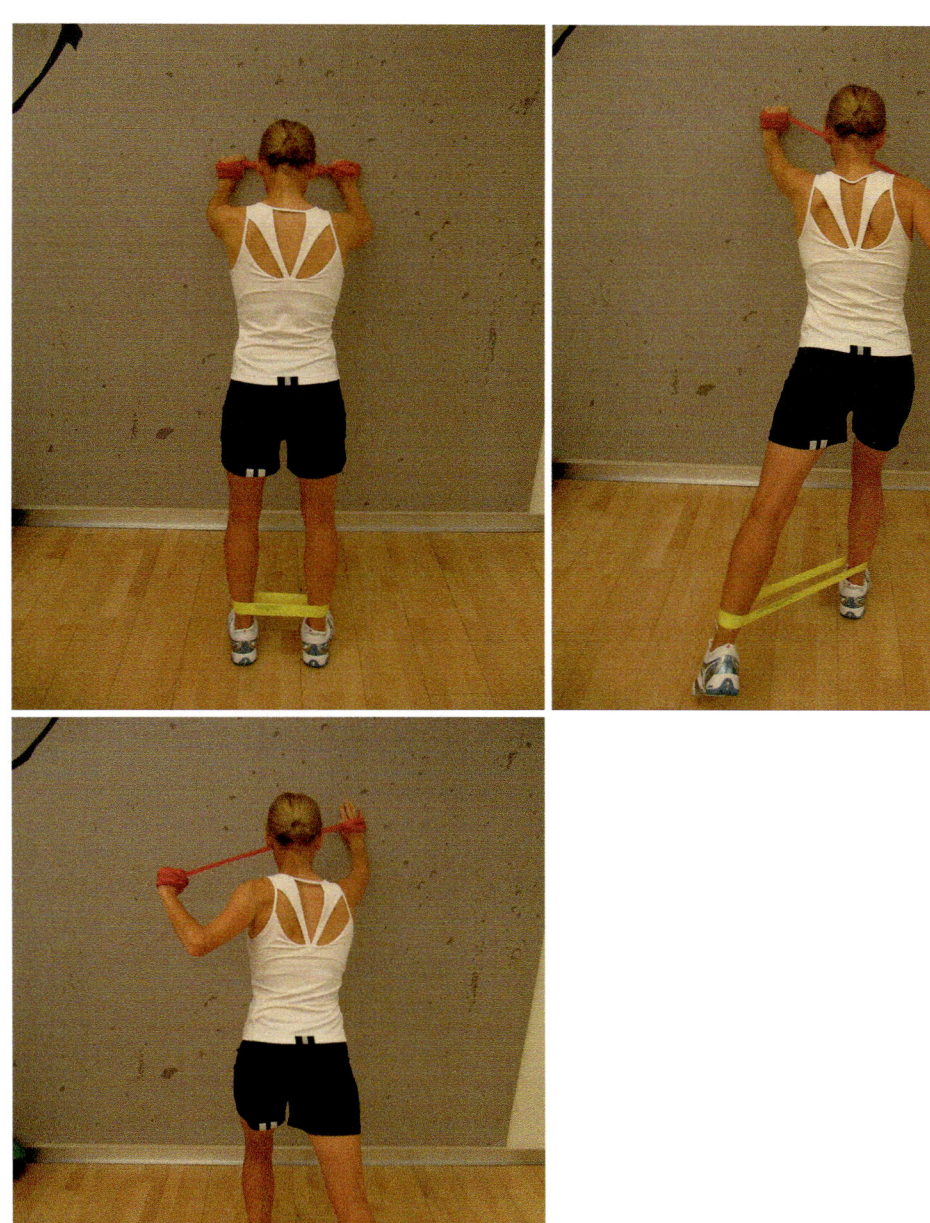

Training tips:

- Stand facing a wall holding two ends of a stretch band against a wall and a light stretch band around ankles.
- Switch on your core muscles.
- Do a shoulder retraction with one arm while doing a hip extension on the opposite side.

Reps, 10–15; sets 1–2; tempo, 2-0-1 or 1-0-1.
Split squat with shoulder press and torso rotation

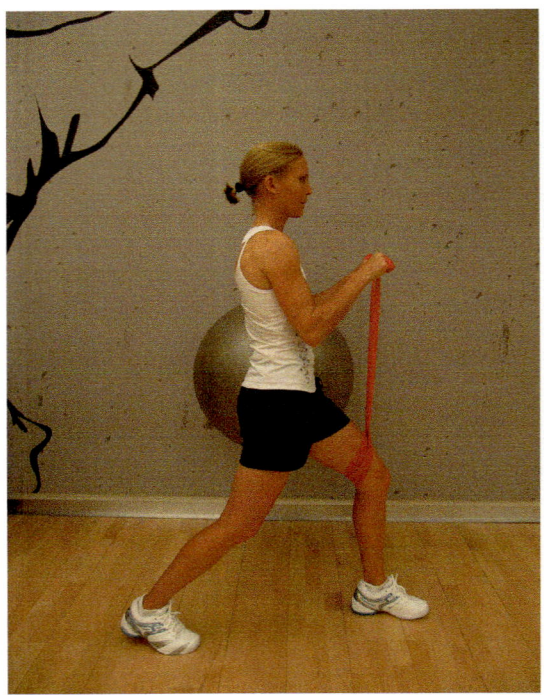 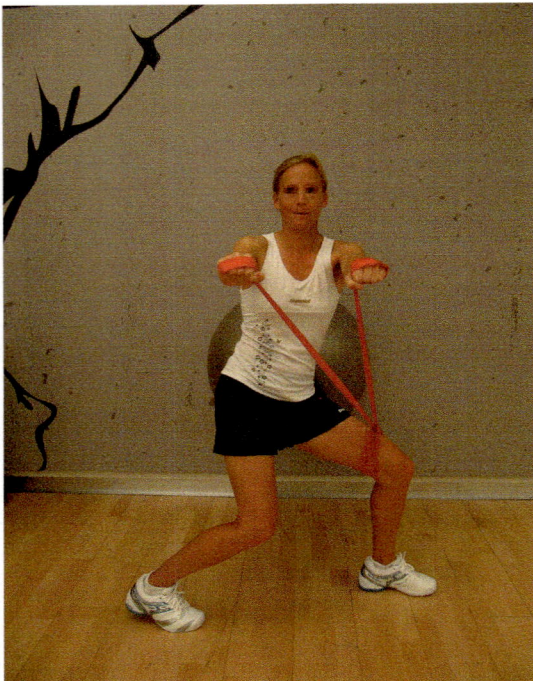

Training tips:

- Start in a split squat position with a physio/exercise ball at your side.
- Hold a stretch band in both hands firmly anchored to your thigh.
- Switch on your core muscles.
- Do a split squat down pushing stretch band out into a shoulder press and rotating torso.

Reps, 10–15; sets 1–2; tempo, 2-1-1 or 1-1-1.

Split squat and shoulder press

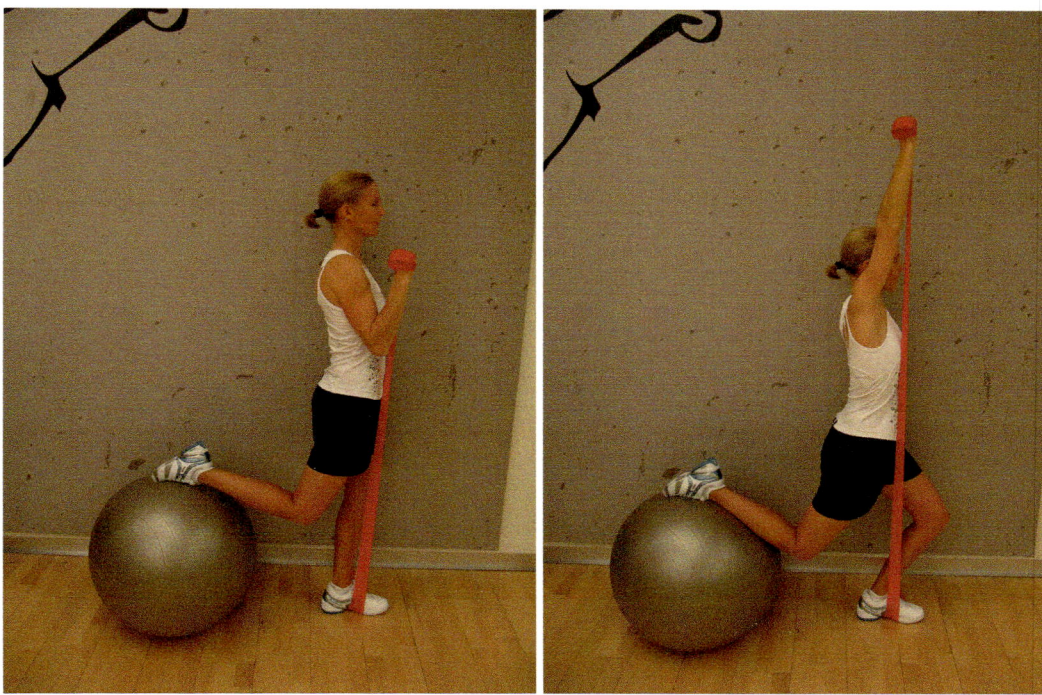

Training tips:

- Start in a split squat position in front of a physio/exercise ball with lower leg on ball.
- Hold a stretch band in the right hand with the other end firmly anchored.
- Switch on your core muscles.
- Do a split squat down pushing stretch band up into a shoulder press.

Reps, 10–15; sets, 1–2; tempo, 2-1-1 or 1-1-1.

39.29 Throwing Drill Series

39.29.1 Tennis Relevance

These exercises help to develop deceleration and rotational power specifically focusing on serve, overhead, and groundstroke explosive movement patterns. Work on sequencing the loading phase of both forehand and backhand movements. Varying the position and stability you work in helps to augment and develop upper and lower core musculature and improve balance. Exercises in hip-extended positions augment tennis-specific movements for open, closed, and varied stance strokes.

Double arm overhead throws

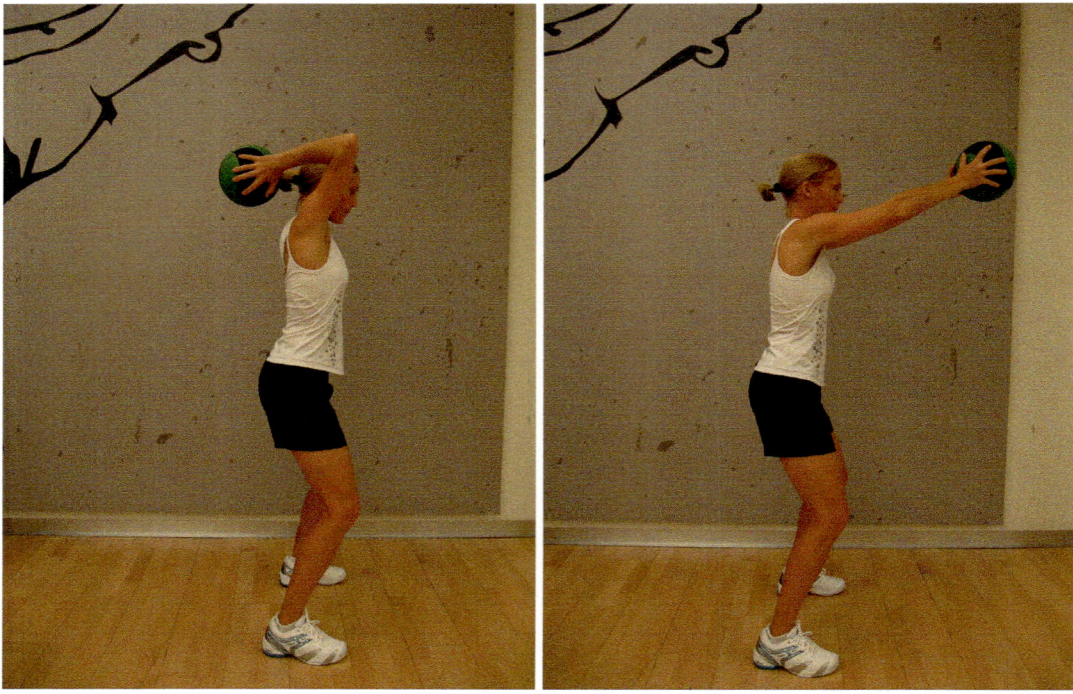

Training tips:

- Stand facing a wall in a good athletic stance holding a sports ball or medicine ball.
- Switch on your core muscles.
- Throw the ball overhead to the wall and catch.

Variation:

- Can also be done in a split or stride step position to encourage weight transfer and power

Reps, 5–10–15; sets, 1–2; tempo, 1-0-*.

Forehand and backhand throws training tips

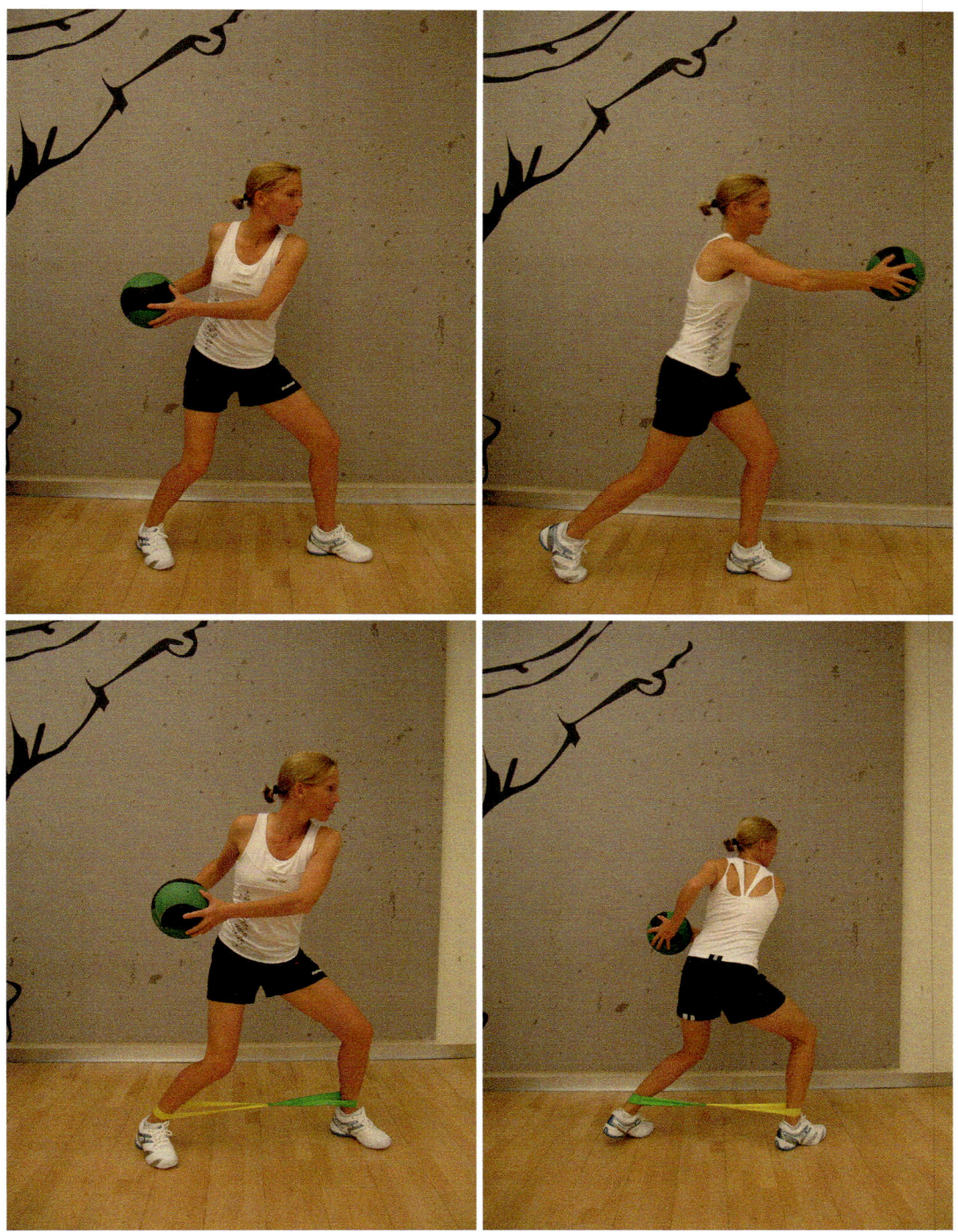

- Stand facing the wall in a good athletic stance holding a sports ball or medicine ball.
- Switch on your core muscles.
- Do forehand and backhand throws against the wall and catch.

Variation:

- Can be done in open stance, closed stance, and semi-closed stance.
- Adding resistance bands around ankles increases the challenge.

Single arm overhead throws

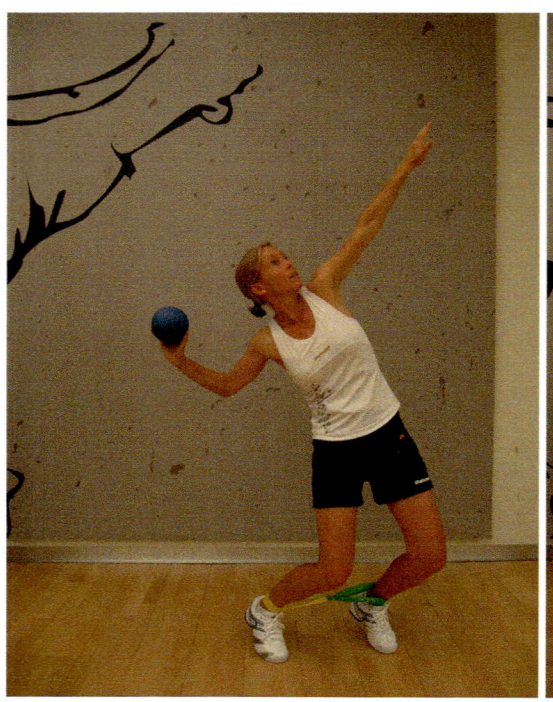 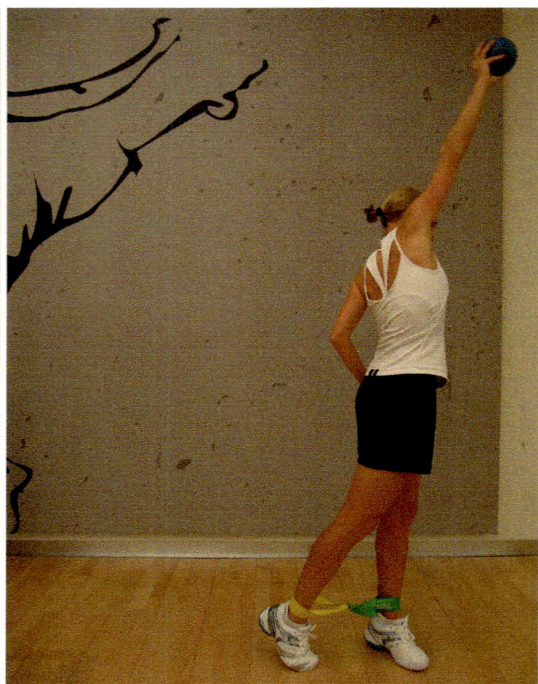

- Start in a service stance position with a light-weighted ball.
- Switch on your core muscles.
- Do a single arm overhead throw mimicking the service motion.

Variation:

- Adding resistance bands around ankles increases the challenge.

Reps, 5–10–15; sets, 1–2; tempo, 1-0-*.

Conclusion

This selection of hip and core strength and stability exercises is chosen for their variability and tennis-specific focus. They promote strength in regions of musculature that are often weak as a result of the training and playing overuse that results in fatigue, active trigger points, and palpable tissue tension. This includes the hip abductors (gluteus minimus and medius) [30] and the local "inner unit" muscles of the core (multifidus, quadratus, and transverses abdominis) [31]. As well, it includes muscles of the peri-scapular region (lower trapezius, serratus anterior, and major and minor rhomboids) [32]. By utilizing easily found and transportable equipment like balls, bands, balance equipment, and weights, we can challenge and augment the functional slings. This will improve player's development of a stable lower and upper core platform to generate speed and execute powerful strokes with precision and endurance.

References

1. Pluim B, Safran M. From breakpoint to advantage. Vista, CA: Racquet Tech Publishing; 2004. p. 33.
2. Maquirriain J, Ghisi JP, Kokalj AM. Rectus abdominis muscle strains in tennis players. Br J Sports Med. 2007;41:842–8.
3. Baechle TR, Earle RW, Wathen D. Resistance training. In: Baechle TR, Earle RW, editors. Essentials of strength training and conditioning. 2nd ed. Champaign, IL: Human Kinetics; 2000. p. 395–425.
4. Putnam CA. Sequential motions of body segments in striking and throwing skills. J Biomech. 1993;26:125–35.
5. Bergmark A. Stability of the lumbar spine. A study in mechanical engineering. Acta Orthop Scand. 1989;230(Suppl):1–54.
6. Richardson CA, Jull GA, Hodges PW, Hides J. Therapeutic exercise for spinal segmental stabilization in low back pain. Edinburgh: Churchill-Livingstone; 1999.
7. Richardson CA, Jull GA. Muscle control-pain control. What exercise would you prescribe? Man Ther. 1995;1:2–10.
8. Comerford MJ, Mottram SL. Functional stability retraining: principles & strategies for managing mechanical dysfunction. Man Ther. 2001;6(1):3–14.
9. Snijders CJ, Vleeming A, Stoeckart R. Transfer of lumbosacral load to iliac bones and legs. 1: biomechanics of self-bracing of the sacroiliac joints and its significance for treatment and exercise. Clin Biomech. 1993;8:285.
10. Vleeming A, Pool-Goudzwaard AL, Stoeckart R, Wingerden JP, van Snijders CJ. The posterior layer of the thoracolumbar fascia: its function in load transfer from spine to legs. Spine. 1995;20:753–8.
11. Kibler WB, Sciascia A, Ellenbecker TS. Musculoskeletal aspects of recovery for tennis. In: Kovacs MS, Ellenbecker TS, Kibler WB, editors. Tennis recovery – a comprehensive review of the research. White Plains, NY: United States Tennis Association; 2010. p. 130.
12. Steindler A. Kinesiology of the human body. Springfield, IL: Charles C. Thomas; 1955.
13. Goldbeck TG, Davies GJ. Test-retest reliability of the closed kinetic chain upper extremity stability test. J Sports Rehabil. 2000;9:35–45.
14. Petersen C. The ABC's of smart training. In: Petersen C, Nittinger N, editors. Fit to play-tennis, high performance training tips. Vista, CA: Racquet Tech Publishing; 2006. p. 26.
15. Petersen C, Sirdevan M, Nittinger N. Upper and lower core training in 3-D. In: Petersen C, Nittinger N, editors. Fit to play-tennis, high performance training tips. Vista, CA: Racquet Tech Publishing; 2006. p. 99–100.
16. Roetert EP, Kovacs MS. Tennis anatomy-your illustrated guide for tennis strength, speed, power and agility. Champaign, IL: Human Kinetics; 2011. p. 1.
17. Weber K, Pieper S, Exler T. Characteristics and significance of running speed at the Australian Open 2006 for training and injury prevention. Med Sci Tennis. 2007;12(1):14.
18. King I. How to write strength training programs. Toowong: King Sports Publishing; 1988.
19. Harris RT, Dudley G. Neuromuscular anatomy and adaptations to conditioning. In: Baechle TR, Earle R, editors. Essentials of strength training and conditioning. Champaign, IL: Human Kinetics; 2000. p. 19–20.
20. Petersen C, Sirdevan M. Core training to hold neutral. In: Petersen C, Nittinger N, editors. Fit to play-tennis, high performance training tips. Vista, CA: Racquet Tech Publishing; 2006. p. 351.
21. Alyas F, et al. MRI finding in lumbar spine of asymptomatic, adolescent elite tennis players. Br J Sports Med. 2007;41:836–41.
22. Akuthota V, Nadler SE. Core strengthening. Arch Phys Med Rehabil. 2004;85(3 Suppl 1):S86–92.
23. Ireland ML, Willson JD, Ballantyne BT, McClay DI. Hip strength in females with and without patellofemoral pain. J Ortho Sports Phys Ther. 2003;33(11):671–6.
24. Leetun DT, Ireland ML, Wislon JD, et al. Core stability measures as risk factor for lower extremity injury in athletes. Med Sci Sports Exerc. 2004;36(6):926–34.
25. Burkhart SS, Morgan CD, Kibler WB. Throwing injuries in the shoulder: the dead arm revisited. Clin Sports Med. 2000;19:125–58.
26. Maenhout A, Van Praet K, Pizzi L, VanHerzeele M, Cools A. Electromyographic analysis of knee push up plus variations: what's the influence of the kinetic chain on scapular muscle activity? Br J Sports Med. 2010;44(14):1010–5. https://doi.org/10.1136/bjsm.2009.062810.
27. De Mey K, Danneels L, Cagnie B, Lotte VD, Johan F, Cools AM. Kinetic chain influences on upper and lower trapezius muscle activation during eight variations of a scapular retraction exercise in overhead athletes. J Sci Med Sport. 2013;16(1):65–70.
28. Knott M, Voss DE. Proprioceptive neuromuscular facilitation-pattern & techniques. New York, ny: Harper & Row; 1968.

29. Huston LJ, Wojtys E. Neuromuscular performance characteristics in elite female athletes. Am J Sports Med. 1996;24:427–36.
30. Ludewig PM, Cook TM. Alterations in shoulder kinematics and associated muscle activity in people with symptoms of shoulder impingement. Phys Ther. 2000;80(3):276–91.
31. Chandler TJ, Kibler WB. Strength, power and endurance in college tennis players. Am J Sports Med. 1992;20(4):455–8.
32. Kibler WB, Press J, Sciasia A. The role of core stability in athletic function. Sports Med. 2006;36(3):189–98.

The Role of Scheduling and Periodization in Competitive Tennis Players

40

Mark Kovacs

The greater the distance between the demands of training and the resources for recovery, the greater the risk of overtraining [1].

40.1 Introduction

Periodization for tennis refers to the manipulation of training variables over specific periods of time for the purpose of promoting maximal performance at the appropriate time and decreasing the risk of overtraining/injury [2]. Well-organized and planned programs have been shown to lead to greater performance improvements than non-periodized programs [3, 4]. To effectively design a periodized program, the following areas of each athlete need to be measured and assessed: speed, agility, power, strength, flexibility, tennis technique, tactical proficiency, anticipation/reaction time, recovery capabilities, and other time constraints (school, work, family, etc.). Before determining appropriate periodization, it is valuable to understand the process and timeline to achieve professional success. The average age of the Top 100 ATP World Tour tennis players in a 2014 study was 27.9 (±3.55), and the age when the athlete first reached a Top 1000 ranking was 18.00 (±2.01); Top 500, 19.06 (±2.22); Top 300, 19.75 (±2.35); Top 200, 20.56 (±2.59); and Top 100, 21.96 (±2.98) [5]. The Tennis Evolution Time (TET) is the time it takes an athlete to improve his ranking from the Top 1000 to Top 100. The TET was 205.92 weeks ±154.96 (or approximately 4 years). The TET takes an average of 4 years for a male professional tennis player [5].

In comparison to the data presented for males on the ATP World Tour, the average age of female players inside the Top 100 WTA rankings in 2014 was 25.21 years (±4.12), height 174.08 cm (±6.93), and weight 63.75 kg (±5.25) [6]. The age when the athlete first reached Top 1000 was 15.91 (±0.95); Top 500, 16.84 (±1.10); Top 300, 17.64 (±1.23); Top 200, 18.60 (±1.57); and Top 100, 19.75 (±1.90). Differences were seen in the age when achieved the first Top 100 between the Top 10 compared to the Top 100 [6]. It takes an average of approximately 4 years for a female professional tennis player to progress to the Top 100 in the world. The top ten players in the world have a significantly different pathway to achieve a Top 100 ranking [6].

Two principles govern how the body responds to exercise:

1. Specific adaptation to imposed demands (SAID) principle. This principle states that the body will respond, and adapt, to the demands that are placed on it. Simply put, if you train

M. Kovacs
International Tennis Performance Association (iTPA), Marietta, GA, USA

Kovacs Institute, Kennesaw, GA, USA

Life Sport Science Institute, Life University, Marietta, GA, USA

by lifting heavier weights or performing more explosive exercises, your body will respond by becoming stronger or more powerful, respectively.
2. General adaptation syndrome (GAS) principle. The GAS principle states that training effects do not occur overnight, and in fact, the body adapts gradually over time, if given adequate time to rest and recover. The body needs time to recover from the stress you put upon it.

Taken together, these two principles can be used to shape the quantity and intensity of training for tennis. More often than not, the recovery portion of the equation is missed, resulting in players who train or compete in a less than optimal state. Incorporating this balance between work and rest is the foundation of what we call periodization training.

Linear (staired) periodization (sometimes referred to as *traditional periodization* or *block periodization*) is a method of manipulating training intensity by systematically increasing intensities while manipulating volume over a predetermined time period. Linear periodization attempts to initiate a physiological state known as *supercompensation*. When a tennis player receives a training stimulus at the beginning a training block (cycle) that is higher than the previous load, fatigue will occur. If the same load is maintained over the period of this same training block (cycle) during following training sessions, the body will begin to adapt to this new training intensity. This new level is referred to as a new *ceiling of adaptation* [7].

The unloading period should not return to initial levels of intensities; rather, it should be reduced to the level of intensity reached at the midpoint of the staired progression phase. Scheduling an unloading period allows for tissue regeneration and protein synthesis as well as the replenishment of energy stores that will have been depleted over the period of staired progression. The energy replenishment above the initial levels is commonly referred to as supercompensation, and it should leave the athlete in a heightened state of training preparedness for another successive series of increasing training intensities [8]. The linear model of periodization is characterized by initial training volume with low levels of intensity. As training progresses toward major competitions, volume decreases and intensity increases in order to maximize strength, power, endurance, or other training variables (such as tactical and technical readiness).

The *nonlinear (undulating) periodization* approach allows for more variation in intensity and volume within each training block (cycle) by alternating different training protocols to prioritize various components of the neuromuscular and metabolic systems (strength, power, speed, endurance, etc.). For the tennis player who has an ever-changing schedule due to success or failure at tournaments, total match counts per year is ever-changing; for changes in training routines and other factors that are inherent to a year-round sport, an undulating periodization schedule is usually the preferred periodization model for a competitive tennis athlete.

Here is an example of an 8-week block of training that involves 2 download weeks. The X-axis highlights the maximum volume the athlete can handle per week. It is important to include download weeks every 3–4 weeks to allow for increased improvement and also to reduce the chance of overtraining, psychological burnout, and increased risk of musculoskeletal injury.

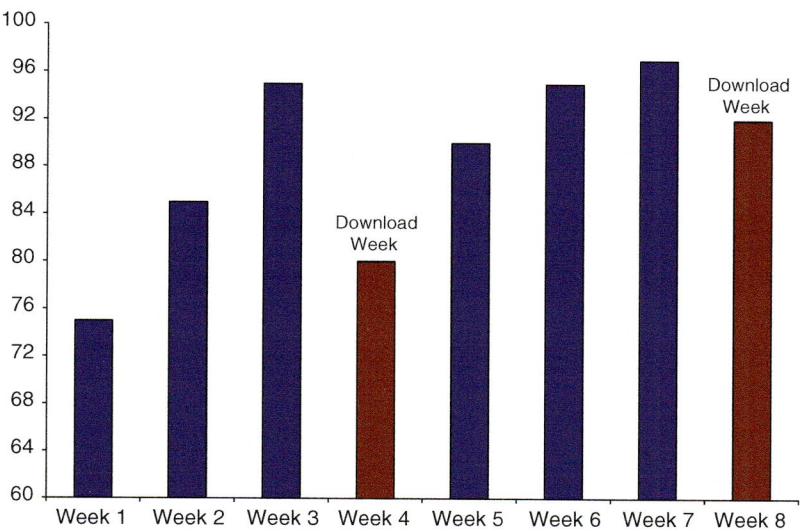

Below is an example of simple weekly outline for a 5-day cycle of off-season tennis-specific training. It highlights a simple way to plan a training week that involves all the major aspects involved in training a tennis athlete from the physical perspective.

MONDAY	TUESDAY	WEDNESDAY	THURSDAY	FRIDAY
Dynamic Stretching	Dynamic Stretching	Dynamic Stretching	Dynamic Stretching	Dynamic Stretching
SAP	SAP	SAP	SAP	SAP
MORNING PRACTICE				
TSE	Recovery	TSE	Recovery	TSE
SAP	SAP	SAP	SAP	SAP
Dynamic Stretching	Dynamic Stretching	Dynamic Stretching	Dynamic Stretching	Dynamic Stretching
AFTERNOON PRACTICE				
UL	LH	RECOVERY	UH	LL
Static Stretching	Static Stretching	Static Stretching	Static Stretching	Static Stretching

SAP	On-Court Speed Agility and Power (10-15 minutes)
TSE	Tennis Specific Endurance (30-45 minutes)
UL	Upper Body Light (Strength Training)
LH	Lower Body Heavy (Strength Training)
RECOVERY	Structured Recovery (Stretching, Foam Rolling, Ice Baths)
UH	Upper Body Heavy (Strength Training)
LL	Lower Body Light (Strength Training)

Information adapted from [1].

40.2 Traditional Periodized Training

Most books and articles on periodization will tell you that a well-designed plan should include a preparation phase, a precompetitive phase, a competitive phase, and an active rest phase [9, 10].

40.2.1 Preparation Phase

The focus of the preparation phase is on developing a base level of fitness and strength, what we'll call foundational conditioning and strength.

The training components of the preparation phase include the following:

- Challenge the aerobic energy system, for example, 20–40 min of aerobic training at 70–85% of maximum heart rate 3–4 times per week.
- Establish a strength base, for example, strength training using a high-repetition (10–15 repetitions per set for 2–3 sets), low-resistance training program.
- Include technical and tactical training, for example, on-court training that incorporates changes in stroke mechanics, develops new shots, and so on (adapted from [10]).

40.2.1.1 Precompetitive Phase

The precompetitive phase is a period of time leading up to the competitive season in which the training shifts from general training to training for power and activities more closely related to the demands of the sport.

In the precompetitive phase, the intensity level increases and the theme becomes more tennis-specific:

- Challenge the anaerobic energy system, for example, on-court training drills, interval training using tennis-specific work/rest intervals.
- Improve speed and power, for example, sprinting and explosive on-court exercises, plyometrics.
- Improve muscular strength, for example, perform 2–4 sets with 8–10 repetitions, decrease the training volume, and increase the intensity of the resistance exercise.
- Maintain aerobic status, for example, perform aerobic exercise two times per week for 20–30 min.
- Improve tennis-specific skill, for example, on-court training focusing on tennis-specific drills, practice matches, and simulated points in preparation for competition (adapted from [10]).

40.2.1.2 Competitive Phase

During the competitive phase, players look to maintain their conditioning and strength over a period of competitions or peak for a specific competition. Here again, training is very sport specific:

- Peak performance
- High-intensity workouts
- Tennis competition or tennis-specific training

Adapted from [10].

40.2.1.3 Active Rest Phase

During the active rest phase, the athlete takes a mental and physical break from the sport. This is not a time when the athlete just does nothing, however, but gives the athlete time to cross-train:

- Rest from tennis.
- Cross-train to maintain fitness levels.
- Emphasize fun, low-intensity workouts.
- Rest for 1–4 weeks.

Adapted from [10].

Tennis tends to reward more successful players, allowing them more time to recover between peak performances. Top professional players have the luxury of not having to play every event to win enough money to make a living or earn ranking points. Similarly, top junior players do not have to chase points across the country or around the world. The players who are trying to make it to that next level feel they have to play more to earn ranking points and consequently have little or no downtime between events.

Even in light of these factors, periodization is still important for the tennis player. Training just has to be approached a bit differently than for say a football player, a swimmer, or a soccer player.

40.3 Obstacles in the Way of Ideal Periodization and Planning for Tennis

40.3.1 Length of the Season

A player will be best served if he or she can devote a period of time within the competitive season, ideally 6–8 weeks, to focus on building a base of fitness and strength. While the player can still compete during this time, he or she should recognize that performance may be less than optimal. However, this base will allow the player to improve in the areas of fitness or strength and serve as the foundation of fitness from which the player will draw late in the season when other players are faltering. This is the time when players will do high volumes of work—high repetitions with low weights—and work hard to build cardiovascular endurance.

40.3.2 Not Knowing When the Tournament Will End

This is a tough one, as every week can be different. However, recognize that training does not necessarily require a weight room or fancy equipment. The International Tennis Performance Association recommends players to travel with equipment such as stretch tubing, a small medicine ball, several cones for movement drills, and a plan for what will happen if they lose in the first round or the second round or make it to the finals so they can start training without missing a beat. Remember when you aren't maintaining or improving fitness or strength, you are losing it.

40.3.3 Lack of Rest for Players Chasing Money or Ranking Points

Rest is key for any player, and it is important to incorporate it into your training plan. Those who train or compete day after day, with no breaks, don't give their bodies any chance to recover, adapt, or grow. We typically recommend that in a 7-day training week, one day be devoted to complete rest with little or no intense physical activity and one day involve active rest. Active rest means doing something other than tennis or other than training for tennis (in the weight room, on-court conditioning, etc.). One day a week, we recommend going for a bike ride, playing soccer, swimming, and doing something that still involves activity but relieves the body of the stresses it experiences when training for tennis.

Additionally, there needs to be a period, or periods, during the year in which the player takes time away from serious tennis training. Again, this is a time for recovery from the demands of a competitive season, a phase of intense training, etc. This provides not only a physical break but a mental break, allowing the player to recharge the battery.

Rest is a vital part of any training plan and is a necessity for any athlete, tennis players included, to reach his or her full potential. It is very easy for a tennis player to become overtrained, a phenomenon exemplified by sluggishness, tiredness, and feelings of apathy, because of all the training players typically engage in. While this is especially true for high-performance players, it is also possible for recreational players to fall into this trap, especially if a player is rededicating herself to fitness or training and makes drastic changes to her training plan.

40.4 Building Your Periodized Training Plan

1. Start by identifying the most important tournaments on the calendar.
2. Identify a period (or several periods) of 6–8 weeks that you are willing to devote your-

self to building your strength and conditioning base.
3. Identify a period of time (or several periods of time) that you will take off from tennis (active rest phase).
4. Develop a chart or table and select an emphasis for each week of the year. For example, during the base strength phase, the emphasis may be on building endurance. However, 2 weeks before the main competition, the emphasis may be on maximizing power or improving on-court movement.
5. Become even more detailed and outline exercises, sets, and repetitions for each day. You do not have to lay out every day of the year on January 1, but some foresight should go into your planning, and you should know what you are going to be doing several weeks or months down the line [10].

40.4.1 Sample Periodized Plan for Tennis

A player could structure a season in many possible ways in terms of the number of tournaments to be played and the times in which the player wants to peak during the year. Keep in mind the guidelines set forth earlier in regard to the amount of time that should be dedicated to each phase of training and the ability to peak.

While the specific exercises, weights, reps, and sets used may differ, the overall structure of the plan will look very similar. Pay attention to the following:

- Training volume should be high in the preparation phases, with low to moderate intensity.
- In the precompetition phase, shift to lower training volumes, but increase the training intensity.
- During competition, the volume should be very low but the intensity should be high.
- During the active rest phases, back off on the volume and intensity.

40.4.2 Steps to Create a Periodization Plan

Step 1. Decide numbers of tournament plays and write down on the calendar.
As mentioned previously, it is very possible to play tournaments every week (even though not recommended). It is critical to schedule the tournaments to minimize the chance of injuries and potential burnout. The general idea of training vs. competition ratio for the set 3 is 40–60% training and 60–40% competition. The United States Tennis Association Player Development has suggested maximum of 60 matches per year at age 14 and maximum of 90 matches per year at the age 16 and older [11]. Professional players range in matches per year from as few as 50 singles matches per year during a full schedule to over 100 singles matches per year [6]. This variability results in challenges for recommendations about appropriate number of matches. Many players can succeed with high-volume match counts. However, Jayanthi et al. studied training and competition volumes for junior tennis players. The recommendations are as follows: (1) consider playing <2 tournaments per month to reduce injury risk and (2) consider playing <18 tournaments annually in the 18 and under division (and potentially less tournaments per year than age) [12].

Step 2. Select tournaments that the athlete needs to be at peak.
As a player prospective, all of the tournament is equally important. Again, especially for young tennis athletes, they are still developing overall physical fitness level as an athlete and tennis skills as a tennis player. It is a long process, so players and coaches need to be on the same page what their goal is. Because of the long season of tournaments, it is

important to prioritize the tournament and decide which tournament(s) to be peak at. Also, by deciding which tournament to peak at, it decides how many training cycles (periodization cycles) are per year. On most of the players, 2–3 peaks per year are realistic and practical.

Step 3. Select day(s)/week(s) for rest/recovery and unload.

This is probably the most important step when creating an annual periodization plan; however, at the same time, it is probably the most forgotten step. After deciding on the tournament schedules, recovery days and weeks are usually assigned after each tournament. It is also important to consider building in recovery/unloading day(s) or week for each mesocycle and microcycle. For a mesocycle, the three-to-one (3:1) split is one of the popular methods to build in an unloading week. With this method, after 3 weeks of training, an athlete will take a week of unloading week. During the unloading week, normal training routine will continue; however, volume or intensity may reduce down to about a half of the previous training week.

Step 4. It is recommended to take off one or more days per week from tennis training if training over 16 h per week. So each microcycle (1 week) should consist of a total of 2 days off from tennis training. One of the popular methods is to take 1 full day off (usually on Sunday if there is no tournament) and take 2 and a half days off.

Step 5. Assign mesocycles and decide training objectivities and goals for each mesocycle.

There should be an overall theme and goal for an athlete. Each mesocycle plan has more specific goal, for example, tennis-specific movement as precompetition phase or muscle hypertrophy as off-season training. Of course, an individual development stage as a tennis player (training age) and person (biological age) will affect actual training goals and programs. As previously mentioned, two same chronological age children might have different biological or training ages.

Step 6. Testing and assessment is another important aspect of periodization planning. It will give a good baseline idea for the athlete, especially at the beginning of the year or off-season, to help create realistic goals. Testing should be scheduled at least twice (ideally 3–4 times) per year to see the athlete's progress and make adjustments on the goals and programs based on the progress. At the beginning or end of some of the mesocycles is usually a good time to schedule testing and assessment. Also, for a young athlete, it is important to monitor their growth by measuring the height and weight at least monthly (ideally weekly) because it helps to identify an athlete's growth and development stage to apply appropriate training programs and not to miss the optimal windows of opportunity.

Step 7. Design each microcycle program.

When designing microcycle (weekly) program, some of the predetermined factors must be considered. As previously mentioned on step 3, recovery days should be built in. Tennis practice schedules are usually set for the week based on the court availabilities, coaches' schedules, etc. Therefore, communication with tennis coaches to discuss available days and times for off-court training is critical; as also previously mentioned, the higher the athlete level is (more tennis training), demand for off-court training is greater to not only improve performance but also prevent overused injuries. Also, if a child goes to a normal traditional school, majority of the days are preoccupied with school schedules.

Step 8. Review and be ready to make adjustments day by day and week by week.

Periodization is a great way to organize a tennis player's annual and monthly plans and on- and off-court training weekly plans and provide a clear direction of a player's development pathway as a tennis player. However, it is important to recognize that the plan requires constant review and adjustments. A tournament might be scheduled for a week, but a player may lose in the first round. There is a great difference in physical fatigue levels between 6-0, 6-0 h-long match win and 7-6, 6-7, 7-6 over 3-h match. It will affect a great deal for recovery method and training and practice for the next day or for next match preparation. Weather will affect practice and training schedules. A coach may plan for a tough day of practice. However it rained out and turned into a full day of fitness when a strength and conditioning coach originally planned for a light day of fitness. School and social stresses will affect an athlete's fatigue and motivation levels. The plan must be adjusted based on an athlete's day-to-day condition.

40.5 Summary

Training for tennis is complex and each athlete has a different tournament and training schedule. These factors do impact how to appropriately set up a periodized training program based on appropriate scheduling. It is a long process of development and requires patience, and constant reviews and adjustments are necessary. Recovery is a key component of the periodization plan. It is always important to remember that training does not improve an athlete without appropriate recovery. The information covered in this chapter provides an appropriate framework to better execute a functional and practical periodization program for tennis with a specific link to appropriate scheduling.

References

1. International Tennis Performance Association, editor. ITPA, Certified Tennis Performance Specialist (CTPS) workbook and study guide. Atlanta, GA: International Tennis Performance Association; 2012.
2. Stone MH, O'Bryant HS. Weight training, a scientific approach. Minneapolis, MN: Burgess; 1987.
3. Kraemer WJ, et al. Physiological changes with periodized resistance training in women tennis players. Med Sci Sports Exerc. 2003;35(1):157–68.
4. Rhea M, Alderman B. A meta-analysis of periodized versus nonperiodized strength and power training programs. Res Quart Exerc Sports. 2004;75:413–22.
5. Kovacs M, et al. How did the top 100 professional tennis players (ATP) succeed: an analysis of ranking milestones. J Med Sci Tennis. 2015;20(2):50–7.
6. Kovacs MS, et al. How did the top 100 Women's Tennis Association (WTA) players succeed: an analysis of player rankings. J Med Sci Tennis. 2015;20(3):122–8.
7. Bompa TO. Periodization of strength. Don Mills, ON: Veritas Publishing; 1993.
8. Zatsiorsky V. Science and practice of strength training. Champaign, IL: Human Kinetics; 1995.
9. Kovacs M, Chandler WB, Chandler TJ. Tennis training: enhancing on-court performance. Vista, CA: Racquet Tech Publishing; 2007.
10. Kovacs M, Roetert EP, Ellenbecker TS. Complete conditioning for tennis. 2nd ed. Champaign, IL: Human Kinetics; 2016.
11. USTA, editor. *USTA, table 6 – scheduling guidelines for junior divisions: maximum number of matches per day*, in *2009* Edition friend at court: rules and regulations handbook. White Plains, NY: USTA; 2009.
12. Jayanthi NA, O'Boyle J, Durazo-Arvizu RA. Risk factors for medical withdrawals in United States Tennis Association junior national tennis tournaments: a descriptive epidemiologic study. Sports Health. 2009;1(3):231–5.

Printed by Printforce, the Netherlands

YALE HISTORICAL PUBLICATIONS

LEONARD WOODS LABAREE · EDITOR

MISCELLANY

XLVI

PUBLISHED UNDER THE DIRECTION OF
THE DEPARTMENT OF HISTORY
FROM THE INCOME OF
THE FREDERICK JOHN KINGSBURY
MEMORIAL FUND

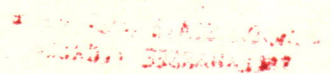

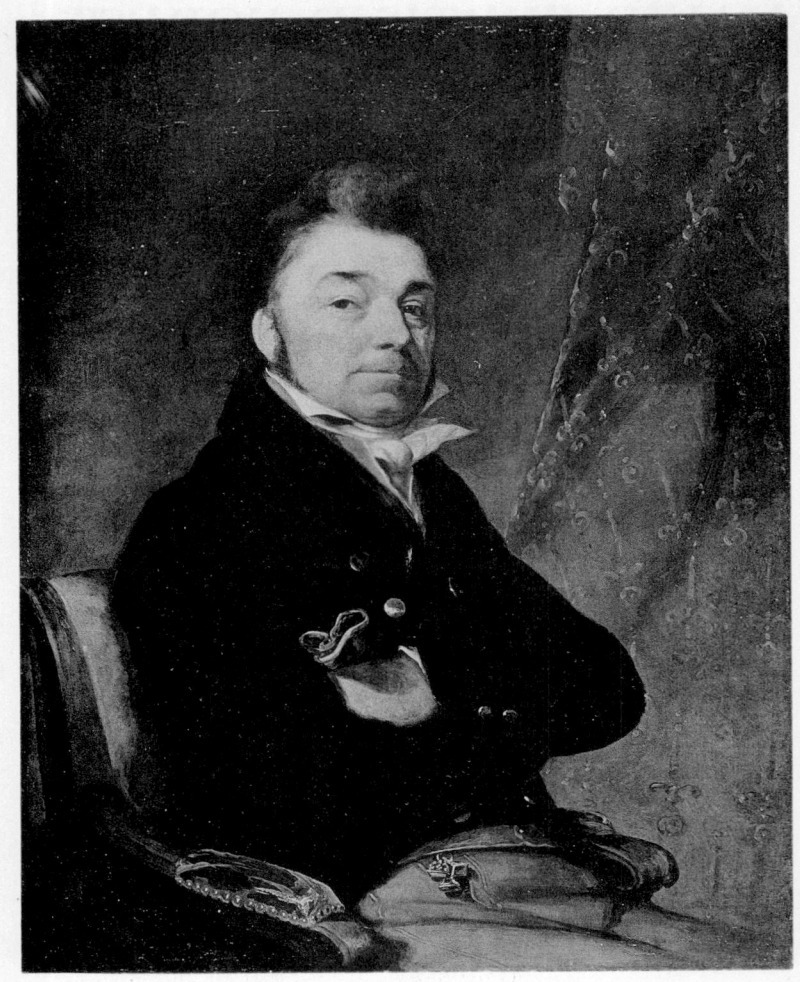

DAVID CURTIS DeFOREST
From a Portrait by Samuel F. B. Morse.
Courtesy of Yale University Art Gallery.

DAVID CURTIS DeFOREST
AND THE REVOLUTION
OF BUENOS AIRES

BY

BENJAMIN KEEN

ASSOCIATE PROFESSOR OF HISTORY
WEST VIRGINIA UNIVERSITY

NEW HAVEN
YALE UNIVERSITY PRESS
LONDON · GEOFFREY CUMBERLEGE · OXFORD UNIVERSITY PRESS
1947

COPYRIGHT, 1947, BY YALE UNIVERSITY PRESS

Printed in the United States of America

All rights reserved. This book may not be reproduced, in whole or in part, in any form (except by reviewers for the public press), without written permission from the publishers.

To
MY MOTHER

PREFACE

THE life of David Curtis DeForest richly documents the contribution of the United States to the movement of Spanish-American emancipation. His colorful career, spanning a quarter-century of revolutionary upheavals along the shores of the Río de la Plata, shows how North American ideological influence and illegal military assistance, and the astute diplomacy of the United States government, helped to inspire, sustain, and bring to a successful conclusion the Argentine struggle for independence. It demonstrates how numerous and varied were the contacts between the United States and Buenos Aires in this formative period of inter-American relations. These historical lessons emerge from a study of the life of one of the greatest of Yankee adventurers, recorded in his own vigorously written journals and letters.

In quoting from the DeForest papers, the principal source for this study, I have modernized the punctuation for the sake of greater clarity, but have retained the original capitalization and spelling. Books and articles have been cited in full at the first reference, but thereafter in abbreviated form.

To all who have helped me in the completion of this work I express my appreciation. In particular, I am deeply indebted to Samuel Flagg Bemis, Sterling Professor of Diplomatic History and Inter-American Relations at Yale University, for his constant advice and encouragement. Professor Leonard Woods Labaree, Editor of the Yale Historical Publications, has offered valuable suggestions and criticisms. I also wish to thank Richard Blanc and Byron Fairchild, who have read and commented on particular chapters. The custodians and staffs of the Yale University Library, the Library of Congress, the National Archives, the Columbus Library of the Pan-American Union in Washington, and the Connecticut State Library at Hartford, have shown me many friendly courtesies. The assistance and inspiration of my wife were invaluable.

B. K.

Amherst, Mass.
February 2, 1946.

CONTENTS

	Preface	vii
I.	"Fortune Is a Slippery Jade"	1
II.	"Doing Business in the Smuggling Way"	14
III.	"A Highly Dangerous Trade"	27
IV.	"Reign of Terror and Confusion"	41
V.	"On Very Safe Ground"	53
VI.	"The Ides of March"	61
VII.	"The Downfall of My Enemies"	77
VIII.	"Adopted Citizen of Buenos Ayres"	91
IX.	"A Dash at the Dons"	103
X.	"The Great South American Witchery"	129
XI.	Epilogue	158
	Bibliographical Note	170
	Index	179

ILLUSTRATIONS

DAVID CURTIS DEFOREST   *Frontispiece*
JULIA WOOSTER DEFOREST   86
    Paintings by Samuel F. B. Morse
    Courtesy of the Yale University Art Gallery

I
"FORTUNE IS A SLIPPERY JADE"

DAVID CURTIS DeFOREST occupies a leading place among the adventurous Yankee traders who in the epoch of Spanish-American emancipation established the first commercial and political relations between the United States and the new states of Spanish America. Merchant, prince of privateers, and diplomat, he took an active part in the revolutionary struggles of the people of Buenos Aires, capital of the provinces known today as the Argentine Republic. His career is a veritable embodiment of the contribution of the United States to the winning of Argentine independence.

The beginnings of DeForest's career are closely linked to the great outward thrust of American commerce after the Revolutionary War. Spurred by their loss of markets in the British Empire, New England's mariners then pushed across the seas in search of trade. Their quest led to the Northwest Coast for otter skins, to Hawaii for sandalwood, to the coasts of Spanish America for the profits of a contraband traffic, and to the seal fisheries of the Antarctic. At the great Chinese port of Canton they exchanged pelts, sandalwood, and specie for silks and teas. From Canton they began the long voyage home, half way around the world.

On such a "circumnavigating voyage" the young DeForest embarked from Boston port on the last day of the year 1800. But he was not to see the wonders of old Canton. Parting company with his domineering captain on the bleak coast of Patagonia, he traveled by devious routes to the town of Buenos Aires, capital of the Spanish province of the Río de la Plata. There he learned to trade "in the smuggling way." As a resident merchant in Buenos Aires he observed the preliminaries of the Argentine *Revolución de Mayo*, and himself stimulated the spirit of creole discontent by his preachment of republican doctrine. On the eve of the revolution, Viceroy Cisneros expelled him from the province. Returning after the events of May 25, 1810, DeForest became an outfitter of patriot privateers that made heavy inroads on Spanish commerce. Later, as diplomatic representative of his adopted country in the United States, he matched wits with Secretary of State John Quincy Adams in an effort to gain recognition of the independence of Buenos Aires. Defeated by the redoubtable secretary, he retired to the town of New Haven in his native Connecticut, where he devoted his last years to philanthropy, to the promotion of cultural relations between the United States and Buenos Aires, and to the annual celebration of the birthday of Argentine independence, the *veinte-cinco de mayo*.

DeForest's European forebears were wool merchants of the little walled town of Avesnes, in the Belgian province of Hainaut. The Religious Wars of the sixteenth century laid waste this once flourishing region, and by the thousands Walloon Huguenots emigrated to neighboring Holland. Among them was one Jesse de Forest, who in 1615 lived in the "goodly and pleasant citie" of Leyden.

Discontent with economic conditions in Leyden evidently inspired Jesse de Forest and a number of his countrymen to try their fortunes in the New World. With the backing of the Dutch West India Company, then engaged in an ambitious program of overseas expansion, the exile from Avesnes in 1623 led a band of Walloon pilgrims on a voyage to the mouth of the Amazon River. On the Oyapok, a stream that separates present-day French Guiana from Northeastern Brazil, they made a settlement. Jesse was exploring the surrounding country when a fever struck him down. "On the 22nd of October 1624," reads an entry in the journal of the expedition, "our said captain died, much regretted by the Indians who had taken a great liking to him. This day we caused him to be buried as honorably as was possible for us, accompanying his body with arms, which we each discharged three times over his grave and our cannon as well."[1] Disheartened by this heavy loss, the survivors soon returned to their families in Holland.

Twelve years later two sons of Jesse de Forest, Henry and Isaac, left their Leyden home to settle in New Netherland. Henry died shortly after his arrival in America, but Isaac lived to become a wealthy merchant and landowner of New Amsterdam. His

---

1. "Journal of the Voyage Made by the Fathers of Families Sent by the Honorable the Directors of the West India Company to the Coast of Guiana," in Mrs. Robert W. de Forest, *A Walloon Family in America* (2 vols., New York, 1914), II, 249.

son, David, founded the Connecticut line of DeForests. About 1694 he left New York and made his way to the growing settlement of Stratford situated a few miles up the Housatonic River. There he met and married Martha Blagge, daughter of a local merchant, and in time acquired a considerable holding of land. He left behind him a large progeny—plain farmer folk, diligent churchgoers, exemplary members of the ecclesiastical societies and military train-bands of Stratford.

His grandson, Benjamin DeForest or Deforest, as he sometimes wrote his name, came to manhood on the eve of the War for Independence. The violence of the great struggle reached perilously close to Stratford; the British burned Fairfield, eight miles to the west, and plundered New Haven twelve miles to the east. Poor health prevented DeForest from bearing arms in the war, as did twenty-five men of his name, but he was active on local relief committees aiding the patriot cause. The care of his land and the rearing of his six children, however, were his chief preoccupations. His eldest child, a son called David Curtis DeForest, was born on January 10, 1774, in the parish of Ripton[2] in Stratford.

David was nearing his tenth year when the Revolutionary War came to an end. The peace that followed was an uneasy one. The long, exhausting conflict had disrupted the colonial economy and had given a severe shock to accepted religious and moral ideas. Even steady-going Connecticut, of which Aaron Burr is reported to have said that one might "as soon attempt to revolutionize the kingdom of heaven," [3] experienced profound change in the post-war years.

There was no Shays' Rebellion in Connecticut to alarm the better sort, but other signs of unrest grieved those who held to the ancient order of things. In the town of Windham, "it was a transition period—a day of upheaval, over-turning, uprootal. Infidelity and Universalism had come in with the Revolution and drawn multitudes from the religious faith of their fathers. Free thinking and free-drinking were alike in vogue; great looseness of manners and morals had replaced the ancient Puritanic strictness." [4] As

2. Incorporated in 1789 as the town of Huntington. In 1919 the name was changed to Shelton.
3. William A. Robinson, *Jeffersonian Democracy in New England* (New Haven, 1916), p. 28.
4. Quoted in Richard J. Purcell, *Connecticut in Transition* (New Haven, 1918), p. 10.

for New London, "all accounts agree in speaking of the *manners* of the inhabitants as belonging to the *free* and *easy* style. Jovial parties of all kinds, hot suppers, tavern dinners, card playing, shooting matches, and dancing assemblies were popular. Merchants and other citizens congregated around the coffee houses, told stories, cracked jokes, and complimented each other with brandy, ginsling and old Jamaica, as matters of course every day of the week, Sundays . . . not wholly excepted." [5]

At Yale College, a stronghold of Congregationalist orthodoxy, students dismayed President Timothy Dwight by taking the names of Voltaire and Rousseau. The Reverend William Bentley, noting the degeneracy of the times, observed that Thomas Paine was universally read in Connecticut. Toward the close of the century, Federalist oligarchs perceived even more ominous portents in the rise of Jeffersonian heresy, recruiting its first disciples among the merchants and workmen of the shore and river towns.

In this era of transition DeForest passed his formative years. The new climate of opinion nourished a lively intellectual curiosity, fostered indifference to religious dogma, engendered a worldly and acquisitive temper. In time of adversity DeForest's forebears had searched their consciences and their Bibles to learn wherein they had offended their stern and jealous God. David, who had read *The Age of Reason*, would instead rail at fortune, that "fickle Damned Bitch of a Goddess," or would compare himself to another roving pagan, the famed Ulysses, and lament his vain search for "darling Penelope: 30 or 40,000 dollars." Disciple of Paine and Jefferson, talk of the rights of man would fall naturally from his lips; and to the rulers of revolutionary Buenos Aires he would teach the maxim of "the patriotic sages of North America . . . *that an uninstructed cannot long be a free people.*"

The economic life of Connecticut was also adjusting itself to new conditions. The return of peace found agriculture in a sorry plight. Loss of the vital West Indies trade, sharply curtailing the market for farming and domestic produce, made the burden of taxation unbearably heavy for the small farmers of the state. Their dissatisfaction was reflected in the steady exodus of emigrants from Connecticut, an occurrence common to all New England. It has been estimated that between 1790 and 1820 approximately 800,000 persons departed from the three states

5. Frances M. Caulkins, *History of New London* (New London, 1895), p. 581.

of Massachusetts, Rhode Island, and Connecticut. Before the Revolution the population of Connecticut had been growing at the rate of 28 per cent in every decade; between 1790 and 1800 it increased only 5½ per cent.[6]

Some of DeForest's generation abandoned the exhausted and tax-burdened acres of their fathers for the more abundant, cheap, and fertile lands of the frontier. Others, no less enterprising, entered the counting-room or took service before the mast. The increased protection given United States commerce by the establishment of the Federal Government, and this country's neutrality during a cycle of European wars, presently stimulated Connecticut shipping. Despite frequent seizures and adverse admiralty decisions, profits were large. The towns of the lower Connecticut Valley and Long Island Sound once again drove a thriving trade with the West Indies, their vessels taking grain, butter, meat, tobacco and other products to be exchanged for sugar and molasses which were later turned into rum.

The coastwise, West Indies, and European commerce did not afford employment for all the available capital, seamen, and mounting tonnage. Enterprising merchants and mariners traced out new trade routes. In 1785 the New London *Gazette*, noting the return of two Sag Harbor ships from successful whaling voyages to the Brazil Banks, boisterously exhorted: "Now, my horse jockeys, beat your horses and cattle into spears, lances, harpoons and whaling gear, and let us all strike out: many spouts ahead! Whales plenty, you have them for catching." [7] Before 1800 New Haven had a South Sea Fleet of about twenty ships engaged in seal fishing in the Antarctic. The skins were sold at Canton, and the vessels returned home laden with silks and teas. On the barren coast of Patagonia was a tract of land two miles long, known to mariners as "New Haven Green," a rendezvous where sealers from that city dried the skins of slaughtered animals.[8] Connecticut sealers and whalers, like their comrades of Massachusetts, smuggled goods into lonely coves on the east and west coasts of South America, gaining valuable specie for the Canton trade as well as the disfavor of Spanish officials. Occasionally they introduced the no less contraband commodity of repub-

6. The above figures are taken from James T. Adams, *New England in the Republic, 1776–1850* (Boston, 1926), pp. 191–192.
7. F. M. Caulkins, *History of New London*, p. 640.
8. Edward E. Atwater, *History of the City of New Haven* (New York, 1887), pp. 497–498.

lican ideas. These activities tended to undermine the Spanish colonial system and furthered the rise of the spirit of independence in South America.

The town of Stratford, DeForest's birthplace, and neighboring Newfield (modern Bridgeport), where he first engaged in business, shared in this general expansion of commerce. When David and his brother John came to Newfield in 1796, Water Street was lined with stores and wharves, and local merchants were carrying on a brisk trade with Boston, New York, and the West Indies.[9] Newfield's skippers occasionally ventured far from the beaten sea paths. The redoubtable Captain Ezekiel Hubbell sailed his ship *Enterprise* to Chile, and narrowly escaped imprisonment in a Spanish dungeon after a daring effort to smuggle his cargo ashore. Then he made for Canton, calling and trading at Nootka Sound, the Sandwich Islands, and the Russian settlements near Kamchatka on the way. Clearing from Canton in January, 1802, the *Enterprise* came to anchor in the Sound off Newfield on June 27, with a valuable freight of Bohea tea and silks, after an absence of nearly three years.[10]

Similar odysseys of the sea, with their exciting themes of high adventure, travel to distant lands, and fabulous profits, were told and retold on the wharves and in the counting-rooms and inns of maritime Connecticut. "Such a romance was there regarding those South Sea ships," remarks the historian of New Haven's commerce, "that very many of the young men of the town were lured to enrol themselves among the companies which manned the sealing fleet, not only to add to their worldly store, but to be able to say to their friends at home that they had been 'round the Horn,' and to 'the place where Captain Cook was murdered'; and such a voyage was . . . something to boast of in New Haven, and none of the ships which left our port for the Pacific but carried representatives of the most respected families of the town." [11]

Merchant princes and sea captains now rivaled Connecticut's ancient ruling class of country squires and parsons in prestige and influence. An expanding money economy, creating new wants and

9. Samuel Orcutt, *A History of . . . Stratford and Bridgeport* (New Haven, 1886), p. 493.
10. *Ibid.*, pp. 612–615.
11. Thomas R. Trowbridge, Jr., "History of the Ancient Maritime Interests of New Haven," in *Papers* of the New Haven Colony Historical Society (New Haven, 1882), III, 148.

aspirations, caused discontent with the rural folkways of the past. Widening horizons of commercial opportunity beckoned young men of parts and ambition. The economic drift of the times and the social values which it generated alike impelled DeForest to turn to a life of trade and to the sea. Thus, all unknowingly, he would revert to an earlier family pattern, to the ways of his long dead and forgotten ancestor Jesse de Forest, wool merchant of Avesnes, who also roved, traded, and sought his fortune in distant lands beyond the seas.

Benjamin DeForest died in 1784, aged only thirty-five, leaving to his wife Mehitable Curtis eighty-five acres of land, a large well-built house, two barns, and a home lot, the estate of a farmer of fair means of that period. With the proceeds of this property the widow could maintain herself and her brood of six young children in what appears to have been modest comfort.

Little information has come down to us concerning the childhood of David C. DeForest. His bold and adventurous temper manifested itself at an early age. A few months after his father's death, according to family tradition, David ran off to become a sailor, was brought back, but some years later ran off again to sea.[12] Complete obscurity surrounds these youthful escapades.

We do not know the extent of DeForest's formal education. He very likely attended the district school at Ripton, a one-story cellarless structure where the children sat on long benches in the middle of the room and the teacher before them, his back to the blazing, crackling fire. Here Dilworth's ancient *Spelling Book* and *Arithmetic* were the standards of instruction. It appears doubtful that David's formal schooling ever advanced beyond this point, for the pretentious Academy at Stratford was not erected until 1804. There is good reason to believe that as a lad DeForest served an apprenticeship in a mercantile establishment; in a letter to his brother John he speaks of himself as having been bred to common commercial pursuits.[13]

A list of books in the possession of David and John DeForest in 1798 points to the early formation of intellectual and literary tastes along well defined lines. Here is found no ponderous work

---

12. John W. De Forest, *The de Forests of Avesnes, and of New Netherland* (New Haven, 1900), p. 112.
13. DeForest to John H. DeForest, Boston, Dec. 29, 1800, DeForest Journal, Vol. 1, Yale University Library.

of divinity, such as might have graced the small library of their parents, but rather such flowers of eighteenth century skepticism and social criticism as Paine's *Age of Reason* and Volney's *Ruins of Empire*. On the lighter side, the collection included Sterne's *Sentimental Journey* and Goethe's *Sorrows of Young Werther*. A *History of South America* (perhaps William Robertson's *History of America*), may have stimulated a youthful desire to see the lands conquered by Spanish valor and treachery. There were works too of a practical nature, the *Seaman's Assistant* and the *Lex Mercatoria*, useful possessions for the prospective merchant and mariner.

Upon reaching his majority, David received his share of the paternal estate and promptly decided on a commercial career. His brother John, then nineteen, had similar notions, and the result was that they merged their slender resources and efforts. In August, 1796, the brothers established a business in Newfield. The only available information concerning the nature of the enterprise is that it was a "dry goods and grocery store." [14]

Hardly had a month gone by, when disaster struck the nascent firm. Robbers entered the store, murdered the clerk, a country lad named Shelton Edwards, and set the building on fire. A New Haven paper gave the following account of the incident under a Newfield date line:

"About ten o'clock on the evening of Thursday last, the store of Messrs. David and John DeForest of this place was discovered to be on fire. The neighborhood was immediately aroused, the store opened, and after considerable exertions of the inhabitants, the fire was extinguished; tho' not until the greater part of the goods in the Store were destroyed. The lad who slept in the Store was then searched for, and was discovered to be murdered, and mangled in a most shocking manner; and cash to the amount of almost nine hundred dollars was missed from the desk." [15]

Recovering from the shock of this catastrophe, the brothers somehow managed to raise the means for a new venture. The first months of 1798 found them at Sullivan, a pioneer settlement on Penobscot Bay, Maine, then a district of Massachusetts. There they kept a store, and shipped lumber and other products to the West Indies.

14. S. Orcutt, *A History of Stratford . . . and Bridgeport*, p. 594.
15. *Connecticut Journal* (New Haven), Sept. 21, 1796.

Misfortune dogged the young partners. Their vessel was condemned at Cap Français in Haiti as unfit for sea, and was sold for the benefit of the underwriters. An auction of their property failed to cover the firm's debts. Among the first entries in DeForest's letterbooks are pleading, cajoling letters to importunate creditors. To one the brothers wrote, "We beg of you not to urge the taking of our bodies, for we are in a distant country from home, and must go to Gaol of necessity." [16] To another they complained whimsically, "Fortune is a damned Slippery Jade, and we hardly know how to manage her; however, honesty shall be our guide under any circumstances, whatever may be said to our disadvantage in your part of the world." [17] In order to fend off sheriff's deputies the brothers barricaded themselves in their house, and kept spies on the lookout for unwelcome visitors. On one occasion a deputy ran three miles to catch his quarry unawares, "but a friend who discovered him and guessed his business was more nimble of foot and arrived at our house about 5 minutes first." [18]

While David stayed in Maine to salvage what he could from his shattered fortunes, he packed his young brother off to Salem to study French and prepare himself otherwise for a mercantile career. To a Connecticut friend he wrote dejectedly, "I shall probably have my Business in this country closed by the 1st of October, which will complete four years' race after wealth, honor and happiness, and so disagreeable is my Situation that I cannot promise myself better." [19]

To his brother John the twenty-four year old DeForest addressed grave homilies, urging the student to make the most of his opportunities. "Time is Cash," he wrote sententiously, "Credit is Cash, Knowledge of Business is Cash. Who would be destitute of Cash, if in their power to obtain it, but such as have no pride, no ambition, no thought for the morrow. From daylight to 9 o'clock at night, an ambitious Young Man will never spend an Idle moment, when all that he can value himself upon is a three months'

---

16. David and John DeForest to Job Nelson, Sullivan, March 31, 1798, DeForest Letterbooks, Vol. 1, Yale University Library.

17. David and John DeForest to Messrs. Hull and Mansfield, Sullivan, March 31, 1798, *ibid.*

18. David and John DeForest to General R. Hunnewell, Sullivan, March 31, 1798, *ibid.*

19. DeForest to Daniel Allen, Sullivan, May 21, 1798, *ibid.*

Opportunity of gaining that Knowledge by which he is to be supported through life." [20]

DeForest now looked about for new roads to "wealth, honor and happiness." The gathering conflict between the United States and France caused him to speculate concerning the merits of a military career. Publication of the "X Y Z dispatches" in the spring of 1798 fanned the flames of Federalist war agitation. Congress hastily prepared for war, levying taxes, creating an army and a navy. Early in August, DeForest called on General Henry Knox of Boston, a stout, rubicund veteran of the Revolution, to apply for a commission in the new army. The general was friendly, and complimented the young man on his excellent appearance.[21] DeForest's application met with moderate success. He did not obtain the captaincy to which he ambitiously aspired, but the records of the War Office show that on March 3, 1799, he was appointed first lieutenant in the 15th Regiment, United States Infantry.[22] In May of that year he received equally cheering news from Connecticut. The general assembly of that state, acting upon a prayer for an act of insolvency for the DeForest brothers, had resolved that after delivering to their creditors all their estate both real and personal, "except such Wages and Emoluments as the said David may be entitled to providing he shall join the Army of the United States . . . the Persons of the said David and John, and all the property which they shall in future acquire be, and the same are hereby discharged and exonerated from all liability for said Debts contracted as aforesaid." [23]

DeForest's hopes for a career of military glory were of course doomed to failure. He spent the greater part of his year of bloodless service in an encampment at Oxford, Massachusetts. Meantime "honest little John Adams," increasingly suspicious of Hamilton's desire for war and of his influence in the presidential cabinet, kept the door open for a peaceful settlement of the imbroglio with France. The tide of public opinion rose rapidly against the war; recruiting lagged; and in later years Adams recalled that the army was as unpopular "as if it had been a

---

20. Charles D. Gray to George D. Gray, Sullivan, (?) 1798, *ibid*. These names were doubtless assumed by the brothers in order to mislead their creditors.

21. DeForest to Isaac Mills, Boston, Aug. 7, 1798, *ibid*.

22. F. B. Heitman, *Historical Register and Dictionary of the United States Army* (2 vols., Washington, 1903), I, 364.

23. Records of the State of Connecticut, Vol. 6, 1797–1801, Connecticut State Library, Hartford.

ferocious beast let loose upon the nation to devour it." [24] In the fall of 1799, after receiving assurances from Talleyrand that good treatment and respect would be accorded to American plenipotentiaries, the President resumed negotiations with France, a treaty settled the quarrel, and the new army was soon disbanded. On June 11, 1800, the encampment at Oxford broke up, and one week later Lieutenant DeForest was honorably discharged from the service.

David set out for Boston, where in the company of some brother officers he celebrated his release from the tedious routine of camp life. High spirits soon gave way to depression, however, as he reflected on his dubious prospects in "this World of dangers and difficulties." Walking the streets of Boston, he ruminated on his hard lot.

"I thought, I pondered, I knew not which way to turn. Already past the time of life when the young men of our country usually begin business, I considered time as precious indeed. A year, a month, or even a day, was worthy of my particular notice and should be used with the greatest prudence and economy. To have thought or done otherwise would have been a crime."

At last he came to a decision that was to shape his career in an unpredictable way.

"I concluded to go to Sea, to engage as a common Sailor, and depend only on my own exertions, for future promotions. It was a singular conclusion for one who had never labored, and perhaps will cause some of my friends many mortifications when thinking on the subject. I can easily anticipate their thoughts and the remarks many of them will make respecting my conduct, but I hope there are some who are not altogether so unsensible, and whose friendship for me is never the less, than when the Sphere in which I move[d] was far more exalted than at present." [25]

He had no difficulty in securing a place before the mast in that heyday of American commerce. On August 28, 1800, he sailed from Boston in the merchant ship *Orislow* bound for Liverpool, England. They anchored in the Mersey River on the last day of September. DeForest was amazed at the multitude of vessels that thronged the great port. "Here," he wrote, "you may see ships belonging to any commercial Nation in the World, ex-

24. Claude G. Bowers, *Jefferson and Hamilton* (New York, 1925), p. 421.
25. DeForest to John H. DeForest, Boston, Dec. 29, 1800, DeForest Journal, Vol. 1.

cepting of such as are at war with England." Great Britain was then at war with Napoleonic France and her satellites. Eager to gain knowledge of the "Manners, customs, and particularly of the Manufactures of this Country, which to any American, is a subject of very great curiosity," DeForest took advantage of his ship's stay in port to make a tour of the counties of Lancashire and Cheshire.

The intensive cultivation of the English countryside won his admiring comments. He plied farmers along the road with questions concerning "the manner in which they cultivated their Lands, the quantity of produce raised, their grazing fields, their Herd of Cows, on what kind of grass fed, their manner of manufacturing Cheese, how it is colored and with what, etc. etc." He had words of praise for English agricultural technique, but the parochial spirit and ignorance of the English countryman elicited his censure. "The people of England," he observed, "do not possess the hospitality of Americans, nor do the peasantry of that Country possess knowledge of Men and things in any proportion to that which American Farmers and tradesmen possess." The reason for this state of affairs, he thought, was the heavy duty laid on newspapers. "Poor people, of course, cannot be at the expense of reading the News of the Day. They have it (if they know it at all) from the Noble and the rich, who put such a coloring on it as they wish it to have, consequently it is not to be wondered at that the peasantry of the Country are so little informed." [26]

Manchester, center of English cotton manufacture, seemed to DeForest an "immense workshop." He marveled at the great height of the five-, six-, and seven-story structures in which carding, spinning, and reeling operations were carried on. From the cellar dwellings of the wretched weavers rose the hum of looms. Questioning of these workers revealed bitter discontent with their conditions. "They will readily tell you," DeForest wrote his brother, "that 'tis with difficulty they support themselves and families, that they have no other mode of obtaining a livelihood, that they would willingly embark on any enterprise, however desperate, to rid themselves of hard hearted poverty. Should they wish to leave the country, Government would say, No. Should they ask redress of grievances, Government turns a deaf Ear.

26. DeForest to John H. DeForest, Cape Verde Islands, Feb. 6, 1801, DeForest Letterbooks, Vol. 1.

They impute their wants to the War, they groan for peace. Unhappy people, how unpleasant does [their] condition appear when compared with that of the mechanics or peasantry of America." [27]

The approaching departure of the *Orislow* made DeForest end his tour and return to Liverpool. At the close of December, 1800, he was back in Boston, and well content with his decision to follow the sea. He wrote brother John that Captain Owen F. Smith of the *Diana* had invited him to come as second mate on a voyage to Canton, that he had considered the matter, decided to accept, and would sail the next day. From Israel Munson and Company of Boston, he secured on credit a stock of watches, knives, and other notions with which to trade on the way.

On the afternoon of December 31, 1800, a large number of persons gathered on Boston's Long Wharf to see the *Diana* set sail for China. The start of a "voyage of circumnavigation" was no ordinary event, and must be attended by some ceremony. At two of the afternoon the *Diana* weighed anchor; the crew gave three cheers, returned by the crowd on the end of Long Wharf; the ship stood down the harbor, was abreast of the lighthouse at six in the evening, discharged her pilot, and proceeded to sea "with a fine breeze from the northwest."

27. *Ibid.*

II

"DOING BUSINESS IN THE SMUGGLING WAY"

THE *Diana* had a complement of twenty-four men, most of them Massachusetts lads in their 'teens or early twenties. Oldest of the crew was Captain Owen F. Smith, thirty years of age, followed by First Mate Reuben Glover, twenty-seven, and Second Mate DeForest, twenty-five years old. Jeremiah C. Barker, a youth of twenty-two, filled the post of ship's doctor.

Their first destination was the Cape Verde islands, where sealers customarily broke voyage to obtain salt for the treatment of sealskins, and fresh provisions as a precaution against the dreaded scurvy. The lookout sighted land on January 31, 1801. Two days later the ship dropped anchor in English Road, under the lee of the island of Mayo. There they stayed six days, taking on provisions and overhauling the vessel. From the Cape Verdes the *Diana* squared off in a southerly direction, making for the sealing grounds off the coast of Patagonia. Favorable trade winds sent the ship scudding along her course. Soon all hands were industriously whittling great numbers of wooden pegs to be used in the drying of sealskins.

Toward the end of February, while still on the high seas, a violent dispute arose between Captain Smith and his second mate. To his journal DeForest confided that the master of the *Diana* was a drunkard and a tyrant. Wearying of alleged persecution, on February 21 he proposed to quit his post and pay for a passage to Rio de Janeiro. Captain Smith would not hear of it. He swore savagely at DeForest, charged him with mutiny, and threatened to confine him to his stateroom should he renew his request.

Remonstrance was useless; DeForest maintained a prudent silence. But bad feeling between the two men persisted. Efforts at mediation by First Mate Glover and Dr. Barker only achieved a brief, uneasy truce. Nursing his grievances, DeForest set down in his journal an ancient maxim of the sea: "So considerable is the power and influence of a Ship's Commander that persons while under them and at Sea, ought to be cautious how they quarrel with them, for very few who are present will remember anything wrong on the Capt's side and everything on the side of his opponent." [1]

The *Diana* was drawing near the coast of Patagonia. Early in March the ship was on soundings, and DeForest had his first glimpse of hair-seals, sporting in the water. Moving leisurely down the coast, they sent out parties to search the shore line for the little rock islands that were the favorite resorts of these animals. In the Bay of Camarónes they found their first prey. DeForest and a party of four men landed on a rock island and killed about 100 hair-seals in forty minutes. A single blow on the head with a stout club crushed the frail skulls of the animals. Later came the arduous task of skinning the seals and cleaning off the blubber, a grueling chore performed with a "beaming knife," after which the skins were pegged out to dry.[2]

Moving southward, the *Diana* came to anchor off Puerto Deseado, an isolated Spanish frontier post with a garrison of thirty-two men. There DeForest saw Patagonian Indians, large and well made men, but not the giants of whom he had read in the works of early travelers. The Americans received a cordial welcome from the local *comandante*, who came to dine on board their vessel and closed his eyes to a brisk contraband trade between the intruders and the inhabitants of the place. The ancient Laws of the Indies were little regarded in this remote borderland of the viceroyalty of La Plata. Zorilla, guanaco, and lion skins were bartered for Yankee rum and dry goods. Such was DeForest's introduction to "doing Business in the Smuggling Way."

Casual and illicit contacts of this kind established the first commercial relations between the United States and the viceroyalty of La Plata. Contraband traffic carried on by English and American sealers and whalers on the east and west coasts of South America was a perennial source of annoyance to higher Spanish

1. DeForest Journal, Vol. 1.
2. For the early days of the sealing industry, see A. Howard Clark, "The Antarctic Fur-Seal and Sea-Elephant Industry," in G. B. Goode and others, *The Fisheries and Fishing Industries of the United States* (Washington, 1887), Section 5, Vol. 2, 400–467.

authorities during the last decades of the colonial era. The mode of its operation is suggested by a royal order of January 20, 1784, which complained of "the clandestine commerce plied by foreigners in our American ports, which they enter on the pretext of stress of weather and the necessity of repairing their ships; and flouting the laws of hospitality and the Law of Nations they introduce their goods despite all the precautions that prudence dictates." This order enjoined that foreign vessels be forbidden entrance on any pretext whatever.[3]

In the closing years of the eighteenth century Spain's distresses in Europe compelled a temporary liberalization of her colonial trade policies, making possible the establishment of United States commerce with La Plata on a more regular and extensive basis. In 1796 Spain became an ally of France; British naval power promptly drove her shipping from the seas; and her communications with the American colonies were almost completely disrupted. Hard necessity drove the Spanish court to promulgate the royal order of November 18, 1797, permitting peninsular merchants to trade with the overseas provinces in neutral ships from national or foreign ports, provided that the goods carried were non-contraband in character (only slaves, specie, and produce were allowed), and that the ships made a return voyage to Spain.[4]

These restrictions, absurd in the face of the British blockade of the peninsula and the unlimited demand of the colonies for all manner of goods, were ultimately disregarded. Even the conservative *consulado* or tribunal of commerce of Buenos Aires concluded that the return voyage to Spain should not be insisted upon, because the requirement could not be adequately enforced; and declared that compliance with the spirit of the royal order demanded the free export of the produce of the country and the import of needed commodities.[5]

By reason of "the location of its ports, the abundance of its merchant marine, and its neutrality toward the two most formi-

3. Facultad de Filosofía y Letras, *Documentos para la historia argentina, comercio de Indias, 1713–1809* (Vols. V, VI, and VII, Buenos Aires, 1915–1916), VI, 269.

4. Ricardo Levene, *A History of Argentina,* translated and edited by William S. Robertson (Chapel Hill, N. C., 1937), pp. 110–111. For the text of the order, see *Documentos para la historia argentina,* VII, 134.

5. Archivo General de la Nación, *Documentos referentes a la guerra de la independencia y emancipación de la República Argentina* (2 vols., Buenos Aires, 1914–1917), I, 293.

dable powers, France and England," in the words of a contemporary colonial observer, the United States was particularly favored by the new dispensation.[6] Yankee merchants were quick to take advantage. The Spanish minister to the United States wrote in 1799 that about five American vessels had already made trading voyages to La Plata. The lucrative nature of this traffic can be gauged from his statement that these ships purchased jerked beef in La Plata at a dollar and a half per quintal, and sold it in Cuba for ten.[7]

At the same time that American trade with La Plata increased, numerous English vessels, flying the American flag and pretending United States registry, came to share in the profitable neutral commerce.[8] These developments aroused Spanish mercantile jealousy, and governmental fears that the supposedly neutral trade was actually strengthening Spain's powerful enemy. Consequently, on April 20, 1799, a new order went forth, revoking that of November 18, 1797, because, "far from experiencing the favorable effects toward which this sovereign dispensation was directed, . . . it has redounded entirely to the private injury of our vassals of America and Spain, and to the increase of the industry and commerce of the enemy." [9]

American vessels nevertheless continued to arrive in the Plate estuary, bringing cargoes that had been ordered before revocation of the permissive edict, and pleading ignorance of the new state of affairs. So lax was the enforcement of the new decree that on July 18, 1800, the Spanish king addressed a vigorous reprimand to the viceroy of La Plata, asserting that the introduction of foreign goods into the colony continued with complete freedom, and insisting on more effective compliance with the law.[10]

This admonition was evidently heeded. At the time of DeForest's first visit to La Plata in 1801 the ban on neutral trade was being enforced with considerable vigor. The net result was to turn this commerce back into illicit channels, in which it henceforth moved, with few exceptions, until the decree of November 6, 1809,

---

6. *Documentos para la historia argentina*, VII, 175.
7. [Carlos Martínez de Irujo], *Observations on the Commerce of Spain with Her Colonies, in Time of War* (Philadelphia, 1800).
8. Emilio Ravignani, "El virreinato del Río de la Plata, 1776–1810," in Academia Nacional de la Historia, *Historia de la nación argentina* (Buenos Aires, 1936–   ), IV, Section 1, pp. 172–173.
9. *Documentos para la historia argentina*, VII, 158.
10. *Ibid.*, pp. 181–182.

issued by Viceroy Cisneros on the eve of the Argentine Revolution, opened the ports of La Plata to allied and neutral vessels bringing cargoes of any kind.[11]

Leaving Puerto Deseado, the *Diana* moved slowly down the coast in search of seal rookeries. Presently there arose a new controversy between Captain Smith and his second mate. The captain determined to land a sealing party on an island that appeared to DeForest to be privately owned. His objections to the undertaking provoked an explosion of wrath. "Captain Smith was in a passion with me and agreed to set me and my effects on Shore, but at about 10 at night he weighed Anchor and put to Sea, altering his plan of Sealing and forfeiting his word with me. On my remonstrating against it he said he should keep me, but that I might do duty or not as I chose. I made my election and determined to do no more duty on board the Ship, but consider myself detained here as a prisoner." [12]

Arrival on the scene of the sloop *Prudence* of Nantucket, Captain John Paddock, broke this awkward deadlock. The newcomers had been sealing at South Georgia, a mountainous, perpetually snow-covered island several hundred miles east of Cape Horn, and were bound for La Plata for repairs and provisions. Captain Smith grudgingly agreed that DeForest might transfer to the sloop and take passage for the Plate estuary. He was not yet to quit the coast of Patagonia, however, for the two commanders decided to pool their crews and take the *Diana* southward in search of better sealing, leaving the smaller vessel in James Harbor. There DeForest and two others remained, keeping guard over the sloop until the return of the sealers from the south.

Early in June the *Diana* returned, with a catch of 500 hair- and fur-seal skins, and a story of narrow escape from foundering on rocks. It was July 2, 1801, before the *Prudence* set sail for La Plata, DeForest on board. They anchored off Montevideo on the nineteenth of the month. In his journal DeForest recorded his

11. There is much useful information on early American commerce with La Plata in Harry Bernstein, *Origins of Inter-American Interest, 1700–1812* (Philadelphia, 1945), pp. 33–51. See also Arthur P. Whitaker, *The United States and the Independence of Latin America, 1800–1830* (Baltimore, 1941), pp. 14–16, and Charles L. Chandler, "United States Merchant Ships in the Rio de la Plata (1801–1809) as Shown by Early Newspapers," *Hispanic-American Historical Review*, II (1919), 26–54.

12. DeForest Journal, Vol. 1.

first impressions of the Platine landscape. "What little of the country I saw appeared to be as delightful as I have ever seen. There are no fences. The Ground is almost perfectly level and productive of almost every luxury of life. It is covered with innumerable Herds of Cattle, Sheep and Horses, and fruit trees in abundance. The Town consists of Houses uniformly one story high, and appears like a very neat little place." [13] Less inviting was the reception accorded by the Spanish authorities to the American visitors. When Captain Paddock and DeForest attempted to go on shore, they were stopped at the head of the pier and ordered out of port.[14]

Through the intercession of a more fortunate countryman, Captain Ray of the *Hope*, they were permitted to take on some sorely needed provisions before leaving. From him they learned that the reason for the official hostility was the large-scale smuggling which American vessels had lately engaged in at Montevideo and Buenos Aires. Such were the proportions of this traffic, he declared, that an order had been received to admit no more United States ships unless actually in such distress that they could not proceed without repairs.

Quitting inhospitable Montevideo, Captain Paddock lifted anchor and set sail for Rio de Janeiro. On July 31 the *Prudence* was hailed and stopped by a Buenos Aires brigantine, the *Volcán*, cruising in search of Portuguese enemy vessels.[15] During the search the captain of the boarding party, a hectoring, swaggering brute, according to DeForest, stole a watch from Captain Paddock's trunk and compelled him to sell a hand organ for half its price.

A few days later, the *Prudence* rode at anchor in the blue and sparkling waters of the bay of Rio de Janeiro. Over these waters, circling the bay, towered lofty and strangely shaped mountains.

13. *Ibid.*
14. The *Telégrafo Mercantil* (facsimile edition, Buenos Aires, 1914) of Buenos Aires, July 22, 1801, carried the following news item, apparently referring to the *Prudence*: "Montevideo, July 22. On the 19th instant an American sloop entered this port, coming from Puerto Deseado, whose garrison she had aided with provisions which were immediately replaced, and yesterday afternoon she sailed for her destination."
15. The farcical "War of the Oranges" between Spain and Portugal was ended in Europe by the Treaty of Badajoz, June 8, 1801, but news of the treaty did not reach La Plata until December of that year. Diego Luis Molinari, "La política lusitana y el Río de la Plata," in *Historia de la nación argentina*, V, Section 1, p. 439.

On the narrow strip of land between the shore and the mountains stood the capital of the Portuguese viceroyalty of Brazil. "The most squalid and filthy abode of humans under the sun," according to an English traveler of the period, the shabby, ugly houses and dirty, narrow streets formed a striking contrast to the magnificent natural surroundings.

DeForest went ashore intent on gaining as much information of the country and its trade as he could. He took lodgings in the city with another newly arrived American, Thomas Halsey of Providence, Rhode Island, with whom many years later he was to have far from friendly dealings. Early in September arrived the ship *Monticello* of Philadelphia, one of whose crew conveyed to DeForest the pleasing news that his brother John had lately been seen at Santiago de Cuba, in good health and making a profitable voyage.[16]

The foreign trade of Brazil, a monopoly of the mother country, was largely in the hands of English merchants whose ships, laden with European manufactures, came to Rio after supposedly touching at Portuguese ports.[17] Despite all precautions to prevent smuggling, DeForest observed, "a person who speaks the language and understands the business may effect it." He could not dispose of his own little adventure, however, for the city was glutted with European goods, chiefly because the war in progress between the Spanish and Portuguese colonies hindered the customary contraband trade with La Plata.

DeForest resolved to seek a more promising field for his enter-

16. In the Dyer White Papers, Yale University Library, there is a letter from John H. DeForest to Dyer White at New Haven, dated Santiago de Cuba, September 25, 1800, that graphically depicts the woes of a neutral trader in the era of the Napoleonic Wars. "In our passage from St. Croix to this port, we were gratified with being taken under the parental care of one of his 'Sovereign Majesty's' servants; who, from his tender affection for us, came near granting us a safe conduct to Jamaica: indeed, nothing but our being destitute of a *valuable* cargo, prevented him from doing that generous office. After *protecting* our vessel for 18 or 20 hours with an officer and arm'd soldiers, and finding we had nothing on board, but a little *salt,* he inhumanly withdrew his paternal care, and oblig'd us to shift for ourselves. 'Twould be ingratitude in me, however, not to acknowledge that this generous minded *Chevalier* assured me, on his taking leave, 'that, should providence permit us to fall in his way on our return home (at which time we should undoubtedly be more worthy his notice) he would certainly renew his fraternal embrace; and, enfolding us in his arms, would not let go his grasp until we were safely lodg'd in the *pure* and uncorrupted bosom of some vice Admiralty Judge.'"

17. For the commerce of colonial Brazil, see Roberto C. Simonsen, *Historia economica do Brasil* (2 vols., Rio de Janeiro, 1937), II, Ch. 4.

prise. He thought of going to Buenos Aires in the *Prudence*, chartered by a Spanish merchant to take a cargo to La Plata. But the merchant, learning that the American planned to bring his wares, would not admit him on board. Next he planned to try the market at Rio Grande, a port near the disputed Spanish border. Formidable obstacles barred this project. Foreigners might not travel in Brazil without passports, very infrequently granted, and no Portuguese would risk imprisonment and confiscation of property to give DeForest passage to Rio Grande. "While at Rio de Janeiro I learned thoroughly the mode of doing business there in the Smuggling way, but I found great difficulty in getting away from there in a Portuguese vessel."

At last he came upon a skipper who would brave the dangers of carrying DeForest to Rio Grande. He was one André da Cunha Rego, the young owner of a *zumaca* or smack about to sail for Rio São Francisco. "I felt very much relieved indeed for I had worried myself exceedingly for a passage away to sell my goods and learn the business of the country."

They took furtive leave of Rio de Janeiro on September 24, 1801. To avoid suspicion DeForest stayed on board an English vessel putting out to sea until they were six or eight leagues from port; then he transferred to Cunha Rego's tiny bark. After fourteen days at sea and three "Gales of Wind," which the superstitious crew sought to conjure by attaching a sacred image to the quarter rail, to DeForest's great amusement, they dropped anchor at Rio São Francisco. Presently André returned from a visit ashore with a disturbing report. The *comandante* of the place was a gloomy fellow who showed no mercy to foreigners found in his domain. Recently he had imprisoned two such intruders and the captain of the ship that brought them.

It was decided to keep DeForest hidden in the boat while Cunha Rego transacted his business in town. Three weeks the smuggler remained pent up in the ship's tiny cabin, much of the time rolled up in a blanket to prevent recognition, and subsisting on an unpalatable diet of jerked beef and the Brazilian preparation of ground cereal known as *farinha*. Meanwhile André attempted to sell some of his friend's wares. The results were not gratifying. "Not only the Rulers of the place," complained DeForest, "but some of the Merchants at this infernal Hole appeared disposed to strip me of everything I had." [18]

18. DeForest to Israel Munson and Co., Rio Grande, Dec. 25, 1801, DeForest Journal, Vol. 2.

Cunha Rego finally wound up his affairs at Rio São Francisco, and they bore away south for Santa Catharina, the next port of any size on the coast. DeForest was in a mood to throw discretion to the winds. On arrival at Santa Catharina he resolved "to make a bold push for a passport, and either get in Prison or my Liberty." Cautious inquiry by the helpful André yielded the information that the governor of the place, Curado by name, was a man of liberal principles, possessed of an excellent knowledge of English and French. DeForest promptly dispatched Cunha Rego with the message that an "English Gentleman of distinction" was in the harbor without a passport, and desired to speak with his Excellency.

Governor Curado sent back a favorable reply. That evening, no doubt wearing his finest garments: coat of broadcloth, swansdown vest, cashmere breeches, and silk hose, DeForest called at the governor's residence. Assuming the consequence of a gentleman of fortune on his travels, a pretension which he supported by display of his old officer's commission, he regaled the Portuguese official with an account of his adventures, with certain judicious omissions and deviations from the facts. In conclusion, he requested the governor to grant him a passport to Rio Grande.

Curado listened, smiled graciously, but probably was not deceived. Fortunately for the impostor, the governor of Santa Catharina was not in sympathy with the exclusive policies of Lisbon. He reminded DeForest that the Portuguese government was very suspicious of foreigners, and its officers generally shared the principles of their government. As for himself, he had been educated in Paris, and was free from those jealous feelings. He invited DeForest to be his guest for the duration of his stay in Santa Catharina. Should he wish to depart, however, his passport to go to Rio Grande by land or sea would be ready on the morrow.

The next morning Governor Curado handed DeForest his passport, and the two men parted with expressions of mutual respect and an exchange of gifts. After settling accounts with the faithful André, the smuggler boarded a vessel bound for Rio Grande, taking leave of Santa Catharina with the comment that the women of the place were "handsomer than I have seen elsewhere in Brasil, but . . . they do not look like the pretty Girls of Connecticut."

He landed at Rio Grande, southernmost port of Brazil, on November 16, 1801. In time of peace, he learned, the port was a center of contraband trade with La Plata, to the amount of $200,000 a year. War between Spain and Portugal had interrupted this traffic, and markets were extremely dull. Failing to sell his goods, DeForest resolved to cross into Spanish territory. Suspension of hostilities on the frontier at the end of December, upon announcement of the treaty of peace of June 8, 1801, aided his plan. On January 13, 1802, in company with a number of Spanish merchants, lately prisoners of war, he set off across the plains for Buenos Aires, some 500 miles away. A priest of Rio Grande, "my good old friend, Padre José Alves Chaves," had provided him with letters of introduction to influential personages on the Spanish side of the border.

In high spirits, the party moved southward over the grassy plains of Rio Grande do Sul. While the older and more sedate travelers rode in carts, DeForest and a young merchant, Don Francisco Galup, generally rode on horseback, desiring "to visit every house we saw within two miles of our road, to converse with the inhabitants, to get every information relative to the country in our power, to eat bread and milk, and make love to the buxom wenches, who uniformly gave preference to the Inglez, as they are pleased to call me, all having a high regard for the English nation." [19]

On January 22 they came to the Spanish frontier post of Santa Teresa, where DeForest presented letters of introduction to the *comandante* and to a local merchant, both of whom treated him with much politeness and attention. A few days later he arrived in Montevideo, where another letter of introduction secured him an invitation to stay at the home of an unidentified merchant.

From Montevideo he sent home a boastful account of his prodigious wanderings, "never before made by a stranger, and an infidel."

"Picture to yourself," he wrote, "a young man deserting his ship, on board of which he was but a petty officer, on the uninhabited coast of Patagonia; arriving in Brasil, where he could neither speak nor understand a word that was spoken by the inhabitants, and where he had not a friend to look to for advice or assistance; flying from Rio de Janeiro without a passport, and contrary to the laws of the country; traversing all the Southern

---

19. DeForest to Isaac Mills, Montevideo, March 10, 1802, in Louis E. de Forest, ed., "A Trip through Brazil in 1802," *Brazil* (New York), Year IX, no. 101, March, 1937.

part of Brasil; introducing himself to the Governador of St. Catherine who speaks English and French, as a young Gentleman of fortune on his travels, and by him invited to live at the Palace all the time he should be there; arriving in this province, introduced to people of the first respectability, received by the Comandant of S. Teresa, and Governor of Maldonado, as a companion, and as such introduced to their families and friends, and in two days going to Buenos Aires, the capital of the viceroyalty, with some excellent letters, and an increased share of assurance." [20]

As he reflected on these experiences, it became clear to DeForest that society bestowed its favors on those who professed to be least in need of them.

"I suppose you will conclude that I possess as much impudence as vanity and that a man of twenty-eight years of age, without property or very particular friends, ought to reduce his feelings, and his actions, to a level with that of his circumstances. I think differently. He who has a good opinion of himself is sure to have the good opinion of others. If a man is poor, he may travel through all parts of the world, at less expense, by assuming the character of a Gentleman, than that of a blackguard. 'Tis ingrafted in our nature to do, unasked, a thousand favors to a man who appears not to be in want of them. But the poor devil who comes modestly before us, and tells us by his actions that his property, or family, does not entitle him to the rank of Gentleman, receives no favors." [21]

DeForest wrote that he would come home by way of Spain as second mate of an unidentified ship. By the time of his return he expected to be possessed of a considerable knowledge of trade and navigation. He suggested that his friends have ready for him a vessel of 400 tons, completely equipped and furnished for a two-year voyage—presumably to La Plata. He closed in a vein of whimsical gaiety. "I ought to be making money, but fate has decreed otherwise. Like Ulysses, I expect I must yet be tossed about a considerable time longer before I shall be able to see and possess my darling Penelope: 30 or 40,000 dollars." [22]

The Yankee Ulysses noted the presence of thirty-two American merchant ships detained in the Río de la Plata. Some had been

20. *Ibid.*
21. *Ibid.*
22. *Ibid.*

there as long as eight months, awaiting permission from Spain to load cargo and leave the river. DeForest thought that failure to secure such permission would prove disastrous to the outfitters. "I am confident the merchants on whose account the ships have come will never be able to make good the damage." [23]

On March 16, 1802, the smuggler boarded a Buenos Aires-bound sloop, without a passport or other official sanction. The capital of the viceroyalty lay some 200 miles from the mouth of the river, on its southwest shore. Twenty-four hours after leaving Montevideo, the sloop anchored in the harbor of Buenos Aires. A rude cart drawn by oxen took DeForest and his baggage from the shore to the inn of the Three Kings.

An almost complete gap in his journal and letterbooks obscures DeForest's movements during the next four months. Much of this time he presumably passed in doing business and in gaining a knowledge of the language and trade of the country. He was confined to his lodgings for several weeks with a severe cold. He evidently suffered no molestation from local authorities, despite the time-honored ban against the residence of foreigners in Spain's colonies.

When his diary resumes, on July 13, 1802, DeForest is most startlingly installed as a guest in a monastery of the Franciscan Order, called *el Regulador*.[24] He evidently wished to improve his knowledge of Spanish by avoiding contact with English-speaking friends in the city. Perhaps he also thought to court the favor of the influential Catholic clergy by display of interest in the "*santa fé romana, católica, y apostólica*." At any rate, the simple regimen of the monastery appears to have been to his liking. "Peace and quietness reign here, Poverty is the order of the day, of course no cause of envy exists to lessen the enjoyment of their humble Meal and still more humble apparel."

The pious brethren regarded DeForest in the light of a prospective convert and spent much time with him in religious discussion. When in early August he announced his intention of leaving the monastery, without having embraced the faith, they sorrowed for him as for a lost soul. "Poor Don David," he quotes

23. DeForest to Isaac Mills, Montevideo, March 12, 1802, in L. E. de Forest, ed., "A Trip through Brazil in 1802." For a list of these ships, see C. L. Chandler, "United States Merchant Ships in the Rio de la Plata (1801–1809)," pp. 26–28.

24. According to DeForest, this name was applied to monasteries of the Franciscan Order whose regimen followed the precepts and example of St. Peter of Alcantara.

them as saying, "he for whom we have such a great respect, and whom it was our expectation to have seen made a Christian before his departure, is now going out into the World, to mix with his Countrymen who have no regard for Religion, and who will undoubtedly turn to ridicule everything they may discover in him appertaining to Religion. He is lost forever, we very much fear, but our Prayers shall daily be offered up for him, that he may be convinced of the necessity of embracing our Holy Religion; that he may embrace it, and finally, that he may be received into heaven, and with all other Good Catholics enjoy happiness for ever and ever." [25]

DeForest took cheerful leave of his kind hosts on August 11, 1802. From the Father Superior, Padre Montero, he carried letters of introduction to a wealthy merchant of Buenos Aires, Francisco Ignacio de Ugarte, and to a "very respectable clergyman of Montevideo." Preparing to depart from La Plata, he invested the proceeds of the sale of his goods in a stock of nutria skins and ostrich feathers. He did not sail for Spain, as he had planned, but instead took ship for England. On December 6, 1802, he embarked from Montevideo in the *Three Sisters* of Philadelphia, Captain John Ansley, "laden with hides and bound to Falmouth and a market."

25. DeForest Journal, Vol. 2.

III

"A HIGHLY DANGEROUS TRADE"

THE *Three Sisters* anchored in Falmouth port on March 6, 1803. While the ship discharged cargo, DeForest went ashore to view the countryside of Cornwall and inspect the famous tin and copper mines of this region. He visited the rotten borough of St. Mawes, boasting some 600 inhabitants, and was amazed to learn that this little town sent two members to parliament. "And what is still more extraordinary, there are but Five Votes given in. Very unequal representation." [1]

At Redruth, he descended into one of the mines. "We were underground about three Hours, in which time we went under houses and Streets. Saw a great Number of People at Work, sometimes going on perpendicular Ladders, then crawling down the rocks, then on slanting Ladders, then on Planks laid across deep caverns, then walking a subterraneous road horizontally, then wading in Channels of Water, then over shoes in Mud and Gravel, till we arrived at the, or nearly, to the lower end of the Water Engine, about 500 feet, perpendicular height. Here we saw two poor, though apparently happy, Devils, who were driven from some 50 feet below by the Water and were waiting for the Engine to clear it. On our return we took various other roads and directions till we arrived by another outlet at the surface where we once more had Daylight. Mudded from head to foot, and most intolerably fatigued, I ran to the Office, stripped, washed and redressed myself. The Miners gave me what they called Cornish wine, made of Rum and molasses." [2]

Some days later the *Three Sisters* sailed for London, DeForest on board. They came into the Thames River on March 19, and that evening the trader dismounted from a "caravan coach" in the English capital. He found lodging at the Virginia and Maryland Coffee House in Cornhill. The next day he consigned his stock of nutria skins and ostrich feathers for sale to Thomas Wilson, merchant of the City.

1. DeForest Journal, Vol. 2.
2. *Ibid.*

Portents of war clouded the English spring of 1803. Formal hostilities with France had ceased in 1801, but bitter commercial warfare between the two countries and British alarm over the advancing tide of Napoleonic power on the continent threatened a rupture of the Peace of Amiens. In Plymouth harbor DeForest had seen a great array of the "wooden walls of old England," guns on board and drawing one tier of water, "a thing uncommon in time of Peace, which plainly shows that the Government are jealous of the French." He found the business world of London sensitive to every turn in the developing crisis. On March 29 it was reported that Pitt and Dundas were coming back into power, "which plainly shows that war is inevitable." Stocks immediately fell 5 and 6 per cent.

In Paris the British ambassador, Lord Whitworth, was engaged in weighty negotiations with the government of the first consul. Stubbornly he resisted the French demand that Britain evacuate the strategic island of Malta. Rumors concerning the progress of these discussions ran in the English capital, exciting alternate fears and hopes. On the morning of May 5, DeForest noted in his diary, "Notice was up at the Mansion House that Lord Hawksbury [British foreign minister] had written to the Lord Mayor that the dispute with France was amicably adjusted. Before 12 o'clock, however, the Letter was found to be a Forgery. All London was in an uproar. Stocks had risen all at once to 7¾–8% higher than yesterday." In a thronged House of Commons he heard Fox, Canning, Addington, and other political leaders discuss the great question of the day until debate waxed so warm that visitors were ordered to withdraw. On May 14 came word that Lord Whitworth had left Paris. "THE DIE APPEARS TO BE CAST," was DeForest's comment. Two days later the British king announced the rupture of negotiations, proclaimed an embargo and the issue of letters-of-marque against French commerce.

Meanwhile Napoleon's embarrassments in Europe had brought a gigantic windfall to the Young Republic across the seas. Fearing that his recently acquired province of Louisiana would fall into British hands at the outbreak of hostilities, Napoleon decided to sell it to the United States and use the proceeds for his military campaigns. Our plenipotentiaries in France, James Monroe and Robert Livingston, hastened to seal the magnificent bargain. They purchased the vast and ill-defined territory for 60,000,000 francs plus the assumption by the United States of claims of its citizens not to exceed 20,000,000 francs. DeForest gave scant attention to this epochal event. "A second report," he noted briefly in his diary on May 17, "that Louisiana has been ceded to the United States by the French Government, in consideration of a certain sum of Money, said to be $6,000,000, payable in Debts due from the French Government, and money."

Time passed swiftly for DeForest as he roamed through London, center of world commerce and industry, repository of innumerable historic monuments and landmarks. He made the customary visits to St. Paul's, Westminster Abbey, and the Tower of London. He browsed in Lackington's book store, reputed the largest collection of books in the world, and jotted in his diary the edifying fact that Lackington was once a very poor man and began by peddling songs and pamphlets. He strolled into "Pidcock's Collection of Wild Beasts," and regarded with curiosity "a very singular animal, Elephant." From the din and bustle of the roaring city he found relief by excursions to the neighboring countryside. At Twickenham he came to the house built by the "so justly celebrated Alexander Pope." Strangers were forbidden entrance, but "the Watch Words, Potosi, or Mexico, overcome in this Country, all such Mandates." DeForest left the hallowed spot with a tribute to the philosopher-poet. "Farewell Pope, I revere and respect your Memory."

Early in August, his nutria skins and ostrich feathers sold, DeForest sailed for America in the ship *Gosport*. He landed at Norfolk, Virginia, on September 24, and from there proceeded by water to New York. Yellow fever raged in the city when he arrived, and many inhabitants had fled. "Gloomy looks the Morn," the traveler wrote in his journal. "No one moving, this beautiful City deserted, silent as the Grave, not a Boy hallooing, or a Sailor quarreling, nor a single ring of a Bell." Some days later he disembarked at New Haven from a New York packet boat, to be warmly greeted by his brother John, now a rising country merchant of Watertown, Connecticut.

The brothers set out by stagecoach for this inland town, the home of their mother and step-father, Edward Lockwood, Sr. As they rode over the rolling Connecticut countryside, David's mind turned back to the flat, treeless, and sky-filled plains of La Plata and Rio Grande do Sul. "I was much surprised that the Country should appear so beautifully, when considering its roughness.

The Craggy Hills, the Groves of Timber, the Rivers and the Brooks—all appeared to possess charms innumerable." They arrived at Watertown on the afternoon of October 14, and the returned wanderer was soon regaling his parents and brothers with accounts of his South American exploits.

DeForest's experiences and observations in La Plata had convinced him that this region offered a rich field for American commercial enterprise. Lacking the means for an independent venture, he broached the subject of a trading voyage to the Plate estuary to several merchants. His overtures met with a cool reception. Established firms, basking in the sun of a lucrative neutral trade with Europe and the West Indies (undiminished until the *Essex* decision of 1805 inaugurated a new restrictive policy on the part of the European belligerents), were not disposed to embark on hazardous expeditions to the forbidden Plate ports. Reports of the prolonged detention of American vessels in the river in 1801–1802 heightened skepticism about the prospects of the Plata trade. Unable to gain support for his cherished scheme, DeForest cast about for other ways to fill a depleted purse.

Organization of the Louisiana territory, then under discussion in Washington, suggested the possibility of an interesting employment. DeForest wrote to Secretary of the Treasury Gallatin, expressing gratification with an administration "so well in accord with my own sentiments of propriety," and conceiving "the acquisition of Louisiana, and consequently the entire command of the Mississippi and all its branches" to be almost invaluable to the United States. He closed by requesting the office of surveyor in the new possession.[3] Despite the support of Pierpont Edwards and Abraham Bishop, Republican party leaders in Connecticut, his application seems to have been denied.

DeForest went to New York in May, 1804, in search of commercial employment. He had not abandoned hope of revisiting La Plata. An entry in his diary notes that on May 5 he wrote to the American consul at Santiago de Cuba, requesting that he "inform me by Letter to Buenos Ayres (directed to care of Don Francisco Ignacio de Ugarte) what are the prices of Slaves, Beef, Tallow, Flour and the probable Markets for Months." In New York he discussed a trading voyage to La Plata for nutria skins with several firms, including the prominent New Haven merchant, Ebenezer Townsend. Nothing came of these negotia-

---

3. DeForest to Albert Gallatin, New Haven, Jan. 10, 1804, *ibid.*, Vol. 3.

tions. At the end of June, DeForest was dispirited and morose. In his diary he inveighed against rich merchants who calculated that "others must dance attendance at their will." Everything relating to him, he complained, went wrong-end first.

A sudden stroke of fortune revived his spirits. On July 2 he received an offer to take command of the schooner *Daphne* on a trading voyage to the Guianas and West Indies. In his capacity of captain and supercargo he would receive wages of twenty-two dollars a month, 5 per cent commission on all property sold, 21½ per cent on all bought for the owners' account. DeForest accepted the offer with alacrity. "Pleasant times in a gloomy season," he wrote in his diary, "I have been so accustomed to disappointments that I fear all will miscarry."

Laden with beef, pickle, and codfish, the *Daphne* sailed out of New York harbor on July 5, her destination the French colony of Cayenne. East of the Bermudas they caught the regular trade winds and ran them down to Cayenne, casting anchor in port after a passage of thirty-three days. DeForest found little demand for his articles, and decided to try the markets of neighboring Dutch Surinam and British Guiana. He touched in turn at Paramaribo and Demerara, but came away almost empty handed. Bewailing his luck, he continued northward, entered the Caribbean, and ran for Tobago in the Windward Islands. He found three American vessels in the harbor of Scarsborough, all complaining of poor sales. Nothing remained, he decided, but to make a dash for Martinique, braving the numerous British cruisers that roamed these waters.

In the early dark hours of September 7, the shadowy bulk of Martinique came in sight. At sunrise they slipped into the great bay of Fort Royal without incident and came to anchor off the town. DeForest went ashore resolved to sell his cargo at whatever price it would bring. In the course of the day he bargained it away for "somewhere about New York prices," investing the proceeds in molasses. He consoled himself with the thought that he had done as well as he could, for indisputably markets in the West Indies were all very bad.

Damning all Fort Royal, DeForest stood out to sea in the middle of the hurricane season. Two days out, a British privateer stopped the *Daphne* and sent her into Tortola for examination. No cause for detention was found, and they were permitted to go on. Cape Hatteras was astern on September 24; the next day they ran into a heavy gale. The heavily loaded craft rolled precariously in the troughs of great seas; their foresail was soon blown to pieces. On the twenty-sixth the gale abated, but it was a momentary respite.

"We poor Devils who cannot see the length of a Man's Nose consoled ourselves by saying, 'to be sure we have lost our Foresail, our most valuable sail, yet we have a fine S. W. breeze, we know exactly our Longitude and will be in New York in Three days.' Little did we know what was then brewing—that all the Infernal Spirits were laying their heads together and plotting a Jig for us to dance—and a hell of a Jig it proved indeed.

"For at 2 P. M. a Black Cloud appeared at the S. W. It flew like lightning from the Place of its Birth to where we were, and much ado. We got in our sail, except our Jibs Bonnet, under which we scudded all the afternoon, the wind whistled, the Seas were mountain high. At Dark, not daring to scud any longer, because we could not see to avoid the Seas that every moment threatened us with destruction, we hove to again under our little Bonnet. She lay to but poorly, her head constantly knocking off, and we rolling in the Troughs of the Seas. 'Twas a situation, in my opinion, very dangerous. We feared to set our reefed Mainsail for 'twas worn so thin that I was confident 'twould immediately blow to pieces, but something must be done. We of course set Just the Peak of the Balanced reefed Mainsail (about one third). She came to better but still it would not do so that we could feel safe and free from the dangers of the immensely heavy Seas by which we were surrounded." [4]

Hurried consultation with the mate and crew revealed general agreement that the ship must be lightened if she were to outlive the gale. With a heavy heart, DeForest gave orders to pump the contents of ten hogsheads of molasses overboard. The *Daphne* immediately came to the wind much better, became more lively in the water. All evening and until late the next morning it blew tremendously from various points, then gradually abated until they could make some small sail. The following day (October 28) the sea was smooth, the weather pleasant. In his cabin, dining on beef and spiced meats, washed down with excellent brandy and port wine, DeForest mourned the eternal loss of ten hogsheads of molasses.

"Don't trouble me no more," he wrote in his diary, "ye spirits

---

4. *Ibid.,* Vol. 4.

of Bad Sales, Molasses and Foresail. If I have not done as I ought, 'tis the best I could, and if I am to be censured, let those who do it, consider every circumstance relating to the business of this very unpleasant Voyage, and I am sure I cannot suffer much in their opinions."

They came safely into New York port, November 3, 1804. For all DeForest's misgivings, his employers professed to be satisfied with his management of the voyage. Settlement of accounts found him richer by several hundred dollars. Fortified with this inconsiderable capital, supplemented by a loan from the firm of Dunham and Lord of Boston, he immediately set about preparing for a smuggling voyage to Brazil and La Plata. He chartered a small schooner, the *Jefferson* of Vinalhaven, Captain Nathaniel Mitchell, and loaded her down with naval stores, in great demand at Buenos Aires.[5]

On the eve of his departure, DeForest wrote to President Jefferson a letter of application for the post of United States consul to the "Vice Kingdom of Buenos Ayres." [6]

"Having passed some time in South America near the close of the French Revolutionary War," he set forth, "more particularly in Brasil and La Plata, and having witnessed many of the difficulties into which our Countrymen plunged themselves from their ignorance of the customs and trade of La Plata, and being satisfied that the carrying trade of the Country must devolve on neutrals should Spain be again engaged in war with England as appears highly probable,[7] I have thought of Establishing myself in mercantile business at Buenos Ayres immediately after the expected war shall have been declared." He closed by assuring the President that his appointment as consul would enable him to render important services to American commerce with La Plata.[8]

DeForest took the *Jefferson* out of New York port on February 2, 1805, his destination the Cape Verdes. After a brief stop there

---

5. In 1799, pitch cost $2 or $3 a barrel in the United States, but sold in Buenos Aires at $40 a barrel. [C. M. Irujo], *Observations on the Commerce of Spain with Her Colonies*.

6. The names *virreinato de Buenos-Ayres* and *virreinato del Río de la Plata* were used without distinction in reference to the colony.

7. Hostilities between Great Britain and Spain, halted by the Treaty of Amiens of March 27, 1802, were renewed in December, 1804.

8. DeForest to President Thomas Jefferson, New Haven, Jan. 25, 1805, DeForest Journal, Vol. 4.

for provisions, they set course for Brazil. On April 22 the schooner dropped anchor in the harbor of Rio de Janeiro, described by DeForest as "the most grand and romantic in nature." Employing the traditional formula of Yankee smugglers in South American waters, he pleaded the need of repairs to his ship in order to secure permission to remain in port. Judicious management of the officials who came on the customary visit of inspection ensured approval of his request. Before long he had smuggled forty barrels of tar aboard a Portuguese vessel, "and could have smuggled another thousand with equal security." He discovered that with proper measures any kind of contraband trade could be plied at Rio. "Everything is bought and sold for Money—Men, Merchandise, and some Women." With an eye to future trading ventures to Brazil, DeForest noted in his diary that cotton cambrics were gaining popularity in the country, and promised to become an article of great consumption.

The *Jefferson* slipped out of Rio harbor on May 30, bound for a rendezvous in the bay of Ilha Grande, a day's sail to the south, where DeForest was to secure an unidentified freight from one Manos da Costa Guimaraes. This obscure transaction miscarried, but a visit ashore netted the smuggler 150 pieces of valuable brazilwood. He hastened to put to sea, "apprehending difficulty and danger on account of my being near the bottom of a deep bay engaged in a highly contraband trade." As they neared the entrance to the bay a Portuguese government brig stood for them, causing DeForest extreme disquiet. Fortunately a fine breeze sprang up and permitted them to evade the inquisitive vessel and get into the open sea.

Moving south, the *Jefferson* reached Montevideo on June 27, 1805. Again DeForest pleaded distress, and, strange to say, inspection by Spanish officials found the schooner in a pitiful condition, with water in the hold and sails and riggings torn. Her master was sent to the governor of Montevideo, Pascual Ruíz Huidobro, who treated DeForest with politeness, but asked that he make all possible haste in getting ready for sea. "Thus ended this very important day," the smuggler wrote in his diary, "and I returned on board much fatigued, went to Sleep, and was as quiet as a Lamb."

The next day he offered his cargo of pitch and boards for sale to the government. He proposed to use the money thus obtained to pay for his ship's repairs, and requested permission to expend any surplus for the purchase of jerked beef. After interminable parleys and inspections his offer was accepted. But first the viceroy must approve the transaction. By dint of great exertions and some bribing DeForest had his petition forwarded to Viceroy Rafaél de Sobremonte at Buenos Aires. Meantime the cargo of the *Jefferson* had been unloaded and stored in the warehouse of one Villardebo, a *regidor* or councilman of Montevideo.

Six weeks went by without any word from Buenos Aires. DeForest grew impatient, and called on Governor Ruíz Huidobro to plead for greater dispatch in the matter. "You have nothing to complain of," brusquely replied the Spaniard. "In my opinion you left Brasil to come here on commercial reviews, your pretended distress is all a hoax." No amount of disavowals could shake the governor's well founded suspicions.[9]

DeForest wrote an English correspondent that the Buenos Aires government had lately grown very severe in its treatment of foreigners. There was a widespread suspicion that British ships were intervening in the neutral trade to La Plata under cover of the United States flag. Americans in the Plate ports resented this trickery and did all in their power to expose the impostors. United States trading voyages to the river had of late been attended by a singular fatality. A notable exception was the voyage of the *Rufus* of Boston, just arrived with a cargo of 396 slaves, with only ten deaths on the passage. "The profits on

---

9. The technique of illicit trade to the Spanish-American colonies had not changed radically in more than half a century, as shown by the following description of smuggling procedure, written in 1741: "Ships frequently approach the *Spanish* coasts under pretense of wanting water, wood, provisions, or more commonly to stop a Leak. The first Thing that is done in such a Case, is to give Notice to the Governor of their great Distress, and as a full Proof thereof, to send a very considerable Present. By this Means Leave is obtained to come on Shore, to erect a Warehouse, and to unlade the Ship; but then all this is performed under the Eye of the King's Officers, and the Goods are regularly enter'd in a Register as they are brought into the Warehouse, which when full is shut up, and the Doors sealed. All these Precautions taken, the Business is effectually carried on in the Night by a Back-door, and the *European* Goods being taken out, Indigo, Cochineal, Vinellos, Tobacco, and above all Bars of Silver and Pieces of Eight are very exactly packed in the same Cases, and placed as they stood before. But then, that such as have bought may be able to sell publickly. . . . A Petition is presented to the Governor, setting forth the Stranger's Want of Money to pay for Provisions, building the Warehouse, Timber for repairing the Ship . . . ; in Consideration of all which, Leave is desired to dispose of some small Part of their Cargo, in order to discharge these Debts." John Campbell, *A Concise History of the Spanish America* (London, 1741), quoted in Madaline W. Nichols, *The Gaucho* (Durham, N. C., 1942), pp. 29–30.

them and her return Cargo will undoubtedly be great, and I heartily congratulate the fortunate Owners." [10]

At last came the long awaited permission for DeForest to load a cargo of jerked beef. On September 14, 1805, he sailed the *Jefferson* out of Montevideo, happy at the prospect of "making so much by my little Voyage as to be able . . . to Kick Poverty out of doors. Should such an event happen, I swear I will conduct with prudence and make myself and friends as happy as possible." Off the Brazil Banks they ran into shallow, rock-strewn waters, and narrowly escaped destruction when a squall came up. They made the ship fast, and prepared to take to their single boat if the cables should part and the *Jefferson* go on the rocks. The next morning the tide came to their assistance, and by dodging some rocks and running over others they got into a clear open channel which led to the sea. They cast anchor near some small islands (the Abrolhos group), and from the master of a Portuguese sailing boat they had information how to escape from this perilous coast. "God is good," exclaimed their informant, "or you never would have got clear."

Steering to the north, they rounded the bulge of Brazil and made for the Caribbean. At Trinidad, DeForest learned that the ports of Cuba had been thrown open to neutral trade because of the renewal of hostilities between Spain and Great Britain.[11] He had planned to take his cargo to New Orleans, but now decided to go to Habana instead. Off Santo Domingo they witnessed a running fight between an English packetboat and a French privateer. At dawn a party from the corsair boarded the *Jefferson*. They reported that they had attempted to board the British craft, but found her too heavy, losing five men killed and six

10. DeForest to Thomas Wilson, Montevideo, August 25, 1805, DeForest Journal, Vol. 4. A Spanish royal order of November 24, 1791, permitted foreigners to engage in the slave trade to the Indies on an equal footing with Spaniards. This permission was prolonged down to 1810 by the royal orders of September 4, 1800, and April 22, 1804. For the slave trade to La Plata, see the erudite introduction of Diego Luis Molinari to Vol. 7 of *Documentos para la historia argentina*. A. P. Whitaker, *The United States and the Independence of Latin America*, pp. 15–16, discusses the importance of the slave trade as a factor in the development of United States commerce with La Plata. Georges Scelle, *Histoire politique de la traite négrière aux Indes de Castille* (2 vols., Paris, 1906), is indispensable for the first two centuries of the slave traffic in Spanish America.

11. For a careful study of United States commerce with Cuba in the period 1779–1809, see Roy F. Nichols, "Trade Relations and the Establishment of United States Consulates in Spanish America," *Hisp. Am. Hist. Rev.*, XIII (1933), 289–313.

wounded in the action. The boarding officers conducted themselves with much civility, DeForest noted in his diary, but their men stole a few things. Two days later a privateer of unknown nationality stood for the *Jefferson*, but drew off when the American ship maneuvered in the manner of an armed vessel. "Oh how I hate these Plundering Rascals," DeForest fretted, "of whatever nation they may be." He did not foresee his own future as a promoter of privateering enterprise.

They came to the Cuban port of Batabano, some fourteen leagues distant from Habana, on December 8, 1805. The *comandante* of the place, a "crabbed, drunken Rascal," would not permit DeForest to go overland to the capital until appeased with a bribe. Leaving Captain Mitchell in charge of the vessel, the trader set out for the "famous City of Havanna," two days' journey. On arrival he consigned his cargo of beef for sale to José Matías de Acebal, merchant of the capital. A purchaser was soon found, and on December 16 DeForest began to discharge cargo, "a very pleasant thing, as I had long wished to do it." His voyage gave him, after paying every charge, a profit of more than 1,000 per cent on his investment of less than $1,000.[12]

DeForest sailed from Habana for the United States on January 20, 1806, in the brigantine *Actress*. He landed at Baltimore on February 11, and there discussed the prospects of a trading voyage to La Plata with Captain Thomas Tenant, a prominent merchant. He went on to Washington, and like other travelers of the time was struck by the forlorn and formless appearance of the capital. "Washington," he noted in his journal, "is by nature as well situated as a City could possibly be, but it is nothing but Country as yet, made up of two or three little Clusters of Houses in different parts of the City Plot. Lots and buildings are very low indeed, and no Purchasers. Not a single Vessel of any description is owned here, every necessary of life is said to be very high. Each settlement in the City is contending with the others. On the whole, it is at present a place of no business of any kind except Quarrels and Law Suits."

Congress was in session, with much debate over President Jefferson's foreign policies. "Attending Congress almost every day," DeForest jotted in his diary, "but have a most contemptible opinion of their abilities, as a body."

12. DeForest to John R. Wheaton, Baltimore, Feb. 17, 1806, DeForest Letterbooks, Vol. 2.

He had a conference with the President, and was much chagrined to learn that Jefferson had not received any letters in support of his application for a commission as consul to Buenos Aires. The President asked his caller many questions about South America. Lately he had received and dined a more celebrated adventurer, the swarthy Venezuelan Francisco de Miranda, who doubtless unfolded to Jefferson his plans for the liberation of his homeland from Spanish rule. Now Miranda's New York-based expedition was on the high seas, headed toward the coasts of Venezuela and disaster, while the Spanish minister to the United States, the Marqués de Casa Irujo, was proclaiming to all the world the perfidy of the American government in conniving with desperate adventurers at subversion of the provinces of a friendly power.[13]

DeForest's attitude toward the Miranda affair is not without interest. In February, 1806, he received a number of letters from a New York friend, Dr. John H. Douglass, who appears to have been an enthusiast for the cause of Spanish-American liberation, and to have acted as a kind of recruiting agent for Miranda's expedition.[14] These messages evidently invited DeForest's participation in the filibustering venture. His reply was guarded and cool. "I hardly know how to address you on the subject of *that* Expedition, not being sufficiently informed, but can assure you that I should not like to engage in any warlike enterprise, however plausible it might appear, except under the banners of some Established Government, and I certainly have no disposition to change my character as a Neutral American. However, being totally ignorant of your plan, I cannot judge of its Quality, of course, shall not hazard a doubt of its propriety." [15] About the

---

13. For Miranda, see the classic biography by William S. Robertson, *The Life of Miranda* (2 vols., Chapel Hill, N. C., 1929), and an earlier but still useful work by the same author, *Francisco de Miranda and the Revolutionizing of Spanish America* (American Historical Association *Annual Report, 1907*, Washington, 1909, I, 189–540). For the diplomatic aspects of the Miranda affair, see Henry Adams, *History of the United States of America* . . . (9 vols., New York, 1891–1898), III, 189–196.

14. A "John H. Douglass, physician," is listed in *Jones's New-York Mercantile and General Directory for* . . . *1805–6*. For his testimony in the trial of Colonel William S. Smith, Miranda's chief American aide, see *The Trials of William S. Smith and Samuel G. Ogden* . . . (New York, 1807), pp. 126–128.

15. DeForest to Dr. John H. Douglass, Washington, Feb. (?), 1806, DeForest Letterbooks, Vol. 2.

same time he wrote friends in Baltimore of a "secret expedition supposed to be bound for La Guaira," and expressed strong disapproval of the project.[16]

Why did the adventurous DeForest frown upon a plan to bring the blessings of independence and free trade to the Spanish-American colonies? The reasons are not far to seek. First, the participation of United States citizens in Miranda's expedition was bound to impair the standing of all American traders in Spain's colonial ports, rendering more hazardous and difficult DeForest's future ventures to La Plata.[17] Second, should the filibusters succeed and one or more of the colonies achieve their independence, an unlikely event, the special conditions favoring United States commerce with Spanish America at this period would disappear. The new states would at once make peace with Britain and open their ports to the world, and England, by virtue of her immensely superior trading position, would soon replace the United States as the chief carrier to their markets.

DeForest voiced fears of this kind in two letters written in the spring of 1806. "The Opposition in this Country," he informed an American firm in Habana, "have taken much pains to make it appear that our Government ought to be implicated in the Expedition of Miranda. They have failed, in my opinion, and I cannot suppose that Spain will consider it aggression on our part, whatever may be the depredations of Miranda. I am very sorry, however, that the expedition was ever undertaken, for I think it will be injurious to the Interests of this Country to have another Independent Nation on the American Continent." [18] To an English correspondent he expressed the view that Miranda's enterprise would not affect adversely United States commerce with Spanish America, "unless Miranda should succeed and establish

16. DeForest to Robert and John Oliver, Feb. 21, 1806, *ibid.*
17. Spanish anger at alleged United States complicity in the Miranda affair is reflected in the royal order of July 29, 1806, advising the viceroy of Buenos Aires "concerning the conduct that should be observed with the American ships that attempt to carry on contraband trade." The order called for an end to toleration of "the insults of these strangers on our American coasts, for heartened by impunity they do not cease to repeat them, as we have seen recently in the case of the expedition projected by the traitor Miranda, prepared in one of the ports of the United States with the design of attacking one of the provinces of Costa Firme." *Documentos para la historia argentina*, VII, 334–335.
18. DeForest to Gray and Bowen, Boston, May 16, 1806, DeForest Letterbooks, Vol. 2.

another Independent Nation on this Continent, which might possibly injure us in our carrying trade, but what we should lose Great Britain would probably gain." [19]

With the fate of the filibusters still uncertain, DeForest prepared for a second trading voyage to La Plata. He planned to employ a strategy long familiar to foreign intruders in Spain's American possessions: the introduction of contraband wares under cover of the legal slave traffic. In May, 1806, he purchased the brigantine *Jane*, and assembled a cargo of dry goods suitable for the Plate market. The *Jane* cleared from Boston on the twenty-ninth of May, her destination the island of Goree, a notable center of the slave trade on the Gold Coast of Africa. On the eve of his departure, DeForest resolved to remain for several years at Buenos Aires as a commission merchant. This decision, he noted in his diary, was "altogether accidental, and if anything clever grows out of it I shall feel very happy indeed."

19. DeForest to Thomas Wilson, Boston, May 28, 1806, *ibid.*, Vol. 3.

IV

"REIGN OF TERROR AND CONFUSION"

THE passage of the *Jane* to the shores of Africa seems to have been bare of incident. DeForest does not disclose how his polyglot crew of two Swedes, two Scotchmen, a Frenchman, an English boy, and an American cook fared together under the command of Captain John Hooper of Manchester, New Hampshire. His journal notes only that in the vicinity of the Canary Islands the weather grew thick and foggy, the winds baffling, but before they got to the latitude of 18° it hauled westwardly, and so continued until they cast anchor at Goree on July 7, 1806.

A barren rock in the sea, only 900 yards long and 330 yards wide, Goree lies about a mile from the peninsula of Cape Verde, westernmost salient of the Old World. The Dutch purchased the island from its native ruler in 1617 and made it a base for their slave trade with the American colonies. Late in the seventeenth century the French Compagnie du Sénégal acquired this emporium, but during the French Revolution and the Napoleonic Wars it fell into British hands. At the time of DeForest's arrival, an English garrison under the command of a Major Lloyd was stationed on the island.

A population estimated by DeForest to number some 1,500, consisting chiefly of French mulattoes and their numerous slaves, lived on Goree. The former class, he noted, appeared to be the lords of the little island. The slave trade was in their hands; in boats of five, eight, and fifteen tons they ranged along the coast and ventured up into the dim recesses of the great river Gambia to procure their human commodities. Negro chieftains, collecting their commissions in gold and trinkets, often assisted in these manhunts. The shackled captives were brought to Goree, and there, in the *maison des esclaves*, were exhibited to prospective buyers. Numerous ships of United States registry called at Goree for cargoes. The standard price of a human chattel was $120 to

$130, barter price in rum or tobacco, but so many American ships had been coming to the island lately that slaves could not be purchased at that price for cash in hand. The *Rufus* of Boston had sailed for La Plata on June 11 with a cargo of many young slaves. DeForest doubted that they would bring much profit at Buenos Aires, "for most of the slaves sent to that market are transferred to that of Lima for sale, and I have been told that grown slaves there are of much greater value than little ones." [1]

"Not being much acquainted with the Trade," relates DeForest, "nor willing to run about in the Sun, I employed Mr. Ezekiel Madden an American to assist me." This strategic move greatly vexed the mulatto slave traders, who lodged a protest with the governor of the island. Obscurity veils DeForest's further transactions on Goree. Presumably he purchased only a small token number of blacks as a cover for the more profitable contraband trade. His business soon done, he cleared on July 15 for La Plata.

The *Jane* entered the Plate estuary some three weeks later. In the morning of September 14 they made out a number of warships lying off Montevideo. Presently a man-of-war approached the American ship. The English boarders did not allay DeForest's fears. They explained that Sir Home Popham's squadron had the Plate ports under blockade. At the end of June an expeditionary force under Sir William Beresford had captured Buenos Aires. Little more than a month later, in an astounding reversal of fortunes, the Spaniards had rallied under an obscure officer named Santiago Liniers and retaken the town, making prisoners of General Beresford and his men. Having volunteered this information, the boarders ordered DeForest to go down to the commodore's ship, the *Diadem*.

Sir Home, a tall, pleasant-faced man in his middle forties, received DeForest in his cabin. He confirmed that the ports of La Plata were closed to trade; he could not say when the blockade would be lifted. By way of amends he invited DeForest to sit down with him to a dinner of roast lamb and cabbage. The smuggler passed an agreeable hour with his English host, then returned to the *Jane*, much perplexed at this interference with his plans.

1. DeForest to Thomas Wilson, Goree, July 12, 1806, DeForest Letterbooks, Vol. 3.

Unknown to DeForest, the fountainhead of his difficulties was that same Francisco de Miranda of whose ill-starred expedition against Venezuela he had so vigorously disapproved. Miranda had inspired the British effort to wrest La Plata from the supposedly inept hands of Spain. In 1803 the revolutionist was in London, working to secure British support of his plans for the emancipation of Spanish America. There he struck up a friendship with Popham, a naval captain whose conduct was being investigated for alleged financial misdemeanors.[2] Popham soon became a convert to Miranda's cause. In a lengthy memoir (dated October 14, 1804), the promoters outlined to the British ministers their project for the liberation of Spain's American empire. Miranda was to lead English land forces against northern South America; Popham was to command an expedition of three thousand soldiers against the viceroyalty of La Plata. The planners argued that this stroke at Spain would greatly reduce the revenues of her French ally and increase Great Britain's trade and importance.[3] Execution of this program, accepted in principle by the British ministers, was so long delayed that Miranda, losing patience, departed for the United States where he prepared his ill-fated *Leander* expedition against Venezuela.

In the meantime Sir Home had gone to sea in command of naval forces sent against the Dutch colony at the Cape of Good Hope. Soon after the fall of the Cape, Popham determined on his own responsibility to make an attack on Buenos Aires. He was strengthened in his decision by advices from an American sea captain lately come from La Plata who assured him that Montevideo and Buenos Aires were in a defenseless state, and that the natives would welcome their British liberators.[4] Popham evidently believed that success in the enterprise would vindicate his unauthorized conduct. On April 14, 1806, Popham's squadron set sail for La Plata with a regiment of soldiers under the command of Sir William Beresford on board. In the wake of the expedition followed a great number of merchantmen eager to pour a mass of English goods through the prospective breach in the Spanish colonial system.

2. W. S. Robertson, *Life of Miranda*, I, 257.
3. *Ibid.*, pp. 275–276.
4. Carlos Roberts, *Las invasiones inglesas del Río de la Plata* (Buenos Aires, 1938), p. 72.

Victory had come with astonishing ease. The viceroy of La Plata, Rafaél de Sobremonte, fled with great celerity to the provincial town of Córdoba upon the approach of the enemy. On June 27, 1806, Beresford's veterans entered the capital and ran up the British colors over the fort. To revive the feelings of the stunned *porteños*, Beresford immediately issued a proclamation in Spanish and English guaranteeing to the inhabitants the rights of private property, administration of justice, worship of the Roman Catholic Church, and freedom of trade. A great store of public treasure and merchandise fell to the invaders. But Popham and Beresford had mistaken both the temper and the capacities of the people of Buenos Aires. United in a sacred fury against the English *herejes*, creoles and old Spaniards joined in planning the expulsion of their unwanted liberators. Led by the French-born captain of the port of Ensenada de Barragán, Santiago Liniers, a volunteer army fell upon the British occupants on August 12, 1806, and utterly routed them, capturing General Beresford and 1,200 of his troops. On his flagship in the river, Popham, helpless to aid his outnumbered comrades, could do no more than proclaim a strict blockade of the Plate ports and await the coming of reinforcements from England and Cape Colony.

This was the state of affairs when DeForest arrived in the middle of September. After drifting about for three weeks, with the situation unchanged, he resolved to go south to the Patagonian port of Río Negro and dispose of part of his cargo there. He evidently expected Montevideo to be in British hands by the time of his return to the river, and may have anticipated difficulty in marketing his goods in competition with the swarm of English merchantmen awaiting the fall of the key to the viceroyalty. The half-formed idea of running the blockade to Buenos Aires may have also entered into his calculations. In the current state of feeling against English-speaking foreigners, the excitable *populacho* of the capital was likely to treat roughly an *anglo-americano* who possibly came as a spy and almost certainly as a smuggler. Against such a contingency, it would be helpful to bring from Río Negro some proofs of DeForest's friendly disposition to the Spanish cause.

The *Jane* sped southward to the lonely frontier post on the coast of Patagonia, and cast anchor at Río Negro on October 15. "There are here," DeForest noted in his diary, "one friar and two curates and a great plenty of Superstition." There were also Indians, eager to barter guanaco skins, sea elephant oil, and salt for vests and laces. These purchases and his slaves the smuggler left at Río Negro under the watchful eye of Captain Hooper. The brigantine was made fit and trim in preparation for her return voyage. On November 12, 1806, the *Jane* put to sea, bearing on board the secretary of the *comandante* with dispatches for the viceroy of La Plata.

They made the mouth of the river one week later and stood for Montevideo. DeForest soon discovered that the town was still in Spanish hands. The gunboat *Protector* intercepted the *Jane* on November 19, put a youthful midshipman and three sailors on board, and sent her for Maldonado, the recently captured rendezvous of the squadron. The English captain told DeForest that "they were all in the dark respecting Sir Home's instructions, intimating the improbability of ever conquering the Country, which appeared very probable to me." [5]

With Montevideo out of reach, and the prospect of a ruinous detention at Maldonado before him, DeForest saw only one way out of his difficulties. He must run the British blockade into Buenos Aires. A smart easterly gale had blown up, giving good hope of success in the enterprise. DeForest had taken the measure of the youthful midshipman assigned to the *Jane* and anticipated no difficulty in deceiving him concerning the course of the ship. The three English sailors would probably rejoice at being set free from the man-of-war. Feeling some compunction over the fate that awaited the midshipman, "a well educated and apparently amiable Young Man," the blockade-runner privately informed his crew to make sail for Buenos Aires while he kept the guardian of the ship "in play."

Scudding along before the gale, the *Jane* drove up the river and toward safety. On the morning of November 21 they were over the Ortiz Bank and within short distance of their port. Then DeForest summoned the midshipman to his cabin and gave account of his stratagem. The youth vainly pleaded with his captor to return to Maldonado. Seeking to quiet his fears, DeForest assured him that if they arrived safely, "I would render him every possible assistance, that I would furnish him with money to buy

5. DeForest to Alpheus Dunham, Montevideo, Sept. 3, 1807, DeForest Letterbooks, Vol. 3.

the necessary clothing he most stood in need of, and that I would exert myself to have him not considered as a Prisoner of War." As for the three sailors, they displayed great satisfaction "at getting away from the Man of War, and rendered all the assistance they could." That afternoon they anchored outside the bar in the port of Buenos Aires.

In response to the *Jane's* signals for a pilot, a launch in the harbor got under way and came alongside the brigantine. A motley crew of privateersmen and soldiery clambered on board. Some held cocked pistols, others brandished swords. Making great noise and perilous display of their arms, they swaggered fiercely fore and aft in evident enjoyment of their easy prize. At nightfall some withdrew, and the rest undertook to get the vessel into port. Since all were commanders, the *Jane* spent most of the night beating at the bar. DeForest, after two sleepless and anxiety-ridden nights, was past all caring; retiring to his cabin he fell into a sound slumber. He awoke in the morning to find the brigantine anchored in port in three fathoms of water. In the afternoon came the customs officers to make their "great visit." To the vexation of the privateersmen they found all in order. "Hurrah for the Prize, was the topic among these poor Devils."

Buenos Aires, a city of some 40,000 inhabitants, had the appearance of an armed camp. In September Liniers had issued a dramatic call for the formation of a people's militia. Now the narrow, dusty streets were alive with volunteer soldiers. Even the Negro slaves had formed their *cuerpo de esclavos*, and proudly sported knife and lance. Brilliantly uniformed officers dashed by on horseback. Daily the raw levies drilled in the public squares. The nights of Buenos Aires, as of old, were filled with music; strains of gay song issued from the white-washed, flat-roofed houses of adobe. But new martial words had been set to the familiar airs.

DeForest lost no time in calling on Santiago Liniers, hero of the *reconquista*, now military governor of Buenos Aires. Of stately bearing, affable and generous, Liniers was the idol of the populace, whose clamor had compelled the municipal authorities to summon a general congress which invested him with the military functions of the discredited viceroy. The shadows of rivalry had already begun to fall between Liniers and the supremely ambitious Martín Alzaga, influential senior *alcalde*. For all save a small minority, however, he was still the most excellent, the incomparable Liniers; time had not yet brought to light the weakness of character that the brave exterior concealed.[6]

Liniers received DeForest with characteristic warmth, commended him on his blockade-running exploit, and offered to exert his influence in the trader's behalf. Through his intercession, DeForest was able to unload cargo two days later. He was anxious to put his commercial affairs in order before the anticipated second British invasion got under way. The British government had dispatched strong forces to La Plata to consolidate its hold on the Spanish colony. The successive arrival of these reinforcements, numbering some 11,000 men by the beginning of 1807, suggested the seriousness of the approaching effort to recapture Buenos Aires.

Expectantly the city awaited the day of the assault, speculated where the first blow would fall. The answer was given in January when the British laid siege to Montevideo, key to the viceroyalty. Liniers with two thousand men sallied to the relief of the town. The sight of the gallant and tranquil bearing of their *jefe* filled the *porteños* with confidence; they "were making calculations to accommodate such of them [the British] as escaped their swords." [7] The expedition soon returned, their march interrupted by the news that Montevideo had surrendered on February 3. For this disaster Viceroy Sobremonte was again held responsible.

The twice-proved incompetence of the viceroy now led to his complete undoing. Turbulent crowds gathered on the afternoon of February 6 before the doors of the *cabildo*, the municipal council, with cries of "No Vice King, no Royal Audience, down with them, hang them." "God only knows how the business will end here," the alarmed DeForest jotted in his diary, "the Government is extremely weak." [8] Bowing to the popular will, the royal *audiencia*, the high tribunal of the province, decreed the suspension and arrest of the viceroy, itself assumed supreme political and military authority, and confirmed Liniers, the beloved of the people, as commander of all the armed forces. The action against Sobremonte had an unmistakable revolutionary significance: "for

---

6. Paul Groussac, *Santiago Liniers, Conde de Buenos Aires* (Buenos Aires, 1907), is a masterful evocation of Liniers and his times; C. Roberts, *Las invasiones inglesas,* pp. 376–380, brings together numerous characterizations of Liniers by contemporaries and historians.

7. DeForest Journal, Vol. 6, Jan. 29, 1807.

8. *Ibid.*

the first time the American colonies witnessed the deposition and imprisonment of the legal representative of the king." [9]

Hard on the heels of this event came the spectacular escape of the British General Beresford from his captivity in Luján. "The Town in uproar and confusion. No one has full confidence in his Neighbour. Many are suspected who are of high rank." The account in DeForest's journal, otherwise accurate, mentions the rumor that "the Spanish General *Liniers*, Secretary of the War Department," had made his escape together with Beresford—suggesting the suspicions held in some circles of Liniers' loyalty to Spain.[10]

The flight of Beresford heightened the mood of panic created by the fall of Montevideo. Many English-speaking foreigners in the city were arrested and imprisoned. In the evening of March 3, soldiers routed DeForest from bed and escorted him to a militia barracks. Other Americans seized about this time were Captain Tibbet of the *Diana* of Wiscasset, the captain of the *George and Mary* of Newport, and Jeremiah Donovan, supercargo of the *Mary* of Philadelphia.[11] After languishing for five days in the cold and drafty barracks, DeForest was released on the application of Benito Rivadavia, a prominent Spanish merchant and father of Bernardino Rivadavia, future president of the United Provinces of La Plata.[12] DeForest learned that he had been accused of being an Englishman, consorting with Englishmen, and of preparing a quantity of "segars" with the evil intent of sending them to Montevideo.[13]

For his greater safety, DeForest decided to take lodgings in the home of Rivadavia, with whom he had an obscure commercial connection. He also obtained a written protection from the powerful Liniers. "What an infernal rascally Government it must be," he fumed, "that can cooly and deliberately take a Gentleman out of his Bed and order him to Prison without any cause but their having the power to do it." Brooding over his

---

9. Bartolomé Mitre, *Historia de Belgrano y de la independencia argentina* (3 vols., Buenos Aires, 1887, 4th ed.), I, 152.

10. C. Roberts, *Las invasiones inglesas*, p. 221, affirms that Liniers indubitably connived in the escape of Beresford, but at the same time holds that Liniers was completely loyal to the Spanish king.

11. DeForest Journal, Vol. 6, April 23, 1807.

12. Alberto Palcos, *La visión de Rivadavia* (Buenos Aires, 1938), a study of the early years of the Argentine statesman, includes much biographical material concerning his father.

13. DeForest Journal, Vol. 6, March 3, 1807.

wrongs, and those of his imprisoned countrymen, he finally composed and sent a bristling memorial on the subject to the royal *audiencia*.

"We are not beasts my Lords," he wrote, "we are Men (or rather we were Men when we first arrived here), we have come to your Country for the Purpose of Friendly Commerce, if you receive us at all, you are bound to give us every protection and every aid in the prosecution of our business." Did their Lordships conceive the United States to be in a state of infancy and therefore incapable of defending the rights of its citizens? "No one doubts its infancy, but pardon me my Lords when I tell you that 'it is an infant lion' which if roused, has already strength enough to make the Spanish Empire tremble to its foundations." He closed with the demand that the marine court decide immediately the case of his impounded vessel and cargo; that the individuals responsible for his arrest and imprisonment be punished in the most severe and public manner; and that he be accorded protection from further insult or injury until his departure from Buenos Aires.[14] What effect this invocation of the infant North American lion had on the deliberations of the august *audiencia*, we cannot tell. In July, however, DeForest had returned to him the *Jane* and her cargo.

The *cabildo*, for reasons of public safety, ordered in April, 1807, that all foreigners should appear and give account of their identity and occupation. DeForest complied, as evidenced by the following curious notation in the census records: "David Forest, of American nationality, musician in the Squadron of Hussars of Pueyrredón, lives in the house of Don Benito Rivadavia." [15] Fortunately the registering officials did not put DeForest's musical prowess to the test. The shrewd Rivadavia may have devised this unique camouflage for his Yankee guest.

An electrifying report ran through Buenos Aires on June 25: a squadron of British transports had been sighted at anchor off Ensenada de Barragán, twelve leagues from the capital. The next day the invaders were off Quilmes, only four leagues distant from the city. In the afternoon, reads the entry in DeForest's journal, "the General was beat. The Troops were collected and reviewed. The General Santiago Liniers told them the Enemy was

---

14. DeForest to "the Royal Audience of the Vice Kingdom of Buenos Ayres," Buenos Aires, April 15, 1807, *ibid*.
15. *Documentos para la historia argentina*, XII, 218.

in offing and that they would soon have an opportunity to meet them. They were unanimous in their declarations of attachment to their General, and willingness to loose the last drop of their blood in defense of their Country. The night was passed by great numbers of Citizens in Serenading the City with various kinds of music, and in rejoicing that the English had at last appeared. For my own part I kept close to my room preferring the charms of security to music." [16]

Eight thousand red-coats landed at Ensenada de Barragán on June 28 and advanced on the city. The crisis was at hand. Liniers with a force of seven thousand troops sallied to meet the enemy at the little stream of Riachuelo de Barracas. "All Buenos Aires," DeForest jotted in his diary," is sure of beating the English, and if they do to give no quarter. Such is the savage spirit many of them possess." [17] At four o'clock in the afternoon of July 2, an aide of Liniers strode into the hall of the *cabildo* with grave news; a part of the British army had eluded the Spanish defenders and made a crossing of the Riachuelo at the ford of Burgos. At five (relates DeForest) the distant firing of musketry could be heard in the city; by six the British were in the suburbs; by seven they had fought their way to the Corrales de Miserere and there put Liniers' men to rout. "All the town in an uproar, Spanish troops returned to the Great Square in front of the Fort, no boasts of having beaten the English, of course very well know their defeat must have been total." [18]

The rashness of Liniers had left the capital dangerously exposed to attack. The energetic senior *alcalde*, Martín Alzaga, rose to the occasion. He caused fortifications to be thrown up on all sides; soldiers and militiamen took positions at the windows and housetops of the streets through which the invaders must pass. Some of the defenders broke open DeForest's dwelling and swarmed on the roof. "Damn the luck," swore DeForest, "I intended to have been clear of soldiers but have got into the midst of them."

In the morning of July 5, after a demand for surrender had been peremptorily refused, the British troops closed in upon the city. As they advanced through the narrow streets they were met by a murderous hail of fire from every window and roof. The end

16. DeForest Journal, Vol. 6, June 26, 1807.
17. *Ibid.*, July 2, 1807.
18. *Ibid.*

of the day found them short of most of their strategic objectives. "The fortunes of this day appear much in favor of the Spaniards," opined DeForest. "Great numbers of English were killed and wounded from tops of the Houses while passing in the Streets beneath, without the power of killing scarce a single man who fired at them." [19]

The British commander, General John Whitelocke, impressed by the tenacity of the defense and his heavy losses, hesitated to continue the struggle. On July 6, he accepted the Spanish terms for his capitulation. The British agreed to evacuate Buenos Aires within ten days and to relinquish the town and fortress of Montevideo. All prisoners were to be returned. The formal treaty ratifying these terms was signed on July 7.

The battle for Buenos Aires had ended. DeForest cautiously ventured into the streets; recoiled at the sight of naked English dead, their clothing stripped by pillagers; noted the extensive damage to the city's buildings. "Damn war and him who invented it," he pungently commented in his diary. A few days later he looked on as thousands of British troops assembled in Retiro Square and marched down to the beach to take ship for England. Defeat at the hands of raw colonial levies rankled in the English breasts; DeForest could hear some angry officers and men cursing General John Whitelocke "for a fool and a coward." [20]

For the first time in many months the trader could communicate with the outside world. He wrote his brother John that he had experienced many disagreeable revolutions at Buenos Aires, but had finally come out "bright as the morning Sun—have the unlimited confidence of the Government as well as of the Populace which latter have ruled that place for a long time past." [21] "During this reign of Terror and Confusion," he informed a friend in North America, "the Populace . . . have had nearly all the power in their mobist hands." [22]

The people of Buenos Aires had indeed tasted power, and

19. *Ibid.*

20. *Ibid.*, July 11, 1807. Upon his return to England, General Whitelocke was tried by court-martial on four distinct charges, was found guilty of three, and was in consequence "cashiered and declared totally unfit and unworthy to serve his Majesty in any military capacity whatsoever." Quoted in Bernard Moses, *Spain's Declining Power in South America* (Berkeley, Cal., 1919), p. 369.

21. DeForest to John H. DeForest, Montevideo, July 20, 1807, DeForest Letterbooks, Vol. 3.

22. DeForest to Alpheus Dunham, Montevideo, July 20, 1807, *ibid.*

would not willingly relinquish it again. In the difficult school of war the heroic *porteños* had gained knowledge of their strength and a vigorous sense of nationality. "I presume to felicitate the Americans," proudly declared Cornelio de Saavedra, hailing the achievements of his legion of *patricios*, "for this last proof of their valor and loyalty, which adds luster to the merit of those who were born in the Indies, and testifies that their spirits know not dejection, that they are not inferior to the European Spaniards, that in point of valor and loyalty they are second to none." [23] Spain's distresses in Europe, rapidly moving toward a crisis, were to prove the golden opportunity of ambitious creoles in Buenos Aires, eager to become masters of their political and economic destinies. The British invasions were only the prelude to the greater struggle for the independence of La Plata.

23. B. Mitre, *Belgrano*, I, 201.

V

"ON VERY SAFE GROUND"

THE British invasion fiasco caused DeForest the liveliest satisfaction. Persuaded that the trade of La Plata must soon return to its former neutral channels, he prepared to remain in Buenos Aires as a commission merchant for the duration of the European war; a matter, he calculated, of two or three years. He disposed of his brig *Jane* by charter to a departing English merchant for the "modest price" of $10,000. To Captain John Hooper at Río Negro, fretfully drumming his heels at that lonely Patagonian post, he sent word to sail for the United States with all the property in his charge, save the Negro slaves, in the first Nantucket fishing vessel quitting the coast. He warned Captain Hooper not to sell the slaves at a sacrifice, but to leave them in the hands of some dependable Spaniard, subject to DeForest's order.[1]

The Laws of the Indies forbade foreigners to trade or reside in the Spanish colonies. But experience had taught DeForest that in time of war these laws were honored as much in the breach as in the observance. Above all he relied on the enlightened views and easy-going ways of the powerful Liniers.[2] His trust was not misplaced. Liniers tolerated the extensive contraband traffic that sprang up as departing English merchants dumped huge stocks of goods on the Plate market, and even gave these enemy traders permission to remain in Buenos Aires in order to dispose of their merchandise after British troops had evacuated the city.[3] He dutifully proclaimed in force in the province Napoleon's Berlin Decree of 1806, making all British property good prize, but gave

1. DeForest to Captain John Hooper, Buenos Aires, Nov. 3, 1807, DeForest Letterbooks, Vol. 3.
2. At this time Liniers was acting as military and civil governor of La Plata in place of the deposed Viceroy Sobremonte. He was appointed *virrey interino* by the Spanish king in December, 1807, and took office in May, 1808. E. Ravignani, "El virreinato del Río de la Plata," p. 312.
3. Dorothy B. Goebel, "British Trade to the Spanish Colonies, 1796–1823," *American Historical Review*, XLIII (1938), 309.

little effect to the edict of Spain's French ally.[4] To the great scandal of the royal *audiencia*, he released from prison the North American adventurer William P. White, who had openly collaborated with the British invaders.[5] When the *audiencia* undertook to purge the country of all foreigners, ordering them to leave the province in the space of eight days on pain of imprisonment and summary expulsion at the official convenience, DeForest's appeal to the governor resulted in immediate instructions "to the Judge Velano that he must not consider me as included in the general order."[6] With good reason, the merchant commended Liniers as "possessed of that liberality and generosity of Soul, which the civilised and well bred part of Mankind alone possess," and "the Friend and Protector of the Foreigners who are here."[7]

Nevertheless, a cover of legality for DeForest's commission-house business seemed desirable. By this time he was thoroughly familiar with the many ruses employed by foreign traders in Spanish America. For a certain consideration a young Spaniard "of the first mercantile talents and respectability," a particular friend of Liniers, Juan Pedro Varangot by name, agreed to act as the ostensible receiver of DeForest's consignments.[8] The

4. Napoleon's Berlin Decree was proclaimed in Buenos Aires on September 27, 1807, in compliance with a Spanish royal order of February 21, 1807. One month later DeForest wrote: "All however is quiet, and it is not probable that it will ever be enforced, though many of the bigoted vassals here would like to see it executed with vigour." DeForest to Stephen Twyecross, Buenos Aires, Oct. 28, 1807, DeForest Letterbooks, Vol. 3.

5. For a biographical sketch of White, see Edward S. Wallace, "Forgotten Men of Dartmouth: Father of the Argentine Navy, William Porter White, 1790," *Dartmouth Alumni Magazine*, March, 1935; see also Enrique Udaondo, *Diccionario biográfico argentino* (Buenos Aires, 1938). The charges against White are set forth in "Carta de la Real Audiencia de Buenos Aires a S. M. informando sobre las graves y escandalosas occurencias acaecidas con el extrangero Guillermo Withe [sic]," in Facultad de Filosofía y Letras, *Documentos relativos a los antecedentes de la independencia de la República Argentina* (Buenos Aires, 1912), pp. 11–14.

6. DeForest to Stephen Twyecross, Buenos Aires, Oct. 28, 1807, DeForest Letterbooks, Vol. 3.

7. DeForest to the Honorable Charles Stewart, Buenos Aires, April 20, 1808, *ibid.* On January 8, 1808, noting the continued presence of many Englishmen and North Americans in the capital, the *cabildo* rebuked Liniers for a tolerance "so contrary to the laws and prejudicial to the interests of the nation," and threatened to appeal to the Spanish king against this "pernicious abuse." Archivo General de la Nación, *Acuerdos del extinguido cabildo de Buenos Aires, 1589–1820* (45 vols., Buenos Aires, 1907–1934), Fourth Series, III, 16–17.

8. François Depons, *Voyage a la partie orientale de la terre-ferme* (2 vols., Paris, 1808), II, 362–363, notes that this ruse was commonly employed by foreign merchants established at Cadiz.

partners took lodgings together in the home of Francisco Ignacio de Ugarte, one of the wealthiest merchants of the city.

In a circular letter to a large number of merchants in the United States, DeForest announced the establishment of his commission-house. The letter took an optimistic view of the prospects of neutral trade to La Plata. Contrary to a widely held opinion, the writer observed, Spanish colonial ports were not completely closed to foreign commerce. The management of this trade offered difficulties, to be sure, but only enough to deter the ignorant. DeForest mentioned first of all the legal traffic in slaves. "I know of no Voyages," he wrote, "which present so fair a prospect of gain to the undertaker, as these."

Spanish law forbade the introduction of any articles save agricultural implements in slave ships, but DeForest dismissed this apparent difficulty. Let the vessel come in ballast with salt, lumber, wine, or rum, represented as ship's stores, and they could be sold without hindrance. Another type of voyage required a license from the governor of Habana authorizing the bearer to purchase beef in La Plata for the Cuban market. A large variety of articles including spirits, rice, iron, hams, cheese, butter, pickles, fish, and lumber could be brought in ballast to pay for the cargo of beef, and other produce could be exported as well.

Hazardous but extremely lucrative was the direct voyage between Spain and La Plata under Spanish colors. The vessel employed for this purpose should be a small fast-sailing craft capable of eluding the chase of British cruisers. Her cargo must appear consigned from a Spanish merchant to one of his countrymen in Buenos Aires. The voyage could be made in the name of Francisco Ignacio de Ugarte, DeForest's very good friend. Spaniards must compose the crew, save for the American captain who might pass for a mate, but not for a master or supercargo. Barcelona wares were much favored in the Plate markets. Catalonian wines, costing $15 or $20 a pipe in Spain, brought from $150 to $200 in Buenos Aires; olive oil in casks or jars yielded a profit of from 200 to 300 per cent. Before entering the river the ship should call at the near-by port of Rio Grande in Brazil. There lived DeForest's old friend, Father José Alves Chaves, who dispensed not only spiritual advice but useful information on the movements of British cruisers in the estuary. Vessels consigned to DeForest must display on arrival his private signal: a blue jack with a white X at the fore-topgallant masthead. No declaration of cargo should be made before receiving his advice.[9]

Two years before DeForest had unsuccessfully applied to President Jefferson for an appointment as United States consul to Buenos Aires. He renewed his solicitations in a letter to Secretary of State Madison that throws a curious light on the beginnings of Anglo-American trade rivalry in La Plata. He explained that he sought the post because of "the unpleasant situation of Americans and their commerce in this Country." Many English ships entered the river under American colors. These impostors produced papers that frequently were forged or plundered from their rightful owners. Spanish ignorance and venality aided the tricksters to escape, while real Americans were sometimes persecuted and cast into prison on suspicion of being British subjects. If appointed consul or commercial agent in Buenos Aires, DeForest could expose these deceptions and protect his injured countrymen. Spanish law would not admit his formal recognition,[10] but the appointment would please the inhabitants and would be sufficiently countenanced by the government to answer all purposes. With adequate protection the Plate trade could provide steady employment for thirty or forty American vessels. "Notwithstanding the rigid Laws against the introduction of Foreigners," affirmed DeForest, "they are constantly admitted, on some pretence or other and derive much profit from their voyages." [11]

DeForest vainly awaited a favorable reply from Secretary Madison. He could not know that the Jefferson administration had just embarked on policies that tended to extinguish United States commercial contacts with the Spanish-American provinces, leaving our agents there but little employment.[12] In re-

9. Copy of Circular Letter, Buenos Aires, Sept. 15, 1807, DeForest Letterbooks, Vol. 3.

10. A royal order of April 24, 1807, prohibited the residence of foreign agents or consuls in the Spanish colonies. For the text of the order, see *Documentos para la historia argentina*, VII, 363–365.

11. DeForest to the Honorable James Madison, Secretary of State, Buenos Aires, Oct. 1, 1808, DeForest Letterbooks, Vol. 3.

12. At this time the United States had a representative in only one Spanish-American colony, that of Cuba. After 1807 his title of consul was replaced by that of "agent for seamen and commerce" because of Spanish refusal to extend official recognition. Before 1808 the United States had appointed consuls to New Orleans (1798–1803), La Guaira (1800–1807), an agent to Cuba during the American Revolution, and a consul stationed there since 1797. On this subject, see R. F. Nichols, "Trade Relations and the Establishment of United States Consulates in Spanish America, 1779–1809."

sponse to the blockade systems of the great European belligerents (Napoleon's Berlin and Milan Decrees and the British orders-in-council), on December 22, 1807, Congress passed a measure designed to bring France and Britain to terms, the famous Embargo act. By the time of its repeal early in 1809, this enactment had practically destroyed the once lucrative American trade with Spain's Caribbean and South American colonies.[13]

The Embargo blighted DeForest's hopes of attracting United States vessels to the Plate estuary. "There are no American ships come to give us opportunity to ship anything," he complained in April, 1808, "and I fear there will not be any for some time." [14] Yet he vigorously defended the men and measures responsible for this state of affairs. "Americans know little of the distresses of War," he informed his brother John, "or they would not clamour as they do against the only measure by which they can avoid it.... I love my country as well as any of its inhabitants; and perhaps should be as great a gainer as any one of my standing in life, were the Embargo to be raised, and the Government of our Country disposed to place us in the degrading situation of accepting without a murmur such commercial privileges as others may please to confer on us, but I had rather beg my Bread. I hope to hear ere long, that the most rigid Commercial measures are adopted against all Nations who continue against my Country their insolent pretensions." [15]

Despite the effects of the Embargo, DeForest prospered during these years beyond all expectation.[16] His letterbooks and journals give the impression of a diversified commercial activity, including the clandestine introduction of British goods, speculation in nutria skins, and the defense of United States firms in suits at law before the Buenos Aires marine court. The opening of Brazilian ports to neutral and friendly commerce in January, 1808, imparted new

13. Timothy Pitkin, *A Statistical View of the Commerce of the United States of America* (Hartford, 1816), p. 192, estimates the value of American exports to Spanish America in 1807 at $12,341,225; in 1808, at $4,177,053. A. P. Whitaker, *The United States and the Independence of Latin America*, pp. 47–52, discusses the Embargo as a factor in the non-fulfilment of Jefferson's "large policy of 1808" toward Spanish America.
14. DeForest to Thomas Brewer, Buenos Aires, April 15, 1808, DeForest Letterbooks, Vol. 3.
15. DeForest to John H. DeForest, Buenos Aires, Feb. 10, 1809, *ibid.*
16. In letters to his brothers, DeForest complacently cites his large gains, unfortunately in a cipher to which we do not have the key. Nor do we possess his account books for this period.

vigor to the Plata trade. "Come try this plan," DeForest wrote his brother, "they can live without you in Watertown. By coming to Rio de Janeiro we can play into each other's hands to much advantage. I think if we don't get into this cursed war, we are on very safe ground." [17] His eye ever on the main chance, he described to friends in Rio how Spanish navigation laws might be circumvented. Let a vessel with Portuguese colors and crew come to Buenos Aires laden with slaves, and represented as having been purchased by DeForest's partner, Juan Pedro Varangot. After introducing as many slaves as she had tons, the ship would be considered as fully naturalized and would enjoy all the trading privileges of a Spanish-built ship. Calico, muslins, silk hose, and other dry goods might be smuggled in with the slaves.[18]

In March, 1809, DeForest purchased an estate with a portion of his growing fortune. Since foreigners were not permitted to hold land in Spain's colonies, the name of Francisco Ignacio de Ugarte, DeForest's friend, figured in the deed of sale as purchaser.[19] The *chacra* lay near the present-day Rivadavia Station of the Argentine Central Railroad, eight miles above Buenos Aires. Fronting the Plata for 400 rods, it was a league in length. A force of nine slaves worked on the land, graced by an old brick house and numerous fruit trees. To his Negroes, DeForest gave names drawn from the annals of war.[20] "For the first time in my life," he proudly entered in his diary on March 19, 1809, "I have slept in a House belonging wholly to myself."

At this time DeForest, now aged thirty-four, began to consider seriously the subject of matrimony. The idea of a union with one of the daughters of Buenos Aires, famed for their beauty and amiability, does not seem to have occurred to him. "I am anxious to go home *to get married*," he wrote brother John, "but am unwilling to neglect my establishment here, which I wish you to take care of and be interested in, if you desire it. At any rate

17. DeForest to John H. DeForest, Buenos Aires, June 12, 1808, DeForest Letterbooks, Vol. 3.
18. DeForest to Charles Twyecross, Buenos Aires, June 12, 1808, *ibid*.
19. This paragraph is based on notations in the DeForest Journal, Vol. 6, supplemented by information drawn from Horacio Zorraquín Becú, *De aventurero yanqui a consul porteño en los Estados Unidos: David C. DeForest, 1774–1825* (Buenos Aires, 1943) (reprint from the *Anuario de historia argentina*, IV, 1942), p. 41 n. Señor Zorraquín Becú has traced the history of the estate with the aid of title deeds and other documents down to its final dismemberment.
20. They were Alexander, Caesar, Pompey, Hannibal, Scipio, Romulus, Hector, Paris, Napoleon.

you must come here, and immediately." "We have but a short time to stay here," he closed plaintively, "and ought for our own happiness do to others, particularly our brothers, all the good we can." [21]

Don David Cortes DeForest—so he sometimes subscribed himself in letters—now wrote and presumably spoke Spanish with considerable fluency and correctness. His circle of acquaintances included some of the most prominent names in Buenos Aires society: Ugarte, Rivadavia, Castelli, Azcuénaga. Their mode of life he made his own. The happy *porteños* of that day, observes a nostalgic Argentine historian, had few cares, worked little, ate well, and slept even better.[22] Manners were simple, diversions few. Religion played a major role in the life of the colony; from morning till night church bells tolled for devotion. At noon the women of the better sort were to be seen on their way to Mass, long black cloaks drawn over their faces, beads and crucifixes on their arms, each followed by a slave carrying a prayer book.[23]

DeForest passed the morning hours at work in his countingroom. At midday all offices closed for the long dinner and siesta, reopening a few hours before dusk. Evening might find him strolling on the *alameda*, the tree-shaded walk near the beach, or taking refreshment with a few friends in the French Coffee House near La Merced Church. There, on the evening of July 24, 1808, he sits at a table with the aged Don Ventura Llorente, formerly prior of the *consulado*, and discusses politics very moderately, "without giving offense to each other." Politics was very much in the air that mid-summer of 1808, but DeForest, as befitted a foreigner on a very uncertain footing in the country, professed an outward neutrality.

He was not always thus discreet. With his friend Juan Larrea, a young Catalonian merchant steeped in the doctrines of French and Spanish liberal philosophers and economists, he spoke much of the rights of man, the governments of the world, and the inde-

---

21. DeForest to John H. DeForest, Buenos Aires, Oct. 28, 1809, DeForest Letterbooks, Vol. 3.
22. P. Groussac, *Santiago de Liniers*, p. 42.
23. For life and manners in colonial Buenos Aires, see the chapters on social history contributed by José Torre Revello to the *Historia de la nación argentina*, IV, Section 1. Alexander Gillespie, *Gleanings and Remarks; Collected during Many Months of Residence at Buenos Aires and within the Upper Country* (Leeds, Eng., 1818), is an engaging account of conditions in La Plata at the time of the British invasions.

pendence of Buenos Aires.[24] Perhaps he knew that some of his friends, such as the fiery young lawyer, Juan José Castelli, were meeting in unobtrusive *tertulias* to concert revolutionary action. For by the late summer of 1808 the affairs of Spain were in crisis, twilight advanced upon the Spanish Empire in America, and in Buenos Aires formidable factions prepared to contend for mastery of this rich heritage of the Spanish crown.

24. Retrospectively affirmed in DeForest to José Antonio Cabrera and Pedro López, New Haven, Nov. 24, 1811, DeForest Letterbooks, Vol. 5.

VI

"THE IDES OF MARCH"

"BET with Mr. Blodget," DeForest carefully noted in his diary on February 13, 1808, "three ounces of gold that the Government of the King of Spain would not continue at Buenos Ayres longer than six months."

News of the arrival of the Portuguese royal family in Brazil, brought that day by the post from Montevideo, inspired this seemingly reckless wager. Fleeing the approach of French invaders, Prince John and his court had sailed from Lisbon on November 29, 1807, under British escort. After a stop at Bahia, where he proclaimed the ports of Brazil open to foreign trade, the prince regent cruised on to Rio de Janeiro, the new seat of his government. The men of Buenos Aires had good reason to apprehend danger from the proximity of the Portuguese court. Spain had connived with the French emperor at the destruction of her neighbor, permitting French troops to march through Spanish territory toward Lisbon. The threat of a vengeful Brazilian attack across the border from the province of Rio Grande was now joined to the menace of a third British invasion. "We are in some expectation of an attack from the English," wrote DeForest, "and many think they will be assisted by the Brasilians, in which case it is feared they will succeed." [1]

The aggressive diplomacy of the Prince of Portugal gave substance to these fears. Newly installed at Rio, Prince John dispatched an envoy to La Plata with an offer to take the people of the viceroyalty under his royal protection. He promised to respect their rights and liberties, and to establish complete freedom of trade. Should they reject his friendly proposals, however, he would be under the necessity of making common cause with powerful England against Buenos Aires.[2] Liniers and the *cabildo*

---

1. DeForest to José da Costa e Abreu, Buenos Aires, March 23, 1808, DeForest Letterbooks, Vol. 3.
2. Ricardo Levene, "Intentos de independencia en el virreinato del Plata (1781–1809)," in *Historia de la nación argentina,* V, Section 1, p. 620.

vigorously rebuffed the Portuguese pretensions. In their dealings with Prince John, in their preparations for defense, the colonial authorities acted like the heads of an independent state. Indeed, Spain, the helpless prisoner of her French ally, could neither aid her colonies nor relieve her own wretched plight. By March, 1808, nearly 100,000 French troops were inside the kingdom. In Aranjuez a mob rose against Godoy, Prince of the Peace, regarded as the author of Spain's misfortunes. To save his favorite's life the aged Charles IV abdicated in favor of his son Ferdinand, Prince of Asturias. Napoleon chose this moment to intervene in the quarrels of the House of Bourbon. He summoned father and son to confer with him at Bayonne in France.[3]

Intimations of the somber crisis of the Spanish monarchy reached Buenos Aires in July, 1808. "The first and certain news," DeForest recorded in his diary, "that the French Troops had possession of Madrid and other parts of Spain and that Carlos IV the King and his son Ferdinand who had been crowned King, as well as the rest of the Royal Familia was at Bayonne in France, where was also the French Emperor and Court." [4] At the end of July the provincial authorities received official word that Charles IV had abdicated in favor of his son, who should be proclaimed king as Ferdinand VII. The ceremony was fixed for August 12, but was postponed in the light of a report that Charles had withdrawn his abdication. To add to the confusion of the time, on August 13 an emissary of Napoleon, the Marquis de Sassenay, arrived in Buenos Aires with dispatches for Liniers. "This day closes," reads the entry in DeForest's journal, "with the whole town gaping with anxious expectation of hearing something important very soon."

In the citadel, after inviting the attendance of the *cabildo* and the *audiencia,* Liniers received the imperial envoy. Before the assembled dignitaries the dispatches he brought were opened and read. They related that Charles IV and Ferdinand VII had renounced their rights to the throne in favor of Napoleon, who ceded them to his brother Joseph, now to become King of Spain. The assembly resolved to ignore these communications. Sassenay was ordered to return forthwith to Bayonne, the proclamation of Ferdinand VII as king was set for August 21. But the cautious

3. André Fugier, *Napoléon et l'Espagne, 1799–1808* (2 vols., Paris, 1930), is authoritative on Franco-Spanish relations at this period.
4. DeForest Journal, Vol. 6, July 15, 1808.

and ambiguous address issued by Liniers with the advice and consent of the *cabildo* and the *audiencia* failed to answer the questions in the public mind: it spoke respectfully of Napoleon, assured the people of the emperor's good wishes for Buenos Aires, and advised them to imitate their ancestors, who during the War of the Spanish Succession "awaited the destiny of the mother country in order to obey the legitimate authority which occupied the throne." [5]

With traditional pomp and festivity the ceremony of proclaiming the new king was celebrated on August 21. Official efforts to conceal the fate of the Spanish monarchs, prisoners in France, proved vain; the public cry, as recorded by DeForest, was "Hurrah for Fernando 7th! Fernando or no King!" The merchant interpreted popular sentiment to be against the admission of French troops into the province, and for the speediest possible conclusion of peace and establishment of free trade with Great Britain.[6] Two days later a new emissary, the Spanish officer Goyeneche, arrived in Buenos Aires. His dispatches revealed that all Spain was in flames. A supreme *junta* installed at Seville directed the insurrection against the usurper Joseph. Peace was being made with England, which offered all manner of aid to the Spanish patriots. "Every one here," commented DeForest, "appears perfectly happy with this intelligence."

A small coterie of creole leaders headed by Manuel Belgrano, brilliant secretary of the *consulado*, took special interest in the news from Spain. In the disasters of the mother country they perceived an unexampled opportunity to achieve the independence of La Plata. The British invasions had stimulated the growth of a revolutionary climate of opinion among the creole landowners, merchants, and professional men of Buenos Aires. Revelations of creole capacity and Spanish official incompetence and cowardice had sharpened the latent conflict between natives and old Spaniards. English propaganda had extolled the blessings of free government, and the influx of cheap British goods had suggested the benefits of free trade. But the conditions for the achievement of independence were not yet present. The Argentine revolutionaries did not possess the clarity of purpose and energy of their North American counterparts; the *populacho*

---

5. For this episode, see Mario Belgrano, "El emisario imperial el marqués de Sassenay," in *Historia de la nación argentina*, V, Section 1, pp. 85–104.
6. DeForest Journal, Vol. 6, August 21, 1808.

of Buenos Aires, still fanatically loyal to their king and the established order, were not to be compared with the democratic and responsive yeomanry and artisans of the thirteen North American colonies. That is why the revolution of Buenos Aires had to await a more propitious moment, and even then proceed by indirection and subterfuge.[7]

"A year passed," recalled the patriot leader Belgrano, "and we had not yet labored in the sense of independence. God himself presented us the opportunity with the events of 1808 in Spain and Bayonne. Then it was that the ideas of liberty and independence quickened in America, and the Americans began for the first time to speak of their rights." [8] Ardently professing allegiance to the dethroned and imprisoned Ferdinand VII, in their hearts the patriots believed that the "beloved" monarch would never return to rule in Spain. They counted on the certain victory of French arms in the peninsula. Accordingly they prepared to set up a new government, nominally ruling in the king's name but actually independent and serving the interests of the natives. By donning the "mask of Ferdinand" they hoped to gain the support of the monarchically disposed people of Buenos Aires, avert premature conflict with the Spanish royalists, and secure the sympathy and even assistance of Britain—Spain's powerful ally.

The prevailing temper of the creole party in the mid-summer in 1808 is suggested in a letter from DeForest to his English correspondent, Thomas Wilson. "There is nothing wanting I assure you, Sir" he wrote, "but good management on the part of the English to have a free trade to this country. Force and flattery ought in my opinion be united to bring it about, and after it is accomplished, to leave the people here to govern themselves, and treat them as an independent Nation in order to insure continuance. All is quiet as yet, but I consider it possible, though not probable, that a Revolution may take place without the assistance of the English." [9]

The most influential advocates of independence, such as Bel-

---

7. For the antecedents of the Argentine Revolution, see the contributions to Vol. 5, Sec. 1 of *Historia de la nación argentina*, particularly R. Levene, "Intentos de independencia en el virreinato del Plata." B. Mitre, *Belgrano*, I, Ch. 6, describes with great power the gathering conflict between creoles and old Spaniards, the impact of the events of Bayonne and Spain, and the constitutional premises of the *Revolución de Mayo*.

8. "Auto-Biografía" of Manuel Belgrano, in *ibid.*, p. 438.

9. Buenos Aires, August 20, 1808, DeForest Letterbooks, Vol. 3.

grano, Nicolás Rodríguez Peña, and Juan José Paso, recoiled from revolution on the French or North American model. They envisaged a peaceful transition to independence under the auspices of a new monarchy limited by constitutional guarantees. A candidate was at hand: she was the Princess Carlota Joaquina of Portugal, wife of the prince regent and sister of Ferdinand VII. After the events of Bayonne, Carlota proclaimed herself Regent of Spain and the Indies, and through emissaries of her husband laid claim to rule in Buenos Aires in the name of her brother. The patriot leaders opened negotiations with the princess, and carried on an active propaganda in her behalf. They could hardly have made a more unfortunate choice. Carlota was not only morally bankrupt, but of decidedly absolutist views.[10] Divining the true designs of the patriots, she denounced her adherents to Viceroy Liniers, charging that their letters were full of revolutionary principles subversive of the monarchial system and tending toward the establishment of a fanciful and visionary republic.[11] With this the Carlota project went into temporary discard.

Meantime the European Spaniards of La Plata, equally convinced of the impending separation of the colony from the mother country, intrigued to depose Liniers and establish a governing *junta* that would confirm and continue their ancient monopoly of political and commercial privilege. Their leader was the stubborn *chapetón*, Martín Alzaga, senior *alcalde* and hero of the *defensa*. Alzaga and his followers had long been critical of Liniers' alien birth, his tolerance of foreigners, and his evident partiality toward the creole element. With the outbreak of hostilities between Spanish patriots and Napoleon's puppet government, the situation of the French-born viceroy grew precarious. His alleged disloyalty to Spain afforded a pretext for the revolutionary plans of Alzaga and his fellow conspirators of the *cabildo*.

In Montevideo the ultra-royalist Governor Javier de Elío, his

10. P. Groussac, *Liniers*, p. 253, gives a pungent portrayal of the princess. "The elder sister of Ferdinand VII was only thirty-three years old at this time. But she was embittered, prematurely aged, sickly, half-consumptive, consumed with ambition and lust, offering the thrice-repugnant spectacle of feminine vice united with perfidy and ugliness." For a more sympathetic view of Carlota and her pretensions to rule in La Plata, see Julián María Rubio, *La infanta Carlota Joaquina y la política de España en América, 1808–1812* (Madrid, 1920). Enrique Ruiz Guiñazú, *Lord Strangford y la revolución de mayo* (Buenos Aires, 1937), discusses the negative attitude of the British minister at Rio de Janeiro toward Carlota's projects and his relations with the patriots of Buenos Aires.

11. R. Levene, "Intentos de independencia," pp. 638–639.

suspicions aroused by certain equivocal utterances and actions of Liniers, defied the viceroy's authority, charged him with treason, and knocked down an officer sent from Buenos Aires to supersede the governor. A tumultuous *cabildo abierto* supported Elío's actions and chose a governing *junta* (September 21, 1808), composed entirely of European Spaniards. In the capital, meanwhile, Alzaga and his partisans prepared to imitate the example of Montevideo. They fixed the date of their uprising for January 1, 1809, when the *cabildo* should choose its membership for the coming year.

The ceremonies of election began tranquilly on that day. But at a prearranged signal the city bell sounded the alarm, and a turbulent crowd composed mainly of armed European troops poured into the great square. As in Montevideo, their cry was, Down with the Frenchman Liniers! A *junta* as in Spain! A *cabildo abierto*, carefully packed, met and chose a governing *junta* comprising European Spaniards with the exception of two creole secretaries. Successive delegations headed by Bishop Lue informed Liniers of these transactions and urged him to resign. The viceroy, shaken by the sweep of events, offered to comply. But he had barely signed the required document when the commanders of the creole regiments, secretly summoned by Liniers, strode into the hall, Cornelio Saavedra at their head. Informed of the voluntary resignation of the viceroy, Saavedra brusquely addressed the gathering:

"Señores, who empowered his Excellency to yield an office that he legally holds, when the reasons urged upon him for this decision are false and groundless?"

"Señor commander," spoke up arrogant Bishop Lue, "in God's name, the people do not wish his Excellency to remain their ruler."

"That," replied Saavedra, "is one of the many falsehoods brought to play in this comedy. As proof, let Señor Liniers come with us and show himself to the people. If they reject him or declare that they do not want him to continue in command, I and my comrades will endorse his deposition."

Saavedra advanced toward the viceroy and took him by the arm. "Come, Señor," said he, "show yourself to the people and hear their wishes." Liniers and the creole officers went out to the square. Meantime native troops had appeared in force, and the Spanish regiments had melted away. Cheering crowds greeted the popular viceroy with loud *vivas!* and assurances of loyalty.

Punishment for the ringleaders of the conspiracy followed promptly. Alzaga and four other *cabildantes* were arrested and exiled to Patagonia, only to be rescued by a warship dispatched from rebellious Montevideo. Liniers acted to consolidate his power by ordering the dissolution of the Spanish regiments that had turned against him.[12]

"What is extraordinary in this affair," DeForest shrewdly commented in a letter to the American consul at Rio de Janeiro, "is that the old Spaniards were on the side of the cabildo, and the Creoles for the Vice Roy." [13] This assertion is not altogether accurate: on the side of the viceroy were ranged the conservative *audiencia,* numerous other Spanish officials, and some of the European military leaders, while the creole lawyer Mariano Moreno, future tribune of the *Revolución de Mayo,* collaborated with the *cabildo.* But differences of motive separated the Spanish and creole adherents of Liniers. Spanish officialdom supported the viceroy as the legal representative of the crown, as a symbol of the established order threatened by the revolutionary formula of governing *juntas* invoked by Alzaga and the *cabildo.* The creoles, the true party of revolution, rallied to the defense of Liniers because for them he was a symbol of popular sovereignty first asserted in the stormy days of the British invasions; be-

---

12. The above account is based on R. Levene, "La asonada del 1º de enero de 1809," in *Historia de la nación argentina,* V, Section 1. In his journal DeForest gives the following version of the *asonada,* under date of January 1, 1809:

"The day for choosing and qualifying a New Cabildo. The old Cabildo determined to ruin the Vice Roy and establish a junta of Government, and supposing they had secured sufficient strength among the military, began to sound the tocsin of discord and confusion about one o'clock when the Catalan Corps took possession of all the Grand Square and intercepted all communications with the Fort or Montevideo, stopping all People they thought proper and firing on some. Their power continued united with many Biscayans and Galicians for about two hours, during which time they were negotiating with Liniers, and the different Corps took some Prisoners, insulted many and fired on others. But on the arrival of the Patrician Corps in the Grand Square it became known that the Creoles of the Country were determined to support the authority of the Vice King. The Polizones began to fly in every direction. Negotiations still going on and the Cabildo and many of the Authorities endeavouring to persuade Genl Liniers to resign his authority to appear and gratify the populace, which he consented to do believing the Town really in danger of cutting the throats of each other if he did [not]. His friends remonstrated strongly against such a measure and with the Comandant of Patricios at their head took him to the Grand Square, where he was recd with the strongest demonstrations of joy as the friend of the People and the head of the Government.

"All Malcontents were immediately arrested, and some hove into irons. On this occasion some few were wounded."

13. DeForest to Henry Hill, Buenos Aires, Jan. 4, 1809, DeForest Letterbooks, Vol. 3.

cause under his regime they enjoyed unwonted influence and opportunity to work for free trade and independence; and, finally, because Alzaga's conspiracy threatened to restore *chapetón* supremacy in all its former vigor.[14] From this conflict the natives emerged with a practical monopoly of military power and greatly increased prestige. By invoking the formula of governing *juntas*, moreover, the Europeans themselves had established a revolutionary precedent that the patriots would one day use with notable effect.

Liniers, comprehending the true source and bulwark of his authority, now showed himself more than ever well disposed toward the creole party. The patriot leader Belgrano, long an earnest advocate of commercial reform, utilized the complacent mood of the viceroy to urge the opening of La Plata's ports to British trade as a means of diminishing the importance of rebellious Montevideo and relieving the financial distress of the government. Admiral Sidney Smith, commanding British naval forces in the river, seconded these efforts with the suggestion to Liniers that he follow the example of the governor of Habana and open the ports "for mutual convenience and regional benefits, raising revenue from a tolerated commerce." [15]

A potent argument for legalizing trade with England was the swelling volume of contraband traffic, which afforded no revenue to the provincial treasury, and which Liniers appeared unwilling or unable to halt. Indeed, it was charged that the viceroy connived at smuggling operations for personal profit.[16] About this time DeForest observed that with proper management almost anything could be done in the way of contraband.[17] Smuggling, he wrote to one correspondent, had reached the proportions of a regular system, "paying so much p% to one, and so

14. This interpretation of the *asonada* of January 1, 1809, as essentially a conflict between creoles and European Spaniards is accepted by most Argentine historians of past and recent times (Mitre, Lopez, Groussac, Ingenieros, etc.). Cf., however, the somewhat revisionist view of Levene ("La asonada del 1o del enero de 1809," pp. 694–699), who tends to reduce the episode to a factional struggle against the overweening pretensions of the *cabildo*, in which Spaniards were enrolled without distinction on both sides.

15. Smith to Liniers, March 18, 1809, quoted in D. Goebel, "British Trade to the Spanish Colonies," p. 311.

16. William Dunn to Alexander Cunninghame, July 26, quoted in *ibid.*, p. 309. On Liniers' commercial interests, see also C. Roberts, *Las invasiones inglesas*, p. 299.

17. DeForest to Stephen Twyecross, Buenos Aires, Dec. 18, 1809, DeForest Letterbooks, Vol. 3.

much to another."[18] So open was this traffic become that several English shops, familiarly known as *baratillas*, did business in the capital.[19]

Liniers, perceiving no other solution for the grave financial problems of his government, signified his approval of Belgrano's plan for trade reform in June, 1809.[20] Just then word came to Buenos Aires that the newly installed *junta central* of Seville had deposed the viceroy, and that his successor, Baltasar Hidalgo de Cisneros, was at Montevideo. Action on the proposed measure was therefore suspended.

The removal of Liniers, fruit of Spanish intrigue, angered and dismayed the creole party. They apprehended new efforts to restore European predominance and commercial monopoly. "The musty old Laws of the Indies," observed DeForest, "may be hunted up to incommode us, and foreign commerce may be entirely prohibited. It is generally believed that the Govt of Bs As had completed their commercial system on the very day in which the news respecting the Vice Roy arrived, and that commerce was to be perfectly free and taxed only with a moderate duty."[21] An English merchant noted general resentment at the ill treatment of Liniers by his government, and fear that the ports would be closed to British trade.[22]

Belgrano, Saavedra, and other patriot leaders, meeting secretly in the home of Juan Martín Pueyrredón, discussed a project for offering resistance to Cisneros. But they could reach no agreement as to ends: one was for a *junta*, another for bringing Princess Carlota to rule in Buenos Aires.[23] "The figs are not yet

18. DeForest to Nathaniel Lucas, Buenos Aires, Feb. 4, 1809, *ibid.*
19. Same to same, Buenos Aires, March 25, 1809, *ibid.*
20. R. Levene, "Significacción historica de la obra económica de Manuel Belgrano y Mariano Moreno," in *Historia de la nación argentina,* V, Section 1, p. 709.
21. DeForest to Lewis Goddefroy, Buenos Aires, July 8, 1809, DeForest Letterbooks, Vol. 3.
22. William Dunn to Alexander Cunninghame, Buenos Aires, July 15, 1809; same to same, Buenos Aires, July 26, 1809, Public Record Office, Foreign Office, Spain, 90, Hiram Bingham Transcripts, Yale University Library.
23. R. Levene, "Intentos de independencia," pp. 654–655. The renewed vitality of the Carlota project at this time is suggested by a memorial on the subject in the archives of the British foreign office. Written in Spanish and English, and dated August, 1809, it purports to be an "Address by Inhabitants of Buenos Ayres to their Magistrates proposing the election of Princess Charlotte Joaquina of Brazil, Regent of Buenos Ayres." A second memorial, addressed to the British foreign minister (August 22, 1809), solicits Britain's support "in upholding the House of Bourbon." P. R. O., F. O., Spain, 90, Hiram Bingham Transcripts.

ripe," remarked the judicious Saavedra. Cisneros, doubtful of the reception that awaited him, remained at Colonia until Liniers himself came to escort the new viceroy to the capital, where he took quiet possession of his office on July 29, 1809.

Cisneros, a veteran of Trafalgar, soon found himself adrift upon a sea of troubles. He discovered, read his official report, "two formidable parties in the capital; the entire extent of the viceroyalty in convulsion; diversity of opinions; presentiments of independence, and other evils to which the state of Spain had given rise." [24] The revolutionary upheavals of Montevideo and Buenos Aires reverberated in the distant northern reaches of the province. In the town of Chuquisaca differences between Spanish authorities culminated in a struggle for control from which the *audiencia*, supported by the creoles, emerged victorious (May, 1809). The spirit of unrest soon spread to the important provincial center of La Paz. There the natives rose under the banner of independence, with the cry: Death to the *chapetónes!* Under the leadership of a *junta tuitiva* they organized a government composed exclusively of creoles, framed a constitution, and instituted extensive reforms. "It is time," boldly proclaimed the patriots, "to raise the standard of liberty in these unfortunate colonies, acquired without the least title and ruled with the greatest injustice and tyranny." [25]

Against these insurgents Cisneros acted with speed and energy. To the seats of disaffection he dispatched Brigadier Goyeneche, who crushed the uprising of La Paz with great cruelty. But in Buenos Aires the new viceroy walked softly, for he recognized the superior military power of the creoles. He restored Alzaga and other ringleaders in the tumult of January 1 to their former places of honor, but he dissolved the *junta* of Montevideo and stripped the Spanish regiments which had taken part in the *asonada* of their separate identity. Alarmed by the infiltration of suspicious strangers from abroad—notably from Philadelphia and Rio de Janeiro—Cisneros had a census of foreigners made preliminary to their expulsion.[26] In the list of names submitted to the viceroy by *alcalde* José Serra y Valle of the Third Quarter figures that of "Dⁿ David Cortez Laforest

---

24. B. Mitre, *Belgrano*, I, 279.
25. *Ibid.*, p. 285. For the uprisings of Chuquisaca and La Paz, see R. Levene, "Intentos de independencia," pp. 602–669.
26. *Ibid.*, p. 665.

[*sic*], captain of an American ship that went to Patagonia, with which he later came hither, and which he dispatched I know not where, remaining in the land to trade. And the same has purchased a *chacra* on the coast of San Isidro. He is an American." [27]

Cisneros, like his predecessor, pondered the means of solving the grave financial crisis of the colony. The need for additional revenue was great, the viceroy's desire to conciliate the creole party was strong; reluctantly he turned to consider the unorthodox expedient of free trade. Two English merchants applied to him in August, 1809, for permission to sell their cargoes. Cisneros passed this petition to the *cabildo* and the *consulado*, with a favorable recommendation. "The general opinion," commented DeForest, "is that the Ports of the River will soon be opened to general Commerce, and on a fair and liberal plane, for, the Treasury is empty, the Government deeply in debt, the interior in commotion, the Govt both unwilling and unable to use effectual force for driving out the English Vessels, of course unable to prevent the Contraband trade and for a variety of other reasons is this opinion formed." [28]

The *cabildo*, representing the monopolists on both sides of the Atlantic, indicated the grave evils that must flow from trade with foreigners, but grudgingly conceded the necessity of the measure. In the *consulado* the proposal of the viceroy won by a vote of seven to five. With breathless interest DeForest followed the fortunes of trade reform. "A majority of the Cabildo and Consulado," he wrote, "approve of the measure. All the Patrician and landed interest make every exertion to support this liberal and patriotic plan. Its opponents are such as have large quantities of Goods on hand, and some rich and infamous old Spaniards, who wish to continue a Connection with Spain whatever may be its situation and Government." [29]

Now Fernández de Agüero, attorney for the *consulado* of Cadiz, submitted to the viceroy an able brief against free trade. This innovation, he asserted, was contrary to the Laws of the Indies and must prove fatal to the merchant marine of Spain, to the agriculture and industry of the province. "The land holders and respectable Creoles then came forward by their Agent in

27. *Documentos para la historia argentina*, XII, 288.
28. DeForest to Henry Hill, Buenos Aires, Aug. 14, 1809, DeForest Letterbooks, Vol. 4.
29. DeForest to Oliver Jump, Buenos Aires, Sept. 12, 1809, *ibid.*

support of the proposed measure of the Vice Roy, and in an exposition of 24 sheets have lashed the supporters of the Old System of things in a masterly manner." [30]

This was the celebrated *Representación de los hacendados* of the thirty-one-year-old creole lawyer, Mariano Moreno. More than a defense of the viceroy's proposal as a temporary financial expedient, it was an ardent and vigorous argument for the adoption of free trade as necessary to the welfare of the people of La Plata and in conformity with the laws of political economy as expounded by Adam Smith. Free trade would provide an outlet for the productions of the country and relieve the distress of the landowners and laborers, it would stimulate commerce, replenish the provincial treasury, and make possible a greater measure of assistance to the patriots of Spain. Indignantly Moreno spurned Agüero's suggestion that this reform might weaken the bonds between La Plata and the mother country. He cited the observation of the philosopher Filangieri concerning prosperous colonies to prove the contrary. "Happy under their metropolis they would not dream of shaking off so light and mild a yoke in favor of an independence that would deprive them of the protection of their mother, leaving them with no sure defense against the ambition of a conqueror, the intrigues of a powerful citizen, or the perils of anarchy. It was not an excess of riches and prosperity that induced the English colonies to rebel; it was an excess of oppression that caused them to turn against their mother the same arms that they had so often employed in her defense." [31]

Argentine historians are not in accord as to the influence of Moreno's memorial on the course of events leading to the *Revolución de Mayo*. Señor Molinari has sought to demolish the claims made for the *Representación*;[32] Professor Levene, on the other hand, ascribes to this writing a far-reaching significance.[33] DeForest's comments suggest that it was warmly received and widely read in cultured creole circles, although Spanish censorship prevented publication at that time. Manuscript copies of the original

30. DeForest to Henry Hill, Buenos Aires, Oct. 5, 1809, *ibid*.
31. For the text of this document, see Norberto Pinero, ed., *Escritos de Mariano Moreno* (Buenos Aires, 1896), pp. 89–224.
32. Diego Luis Molinari, *La representación de los hacendados de Mariano Moreno, su ninguna importancia en la vida económica del país y en los sucesos de mayo de 1810* (Buenos Aires, 1939, 2d edit.).
33. R. Levene, *Ensayo histórico sobre la revolución de mayo y Mariano Moreno* (2 vols., Buenos Aires, 1920–21), I, 282 ff.; see also by the same author, "Significacción histórica de la obra económica de Manuel Belgrano y Mariano Moreno," in *Historia de la nación argentina*, V, Section 1, pp. 732 ff.

circulated in the capital; DeForest notes that he paid eighteen dollars for one. An interested English merchant forwarded a copy of Moreno's memorial to the British foreign minister with an account of the events which led to its composition.[34]

Delighted by the vigorous style and liberal sentiments of this Argentine *Common Sense*, DeForest resolved to bring Moreno's statement before a wider reading public. Accordingly he sent his manuscript copy to English acquaintances at Rio de Janeiro, requesting them to arrange for its publication in an edition of two or three thousand copies. He assured his correspondents that the pamphlet would have a large sale in Buenos Aires. "Profit however would not be the object of you or myself in putting it forward, but the interest and improvement of the Spanish Americans in which most certainly your Country is very deeply and directly interested." He would assume one-fourth of the costs of publication, and expected British merchants at Rio to advance the remainder. Suggesting that Moreno had been consulted on the project, he promised shortly to send a title and introduction, "with a variety of notes which ought to accompany it." [35]

Unfortunately DeForest soon lapsed into silence concerning the progress of his publishing plans. Presumably he failed to secure the support at Rio which he had anticipated. The first publication of the *Representación* did take place at Rio de Janeiro in the early part of 1810, in a Portuguese translation by the economist José da Silva Lisboa.[36] But there is no evidence that DeForest was linked with this project, which differed substantially from his own.

Meantime the three-months-old debate on the viceroy's proposal for trade reform drew to a close. A *junta* of commerce convoked by Cisneros sanctioned a decree establishing a limited free trade with allied and neutral nations (November 6, 1809). DeForest proudly noted in his diary that the first ship to enter the port of Buenos Aires under the new dispensation was the Portuguese brig *Roquete do Sul*, consigned to him by Henry Glover of Rio de Janeiro. "This brig began to discharge on the 14th November, and had the Goods discharged in the Custom

34. Alexander Mackinnon to George Canning, Buenos Aires, Nov. 2, 1809, P. R. O., F. O., Spain, 90, Hiram Bingham Transcripts.
35. DeForest to Nathaniel Lucas, Buenos Aires, Oct. 20, 1809, DeForest Letterbooks, Vol. 4.
36. R. Levene, "Significaccion histórica de la obra económica de Manuel Belgrano y Mariano Moreno," p. 738, ascribes this publication to the efforts of interested British subjects.

House on the 16th and 17th before any other vessel had begun to discharge."

The decree of November 6 soon justified itself as contraband trade gave way to open commerce, with increased receipts from customs accruing to the treasury. Withal vexatious restrictions upon trade remained. Foreigners could consign only to Spanish merchants, duties were unduly high, and one totally impracticable provision declared that payment for imports must be made one-third in money, two-thirds in produce. About this time Juan Pedro Varangot departed for Spain on a government mission, and DeForest secured a new partner to act as the nominal receiver of his consignments. His choice fell on Juan Larrea, syndic of the *consulado*, a young Spaniard of liberal proclivities.[37] A gentleman of handsome fortune, a well bred merchant, in every particular well qualified for a consignee—so DeForest described his new business associate.[38]

In the winter of 1809 gloomy tidings came to Buenos Aires from mother Spain. Inexorably the armies of Napoleon drove toward total conquest of the peninsula. The colonials anxiously discussed what they must do when Spain fell to the invader. Three courses, observed DeForest, were open to the people of Buenos Aires: independence, union with Brazil under Princess Carlota, or submission to the new rulers of Spain. The old Spaniards, intolerant of all foreigners and warmly attached to the mother country, preferred to maintain the peninsular connection under all circumstances. They filled the principal offices of government and therefore possessed considerable strength. But military power rested in the hands of the creoles, and armed force must ultimately settle the question. Serious differences of opinion and a spirit of vacillation obtained in creole ranks. "The most respectable and best informed Natives tho' they much wish a complete independence, doubt their ability to establish it on a firm basis, and will of course (as I believe) throw their influence into the scale of the Princess of Brasil, whose pretensions I think will prevail." [39]

Cisneros, apprehensive of the furtive intrigues of the patriots, but lacking the material or moral resources to act decisively

---

37. For Larrea, see the sketch in E. Udaondo, *Diccionario biográfico argentino*.
38. DeForest to Balch and Godard, Buenos Aires, Nov. 11, 1809, DeForest Letterbooks, Vol. 4.
39. DeForest to Thomas Wilson, Buenos Aires, Nov. 26, 1809, *ibid*.

against them, pursued a vacillating policy of small concessions to the natives coupled with ineffectual efforts to stamp out sedition. At the end of December, 1809, he moved to purge the province of undesirable foreigners. DeForest was among the first to receive the order of expulsion. He had been singled out for banishment, reflected the merchant, because he had property exposed, had lived in Buenos Aires a long time, received the consignments of others, and possessed "too much liberality of sentiment to live in a Country where individuals have no rights." [40] That the viceroy's motives were primarily political is suggested by the simultaneous expulsion of a number of Portuguese and Frenchmen whose conversation on the relations between Spain and her colonies had made them obnoxious to the government.[41]

"Know ye," DeForest addressed himself to posterity in the pages of his journal, "that the new and brutal Vice Roy Cisneros, influenced by some of my private enemies, ordered me out of the Country within Eight days from the 17th December." Vainly he appeared before the Spanish official to plead for an extension of time; Cisneros drove him forth without deigning to reply. Then the exile retreated to an English ship in the harbor, and from this place of refuge carried on an active correspondence with friends on shore, meanwhile peppering his foes with epistolary abuse. Confident of a speedy return to the capital, DeForest renewed his partnership with Juan Larrea for the year 1810, and by means of a fictitious sale arranged to place his *chacra* in Larrea's safekeeping.

Revolution was in the air. In Buenos Aires the patriots awaited the hour fixed by Saavedra: when Seville should fall to the French.[42] DeForest was evidently in the secret; to an English friend he wrote that he would not seek to have the order of expulsion revoked "till after the Ides of March are over." [43] But life on board ship grew irksome, and he determined to voyage to Rio de Janeiro and there await the great and certain tidings. Armed with letters of introduction from the patriot leader Belgrano, he sailed for Rio on February 13, 1810, in the Portuguese bark *In-*

40. DeForest to Oliver Twyecross, Buenos Aires, Dec. 23, 1809, *ibid.*
41. Alexander Mackinnon to George Canning, Buenos Aires, Dec. 18/23, 1809, P. R. O., F. O., Spain, 90, Hiram Bingham Transcripts.
42. A. Zimmerman Saavedra, *Cornelio de Saavedra* (Buenos Aires, 1909), p. 168.
43. DeForest to Oliver Jump, on board the *Seaton,* Dec. 29, 1809, DeForest Letterbooks, Vol. 4.

dustria. He had a fellow passenger in Juan Larrea's young brother Ramón, bound for Spain by way of England.

They landed at the Brazilian capital on March 5, 1810. Hospitable *cariocas* opened their homes to the travelers from La Plata, until DeForest fell ill from high living, "being invited to parties for 15 and 20 days daily after my arrival." To Belgrano he wrote a long and circumstantial account of the latest news from Spain, relating the fall of Seville, the dissolution of the *junta central,* and the apparently impending fall of Cadiz—last stronghold of the Spanish cause.[44] Two and a half months passed by without a hint of revolution in Buenos Aires. DeForest grew restless, decided to heed the urging of young Ramón Larrea and accompany him on the voyage to England. Perhaps while there he would find "a good daring girl for a wife." They sailed out of Rio harbor on May 20, 1810, in the packet-ship *Dispatch.*

One week earlier, the "Ides of March" had dawned in Buenos Aires. On May 13 an English vessel brought to Montevideo news that French armies had burst across the Sierra Morena and swept over the plains of Andalusia, entered Seville, and were threatening Cadiz. The *junta central,* the provisional government that claimed to rule in the name of the captive Spanish king, had fled and dispersed. This was the event that the secret society of the patriots had fixed upon as the signal for revolutionary action. From the unwilling viceroy and *cabildo* they wrested assent to the calling of a *cabildo abierto* which should decide the future form of government of the colony.

This first Argentine congress, from which many conservative notables were barred by the creole militia, voted overwhelmingly to depose the viceroy and establish a governing *junta.* On the historic twenty-fifth of May the clamor of the people compelled a reluctant *cabildo* to abide by these decisions and confirm a government nominated by the patriots. In the newly erected *junta* of nine sat friends and associates of DeForest: Larrea, Castelli, Azcuénaga, Belgrano. On the same day "the patriot *junta* installed itself in the citadel, residence of the ancient rulers of the colony, and began to act in revolutionary fashion while invoking the name and authority of the King of Spain, Ferdinand VII." [45]

44. DeForest to Manuel Belgrano, Rio de Janeiro, April 27, 1810, *ibid.*
45. B. Mitre, *Belgrano,* I, 346. On the *Revolución de Mayo,* see the chapters by R. Levene on "Los sucesos de mayo" and "El 25 de mayo" in *Historia de la nación argentina,* V, Section 2.

VII

"THE DOWNFALL OF MY ENEMIES"

DeFOREST, his Negro servant Joseph, and young Ramón Larrea landed at Falmouth port on July 19, 1810, after a voyage of sixty days. In his diary the exile expressed delight at the appearance of the English countryside, with its variegated pattern of hedges, fields, hills, and dales. In leisurely fashion, with frequent visits to scenes of interest, they journeyed by stage-coach toward London. At Redruth they inspected mines and machinery, at Plymouth they viewed the great navy yard where the king's ships lay, and at the little village of Ashburton they entered cottages where entire families wove serges that the East India Company would later export to India and China. It was the fourth of August before the travelers set foot in the capital. Two days later, at the counting-house of his old friend and correspondent Thomas Wilson, DeForest received and eagerly perused official accounts of the Revolution of Buenos Aires.

"Never, perhaps," the merchant recorded in his journal, "was there a Person more happily surprised than I to hear of the REVOLUTION OF BUENOS AYRES, of the disgrace and downfall of my enemies, and the complete establishment of the Government of my friends. This is the news, and certain news of the day, and I never felt more overjoyed at any circumstance in my life. Now let the infamous Cisneros grind his Teeth and mourn over his follies. He was a savage Villian while in power, and will be a most contemptible wretch out of it. Let him be so. Huzza! Huzza! Huzza for Buenos Ayres! May it be happy, and may its Enemies be damned. May all those who have had rule there and have conducted themselves in an unjust manner be severely punished. And may the Natives of Old Spain, who have no other crime but being Natives, be treated with a compassionate forgiveness, and become good citizens."

Simultaneously with this welcome intelligence, the first diplomatic representative of the patriot *junta* of Buenos Aires arrived in the English metropolis. He was a young naval officer, Matías

Irigoyen by name, dispatched by the revolutionary régime on a mission to London and Cadiz.[1] His instructions charged him to solicit British protection against the aggressive designs of Portugal and permission to export arms and munitions to Buenos Aires. This accomplished, he should cross over to Spain and present to the Cadiz *junta* a message that affirmed the stainless loyalty of the colonials to their captive king. A British warship brought Irigoyen to Britain's shores. Upon landing he discovered that the Spanish central *junta* had fallen and given way to a council of regency. Digesting this information, he concluded that the new régime did not even remotely "unite the qualities prescribed by law for a legitimately constituted government," and resolved to limit his diplomatic dealings to the British foreign office. The emissary carried letters of introduction to DeForest and Ramón Larrea, and the three *porteños* took lodgings together at No. 7, Southampton Street.

Irigoyen had his first interview with Marquis Wellesley, the British foreign secretary, on August 6, 1810. The English statesman expounded with precision the views of his government on the revolution of Buenos Aires. Britain stood ready to mediate the dispute between Spain and her disaffected subjects of the colonies, and greatly desired a reconciliation in the interests of the common struggle against Napoleon. She offered to the patriot *junta* protection against the aggressions of the Corsican, and her good offices in the quarrel with Portugal. But Britain would not aid or abet any movement tending toward the separation of the colonies from the mother country. Therefore Wellesley declined formally to receive the patriot agent and, tactfully alleging legal impediments and arms shortages, refused permission to export materials of war to Buenos Aires. The foreign secretary had conveyed essentially similar views to a delegation from the supreme *junta* of Caracas, headed by the immortal Simón Bolívar, that arrived in London on July 12 to solicit British aid for revolted Venezuela.[2]

1. Documents bearing on this and other early missions from Buenos Aires to Britain have been published by the Archivo General de la Nación of the Argentine Republic in the first volume of its *Misiones diplomáticas (misiones de Matías Irigoyen, José Agustín de Aguirre y Tomás Crompton)* (Buenos Aires, 1937). On these missions, see Daniel Antokoletz, *Histoire de la diplomatie argentine* (Paris and Buenos Aires, 1914), pp. 117–162.

2. C. K. Webster, *Britain and the Independence of Latin America* (2 vols., London, 1938), contains selected documents bearing on British policy, with an

British official coolness toward the suppliants from Buenos Aires and Caracas represented a significant reversal of attitude toward Spanish America. Cautious interest and encouragement to sundry schemes for Spanish-American emancipation under English auspices had been for two decades a characteristic feature of British policy. That stormy petrel of revolution, Miranda, had enjoyed British financial support while he plotted the subversion of Spain's American dominions, and such responsible statesmen as the great William Pitt had seriously considered his audacious plans. The filibustering expedition of the Venezuelan against his homeland had not been without implied British sanction. But the events of 1808 in Bayonne and Spain sounded the knell of this liberal policy. In January, 1809, Spain became Great Britain's formal ally in the mortal contest with Napoleon, and now it was to English interest that the Spanish Empire remain intact to provide effective aid to the mother country. Moreover, recent developments in the colonies weakened the force of commercial motives for desiring Spanish-American independence. While there is no basis for the commonly accepted view that in 1810 the Spanish government gave Britain permission to trade with the Indies,[3] by that year financial and political exigencies had compelled a number of colonial governments (notably at Habana and Buenos Aires) to open their ports to British ships.[4] Thus even before the first revolutionary outbreaks in Spanish America British merchants effectively enjoyed free trade with some Spanish provinces, while steady diplomatic pressure on the Cadiz régime gave promise of complete relaxation of the Laws of the Indies in return for British succors of all kinds. Under these conditions, there appeared to be "no special reason why British policy should desire the emancipation of the Spanish Colonies." [5]

interpretative introduction by the editor. William S. Robertson has described the first diplomatic reachings of the revolted colonies toward Great Britain and the United States, with special reference to Venezuela, in "The Beginnings of Spanish-American Diplomacy," in *Essays in American History Dedicated to Frederic Jackson Turner* (New York, 1910), pp. 231–267. For a stimulating comparison of British and American policy toward the Spanish-American revolutions, see Samuel Flagg Bemis, *Early Diplomatic Missions from Buenos Aires to the United States, 1811–1824* (Worcester, Mass., 1940, reprinted from the *Proceedings* of the American Antiquarian Society, April, 1939), pp. 89–93.

3. See, for example, C. K. Webster, *Britain,* I, 10. D. Goebel, "British Trade to the Spanish Colonies, 1796–1823," rejects this thesis in her heavily documented study of the status of British trade in the colonies.

4. This question is carefully studied in *ibid.,* p. 298 and *passim.*

5. C. K. Webster, *Britain,* I, 10.

In the light of these facts, British diplomacy in relation to the Spanish-American struggle for independence pursued a consistent yet flexible course. During the first stage of the conflict it diligently strove to reconcile Spain with her revolted dominions on the basis of imperial reforms that would include the admission of British commerce to colonial ports.[6] Later, when Iberian obstinacy and the victories of Bolívar and San Martín had shattered all hopes of reunion, it encouraged as the next best choice the establishment of congenial monarchial régimes under European princes in the new states.[7] At all stages of the struggle, Britain interposed her formidable might to bar armed intervention by a third party in the dispute.

Irigoyen emerged from his parleys with Lord Wellesley convinced that British policy was governed by Machiavellian precepts, and that Britain would not openly favor the South Americans while Spanish resistance to Napoleon continued.[8] He evidently imparted these impressions to his fellow-lodger DeForest. In a letter to Juan Larrea, now an influential figure in Buenos Aires politics, the merchant bitterly assailed the attitude of the British cabinet toward Spanish America. The people of England, he asserted, rejoiced at the liberation of that interesting part of the world. "But of the Government of England I have a very different opinion. It is selfish in the extreme, and while it is possible to keep the people of Old Spain and Portugal in a state of insurrection, I do not believe that they will perform any act of generosity toward the Spanish Americans." On the other hand, "the people of the United States of America and also the Government are enthusiastic in the cause of all oppressed Nations, and unlike the junta of Cadiz are as anxious to see Spanish America liberated from Spain, as to see Spain liberated from the modern Alexander." The patriots of Buenos Aires, however, he advised in closing, must not look for assistance abroad, but should depend solely on themselves and by their sincerity and exertions avoid the necessity of aid from others.[9]

6. On British offers of mediation, see for the first phase of negotiations, John Rydjord, "British Mediation between Spain and Her Colonies, 1811–1813," *Hisp. Am. Hist. Rev.*, XXI (1941), 29–50; for the second phase, C. K. Webster, "Castlereagh and the Spanish Colonies," *English Historical Review*, XXVII (1912), 78–95.

7. C. K. Webster, *Britain*, I, 26–34, discusses British interest in the establishment of monarchical institutions in the New World.

8. D. Antokoletz, *Histoire de la diplomatie argentine*, pp. 123–124.

9. DeForest to Larrea, London, Aug. 15, 1810, DeForest Letterbooks, Vol. 4.

In recognition of "the gallant and consistent conduct" of the people of Buenos Aires "in bringing to a crisis the long wished for change," DeForest sent for presentation to the new government a collection of books that included fittingly enough the works of the Abbé Raynal, Montesquieu, Voltaire, and Rousseau. These offerings were incorporated in the collections of the public library founded in Buenos Aires in 1810 at the initiative of Mariano Moreno, "for the purpose of encouraging reading and to instruct the people." [10]

To an old and honored friend, now a member of the patriot *junta,* the patron of learning wrote in praise of the educational and cultural undertakings of the new régime, particularly the establishment of a school of mathematics and a public library. He urged the further creation of an agricultural institute, furnished a detailed plan of organization, and sent plants and seeds for a projected botanical garden. "It is an undisputed maxim," he observed, "among the patriotic sages of North America (where I had the happiness to be born) *that an uninstructed cannot long be a free people.*" [11]

In Buenos Aires, however, the first preoccupation of the revolutionaries was with arms, sorely needed to repel threatened attacks by the royalists of Montevideo and their Portuguese allies, and to extend patriot authority into the distant northern reaches of the viceroyalty. Irigoyen, we have seen, vainly appealed to the British foreign secretary for permission to export articles of war. In this extremity the distraught agent resolved to seek to "elude the vigilance of a discreet government [*govierno savio*] and its strict laws," [12] secretly purchasing and smuggling arms out of the country. DeForest readily lent himself to these forbidden purposes; in behalf of Irigoyen (who evidently knew little or no English) he corresponded and otherwise negotiated with interested munitions makers.[13] "Your great want of arms is well known," he wrote Larrea, "I assure you that I am making every possible exertion to have your wants supplied." [14] One must con-

---

10. R. Levene, *History of Argentina,* p. 264.
11. DeForest to Miguel de Azcuénaga, London, Jan. 5, 1811, DeForest Letterbooks, Vol. 4.
12. Irigoyen to the *junta gubernativa,* London, Oct. 13, 1810, *Misiones diplomáticas,* p. 22.
13. DeForest to Graham, Riggs, and Co., London, Aug. 23, 1810; DeForest to Simon Walker, London, Jan. 14, 1811, DeForest Letterbooks, Vol. 4.
14. London, Oct. 27, 1810, *ibid.*

clude that the British government deliberately closed its eyes to these endeavors, for presently, without having experienced other embarrassments than his scanty funds occasioned, Irigoyen sailed for Buenos Aires with a cargo of armaments and a letter from Lord Wellesley recommending him to the protection of the British minister at Rio de Janeiro.[15]

Active interest in the patriot cause did not render DeForest oblivious of his personal concerns. Tartly he reproached Juan Larrea for devoting too much time to affairs of state. "You will certainly excuse me," he wrote that budding legislator, "for my interest and character must stand or fall with you, and I cannot forego this opportunity of saying to you: That you have it in your power to be the first Merchant in Buenos Ayres, if you will be content to be only that; but to be so, it is necessary that your whole *Time, Capital* and *Credit* be applied to the object for which your House is established. The moment you divide them you cease to be first." Predicting that the town of Lima in Peru would ere long be opened to foreign trade, the promoter broached a project for establishing Larrea's brother Ramón as their agent in that provincial capital.[16]

Revolutionary upheavals on the shores of La Plata revived DeForest's waning hopes for a consular appointment to Buenos Aires. Spanish authority had departed from the port, and he could see no reason why the United States should not maintain an agent there. Long years of residence in the Plate area, an intimate acquaintance with trade conditions, his friendship with the members of the patriot *junta;* these and other endowments appeared eminently to qualify the merchant for such a post. He resolved to proceed to the United States and make personal application for the office. Confident of success in his mission, DeForest left England on February 22, 1811, in the *George Augustus* of Philadelphia. He had taken the precaution of writing to Abraham Bishop, Republican party leader of New Haven, and to Postmaster General Gideon Granger, soliciting their patronage and influence to delay any appointment to Buenos Aires until his arrival in Washington.

DeForest, it appears, was unaware that in the spring of 1810, following the arrival in the United States of a delegation from the

15. D. Antokoletz, *Histoire de la diplomatie argentine,* p. 131; A. P. Whitaker, *The United States and the Independence of Latin America,* p. 75.
16. DeForest to Larrea, London, Nov. 29, 1810, DeForest Letterbooks, Vol. 4.

supreme *junta* of Caracas in search of succors and a treaty of alliance,[17] Secretary of State Smith had appointed three "agents for seamen and commerce" to as many actual or prospective centers of revolt in Spanish America. To Vera Cruz he dispatched William Shaler (June 16, 1810); to Caracas, Robert K. Lowry (June 26); to Buenos Aires, Joel Roberts Poinsett (June 28).

"You will make it your object," read Poinsett's notable instructions in part, "wherever it may be proper, to diffuse the impression that the United States cherish the sincerest good will toward the people of Spanish America as neighbors, as belonging to the same portion of the globe, and as having a mutual interest in cultivating friendly intercourse: that this disposition will exist, whatever may be their internal system or European relation, with respect to which no interference is pretended: and that, in the event of a political separation from the parent country, and of the establishment of an independent system of National Government, it will coincide with the sentiments and policy of the United States to promote the most friendly relations, and the most liberal intercourse, between the inhabitants of this hemisphere, as having all a common interest, and as lying under a common obligation to maintain that system of peace, justice, and good will, which is the only source of happiness for nations." [18]

Poinsett, a highly conscious protagonist of North American republican ideals, landed in Buenos Aires on February 13, 1811.[19] The initial misgivings of the patriots over the form of his commission, which was not directed to the revolutionary *junta* nor signed by the President, vanished when Poinsett explained that his credentials were identical with those issued to American agents at Habana and La Guaira. From the outset, British political and commercial pretensions on the River Plate gave the United States representative much concern. Soon after his arrival he advised

17. Composed of Juan Vicente Bolívar and Telésforo de Orea. The mission is briefly discussed in Charles C. Griffin, *The United States and the Disruption of the Spanish Empire* (New York, 1937), pp. 50–52.

18. William R. Manning, *Diplomatic Correspondence of the United States Concerning the Independence of the Latin-American Nations* (3 vols., New York, 1925), I, 6–7.

19. On Poinsett, see J. Fred Rippy, *Joel Roberts Poinsett, Versatile American* (Durham, N. C., 1935); Dorothy M. Parton, *The Diplomatic Career of Joel Roberts Poinsett* (Washington, D. C., 1934); and Charles Lyon Chandler and Edwin J. Pratt, "Vida de Joel Roberts Poinsett," in course of publication in the *Revista chilena de historia y geografía* (Santiago), LXVII (mayo-agosto, 1935), 37–52, and LXXXVIII (enero-junio, 1940), 295–309, to date.

the state department to establish a permanent consulate in Buenos Aires to keep the English from securing exclusive trade privileges.[20] James Monroe was now Madison's secretary of state. About this time a group of Baltimore merchants addressed to Monroe a letter of recommendation in behalf of one Louis Goddefroy, a French merchant domiciled for several years at Montevideo, and currently in the United States to apply for the post of consul to Buenos Aires. The signers deplored the languishing state of American commerce because of the European war, and remarked the expediency of maintaining a resident consul on the River Plate in view of our lucrative and important trade with that region.[21] These observations bore fruit; on April 30, 1811, President Madison appointed Goddefroy "Consul for Buenos Ayres and the ports below it on the River Plate," [22] and at the same time made Poinsett consul general to Buenos Aires, Chile, and Peru.

Two days later DeForest arrived in Washington from Baltimore where, suspecting nothing, he had encountered and spent some convivial hours with his old friend and agent at Montevideo, Louis Goddefroy. Without delay he called on Monroe and from the secretary of state learned that his long quest was in vain. The embittered applicant then saw President Madison, but his angry protests only elicited soft words of regret and promises of patronage at a future opportunity. Rancorous at this perverse preference of the Frenchman Goddefroy over his own highly qualified self, DeForest returned to his lodgings, seized pen and paper, and wrote a severe letter of censure to Monroe.

Brooding over his humiliation, DeForest resolved at all costs to defeat the appointment of Goddefroy as consul to Buenos Aires. He persuaded the United States senators from Connecticut, Samuel W. Dana and Chauncey Goodrich, to lead the fight against confirmation at the forthcoming session of Congress. His

20. D. M. Parton, *Poinsett,* p. 6.
21. Robert and John Oliver, and others, to James Monroe, Baltimore, April 1, 1811. National Archives (Washington), Department of State, Appointment Papers.
22. W. S. Robertson has printed Madison's letter to Goddefroy in "Documents Concerning the Consular Service of the United States in Latin America, with Introductory Note," *Mississippi Valley Historical Review,* II (1916), 561–568. On receiving his appointment, Goddefroy immediately departed for Buenos Aires, but on arrival in the river was refused permission by the blockading royalists either to land at Montevideo or to proceed to Buenos Aires. D. M. Parton, *Poinsett,* p. 19.

exertions were so successful that the Senate by unanimous vote rejected the nomination of Goddefroy.[23] This triumph salved DeForest's injured feelings, but furthered his own consular hopes none at all, for the irate Madison reportedly vowed to appoint any applicant in preference to the schemer from Connecticut.[24] The Buenos Aires post ultimately went to William Gilchrist Miller, a candidate recommended by Joel Poinsett. DeForest viewed the appointment with an understandably jaundiced eye. He described Miller as a very young man lately arrived at Buenos Aires from the East Indies without property or mercantile credit. "However," he grudgingly conceded, "Mr. Miller is a gentlemanly young man, has a good education, and perhaps may perform the duties of such an office satisfactorily." [25]

From Washington, still nursing his grievances, DeForest departed for the north. In July, 1811, he came to Watertown, Connecticut, where his parents and brothers fondly received the returned wanderer after an absence of six years. It was on a visit to his birthplace, the village of Ripton, that he found the "good daring girl" he sought for wife. Julia Wooster was distantly related to General David Wooster of Revolutionary War fame, and to that Charles W. Wooster who won distinction on the sea in the War of 1812, later enlisted in the patriot navy of Chile, and by his gifts of leadership rose to the rank of rear-admiral in that service.[26] Only sixteen years old, she was already a notable beauty, "a golden-haired woman with a skin like roseate snow," in the adulatory words of a family historian.[27] DeForest was thirty-seven, swarthy, dark-haired, and dark-eyed. Ardently he courted

23. The Senate rejected the choice of Goddefroy as "inexpedient." *Journal of the Executive Proceedings of the Senate of the United States of America* (Washington, 1828–), Vol. 2, p. 190.
24. DeForest to Samuel W. Dana, New Haven, Dec. 4, 1811, DeForest Letterbooks, Vol. 5.
25. *Ibid.* The *Dictionary of American Biography* contains no account of Miller. Some of his consular reports are printed in W. R. Manning, *Diplomatic Correspondence*, I, 322–331, 333. Miller arrived at Rio de Janeiro in the spring of 1810 as supercargo of the schooner *Juliet*. At Rio he made the acquaintance of DeForest, then an exile from Buenos Aires. It was agreed that Miller should go to Buenos Aires and be associated with Juan Larrea, assisting him in the conduct of his business. In return Larrea was to lend his name to Miller's commercial transactions, receiving half of the North American's commissions. DeForest to Larrea, Rio de Janeiro, March 16, 1810, DeForest Letterbooks, Vol. 4.
26. On Charles Wooster, see the adequate biographical sketch in the *D. A. B.*
27. J. W. De Forest, *The de Forests of Avesnes*, pp. 121–123.

her, quickly won her consent, and presently, feeling some trepidation, set out to obtain the approval of Julia's parents for the match.

"Took a Horse and Gig," reads the entry in DeForest's diary, "and went to Ripton with a view of asking my beloved little Julia of her Parents. The anxiety caused by this novel and to me most important Journey was very great. I sometimes doubted the propriety of my attempt, the Knowledge of my own mind, and, what was greater than everything else, I feared that she might not alter her's. However, on I went, and before twelve o'clock, arrived at Mr. Ephraim Wooster's the Father of my Julia. Told her my errand, with which she seemed highly delighted, and soon after went into conversation with her Mother, who appeared to be much opposed to the proposed connection. The Father was consulted, Julia cried, the Mother cried, all was confusion, and after Dinner I bade them all farewell and left the House with a positive denial from the Mother."

Next day, however, mature reflection had brought Julia's parents to a more favorable view of the matter.

"Towards Evening Julia's brother arrived at Mr. Butler's and informed me that his Father, Mother and Julia were on their way to New Haven with a view of complying with my proposition, to put her to school, Marry her and take her with me to Buenos Ayres.

"Now I felt that it was too late to recede, and that I was about to enter into an engagement which might prove ruinous to my happiness.

"However, the charms of her I loved presented themselves to my Imagination and dispelled my gloomy fears. I waited on Mr. Wooster and Family at the House of Mr. James Prescott, and indirectly gave them assurances of my satisfaction at their arrival with Julia."

Thereupon Julia was sent to an unidentified school in New Haven for instruction in the management of a well-ordered household and the niceties of social routine. Some weeks later DeForest brought her home, "as innocent and virtuous, as I believed, as when she was carried to New Haven to go to school." That learned man of God, Dr. David Ely of Huntington, joined them in wedlock on October 6, 1811.

Disquieting news from La Plata cast a shadow on DeForest's

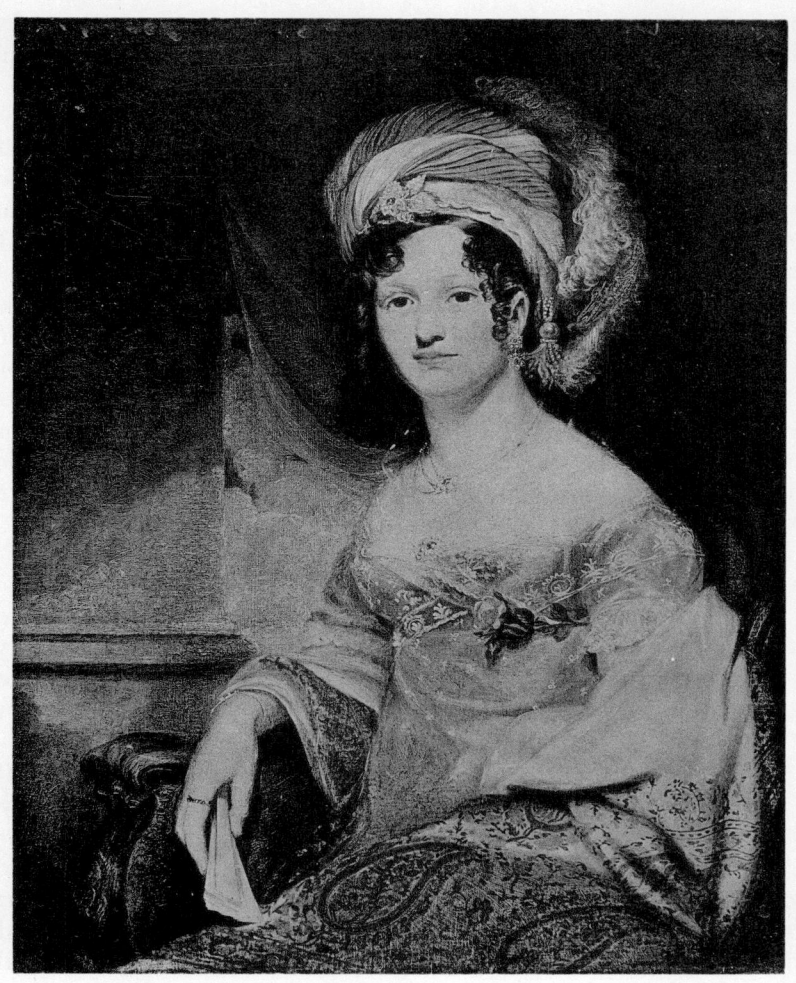

JULIA WOOSTER DeFOREST
From a Portrait by Samuel F. B. Morse.
Courtesy of Yale University Art Gallery.

new-found felicity. A letter from an old friend told of developments that boded ill for the merchant's prospects at Buenos Aires. Discord had early arisen among the creole revolutionaries, with a cleavage into liberal and conservative factions. Cornelio Saavedra, president of the governing *junta*, headed the moderates in the patriot ranks; about Mariano Moreno, fiery secretary of the new government, gathered the enlightened youth who desired sweeping political and social reforms. Admission of conservative provincial deputies into the governing *junta* represented a serious defeat for the fervent secretary and his followers. Moreno resigned and accepted a diplomatic mission to Great Britain, but died on the voyage, March 9, 1811. His passing did not content the friends of Saavedra. On April 5 and 6, 1811, they instigated a tumult in the capital that resulted in the dismissal and banishment from Buenos Aires of Moreno's supporters in the governing *junta*, among them Juan Larrea.

DeForest bore this last stroke of misfortune with philosophic patience. "I have ever considered such a thing possible," he commented, "and of course have in all my letters warned Larrea to return as soon as he could from Governmental affairs. . . . If the banishment of Larrea was necessary or acted as a safeguard to the Revolution, I am glad of it—and should be, even if I had lost one half of my property by it." [28]

A few days later the friend of liberty learned that two agents of the reconstructed *junta* had unobtrusively arrived in the United States in the guise of commercial travelers. They went by the plebeian names of José Cabrera and Pedro López, but these pseudonyms concealed the identity of Diego de Saavedra, son of the president of the *junta*, and the merchant Pedro de Aguirre. They carried instructions to purchase quantities of arms and munitions, pledging the public funds of the new régime for their purchases, and were particularly enjoined not to compromise the government of the United States or any other government. A letter from the *junta* to President Madison revealed the true names and objects of the emissaries, and besought his aid for their enterprise.[29]

28. DeForest to Thomas W. Stansfeld, New Haven, Oct. 22, 1811, DeForest Letterbooks, Vol. 5.
29. The best account of this mission is in S. F. Bemis, *Early Diplomatic Missions from Buenos Aires*, pp. 9–16.

DeForest promptly wrote to these agents, making generous offer of his services.[30] In their reply the commissioners from Buenos Aires evidently alluded to the fate of Juan Larrea, for in his next letter the merchant descanted on the singular virtues of that unlucky statesman. "I have always considered him," observed DeForest, "a man of honor, and a particular friend of that beautiful country. We have often spoken concerning the liberty of men, the governments of the world, and much more concerning the emancipation of Buenos Ayres, and his opinions were so much akin to mine and those of my countrymen in this hemisphere, that he won my heart completely. Notwithstanding my great interest in the fate of Larrea, my friends, I can say to you in all sincerity that if the security and tranquillity of the country were increased by his exile, I am perfectly content with it." [31]

There is no evidence that the patriot agents required or made use of DeForest's proffered aid. Received in most friendly fashion by Secretary of State Monroe in the name of the President, and given every facility to purchase and export arms to Buenos Aires, the only limits upon their procurements were financial ones. They finally sailed for La Plata with a shipment of munitions which they brought safely to the port of Ensenada de Barragán on May 19, 1812. "The liberality with which we have been considered by the government and inhabitants of the United States," they wrote Monroe on the eve of departure, "and their favorable disposition toward the cause we uphold remain graven in our gratitude and respect." [32]

At the beginning of the year 1812, DeForest prepared to depart with his young wife for Buenos Aires. He employed the closing weeks of his stay in North America to good advantage, soliciting business for his commission house. Conditions were propitious, for European blockade systems and our own non-intercourse measures were proving most injurious to American commerce. About this time Stephen Girard of Philadelphia made his entrance into the South American field, sending the *Montesquieu* to Valparaiso and the *Rousseau* to La Plata. The reason he gave for these voyages was "the unpleasant prospect of our European commerce, together with my anxiety to employ my ships as advan-

---

30. DeForest to Pedro López and José Antonio Cabrera, N. Y., Nov. 8, 1811 (in Spanish), DeForest Letterbooks, Vol. 5.
31. Same to same, New Haven, Nov. 24, 1811 (in Spanish), *ibid.*
32. S. F. Bemis, *Early Diplomatic Missions from Buenos Aires,* p. 16.

tageously as possible." [33] Another magnate, John Jacob Astor of New York, ventured into the South American market at this time, perhaps in response to DeForest's solicitations. Astor instructed the commission merchant to purchase for his account four or five thousand dollars' worth of nutria skins at Buenos Aires. DeForest accepted this commission with thanks, but warned the capitalist that if his object was a complete monopoly of the article, "your present order is but illy-calculated to accomplish it." [34] Apparently it was also agreed that in the future DeForest should represent Astor's interests at Buenos Aires.[35]

On February 13, 1812, DeForest, his wife, and his black servant Joseph boarded the ship *Mary*, Captain Edward Garland, bound from New York for Rio de Janeiro. Just seventy days later the mountain-girdled Brazilian capital came into view. There they stayed for several weeks, during which time DeForest satisfied himself that a Spanish squadron maintained a blockade of the River Plate beyond Montevideo. Once before the adventurer had successfully run a blockade of the river, in the days of the British invasions; he resolved to thwart the royalists of Montevideo with equal dexterity. In an ugly little brig, the *Southern Packet*, they sailed for La Plata on May 17. Three weeks later their ship had reached the point where the yellow waters of the great stream merged with those of the Atlantic. At midnight of June 6, 1812, the brig stood off Islas on the southern shore of La Plata. At this appointed spot, under cover of darkness, DeForest and his party took the ship's boat and softly made for shore. They landed about four leagues below Islas and encamped for the night under some willow trees near the bank of the river. In the morning they discovered that a cane swamp more than half a mile wide barred their way to dry land. After passing the entire day in fruitless search of a passage through the bog, they decided to camp another night by the side of the river. At dawn the party began to wade through the marsh, Julia wearing the great coat and boots of the black servant. It was the winter season in these southern latitudes; a two-day frost had covered the swamp with a thick crust that broke under their

---

33. John B. McMaster, *The Life and Times of Stephen Girard, Mariner* (2 vols., Philadelphia, 1918), II, 146.
34. DeForest to Astor, N. Y., Feb. 11, 1812, DeForest Letterbooks, Vol. 5.
35. Kenneth W. Porter, *John Jacob Astor, Business Man* (2 vols., Cambridge, Mass., 1931), II, 650.

tread. The mud and water almost came to Julia's waist. Twice the fatigued and frightened bride, now in the eighth month of her pregnancy, was about to collapse. DeForest and Joseph supported her, and on they went till they finally came to dry ground.

"On our arrival to the hard land," reads the journal, "under the lee of the monte Talas, I stripped my lovely little wife of her wet clothes, wiped her dry, and put her into my Great coat, which I had cautiously preserved dry, wrapped her up and piled on all the things I could find till she began to perspire. I then wiped her dry again, and dressed her from head to foot in flannels which I had purposely brought with me, when she appeared to be as well as ever she was in her life."

Now the weary travelers set out to find a dwelling, and advanced toward the river. Soon they came to a deep, well-nigh impassable marsh, and so had to retrace their steps to the camp hard by the hill of Talas where they had left a great fire.

"I was sick of a fever. Julia began to despair, and the Black Boy looked as though he had lost all his friends. We returned, and much fatigued, sat down in silence near our fire. Julia cried, I doubted of our fate, and all was sadness for 15 or 20 minutes, when the boy astonished us by crying out 'here is a man.' I started up, and beheld a country man on Horseback, surrounded by a Pack of Dogs which had smelt us out, and shewn their Master where we were."

Their deliverer was a *campesino* of the vicinity. Hospitably he offered to assist the bedraggled pilgrims, went home for a cart, and by sundown had brought them to his *rancho*. On the following day they proceeded to the village of Islas, where a friendly curate afforded them lodgings for the night. They reached the port of Ensenada de Barragán on the ninth of June. Loaded into a lumbering cart, the travelers set out on the last lap of their journey to Buenos Aires. Halfway between Ensenada de Barragán and the capital they came to a post house, met a coach "coming on the run," and that evening, safely ensconced in the house of Juan Larrea, rested from the fatigues and perils of their strange homecoming to La Plata.

VIII

"ADOPTED CITIZEN OF BUENOS AYRES"

THE political face of La Plata had greatly altered since DeForest left Buenos Aires for Rio de Janeiro in February, 1810. The ideal of independence which he and Juan Larrea once ardently discussed had become an effective reality. The government of the United Provinces of La Plata yet professed to rule in the name of the captive Ferdinand VII, but this concession was everywhere evaluated at its proper worth. Against the true loyalists of Peru and Montevideo the men of Buenos Aires waged war; against the king's friends in their midst they employed a revolutionary strategy of terror. Already in 1810 the governing *junta*, then dominated by the stern and unbending Mariano Moreno, had sent before a firing squad the former Viceroy Liniers and other Spanish dignitaries implicated in the rising at Córdoba. A few days after DeForest's return, the government discovered and vigorously suppressed the last and most formidable conspiracy against creole rule, planned and directed by the intractable *chapetón* leader, Martín Alzaga. In his journal DeForest noted with satisfaction that "the Robespierre of the America de Sur" was shot in the Great Square "amidst the most unanimous cries of 'Viva la Patria, y muerte a los Traidores.' " Forty others expiated their part in the plot with their lives. Grimly the diarist expressed a hope that this harsh lesson would have a salutary effect on the survivors. "The chastisement they receive will be felt during the lives of those who are on the stage of action." [1]

The wheel of party fortune in Buenos Aires had made a full turn since DeForest learned of the conservative revolution of April 5 and 6, 1811, so ruinous to the interests of his friend Larrea. The military disaster of Huaqui in June of that year, which lost Upper Peru to the revolution, soon provoked widespread discontent with the timid leadership of Cornelio Saavedra and the unwieldy governing *junta*. In September, 1811, popular clamor moved the *junta* to establish a triumvirate of which the

---

1. DeForest Journal, Vol. 8, 1812.

driving force was the youthful but extremely competent Bernardino Rivadavia, in whose father's home DeForest had taken shelter during the difficult days of the British invasions. Between this executive power and the *junta*, now transformed into a legislative chamber (*junta de conservación*), arose a struggle from which the triumvirate emerged victorious; presently it dissolved the *junta*, banished the wretched Saavedra, and assumed dictatorial powers. The ascendancy of Rivadavia betokened a return to the principles of *porteño* centralism and liberalism proclaimed by the martyred Moreno. From exile in the interior the triumvirate recalled Juan Larrea and other lieutenants of the great revolutionary.

The government of Rivadavia accorded a friendly welcome to DeForest. Two months after his arrival, citing the merchant's "distinguished merits, patriotism, and adherence to the liberal system adopted by the peoples," it conferred on him the title of honorary citizen of the United Provinces of the Río de la Plata.[2] Gratified by this official mark of attention, and by numerous calls of old acquaintances who came to pay their respects to the returned exile and his young wife, DeForest expressed belief that it would continue to his "happiness and interest" to stay in Buenos Aires for a few years.

News of the American declaration of war on Britain of June 18, 1812, however, soon nullified these favorable auguries. Already United States trade to La Plata had suffered from unsettled political conditions in Buenos Aires and the forbidding presence of a Spanish squadron in the river.[3] The Anglo-American War of 1812 dealt a mortal blow to this dwindling commerce. British warships patrolled the mouth of the Plate estuary and even seized American vessels within the territorial waters of the United Provinces.[4] English merchants naturally would not consign to an enemy Yankee. Under these conditions, DeForest's business prospects appeared in a dismal light.

His relations with Juan Larrea at this time bore an equally un-

2. *Gaceta de Buenos Aires,* Aug. 22, 1812.
3. Consul Miller described United States commerce to Buenos Aires in the first half of 1812 as very trifling, only seven vessels having arrived during that period. He ascribed this condition to the unsettled state of the country, and asserted that the presence of an American warship in the river would lead to an immediate increase of trade. W. G. Miller to James Monroe, Buenos Aires, July 16, 1812, in W. R. Manning, *Diplomatic Correspondence of the United States,* I, 329.
4. J. R. Poinsett to Monroe, Buenos Aires, June 14, 1812, *ibid.,* I, 336.

satisfactory character. To insistent demands for a settlement of accounts covering the period of DeForest's absence from Buenos Aires, the Catalonian merchant, evidently immersed in political concerns, long gave evasive replies. When, late in 1813, an adjustment was made, the silent partner was dismayed to find that instead of having made money he had lost many thousands of dollars.[5]

With British sea power in effective control of the trade routes to America, DeForest resolved to quit Buenos Aires and commerce for the duration of the war. His *chacra*, conveniently situated seven miles above the capital, offered an ideal site for a rural retirement. With his little family, augmented by the birth of Francisca Tomasa Isabel, born on July 24, 1812, and christened in the great cathedral of Buenos Aires with Doña Tomasa de Larrea as godmother,[6] he departed for the country in September of that year. Under DeForest's direction his Negro slaves soon put the sadly neglected estate in order; flowers, shrubs, and fruit trees bloomed forth. "Having a well chosen little library," he wrote one correspondent, "which engages a considerable share of attention, the days pass by swiftly; and I assure you Sir very pleasantly." [7]

While DeForest reposed on his *chacra* overlooking the broad Plata, "very quietly and stupidly, waiting for a peace and better times," in the debatable mountain province of Upper Peru the patriot troops battled to stem the advance of a royalist army moving southward to an ultimate junction with the Spanish defenders of Montevideo. On September 24, 1812, creole soldiers under General Manuel Belgrano routed the invaders on the plain of Tucumán, and decisively dispelled the danger to the heart of the revolution. DeForest shared the universal sentiment of grati-

---

5. DeForest to James Smith, Buenos Aires, Feb. 8, 1815, DeForest Letterbooks, Vol. 5.

6. It does not appear, however, that any of DeForest's children were reared in the Catholic faith. In a letter written many years later to the director of a Montreal school attended by his son Carlos, DeForest forbade any religious instruction for his son. "You are pleased to intimate," he wrote, "what I feel and have ever professed—viz. to be perfectly liberal on the subject of Religion, and I assure you, my dear Sir, that I would as soon make my Children Catholics, as of any other Christian Persuasion. But I cannot consent, that any one of them should be spoken to respecting Religion till he arrive at years of discretion." DeForest to Monsieur Roque, New Haven, Nov. 13, 1824, DeForest Letterbooks, Vol. 8.

7. DeForest to Gideon Granger, "Plaza de Washington," Jan. 3, 1813, *ibid.*, Vol. 5.

tude and relief. To Belgrano he sent a letter of felicitation and a copy of Washington's Farewell Address. "Although very little," he wrote, "it is worth reading a great many times, and may be a valuable and appropriate model for you, when, after having established the liberties of your Country, you may be disposed to retire from publick affairs and cultivate some beautiful Chacra, in the neighborhood of mine, on the banks of the delightful Plata." [8]

DeForest thus planted a seed of republican propaganda better than he knew. Early in 1813 a Spanish edition of the Farewell Address was published in Buenos Aires. A reverent preface from the pen of Belgrano introduced the North American classic. In this foreword the patriot general related that the Address first came into his hands about 1805; that he had burned it together with all his other papers at the dangerous and hasty battle of Tacuari in Paraguay; and that having received another copy from DeForest, in his eagerness to make known the teachings of Washington among his countrymen he had undertaken to translate it for publication. Belgrano charged the Argentines to read, study, and ponder Washington's words. "Determine to imitate this great man, that we may reach the goal to which we aspire—to constitute ourselves a free and independent nation." [9]

In turbulent Buenos Aires, however, creole politicians were little disposed to heed admonitions against factional strife. Rivadavia's government soon lost support among decisive sections of the people. Clinging jealously to power, it rejected all proposals to broaden the base of the revolution by summoning a representative assembly of the United Provinces. Opposition to the régime centered in the Patriotic Society, a political club on the Gallic model led by the vehement republican Bernardo Monteagudo, inheritor of Moreno's mantle; and in the Lautaro Lodge, a secret revolutionary order founded in Buenos Aires by two newly arrived soldiers come to offer their swords to the cause, Carlos de Alvear and José de San Martín. With the watchwords of independence, constitutional government, and democracy, a revolt spearheaded by the grenadiers of Alvear and San Martín overthrew Rivadavia's tottering régime on October 8, 1812. In its

8. DeForest to Manuel Belgrano, "Plaza de Washington," Dec. 15, 1812, *ibid.*
9. Antonio Zinny, *Bibliografía histórica de las Provincias Unidas del Río de la Plata* (Buenos Aires, 1875), pp. 88–89, relates the circumstances of publication and reprints Belgrano's preface to this pamphlet of thirty-nine pages.

place arose a second triumvirate which proclaimed that the last rights of Ferdinand VII had disappeared and summoned the people to elect delegates to a general constituent assembly.

On his *chacra* DeForest regarded with approval the triumph of the radical wing of the revolutionary party, in whose councils Juan Larrea figured prominently. "Larrea's party," he commented, "is again in power, and appears to have great strength. He of himself has probably more influence than any other Man in the Country; altho he has not any office." [10]

The constituent assembly of the United Provinces of La Plata opened its sessions under hopeful auspices on January 31, 1813. "It is supposed," DeForest had written, "that Independence will be declared; and a Constitution of Government formed on a Plan similar to that of the United States of N. A." [11] The assembly chose to evade these crucial issues, but it suppressed the symbols of royal authority and sanctioned a national anthem that proclaimed the birth of "a new and glorious nation." The congress also enacted a series of important social reforms that reflected the liberal proclivities of its guiding spirits, Alvear and Larrea. The Inquisition, judicial torture, Indian forced labor and tribute, entailment of estates, and titles of nobility were swept away. A memorable law decreed the freedom of all children of slaves born after January 1, 1813. The assembly in conclusion abolished the impractical triumvirate and vested executive power in a supreme director who should rule with the advice of a council of state. They chose Gervasio A. Posadas for this high post, through the intrigues of his nephew Alvear; and in the cabinet of Posadas, Larrea occupied the strategic post of secretary of the treasury. "A rather curious arrangement," observes an Argentine historian. "The management of the public funds was intrusted to a great merchant, a Spaniard to boot, and for many years linked all too closely to all the foreign speculators and merchants of the capital." [12]

It was Larrea, in concert with the Americans William P. White and DeForest,[13] who at the beginning of the year 1814 gave effect

10. DeForest to Thomas W. Stansfeld, "Plaza de Washington," Nov. 21, 1812, DeForest Letterbooks, Vol. 5.
11. DeForest to Gideon Granger, "Plaza de Washington," Jan. 3, 1813, *ibid.*
12. H. Zorraquín Becú, *De aventurero vanqui a consul porteño en los Estados Unidos*, p. 20.
13. C. Roberts, *Las invasiones inglesas*, p. 414, links DeForest with Larrea and White in the creation of the patriot navy, but gives no details. DeForest makes

to a daring plan that changed the face of the Argentine war for independence. At this period the military fortunes of the patriots were at a low ebb. In Upper Peru, General Belgrano was in full retreat after suffering severe defeats at Vilcapugio and Ayohuma. In the Banda Oriental the irrepressible gaucho chieftain Artigas was in open revolt against the authority of Buenos Aires. The siege of Montevideo went ill, for the royalists enjoyed naval supremacy in the river and constantly replenished the fortress with men and supplies. A bold and decisive stroke was necessary to break the ring of Spanish encirclement by land and sea. Larrea's grand design, which won the support of the powerful Carlos de Alvear and of Director Posadas, proposed the creation of a patriot navy which should establish a blockade of Montevideo and thereby compel the capitulation of the royalist stronghold. For this all the elements of a fleet—ships, armaments, crews—had to be assembled in the shortest possible time. As his chief agent in this enterprise of fantastic difficulty Larrea designated an old crony, the American adventurer William P. White, also known to DeForest since the period of the British invasions.

White, aided by DeForest, energetically set about the performance of his assigned tasks. Merchant ships lying idle in the harbor were purchased to make up a naval force mounting 264 cannon. Deserters from English vessels composed the majority of the Argentine crews. A spirited Irish sea captain, William Brown, assumed command of the hastily formed armada. In a series of combats he won undisputed command of the river. The situation of blockaded Montevideo now became hopeless; and in June, 1814, General Vigodet surrendered to a besieging patriot army Spain's last foothold in La Plata.

Great stores of supplies fell to the captors of Montevideo. This booty presented opportunities for private gain that Juan Larrea was quick to apprehend. Mindful of old friends, he offered DeForest a commission for a state auction house in Buenos Aires or, in DeForest's blunt words, "the sales of the possessions plundered at Montevideo by M[r.] L[arrea] who is First Lord of the Treasury and Prime Minister." [14] The merchant quickly ac-

---

no mention of such activity in his letters or journals. The classic history of the Argentine navy is Angel Justiniano Carranza, *Campañas navales de la República Argentina* (4 vols., Buenos Aires, 1914).

14. DeForest to Thomas Wilson, Buenos Aires, Feb. 8, 1815, DeForest Letterbooks, Vol. 5.

cepted this invitation to return to the ways of commerce. In September, 1814, his store, situated next to the municipality, opened its doors. A circular letter to British and American merchants explained his commercial advantages. "I am backed by my intimate friend Larrea, who is secretary of the Treasury, and has already given me a great deal of business in sales of government property." [15]

DeForest's first account book with the Buenos Aires government opened September 21, 1814, and closed April 8, 1815. During this period of six months and fifteen days his sales of state property amounted to $191,704, on which he received 2½ per cent commission. Meantime the Anglo-American War of 1812 had ended, although many months after the Treaty of Ghent, DeForest, styling himself "an adopted citizen of Buenos Aires," complained to the Supreme Director Pueyrredón of British interference with mail coming to American residents of La Plata.[16] In September, 1815, the commission merchant sent his first shipment to the United States since his return to Buenos Aires, a cargo of 2,400 nutria skins consigned to Thomas Tenant of Baltimore with orders to sell immediately on his account.[17] About this time he wrote John Jacob Astor, advising him that nutria skins, though scarce, could be had for $1.75 a dozen, and counseled the New York capitalist to open a trade between Buenos Aires and Calcutta. Three weeks later he offered a $5,000 draft of Astor's to one Broghan, asking him to make the necessary inquiries "about the standing of Mr. Astor." [18] Five out of seven American vessels which had arrived in the river since August, 1815, DeForest boasted in another letter, were consigned to him.[19]

15. Letter dated Dec. 22, 1814, quoted in J. W. De Forest, *The de Forests of Avesnes*, p. 124.
16. "Copy of Memorial presented to his Excellency, the Supreme Director of Buenos Ayres, on the 20th day of September, 1815," in *Niles' Weekly Register* (Baltimore), Jan. 20, 1816.
17. DeForest to John and Benjamin DeForest, Buenos Aires, Sept. 16, 1815, DeForest Letterbooks, Vol. 5.
18. J. W. De Forest, *The de Forests of Avesnes,* p. 129.
19. DeForest to Louis Goddefroy, Buenos Aires, Dec. 28, 1815, abstract of letter in John W. De Forest Papers, Yale University Library. Included is an account of these five vessels, as follows:

William and Charles of Salem, Henry King, master and supercargo, arrived on August 23 with a cargo of quicksilver, gin, codfish, cordage, lumber, etc., valued at $18,000, and sailed for Baltimore on November 18 with 5,000 pesos, 8,000 hides, and other freight.

Schooner *Kemp* of Baltimore, John C. Zimmerman, supercargo, arrived on

An ambitious young creole of Irish ancestry, Patricio Lynch by name, at this time appears in DeForest's counting-room. Their agreement stipulated that Lynch should devote all his "time and attention to the business and interests of the House," turning over to DeForest all the commissions his influence could secure. As junior partner he was to receive a third part of the firm's profits. Presently Patricio's brothers joined him in service. Benito came at nine dollars a month, Manuel at eight, Felix at five dollars a month. This growing force of assistants suggests the mounting proportions of the business. From near and distant lands came wine, indigo, balsam, sugar, tobacco, cochineal, copper and many other articles to rest in the vast and redolent store-rooms. Over these rooms lived DeForest in the ample style of a merchant prince. His household expenses, relates a family historian, amounted to the prodigious sum of $7,000 a year; the table was always set for twenty-four persons.[20] Meantime, keeping pace with waxing prosperity, DeForest's progeny likewise increased. In addition to his first-born, Francisca Tomasa Isabel, there were Carlos María, born September 8, 1813, "a day most glorious in the annals of our family"; Juliana Nicanora, born January 10, 1815; and Jacoba Pastora, born December 30, 1815. All were christened in the great cathedral of Buenos Aires.

At this period, also, Juan Larrea and his party fell on evil days. In January, 1815, the Director Posadas, weary of unprofitable dispute with provincial *caudillos* and insubordinate military, resigned his office. Into his place stepped the youthful and supremely ambitious Carlos de Alvear. For four months he maintained a precarious sway in Buenos Aires. But in the Banda Oriental the gaucho chieftain Artigas ruled contemptuous of Alvear's pretensions, and even took under his protection the

August 29 with a cargo of 500 muskets, gunpowder, cordage, and naval stores valued at $19,000, and sailed for Bordeaux on October 27 with 6,000 hides, etc.

Brig *Expedition* of Baltimore, Captain John Chase, arrived on September 2 with a cargo of 3,000 muskets and other warlike stores valued at $70,000, and sailed on November 9 with 37,000 pesos, 672 bars of copper, 3,200 nutria skins, horse hair, etc.

Brig *Nancy Anne* of Salem, J. B. Osgood, master and supercargo, arrived from Hamburg on December 1 with a cargo of linens, gin, and iron, valued at $36,000, and sailed for Marseilles on January 15 with hides and tallow.

Brig *Favorite* of Boston, Ezra Foster, master and supercargo, ran on shoal near Cape San Antonio on December 17. Came with a cargo of 20,000 Spanish dollars and 100,000 feet of pine boards. "In safety and expected to arrive."

20. J. W. De Forest, *The de Forests of Avesnes*, p. 127.

neighboring provinces of Entre Ríos, Corrientes, and Santa Fé; the army of Upper Peru rejected the new director's authority, proclaiming him suspect and incompetent; and in the distant province of Cuyo, where San Martín was building up and training his army for the fateful campaign of the Andes, Alvear's decrees went unheeded. In April, 1815, national troops dispatched against Artigas mutinied and fraternized with the enemy; in the capital the *cabildo*, long resentful of Alvear's arrogant and headstrong ways, led an uprising against the dictator and proclaimed his downfall. Thus abandoned, Alvear sought safety on an English ship, but his secretary of the treasury did not make good his escape. Thrust into prison and loaded with irons, Larrea had opportunity to meditate on the mutability of power and the vicissitudes of a revolutionary career. Presently the new interim régime of Alvarez Thomas organized a civil commission of justice to sit in judgment on Larrea, among others, charged with misuse of his office for private ends, and also on his colleague William P. White.

Manuel Vicente de Maza, judge of the commission, directed the interrogation of Larrea.[21] What, he inquired at one point in the proceedings, was the motive of public interest that induced Larrea to intrust the sale of state property to the foreigner DeForest, in preference to sons of the country? Lamely the accused explained that DeForest was associated with the creole Patricio Lynch; he, Larrea, had also anticipated certain advantages from this "innovation" (*novedad*). But the prosecutor, unconvinced, on August 18, 1815, listed among other charges against Larrea the sale of government effects with payment of commissions to a foreigner, when the state auction board (*junta de almonedas*) could have done as much with a saving of interest to the necessitous public treasury.

DeForest, meantime, followed the course of the trial from a safe distance. "It is nearly four months," he wrote an English correspondent, "since Mr. Larrea's political fall. He is now in prison, loaded with irons; and when he will be set at liberty is very uncertain. He has several thousand pounds of my money in his hands, which probably I shall never recover." [22]

21. For the trial of Larrea, I have drawn on the account in H. Zorraquín Becú, *De aventurero yanqui a consul porteño en los Estados Unidos,* pp. 22–23.
22. DeForest to Thomas Wilson, Buenos Aires, Aug. 7, 1815, in J. W. De Forest, *The de Forests of Avesnes,* pp. 128–129.

On October 9, 1815, the court passed sentence of exile and confiscation of goods upon Alvear's chief lieutenant. Soon he took ship for Bordeaux in France, assuring DeForest that he had $80,000 there and would repay his debts in full. "I hope it may be so," Larrea's former partner commented doubtfully, "he has not for twelve months paid me a shilling on account." In this manner the Catalonian merchant, in whom political idealism and shrewd practicality were so ambiguously mingled, passed forever out of DeForest's life.

The fall of Alvear had brought no solution for the acute political problems of the distracted country. The United Provinces of the Río de la Plata appeared to be in full process of dissolution. Weak economic ties between the vast regions composing the former viceroyalty, and rural hostility for rich and cultured Buenos Aires, underlay the trend toward disunity. Artigas in the Banda Oriental, Güemes in Salta, lesser potentates in other provinces, under the slogan of "federalism" expressed the suspicion of the rude democracy of the countryside concerning *porteño* designs. For decades this problem, in its constitutional aspect of a balance between the powers of the central government and the provinces, was to engross Argentine political thought and activity.

In a letter written to a friend in New York, an extract from which was published in a leading American newspaper, DeForest gave a sober estimate of the military and political prospects of his adopted country. The patriots had recently fought and disastrously lost the battle of Sipe Sipe in Upper Peru, November 23, 1815. "Our physical force," he affirmed, "as well as our military means, are fully competent to the task of defeating all the attempts of Spain to subjugate the country; but we are unaccustomed to self government, and possess, but very partially indeed, the stubborn virtue and determined patriotism of the North Americans. However, the country must and will be independent, notwithstanding all the follies of its inhabitants, who are rapidly increasing in numbers, and even by their defeats are learning the art of war." [23]

Independence was a crucial issue at the provincial congress of Tucumán, summoned by the provisional government that the *cabildo* of Buenos Aires had established after the fall of Alvear.

---

23. *National Intelligencer* (Washington), May 14, 1816.

As an earnest of its desire to achieve a truly national union and avoid imputations of *porteño* supremacy, the Buenos Aires *junta* had selected a site distant from the capital, and hallowed by Belgrano's great victory of 1812. From all the provinces save the Banda Oriental and the three littoral provinces deputies slowly arrived. Not until March 24, 1816, did the congress begin its sessions. Action on a definitive constitution was again delayed; many members viewed with favor a constitutional monarchy under a European king, but no eligible candidate was immediately available and the scheme was repugnant to the democratic sentiments of the Argentine people. There was general agreement, however, on the desirability of proclaiming the independence that had long been exercised in practice. On July 9, 1816, the congress solemnly declared the United Provinces of South America[24] "a nation free and independent of King Ferdinand VII, of his successors, of the mother country and of any other foreign domination"; and to this end the signers, in obvious imitation of the North American precedent, pledged "the security and guarantee of their lives, their property and their reputation." [25] Possibly some of the members had drawn inspiration from two books that DeForest opportunely advertised in a Buenos Aires newspaper on March 31, 1816, as "worthy of the notice of the people in the present crisis." [26] One contained translations of extracts from Thomas Paine's political writings, under the title, *La independencia de Costa Firme justificada por Thomas Paine treinta años ha;* included in this volume were translations of the Declaration of Independence of July 4, 1776, the Articles of Confederation, the Constitution of the United States, and the constitutions of Connecticut, Massachusetts, New Jersey, Pennsylvania, and Virginia.[27] The translator, a Venezuelan patriot named García de Sena, had written the second book, entitled *Historia concisa de*

---

24. Luis P. Varela, *Historia constitucional de la República Argentina* (4 vols., La Plata, 1910), II, 529 n., affirms that this name was chosen in place of the traditional phrase, "United Provinces of the Río de la Plata," in order to establish a likeness of origins (*paridad de orígenes*) with the United States of North America. Both names, however, were used with little distinction during the revolutionary period.

25. The text of the Declaration (in English translation) may be consulted in F. A. Kirkpatrick, *A History of the Argentine Republic* (Cambridge, Eng., 1931), p. 241.

26. *Gaceta de Buenos Aires,* March 31, 1816.

27. William S. Robertson, *Hispanic-American Relations with the United States* (N. Y., 1923), pp. 70–71.

los Estados Unidos desde el decubrimiento de América hasta el año 1807.[28]

All diplomatic ambiguities cast aside, the Argentine people at last stood forth as a "free and independent nation." A grave danger, however, menaced the infant state. The Bourbon King of Spain, restored to his throne in 1814, had already sent to northern South America a powerful army that soon ended practically all patriot resistance in the provinces of Venezuela and New Granada. A like fate threatened his rebellious subjects of Buenos Aires. It was to ward off the anticipated invasion, by crippling attacks on Spanish convoys and seaborne commerce, that the United Provinces now launched a great privateering campaign with the aid of North American ships, commanders, and crews.

28. A North American visitor to Buenos Aires in 1818 observed that these two books had been read "by nearly all who can read, and have produced a most extravagant admiration of the United States." Henry M. Brackenridge, *Voyage to South America . . . in the Years 1817 and 1818* (2 vols., Baltimore, 1819), II, 214.

IX

"A DASH AT THE DONS"

THREE passengers landed at Annapolis on January 17, 1816, from the brig *Expedition,* Captain John Chase, thirty-three days out of Buenos Aires. They were bound on separate yet not unrelated missions. One was a young and handsome South American patriot, José Miguel Carrera, the most renowned of three brothers of tragic destiny.[1] He came to the United States in search of aid for a liberating expedition to his native Chile, lately reconquered by Spanish arms. In his possession were letters from David C. DeForest, commending "Don José Miguel Carrera, late President of Chile, and now in exile," to the favorable attention of merchants Samuel Carp and John Jacob Astor of New York, Walter and Nixon of Philadelphia, and Robert Oliver and Thomas Tenant of Baltimore.[2]

Captain Marcena Monson was the name of the second passenger; he was the confidential agent of David C. DeForest. Monson came of an old and worthy Connecticut family, and his father dispensed spiritual advice to a flock in the town of Huntington.[3] A letter from DeForest to a merchant of Baltimore introduced Captain Monson as one who for some years past had been employed by a New York firm on "voyages of peculiar

1. Benjamín Vicuña Mackenna, *El ostracismo de los Carreras* (Santiago de Chile, 1857, and later editions), is the classic account of the misfortunes of the Carrera brothers and their tragic end. Miguel Varas Velásquez, *Don José Miguel Carrera en Estados Unidos* (Santiago, 1912), first published in the *Revista chilena de historia y geografía,* 1912, num. 7 y 8, is based on Carrera's diary of his stay in the United States. S. F. Bemis, *Early Diplomatic Missions from Buenos Aires,* pp. 30–33, utilizes fresh archival sources as well as published materials in his summary of Carrera's mission.

2. These letters were all dated November 7, 1815. DeForest's letterbook for the period of his major privateering activity is now missing, but I have been able to use a set of transcripts and abstracts drawn off from this letterbook by Col. George Butler Griffin (the son of one of DeForest's daughters) for the use of J. W. De Forest when he was preparing a family history. These notes, which form part of the J. W. De Forest Papers in the Yale University Library, will hereafter be cited as the G. B. Griffin Notes.

3. Myron A. Munson, *The Munson Record* (2 vols., New Haven, 1896), I, 170–171.

delicacy and confidence." [4] Now he was bound for Baltimore, there to negotiate most secretly for the outfitting of privateers to cruise against Spanish commerce under the flag of Buenos Aires. Captain Monson himself, it had been agreed, was to assume command of one of these vessels.

The third emissary was also a seafaring man. Captain Thomas Taylor hailed from the town of Wilmington in Delaware, but in recent years he had been active in the naval service of the United Provinces of La Plata. He, too, was bound for Baltimore in order to "initiate and encourage (*entablar y propagar*) privateering enterprise against the vassals of the King of Spain," [5] and to this end he brought six blank patents for disposal among interested merchants. Taylor had sailed in the *Expedition* by a very scanty margin, for the brig was two days out of the port of Buenos Aires and about to leave the river when he clambered aboard after a hot pursuit along the shore. The observant Carrera, noting the discomfiture of Captains Chase and Monson, confided to his diary that they were put out because they had agreed with David C. DeForest to sail for the United States without Taylor. Behind this intrigue, he surmised, was the interesting circumstance that everyone concerned had privateering patents to dispose of in the United States: Taylor had six, DeForest four, Monson one, Chase one. [6]

With unerring judgment, the voyagers from Buenos Aires had selected Baltimore as the base for their warlike operations against Spain. During the late conflict with Britain this town had gained

4. DeForest to Robert Oliver, Buenos Aires, n. d., G. B. Griffin Notes.
5. Thomas Taylor to the Supreme Director Pueyrredón, Buenos Aires, Feb. 19, 1818, Archivo General de la Nación (Buenos Aires), S[ala] 1, A[rmario] 2, A[naquel] 4, núm[ero] 3. Charles C. Griffin, "Privateering from Baltimore during the Spanish-American Wars of Independence," *Maryland Historical Magazine* (March, 1940), XXXV, 1–25, is an intensive study of the Baltimore end of the Buenos Aires-Baltimore privateering axis, based on United States court records. Two valuable works on the corsairs of Buenos Aires are Lewis W. Bealer, *Los corsarios de Buenos Aires* (Buenos Aires, 1937); and Theodore S. Currier, *Los corsarios del Río de la Plata* (Buenos Aires, 1929). T. S. Currier, *Los cruceros del "General San Martin"* (Buenos Aires, 1944), a case study in privateering based on United States court records, appeared after most of the work on this book had been completed.
6. Carrera's Diary, Nov. 11, 1815, quoted in Miguel Varas Velásquez, *Don José Miguel Carrera en Estados Unidos* (Santiago de Chile, 1912), p. 15. Carrera's rather vague wording is that Chase and Monson, "de acuerdo con Deforest [*sic*], habian violentado el viaje por llegar sin Taylor a los Estados Unidos."

fame through the exploits of its many privateers. Here resourceful shipbuilders had developed a type of craft ideally suited for such ventures, the Baltimore clipper, fast and rakish, designed for speed and ability to sail close to the wind. Fortunes had been made in those years of Baltimore's privateering glory. Then came peace, and, after a brief flurry of activity in the carrying trade to Europe, a great quiet and sadness descended upon the once roistering town. The swift ships were laid up; their crews, prize money spent, lounged about the docks; and even well-to-do merchants and shipowners felt the pinch of hard times. Upon this sorry scene now entered the agents from Chile and Buenos Aires, bringing promise of employment for idle capital, ships, and crews.

Presently Baltimore felt the stimulating touch of their demand. In December, 1816, after a long siege of failure, José Miguel Carrera sailed away with three ships and a motley band of adventurers, guaranteeing payment by the still inexistent government of Chile to the trusting outfitters, Darcy and Didier. Meantime Captains Monson and Taylor had prevailed upon various merchants to arm and send to sea a number of privateers. Among the first to put out were the *Romp* and the *Orb*, both veterans of the Anglo-American War of 1812. Lest federal authorities interfere in these ventures on the ragged edge of legality, the corsairs cleared as merchantmen with crews of normal size and took on the rest of their complements after leaving port. Once at sea they discarded their prosaic names in favor of the more sonorous *Santafecino* and *Congreso*, hoisted the sky-blue-and-white ensign of Buenos Aires to the mizzen top, fired a salute under the flag amid the cheers of the crew, and set off in search of Spanish prey.

These were the beginnings of a spectacular chapter in the history of North American participation in the winning of Argentine independence. For a space of several years thousands of Americans carried on hostilities against Spanish commerce in privateers built in American shipyards and owned by American citizens. Of this unneutral activity Baltimore was the center, and she gloried in her depravity. When a bill designed to strengthen the neutrality law was introduced into Congress, John Randolph, with his usual acrid wit, called it a bill to make peace between the town of Baltimore and Spain. "We have been informed," exulted a Buenos Aires newspaper, "that the people of Baltimore are the greatest enthusiasts in the United States for the cause of our liberty. Its merchants have reduced Spanish commerce to an unhappy state." [7] Matters came to such a pass that a respectable merchant could not procure a crew for his ship waiting to proceed on a legal voyage: "The universal reply was, *he must wait until another Privateer arrived;* for that every one now in port had shipped on board some one of these cruizers; and the consequence is, our honest merchants are obliged to send to Philadelphia, (where pirates and privateersmen do not meet similar encouragement and facilities,) in order to procure seamen to enable them to send their vessels abroad." [8]

To the American Government, engaged in difficult negotiations with Spain over the Florida question; and above all to Secretary of State John Quincy Adams, who had the onerous task of replying to the well documented charges of the Spanish minister concerning the outfitting of insurgent privateers within the United States, in violation of the Treaty of 1795 between Spain and the United States and the neutrality laws of the United States itself,[9] the privateering issue was a constant source of annoyance and embarrassment. The small force of revenue cutters available for police duties was quite inadequate to patrol the extensive territorial waters of the United States. In the Chesapeake Bay area, the principal seat of outfitting activity, the interest of some public officials in the industry, the tolerance of many citizens for a practice by which numbers of their townsmen gained a living, and the sympathy of others for the insurgent cause, gave rise to few arrests and fewer convictions. Indeed, a letter to a Baltimore newspaper gave notice that "any judge who should presume to condemn the privateersmen under South American colors could not expect to live long, either as a judge or as a man." [10]

Since privateering was at best a business in the twilight zone of legality, extreme precautions were taken to conceal the identity of the solid citizens of Baltimore and other seaboard cities who owned shares in the South American corsairs. Nominal ownership of these craft was vested in the outfitters (*armadores*) of

7. *El Censor,* March 20, 1817, quoted in L. W. Bealer, *Los Corsarios de Buenos Aires,* pp. 36–37.
8. Baltimore *Federal Republican,* in Washington *National Intelligencer,* Dec. 18, 1819.
9. For this legislation, see C. G. Fenwick, *The Neutrality Laws of the United States* (Washington, 1913).
10. Quoted in John Quincy Adams, *Memoirs* (12 vols., Philadelphia, 1874-1877), IV, 186.

Buenos Aires, in the case of vessels sailing under that flag. These men, natives or naturalized citizens of Buenos Aires, secured privateering patents from the patriot government; answered for the good conduct of the corsairs named in these licenses; disposed of prizes when brought to the home port; and generally watched over the interests of the true owners. David C. DeForest, we shall show, was the most active and successful of these agents. Other leading *armadores* were the two Aguirres, Manuel Hermenegildo and Juan Pedro; and a number of Americans, among them Thomas Taylor, William G. Ford, and John Higginbotham.[11] A commission of 10 per cent of the net proceeds of prizes appears to have been the customary share of the Buenos Aires outfitter.[12]

Baltimore rather than Buenos Aires was the fountainhead of that "system of pillage and aggression . . . against the vessels and property of the Spanish nation" of which the Spanish minister to the United States, Luis de Onís, ceaselessly complained.[13] Onís justly charged that "formal companies" had been established in Baltimore to finance privateering operations.[14] The principal syndicate in Baltimore was known as the "American Concern."[15] The typical practice seems to have been for a number of merchants to purchase one or more shares in a privateer. In the case of the Buenos Aires corsair *Tucumán*, DeForest speaks of her "numerous owners."[16] It was admitted on all sides that the firm of Darcy and Didier of Baltimore, whose Buenos Aires representative was DeForest, had the largest single interest in the privateering industry.[17] The customary share of owners, to judge

11. For the privateering patents issued by the government of Buenos Aires during the War for Independence, the authoritative source is *Las presas marítimas en la República Argentina, primera parte, 1810–1830*, in *Estudios editados por la facultad de derecho y ciencias de la Universidad de Buenos Aires*, no. XIII, Buenos Aires, 1927.

12. DeForest to Juan Pedro de Aguirre, Georgetown, Md., Dec. 19, 1818, DeForest Letterbooks, Vol. 6.

13. Onís to J. Q. Adams, Washington, Nov. 16, 1818, in W. R. Manning, *Diplomatic Correspondence*, III, 198.

14. Luis de Onís, *Memoria sobre las negociaciones entre España y los Estados Unidos* . . . (Mexico City, 1826), p. 70.

15. C. C. Griffin, "Privateering from Baltimore," p. 5.

16. DeForest to Lynch and Zimmerman, New Haven, Oct. 14, 1819, DeForest Letterbooks, Vol. 6.

17. Manuel Aguirre to the Supreme Director Pueyrredón, Washington, Aug. 30, 1817 (copy), Archivo General de la Nación (Buenos Aires), S.1 A.2–A.4, no. 9; A. J. Carranza, *Campañas navales*, III, 90 n.

from entries in DeForest's ledgers, was one-half of the proceeds from the sale of prizes.

A murky atmosphere of secrecy, suspicion, and thinly disguised anxiety emerges from such of DeForest's privateering correspondence as has come down to us. Principals in Baltimore complain of the excessive charges of the Buenos Aires *armadores;* these agents in turn darkly hint at misuse of patents in the United States; fear is expressed that aggrieved parties will resort to the courts and bring to light matters that were better hidden.[18] The use of fictitious names (DeForest thus becomes Don Carlos Cortez de Güemes in certain privateering connections),[19] the guarded and reticent language, the sudden disappearance of famous corsairs which presently turn up at lonely *rendezvous* to undergo change of name, patent, and captain, for no clearly apparent reason—these and like circumstances contribute to the prevailing mood of mystery and to the difficulties of the student who would unravel the tangled skein of privateering affairs.

Along the trade routes of the Pacific, in West Indian waters, and off the very shores of Spain, the corsairs of Buenos Aires hunted down their Spanish quarry with prodigious success. It has been estimated that "the damage relative to the total tonnage of Spanish merchant ships must have been much greater than that done by the *Alabama* and other Confederate cruisers to United States shipping."[20] The Spanish minister to the United States, suggesting a plan for the annihilation of these scourges of the sea, indicated an involuntary respect for their prowess. He proposed that Spanish armed ships should cruise in squadrons of six or eight, attacking individual corsairs and avoiding all combats in which they did not enjoy a decisive superiority. What a disgrace, fretted the excitable minister, that a band of wretched pirates in a miserable schooner should dare proclaim a blockade of all the ports of Cuba and make a jest of our navy![21]

The very effectiveness of the patriot privateers contributed largely to their eventual downfall. Once Spanish shipping had been swept from the seas, less scrupulous elements, made desperate by

---

18. Much illustrative material is contained in letters from DeForest to Darcy and Didier, Juan Pedro de Aguirre, John Higginbotham, and others, in the DeForest Letterbooks, Vol. 6.

19. J. W. De Forest, *The de Forests of Avesnes*, p. 133.

20. C. C. Griffin, "Privateering from Baltimore," p. 10.

21. Luis de Onís to Irujo, Washington, Dec. 24, 1818, Archivo Histórico Nacional (Madrid), Estado, Legajo 5643 (L. C. photocopies).

the dearth of prizes, began to attack flags of all nations. Spreading political disintegration in the United Provinces of the Río de la Plata, moving toward the anarchy of the "Year XX," made difficult any strict control over vessels flying the Buenos Aires ensign. In this last degenerate period of privateering activity, the patents issued by the shadowy government of Artigas in the Banda Oriental, at war with Portugal as well as with Spain, became increasingly popular among prize-starved corsairs. Some of the more predatory brethren of the privateering fraternity turned to slave-dealing. Lying in wait in the waters about the Dutch island of St. Eustatius, Danish St. Thomas, or Swedish St. Bartholomew, they fell upon slavers come from Africa, murdered or otherwise disposed of their crews, and sold their human cargoes in "legal" fashion to planters of nearby islands. The United States consul at St. Bartholomew grew vehement in reporting the outrages perpetrated under patriot colors. "Without exaggerating," he asserted, there were "not less than fifteen hundred men" aboard the privateers cruising in these waters, "chiefly *Citizens* of the *United States* one half of which at least, are concern'd in slave dealing, and I may very justly add, that not one of them but considers a *Guinea Man* a very profitable Prize!" [22]

By the year 1819 the privateering industry had come to display all the characteristics of piracy. Horrifying tales of pillage, murder, and mutiny reached the United States, turning the once favorable opinion of patriot corsairs into hostility. An influential Washington newspaper rejoiced that it was no longer fashionable to confound privateering and patriotism, and that even in Baltimore agents could no longer be found to transact any kind of privateering business.[23] Some months later, the same journal had to deplore that there were still seven or eight privateers in Baltimore harbor, and "*encouragement* enough left for them to be fitted out." [24]

The irresponsible and piratical conduct of many privateers cruising under the flags of Buenos Aires and Venezuela moved the United States to make vigorous representations to these governments. Commodore Oliver H. Perry, dispatched on a mission

---

22. Robert Monroe Harrison to J. Q. Adams, St. Bartholomew, Dec. 1, 1820, National Archives (Washington), Department of State, Consular Letters, St. Bartholomew.
23. *National Intelligencer*, July 3, 1819.
24. *Ibid.*, Dec. 4, 1819.

to South America, was instructed to inform the Supreme Director Pueyrredón at Buenos Aires that "many of the privateers commissioned by the South American Governments have become common nuisances to the peaceful commerce of all Nations. That we have seen proclamations from Pueyrredon at Buenos Ayres and from General Arismendi at Margarita themselves declaring some of such Vessels Pirates. That of others the Crews have revolted and murdered or turned on shore their Captains; attacked, plundered and ravaged defenceless islands, robbed indiscriminately every vessel that came within their power; seduced the crews of some, to join them in their depredations, suborned others to make false declarations of property; to alter and disguise the marks upon bales or cases of Merchandise—transshipped whole cargoes, and stranded captured Vessels to escape the detection of their guilt, or evade the redeeming process of the law. . . . That ministers of friendly nations have complained and it was impossible to regard this state of things without effort for effectual interposition." [25]

Perry did not live to lay this formidable catalogue of complaints before Pueyrredón, but his instructions accompanied John M. Forbes when that veteran diplomat departed to take up the post of consul in Buenos Aires. Forbes succeeded where others had failed; on October 6, 1821, largely through his influence, the government of Bernardino Rivadavia abolished privateering under the flag of Buenos Aires. For some years longer, however, pirates thinly disguised as patriot privateers continued to roam the Spanish Main, waging impartial war against the commerce of all nations.

We cannot state with certainty when or how DeForest first became interested in privateering enterprise. Perhaps the successful pioneering cruise of Captain Thomas Taylor in the *Zephyr*, made in the summer of 1815,[26] stimulated his imagination, ever susceptible to projects that combined the elements of hazard and a high rate of profit. About this time a group of foreigners resi-

25. J. Q. Adams to Smith Thompson, Washington, May 23, 1819, National Archives (Washington), Department of State, Domestic Letters, Vol. 17. Extracts from this letter have been printed in W. R. Manning, *Diplomatic Correspondence*, I, 101–102.

26. L. W. Bealer, *Los corsarios de Buenos Aires*, p. 20.

dent in Buenos Aires petitioned the supreme director for permission to outfit privateers to cruise against Spain,[27] and DeForest may have been of their number. At any rate, it is certain that he was one of the first to conceive and act upon the happy notion of "making a fortune by a dash at the Dons."[28] In this endeavor he was notably successful. No less a figure than John Quincy Adams testified, though in a censorious spirit, that DeForest was "among the persons most deeply and extensively concerned in the privateers commissioned by that [Buenos Aires] Government."[29]

Under date of September 20, 1815, the merchant drafted a letter, copies of which were to go to John Jacob Astor of New York, George Crowninshield of Salem, Thomas Tenant and the firm of Darcy and Didier, both of Baltimore. He proposed to these magnates that they should outfit corsairs to cruise against Spanish commerce under the flag of Buenos Aires. "I lend my name to these privateers," he wrote, "and shall expect my reward in a commission of 10% on sales of prizes, holding myself to remit net proceeds as real owners may direct, and under all circumstances will protect and defend to the utmost the interests of the privateers, officers and men. To cover you from any censure by our govt. or prosecution from any irritated subject of his Catholic Majesty, I enclose to you a formal order to purchase for my account, arm and equip a ship or vessel and in my name to send her to sea with orders to capture such Spanish ships as she may meet and send them here for condemnation. Blanks in the commission you will please fill up according to circumstances."[30]

Under this arrangement, Thomas Tenant was to outfit a privateer to be called the *Potosí;* John Jacob Astor, the *Criollo de Buenos Aires;* Darcy and Didier, the *Congreso;* George Crowninshield, the *Tucumán.* Two days later, however, there was a change of plan; DeForest now wrote Tenant that he had decided to send all four commissions to the Baltimore merchant. Tenant and his friend Didier were to keep the whole secret to themselves if they wished to outfit all four vessels; if not they should take their com-

---

27. *Ibid.,* p. 15.
28. DeForest to Thomas Reilly, Buenos Aires, Nov. 9, 1815, G. B. Griffin Notes.
29. J. Q. Adams to Smith Thompson, Washington, May 23, 1819, cited above, note 25.
30. G. B. Griffin Notes.

missions first and send the others to Astor and Crowninshield, respectively.[31] These documents DeForest sent to Baltimore by the *Dorothea*, Captain Adams, sailing October 5, 1815. Presumably they were of an unauthorized, makeshift character, for not until October 23 did the promoter secure from the patriot government patents for the four privateers named above and two others: the *Mangoré* and the *Tupac-Amarú*.[32] These six licenses went to the United States on November 9, 1815, in the *Expedition*, owned by Darcy and Didier of Baltimore. Captain Marcena Monson, it will be recalled, also sailed on this ship, intrusted by DeForest with the management of his privateering interests in the United States.

In a letter to the owners of the *Expedition*, DeForest observed that the government of the United Provinces had granted only two other general privateering commissions, one to the *True Blooded Yankee*,[33] the other to Captain Thomas Taylor's ship, the *Zephyr* or *Céfiro*, since lost at sea. He acknowledged that privateering patents had been given to a number of vessels gone to cruise in the Pacific, but they were strictly forbidden to operate elsewhere.[34] He had not been able to prevail on the government to grant him more than six licenses, ruefully admitted the merchant, but these were "sufficient to make business for any one house." [35]

At this time DeForest also made contracts with "the most Excellent the Director of the State," Ignacio Álvarez Thomas, which governed the mode of disposal of prizes and other routine matters. The privateers were to send their captures for Buenos Aires, together with the papers necessary for condemnation proceedings, but in the event of a blockade of the river they could proceed to the Patagonian port of Río Negro, dispatching the required documents overland to the capital. Prize cargoes would be free from custom-house duties, paying the government only 15

---

31. DeForest to Thomas Tenant, Buenos Aires, Sept. 22, 1815, G. B. Griffin Notes.

32. *Las presas marítimas*, p. 204.

33. Otherwise known as the *Invencible*, Captain David Jewett, which departed on her first cruise in July, 1815, with a patent issued on June 23, 1815. A. J. Carranza, *Campañas navales*, III, 216–221.

34. This presumably refers to the famous expedition of Brown and Bouchard to the Pacific in 1815–1816. Ricardo Caillet-Bois has described this expedition in *Nuestros corsarios*, I, *Brown y Bouchard en el Pacífico, 1815–1816* (Buenos Aires, 1930). There is a convenient account in L. W. Bealer, *Los corsarios de Buenos Aires*, pp. 105–122.

35. DeForest to Darcy and Didier, Buenos Aires, Oct. 30, 1815, G. B. Griffin Notes.

per cent of the auction sales, and the captured vessels, their armament, tackle, and apparel were to pay no duty whatever. The government, however, claimed a preferential right of purchase of these articles, "at fair prices." Privateering patents were valid for one year from the time of leaving port, but could be prolonged if deemed convenient by new and special commissions.[36]

Meantime official instructions were being prepared for the guidance of DeForest's commanders. Article 1 of the instructions to the captain of the *Mangoré* permitted him to "commit hostilities against, capture, or burn" every Spanish vessel, unless there be on board "some person of rank, sent by the Spanish Government in a public character toward that of the United Provinces; in which case you will allow him to proceed on his voyage unmolested." Article 2 warned the corsair to respect Spanish goods not contraband of war, found under neutral flags, "as a convincing proof of the desire of the Government, to preserve friendship and good Harmony with powers in amity and with neutrals." Article 5 reflected the persistent patriot fears of a Spanish military expedition against Buenos Aires. Should the captain learn that such a force was *en route* to the shores of La Plata, his chief care must be to cut off transports, following the route of the enemy "with a view to capture, burn and destroy as many vessels of the Spanish convoy as possible—this service to be considered the most important that can be rendered to the American cause." Article 7 declared that vessels under the Spanish flag trading between the ports of Brazil and La Plata must not be molested, "from political considerations which the Government reserves to itself." Article 9 instructed the commander to obtain, while cruising in the Pacific, "every information you can . . . of the number of regular troops at Lima; those detached throughout the kingdom of Chile; those sent by the Viceroy Abascal to the succour of the army oppressing Peru; the general opinion in Lima concerning the present state of the Peninsula; the opinion of those people of the cause of the United Provinces; of the persons of respectability and character they consider attached to the cause of liberty; the parties of Patriots still existing in Chile.' All these declarations you will insert in your journal." Article 10

---

36. "Contract . . . for the arming in North America of two Privateers under the flag of the United Provinces to cruise against the Spanish Nation. The said vessels to be named the Tupac-Amaru and the Mangore." Jonathan Meredith Papers, Manuscripts Division, Library of Congress.

struck a humanitarian note. "Should you go near the islands of St. Felix and Juan Fernández, you will make signals, so that the colours of the State to which the Privateer belongs may be known: and in case there should be any Patriots exiled there for being such; you will receive them on board if they can effect their escape and forward them to this place by first opportunity." [37]

Instructions of this tenor were issued to the commander of each privateer, together with the vessel's patent, a copy of the privateering ordinance of 1801,[38] a set of officers' commissions, and a covering letter from DeForest. "As a citizen of B[uenos] A[ires]," he wrote Captains Marcena Monson and John Chase of the *Tupac-Amarú* and *Mangoré*, respectively, "I lend my name to the owner of this privateer and take upon myself all responsibility attaching to this situation. You will, therefore, be at all times on your guard as to rendering me liable to vexatious law suits, and have nothing to do with a prize of doubtful character or one that is not of considerable value." [39]

Thus instructed, and fortified with documents that attested the unimpeachable legality of their proceedings, DeForest's captains were ready to take command of the cruisers that one by one cleared from the port of Baltimore, presently to hoist the flag of Buenos Aires, mount the armament that had been stowed in the hold, and make for the Caribbean and other fields of privateering activity. Among the most celebrated of these corsairs were the *Congreso*, the *Potosí*, the *Tucumán*, the *Tupac-Amarú*, and the *Mangoré*.

Captain Joseph Almeida of the *Congreso*, the former *Orb* of Baltimore, was "a rough, open-looking, jovial jack tar," according to John Quincy Adams who met him in 1819, "who can neither write nor read." [40] No mercenary spirit, by his own account, but a sacred thirst for vengeance inspired this native of the Azores and veteran of the Anglo-American War of 1812 to take up arms against Spain. Attempting to run the blockade into patriot Car-

---

37. "Secret Instructions given by the Government of the United Provinces, to the Commander Mr. ——— for the cruize of the ——— named Mangore." Jonathan Meredith Papers, Manuscripts Division, Library of Congress.

38. Until November 16, 1816, when a formal privateering code was promulgated, the United Provinces used the Spanish privateering code of 1801. L. W. Bealer, *Los corsarios de Buenos Aires*, pp. 19–23.

39. DeForest to Marcena Monson and John Chase, Buenos Aires, Oct. 30, 1815, G. B. Griffin Notes.

40. J. Q. Adams, *Memoirs*, IV, 377–378.

tagena in 1815, Almeida had been captured by the Spaniards and thrust into General Morillo's singularly unpleasant dungeons, where he languished until released early in 1816. Swearing to revenge himself upon his jailors, Almeida departed for Baltimore and there assumed command of the *Orb*, outfitted for privateering service under a patent granted to DeForest. The corsair cleared from Baltimore in the guise of a merchantman on May 16, 1816. Thirteen days later she hoisted the flag of Buenos Aires, took the name *Congreso*, and like an avenging fury swept down on the commerce of Spain both in the West Indies and in peninsular waters. No less than six prizes of sufficient value to be sent for condemnation fell to her commander on this first cruise. When the *Congreso* came to anchor at Buenos Aires in October, 1816, her patent was about to expire, whereupon Captain Almeida purchased the vessel at public auction and secured a patent in his own name.[41] One suspects that this change of ownership was fictitious, but the reasons for the manipulation are not apparent. The *Congreso* arrived at Baltimore from a second successful cruise in the West Indies on April 2, 1817. She vanishes from sight after that date; but it appears that under the names of *Tyger* and *Pueyrredón*, with Captain John Daniels in command, this notable corsair continued to sail the seas as late as 1819.[42]

Captain Almeida not only settled some old scores with his first cruise, but enriched himself and the owners of the *Congreso*. He got a 5 per cent commission on the sale of cargoes, twelve shares of prize money as captain at 465 pesos each, and the one and one-half shares of "York Davy his Black Boy," the whole amounting to 19,506 pesos.[43] The true owners in North America received 79,744 pesos. DeForest is credited with thirty and one-half shares of prize money, amounting to 14,184 pesos. Each common sailor got a wage of one peso a day and one share of prize money. Privateersmen, however, sometimes never saw the full amount of their shares; a long time frequently elapsed before captured cargoes were realized and the proceeds distributed, and impatient

41. A. J. Carranza, *Campañas navales*, III, 84–85.
42. See the list of privateers, under *Orb,* in C. C. Griffin, "Privateering from Baltimore," p. 9.
43. All privateering figures are taken (except when other sources are indicated) from the DeForest Ledger, no. 2, where they are embedded in a number of individual accounts. They are given in Spanish pesos or silver dollars. I have omitted fractions of the dollar. Presumably Spanish and American silver dollars were roughly equivalent in value.

or needy sailors occasionally disposed of their prize tickets at a loss. Thus George Cochrane sells his share worth 465 pesos to DeForest for 375 pesos; and prizemaster William Frisby of the *Leona* similarly disposes of his eight shares for 3,200 pesos.

Brief yet spectacular was the career of the *Potosí*, the former *Spartan* of Baltimore. Her commander was Captain John Chase, late of the *Expedition*. The privateer sailed out on her first and only cruise early in 1816. Cruising in front of Cadiz, she fell in with the Spanish armed merchantman *Ciencia*. The Spaniard offered fierce resistance; but was soon humbled and forced to strike his colors. Chase transferred part of the cargo and treasure to the amount of some $20,000 to his ship, sent the prize to Port-au-Prince for condemnation,[44] and incontinently departed for the Chesapeake with his loot. Spain's minions in Baltimore exerted themselves to track down these privateering spoils. The Spanish minister Onís inveighed against the piratical activities of Chase and the complacence of Baltimore customs officers, affirming that in the hands of Henry Didier were more than $20,000 taken from the *Ciencia*.[45] Despite the ministerial fulminations, Chase continued to reside in calm and security at Norfolk, where Spanish agents discovered him enjoying the fruits of his depredations.[46] The great hue and cry raised by Onís, however, was decidedly embarrassing, and the owners of the *Potosí* evidently judged it convenient for the corsair and her captain to drop out of sight, in a manner about to be related.

From a privateering letter of DeForest's, we learn that the value of the captures of the *Potosí* amounted to 81,552 pesos. DeForest acknowledges receipt of 4,077 pesos, perhaps only partial payment of his commission. To General William H. Winder of Baltimore and three other attorneys, he paid 500 pesos for unspecified legal services.[47]

In June, 1817, the *Potosí* sailed out of New Orleans port. In the tranquil waters of the Gulf she came to anchor, and a strange little ceremony was enacted on board. Captain John Chase yielded

---

44. The stipulation in the privateering code of 1816 that required prizes to be sent to Buenos Aires for condemnation was frequently violated on one pretext or other. L. W. Bealer, *Los corsarios de Buenos Aires*, p. 25.

45. Luis de Onís to James Monroe, Washington, Feb. 12, 1817, W. R. Manning, *Diplomatic Correspondence*, III, 1918–1919.

46. Onís to Monroe, Washington, March 11, 1817, *ibid.*, p. 1921.

47. DeForest to Patricio Lynch, New Haven, May 11, 1819, DeForest Letterbooks, Vol. 6.

up his command to Captain George Wilson; the *Potosí* simultaneously became the *Tucumán*.⁴⁸ These formalities completed, the corsair set off to cruise in the Caribbean, then to the Bay of Cadiz, laying effective blockade to that Spanish port. An aggressive and experienced sea fighter, Captain Wilson yet had in his character a touch of idealism and a flair for dramatic expression. From his anchorage in front of Tenerife, he reported to the Buenos Aires ministry of war that he had taken twenty-four Spanish ships, of which he sent four to Buenos Aires, burned four, and returned the others to their owners. "The reason for abandoning these craft was that for the most part they belonged to very poor men: such men as would doubtless shake off the yoke of the imbecile government of Spain, if they but could." ⁴⁹

The *Tucumán* came to anchor at Buenos Aires on December 3, 1817. There is no record of the value of her captures. At this time, William P. Ford, an American who was a naturalized citizen of the United Provinces and had an obscure association with DeForest, purchased the *Tucumán* at public auction together with the unexpired term of her commission.⁵⁰ Clearly this negotiation was linked with the impending departure of DeForest for the United States, and the consequent necessity of finding a new *armador* to pose as the privateer's owner and receive her captures.

The *Tucumán* sailed from Buenos Aires, bound for a cruise in the Bay of Cadiz, on March 6, 1818. Her patent running out on the passage, she took the name *Julia DeForest* on the strength of a commission that Ford had secured on January 10, 1818. Under this winsome appellation, the corsair operated with considerable success in Spanish and West Indian waters. In June, 1819, Captain Wilson brought his ship into the island of Margarita, a favorite *rendezvous* of the privateering brotherhood. Her commission having expired, Captain Joseph Almeida now came forward to purchase the vessel and outfit her for service under the flag of Venezuela and the name *Almeida*, Wilson con-

---

48. For the successive incarnations and movements of the *Potosí*, I have relied principally on an unsigned and undated relation (perhaps a deposition) in the Jonathan Meredith Papers, Manuscripts Division, Library of Congress.

49. A. J. Carranza, *Campañas navales*, III, 235.

50. The patent of the *Tucumán* had been issued to DeForest on October 23, 1815, but remained deposited with the Buenos Aires secretary of war until January 10, 1818, when it was granted to the outfitter for one year, made retroactive to June 3, 1817, the date of the sailing of the *Tucumán* (late *Potosí*) from New Orleans. *Ibid.*, III, 234–235.

tinuing as commander. In August, 1819, the privateer cleared from Margarita on a cruise and in early October fell in with a Spanish armed packet; in the ensuing action Captain Wilson suffered wounds and the corsair's sails and rigging were badly shattered. Shortly after this the *Almeida* limped into the Chesapeake for repairs. Here the manuscript relation on which this account is mainly based abruptly ends; but from another source we gather that as late as December, 1820, Captain Wilson, having recovered from his wounds, operated in West Indian waters in command of the *Bolívar* (presumably the former *Almeida*), a privateer of ten guns and one hundred men.[51] Whether any genuine transfers of ownership accompanied these changes of identity of the old *Spartan* or *Potosí*, it is not possible to determine.

One masterful stroke brought Captain Marcena Monson of the *Tupac-Amarú* such success as this adventurous son of Connecticut had not dreamed of. He took his ship, the former *Regent* of Baltimore, to sea at the end of December, 1816. Twenty-three days later, off Cape Verde, a Spanish sail came in sight. She was the *Triton*, a fine new ship of the Philippine Company, bound for Spain with a precious freight of silks and other Eastern merchandise. Monson swooped down on his quarry; but there was no tame surrender. For two and a half hours the sea resounded with the roar of their broadsides; the *Triton* fighting with her twenty-two guns, the *Tupac-Amarú* with her twelve, eighteen- and six-pounders. The Spaniard fought stubbornly and well: when the *Triton* struck her colors twenty of her crew of eighty-five lay dead upon the deck. The corsair had not gone unscathed; among her fallen was young Lieutenant Francis Bulkley of New Haven.[52]

Captain Monson was done with cruising; he sent his fabulous prize for Buenos Aires with all the speed her shattered sails and rigging could muster. The entire privateering world marveled at the splendor of his windfall. After deducting 83,790 pesos for duties and other local charges, there remained a net product of 640,000 pesos. Captain Monson got a 5 per cent commission on the sales of the *Triton*, twenty shares of prize money, and one-

---

51. Robert M. Harrison to J. Q. Adams, St. Bartholomew, Dec. 1, 1820, National Archives (Washington), Department of State, Consular Letters, St. Bartholomew.

52. The New Haven *Columbian Register*, July 19, 1817, mourned this fatality in an editorial note.

third of the gains from a joint speculation in prize tickets with DeForest, a total of 54,944 pesos. The heirs of Lieutenant Bulkley received ten shares of prize money, and one extra "allowed by Captain Monson on account of the extraordinary gallantry and good conduct of the unfortunate Capt. Bulkley," making 7,122 pesos in all. Each common sailor rejoiced in a prize ticket worth 647 pesos, in addition to wages of one peso a day. To the anonymous owners went the lion's share, 304,189 pesos. It is not clear what part of the proceeds fell to DeForest, but it must have been at least as large as Monson's.

Captain Monson, having made his fortune, now thought only of how to keep it untroubled by attentions from inquisitive grand juries. He retired from privateering practice, made his way back to the United States, and settled down to a secluded existence at Astoria, Long Island. His exploits, however, lived on in the memory of his Connecticut neighbors and associates. Thus in old New Haven it was told that "one Marcena Monson was captain of a privateer . . . that on a certain occasion they encountered a Spanish galleon loaded with treasure, engaged in a bloody battle and brought the wreck of the vessel safely into Buenos Ayres, that after making a fortune at privateering, Monson returned to his native land, and built himself a large and handsome house at Astoria."[53]

Captain Livingston Shannon, a New Yorker who had served as first lieutenant on the first cruise of the *Tupac-Amarú*, commanded the privateer when she sailed from the Río de la Plata on July 9, 1817, with a new patent obtained by DeForest on May 28, 1817.[54] In one hundred and fifteen days of navigation they sighted only one Spanish sail, the *Santo Cristo de la Salud*, taken September 1 near the Azores. Shannon sent this ship with her rich freight of cacao, coffee, and cotton for Buenos Aires; but $50,000 in coin found aboard were divided among the crew in conformity with privateering practice. The subsequent history of the *Tupac-Amarú* contains little of interest. As for Captain Shannon, finding privateering under the flag of Buenos Aires unprofitable, he looked about for greener pastures, and in December, 1820, cruised in the Caribbean in command of the *Invencible*, ten guns, with a patent issued by Artigas.[55]

53. M. A. Munson, *The Munson Record*, I, 171 n.
54. *Las presas marítimas*, p. 204.
55. Robert M. Harrison to J. Q. Adams, St. Bartholomew, Dec. 1, 1820, cited above, note 51.

Like so many of his comrades, Captain James Barnes of the *Mangoré*, the former *Swift* of Baltimore, had obtained his privateering novitiate in the Anglo-American War of 1812. Sailing from Baltimore in the guise of a merchantman at the beginning of August, 1816, the *Swift* entered the service of the United Provinces at Port-au-Prince toward the end of the month. In December the *Mangoré* returned to port laden with Spanish spoils which Captain Barnes declared to custom-house officials in the most natural and routine manner. After repairing and provisioning his ship, Barnes prepared to go to sea again, but at the demand of the vigilant Spanish minister the *Mangoré* was detained and embargoed in port. Legal trammels, however, could not long embarrass a privateering captain in the genial and sympathetic atmosphere of Baltimore. Soon the corsair was free to sail under bond, but now ice in the river impeded her departure. Meantime the angry Onís complained that Barnes was very tranquilly and publicly taking out of his ship "the effects plundered by him, which it is calculated, exceed eighty thousand dollars in value, without any impediment being put to his proceedings by the authorities at Baltimore." [56]

Despite these strictures, the *Mangoré* sailed from port in March, 1817, bound on a cruise in the waters about Cadiz. In four months Captain Barnes took twenty-one prizes; of these the most valuable was *La Esperanza*, a ship of the Philippine Company, captured in collaboration with the privateer *La Independencia del Sud*, Captain James Chayter. From this cruise Barnes put into Buenos Aires in August, 1817. The commission of the *Mangoré* was now about to expire, and DeForest, her nominal owner, had already resolved to leave shortly for the United States. These circumstances probably prompted the sale of the vessel to the *armador* John Higginbotham, who on November 20, 1817, secured from the government of the United Provinces a patent for a privateer to be known as the *Pueyrredón*, in honor of the new supreme director of the state.[57] Under this name, the old *Mangoré* continued to operate against Spanish commerce until November, 1819, when she entered the service of Artigas as the *Tigre Oriental*.[58] As late as December, 1820, a

---

56. Luis de Onís to James Monroe, Washington, Feb. 11, 1817, W. R. Manning, *Diplomatic Correspondence*, III, 1917.
57. A. J. Carranza, *Campañas navales*, III, 231.
58. L. W. Bealer, *Los corsarios de Buenos Aires*, p. 219.

corsair of this name, commanded by one Murray, cruised in the Caribbean.[59] There is no record of the value of the captures of the *Mangoré*, but it is known that Darcy and Didier of Baltimore had a heavy interest in this privateer.[60]

The privateering business had many ramifications, and DeForest utilized all of them to put money in his purse. He had a large interest in the prizes taken; he bought up the shares of officers and men; the "house" bought the cargoes sold by him as auctioneer and speculated in them. In these last years of his stay in Buenos Aires, DeForest's financial affairs assume a rather complicated character. Patricio Lynch, lately head clerk and junior partner, turns into Patricio Lynch and Co.; and still later into Lynch, Zimmerman, and Co.[61] About this time DeForest also aided Lynch's young brother Estanislao to set himself up in business at Santiago de Chile in company with the American Henry Hill, who had come to Buenos Aires as supercargo of the *Salvaje* in José Miguel Carrera's ill-starred expedition.[62] In later years DeForest ever regarded this fomenting of mixed North and South American commercial enterprises as one of his chief claims to honor.[63]

By the close of the year 1817, it would appear, DeForest had attained that goal of "wealth, honor and happiness" to which as a youth of twenty-four he had ingenuously aspired. He was worth a sum conservatively estimated by a family historian at $150,000. The *chacra* or country estate was valued at another $20,000. He was a financial pillar of his adopted country. When the American consul to Buenos Aires, Thomas Halsey, demurred at asking United States merchants resident in the city to make a large loan

---

59. Robert M. Harrison to J. Q. Adams, St. Bartholomew, Dec. 1, 1920, cited above, note 51.

60. L. W. Bealer, *Los corsarios de Buenos Aires*, p. 56.

61. John C. Zimmerman, "a young German gentleman of New York," made his advent in Buenos Aires as supercargo of the schooner *Kemp* from Baltimore, which arrived on August 29, 1815, bringing military and naval stores. The firm-name of "Lynch, Zimmerman & Co." first appears in the DeForest papers in October, 1817. J. W. De Forest, *The de Forests of Avesnes*, p. 126.

62. Henry Hill, many years later, told the story of his South American experiences in his inchoate memoirs, *Recollections of an Octogenarian* (Boston, 1884). Eugenio Pereira Salas has described his career in Chile in *Henry Hill, comerciante, vice-consul y misionero* (Santiago, Chile, 1940). Hill's voluminous business correspondence and other papers are now preserved in the Yale University Library.

63. DeForest to William H. Crawford, Secretary of the Treasury, New Haven, Aug. 1, 1820, DeForest Letterbooks, Vol. 7.

to the hard pressed government, DeForest came forward with the money. "Desirous," he proclaimed, "of maintaining the honor and patriotism of the people of my native country to the best of my ability, I have this day delivered the sum of 6,851 pesos and 6 reals, and assure you as a citizen of these provinces that I will do all I can to assist this government, which I support warmly." [64]

All Buenos Aires knew the North American merchant, Don David of the stocky frame, swarthy features, shrewd dark eyes, and imperious bearing. They told of his prodigious wealth, princely hospitality, and impulsive kindness; of his arbitrary temper and cutting sarcasm. Some remembered the young foreigner who had landed at Buenos Aires at the turn of the century, bringing only his slight baggage of Yankee notions, a ready tongue, and the assurance of youth; and they marveled how far he had come. Now DeForest was on terms of intimacy with the rulers of the state, Pueyrredón, San Martín, Tagle; a secret document of the time listed him among the "individuals who figure in or have some influence on the present affairs of Buenos Aires." [65]

Despite such evidences of prosperity and high social standing, all was not well with this adopted citizen of Buenos Aires. A gnawing anxiety beset him. Now forty-four years old, with a turbulent career behind him, DeForest longed intensely to return to the peace of steady old Connecticut. But what would be the fate of his curiously gotten fortune if he returned to the United States? In more than one case heard in the courts of Baltimore he had ostentatiously figured as owner of privateers that Spain branded as pirates. An American citizen, he had flagrantly violated his country's neutrality law. If the American government were disposed to overlook his offenses, would Spain's agents be equally indulgent? He had a family, hostages to fortune, and dared not risk disaster by one rash, unpremeditated move. Against all contingencies that might arise from his return to the States he must first prepare safeguards. Cares of this sort weighed heavily on DeForest's mind in the closing months of the year 1817.

Two visitors from North America came to know DeForest at this period; but their descriptions of him can hardly be said to

64. DeForest to José D. Trillo, Buenos Aires, Oct. 18, 1816, Archivo General de la Nación (Buenos Aires), S.1–A.2–A.4, no. 8.
65. H. Zorraquín Becú, *De aventurero yanqui a consul porteño en los Estados Unidos*, pp. 39–40 n.

agree. One was Henry Hill, the supercargo of the *Salvaje* mentioned above, who landed in March, 1817, carrying letters of introduction to DeForest from friends in Baltimore. The merchant was not in his counting-room when Hill called; and the traveler, accompanied by young Manuel Lynch, rode out to the *chácra*. "We found Mr. and Mrs. DeForest writing at separate tables; and she said, with a smile, that she was assisting her husband as clerk, and was copying one of his letters. After I had concluded my business with him, it was in vain that I proposed to return to town before dinner. The writing apparatus was laid aside, and we took a walk among his fruit trees. The figs were delicious, and it was the first time I had ever plucked them from the trees. His house is on a rising ground; the river is in full view, and on the right is the city of Buenos Ayres, with an extensive, verdant plain between. He has a large *hacienda*, or plantation; and the Madeira nuts, peaches and other fruit on the table, were part of its produce. On our way home Don Manuel and I found it pretty warm and dusty, but we had a pleasant ride." [66]

DeForest displayed a kindly interest in his young visitor; at the home of General San Martín's father-in-law he introduced him to the great soldier, just returned from a victorious campaign in Chile; he also gave Hill valuable letters of introduction to correspondents in that country. "Mr. DeForest," wrote Hill many years after this encounter, "was a man of commanding form and fine personal appearance, and naturally was high-spirited, imperious, yet dignified, gentlemanly, affable and very interesting in conversation." [67]

Jeremy Robinson of Massachusetts, who called on DeForest almost one year later, had obtained a commission as special agent of the United States in Lima from President Monroe, only to have his appointment abruptly revoked just before his departure.[68] Robinson nevertheless decided to travel in South America for his health, and also to study the progress of the sciences and letters in that little known part of the world. He sailed for La Plata in November, 1817, in the brig *Columbus*, commanded by

66. H. Hill, *Recollections of an Octogenarian,* pp. 111–112.
67. *Ibid.,* pp. 113–114.
68. On Robinson's travels in South America, see Eugenio Pereira Salas, "Jeremías Robinson, agente norteamericano en Chile (1818–1823)," *Revista chilena de historia y geografía,* LXXXII (1937), 201–236, based on the Jeremy Robinson Papers, Manuscripts Division, Library of Congress. I have made independent use of these papers, particularly of Robinson's Diary.

the future rear-admiral of Chile, Charles W. Wooster. Robinson carried a letter of introduction to DeForest from Darcy and Didier of Baltimore.

The *Columbus* anchored in the port of Buenos Aires on February 4, 1818. Her arrival coincided with the rise of a crisis in the affairs of the American consul to La Plata, Thomas L. Halsey. The Pueyrredón régime, accusing Halsey of furnishing munitions to Artigas and of accepting privateering commissions from the gaucho chieftain, decreed the consul's banishment.[69]

The ruined Halsey met Robinson shortly after his arrival in Buenos Aires, and poured into his sympathetic ear a story of unmerited sufferings. He denied having assisted Artigas or having received privateering commissions from that wandering ruler of the pampas. The author of his downfall, he affirmed, was David C. DeForest, who from motives of commercial jealousy had prevailed upon the Supreme Director Pueyrredón to banish him (Halsey) from the country.

The credulous Robinson listened, believed, and was properly incensed at this insult to the dignity of the United States and at the malignity of DeForest. He did not know that an order from Washington for Halsey's dismissal, based on his well substantiated privateering activities and other charges, was on its way, crossing Pueyrredón's demand for the consul's recall. It was in a hostile mood that Robinson made the acquaintance of the much abused DeForest. In his diary he recorded some impressions of this meeting.

"Dined with Mr. DeForest. He is assuming inflated and impudent in the extreme. A few years ago this gentleman came to this country poor. He acquired some little wealth and applied rather indecorously to the President of the U S for the consular appointment to this place. His rudeness offended the President and he would not listen to Mr. DeForest's application. The consequence has been that he hates and will annoy the Government of the United States by every means in his power. The person who had been appointed to the office was negatived by the intrigues of D[e]F[orest], and his friends in the Senate of the United States, at the same time that D[e] F[orest] professed for him the warmest friendship and esteem. Here we perceive that interest and mercantile habits prostrate every generous principle to their advance-

---

69. On Halsey and his relations with Artigas, see C. C. Griffin, *The United States and the Disruption of the Spanish Empire*, pp. 151–154.

ment. In fine, this man is a vain, conceited purse proud arrogant arbitrary designing being who has renounced allegiance to his country and disrespects that which gives him subsistence. He has been largely concerned in Privateering as have several other Americans who are citizens of the U S in name [crossed out] in sentiment. Captain M[onso]n has imbibed the same spirit. They live together and like the other Americans here amuse themselves in gossiping and in forming machinations against each other. They all hate Mr. H[alsey] the Consul." [70]

DeForest, Robinson jotted in his journal, had been deeply engaged in the privateering business, and had accumulated so much money that he exacted "homage from every person who approaches him. He at present contemplates returning to the U States but not without fear of being troubled through the cordial but mild embrace of the law. Captain M[onson] is likewise apprehensive of similar danger and inconvenience."

From an undisclosed source Robinson learned that DeForest daily expected to be appointed consul general from the United Provinces to the United States. This intelligence elicited from the peevish tourist the observation: "Very disinterested. Invested with a new nominal allegiance to and a publick function from an unacknowledged Gt. Perhaps it will enable him to avoid the penalties due to a violation of the laws of the U S while a citizen."

One day later DeForest called on Robinson at his lodgings. The merchant confirmed the report that the government of Buenos Aires had appointed a consul general who would shortly depart for the United States. "I am anxious to know," was his tactful query, "whether he will be received or not." Robinson suggested that such an emissary might be received but not formally recognized. "I objected to it the indecent and barbarous banishment of the [U. S.] Consul General Halsey. Mr. DeForest is doubtless the person in question." [71]

DeForest was indeed the person in question. Whether his appointment was suggested by the Supreme Director Pueyrredón or by the merchant himself is not clear. But the arrangement offered obvious advantages to all concerned. For DeForest a diplomatic status signified protection from the meddlesome attentions of American courts. For Pueyrredón and his foreign minister,

70. Jeremy Robinson Diary, Feb. 19, 1818, Manuscripts Division, Library of Congress.
71. *Ibid.,* Feb. 21, 1818.

Gregorio Tagle, it presented an opportunity to send to Washington, where a heated congressional struggle over recognition of the revolted colonies was in progress, an able and resourceful agent to further their cause. Nor would there be any question of remuneration involved. Was not DeForest one of the wealthiest men in Buenos Aires?

Already the amateur diplomat had sent his wife and children to North America in the brig *Aurora*, Captain Searl, which sailed for New Haven in the spring of 1817. Now he prepared to take leave of Buenos Aires, to which he was bound by many strands of experience and recollection. He had first come to this city of azure skies, imposing churches, and white, flat-roofed homes in the remote days of the viceroys, smuggling himself and his little "adventure" across the border from Brazil. He had known here the stormy season of the British invasions, when the *porteños* first gained awareness of their strength and nationality. He had witnessed the uneasy preliminaries of the *Revolución de Mayo;* and from exile he had rejoiced at the downfall of his Spanish enemies. He had contributed to the establishment and consolidation of an independent Argentine state by word and by deed; by the diffusion of republican propaganda, by financial support to the struggling patriot government, and by his leading rôle in the promotion of privateering enterprise against Spanish commerce. In return, his adopted country had afforded him the means of achieving "wealth, honor and happiness."

Preparing to depart for the United States, DeForest gave a notable proof of his gratitude to the people and government of the United Provinces. He presented to the state his *chacra*, to be used for the endowment of the first institution of higher learning in independent Buenos Aires, the Academy of the Union of the South. His communication on this subject, and the letter of acceptance from the government, appear together in a handsomely printed folder evidently published by DeForest. On November 22, 1817, the patron of learning wrote as follows to the *gobernador intendente* of Buenos Aires, Manuel Luis de Oliden:

> More than seven years ago I bought an estate [*chacra*] pleasantly situated on the coast of San Isidro, two and a half leagues distant from this Capital, on which I have expended much money, for it served me regularly as a retreat during the summer. For this reason I have a great regard for the said estate, and cannot bring

myself to sell it to any private individual, no matter how attractive the offer. But this regard and every other consideration cede to the gratitude which this generous people has always inspired in me by its hospitality and the many other benefits for which I am indebted to it. It is well known that the leaders and public authorities are at present engaged in reestablishing the ancient college [*estudios*] under more liberal and beneficial principles. At the time of the establishment of the Library, which today does so much honor to Buenos Aires, I had the pleasure of collaborating by the donation of some classical works. Since the advantages of reestablishing the college among this great people are even more important, I cannot refrain from taking part in this admirable work as well. Therefore I publicly present this estate to your Lordship, with the accompanying documents of ownership, excepting only two slaves whom I have determined to set free. One only interest moves me—that of making my memory cherished by the sons of this city, and of giving one more proof of my adherence to the cause which it defends. I pray you, therefore, to accept this estate, considering only the motives that inspire this action; and to bring it to the attention of the commissioners for the reestablishment of the college, that they may make use of it in good time.

I hope soon to be reunited with my family in North America, where my concerns have called me for some time. On all occasions it will be highly pleasing for me to perform services for this city, or for its good citizens; and I hope that they will frankly consider me their most sincere friend and fellow-citizen, interested in the glory of this country.

On November 25, 1817, the government of Buenos Aires made the following reply:

This Government has the pleasure of transmitting to you the decree which I affixed yesterday to your representation offering to this country an unequivocal proof of the respect and gratitude that it deserves. The contents of this decree are of the following tenor.

"Acknowledgement is made to Citizen DAVID CORTES DEFOREST of the donation that he freely makes in favor of this city with specific application to the college which it has been ordered to reestablish. The secretary of this Government will go to the home of this worthy Citizen and will thank him for his generous display of gratitude and solicitude for this city, assuring him that this Government will inscribe the names of his esteemed children in the records of the municipality, and will obtain from the most Excellent Supreme Director an order that his portrait be placed in one of the principal halls of the college in order to perpetuate his memory as a benefactor of that establishment. There shall also be established in the new college a scholarship, to be assigned with preference to the children of the donor, and in their absence, to the sons of this country who are descendants of citizens of the United States of North America. For this purpose let there be issued a corresponding order to the Minister of State charged with the reestablishment of the college, transmitting it to the donor for his intelligence and satisfaction." [72]

In these days of his departure from Buenos Aires, DeForest performed another act of sweeping generosity. He freed all his slaves, and gave to each a small sum of money with which to begin life anew. In early March, 1818, he sailed by the *Plattsburg* for the United States, where difficult official duties awaited him. No ordinary test of strength lay before DeForest, but a diplomatic duel with a statesman of great dialectical skill. After meeting and besting all obstacles as smuggler, merchant, and promoter of privateering enterprise, he was about to meet his first serious check at the hands of Secretary of State John Quincy Adams.

[72]. A copy of this published exchange of letters is preserved in the National Archives (Washington), Department of State, Despatches from Consuls, Buenos Aires, I, Part II.

X

"THE GREAT SOUTH AMERICAN WITCHERY"

A SUCCESSION of emissaries had voyaged from the Río de la Plata to North American shores in quest of aid for their cause since the historic twenty-fifth of May, 1810, birthday of Argentine independence.[1] We have already told of the first mission of this kind, that of Diego de Saavedra and Pedro de Aguirre, sent by the patriot *junta* of Buenos Aires to purchase arms in the United States. It will be recalled that these commissioners at last sailed for home with a sorely needed cargo of munitions, showering blessings upon the friendly neighbor of the North.

The Anglo-American War of 1812 interrupted the flow of envoys from Buenos Aires to Washington. The first visitor with any pretensions to an official character to arrive in the United States after the close of those hostilities was the redoubtable privateering captain, Thomas Taylor, who brought a letter of introduction to President Madison from General Álvarez Thomas, then supreme director of the United Provinces. As we know, Taylor came primarily to foster the progress of his interesting profession, but he also made it his business to inquire into the state of American public opinion on the insurgent cause. His researches led to the conclusion that all classes of the population sympathized with the Spanish American patriots, and that it only required an individual of "brilliance and imagination," invested with an official character by the Buenos Aires government, to set on foot a great movement in support of the revolted colonists. Such a person, Taylor suggested on his return to La Plata, was General William H. Winder of Baltimore, a prominent lawyer whose generous enthusiasm for the cause of freedom knew no bounds. Winder had publicly caned the Spanish consul in

---

1. For this chapter I have drawn heavily on S. F. Bemis, *Early Diplomatic Missions,* particularly on the excellent account of DeForest's mission, pp. 70–89. Professor Bemis used DeForest's personal papers, and also employed archival materials in the United States, Spain, and the Argentine. There is a brief but appreciative discussion of DeForest's consular activity in A. P. Whitaker, *The United States and Latin America,* pp. 256–259.

Baltimore for outrageous interference with the outfitting of patriot privateers; Winder proposed to leave home, family, and a secure station in life to lead patriot armies in battle against Spanish tyranny.[2] These observations were shortly to bear fruit.

Even before Captain Taylor set foot on North American shores, the Supreme Director Álvarez Thomas had designated Colonel Martín Thompson as agent to the United States (January 16, 1816). His instructions enjoined strict secrecy as to the nature of his mission, which he might divulge only to the President. He should endeavor to secure all possible material assistance, and should urge the government of the United States to use its influence with European powers in favor of the patriot cause. Thompson's mission turned out badly; he entered into unauthorized contracts with army officers for service in Buenos Aires, violated the injunction concerning secrecy, and was finally removed by the new Supreme Director Pueyrredón. Be it from this or other causes, the unlucky agent's mind became completely deranged: his successor reported him in a hospital, "hopelessly crazy." [3]

The next mission from Buenos Aires was directly related to General San Martín's strategy for the winning of continental independence. The Argentine Liberator had already crossed the Andes with his army and gained an important victory over the Spanish royalists at Chacabuco (February 12, 1817); an invasion of Peru from the sea was to follow the complete emancipation of Chile. Accordingly, San Martín, representing the government of Chile, and the Supreme Director Pueyrredón, on behalf of the United Provinces, commissioned Manuel Hermenegildo de Aguirre as chief of mission, and Gregorio Gómez as second, to proceed to the United States and purchase or have constructed there a fleet of armed vessels. By this time the historic congress of Tucumán had formally proclaimed the independence of the United Provinces of South America from Spain (July 9, 1816), but Aguirre's instructions did not direct him to solicit a recognition of independence. A letter from Pueyrredón to President Monroe described its bearer as deputed to the American Chief

2. Thomas Taylor to the Supreme Director Pueyrredón, Buenos Aires, Feb. 19, 1818, Archivo General de la Nación (Buenos Aires), S.1–A.2–A.4, no. 8. Had Taylor known of General Winder's military incompetence, strikingly manifested in the late war with Britain at the battle of Bladensburg and the capture of Washington, he would doubtless have been terrified at this last prospect.

3. S. F. Bemis, *Early Diplomatic Missions*, p. 39.

Executive "in the character of the agent of this Government," and sought for him "all the protection and consideration required by his diplomatic rank and the actual state of our relations." Another missive from San Martín to Monroe stressed the importance of Aguirre's mission to the success of his military projects and compared the struggles of the South American patriots to the trials of the North American revolutionists.[4]

Arrived in Washington, where he found President Monroe absent on a "good feeling" tour of the country, Aguirre was received in a cordial albeit informal manner by Acting Secretary of State Richard Rush. The American official assured his visitor of the sympathy with which the President and people of the United States regarded the independence struggle of the Spanish Americans. He explained that his government, pursuing a policy of strict neutrality, and bound by its treaty of commerce and amity with Spain, must remain aloof from this struggle. At the same time Rush adverted strongly to the advantages which flowed to the patriots from this policy of neutrality. Finally, the secretary advised Aguirre that within the limits of United States law he was free to purchase or have built ships and engage in every other private commercial transaction.

Despite a three day confinement in a New York jail on charges of violating American neutrality legislation—an experience that set the proud creole fairly dancing with rage—Aguirre was moderately successful as concerned the legitimate object of his mission. He had two frigates constructed and dispatched to Chile by way of La Plata. The *Curiacio* later participated in the campaign for the liberation of Peru. Not so the *Horatio*. On arrival at Buenos Aires her suspicious captain refused to hand over the ship until he received payment for a note of 69,541 pesos. Before port officials could seize the vessel he had bolted for Rio de Janeiro, where he sold the frigate to the Portuguese government to satisfy the debt.

An unauthorized adventure in diplomacy turned out less auspiciously for Aguirre. At the opening of Congress in December, 1817, Henry Clay and his partisans launched a spirited attack on the Spanish and South American policies of the administration. They railed against the neutrality act of March 3, 1817, as unfair to the patriots; they protested against the

4. These letters are printed in W. R. Manning, *Diplomatic Correspondence*, I, 352–353.

occupation by United States forces of Amelia Island, a haunt for insurgent privateers, slave-traders, and smugglers off the Florida coast and near the American border; and finally they set up a cry for the immediate recognition of the United Provinces. Aguirre, delighted at this outburst of enthusiasm for his country, hastened to confer with Secretary of State John Quincy Adams, who had taken over the duties of his office from Acting Secretary Rush on September 22, 1817.

In imitation of Clay and his followers, the rebel agent asserted the claim of Buenos Aires to recognition, and complained of the inequalities of the neutrality law and of American occupation of Amelia Island. The imperturbable Adams speedily demolished the groundwork of Aguirre's pretensions. He extracted from the tactless diplomat the confession that he had no new instructions to request recognition;[5] and asked embarrassing questions as to the exact extent of the territory under control of the Buenos Aires government (at this time the Portuguese were in possession of Montevideo and the gaucho chieftain Artigas ruled over the remainder of the Banda Oriental or present-day Uruguay). When Aguirre protested against the occupation of Amelia Island, Adams retorted with the query: Did the government of the United Provinces mean to assume a "superintendency" of all Spanish provinces in both of the continents of America? The United States should be given explicit notice of this fact, that they might regulate their policy toward that government accordingly. Aguirre realized that he had overreached himself, and beat a hasty retreat, assuring the secretary that he spoke for himself only, and without official authority.[6]

In Congress, meantime, Clay was riding hard his "South American great horse."[7] The House, stirred by his persuasive oratory, called on the President to send in all documents relating to Amelia Island and the revolted colonies. Aguirre's representations to the secretary of state, which the agent had carefully

---

5. Aguirre did tell Adams that he had instructions to urge the recognition of Buenos Aires "as circumstances might occur to favor the demand," but was expressly ordered not to urge it "at the hazard of embroiling the United States with any of the powers of Europe." J. Q. Adams, *Memoirs,* IV, 30, under date of December 24, 1817. But there is nothing of this tenor in the credentials and instructions carried by Aguirre as given in S. F. Bemis, *Early Diplomatic Missions,* pp. 42–45.

6. J. Q. Adams, *Memoirs,* IV, 47, under date of Jan. 22, 1818.

7. The phrase is Adams', *ibid.,* p. 28.

restated in written notes to Adams, would thus find their way into the public prints. The secretary, submitting the required papers to Monroe, appended a statement in which he emphasized that "Aguirre had no diplomatic title, no powers to treat, and that all his demands for recognition had arisen since the assembly of Congress." [8] When, after much debate, the issue of recognition came to the test in the House on March 28, 1818, on a motion by Clay to appropriate $18,000 for a minister and legation in Buenos Aires, it was beaten down by the decisive vote of 45–115. Aguirre's unauthorized and injudicious approaches to Adams had doubtless stiffened administration resistance to the recognition proposal and thereby ensured its defeat.

President Monroe and his secretary of state, it hardly needs to be said, were not unfriendly to the cause of Spanish-American independence. Adams, who on occasion voiced gloomy distrust of the patriots' capacity for self-government and questioned the supposed affinity between the peoples and revolutions of the two continents, was as solicitous as Clay to acknowledge the new states, but only when the fact of their independence and internal stability had been fully established, and when such recognition would not imperil the security of the United States. To satisfy itself completely on the first of these conditions as it concerned the United Provinces, the American government had just despatched a commission of inquiry to Buenos Aires to report on the state of affairs there.[9] Only a few weeks after Clay's crushing defeat, the secretary wrote the United States minister in Spain that if the government of Buenos Aires "should maintain that stability which it appears to have acquired since the Declaration of Independence of July 9, 1816, it cannot be long before they will demand that acknowledgment of right." [10]

The relation of the problem of recognition to the diplomatic interests and security of the United States was more complicated. It was the considered judgment of Adams that from this point of view the time for acknowledgment of the new states had not yet arrived. Delicate negotiations with Spain over Florida and the Western boundary question were in progress; the occupation of

8. S. F. Bemis, *Early Diplomatic Missions*, p. 57.
9. It was composed of Theodorick A. Bland, Caesar A. Rodney, and John Graham. For the mission, see Watt Stewart, "The South American Commission, 1817–1818," *Hisp. Am. Hist. Rev.*, IX (1929), 31–59. The reports of the commissioners are printed in W. R. Manning, *Diplomatic Correspondence*, I, 382–438.
10. Adams to George W. Erving, Washington, April 20, 1818, *ibid.*, p. 61.

Amelia Island had exacerbated the already inflamed peninsular sensibilities; and Adams still feared that if Spain should go to war with the United States over recognition of her revolted provinces, she might find European support. The dangers to which premature recognition might expose the United States became plain from the information which the secretary obtained by circuitous channels in May, 1818, that Great Britain had consented to a general mediation by the European powers to bring about the pacification of Spanish America.[11] To draw England away from collaboration with her reactionary allies on this issue and into a joint acknowledgment with the United States of the independence of the revolted colonies, meantime preserving a posture of strict official neutrality toward the struggle as the best means of averting European armed intervention on the side of Spain, was the prudent course of diplomatic action adopted by the Monroe administration at this juncture. It was a course of policy, as Adams never wearied of reminding importunate South American emissaries, that fully conformed to the true interests of their countries.

The indiscretions of an American special agent to South America were directly responsible for the decision of the Buenos Aires authorities to appoint David C. DeForest as Aguirre's successor at Washington. William G. D. Worthington was sent to Buenos Aires in 1817 to disavow a loan agreement made with the Supreme Director Pueyrredón in the name of the United States government by an earlier agent, Colonel John Devereux, and to promote trade relations between the two countries. Arrived at the Río de la Plata, however, Worthington "swelled upon his agency" until he broke out "into a self-accredited Plenipotentiary," in the words of the angry Adams,[12] and drew up with Pueyrredón a set of articles that amounted to a provisional treaty of amity and commerce.

Encouraged by this seeming portent of recognition by the United States, the supreme director now for the first time addressed a formal request for acknowledgment of independence to President Monroe.[13] At the same time the Buenos Aires government arranged for a more adequate diplomatic representation at

11. A. P. Whitaker, *The United States and Latin America*, p. 251.
12. *Memoirs*, IV, 158–159.
13. This letter is printed in W. R. Manning, *Diplomatic Correspondence*, I, 370–371.

Washington. To DeForest, who had his private reasons for wishing to return to North America covered by the immunities of a diplomatic character, Pueyrredón tendered, as we already know, the post of consul general. On the recommendation of Captain Thomas Taylor, the supreme director also appointed General William H. Winder of Baltimore as special deputy of the United Provinces near the government of the United States. A letter from Pueyrredón to the "hero of Canada" besought him to accept the appointment, or, at least, to lend his protection to DeForest, the bearer of Winder's credentials.[14]

DeForest's own instructions (dated February 24, 1818) embodied six articles. The first three placed him under the general obligations of consuls, empowered him to appoint vice-consuls, and declared that until an ambassador or other emissary should be sent to the United States, he was to endeavor to obtain recognition of independence by the United States and all other manner of assistance. Article 4 enjoined DeForest to make every effort to refute the slanders (*especies*) circulated in North America by a group of political exiles from Buenos Aires that included José Agrelo, Manuel Dorrego, and Manuel Moreno, the brother of the famous revolutionary leader.[15] The consul general should not imitate these "detractors," but must seek to win them over to the Pueyrredón régime. The next article authorized DeForest to issue privateering patents in the United States; accordingly, on March 2, 1818, he was given blank commissions for two frigates, six corvettes, twenty brigs, and twenty schooners, with the corresponding officers' commissions, including one made out to our old acquaintance Marcena Monson, now become "colonel and commander-in-chief of the squadron of this state in the North Atlantic." [16] Article 6 suggested a major object of DeForest's mission. "In case our corsairs should occupy some island suitable as a base and to which none of the recognized nations have any right, the said consul is empowered to set up such a municipal government there as may seem best to him, taking possession of the island in the name of this government." [17]

14. Buenos Aires, Feb. 25, 1818, Archivo General de la Nación (Buenos Aires), S.1–A.2–A.4, no. 8.
15. C. C. Griffin, *The United States and the Spanish Empire,* pp. 127–128, describes the activities of this group.
16. A. J. Carranza, *Campañas navales,* III, 242.
17. Confidential instructions for DeForest as consul general in the United States, draft, Buenos Aires, Feb. 24, 1818, Archivo General de la Nación (Buenos Aires), S.1–A.2–A.4, no. 8.

An accompanying letter from Pueyrredón to President Monroe stated that in conformity with the articles agreed upon with the United States agent William G. D. Worthington, he had appointed David C. DeForest as consul general to the United States, with the powers specified in his commission and instructions respectively.[18] "DeForest's credentials," observes Professor Bemis, "were thus based on the unsafe authority of Worthington's unauthorized agreement, and we may presume that the alert John Quincy Adams would not fail to note this, should he find it convenient to do so." [19]

Accompanied by young Manuel Lynch, bound for the United States to learn English and obtain a commercial education, the amateur diplomat sailed from Buenos Aires in the first days of March, 1818, in the United States frigate *Plattsburg*. From this vessel had just disembarked a commission of inquiry despatched by President Monroe to report on the progress of the revolution in the Río de la Plata. DeForest and his companion landed at Baltimore on April 28.

Arrived at that thriving center of privateering enterprise, the envoy placed in the hands of General Winder his appointment as deputy from the United Provinces near the government of the United States. The lawyer, much gratified at the honor thus thrust upon him, asked for time to consider the propriety of acceptance. He immediately notified President Monroe of the designation and sought his opinion on the subject. Monroe unhesitatingly encouraged his old friend to accept the post, and appended a brief but vigorous defense of the administration's South American policy, presumably for the edification of the Buenos Aires authorities.[20] Winder nevertheless finally turned

18. W. R. Manning, *Diplomatic Correspondence*, I, 377–378.
19. S. F. Bemis, *Early Diplomatic Missions*, pp. 73–74.
20. "I have no hesitation to state to you, that the sincere desire of this government, is, that the Spanish Colonies may achieve their independence, and that we shall promote it, by our councils and interest, with other powers, when we have any, and by every honourable and impartial measure, which we can adopt, consistently, with our neutrality, and without compromising, the highest interests of our country. I am satisfied that the true interest of the Colonies, consists, in leaving us perfectly free, to pursue, such course, in regard to them, as we think proper, and that on the ground of interest, there can be no disagreement much less collision between us. It is a miserably shortsighted, and contracted policy, in those who represent the Colonies, or patronize their interest, to pursue a different course, since its tendency is to deprive them of the friendship, of the only power on earth, sincerely friendly to them, and of the immense advantages which they derive, by the supplies, which they receive from us, and from the

down the offer, and in his letter of declination set forth as emanating from himself the substance of Monroe's cogent remarks. He also affirmed that DeForest appeared to have the needful qualifications for his office, and promised to aid the consul general with his advice.[21]

After his visit to Winder, DeForest departed for Washington. At the Department of State, where he left his credentials, he learned that the President had just set out for his home in Virginia and would not return till the following week. This the envoy from Buenos Aires soon found to be a fortunate circumstance, for in the intervening days he could orient himself politically and discover that the campaign launched in Congress for the recognition of the United Provinces by "our own warm friends," meaning Clay and his group, had embarrassed and irritated the President.[22] Shrewdly DeForest concluded that for the present it would be prudent to conceal his intention of soliciting recognition. Meanwhile he lost no time in making the acquaintance of Clay, to whom he presented a letter of introduction from John Graham, one of the commissioners sent by the President to Buenos Aires.

Responding to a note from Secretary of State Adams, DeForest appeared for an audience at the department on the afternoon of May 7, 1818. Adams must have eyed his visitor with a peculiar interest. He knew more of the privateering past of this adventurer from Connecticut than DeForest suspected. Thomas L. Halsey, ex-consul of the United States in Buenos Aires, had lately furnished the secretary with some gratuitous information on that subject.[23]

After the customary exchange of civilities, Adams turned to the business at hand. He explained to DeForest that the treaty which Worthington had presumed to make with the Supreme

---

countenance which we give them and for what purpose encounter this danger? Equally satisfied I am, that were we ever to engage in the war, in their favour, they would be losers by it." Monroe to Winder, Washington, May 11, 1818. This correspondence between Monroe and Winder has been printed in the *Hisp. Am. Hist. Rev.*, XII (1932), 457–461.

21. Winder to Gregorio Tagle, Baltimore, June 5, 1818, Archivo General de la Nación (Buenos Aires), S.1–A.2–A.4, no. 8.

22. DeForest to Tagle, Baltimore, May 17, 1818, Archivo General de la Nación (Buenos Aires), S.1–A.2–A.4, no. 8.

23. See Halsey to Adams, Buenos Aires, Jan. 25, 1818, National Archives (Washington), Department of State, Despatches from Consuls, Buenos Aires, I, Part 2.

Director Pueyrredón at Buenos Aires, and on which DeForest's appointment was based, had been made without authority and was therefore wholly null and void. Under existing circumstances, he went on, it was not deemed prudent to acknowledge the independence of the United Provinces, and consequently DeForest could not be formally received in the capacity of consul general, since that would be tantamount to a recognition of his government. He was free, however, to reside anywhere in the United States and to act in his official character as if he were received in due form. He might hold correspondence with the Department of State and would receive all proper attentions and respect from the American government.

DeForest mildly rejoined that his agency was only commercial in nature, and should not be regarded as bearing a political character. The United States had sent a similar agent to Buenos Aires, where he was duly accredited; and the government of the United Provinces had not thought there would be any objection to granting a like status to DeForest. It was an appointment of very little consequence, to be sure; he, DeForest, had not solicited it; it had been given to him on the eve of his return to the United States, where he intended to remain, in order to prevent the irregularities committed by privateers flying the flag of Buenos Aires, irregularities of which the Supreme Director Pueyrredón entirely disapproved. After these cautious and self-deprecatory remarks, DeForest asked whether he should show his commission to Adams, and whether he would receive an answer to his written application for an *exequatur*.

The secretary readily perceived the purport of DeForest's clever and plausible suggestion that an exchange of commercial agents could be made by the two countries without a formal recognition of the independence of Buenos Aires by the United States. He immediately rebuffed this ingenious effort to smuggle recognition in by the back door. The United States, Adams pointed out, had appointed many consuls to reside at colonial establishments. They were seldom received with their regular titles, but were generally allowed to act as commercial agents. At Buenos Aires, it was true, Consul Halsey had been formally received. But this was a wholly voluntary act on the part of the Buenos Aires government, which might have declined to do so without any offense to the United States. DeForest's appointment as consul general, on the other hand, was expressly based on the Worthington agreement, which was entirely disavowed. As to writing, the cautious Adams thought it unnecessary; it would be more consistent with delicacy if they understood each other verbally. If DeForest should apply in writing for an *exequatur*, however, he would receive an answer in the same manner.

DeForest hastened to assure the secretary that his government was not disposed to urge any point which might be disagreeable to the United States; he would be careful not to take any step which might embarrass the administration. In reply to a question from Adams, he observed that his commission did not interfere with that of Aguirre, which was merely to procure arms, naval stores, and an armed vessel. In this connection, he confirmed that Aguirre had no authority to ask for recognition, had flouted the supreme director's wishes not to press the United States government on that subject, and had been instigated to his actions by other parties.[24]

The consul general from Buenos Aires had not ventured to broach in this initial conference a major object of his mission: the occupation of an island in the Gulf of Mexico as a base of privateering operations, similar to the lately extinguished establishment at Amelia Island. The next day, in the course of a second conversation with Adams, he skirted rather undiplomatically about the subject. If the government of the United Provinces should send an expedition to take Florida, he asked, would the American government take any measure to prevent it?

The secretary stiffly replied that the same law by virtue of which the United States had lately taken possession of Amelia Island [25] would apply in such a contingency to the remainder of Florida. The United States had a claim upon that province for indemnities long due from Spain, and could not suffer its occupation by a third party.

DeForest assured the secretary that the government of Buenos Aires had no part in the dubious proceedings of the adventurers who had established themselves at Amelia Island, and was entirely content with the recent occupation of the place by the United

24. The sources for this conference are the entry in J. Q. Adams, *Memoirs,* IV, 88–89, under date of May 7, 1818; and DeForest to Tagle, May 17, 1818, cited above, note 22.

25. The reference is to the act of Congress of January 15, 1811, voicing the famous "non-transfer" principle. In his interview with DeForest, Adams inadvertently stated that the law had been in existence "ever since 1815."

States. But the possession of a port in the Gulf of Mexico would greatly aid the United Provinces in privateering operations against Spain, and if they could not take Florida there was no port in the Gulf to which their corsairs could resort.

Adams drily replied that the law of 1811 had been made without any intention to injure the interests of Buenos Aires, but while it remained in force the President was bound to execute it. He added that the commissioners sent to South America had been instructed to give suitable explanations on this subject to the supreme director at Buenos Aires.

DeForest wisely decided not to press the matter further. He informed the secretary that he would let his reception as consul general rest on these conversations without any exchange of notes.[26] Then, by prior arrangement with Adams, he went to call on the President.

The disciple of Jefferson did not scruple to show his ardent sympathy with the patriots of Buenos Aires. He lamented the cause which prevented a formal recognition of DeForest, and hoped for a speedy removal of these obstacles. "He observed that the world was in such a state that much caution was required; and that, having our commercial relations placed on an equal footing with those of Spain, was as much as could be done for us at this moment." [27]

After these unpromising exchanges with Adams and Monroe, DeForest returned to Baltimore. There Manuel Moreno, brother of the revolutionary apostle, and an exiled opponent of Pueyrredón, sought him out. The refugee, evidently in straitened circumstances, was eager to be permitted to return to Buenos Aires. As directed by his instructions, DeForest received the repentant Moreno in friendly fashion, and accepted his professions of renewed allegiance to the supreme director at their face value. He introduced the exile to General Winder as one who might be usefully employed "in any business relating to our country," meaning of course privateering business; and wrote home a favorable report on Moreno's attitude and actions.[28]

26. The source for DeForest's second interview with Adams is the entry in Adams' *Memoirs,* IV, 89–90, under date of May 8, 1818. DeForest does not mention it in his letter to Tagle of May 17, cited above, note 22.

27. DeForest reported on this interview in his letter to Tagle of May 17, 1818, cited above. He mentions the conference as held on May 9; Adams, in his *Memoirs,* gives the date as May 8.

28. DeForest to Tagle, May 17, 1818, cited above.

At Buenos Aires, where the authorities had built great hopes on the weak foundations of the Worthington agreement, DeForest's report on his seemingly barren conferences with Adams and the President caused disappointment. The supreme director informed the congress of the United Provinces in secret session that the planned dispatch of a commissioner to the United States should be deferred, for he would probably suffer the same slights as had the consul general sent there.[29] Gregorio Tagle, Pueyrredón's secretary of foreign affairs, was also vexed by what he considered the unreasonable refusal of the government of the United States to receive DeForest.[30]

In reality, DeForest's mission had not been altogether futile up to this point. His discreet approaches to Adams and Monroe had been in refreshing contrast to the importunities of his predecessor, Aguirre, and had contributed to a more favorable opinion of the Buenos Aires government on the part of the administration. To this kindlier disposition can probably be ascribed the moves toward acknowledgment of the United Provinces made by Adams in the summer of 1818. Thus, in mid-August, the secretary instructed the ministers of the United States at the courts of England, France, and Russia to inquire of these governments how they would regard a recognition of the independence of Buenos Aires by the United States, and what position they would take if Spain declared war on the United States in consequence of such recognition. Later that month, he wrote to Monroe that if the Buenos Aires government would moderate its territorial claims and agree to place the United States on the most-favored-nation footing (as Pueyrredón had declined to do in the disavowed agreement with Worthington), he would think the time had come when such acknowledgment could be made without breach of neutrality.[31]

Unaware of these hopeful developments, with the advent of summer the unrecognized consul general had set out on a tour through the "Northern and Eastern States of this great and

---

29. Emilio Ravignani, ed., *Asambleas constituyentes argentinas* . . . (7 vols., Buenos Aires, 1937–1939), I, 536. Pueyrredón also advanced as reasons for delaying the appointment the lack of a person with suitable qualifications and the difficult situation of the treasury.

30. Tagle to Bernardino Rivadavia, Buenos Aires, Sept. 10, 1818, in Universidad de Buenos Aires, *Comisión de Bernardino Rivadavia ante España y otras potencias de Europa* (2 vols., Buenos Aires, 1933–1936), I, 303–304.

31. In this appreciation of DeForest's mission, I have followed A. P. Whitaker, *The United States and Latin America*, pp. 258–259.

growing Republic." [32] At New Haven he rejoined his family, and arranged for the construction of a large and stately home on the Green by David Hoadley, the "self-taught architect" of Connecticut.[33] After a festive reunion with his parents at Watertown, DeForest journeyed across the land of steady habits to the town of Boston. There the arrival of an envoy from distant Buenos Aires attracted some attention. By official invitation, DeForest attended a "visitation of schools," and afterwards dined in the company of the selectmen of Boston.[34] William L. Shaw, secretary of the Boston Athenaeum, who proposed to visit Buenos Aires in search of "Coins, Medals and other curiosities peculiar to South America," called to ask for letters of introduction; and Captain John Downes of the United States frigate *Macedonian*, bound for the Pacific "with a view to protecting the trade of the U. S. from marauding Spaniards on the coast of Chile," made the same request.[35]

When Congress opened, in November, 1818, DeForest was in Washington, now joined by his handsome young wife. By this time the commissioners sent to Buenos Aires had returned with reports that agreed that Spain could never reconquer the former viceroyalty, though they were divided on the virtue and stability of Pueyrredón's government. On the plains of Maipú, San Martín had won a great victory over the royalists of Chile. General Andrew Jackson had made his famous incursion into Florida in the summer of 1818, provoking a fresh crisis in the relations between the United States and Spain. From the congress of Aix-la-Chapelle, meeting that autumn, came the report that the European allies had agreed not to use force in the mediation under way between Spain and her revolted colonies.[36] Contemplating these diverse events, DeForest gathered renewed hope for his formal reception by the Washington authorities.

32. DeForest to Gregorio Tagle, Boston, Aug. 20, 1818, Archivo General de la Nación (Buenos Aires), S.1–A.2–A.4, no. 8.

33. On Hoadley, see George Dudley Seymour, *New Haven* (New Haven, 1942), pp. 239–243. The DeForest house stood on the northwest corner of Church and Elm streets, facing the Green. It was remodeled in 1878–1879 for Mayor Joseph B. Sargent. In 1910 it was demolished to provide a site for the new county court house. For views of the house, see *ibid.*, pp. 711–713.

34. DeForest to the selectmen of the town of Boston, Exchange Coffee House, Aug. 17, 1818, DeForest Letterbooks, Vol. 6.

35. DeForest to Lynch, Zimmerman and Co., Boston, Aug. 24, 1818; DeForest to General José de San Martín, Boston, Aug. 24, 1818, *ibid.*

36. DeForest to Tagle, Dec. 12, 1818, Archivo General de la Nación (Buenos Aires), S.1–A.2–A.4, no. 8.

Having already learned, perhaps from Aguirre with whom he had several conferences during the summer, that the question of Spanish-American independence was much mixed up with the party politics of the country,[37] DeForest now rashly undertook to follow Aguirre's mischievous example of collaborating with the opposition in Congress. He conferred with Henry Clay, leader of the anti-administration group, and with that skillful politician contrived a plan of action. They agreed that DeForest should renew his solicitations for a formal reception as consul general from the United Provinces, but in writing, so that Congress could call for the record and DeForest's notes be printed for their effect on public opinion.

In conformity with this plan, in early December, 1818, the Buenos Aires agent addressed to Secretary Adams a note requesting that he be accredited as consul general from the United Provinces of South America. DeForest submitted that his unofficial standing prevented him from protecting the commercial interests of his countrymen in American courts, thus placing him on an unequal footing with the consuls of Spain. Though he made no direct claim to a recognition of the independence of Buenos Aires, he affirmed that the reports of the commissioners lately returned thence established beyond a doubt that the United Provinces were truly independent; that their inhabitants possessed capacity for self-government; and that "they look up to this great republic as a model, and as to their elder sister, from whose sympathies and friendship they hope and expect ordinary protection at least." [38]

This communication led to a long conference with Adams on December 14. The secretary again set forth the view that to accredit DeForest as consul general would constitute a formal recognition of the government of the United Provinces. The United States, earnestly asserted Adams, was using its influence to produce a simultaneous acknowledgment of that government by other powers as well as the United States. There was reason, he continued, to believe that this influence had produced favorable effects; when the proper time came, "recognition would not be withheld." The patriots of Buenos Aires, he avowed, would one

---

37. DeForest to Tagle, Boston, Aug. 20, 1818, cited above, note 32.

38. DeForest to Adams, Washington, Dec. 9, 1818, in W. R. Manning, *Diplomatic Correspondence,* I, 515.

day be more distinctly aware of the exertions made by the American government in their behalf.

DeForest grew impatient with these diplomatic subtleties. "I am not a negotiator," he brusquely reminded Adams, "but a merchant, and my commission is only that of a Consul; should I recommend to the Supreme Director to send out here a Minister with full powers?"

"Not at present," replied the secretary, "because the objections to his reception would probably still exist." Adams then informed DeForest that the act of recognition, when made, would not involve the United States in controversy over the Banda Oriental, Santa Fé, Paraguay, or any other provinces contesting the authority of the Buenos Aires government. Further, the reported refusal of the Supreme Director Pueyrredón to accord the United States most-favored-nation treatment, on the ground that certain privileges must be reserved for Spain as a possible reward for renunciation of her claims to rule over the Río de la Plata, cast serious doubt on the integrity of the independence which the United Provinces professed to enjoy. The United States, declared Adams, would not ask any commercial favors as the price of recognition, and would regard the concession of such exclusive privileges to any other nation as "evidence rather of dependence transferred than of independence."

At DeForest's request, the secretary agreed to embody these ideas in a written answer to his caller's notes.[39] This Adams did,[40] and in a second note sharply protested against the excesses of Buenos Aires privateers and the outfitting of such vessels in North American ports in violation of the neutrality laws.[41] Even as he administered this rebuke to the Buenos Aires government, however, the secretary was drafting instructions to the United States minister in England to inform the British government that the United States would probably recognize the independence of the United Provinces "at no remote period." Only the objections of the President and other members of the cabinet ultimately caused

---

39. The sources for this interview are the account in Adams, *Memoirs*, IV, 190–192, under date of December 14; and DeForest to Tagle, Georgetown, Dec. 18, 1818, Archivo General de la Nación (Buenos Aires), S.1–A.2–A.4, no. 8. At one point I have altered the indirect discourse of Adams' entry to direct discourse, making no other change in the text.

40. Adams to DeForest, Washington, Dec. 31, 1818, W. R. Manning, *Diplomatic Correspondence*, I, 82–85.

41. Jan. 1, 1819, *ibid.*, pp. 88–89.

this statement of intention to be qualified by the phrase, "should no event occur which will justify a further postponement." [42]

On Christmas Day, 1818, with Monroe's previous consent, DeForest and his wife appeared at the President's drawing room. Monroe's republican court unstintingly admired the Connecticut beauty. DeForest did not resent the attentions lavished on his Julia. He wrote little Pastora that all the world admired her mother so much that he was afraid of losing her. "May you excel your mother in everything, my little Darling," wrote the loving parent.[43]

But the Spanish minister Onís was sorely vexed by the presence at this official reception of the unrecognized agent of a revolted province. "Last Wednesday," wrote Don Luis to his government, "finding myself at what is called here the Drawing Room, where the President and his wife hold court together, I saw a rather handsome woman in the *salon* standing beside one of my daughters next to the fireplace, which is the spot of most distinction at this time of the winter. I observed that she seemed to feel at home, and that a great many people were paying homage to her. When I asked who she was, I was told that she was Mrs. Forest, the wife of the Consul General from Buenos Ayres, and they pointed out to me, near her, an uncouth, coarse-looking man, six feet six in height,[44] saying that he was her husband, a millionaire, who a few years ago was a stableboy in this country. Without saying anything, I immediately picked up my daughters and went home, with the British Minister and his wife following me, although this might have been by chance and not for the same reason. This is the second time that I have found such gentry in this court. The first was in the time of the previous President, Mr. Madison, when I met up with the famous Gual, who then called himself Minister of Cartagena and Caracas, but having indicated my displeasure to those who could suggest to the President that he should not return, I did not see him any more. I do not think this will be the case now, because DeForest enjoys a high degree of protection, above all from Clay's party, and the Government

---

42. A. P. Whitaker, *The United States and Latin America*, p. 264; Adams to Richard Rush, Washington, Jan. 1, 1819, W. R. Manning, *Diplomatic Correspondence*, I, 87.

43. Washington, Dec. 30, 1818, G. B. Griffin Notes. This excerpt was first printed in S. F. Bemis, *Early Diplomatic Missions*, p. 81.

44. DeForest was actually 5 feet 11½ inches in height, as shown by his military record, contained in a Memorandum Book among his papers.

does not care to collide with him. Nevertheless . . . I shall continue to leave any social gathering where I find myself together with gentry of this kind, for it does not seem proper that the King's Minister should sanction with his presence the tacit recognition of these revolutionaries." [45]

A few days after this episode, the French minister Hyde de Neuville, happening to be at Adams' office, complained to the secretary of the inconvenient social aspirations of the agent from Buenos Aires and his lady. He said that DeForest had called on him, and that Mrs. DeForest had paid a visit to Madame de Neuville. "He did not know why. They must be sensible that neither he nor Madame de Neuville could return their visits." Adams assured the perplexed Frenchman that his concern was unfounded. "De Forrest was a citizen of the United States, and as such had been received at the President's. But he was not recognized as Consul from Buenos Ayres, and I myself had not returned his visit." [46]

In following the story of DeForest's efforts to secure formal recognition of his diplomatic character, and thus of his government, we must not lose sight of his interest in wresting from Spain an island in the Gulf of Mexico that should serve as a base for privateering operations, as authorized by his instructions. Although the project by which he hoped to achieve this purpose proved abortive, it illustrates in a most suggestive manner the close and complex interplay between the movement for Spanish-American independence and the steady pressure of the United States to gain strategic security and round out its borders at the expense of the dissolving Spanish empire.

In the letter from which I have just quoted, the Spanish minister Onís had more to relate concerning the activities of the troublesome agent from Buenos Aires. He informed his government that DeForest, Manuel Moreno ("a man of the greatest talents"), the Venezuelan agent Lino Clemente, and the adventurer Pierre Laffite were planning to hold one or more secret meetings with Clay and other persons "in this government." In these conferences the conspirators would discuss what must be done to secure recognition of the independence of Buenos Aires

---

45. Onís to Casa Irujo, Washington, Dec. 29, 1818, Archivo Histórico Nacional (Madrid), Estado, legajo 5643, apartado 1. This extract from Onís' despatch was first printed in S. F. Bemis, *Early Diplomatic Missions,* pp. 81–82.

46. Adams, *Memoirs,* IV, 210.

by the United States, and would also prepare a plan of attack against the possessions of his Catholic Majesty on the North American continent. This last project had the approval of the American government, because it knew that Great Britain was meditating the seizure of a port on the coast of Venezuela, or perhaps the islands of Puerto Rico and Santo Domingo, with the aid of Spanish-American corsairs; and it wished to use the rebel forces for its own ends (*trata de sacar partido del mismo plan*). The administration had therefore proposed to the filibusters that immediately after the return of Pensacola and St. Marks to Spain,[47] they should fall upon and occupy these posts and St. Augustine as well, and then turn them over to the United States! At the head of this enterprise American officials wished to install Pierre Laffite, in whom they placed great confidence, remembering his notable services at the defense of New Orleans. Yet it was Laffite, repenting his past misdeeds against Spain and avowing his sincere love for *la Patria*, who had revealed this intrigue to Onís, offering at the same time to assist in trapping and destroying the filibusters.[48]

The alarm which this cloudy report of the dubious adventurer Laffite inspired in the Spanish minister is more understandable than may appear at first view. At the close of the year 1818 the painfully protracted negotiations between Adams and Onís were at a standstill, with the two diplomatists deadlocked over the question of the international western boundary.[49] Under the circumstances, it was not unreasonable for Onís to believe that Monroe's government, despairing of a satisfactory adjustment of the dispute with Spain, might resort to measures roughly analogous to those by which President Madison, having stirred up revolt in West Florida, had been enabled to proclaim the occupation of that province in 1810, and which Monroe, then secre-

47. General Andrew Jackson had captured these places during his campaign against the Florida Indians in the spring of 1818.
48. Onís to Casa Irujo, Dec. 29, 1818, cited above, note 45. On the Laffites and their secret connections with Spain, see Harris Gaylord Warren, *The Sword Was Their Passport: A History of American Filibustering in the Mexican Revolution* (Baton Rouge, La., 1942), especially Chapters 5, 6, 9, and 10. My account of the filibustering project in which DeForest figured is largely taken from this work, pp. 214–232, and from H. G. Warren, ed., "Documents Relating to George Graham's Proposals to Jean Laffite for the Occupation of the Texas Coast," *Louisiana Historical Quarterly*, XXI (1938), 212–219.
49. Philip C. Brooks, *Diplomacy and the Borderlands: the Adams-Onís Treaty of 1819* (Berkeley, Cal., 1939), covers these negotiations authoritatively.

tary of state, had employed less successfully through the agency of General George Mathews in East Florida in 1811.[50] As a matter of fact, Laffite's allegations and Onís' fears were not entirely unfounded. The indiscretions of a presidential agent, about to be related, gave color to the belief that the United States government was conniving in rebel schemes to seize Spain's possessions in North America. In these schemes DeForest was designed to play a certain part.

A group of Napoleonic officers, ostensibly seeking a refuge for the exiled officers of the fallen emperor, made a settlement early in 1818 on the Trinity River above Galveston, thus within territory in dispute between Spain and the United States. To this colony they gave the hopeful name of Le Champ d'Asile. The French lodgment gave concern to both claimants of the debatable ground between the Sabine and the Rio Grande. It was feared that the exiles aspired to place Joseph Bonaparte on a Mexican throne. The viceroy of New Spain organized a military expedition against the French settlement. About the same time Monroe's government resolved to send an agent, George Graham, who should protest to the colonists against their occupation of American territory and ascertain the real ends of their venture. Adams suspected that the Frenchmen might actually be instruments of Spanish policy in Texas. The Graham mission also offered an opportunity to warn off the celebrated brothers Laffite. These adventurers of shifting allegiance, ousted from their smuggling and privateering establishment at Barataria by American troops in 1814, had lately installed a new seat of lawless enterprise on Galveston Island. But Adams' written instructions to Graham were silent on this subject.

The agent, arrived at Galveston on August 24, 1818, discovered that the French exiles had already fled thither from Le Champ d'Asile before the threat of a Spanish attack. Graham nevertheless made known to General Charles Lallemand, leader of the hapless settlers, his government's views as to their alleged encroachment on American territory. Lallemand proved properly submissive, and Graham, relenting, assured the Napoleonic veteran that in the event of an occupation of Galveston by the

50. On the West Florida question, see Isaac J. Cox, *The West Florida Controversy; 1798–1813, a Study in American Diplomacy* (Baltimore, 1918); on East Florida, see R. K. Wyllys, "The East Florida Revolution of 1812–1814," *Hisp. Am. Hist. Rev.*, IX (1929), 414–445, and the careful study of the Mathews affair in Julius W. Pratt, *The Expansionists of 1812* (N. Y., 1925), pp. 76–115.

United States, the members of his expedition and their property would not be harmed. Monroe's emissary then decided to seek explanations from Jean Laffite. The master of Galveston ruled over his island domain from a large, mastless brig grounded in the bay, his "dwelling, storehouse and arsenal," reported Graham to Secretary Adams.[51] In the ensuing exchange of views, Laffite avowed most disinterested motives for having come to Galveston: "that of offering asylum to the armed vessels of the revolution and that of being able . . . to fly to the aid of the United States if circumstances should demand." [52] He had not known that the United States laid claim to the entire coast from the Sabine to the Rio Grande, asserted the affable corsair, but was ready to quit Galveston as soon as he could assemble his forces.

Beguiled by these fair words, Graham now made to Jean Laffite and General Charles Lallemand a series of proposals for which his instructions gave not the least warrant. He allegedly suggested that the Laffites, the noted privateersman Louis Aury, and Lallemand should unite their forces to defend Galveston against Spanish attack. The United States would assist these filibusters in occupying successively all the points on the coast from Galveston to the Rio Grande. American forces would then go through the motions of attacking these places, which the corsairs should surrender to the United States for a suitable compensation. When Laffite observed that his privateering commissions were from the shadowy patriot government of Mexico, Graham advised him to take out patents from the more stable régime at Buenos Aires, and helpfully supplied him with a letter to Consul General DeForest at New York. All these proposals Laffite pretended to embrace, but took good care to relay them to his Spanish employers.

On his return to Washington, Graham reported to the secretary of state on his mission. He apparently failed to reveal the full scope of his negotiations with the adventurers at Galveston. Adams nevertheless registered his serious concern over the agent's proceedings in his diary.

"He had a sort of negotiation, it seems, with Lallemand and Lafitte, from which it appears that Lallemand's case is desperate. Graham's transactions with Lafitte, as related by himself, did not exactly tally with my ideas of right, and they were altogether

51. H. G. Warren, *The Sword Was Their Passport*, p. 218.
52. *Ibid.*, p. 219.

unauthorized. He says Lafitte told him that he had commissions from the Mexican Congress, but they were like Aury's commissions, and he [Graham] advised him to take a commission of Buenos Ayres, and gave him a letter to De Forrest, at New York, to assist him in obtaining one, and that Lafitte took his advice, and immediately dispatched a man to New York for that purpose. Now, I should not be surprised if we should hear more of this hereafter, and not in a very pleasant manner. But it was all of Graham's own head, and, in my opinion, not much to the credit of its wisdom. He is for taking immediate possession of Galveston, and so am I." [53]

Jean Laffite had indeed taken Graham at his word and sent an emissary, one V. Garrot, to negotiate with DeForest. Their conference took place on November 16, 1818, in Philadelphia. Since DeForest did not speak French, an interpreter was present. After reading the letter from Graham, which asked him to give Pierre Laffite "the flag with the dispatches from Buenos Aires," and to name the authorities who should head the government to be established by the corsairs in the Gulf of Mexico, the rebel agent displayed a lively interest in the filibustering project. He asked Garrot on what point of the Spanish dominions Laffite planned to make his establishment.

The messenger replied that no decision had been reached on that subject. Operations of such importance required mature deliberation. He presumed that Laffite had fixed his attention more particularly on the Gulf of Mexico, but about the rest nothing could be said with certainty. If DeForest could obtain from President Monroe a promise that the United States would postpone the occupation of Galveston for one year, suggested Garrot, during that time the corsairs could be engaged in selecting another convenient port.

DeForest agreed to make this request of the President. Learning from Garrot that Laffite had six ships at his command, the Buenos Aires agent seemed impressed, and observed that if these forces were joined with Aury's it would be possible to take possession of Puerto Rico or Santo Domingo. After giving assurances of his full support to Laffite's enterprise, DeForest informed Garrot that he would leave for Baltimore in a few days to arrange with the merchant Thomas Tenant for the necessary arms and supplies. Then he would go to Washington, where he hoped to

53. Adams, *Memoirs*, IV, 175–176.

"SOUTH AMERICAN WITCHERY"   151

meet with Pierre Laffite.⁵⁴ Pierre was then in the capital, conferring with Onís.

The affair made progress, and by the end of December, 1818, DeForest could send the following note to Manuel Moreno, now his trusted lieutenant:

"The time has now arrived when I shall probably be able to come to a determination to relate the plan I spoke to you about when I last saw you. The Gentlemen who have the power to carry the plan into Execution, arrived here last evening; and if you will come up here on Monday I have no doubt something will be done very much to your advantage, for, my object will be to chasten the enemies of Buenos Ayres in a honorable way; and to place you where you can make a fortune rapidly." ⁵⁵

Gathered in secret conclave at Washington, as foretold by Pierre Laffite to Onís, Pierre, DeForest, Moreno, and possibly others, concerted their plans. They agreed that Moreno should take command of the projected expedition against "some port or place in or near the Gulf of Mexico." The precise point of attack was apparently left for later determination, but DeForest seems to have contemplated a descent on Florida. The size of the armada to be employed is suggested by a letter from DeForest to Manuel Lynch in New York, directing him to deliver to Moreno twenty privateering patents for craft of the following description: one ship, seven brigs, and twelve schooners.⁵⁶ Moreno, acting as representative of the Supreme Director Pueyrredón of Buenos Aires, would hold the occupied territory as a colony of the United Provinces, "under whose laws it should be governed as a rendezvous for the privateers of that country." ⁵⁷ The promoters even settled the mode of division of the anticipated spoils. "Moreno and No. 19 [Pierre Laffite] will have a part of all the cargoes taken by them, all the payments incurred for anchorage, condemnation, and other charges which they will divide between them; one per cent will be given to Consul Forestt, who will issue corsair commissions, and one per cent will be for the Minister of Buenos Ayres who has signed said commissions." ⁵⁸

54. Garrot to Pierre Laffite, Philadelphia, Nov. 17, 1818, in H. G. Warren, ed., "Documents Relating to George Graham's Proposals to Pierre Laffite."
55. DeForest to Manuel Moreno, Georgetown, Dec. 26, 1818, DeForest Letterbooks, Vol. 6.
56. DeForest to Manuel Lynch, Washington, Jan. 6, 1819, *ibid.*
57. DeForest to Henry Didier, Washington, Jan. 4, 1819, *ibid.*
58. H. G. Warren, *The Sword Was Their Passport*, p. 228.

As late as the middle of January, 1819, DeForest buoyantly envisaged the rise of a new and more successful Amelia Island, a privateering paradise whither the corsairs of Buenos Aires could conveniently bring Spanish prizes for summary condemnation by Laffite's henchman Garrot, designated in the plan as prize-court judge. He brushed aside certain objections advanced by the more cautious Henry Didier of Baltimore. "The negotiations between this Country and Spain," argued DeForest, "appear to be pretty much at an end: and the U. S. cannot consider it any interference with her affairs, if any enemy of Spain should take possession of Florida. The thing is practicable; and I am confident the U. S. would not complain in the least. If effected, and the War with Spain ended, a cession of it might be profitably made to the U. States . . ."[59]

These rash assertions of course overlooked Secretary Adams' emphatic warning to DeForest, given in his second interview with the Buenos Aires agent, that the United States would not tolerate a rebel occupation of Florida. Nor were the negotiations between Adams and Onís as moribund as DeForest believed. On January 11, 1819, after receiving authority from his government to reopen the suspended treaty negotiations, Onís wrote to the secretary proposing to renew their conversations with a view to further compromise.[60] Thereafter negotiations proceeded at an accelerated pace, and on February 22, 1819, Adams scored his greatest diplomatic triumph with the signing of the treaty by which Florida became American territory and the boundary of the United States was drawn clear across the continent to the Pacific Ocean.

This happy and unexpected consummation immediately destroyed DeForest's filibustering hopes. He forthwith severed his connections with the Laffites, whose integrity he had evidently begun to doubt, and fixed his attention again on the central struggle for his official reception by the government of the United States as consul general from the United Provinces.

Early in January, 1819, DeForest sent a carefully prepared reply to Adams' two notes of December 31, 1818, and January 1, 1819. He reiterated his contention that the reception of a

59. DeForest to Henry Didier, Georgetown, Jan. 13, 1819, DeForest Letterbooks, Vol. 6.
60. P. C. Brooks, *Diplomacy and the Borderlands*, p. 155.

consular agent from Buenos Aires was a distinct and separate question from an acknowledgment of independence. "I do not profess to be skilled in the laws of nations, nor of diplomacy . . .; yet I must say, that I cannot understand the difference between the sending of a consular agent duly authorized to Buenos Ayres, where one was accredited from this country, four or five years ago, and has continued ever since, in the exercise of the duties of his office, and the reception of a similar agent here." He only sought to be received as a consular agent, "having never agitated the question of an acknowledgment of our independence as a nation, which most certainly is anxiously desired by the Government and people of South America, but which, being a political question, I have never asked." [61]

This note was clearly timed to accord with an appropriate move by anti-administration forces in Congress. On January 14, 1819, Clay's group pushed through a resolution requesting information as to whether any independent government in South America had asked for recognition of a minister or consul general, and what reply had been made.

This latest attempt to embarrass the administration with the "great South American witchery" moved the harassed Adams to bitter reflection. "In this affair," he confided to his diary, "everything is invidious and factious. The call is made for the purpose of baiting the administration, and especially in fastening upon the Secretary of State the odium of refusing to receive South American Ministers and Consul-Generals. I am walking on a rope, with a precipice on each side of me, and without human aid beyond myself upon which to rely. . . . DeForrest's notes are cunning and deceptive. To the last and longest of them I have not replied. It must be sent in under the call, and if unaccompanied by a refutation of its contents, advantage will be taken of it to censure the course of the Executive, and perhaps even to force the recognition of the Southern independents. I must, therefore, demolish the arguments in De Forrest's last note, which is indeed not a difficult task, but which must take time and many words." [62]

Thereupon the sturdy little secretary set himself to the task of replying to DeForest's "cunning and deceptive" note. This state-

61. DeForest to Adams, Georgetown, Jan. 8, 1819, W. R. Manning, *Diplomatic Correspondence*, IV, 516–519.
62. Adams, *Memoirs*, IV, 223–224, under date of Jan. 20, 1819.

ment, together with the correspondence he had exchanged with DeForest and Lino de Clemente of Venezuela, Adams sent in to the President for transmission to Congress.

The secretary of state explained that the government had declined to have further communication with Clemente because he had been one of those who signed the commission of the adventurer Gregor MacGregor to take possession of Amelia Island. DeForest was charged with no offense, but his credentials were void because they were founded on Worthington's unauthorized treaty. "Mr. De Forest's credential letter asks that he may be received by virtue of a stipulation in supposed articles concluded by Mr. Worthington, but which he was not authorized to make; so that the reception of Mr. De Forest, upon the credential on which he founds his claim, would imply a recognition, not only of the Government of the Supreme Director, Pueyrredón, but a compact as binding upon the United States, which is a mere nullity." Adams also noted that in the previous May the agent had declared himself entirely content with his informal reception, but that "shortly after the commencement of the present session of Congress" he had renewed his solicitations.[63] The secretary thus indicated his suspicion that DeForest was collaborating with Clay's opposition group.

Adams was now resolved to rid himself forever of the troublesome envoy from Buenos Aires. When DeForest called at his office again, on January 22, 1819, Adams found occasion to remind his visitor that he was still a citizen of the United States and hence liable to prosecution for violation of the neutrality laws.

Disquiet was suddenly written on DeForest's face. "When I informed you that I had no intention of returning to Buenos Aires, but had come finally to settle here," he said, "I did not expect the information would ever be used against me. Would I be considered by law to have been a citizen of the United States while at Buenos Aires?"

"It is unnecessary for me to give you an opinion on that point," replied Adams. "You had better consult a lawyer upon it. It is not my intention to make any use to your disadvantage of anything you have said to me. Although the information you gave me was voluntary, under no injunction of secrecy or intimation of confidence, I have never mentioned it to any other person than the

---

63. Adams to President James Monroe, Washington, Jan. 28, 1819, W. R. Manning, *Diplomatic Correspondence*, I, 89–94.

President, and shall never notice it publicly unless it should be necessary in the discharge of my public duties. But it is in candor due to you to let you know that the recognition of yourself as Consul General of Buenos Aires, should it hereafter be granted, will in no wise divest you of your character as a citizen of the United States."

Somewhat reassured by Adams' words, DeForest unburdened himself to the secretary. "For the last seventeen years," he said, "I have resided principally at Buenos Aires, and have become a citizen of that country. In their revolutionary struggle with Spain I have taken a very decided and active part, particularly in the business of privateering. I have now returned to this country with the view of remaining here, and am building a house at New Haven. But if Spanish subjects can molest me here for what I did while an inhabitant of Buenos Aires my situation will be very perilous."

DeForest also confirmed what Adams had suspected—that he had conferred with Clay on the question of recognition. He assured the secretary, however, that he was now convinced that Clay's proceedings had injured rather than aided the patriot cause; he, DeForest, was entirely satisfied with the Spanish-American policy of the administration.[64]

Adams' veiled threat had served its purpose. DeForest beat a precipitate retreat from Washington, settled down in New Haven, and never again crossed the path of the formidable secretary of state. The shadows of his privateering past already hung darkly about him. "You do not appear to know," he was soon writing to former associates in Buenos Aires, "how much anxiety I have had on account of my fears of suits brought by Spanish claimants, although I have openly pretended to the contrary. Captain M[arcena] Monson, however, has always shown his fears, and even to this day keeps very retired, and has no property except what is covered by some friend." [65]

In its own good time Monroe's government accorded to the new Spanish-American states that recognition for which De-Forest had unsuccessfully labored. When the President sent his

---

64. This account of DeForest's last interview with Adams is based on the entry in the latter's *Memoirs*, IV, 225. I have altered indirect to direct discourse, but have made no change in the original sense of this material.

65. DeForest to Lynch and Zimmerman, New Haven, July 2, 1820, DeForest Letterbooks, Vol. 7.

celebrated message to Congress of March 8, 1822, recommending an appropriation for the dispatch of diplomatic missions to five of these states—the United Provinces of Río de La Plata, Chile, Peru, Colombia, and Mexico—he did so not in consequence of partisan political pressure but from a variety of considerations in which the decisive victories of patriot armies, the final ratification of the Adams-Onís Treaty by Spain, the passing of the danger of European intervention, the desire to strengthen the influence of the United States in Spanish America, and Adams' belief that the legal conditions for recognition had at last been satisfied, all played a certain part. Congress, almost without a dissenting voice, voted the required appropriation on May 4, 1822.

Monroe's message encouraged DeForest to write to Secretary Adams, claiming for Buenos Aires the honor of being the first state to be recognized, with himself as *chargé d'affaires* and consul general. Adams replied that as an American citizen he could not serve as *chargé d'affaires*; that his invalid credentials did not entitle him to be received as consul general; and that the department had been notified of the intention of the new government of Buenos Aires to revoke DeForest's commission.[66] Manuel Torres, the aged and infirm representative of Colombia, had the distinction of being first to be received. Formal diplomatic relations with the United Provinces of La Plata were established by the appointment of Caesar A. Rodney as first United States minister to that country (January 27, 1823).

In June, 1823, DeForest received official notification from the new Rivadavia government of the recall of his commission as consul general. He was to send to Buenos Aires his archives, together with any remaining privateering patents and an explanation of the status of those he had used.[67] In a belated reply to Rivadavia, DeForest pleaded the want of a "convenient opportunity" for not having written earlier. Perhaps he feared to send the incriminating privateering material in his possession by ordinary channels. There is evidence that Spanish agents intercepted at least one letter directed to him.[68] DeForest complained

66. W. R. Manning, *Diplomatic Correspondence,* I, 159–160.
67. Bernardino Rivadavia to DeForest, March 13, 1823, in *Documentos para la historia argentina,* XIV, 202–203.
68. In the Archivo Histórico Nacional (Madrid), Estado, legajo 5567, expediente 13, there is an intercepted letter from the noted Argentine patriot Tomás Guido to DeForest, sent from Guayaquil, Jan. 3, 1821. Guido wrote that he would continue to keep DeForest informed concerning developments in "this important

that Rivadavia's communication was the first he had received from the government of Buenos Aires since the establishment of the new régime in 1821; and that this note did not even acknowledge receipt of any dispatches from him, "of which I have made many, most of them in triplicate. Nor does it intimate to me how and when, I am to be rewarded for my services, during the time I have been in their employ." He bore his adopted country no ill will, however, on that account. "With my best wishes for the happiness of Buenos Aires, I have the honor to remain . . . David C. DeForest." [69]

It was not until September 23, 1824, one year later, that a messenger turned over DeForest's official archives to the first recognized minister to the United States from Buenos Aires, Carlos de Alvear.[70] They included, in addition to the exchanges of notes with Secretary Adams, 432 unused privateering patents and officers' commissions that had been issued to DeForest in connection with his mission to North America, and two used and surrendered patents.[71] With this action DeForest wrote *finis* to the diplomatic chapter of his career. His qualities of a pertinacious, bold, and resourceful fighter had not availed to change the set course of the Spanish-American policy of the United States, guided by the firm and skillful hand of John Quincy Adams.

section of the globe, in whose fate you have always displayed such a lively interest."

69. DeForest to Bernardino Rivadavia, New Haven, Sept. 7, 1823, Archivo General de la Nación (Buenos Aires), S.1–A.2–A.4, no. 8.

70. Dr. Thomas B. Davis, Jr., is preparing for publication a study of Alvear's mission to the United States. For an important aspect of this mission, see T. B. Davis, Jr., "Carlos de Alvear and James Monroe: New Light on the Monroe Doctrine," *Hisp. Am. Hist. Rev.*, XXIII (1943), 632–649.

71. Memorandum of Carlos de Alvear, acknowledging receipt of DeForest's official archives, New York, Sept. 24, 1824 (copy), Archivo General de la Nación (Buenos Aires), S.1–A.2–A.4, no. 10.

XI

EPILOGUE

SINCE the early months of 1819, conforming with the broad hint of Secretary Adams not to annoy the administration any more with his diplomatic attentions, DeForest had quietly resided in the town of New Haven. With commerce he had no further concern. Until the middle of 1823 he continued to style himself consul general of the United Provinces of South America, a title flattering to his vanity, but this shadowy office imposed no serious duties. For the rest, he had only to enjoy the leisure that his ample means made possible. One of his first actions on returning to New Haven was to search out and reimburse with interest the creditors of his youthful venture in Maine. In his prosperity he was mindful of his brothers and other kinsmen; among his relatives DeForest divided $15,000, no inconsiderable fortune for those days.[1]

The stately house on the Green that David Hoadley had built was ready for occupation on July 1, 1820. Contemporaries of DeForest regarded his house as "the handsomest residence in the state."[2] In the basement of his home the envoy from Buenos Aires placed a marble tablet engraved on both sides. On one side was an inscription recording the names, with dates and places of birth, of himself, his wife, and his five children. On the other side was a whimsical injunction to future owners of the house ever to honor the anniversary of the Revolution of Buenos Aires.

"To the owner of this House.
David C. DeForest,
A native citizen of Huntington in this state; and at present Consul General of the United Provinces of South America, of which Buenos Ayres is the Capital, where he

---

1. J. W. De Forest, *The de Forests of Avesnes,* p. 156.
2. Henry Howe, "New Haven's Elms and Green," Chap. 20, *Daily Morning Journal and Courier* (New Haven), Jan. 1, 1884.

resided for many years; and
assisted in establishing its
Independence. greeting.
I have caused this
beautiful building to be erected
for your use, as well as mine; &
have taken much pains to accom
odate you, for which you will
never pay; & being no relative of
mine, I demand: that you assemble
your friends together on every
25th day of May in honor of
the Independence of South
America; it being on that day
in the year 1810, that the
Inhabitants of
Buenos Ayres
established a free Government
New Haven, 1820

David Hoadley, Arch't.
Horace Butler, Mason   D. Ritter, Sculp." [3]

The coming of the Don, as New Haveners were quick to call the swarthy man from Buenos Aires, was a memorable event in the life of the little town. The mystery of DeForest's reputedly vast fortune excited speculation; and about him gossip weaved tales that grew in the telling. In this wise the Don acquired the fame of having been a pirate. A genial story-teller of the last century who spent some youthful years in "getting learning" at Yale College attests to the persuasive power of this legend. Recalling DeForest as a stern man with black-eyed lovely daughters and a son called Carlos who was handsome but effeminate, he comments: "I never saw him that I did not dream of bloody decks, fierce sea fights, a pirate's doom, and I had a general idea that his cellar, instead of containing barrels of cider, metheglin, and bins of apples, was filled with kegs of Spanish gold coin, diamond necklaces, finger rings, and breast-pins, in barrels. To me the Don was a mystery never solved." [4]

3. This tablet is now in the possession of the New Haven Colony Historical Society of New Haven.
4. [Joseph A. Scoville], *The Old Merchants of New York City,* by Walter Barrett, clerk (5 ser., N. Y., 1863–1870), IV, 204–205.

In recital to the youngest and most credulous sort, this fable was appropriately embellished. Imaginative parents told their offspring that in the cellar of DeForest's mansion was a deep sink or well containing hogsheads of doubloons. Monstrous serpents, kept there for the purpose, guarded the treasure. "So great was the terror inspired by this statement that often small children on their way to school avoided passing by the house for fear those snakes would be out after them." [5] Yet the Don was kind to children, and his friendliness sometimes conquered the dread that his fame inspired. "He was a pompous, arbitrary man," recalled one contemporary, "but I loved as well as feared him, as he always had a playful word or a ready joke for children who he knew." [6]

In New Haven, as in Buenos Aires, DeForest practiced a hospitality that also became legendary. His great house, says one account, was open to "the wise, the witty, the struggling scholar, and the grace and fashion of town." [7] To his receptions at seven o'clock in the evening came many distinguished folk, among them James Gates Percival, the shy poet-geologist and New Haven's literary lion; DeForest's counsel and particular friend Judge David Daggett; and the learned lexicographer Noah Webster. When General Lafayette came to New Haven in August, 1824, it was at the home of "David C. DeForest, esquire, late consul general from Buenos Ayres and the provinces of the Rio de la Plata," that he paused to take refreshment and rest from his triumphal procession through the town. DeForest was then away, placing one of his daughters in a Montreal school, and it was his wife who received the comrade of Washington at the door, no doubt with three profound curtsies, an importation from Spanish America not wholly approved by the sober people of New Haven. The editor of the *Columbian Register* duly noted the impressions of the revolutionary hero. "No such splendid mansion, with its brilliant furniture, was here in 1778. From the portico in front he surveyed the beautiful Green, full of people, with the long line of troops, the buildings around, and the fine foliage of the trees. A lively sensibility at once appeared. He was struck with the beauty of the scene. Such another prospect can

---

5. Henry Howe, "New Haven's Elms and Green," Chap. 20, *Daily Morning Journal and Courier* (New Haven), Jan. 1, 1884.
6. "New Haven in Old Times," *Daily Palladium* (New Haven), Feb. 24, 1869.
7. "A Former Townsman," *Daily Morning Journal and Courier* (New Haven), Feb. 21, 1873.

hardly be presented in America." [8] Later, standing under the portrait of DeForest by Samuel F. B. Morse, Lafayette drank a toast to the absent master of the house.

Morse painted two portraits of DeForest in 1823. At that period the "American Leonardo" [9] was living with his father Jedidiah, the celebrated geographer, on Hillhouse Avenue in New Haven. Morse's attention was already divided between art and inventions, with neither pursuit proving very profitable, and he undoubtedly rejoiced to receive this message from the local magnate:

"Mr. D. C. DeForest's compliments to Mr. Morse. Mr. DeForest desires to have his portrait taken such as it would have been six or eight years ago, making the necessary calculations for it, and at the same time making it a good likeness in all other respects. The reason is not to make himself younger, but to appear to children and grandchildren more suitably matched as to age with their mother and grandmother." [10]

For this portrait DeForest sat in a riding dress of blue coat and red vest that heightened the desired youthful appearance. Morse painted a spruce and vigorous gentleman whose features express energy, shrewdness, and good humor. About this time Morse also painted a companion portrait of Mrs. DeForest in the yellow satin dress she wore at President Monroe's drawing-room in 1818. This canvas brilliantly communicates the classic beauty that Monroe's republican court so greatly admired. These portraits now hang in the Yale University Art Gallery.

For presentation to the Academy of La Unión del Sud in Buenos Aires, which his donation had helped to found, DeForest commissioned Morse to paint a second and more authentic likeness of himself. In this picture DeForest is dressed in a formal suit of black. From the lapel of his coat hangs what appears to be a badge decorated with the blue-and-white Argentine colors. The head, observes a student of this canvas, is a superb pictorial and psychological synthesis, in which the prematurely gray hair contrasts with the face, still smooth and ruddy "in that intensive second youth which Providence is wont to bestow on generous natures as they near the fifty year mark." The heavy eyebrows,

8. J. W. De Forest, *The de Forests of Avesnes*, p. 155.
9. Carleton Mabee, *The American Leonardo, A Life of Samuel F. B. Morse* (N. Y., 1943).
10. Letter dated New Haven, March 30, 1823. Edward Lind Morse, *Samuel F. B. Morse: His Letters and Journals* (2 vols., Boston, 1914), I, 243.

the compressed lips, the solid and obstinate chin, bespeak energy and daring. But this effect is softened by a cordial, almost benign expression: "Neither gravity nor ostentation; a frank, affectionate, and absolute simplicity." [11]

This portrait DeForest sent to Buenos Aires together with a number of other artistic pieces: an engraving of a symbolic representation of the independence of the United States, with the coats of arms of the thirteen original states and a copy of the Declaration of Independence of July 4, 1776, with "facsimiles of the signatures of the great and good men who constituted the Congress that made it"; an engraving by Asher B. Durand of John Trumbull's painting of the signing of the Declaration, "containing the portraits of the members of the North American Congress of 1776"; and a landscape by Henry C. Pratt, a pupil of Morse, depicting the DeForest mansion in New Haven and some adjacent buildings. "Of these paintings," wrote DeForest with patriotic pride, "permit me to assure you, Sir, that all, and every part thereof, is the work of Americans. The landscape is sent to show the style of Architecture in this part of the New World, and a Mansion on which waves the Flag of South America on every twenty-fifth of May, surrounded and cheered by the inhabitants of the little city in which it stands." [12]

These tokens of his friendship DeForest sent to Buenos Aires in charge of the first United States minister to the provinces of the Río de la Plata, Caesar A. Rodney, who duly delivered them to President Achega of the Academy of La Unión del Sud. The portrait of DeForest by Morse, unsigned by the artist, hung in the halls of the University of Buenos Aires until the close of the nineteenth century, when it was placed in the newly founded Museo Nacional de Bellas Artes. About 1910 the then director of the Museo officially ascribed the unknown masterpiece to the Spanish painter Goya; and this attribution was accepted until 1921, when a letter of inquiry from Dr. Louis S. de Forest, a relative of DeForest, reopened the question. Subsequently evidence sent from the United States conclusively established that Morse had painted the anonymous canvas. The whereabouts of the other art objects sent by DeForest is unknown.

11. Atilio Chiáppori, *Maestros y temperamentos* (Buenos Aires, 1943), "Un Goya yanqui y un yanqui porteño," pp. 105–106.
12. DeForest to Domingo Vicente de Achega, President of the University of La Unión del Sud, New Haven, April 10, 1823, DeForest Letterbooks, Vol. 8.

EPILOGUE

As mentioned in his letter to President Achega, DeForest had already begun annual celebrations in New Haven of the Argentine Independence Day, the twenty-fifth of May. The first such commemoration was held in 1821. "On Friday the 25th inst.," reported the *Columbian Register*, "the anniversary of the independence of Buenos Ayres was celebrated in this city in handsome style. The day was ushered in by the discharge of a national salute. At about 11 o'clock, a. m., a large company of gentlemen assembled at Butler's County Hotel, agreeably to a general invitation which had been publicly given in the newspapers; but the concourse was so great that it was found necessary to adjourn to the State House, where a neat and appropriate address was delivered by Robert Lockwood, Esq. After which the company returned to Butler's Hotel, and drank a number of patriotic toasts, and partook of some refreshments which had been prepared for the occasion. At noon and sunset the national salute was repeated. Soon after 8 o'clock, p. m., a very numerous company of ladies and gentlemen convened at the elegant mansion of Don David C. DeForest, and passed the evening in great hilarity."

The friends of South American liberty drank to "the city of Buenos Ayres," to "General San Martín and the Army of Peru," to "the gallant little navy of Chile," and finally a fervent toast went up to "the Holy Alliance and the Devil—may the friends of liberty check their career, and compel them to dissolve partnership." [13]

DeForest held a similar observance in 1822. Before the next twenty-fifth of May he had been divested of his consular office, but during the brief years of life that remained to him he continued to commemorate, more simply and privately, the day that had marked a turning point in the history of the Río de la Plata and in his personal fortunes.

The Don gave one more proof of loyalty and attachment to his adopted country. At his suggestion, six young Argentines came to the United States, intrusted to his care, in order to study English and otherwise prepare themselves for mercantile careers. First to come was Manuel Lynch, a brother of DeForest's former partner in Buenos Aires. Manuel went to school at an academy in Hudson, New York, served an apprenticeship in the counting-

---

13. *Columbian Register* (New Haven), May 26, 1821; see also *Connecticut Herald* (New Haven), May 28, 1821.

house of Lockwood De Forest in New York City, and having completed his training sailed for home at the end of 1819.[14] Other youthful *porteños* followed him to North America: Pedro Martínez y García, José María and Francisco Rodríguez de Vida, Patricio Basabilbaso, and Pedro J. Trellechea. Some DeForest placed in the academy at Hudson; others he sent to a nearby school in Huntington.[15] After gaining a competent knowledge of English, these lads were expected to acquire practical commercial experience in a counting-house. Although their relations were generally harmonious, some sharp clashes of wills occurred between DeForest and his charges. Of Pedro Martínez y García, "a very gentlemanly and well behaved young man," he wrote that "we have never differed except on the amount of money he ought to spend. He feels much hurt at my foolish ideas." [16] It is worthy of note that young Patricio Basabilbaso took advantage of his sojourn in the United States to court and marry a North American bride before returning to Buenos Aires where he became a prosperous merchant.[17] Many years were to pass before DeForest's pioneering conception would be taken up by governments, universities, and private foundations to become an accepted and integral feature of inter-American cultural relations.

Having assisted in the foundation of the first seat of higher learning in the land of his adoption, DeForest fittingly enough became a benefactor of Yale College in the town of New Haven where he had made his home. In 1821 he offered to the college a donation of $5,000, to be held at 6 per cent interest until January 1, 1850, when the principal, amounting to $25,941, should yield an annual interest of $1,556, to be expended as follows: $1,000 for the support and education of DeForest's assigns at the college; $500 for the purchase of books, maps, and charts to be placed in an alcove of the college library, with the name of DeForest written thereon and on each volume or other item thus purchased; and $56 to purchase a gold medal to be awarded to the best orator of the senior class, and to be called the DeForest medal.[18]

14. DeForest to Patricio Lynch, New Haven, Oct. 14, 1819, DeForest Letterbooks, Vol. 7.
15. DeForest to José Rodríguez de Vida, New Haven, Oct. 13, 1819, *ibid.*
16. DeForest to Manuel Martínez y García, New Haven, Oct. 2, 1819, *ibid.*
17. E. Udaondo, *Diccionario biográfico argentino,* p. 129.
18. DeForest to his Excellency Ethan A. Brown, Governor of the State of Ohio, New Haven, Nov. 5, 1821, DeForest Letterbooks, Vol. 8.

EPILOGUE

When this proposal was laid before the corporation of Yale College, in meeting assembled, it appears to have raised a storm of controversy. According to DeForest himself, several of the trustees opposed acceptance of the gift, "principally on the ground of its having a tendency to the establishment of an aristocracy; and although a majority was in favor of it they did not press a vote then, but adjourned its further consideration till the next commencement." [19] J. W. De Forest, in his family history, affirms that the opposition was led by a certain unnamed trustee, "a locally illustrious gentleman," who had just donated $1,000 to the college library and whose feelings were hurt by the magnitude of DeForest's offering.[20] The records of Yale College, silent on this point, disclose only that on September 11, 1821, the president and fellows of the college "voted that the Proposal of David C. DeForest to deposit $5,000 in the Treasury of this Corporation on certain terms and conditions be [laid over to] the next meeting of the Board, and that James Hillhouse and Elizur Goodrich, Esq.ˢ be a committee to confer with Mr. DeForest on the subject of said Proposal." [21] According to DeForest's biographer-nephew, this committee requested the would-be benefactor to withhold his donation until the dissenting minority of the board could be reconciled to it.[22]

DeForest, never one to bear slights with equanimity, was understandably resentful of this rebuff. In his anger he considered offering his $5,000 on the same terms to the projected State University of Ohio, and actually began negotiations toward that end.[23] But he may have thought better of it, or perhaps the legislature of Ohio was equally suspicious of aristocratic influences, for when Secretary Goodrich and Treasurer Hillhouse called on DeForest again in 1823 he was ready to renew his tender to Yale College with somewhat altered conditions. Now he proposed that $1,000 of the anticipated annual income of the fund, amounting to $1,556 in 1852, should be devoted for the education and support at Yale College of four direct male descendants of his mother, Mrs. Mehitable Lockwood, and "in default of such descendants the same sum to be applied to the education of others

19. *Ibid.*
20. J. W. De Forest, *The de Forests of Avesnes*, p. 157.
21. DeForest Fund Records, Yale College 1823 to ———, in Yale Memorabilia Room, Yale University Library.
22. J. W. De Forest, *The de Forests of Avesnes*, p. 157.
23. DeForest to his Excellency Ethan A. Brown, New Haven, Nov. 5, 1821, cited above, note 18.

of the name of DeForest, giving preference to the next of kin of the donor," or, in default of candidates of that name, to indigent young men of good talents who would assume the name of DeForest. The donor assumed that $1,000 would support and educate four scholars each year, but "as this may depend on the value of money and other articles, nothing definite can be determined." He further stipulated that "in the selection of candidates for the bounty herein provided, the Religious or Political opinions of themselves or their families should not operate against or for them, in any case; but a preference shall always be given to those who are of moral and virtuous conduct; and it is left wholly at the discretion of the Corporation of Yale College to make the selection." In addition, there should be presented an annual gold medal worth $100, for superiority in English composition and declamation, the president and professors being judges, and every member of the senior class a candidate for the prize.[24]

The lone trustee mentioned above, supported by one member of the faculty, again opposed accepting DeForest's gift. He is reported to have denounced it as un-American: "It is contrary to the spirit of our American institutions. It is an attack upon republican equality. Here is a family which is to have special privileges; its young men are to be made literary aristocrats. As an American, I protest against it." [25] But on September 9, 1823, the corporation overrode his protests and voted to accept DeForest's offer. The fund finally accumulated and became available in 1852. In 1864 the DeForest heirs agreed to an alteration in the terms of the scholarships fund, so that—in default of DeForests—other qualified candidates need not change their names. To this day the David C. DeForest Scholarships and gold medal for oratory are coveted prizes at Yale University.

The Don continued to give generously of his time and money to liberal causes and to charitable works. When the citizens of New Haven assembled at the county house on December 17, 1823, "for the purpose of concerting measures to aid the Greeks in their glorious struggle for independence," David C. DeForest was elected along with his friends David Daggett and Noah Webster to the committee on resolutions.[26] Two months later the

24. *A Copy of the Acts and Doings Respecting the DeForest Fund at Yale College in New Haven (Conn.), Established in the Month of September, 1823.* New Haven, S. M. Dutton, printer, 1823.
25. J. W. De Forest, *The de Forests of Avesnes,* p. 157.
26. *Columbian Register,* Dec. 20, 1823.

EPILOGUE

Register carried an account of a feast "given at the Alms-House in this town, to the poor, in commemoration of Washington's birth day, by David C. DeForest, Esq. which is the third and not the least dinner served up in style at 4 o'clock, and abundant."[27] Hospitable as ever, DeForest's "feasts of grapes" attracted particular mention. The discriminating editor of the *Register* reported of one of these affairs that "the grapes were all excellent of their kind, but those denominated the La Fayette, were very superior in flavor and richness."[28]

New Haveners did not suspect that this worthy citizen and pleasant host was beset by tormenting fears that very likely contributed to his prematurely gray hair and hastened his death. The lawsuits that he had sought to avoid, threatening disgrace and the forced restitution of his privateering profits, became painful reality by 1821. One suit concerned the Spanish merchantman *Sereno*, taken by the patriot corsair *Congreso* in 1816, and illegally condemned by the Buenos Aires prize court.[29] The Royal Philippine Company commenced another action for the value of their ship *Triton* and its cargo, taken by Captain Marcena Monson of the *Tupac-Amarú*.[30] Against these attempts on his fortune and honor, for so he regarded them, DeForest conducted a vigorous legal defense. He was immersed in these affairs when, on a wintry evening in February, 1825, he fell ill. The next day he was waging a losing struggle with pneumonia; and on February 22 he died, aged fifty-one. He was buried in the Grove Street Cemetery of New Haven, in the presence of a great number of mourners. "There were so many country wagons hitched along the fences of the Green," wrote an eye-witness, "that one was reminded of the fourth of July."[31] From the poor of the town came a laboriously worded message of sympathy for DeForest's wife and children.

Of the eight children born to DeForest in Buenos Aires and

27. *Ibid.*, Feb. 28, 1824.
28. *Ibid.*, Oct. 9, 1824.
29. There is a docket on the case of the *Sereno*, containing proceedings from 1816 to 1818, in the archives of the United States district court at Baltimore. In the Spanish archives is a memorandum or note on the case which indicates that in 1827 it was settled in favor of the Spanish claimants, who collected $25,000 from DeForest's heirs. Archivo Histórico Nacional (Madrid), Estado, legajo 5561, expediente 13.
30. J. H. DeForest to John Wells, New Haven, May 29, 1821, DeForest Letterbooks, Vol. 8.
31. J. W. De Forest, *The de Forests of Avesnes*, p. 160 n.

New Haven, only three daughters and two sons lived to maturity. The three girls, all acclaimed for their beauty, made excellent marriages.[32] David Curtis, bold and adventurous like his father, took to the sea; in January, 1838, aged only eighteen, he fell to his death from the masthead of a sealing vessel in the south Pacific. Carlos María, less vigorous in body and temper, left New Haven at an early age and settled in Bradford County in Western Pennsylvania, where he lived and died obscurely. Julia DeForest did not marry again. A visitor to Saratoga Springs in the summer of 1833 often saw "the accomplished widow" on the arm of the courtly Vice-President of the United States, Martin Van Buren.[33] She died in New Haven at the dawn of New Year's Day, 1873, aged seventy-seven, having survived her husband almost forty-eight years.

The career of David C. DeForest spans and embodies a quarter-century of relations between the United States and Buenos Aires in the great epoch of Spanish-American emancipation. That quarter-century witnessed, to use the happy phrase of Professor Arthur P. Whitaker, the discovery of Latin America by the people of the United States. The progressive disintegration of the Spanish Empire in America opened the way for a notable increase of commercial, ideological, and political contacts between the republic of the North and the former Spanish colonies. The consciousness of a common opportunity and a common peril in the face of a hostile monarchical Europe inspired sentiments of hemispheric solidarity and yearnings for inter-American collaboration in the struggle against Spanish tyranny. A multitude of North Americans actually foreswore neutrality and rendered effective military assistance to the rebels. The friendly government of the United States opened its ports to rebel cruisers, permitted the free flow of munitions to the patriots, and conducted a vigorous diplomatic defense of the new states against the menace of an armed European intervention. An outpouring of books, pamphlets, and newspaper articles in the United States informed interested readers concerning the progress of the revolutionary struggle in Spanish America. Cultural relations multiplied as

32. Francisca Tomasa Isabel, the eldest daughter, married a son of Judge Van Ness of Columbia County, New York; Julia Nicanora married a son of Hiland Hill, a banker of Catskill, New York; and the youngest daughter, Pastora Jacoba, married a son of the prominent New York City lawyer, George Griffin.

33. Henry Wikoff, *The Reminiscences of an Idler* (N. Y., 1880), p. 59.

learned societies in the United States entered into correspondence with Spanish-American savants and the first students from Chile and Buenos Aires arrived in North America.

DeForest's life provides a remarkably complete record of this process of inter-American acquaintance and coöperation in the first great international crisis of the Americas. It mirrors the course of the early relations between the United States and Buenos Aires from the first furtive contacts in the days of the viceroys to the formal exchange of diplomatic representatives a quarter-century later.

DeForest himself shaped those relations in a large measure. At the dawn of the nineteenth century he helped to blaze a trail for United States commerce to the Plate ports; as early as 1805 he urged President Thomas Jefferson to establish a consulate in Buenos Aires. As a resident merchant in the provincial capital he drew on an arsenal of ruses to evade Spain's restrictive laws, and diligently taught the use of these devices to other North American traders. He also became a carrier and interpreter of North American republican doctrine to discontented creoles: mingling with such fathers of the *Revolución de Mayo* as Juan Larrea and Juan José Castelli he spoke to them of the rights of man, the governments of the world, and the independence of Buenos Aires. Expelled from La Plata by Viceroy Cisneros, allegedly for his liberal sentiments, DeForest returned after the *veinte-cinco de mayo* to become a promoter of privateering enterprise against Spanish commerce. The exploits of the *Congreso*, the *Tupac-Amarú*, the *Mangoré*, and other corsairs outfitted in Baltimore through DeForest's initiative attest to the important military contribution of the United States to the winning of Argentine independence. His mission as consul general of the United Provinces of La Plata at Washington was a milestone in the establishment of diplomatic relations between the United States and his adopted country. Finally, by his generous donation for the support of the first institution of higher learning in independent Buenos Aires; by his presentation of North American art objects to that institution; and by his encouragement to young *porteños* to study in the United States, DeForest broke new ground in the field of cultural relations between the two countries.

BIBLIOGRAPHICAL NOTE

Bibliographies and Guides

Cecil K. Jones, *A Bibliography of Latin American Bibliographies* (2nd ed., Washington, 1942), is of broader scope than the title indicates; the section on Argentina yielded many useful historical titles and clues for research. Samuel F. Bemis and Grace G. Griffin, *Guide to the Diplomatic History of the United States, 1775–1921* (Washington, 1935), was indispensable for the diplomatic relations between the United States and revolutionary Buenos Aires. An informing discussion of authorities and sources introduces the section on "La revolución en el Río de la Plata" in the monumental work of Antonio Ballesteros y Berreta, *La historia de España y su influencia en la historia universal* (8 vols., Barcelona, 1919–1936), VII, 318–321; there is a supplementary list of titles on pp. 467–468. The "principal bibliographies" appended to the chapters of the *Historia de la nación argentina*, discussed below, have also been useful. Two publications largely devoted to historical bibliography, the *Boletín* of the Instituto de Investigaciones Históricas of the University of Buenos Aires (Buenos Aires, 1922–), and the *Anuario de historia argentina* (Buenos Aires, 1940–), published by the Sociedad de Historia Argentina, were of value for the annual increment of writings on the colonial and revolutionary periods in La Plata. The best guide to the minor figures of the Argentine revolution is Enrique Udaondo, *Diccionario biográfico argentino* (Buenos Aires, 1938). I have consulted numerous published guides to the manuscript collections of the Library of Congress, the National Archives (Washington), and other depositories in the United States; similarly full analyses do not yet exist for the archives of the Argentine Republic.

Manuscripts

The manuscript material on which this work is based has been obtained from the manuscript collections of the Yale University Library, the Library of Congress, and the National Archives in Washington, and the United States District Court in Baltimore.

The richest and by far the most useful source for this study has been the David C. DeForest Collection in the Yale University Library. The eight letterbooks, seven journals or diaries, and five account books which form the bulk of this collection allow a comprehensive reconstruction of DeForest's life from 1798 to his death in 1825. These papers also constitute a rich and hitherto untapped source for the commercial and political history of the Río de la Plata in the late colonial and revolutionary periods. They appear to be fairly complete; the most important missing item is a letterbook for the years 1815–1817, containing much correspondence on privateering affairs. It should be noted that while we have almost all of DeForest's outgoing letters, copies of which he entered in his letterbooks, we do not have any of the letters sent to him. This is a pity, for among DeForest's friends and correspondents were such *próceres* of the Argentine revolution as Juan Larrea, Juan José Castelli, Manuel Belgrano, and Bernardo Monteagudo.

In the John W. De Forest Collection, also in the Yale Library, I found among the papers of this distinguished novelist, a nephew and biographer of DeForest, a folder of notes and transcripts drawn off for him from family papers by Colonel George Butler Griffin, the son of one of DeForest's daughters. Particularly useful here were transcripts from the now missing letterbook containing DeForest's privateering correspondence. In the Hiram Bingham Collection in the Yale Library, I consulted profitably a set of abstracts and transcripts made by Professor Bingham from British Foreign Office material in the Public Record Office (London), relating to the Spanish-American Wars of Independence. They were valuable for evidence of early Anglo-American commercial rivalry in La Plata and the reports of British merchants on conditions in Buenos Aires on the eve of the *veinte-cinco de mayo*.

Two collections of personal papers in the Division of Manuscripts in the Library of Congress were especially helpful. The Jonathan Meredith Papers yielded documentary material (a privateering contract between DeForest and the government of Buenos Aires, instructions to privateering captains, and the like) that usefully supplemented information obtained from other sources. In this collection there is also much evidence of the privateering interests of DeForest's arch-foe, Thomas L. Halsey, sometime United States consul in Buenos Aires. The Jeremy Robinson Papers contributed the interesting diary of the traveler in South America of that name, with its acid characterization of DeForest and his motives for desiring a consular appointment in the United States.

For DeForest's diplomatic career, the most valuable source in the Manuscripts Division of the Library of Congress was photocopies of material from the Archivo General de la Nación (Buenos Aires), sección Gobierno, Estados Unidos, S[ala] 1, A[rmario] 2, A[naquél] 4, Núm[eros] 8, 9, and 10. This material comprises correspondence between United States consuls and the government of Buenos Aires; the file of instructions and reports of DeForest and other early missions from Buenos Aires to the United States; and correspondence between DeForest and the first recognized minister from Buenos Aires, Carlos de Alvear. Comparison with DeForest's letterbooks, in which he entered copies of all his official despatches, shows that the reports from him in the Buenos Aires archives are fairly complete. In the Library of Congress I have also made use of photocopies of material in the Archivo Histórico Nacional (Madrid), Estado, legajos 5552–5576, 5636–5648 inclusive; scattered information obtained here is cited in my footnote references.

In the Department of State Division of the National Archives (Washington), the following series were of limited assistance: Consular Letters, Buenos Aires, Vol. 1, parts 1 and 2, for occasional references to DeForest in consular despatches from Buenos Aires; Consular Letters, St. Bartholomew, for the excesses of patriot privateers in West Indian waters; and Domestic Letters, for a remonstrance from Secretary of State Adams to Spanish-American governments concerning these excesses.

The Admiralty Records of the United States District Court in Baltimore contain much material on privateering under the flag of Buenos Aires. The most important material consulted here was the docket of the case of the *Sereno,* which DeForest finally lost to Spanish claimants, to the great financial loss of his heirs. There are scattered references to DeForest in other privateering cases recorded here.

Newspapers

La Gaceta de Buenos Aires (facsimile edition, 6 vols., Buenos Aires, 1910–1915), published by the Junta de Historia y Numismática Americana of Buenos Aires, was useful for some details of DeForest's commercial activity in Buenos Aires, 1812–1818. For his New Haven years (1818–1825), I have relied chiefly on the *Columbian Register* and the *Connecticut Journal,* both published in New Haven. I am indebted to many other newspapers for scattered information cited in footnote references.

Printed Sources

In the notable continuing series, *Documentos para la historia argentina* (Buenos Aires, 1913–), published by the Facultad de Filosofía y Letras of the University of Buenos Aires, the following volumes were of particular value: Vol. 7, *Comercio de Indias; consulado, comercio de negros y de extranjeros, 1791–1809,* for contraband trade between the United States and the viceroyalty of the Río de la Plata, and commercial matters generally; Vol. 12, *Territorio y población; padrón de la ciudad de Buenos Aires,* for the dates and places of DeForest's residence in Buenos Aires; and Vol. 14, *Correspondencias generales de la provincia de Buenos Aires,* for DeForest's diplomatic mission to the United States. *Documentos relativos a los antecedentes de la independencia de la República Argentina* (Buenos Aires, 1912), a publication of the Facultad de Filosofía y Letras, was helpful for political conditions in Buenos Aires after the British invasions.

BIBLIOGRAPHICAL NOTE

William R. Manning, ed., *Diplomatic Correspondence of the United States Concerning the Independence of the Latin American Nations* . . . (3 vols., N. Y., 1925), was indispensable for the early missions from Buenos Aires to the United States; Vol. 1 contains the exchange of notes between DeForest and Secretary of State Adams. In his *Memoirs,* edited by Charles F. Adams (12 vols., Philadelphia, 1874–1877), the secretary made fairly detailed entries of his interviews with DeForest; these accounts usefully supplement DeForest's own reports in the Buenos Aires archives. The *Writings of John Quincy Adams* (7 vols., N. Y., 1913–1917), edited by Worthington C. Ford, supplement the *Memoirs* as a helpful source for Adams' Spanish-American policy. C. K. Webster has illustrated British policy, a constant factor in Adams' diplomatic calculations, with selected documents from Foreign Office archives bearing on *Britain and the Independence of Latin America* (2 vols., N. Y., 1938).

Louis Effingham de Forest printed two early letters of DeForest in "A Trip Through Brazil in 1802," *Brazil* (N. Y.), Year IX, no. 101, March, 1937. These are the only DeForest papers that have appeared in print.

Secondary Works

For the ancestry of David C. DeForest I have drawn on two family histories: John W. De Forest, *The de Forests of Avesnes (and of New Netherland)* (New Haven, 1900); and Mrs. Robert W. de Forest, *A Walloon Family in America* (2 vols., N. Y., 1914). Jane DeForest Shelton, *The Salt-Box House* (N. Y., 1929), is a charming evocation of eighteenth-century life in DeForest's birthplace, the town of Stratford. W. A. Robinson, *Jeffersonian Democracy in New England* (New Haven, 1916); and Richard J. Purcell, *Connecticut in Transition* (New Haven, 1918), depict the economic changes and shifting climate of opinion that moulded the thoughts and aspirations of the young DeForest.

Samuel E. Morison, *Maritime History of Massachusetts, 1783–1860* (N. Y., 1921), is a vigorous account of the great outward thrust of American commerce of which DeForest's early ventures formed an incident. Harry Bernstein, *Origins of Inter-American Interest, 1700–1812* (Philadelphia, 1945), illustrates with the aid of numerous printed sources and some manuscript material an unsuspected wealth of early contacts between North and Spanish America; trade with La Plata is discussed on pp. 33–51. A pioneering little work, rich in information but lacking the apparatus of scholarship, is Charles L. Chandler, *Inter-American Acquaintances* (Sewannee, Tenn., 1915); there are a number of references to DeForest. Three articles by the same author are useful for the proportions and character of early United States trade to La Plata: "The River Plate Voyages," *American Historical Review,* XXIII (1918), 816–826; "United States Merchant Ships in the Río de la Plata (1801–1809) as

Shown by Early Newspapers," *Hispanic-American Historical Review,* II (1919), 26–54; and "The United States Shipping in the La Plata Region, 1809–1810," *ibid.,* II (1920), 159–176. Roy F. Nichols, "Trade Relations and the Establishment of the United States Consulates in Spanish America, 1779–1809," *ibid.,* XIII (1933), 289–313, shows how Spain's maritime distresses during periodic wars compelled the opening of her colonial ports to United States trade; commerce with La Plata is only briefly discussed. Dorothy B. Goebel, "British Trade to the Spanish Colonies, 1796–1823," *American Historical Review,* XLIII (1938), 276–318, reveals with the aid of British archival material how financial exigencies and the rise of revolutionary crises in the Spanish colonies furthered English trade penetration unsanctioned by the Spanish government; the discussion of trade to La Plata, while helpful, suggests only slight familiarity with Argentine printed material. Roberto C. Simonsen, *Historia economica do Brasil* (2 vols., São Paulo, 1937), provided background information for DeForest's smuggling activity in Brazil.

Two standard works, Ricardo Levene, *A History of Argentina* (Chapel Hill, N. C., 1937), translated and edited by William S. Robertson; and F. A. Kirkpatrick, *A History of the Argentine Republic* (Cambridge, Eng., 1931), were useful for general reference as concerned the Argentine struggle for independence. For particular episodes, however, I have relied in the main on the pertinent contributions to the coöperative *Historia de la nación argentina* (Buenos Aires, 1936–   ), under the general editorship of the erudite Professor Ricardo Levene. This vast and continuing enterprise is planned to cover in ten volumes the course of Argentine history from its beginnings to the definitive organization of the nation in 1862. Two supplementary volumes will bring the history down to the 1912 electoral reform. Vol. IV, *El momento histórico del virreynato del Río de la Plata;* and Vol. V, *La revolución de mayo hasta la asamblea general constituyente,* have been most useful in the writing of this study.

The British invasions of 1806–1807, of which DeForest became an unwilling observer, gave a powerful stimulus to the movement for independence in Buenos Aires. The best account in English, based on the then available printed material, is by Bernard Moses, "The British in Buenos Aires," in *Spain's Declining Power in the New World* (Berkeley, Cal., 1919), pp. 337–371. Juan Beverina, "Las invasiones inglesas," in *Historia de la nación argentina,* IV, section 2, is a convenient summary of the military operations. Paul Groussac, *Santiago de Liniers, conde de Buenos Aires* (Buenos Aires, 1907), is a wise, witty, and learned biography of the French-born hero of the *reconquista.*

Napoleon's seizure of the Spanish throne in 1808 precipitated a crisis of the old régime in the Spanish-American colonies. Bartolomé Mitre, *Historia de Belgrano y de la independencia argentina* (4th ed., 3 vols.,

Buenos Aires, 1887–1888), is a broad study of the process of Argentine independence, based on extensive archival research, and framed about the life of the patriot leader Manuel Belgrano. For particular trends and events leading to the *veinte-cinco de mayo,* the following contributions to the *Historia de la nación argentina,* V, section 1, have been most helpful: Ricardo R. Caillet-Bois, "Las corrientes ideológicas europeas del siglo XVIII, y el virreinato del Río de la Plata"; Ricardo Levene, "Intentos de independencia en el virreinato del Plata (1781–1809)"; and by the same author, "La asonada del 1º de enero de 1809." Argentine historians are not in accord as to the influence exerted on the course of revolutionary events by Mariano Moreno and his famous memorial on the advantages of free trade. Diego Luis Molinari, *La representación de los hacendados de Mariano Moreno, su ninguna influencia en la vida económica del país y en los sucesos de mayo* (2d ed., Buenos Aires, 1939), subjects the original documents to searching analysis and vigorously rejects any suggestion of such influence; an affirmative and probably more widely accepted position, embodying conclusions based on many years' research in the subject, is taken by Ricardo Levene, "Significación histórica de la obra económica de Manuel Belgrano y Mariano Moreno," in *Historia de la nación argentina,* V, section 1. The same author contributes two masterly surveys of the *Revolución de Mayo* to Vol. V, section 2 of the *Historia:* "Los sucesos de mayo," an authoritative statement of the train of events; and "El 25 de mayo," a thoughtful essay on the nature and ends of the revolution. Other contributions to this volume, narrating the rise and fall of successive patriot governments down to the *asamblea general constituyente* of 1813, have been useful for general reference. Volume VI of the *Historia,* which continues the story of the revolution, had not appeared at the time of this writing.

With the aid of ships and crews supplied by merchants in the United States, the Buenos Aires government launched an effective privateering campaign against Spanish commerce. North American investigators have delved deeply into this picturesque theme. Theodore S. Currier, *Los corsarios del Río de la Plata* (Buenos Aires, 1929), is a useful preliminary account based exclusively on printed material in the United States. Lewis W. Bealer, *Los corsarios de Buenos Aires* (Buenos Aires, 1937), exhausts published sources in Argentina and the United States, but does not exploit archival sources in either country. Charles C. Griffin, "Privateering from Baltimore during the Spanish American Wars of Independence," *Maryland Historical Magazine,* XXXV (1940), 1–25, illuminates the organization and practice of privateering industry with the aid of admiralty records in the federal court archives of Baltimore and other seaboard cities. Theodore S. Currier, *Los cruceros del "General San Martín"* (Buenos Aires, 1944), a case study in privateering also based on United States court records, appeared after most of the work on this book had been completed. Angel Justiniano Carranza, *Campañas navales de la República Argentina, cuadros históricos* (4 vols., Buenos Aires, 1911–1914), a eulogistic history based largely on archival sources, was helpful for scattered information on DeForest's privateers.

To the United States the patriots of Buenos Aires early turned for support and encouragement. Samuel Flagg Bemis, *Early Diplomatic Missions from Buenos Aires to the United States, 1811–1824* (Worcester, Mass., 1940) (reprinted from the *Proceedings* of the American Antiquarian Society for April, 1939), a definitive study founded on exhaustive research in United States, Argentine, and Spanish archival material, as well as the DeForest papers, was invaluable for DeForest's consular mission to the United States. Of the voluminous literature on the relations between the United States and the new Spanish-American states, only three works need be mentioned here. Frederic L. Paxson, *The Independence of the South-American Republics; A Study in Recognition and Foreign Policy* (Philadelphia, 1903), a pioneer monograph that exploits United States and British archives, contains the first scholarly though brief account of DeForest's diplomacy. Charles C. Griffin, *The United States and the Disruption of the Spanish Empire* (N. Y., 1937), a multi-archival study, places in useful focus the intimate interplay between United States boundary disputes with Spain and the Spanish-American struggle for independence; there is only brief mention of DeForest's mission. Arthur P. Whitaker, *The United States and the Independence of Latin America, 1808–1830* (Baltimore, 1941), a broad survey founded on prodigious research in United States, European, and South American archives, has for its main theme the retreat from Jefferson's "large policy of 1808" to the more cautious policies of Madison and Monroe; it contains a judicious appraisal of DeForest's efforts to gain recognition for Buenos Aires. Harris G. Warren, *The Sword Was Their Passport: A History of American Filibustering in the Mexican Revolution* (Baton Rouge, La., 1942), a monograph based on Spanish and United States archival material, was invaluable for DeForest's projects to establish a base in Florida for the privateers of Buenos Aires.

There are a few slender writings that seek to encompass the life of DeForest as a whole. J. W. De Forest devoted two chapters to his uncle in a family history, *The de Forests of Avesnes (and of New Netherland)* (New Haven, 1900). Within its limitations (source material was apparently confined to a few early letters of DeForest, a number of extracts from DeForest's letterbooks and account books, and the *Memoirs* of John Quincy Adams), this is a useful preliminary sketch, but the historical observations are practically worthless. Atilio Chiáppori, "Un Goya yanqui y un yanqui porteño," *La Nación* (Buenos Aires), May 20, 1934, 2ª sección, p. 2 (reprinted in a collection of essays by the same author, *Maestros y temperamentos*, Buenos Aires, 1943, pp. 105–135), weaves a highly impressionistic account of DeForest's life about the Morse portrait of DeForest in Buenos Aires; aside from information on this painting it was of no value. Horacio Zorraquín Becú, *De aventurero yanqui a consul porteño en los Estados Unidos: David C. DeForest, 1774–1825* (Buenos Aires, 1943) (reprint from the *Anuario de historia argentina,* IV, 1942), has diligently combed printed material in the United States and Argentina, but did not avail himself of archival sources close at hand; this pleasantly written little study was helpful for some sections of my narrative. Señor Zorraquín Becú promises a closer analysis of DeForest's mission to the United States in a work as yet unpublished, "Inglaterra, la diplomacia norteamericana y el reconocimiento de la independencia argentina." Madame Courtney Letts de Espil has published a series of four popular articles on DeForest in *La Nación* (Buenos Aires), Nov. 12, 26; Dec. 10, 24, 1944, with the aid of some Argentine printed sources and a few extracts from the DeForest papers. Mention should also be made of the brief but accurate biographical sketch of DeForest in the *Dictionary of American Biography.*

INDEX

ABASCAL, José de, viceroy of Peru, 113
Abrolhos Islands, 36
Academy of the Union of the South, 126, 161–162
Acebal, José Matías de, merchant of Habana, 37
Achega, Domingo Victorio de, president of the Academy of the Union of the South, 162–163
Adams, Captain, 112
Adams, John, President, 10
Adams, John Quincy, secretary of state, 106, 111, 114, 132, 136, 140–141, 146–147, 152, 157; on recognition of Spanish-American independence, 133–134; confers with DeForest, 137–140, 143–144; quoted on Graham's mission, 149–150; replies to DeForest's notes, 153–154; warns DeForest of violation of neutrality laws, 154–155
Adams-Onís Treaty (1819), 156
Age of Reason, Thomas Paine's, 4
Agrelo, José, 135
Agüero, Fernández de, advocate of the *consulado* of Cadiz, 71–72
Aguirre, Juan P., 107
Aguirre, Manuel H. de, Buenos Aires agent to U. S., 107, 130–134, 139, 141, 143
Aguirre, Pedro de, Buenos Aires agent to U. S., 129
Aix-la-Chapelle, congress of, 142
Almeida, ship, 117–118
Almeida, Captain Joseph, 114–117
Álvarez Thomas, I., supreme director of La Plata, 99, 112, 129–130
Alvear, Carlos de, supreme director of La Plata, 94–96, 98–100, 157
Alzaga, Martín, *alcalde* of Buenos Aires, 46–50, 65–70, 91
Amelia Island, 132–134, 139, 152
"American Concern," 107
Ansley, Captain John, 26
Artigas, José, Uruguayan patriot, 96, 98, 100, 109, 119–120, 132
Ashburton, village of, 77
Asonada of Jan. 1, 1809, 66–68, 70
Astor, John J., merchant, 89, 97, 103, 111–112

Audiencia of Buenos Aires, 47, 49, 54, 63, 67, 70
Aurora, ship, 126
Aury, Louis, 149–150
Avesnes, town of, 2, 7
Ayohuma, battle of, 96
Azcuénaga, Miguel de, patriot leader, 59, 76

BAHIA, 61
Baltimore, 37, 39, 97, 114, 120; center of privateering enterprise, 104–107
Banda Oriental (Uruguay), 96, 98, 100, 109, 144
Barker, Dr. Jeremiah C., 14
Barcelona, 55
Barataria, 148
Baratillas, 69
Barnes, Captain James, 120
Basabilbaso, Patricio, 164
Batabano, 37
Bayonne, 62, 64–65, 79
Bay of Cadiz, 117
Bay of Camarónes, 15
Belgrano, Manuel, patriot leader, 60, 63–64, 69, 75–76, 93–94
Bentley, Reverend William, 4
Beresford, Sir William, 42–44, 48, 50
Berlin Decree, Napoleon's, proclaimed in Buenos Aires, 53–54
Bishop, Abraham, Connecticut politician, 30, 82
Blagge, Martha, 3
Bland, Theodorick A., 133 n.
Blodget, Mr., 61
Bonaparte, Joseph, King of Spain, 62–63, 148
Boston, 6, 10–11, 13, 33, 35, 40
Boston Athenaeum, 142
Bolívar, Simón, liberator of northern South America, 78, 80, 118
Brackenridge, Henry M., visitor to Buenos Aires, quoted, 102 n.
Brazil, 20–24, 33–36, 61–74, 113, 126
Brazil Banks, 5, 36
Bridgeport (Conn.), 6
British Guiana, 31
British invasions of La Plata, 42–52
Brown, Captain William, 96

Buenos Aires, colonial, life in, 59; preliminaries of revolution in, 61–75; revolution of May, 1810 in, 76; first diplomatic missions of, to Great Britain, 77–82; first diplomatic missions of, to the U. S., 87–88, 129–157; royalist conspiracy in, 91; political struggles in, 91–92, 94–95, 98–101; privateering under the flag of, 104–121
Buenos Aires Marine court, 57
Bulkley, Lieutenant Francis, 118–119
Burr, Aaron, 3
Butler, Horace, 159

Cabildo of Buenos Aires, 47, 49, 61, 63, 67, 71, 76
Cabildo abierto, 66, 76
Cadiz, 78–80, 116
Canary Islands, 4
Canton, 5–6, 13
Cape Horn, 18
Cape Verde Islands, 14, 33, 41
Cap Français, 9
Caracas, 78–79, 83
Carlota, Joaquina, Princess of Brazil, 6, 9, 65, 74
Carp, Samuel, merchant, 103
Carrera, José Miguel, Chilean patriot, 103–105, 121
Casa Irujo, marquis of, Spanish minister to U. S., 38
Castelli, Juan José, patriot leader, 59–60, 76
Cayenne, 31
Céfiro. See *Zephyr*
Chacabuco, battle of, 130
Charles IV, King of Spain, 62
Chase, Captain John, 98 n., 103, 114, 116
Chayter, Captain James, 120
Chapetones, 70
Chaves, Padre José Alves, 23, 55
Chile, 6, 84, 113, 123, 130, 142, 156
Chuquisaca, 70
Ciencia, ship, 116
Cisneros, Baltasar Hidalgo de, last viceroy of La Plata, 18, 69–75, 77
Clay, Henry, champion of Spanish-American independence, 131–133, 137, 143, 145, 153–155
Clemente, Lino, Venezuelan agent to U. S., 146, 154
Cochrane, George, 116
Colombia, 156
Colonia, 70
Columbus, ship, 123–124

Compagnie du Sénégal, 41
Congreso, ship, 105, 111, 114–115, 167
Connecticut, 3–6, 9–10
Consulado of Buenos Aires, 16, 59, 71
Constitution of the U. S., read in Buenos Aires, 101
Contraband trade, to La Plata, 15–17, 19–20, 34–36, 39 n., 53–54, 57–58, 68–69; to Brazil, 20–23, 34. See also Neutral trade; Slave trade
Cook, Captain James, 6
Córdoba, 44
Cornhill (London), 27
Cornwall, 27
Corrientes, province of, 99
Costa Guimaraes, Manos da, 34
Costa Firme, 38 n.
Crowninshield, George, merchant, 111–112
Criollo de Buenos Aires, ship, 111
Cuba, 17, 36, 56 n., 108
Cunha Rego, André da, 22
Curado, governor of Santa Catharina
Curiacio, ship, 131
Cuyo, province of, 99

Daggett, Judge David, 160, 166
Dana, Samuel W., U. S. senator, 84
Daniels, Captain John, 115
Daphne, ship, 31–32
Darcy and Didier, merchants, 105, 107, 111, 121
Davy, York, 115
Declaration of Independence of the U. S., read in Buenos Aires, 101
Decree of Nov. 6, 1809 establishes limited free trade to La Plata, 73–74
DeForest, Benjamin, 7
DeForest, Carlos María, 93, 98, 159, 168
DeForest, David, 3
DeForest, David Curtis, ancestry, 2–3; birth, 3; first years and schooling, 7; literary tastes, 7–8; early business misfortunes, 8–9; enters U. S. army, 10–11; voyage to England, 11–12; voyage of circumnavigation, 13; quarrels with Captain Smith, 14, 18; travels in Brazil and La Plata, 19–25; enters monastery in Buenos Aires, 25–26; second voyage to England, 26–30; voyage to the Guianas and West Indies, 31–33; letter to Jefferson, 33; voyage to Brazil and La Plata, 33–36; confers with Jefferson, 38; views on Miranda's expedition, 38–40; voyage to Goree and La Plata, 40–42; runs Brit-

INDEX

ish blockade of Buenos Aires, 45–46; arrest and imprisonment, 48; protests to *audiencia* against ill-treatment of Americans, 49; establishes commission-house in Buenos Aires, 53–54; circular letter on neutral trade with La Plata, 55–56; applies for post as U. S. consul, 56; on the Embargo Act, 57; purchases estate, 58; mode of life in Buenos Aires, 59; discussions with Larrea, 59–60; comments on *asonada* of Jan. 1, 1809, 67; proposes publication of Moreno's *Representación*, 73; analysis of political situation in La Plata, 74; expelled by Cisneros, 75; goes to Rio de Janeiro, 75–76; voyage to England, 76–77; attacks British policy toward Spanish America, 80; aids Irigoyen in obtaining munitions, 81; returns to the U. S., 82; defeats Goddefroy's appointment as consul to Buenos Aires, 84–85; courtship and marriage, 85–86; strange homecoming to La Plata, 89–90; honored by Rivadavia's régime, 92; retires to estate, 93; religious views of, 93 n.; presents Washington's Farewell Address to Belgrano, 94; assists in creation of patriot navy, 95–96; opens store in Buenos Aires, 96–97; advertises North American political writings, 101–102; outfits Buenos Aires privateers, 110–114; aids in establishment of mixed North and South American businesses, 121; makes loan to Buenos Aires government, 121–122; description of, by Henry Hill, 123; description of, by Jeremy Robinson, 124–125; appointed consul general to the U. S., 125; endows Academy of the Union of the South with estate, 126–127; departs for the U. S., 128; confers with Adams and Monroe, 137–140, 144–145; builds home at New Haven, 142; consults with Clay on demands for recognition, 143; appears at Monroe's Drawing Room, 145–146; projects attack on Spanish Florida, 150–152; sends notes to Adams, 152–153; warned by Adams, 154–155; retires to New Haven, 155; consular commission recalled, 156; hospitality, 160–161; portraits of, by Morse, 161–162; sends art objects to Buenos Aires, 162; celebrates Argentine Independence Day, 163; sponsors visits of Argentine students to the U. S., 163–164; establishes scholarships at Yale College, 165–166; concern over lawsuits, 167; illness and death, 167

DeForest, Francisca Tomasa Isabel, 93, 168 n.
De Forest, Henry, 2
De Forest, Isaac, 2
DeForest, Jacoba Pastora, 98, 168 n.
De Forest, Jesse, 2, 7
De Forest, John H., 6–8, 13, 57–58
De Forest, John W., 103 n., 165
DeForest, Julia (Wooster), 145, 161, 168
DeForest, Juliana Nicanora, 98, 168 n.
De Forest, Lockwood, 164
DeForest, Mehitable (Curtis), 7
De Forest, Dr. Louis S., 162
Demerara, 31
Devereux, Colonel John, U. S. agent to Buenos Aires, 134
Diadem, ship, 42
Diana, ship, 13–15, 18, 48
Didier, Henry, merchant, 116, 152
Dilworth's *Spelling Book* and *Arithmetic*, 7
Dispatch, ship, 76
Donovan, Jeremiah, 48
Dorothea, ship, 112
Dorrego, Manuel, 35
Douglass, Dr. John H., and Miranda's *Leander* expedition, 38
Downes, Captain John, 142
Dunham and Lord, merchants, 33
Durand, Asher B., artist, 162
Dutch West India Company, 2
Dwight, Timothy, president of Yale College, 4

EDWARDS, PIERPONT, Connecticut politician, 30
Edwards, Shelton, 8
Elío, Javier de, governor of Montevideo, 65–66
El Regulador, monastery, 25
Ely, Dr. David, 86
Embargo Act, 57
England, 12, 17, 26, 33, 63, 68
English Road, 14
Enterprise, ship, 6
Ensenada de Barragán, 49–50
Entre Ríos, province of, 99
Essex decision of 1805, 30
Expedition, ship, 98 n., 103, 104, 112

FAIRFIELD (Conn.), 3
Falmouth, 26–27
Favorite, ship, 98 n.

Ferdinand VII, King of Spain, 62, 64–65, 76, 91, 95, 101
Filangieri, Gaetano, 72
Florida, 106, 133, 139, 140, 142, 151–152
Florida, East, 148
Forbes, John M., U. S. consul to Buenos Aires, 110
Ford, William G., 107, 117
Fort Royal, 31
France, 10–11, 16–17, 28, 62
Franciscan Order, 25
French Coffee House, 59
French Guiana, 2
Frisby, William, 116

GALLATIN, ALBERT, secretary of the treasury, 30
Galup, Francisco, merchant, 23
Galveston, 148–150
Gambia River, 41
Garland, Captain Edward, 89
Garrot, V., 152
Gazette (New London), 5
George and Mary, ship, 48
George Augustus, ship, 82
Girard, Stephen, merchant, 88
Glover, Henry, merchant, 73
Glover, Reuben, 14
Goddefroy, Louis, merchant, 83, 85
Godoy, Prince of the Peace, 62
Gold Coast, 40
Gómez, Gregorio, Buenos Aires agent to U. S., 130
Goodrich, Chauncey, U. S. senator, 84
Goodrich, Elizur, 165
Goree, island of, 40–42
Gosport, ship, 29
Goyeneche, José M. de, Spanish officer, 63
Graham, George, mission of, to Galveston, 148–150
Graham, John, 133 n., 137
Granger Gideon, postmaster general, 82
Great Britain, trade of, to La Plata, 17, 35, 53, 68–69, 71; trade of, to Brazil, 20; policy of, toward Spanish America, 78–80
Griffin, George, 168 n.
Griffin, George Butler, 103 n.
Güemes, Carlos Cortez de (DeForest's privateering pseudonym), 108
Guianas, 31
Guido, Tomás, Argentine patriot, 156 n.

HABANA, 36–37, 55, 68, 79, 83

Haiti, 9
Halsey, Thomas L., U. S. consul to Buenos Aires, 20, 121, 124–125, 137–138
Hamilton, Alexander, 10
Hawkesbury, Lord, 28
Higginbotham, John, 107, 120
Hill, Henry, merchant, 121, 123
Hill, Hiland, 168 n.
Hillhouse, James, 165
Historia concisa de los Estados Unidos desde el descubrimiento de América hasta el año 1807, García de Sena, 101–102
Hoadley, David, architect, 142, 158–159
Hooper, Captain John, 41, 53
Hope, ship, 19
Horatio, ship, 131
Housatonic River, 3
Huaqui, battle of, 91
Hubbell, Captain Ezekiel, 6
Hudson (N. Y.), 163–164
Huntington (Conn.), 3 n., 86, 103, 158, 164

ILHA GRANDE, bay of, 34
Independencia de Costa Firme justificada por Thomas Paine treinta años ha, García de Sena, tr., 101
Industria, ship, 75–76
Invencible, ship, 119
Irigoyen, Matías, Buenos Aires agent to Great Britain, 78, 80–82
Islas, 89–90

JAMAICA, 20 n.
Jane, ship, 40–42, 44–46, 49, 53
Jackson, General Andrew, 142
James Harbor, 18
Jefferson, Thomas, President, 4, 33–38, 56
John, Prince, John VI of Portugal and Brazil, 61–62
Joseph, 77, 89–90
Juan Fernández, island of, 114
Julia DeForest, ship, 117
Junta de conservación, 9
Junta of Buenos Aires, 76–78
Junta of Cadiz, 78
Junta of Caracas, 78
Junta of Montevideo, 70
Junta tuitiva of La Paz, 70

KAMCHATKA, 6
Kemp, ship, 97 n.
King, Henry, 97 n.
Knox, General Henry, 10

INDEX 183

Lackington's book store, 29
La Esperanza, ship, 120
Lafayette, General, 160–161
Laffite, Jean, smuggler and privateersman 149, 152
Laffite, Pierre, 146–148, 151
Laffite brothers, 148
La Guaira, 39, 56 n., 83
La Independencia del Sud, ship, 120
Lallemand, General Charles, 148–149
La Merced Church, 59
Lancashire, 12
La Paz, 70
La Plata, United Provinces of, 91, 92, 95, 100, 104, 109
La Plata, viceroyalty of, 15–18, 23–24, 26, 29–30, 33, 35, 37, 39–40, 42–43, 47, 53, 55–56
"Large policy of 1808," Jefferson's, 57 n.
Larrea, Juan, patriot leader, 59, 74, 76, 85 n., 80–82, 87–88, 90–91, 95–100
Larrea, Ramón, 76–78, 82
Larrea, Tomasa de, 93
Lautaro Lodge, 94
Laws of the Indies, 15, 53, 69, 71, 79
Leander expedition, Miranda's, 43
Le Champ d'Asile, 148
Leona, ship, 116
Leyden, 2
Levene, Ricardo, on Moreno's *Representación de los hacendados*, 72
Lima, 42, 82, 113, 123
Liniers, Santiago, viceroy of La Plata, 42, 44, 46–50, 53–54, 61, 63, 65–70
Lisbon, 22, 61
Liverpool, 11, 13
Livingston, Robert, American minister to France, 28
Llorente, Ventura, syndic of the *consulado* of Buenos Aires, 59
Lloyd, Major, 4
Lockwood, Edward, Sr., 29
Lockwood, Mehitable, 165
Lockwood, Robert, 163
London, 27–29, 43, 77–78
Long Island Sound, 5
López, Pedro. *See* Aguirre, Pedro de
Louisiana, 28–30
Lowry, Robert K., U. S. agent to Caracas, 83
Lue y Riego, Benito de, Bishop of Buenos Aires, 66
Luján, 48

Lynch, Benito, 98
Lynch, Estanislao, 121
Lynch, Felix, 98
Lynch, Manuel, 98, 123, 136, 151, 163
Lynch, Patricio, merchant, 98, 99, 121
Lynch and Co., Patricio, 121
Lynch, Zimmerman, and Co., 121

MacGregor, Gregor, adventurer, 154
Macedonian, ship, 142
Madden, Ezekiel, 42
Madison, James, secretary of state, President, 56, 84, 87, 145, 147
Madrid, 62
Maine, district of, 8–9
Maipú, battle of, 142
Maldonado, 24, 45
Malta, 28
Manchester (Eng.), 12
Manchester (N. H.), 41
Mangoré, ship, 112–114, 120–121
Margarita, 110, 117–118
Martínez y García, Pedro, 164
Martinique, 31
Mary, ship, 48, 89
Massachusetts, 5, 8, 14, 101
Mathews, General George, 148
Mayo, island of, 14
Maza, Manuel Vicente de, 99
Mersey River, 11
Milan Decree, Napoleon's, 57
Miller, William G., U. S. consul to Buenos Aires, 85
Miranda, Francisco de, Venezuelan patriot, 38–40, 43, 79
Mitchell, Captain Nathaniel, 33, 37
Molinari, Diego L., on Moreno's *Representación de los hacendados*, 72
Monroe, James, secretary of state, President, 28, 84, 88, 123, 135, 155, 167
Monson, Captain Marcena, 103–105, 114, 118–119, 125, 135, 155, 167
Monteagudo, Bernardo, revolutionary leader of Buenos Aires, 94
Montero, Padre, 26
Montevideo, 18–19, 23, 25–26, 34, 42–43, 45, 47–48, 51, 61, 65–70, 76, 81, 89, 91, 93, 96, 132
Monticello, ship, 20
Moreno, Manuel, 135, 140, 146, 151
Moreno, Mariano, revolutionary leader of Buenos Aires, 67, 81, 87, 91–92, 94
Morillo, General Pablo, 115

Morse, Jedidiah, geographer, 161
Morse, Samuel F. B., artist and inventor, 161–162
Munson and Co., Israel, 13

Nantucket, 18, 53
Nancy Anne, ship, 98 n.
Neuville, Hyde de, French minister to U. S., 146
New Amsterdam, 2
New England, 4
Newfield (Conn.), 6, 8
New Granada, 102
New Haven, 3, 6, 8, 29, 82, 86, 126, 142, 155
New Jersey, 101
New Netherland, 2
New Orleans, 36, 56 n., 116
Newport (R. I.), 48
New Spain, 148
New York, 3, 6, 29–30, 89, 111
Nootka Sound, 6
Norfolk, 29

Oliden, Manuel L. de, 126
Oliver, Robert, 103
Onís, Luis de, Spanish minister to U. S., 116, 120, 145–148, 151
Orb, ship, 105, 114–115
Orders-in-council, British, 57
Ortiz Bank, 45
Osgood, H. B., 98 n.
Oxford (Mass.), 10–11
Oyapok River, 2

Paddock, Captain John, 18–19
Paine, Thomas, influence on DeForest, 4
Paraguay, 98, 144
Paramaribo, 31
Paris, 28
Paso, Juan José, patriot leader, 65
Patagonia, 5, 14–15, 18, 23, 67
Patriotic Society, 94
Peace of Amiens (1802), 28
Pennsylvania, 101
Penobscot Bay (Me.), 8
Pensacola, 147
Percival, James Gates, 160
Perry, Commodore Oliver H., 109
Peru, 84, 91, 130, 156
Philadelphia, 20, 26, 48, 70, 82, 88
Philippine Company, 118, 120
Pitt, William, British statesman, 28, 79

Plattsburg, ship, 128, 136
Plymouth (Eng.), 28, 77
Poinsett, Joel Roberts, U. S. consul to Buenos Aires, 83–85
Pope, Alexander, 29
Popham, Sir Home, British naval officer, 42–45
Port-au-Prince, 116
Portugal, 23, 78, 109
Posadas, Gervasio A., director of the United Provinces, 95–97
Potosí, ship, 111, 114, 116–118
Pratt, Henry C., artist, 162
Prescott, James, 86
Privateering code of 1816, 116 n.
Privateering, under the flag of Buenos Aires, 103–121
Protector, ship, 45
Providence (R. I.), 20
Prudence, ship, 18, 20
Puerto Deseado, 15, 18, 19 n.
Puerto Rico, 147, 150
Pueyrredón, ship, 115, 120
Pueyrredón, Juan Martín de, director of the United Provinces, 49, 69, 97, 110, 122, 124–125, 130, 134, 136, 138, 140–141, 144, 151, 154

Quilmes, 49

Randolph, John, 105
Ray, Captain, 19
Raynal, Abbé, 81
Redruth, town of, 27, 77
Regent, ship, 118
Representación de los hacendados, Moreno's, 72–73
Retiro Square, 51
Revolución de Mayo, 67, 72, 126
Rhode Island, 5
Riachuelo de Barracas, 50
Ripton (Conn.), 3, 7, 85–86
Rio de Janeiro, 14, 19–21, 23–24, 58, 61, 67, 70, 73, 75, 89, 91
Rio Grande, province of, 23, 29, 61
Rio Grande, town of, 21–23
Río Grande River, 148–149
Río Negro, 44–45, 53, 112
Rio São Francisco, 21
Ritter, D., 159
Rivadavia, Benito, merchant, 48–49, 59
Rivadavia, Bernardino, Argentine statesman, 48, 92, 110, 156

INDEX 185

Robinson, Jeremy, 123-125
Rodney, Caesar A., U. S. minister to Buenos Aires, 133 n., 156, 162
Rodríguez de Vida, Francisco, 164
Rodríguez de Vida, José María, 164
Rodríguez Peña, Nicolás, patriot leader, 65
Romp, ship, 105
Roquete do Sul, ship, 73
Rufus, ship, 35, 42
Ruíz Huidobro, Pascual, governor of Montevideo, 34
Rush, Richard, acting secretary of state, 131-132

S AAVEDRA, CORNELIO DE, revolutionary leader, 52, 66, 75, 87, 91-92
Saavedra, Diego de, Buenos Aires agent to U. S., 129
Sabine River, 148-149
Sag Harbor (L. I.), 5
St. Augustine, 47
St. Bartholomew, 109
Saint Croix, 20
St. Eustatius, 109
St. Felix, island of, 114
St. Marks, 147
St. Mawes, 27
St. Thomas, 109
Salem, 9, 97 n., 111
Salta, province of, 100
Salvaje, ship, 123
Sandwich Islands, 6
San Isidro, 71
San Martín, José de, liberator of southern South America, 80, 94, 122-123
Santa Catharina, 22, 24
Santa Fé, province of, 99, 144
Santefecino, ship, 105
Santa Teresa, frontier post, 23-24
Santiago de Chile, 20, 121, 130
Santo Cristo de la Salud, ship, 119
Santo Domingo, 136, 147, 150
Saratoga Springs, 168
Sargent, Mayor Joseph D., 142 n.
Sassenay, Marquis de, 62
Scarsborough, 31
Searl, Captain, 126
Sena, García de, 101
Sereno, ship, 167
Serra y Valle, José, 70
Seville, 63, 75-76
Shaler, William, U. S. agent to Vera Cruz, 83
Shannon, Captain Livingston, 119

Shays' Rebellion, 3
Shaw, William L., 142
Shelton (Conn.), 3 n.
Sierra Morena, 76
Silva Lisboa, José da, Brazilian publicist, 73
Sipe Sipe, battle of, 100
Slave trade, to La Plata, 16, 35, 40-42, 53, 55, 58
Smith, Adam, English economist, 72
Smith, Captain Owen F., 13-14
Smith, Robert, secretary of state, 83
Smith, Admiral Sidney, 68
Smith, Colonel William S., 38 n.
Smuggling. *See* Contraband trade; Neutral trade; Slave trade
Sobremonte, Rafaél de, viceroy of La Plata, 35, 44, 47, 53 n.
Southern Packet, ship, 89
South Georgia, island of, 18
South Sea Fleet, of New Haven, 5
Spain, 16-17, 23-26, 33, 55, 60, 62-64, 109
Spartan, ship, 116, 118
Stratford (Conn.), 3, 6-7
Sullivan (Me.), 8
Surinam, 31
Swift, ship, 120

T ACUARI, BATTLE OF, 94
Tagle, Gregorio, foreign minister of Buenos Aires, 122, 126, 141
Taylor, Captain Thomas, 104, 107, 112, 129, 135
Tenant, Captain Thomas, merchant, 37, 97, 103, 111-112, 150
Tenerife, 117
Thames River, 27
Thompson, Colonel Martin, Buenos Aires agent to U. S., 130
Three Kings, Inn of the, 25
Three Sisters, ship, 26-27
Tibbet, Captain, 48
Tigre Oriental, ship, 120
Tobago, 31
Tortola, 31
Torres, Manuel, Colombian minister to U. S., 156
Townsend, Ebenezer, merchant, 30
Trade. *See* Contraband trade; Neutral trade; Slave trade
Trafalgar, battle of, 70
Treaty of Amiens (1802), 33 n.
Treaty of Ghent (1814), 97
Trellechea, Pedro J., 164
Trinidad, 36

Trinity River, 148
Triton, ship, 118, 167
True Blooded Yankee, ship, 112
Trumbull, John, 162
Tucumán, battle of, 93
Tucumán, congress of, 100–101, 130
Tucumán, ship, 107, 111, 114, 117
Tupac-Amarú, ship, 112, 114, 118–119
Twickenham, village of, 29
Tyger, ship, 115

Ugarte, Francisco Ignacio de, merchant, 26, 30, 55, 58–59
United States, trade of, with La Plata, 15–17, 19, 24–25, 30, 33, 35–36, 39–40, 42, 55–57, 84, 88–89, 92, 97–98 n; first diplomatic missions of, to La Plata, 83–84, 109–110, 134, 156
Upper Peru, 90, 93, 99–100

Van Buren, Martin, Vice-President, 168
Van Ness, Judge, 168 n.
Valparaiso, 88
Varangot, Juan Pedro, merchant, 54–58, 74
Varela, Luis P., quoted, 101 n.
Velano, Judge, 54
Venezuela, 38, 78, 102, 109, 117, 147
Vera Cruz, 83
Vigodet, General, 96
Vilcapugio, battle of, 96
Villardebo, *regidor* of Montevideo, 35
Vinalhaven, 33
Volcán, ship, 19
Virginia, 10
Virginia and Maryland Coffee House, 27

Walter and Nixon, merchants, 103
"War of the Oranges" (between Spain and Portugal), 19 n.
War of the Spanish Succession, 63
Washington, 37
Washington's Farewell Address, 94
Watertown (Conn.), 29–30, 58, 85, 142
Webster, Noah, lexicographer, 160, 166
Wellesley, Marquis, British foreign secretary, 78, 80
West Florida, 147
West Indies, 4–6, 8, 30–31
White, William P., North American merchant and adventurer, 54, 95–96, 99
Whitelocke, General John, 51
Whitworth, Lord, 28
William and Mary, ship, 97 n.
Wilmington (Del.), 104
Wilson, Captain George, 117–118
Wilson, Thomas, merchant, 27, 64, 77
Winder, General William H., 116, 129–130, 135, 136–137, 140
Windham (Conn.), 3
Windward Islands, 31
Wooster, General David, 85
Wooster, Charles W., rear-admiral in Chilean navy, 85, 124
Wooster, Julia, 85–86
Wooster, Ephraim, 86
Worthington, William, G. D., U. S. special agent to Buenos Aires, 134, 136–137

"XYZ" dispatches, 10

Yale College, 4, 164–166

Zephyr, ship, 110–111
Zimmerman, John C., merchant, 121 n.